Practical Nephrology

Mark Harber
Editor

Practical Nephrology

Springer

Editor
Mark Harber, MBBS, PhD, FRCP
UCL Department of Nephrology
Royal Free London NHS Foundation Trust
Hampstead
London
UK

This book contains electronic supplementary material which is available on Springer Images http://www.springerimages.com/. In addition, the Resources for Patients and Carers and, Physicians appendix can be downloaded from Extra Materials http://extras.springer.com/

ISBN 978-1-4471-5546-1 ISBN 978-1-4471-5547-8 (eBook)
DOI 10.1007/978-1-4471-5547-8
Springer London Heidelberg New York Dordrecht

Library of Congress Control Number: 2014936595

Printed on acid-free paper

Springer is part of Springer Science+Business Media (www.springer.com)

Preface

Nephrology is a fascinating, complex speciality that will keep most of us challenged, entertained and stretched until retirement beckons. Beyond the complexity of the subject, there are particular challenges facing nephrologists including an aging patient base, often with significant comorbidities, transient populations with chronic disease and often fragmented care. The global pandemic of chronic kidney disease and frequently superimposed acute kidney injury presents us with some very challenging practical, ethical and financial issues in the pursuit of delivering excellent, holistic patient centred medical care.

The aim of this practical nephrology book is to take a fresh look at the topics in this speciality, covering the core subjects and emphasizing strategies for improving the management of complex conditions and support for patients. To this end there are several themes that recur throughout the book including patient safety, improving the patient pathway and systems of care. Integral to all of these is the quality of communication in particular with patients but also with other specialities that may see patients who have underlying renal disease. The emergence of multidisciplinary team meetings has greatly assisted the governance of multidisciplinary care and the sharing of protocols (such as AKI management). However, in any nephrologist's patch, there are likely to be many specialities dealing with renal patients or diseases with a potential for renal involvement that have not yet established reliable links, agreed referral patterns and joined-up reviews. Yet such links and protocols are often easy to establish, facilitating early diagnosis and integrated care, with the patient at the centre. Similarly, patients with renal disease often have complex histories and need lifelong follow-up, yet transition of patient care and data from one renal unit to another can be poor unnecessarily compromising patient care. Again, with some thought, systems to facilitate smooth transition are not difficult to establish and are likely to be mutually beneficial. Renal information technology has, in general, underperformed in nephrology to date, but intelligent design in IT has huge potential to drastically reduce errors, improve communication with patients and colleagues, facilitate timely intervention and encourage reference to protocols and guidelines.

In this book we have tried to generate useful lists that help in the differential diagnosis, investigation and treatment of conditions; links to patient information; and guidelines that hopefully will be useful resources for the patient and doctor. The videos aim to help trainees bypass the first ascent of the learning curve and assist their patients through these procedures with comfort and safety. Tips and tricks based on the experience of the authors are scattered throughout the book with the hope of providing useful suggestions and avoiding common errors.

Finally, the last chapter discusses the benefits and practicalities of establishing health care partnerships with other units. Such partnerships as championed by, among others, the International Society of Nephrology can be incredibly rewarding and mutually beneficial.

This book only scratches the surface of practical improvements that might be made to renal patient care, but I hope that it will at least inspire a fresh look at some aspects of practice, as editing the book has done for me.

Hampstead, London, UK — Mark Harber, MBBS, PhD, FRCP

Acknowledgments

First and foremost I wish to thank the generosity of the contributing authors, all of whom are busy, dedicated clinicians and were too polite to say no when asked to contribute, although perhaps it is not a mistake that they would repeat again. Many of the authors have over the years taught me much of the nephrology I know and are equally committed to teaching and improving patient care, and I am indebted to them for their effort and tolerance.

I am also particularly grateful to those who have very generously contributed to the additional material used in the book especially Sue Car and Peter Topham, Steve Holt and Michael Cai, Mr Peter Veitch, Arundi Mahendran, Justin Harris, Dominic Yu, Shella Sandoval, Ramesh Batra, Hannah Deltrey-King, Amanda Rea and David Bishop who have produced videos that demonstrate procedures with much greater clarity than I could have achieved in prose and that I hope will assist doctors in carrying out these procedures with safety and confidence. I would particularly like to thank Paul Sweny for the gift of his collection of clinical images accumulated over the years of front-line service and Paul Bass, Alec Howie, Catherine Horsfield and Mared Casey-Owen for their patience and assistance in matters pathological.

Perhaps most significantly, patients have contributed extensively to this book not only by participating in videos and clinical material but by generally being the life and soul of nephrology, the reason for coming to work and the key motivation behind this book.

Finally my thanks go to Elina, Oskar and Kasper for their good humour, support and encouragement.

Contents

1 **Assessment of the Renal Patient** 1
Maryam Khosravi, Edward Kingdon, and Ben Caplin

2 **Urine Analysis** 19
Scott R. Henderson and Mark Harber

3 **Imaging in Nephrology** 29
Benjamin Salt and Antony Goode

4 **Kidney Biopsy** 39
Nick Woodward and Mark Harber

5 **Acute Kidney Injury: Epidemiology and Assessment** 47
Rachel M. Hilton

6 **Acute Kidney Injury: Management and Prevention** 63
Yogita Aggarwal, Mark Harber, and Christopher M. Laing

7 **Acute Renal Replacement Therapy** 75
Andrew Davenport

8 **Hepatorenal Syndrome** 91
Aisling O'Riordan

9 **Common Electrolyte Disorders** 101
Antje Fürstenberg, Stephen B. Walsh, and Christopher M. Laing

10 **Acid-Base Disorders** 123
Stephen B. Walsh

11 **Diagnosis and Investigation of the Hypertensive Patient** 135
Marc Jonathan George, Reecha Sofat, Aroon D. Hingorani, and Raymond MacAllister

12 **Management of High Blood Pressure** 147
Reecha Sofat, Marc Jonathan George, Aroon D. Hingorani, and Raymond MacAllister

13 **Podocytopathies** 157
Peter W. Mathieson

14 **Management of the Nephrotic Patient: The Overall Approach to the Patient with Nephrotic Syndrome (NS)** 161
Mark Harber

15 **Management of the Nephrotic Patient: Treatment of ECF Volume Expansion Due to Nephrotic Syndrome in Adults** 165
Liam Plant

16 **Minimal Change Disease and Focal Segmental Glomerulosclerosis** 171
Philip David Mason

17 **Membranous Nephropathy** 183
Peter W. Mathieson

18 **Membranoproliferative Glomerulonephritis and C3 Glomerulopathy** 189
Daniel P. Gale and Mared Owen-Casey

19 **IgA Nephropathy and Henoch-Schönlein Purpura** 203
Chee Kay Cheung, Joanna K.F. Boyd, and Jonathan Barratt

20 **Systemic Small Vessel Vasculitis** 215
Tabitha Turner-Stokes and Mark A. Little

21 **Goodpasture's or Anti-glomerular Basement Membrane (GBM) Disease** 227
Alan D. Salama

22 **Systemic Lupus Erythematosus, Antiphospholipid Syndrome and the Kidney** 235
Neeraj Dhaun (Bean)†, Christopher O.C. Bellamy, and David C. Kluth

23 **Practical Immunosuppression Guidelines for Patients with Glomerulonephritis** 249
Ruth J. Pepper and Alan D. Salama

24 **Infectious Diseases and the Kidney** 257
Elizabeth Williams, Sanjay Bhagani, and Mark Harber

25 **Blood-Borne Viruses and the Kidney** 269
John W.R. Booth, Sanjay Bhagani, and Mark Harber

26 **Tubulointerstitial Nephritis** 281
Simon Ball

27 **Rheumatological Conditions and the Kidney** 291
Bernadette Lynch and Aine Burns

28 **Multiple Myeloma and the Kidney** 303
Paul Cockwell and Stephanie Stringer

29 **Amyloidosis** 311
Julian David Gillmore and Helen J. Lachmann

30 **Thrombotic Microangiopathies** 323
Neil S. Sheerin

31 **Sickle Cell Disease and Other Haematological Disorders Involving the Kidney** 331
Claire Sharpe, Catherine J. Horsfield, and Mark Harber

32 **Diabetes and the Kidney** 345
Bryan Conway, Jane Goddard, Alan J. Jaap, and Alan W. Patrick

33 **Pregnancy and the Kidney** 359
Graham W. Lipkin, Clara J. Day, Nerissa Jurawan, Tracey A. Johnston, and Ellen M. Knox

34 **Disease of the Renal Vessels** 381
James P. Ritchie, Darren Green, and Philip A. Kalra

35 **Urinary Tract Infection** 395
Gayathri K. Rajakaruna and Mark Harber

36 **Renal Stone Disease** 413
Shabbir H. Moochhala and Robert J. Unwin

37 **Congenital Anomalies of the Kidneys and Urinary Tract** 429
Angela D. Gupta, Dan Wood, and John O. Connolly

38 **Acquired Urinary Tract Obstruction** 439
Gillian Smith and Mark Harber

39 **Kidney Cancer** 453
David Nicol and Ekaterini Boleti

40 **Inherited Renal Tumour Syndromes** 469
Thomas M.F. Connor and Patrick H. Maxwell

41 **Polycystic Kidney Disease** 481
Gareth Lewis and Alexander P. Maxwell

42 **Other Cystic Kidney Diseases** 491
Daniel M. McGuinness, Mark Harber, and Stephen D. Marks

43 **Genetic Disorders of the Glomerular Basement Membrane** 497
A. Neil Turner and Eleri Williams

44 **Anderson-Fabry Disease and Other Inherited Lipid Disorders of the Kidney** 509
Edward Stern and Mark Harber

45 **Inherited Metabolic Disease** 515
Sally-Anne Hulton

46 **Dermatology in Kidney Disease** 525
Ferina Ismail

47 **Chronic Kidney Disease: Epidemiology and Causes** 537
Dorothea Nitsch

48 **Chronic Kidney Disease: Management** 547
Charles R.V. Tomson and Shona Methven

49 **Transition** 563
Stephen D. Marks

50 **Anaemia Management in Chronic Kidney Disease** 569
Iain C. Macdougall

51 **Chronic Kidney Disease: Mineral and Bone Disorder (CKD-MBD)** 581
Richard S. Fish and John Cunningham

52 **Chronic Kidney Disease: Cardiovascular Complications** 589
Ben Caplin and David C. Wheeler

53 **Coagulation in Kidney Disease** 603
Duncan Brian and Pratima Chowdary

54 **Symptom Control and Palliative Care in Advanced CKD** 613
Fliss E.M. Murtagh and Sara N. Davison

55 **Nutrition and Kidney Disease** 621
Peter Choi and Jessica Stevenson

56 **Pharmacology and the Kidney** 629
Caroline Ashley

57 **Prevention of Infection in Kidney Patients** 635
Sophie Collier and Susan Hopkins

58 **Setting Up and Running a Haemodialysis Service** 647
Roger N. Greenwood and Hugh Feidhlim Woods

59 **Vascular Access: Improving Outcomes for Haemodialysis Patients** 657
Lindsay Chesterton, Ben Lindsey, and Richard J. Fluck

60 **Vascular Access: Fistulae and Grafts** 675
Madhu Kalyan Potluri, Dominic Yu, Justin Michael Harris, and Jennifer M. Cross

61 **Complications of Maintenance Haemodialysis and How to Avoid Them** 685
Nigel Suren Kanagasundaram

62 **Providing a Peritoneal Dialysis Service** 705
Stephen G. Holt, Michael X. Cai, Annabel H. Ryan, and Lawrence P. McMahon

63 **Peritoneal Dialysis Prescription** 717
Stanley L. Fan and Nasreen Samad

64 **Complications of Peritoneal Dialysis and How to Avoid Them** 725
Sarah Jenkins, Badri M. Shrestha, and Martin E. Wilkie

65 **Assessment of the Potential Transplant Donor** 739
Gareth Jones

66 **Assessment of the Potential Transplant Recipient** 755
Albert Power and Peter J. Dupont

67 **Tissue Typing, Crossmatch and Antibody Incompatibility in Kidney Transplantation** 767
Henry Stephens, Peter J. Dupont, and Mark Harber

68 **Surgical Aspects of Kidney and Pancreas Transplantation** 783
Chris J. Callaghan and Christopher J.E. Watson

69 **Management of the Acute Transplant** 797
Rawya Charif, Jack Galliford, David Game, and Adam McLean

70 **Immunosuppression for Kidney Transplantation** 813
Iain A.M. MacPhee

71 **Infectious Complications of Transplantation** 829
Rhys Evans, Sanjay Bhagani, Tanzina Haque, and Mark Harber

72 **Long-Term Management of Kidney Transplant Recipients (KTRs)** 857
Richard J. Baker

73 **International Health Partnerships** 877
Stacey Mearns

Appendix: Resources for Patients and Carers and Physicians 881

Index 887

Contributors

Yogita Aggarwal, MBCHB, Pg.Cert, Med. Edn, MA Renal Department, Royal Free Hospital, London, UK

Caroline Ashley, MSc, BPharm (Hons) Department of Pharmacy, Royal Free London NHS Foundation Trust, London, UK

Richard J. Baker, MBBChir, MA, FRCP, PhD Renal Medicine, St James's University Hospital, Lincoln Wing, Leeds, UK

Simon Ball, MA, PhD, FRCP Department of Nephrology, Queen Elizabeth Hospital Birmingham, Birmingham, UK

Jonathan Barratt, PhD, FRCP John Walls Renal Unit, Leicester General Hospital, Leicester, UK

Christopher O.C. Bellamy, MBBS, PhD, FRCPath Department of Pathology, Royal Infirmary of Edinburgh, Edinburgh, UK

Sanjay Bhagani, BSc (Hons), MBChB, FRCP (UK) Department of Infectious Diseases/HIV Medicine, Royal Free Hospital, London, UK

Ekaterini Boleti, MD, PhD, MRCP Academic Oncology, Royal Free London NHS Foundation Trust, London, UK

John W.R. Booth, MA, MRCP UCL Centre for Nephrology, Royal Free Campus, London, UK

Joanna K.F. Boyd, MBChB John Walls Renal Unit, Leicester General Hospital, Leicester, UK

Duncan Brian, MBBS, MRCS, MRCP (Lond) Thrombosis Unit, Katharine Dormandy Haemophilia Centre, Royal Free London NHS Foundation Trust, London, UK

Aine Burns, MD, FRCP, MSc Med Ed UCL Department of Nephrology, Royal Free London NHS Foundation Trust, London, UK

Michael Cai, MBBS Department of Nephrology, Royal Melbourne Hospital, Parkville, Melbourne, VIC, Australia

Chris J. Callaghan, PhD, FRCS Renal and Transplant Surgery, Guy's Hospital, London, UK

Ben Caplin, BSc (Hons), MBChB, PhD Centre for Nephrology, UCL Medical School, London, UK

Rawya Charif, MRCP, MD(Res) Imperial College Kidney and Transplant Centre, Imperial College Healthcare NHS Trust, Hammersmith Hospital, London, UK

Lindsay Chesterton, BMBS, MRCP, DM Department of Renal Medicine, Royal Derby Hospital, Derby, UK

Chee Kay Cheung, BSc, MBChB The John Walls Renal Unit, Leicester General Hospital, Leicester, Leicestershire, UK

Peter Choi, MBBChir, PhD, FRCP(UK) Department of Nephrology, John Hunter Hospital, New Lambton Heights, NSW, Australia

Pratima Chowdary, MBBS, FRCPath Thrombosis Unit, Katharine Dormandy Haemophilia Centre, Royal Free London NHS Foundation Trust, London, UK

Paul Cockwell, MBBCh, MRCP, FRCP, PhD Department of Renal Medicine, Queen Elizabeth Hospital Birmingham, Edgbaston, Birmingham, UK

Sophie Collier, BMBCH, MA, MRCP, FRCPath Department of Microbiology, Royal Free London NHS Foundation Trust, Royal Free Hospital, London, UK

John O. Connolly, PhD, FRCP UCL Centre for nephrology, Royal Free Hospital, London, UK

Thomas M.F. Connor, MRCP, BM, BCh UCL Division of Medicine and Centre for Nephrology, University College London, London, UK

Bryan Conway, PhD, MRCP Department of Renal Medicine, Royal Infirmary of Edinburgh, Edinburgh, UK

Jennifer M. Cross, MBChB, FRCP, PhD Department of Nephrology, UCL Centre For Nephrology, Royal Free Hospital Foundation Trust, London, UK

John Cunningham, DM, FRCP UCL Centre for Nephrology, University College London Medical School, London, UK

Andrew Davenport, MD UCL Centre for Nephrology, Royal Free Hospital, London, UK

Sara N. Davison, MD, MSc Department of Medicine, University of Alberta, Edmonton, AB, Canada

Clara J. Day, BMBCh, MA, PhD, FRCP Department of Nephrology, Queen Elizabeth Hospital Birmingham, Birmingham, UK

Neeraj Dhaun (Bean), MB, PhD Department of Renal Medicine, Royal Infirmary of Edinburgh, Edinburgh, UK

Peter J. Dupont, PhD, FRCPI UCL Centre for Nephrology, Royal Free Hospital, London, UK

Rhys Evans, MBBS, MRCP UCL Centre for Nephrology, Royal Free Hospital, London, UK

Stanley L. Fan, DM and MBBChir (Cantab), FRCP(UK) Renal Unit, Barts Health NHS Trust, London, UK

Richard S. Fish, MRCP, BMBS, BMedSci (Hons) UCL Centre for Nephrology, UCL Medical School, London, UK

Richard J. Fluck, FRCP, MA (Cantab), MBBS Department of Renal Medicine, Royal Derby Hospital, Derby, UK

Antje Fürstenberg, SpR UCL Centre for Nephrology, Royal Free Hospital, London, UK

Daniel P. Gale, MA, MBBChir, MRCP(UK) PhD UCL Centre for Nephrology, Royal Free Hospital, London, UK

Jack Galliford, MBBS, FRCP Imperial College Kidney and Transplant Centre, Imperial College Healthcare NHS Trust, Hammersmith Hospital, London, UK

David Game, MA, PhD, FRCP Department of Nephrology and Transplantation, Guy's Hospital, London, UK

Marc Jonathan George, MBChB (Hons), BSc (Hons) Department of Clinical Pharmacology and Therapeutics, University College London Hospital, London, UK

Julian David Gillmore, MBBS, MD, PhD, FRCP National Amyloidosis Centre, UCL Medical School, London, UK

Jane Goddard, PhD, FRCPE Department of Diabetes, Royal Infirmary of Edinburgh, Edinburgh, UK

Antony Goode, BSc (Hons), MBBS, MRCP, FRCR Radiology Department, Royal Free London NHS Foundation Trust, London, UK

Darren Green, MBChB Department of Renal Medicine, Salford Royal Hospital, Salford, Greater Manchester, UK

Roger N. Greenwood, MSc, ACGI, MD, FRCP Renal Unit, Lister Hospital, East and North Herts NHS Trust, Stevenage, UK

Angela D. Gupta, MD Urology, Johns Hopkins Hospital, Baltimore, MD, USA

Tanzina Haque, MBBS, PhD, FRCPath Department of Virology, Royal Free Hospital, London, UK

Mark Harber, MBBS, PhD, FRCP UCL Department of Nephrology, Royal Free London NHS Foundation Trust, Hampstead, London, UK

Justin Michael Harris, BSc(Hons), MBBS, FRCR Department of Radiology, Conquest Hospital, St Leonards-on-Sea, Hastings, East Sussex, UK

Scott R. Henderson, MBChB, BScMedSci (Hons), MRCP UCL Centre for Nephrology, Royal Free Hospital, London, UK

Rachel M. Hilton, MA, PhD, FRCP Department of Nephrology and Transplantation, Guy's and St Thomas' NHS Foundation Trust, London, UK

Aroon D. Hingorani, MA, FRCP, PhD Institute of Cardiovascular Science, University College London and University College London Hospitals NHS Foundation Trust, London, UK

Stephen Geoffrey Holt, BSc, MBBS, PhD, FRCP, FRACP Department of Nephrology, Royal Melbourne Hospital, Parkville, Melbourne, VIC, Australia

Susan Hopkins, BA, MBBCh, BAO, MSC, FRCPI, FRCP Department of Infectious Diseases and Clinical Microbiology, Royal Free London NHS Foundation Trust, London, UK

Catherine J. Horsfield, FRCPath Department of Histopathology, Guy's & St Thomas' NHS, St Thomas' Hospital, London, UK

Sally-Anne Hulton, MD, FRCP, FRCPCH, MBBCh Department of Nephrology, Birmingham Children's Hospital, Birmingham, UK

Ferina Ismail, BSc, MBBS, MRCP, PhD Department of Dermatology, Royal Free London NHS Foundation Trust, London, UK

Alan J. Jaap, MD, FRCPE Department of Diabetes, Royal Infirmary of Edinburgh, Edinburgh, UK

Sarah Jenkins, MA, MBBChir, FRCP Sheffield Kidney Institute, Northern General Hospital, Sheffield Teaching Hospitals NHS Foundation Trust, Sheffield, South Yorkshire, UK

Tracey A. Johnston, MD, FRCOG Department of Obstetrics, Birmingham Women's NHS Foundation Trust, Birmingham, UK

Gareth Jones, MBBS, FRCP, PhD UCL Centre for Nephrology, Royal Free London NHS Trust, London, UK

Nerissa Jurawan, MBBS, MRCP (UK) Renal Medicine, University Hospital Birmingham, Birmingham, UK

Philip A. Kalra Department of Renal Medicine, Salford Royal Hospital, Salford, Greater Manchester, UK

Nigel Suren Kanagasundaram, MBChB, MD, FRCP (Lon) Renal Services, Newcastle upon Tyne Hospitals NHS Foundation Trust, Freeman Hospital, High Heaton, Newcastle upon Tyne, Tyne and Wear, UK

Maryam Khosravi, BSc, MRCP UCL Centre for Nephrology, Royal Free Hospital, London, UK

Edward Kingdon, FRCP Sussex Kidney Unit, Royal Sussex County Hospital, Brighton, UK

David C. Kluth, MB, PhD Department of Renal Medicine, Royal Infirmary of Edinburgh, Edinburgh, UK

Ellen M. Knox, MD, MRCOG Department of Obstetrics, Birmingham Women's NHS Foundation Trust, Birmingham, UK

Helen J. Lachmann, MA, MBBChir, MD, FRCP National Amyloidosis Centre, University College London School of Medicine and Royal Free London NHS Foundation Trust, London, UK

Christopher M. Laing, MBChB, MRCP, MD (Res) UCL Centre For Nephrology, Royal Free London NHS Foundation Trust and University College London Hospitals, London, UK

Gareth Lewis, MB, PhD Regional Nephrology Unit, Belfast City Hospital, Belfast, Antrim, UK

Ben Lindsey, FRCS Department of Vascular Surgery and Department of Renal Surgery, The Royal Free London NHS Foundation Trust, London, UK

Graham W. Lipkin, MD, FRCP Department of Nephrology, Queen Elizabeth Hospital Birmingham, University Hospital Birmingham NHS Foundation Trust, Birmingham, UK

Mark A. Little, FRCP, PhD UCL Centre For Nephrology, Trinity Health Kidney Centre, Tallaght Hospital and Trinity College Dublin, Tallaght, Dublin, Ireland

Bernadette Lynch, MD, MRCPI, BA Physiology Rheumatology Department, Royal Free Hospital, London, UK

Raymond MacAllister, FRCP, MD Division of Medicine, Centre for Clinical Pharmacology, University College London, London, UK

Iain C. Macdougall, BSc, MD, FRCP Renal Unit, King's College Hospital, London, UK

Iain A.M. MacPhee, DPhil, FRCP Division of Clinical Sciences: Renal Medicine, St. George's, University of London, Cranmer Terrace, London, UK

Stephen D. Marks, MD, MSc, MRCP, DCH, FRCPCH Department of Paediatric Nephrology, Great Ormond Street Hospital for Children NHS Foundation Trust, London, UK

Philip David Mason, BSc, PhD, MBBS, FRCP Oxford Kidney Unit, The Churchill Hospital, Oxford, UK

Peter W. Mathieson, PhD, FRCP, FMedSci Academic Renal Unit, University of Bristol and Southmead Hospital, Bristol, UK

Patrick H. Maxwell, DPhil, FRCP, FMedSci University of Cambridge School of Clinical Medicine, University of Cambridge, Cambridge, UK

Alexander P. Maxwell, MD, PhD, FRCP Regional Nephrology Unit, Belfast City Hospital and Queens University Belfast, Belfast, Antrim, UK

Daniel M. McGuinness, MBBS, BSc, MRCP UCL Centre for Nephrology, Royal Free Hospital, London, UK

Adam McLean, MA, MBBS, FRCP, DPhil Imperial College Kidney and Transplant Centre, Hammersmith Hospital, Imperial College Healthcare NHS Trust, London, UK

Lawrence P. McMahon, MBBS, MD Department of Renal Medicine, Eastern Health and Eastern Health Clinical School, Monash University, Box Hill, Melbourne, VIC, Australia

Stacey Mearns, BSc, MBChB, DTMH, MRCP General Medicine, Royal Free Hospital, London, UK

Shona Methven, BSc (Med Sci) (Hons), MD, MRCP(UK) Academic Renal Unit, University of Bristol, Southmead Hospital, Westbury-on-Trym, Bristol, UK

Shabbir H. Moochhala, MRCP, PhD UCL Centre for Nephrology, Royal Free Hospital, UCL Centre for Nephrology Royal Free, London, UK

Fliss E.M. Murtagh, PhD, MRCGP, MBBS Department of Palliative Care, Policy and Rehabilitation, King'd College London, Cicely Saunders Institute, London, UK

David Nicol, MBBS, FRACS Department of Urology, The Royal Marsden NHS Foundation Trust, London, UK

Dorothea Nitsch, MD, MSc Department of Non-Communicable Disease Epidemiology, Faculty of Epidemiology and Population Health, London School of Hygiene and Tropical Medicine, London, UK

Aisling O' Riordan, MBBCh, BAO, MRCPI, MD Renal Department, Royal Free NHS Foundation Trust, London, UK

Mared Owen-Casey, MBBCh, FRCPath Histopathology Department, Betsi Cadwaladar University Health Board, Wrexham, UK

Alan W. Patrick, MD, FRCPE Department of Diabetes, Royal Infirmary of Edinburgh, Edinburgh, UK

Ruth J. Pepper, MRCP, PhD Department of Nephrology, Royal Free Hospital, London, UK

L. Plant Cork University Hospital, University College Cork, Ireland

William D. Plant, BSc, MB, FRCPI, FRCPE Department of Renal Medicine, Cork University Hospital & University College Cork, Cork, Ireland

Madhu Kalyan Potluri, MBChB, BSc MedSci, MRCP (UK) Renal Department, Royal Free Hospital, London, UK

Albert Power, MB, BChir, MRCP, MD Department of Medicine, Imperial College London, London, UK

Gayathri K. Rajakaruna, MBBS, MRCP (UK) Department of Nephrology, Royal Free Hospital, London, UK

James P. Ritchie, MB, ChB Department of Renal Medicine, Salford Royal Hospital, Salford, Greater Manchester, UK

Annabel H. Ryan, RN Div 1 Department of Nephrology, Western Health Sunshine Hospital, St. Albans, VIC, Australia

Alan D. Salama, MA, PhD, FRCP UCL Centre for Nephrology, Royal Free Hospital, London, UK

Benjamin Salt, MBBS, MA Department of Radiology, Royal Free Hospital, London, UK

Nasreen Samad, FRCP (UK), MBBS Renal Unit, Barts Health NHS Trust, London, UK

Claire Sharpe, MBBS, PhD, FRCP Department of Renal Medicine, King's College London and King's College Hospital NHS Foundation Trust, London, UK

Neil S. Sheerin, BSc, MBBS, PhD, FRCP Institute of Cellular Medicine, Newcastle University, Newcastle upon Tyne, UK

Badri M. Shrestha, MD, FRCS(Eng, Edin and Gen), FICS Department of Renal Transplantation, Sheffield Kidney Institute, University of Sheffield, Sheffield, South Yorkshire, UK

Gillian Smith, MD, FRCS(Urol) Department of Urology, Royal Free London NHS Foundation Trust, London, UK

Reecha Sofat, BSc, MBBS, MRCP, MSc Department of Metabolism and Experimental Therapeutics, Divison of Medicine Faculty of Medical Sciences, London

Henry Stephens, BSc, PhD UCL centre for Nephrology and the Anthony Nolan Trust, Hospital Royal Free London NHS Foundation Trust, London, UK

Edward Stern, BA (Hons), MBBS Centre for Nephrology, Royal Free London, London, UK

Jessica Stevenson Nutrition and Dietetics Department, John Hunter Hospital, New Lambton, NSW, Australia

Stephanie Stringer, MBChB, MRCP, PhD Department of Renal Medicine, Queen Elizabeth Hospital Birmingham, Edgbaston, Birmingham, UK

Charles R.V. Tomson, MA, BMBCh, FRCP, DM (Oxon) Department of Renal Medicine, Southmead Hospital, Bristol, UK

A. Neil Turner, PhD, FRCP Department of Renal Medicine, Edinburgh Royal Infirmary, Edinburgh, UK

Tabitha Turner-Stokes, MA (cantab), MBBS Imperial College Kidney and Transplant Centre, Imperial College Healthcare NHS Trust, Hammersmith Hospital, London, UK

Robert J. Unwin, BM, FRC, PhD, FSB, CBiol UCL Centre for Nephrology, Royal Free London NHS Foundation Trust, London, UK

Stephen B. Walsh, MBBS, PhD UCL Centre for Nephrology, Royal Free Hospital, London, UK

Christopher J.E. Watson, MA, MD, BChir, FRCS University Department of Surgery, Addenbrooke's Hospital, Cambridge, UK

David C. Wheeler, MD, FRCP Centre for Nephrology, UCL Medical School, London, UK

Martin E. Wilkie, BSc, MBChB, FRCP, MD Sheffield Kidney Institute, Sheffield Teaching Hospitals NHS, Sheffield, South Yorkshire, UK

Elizabeth Williams, MBBS, MRCP Genito-Urinary Medicine, Royal London Hospital, London, UK

Eleri Williams, MB BChir MRCP Department of Renal Medicine, Royal Infirmary of Edinburgh, Edinburgh, UK

Dan Wood, PhD, FRCS (Urol) Adolescent Urology, University College London Hospitals, London, UK

Hugh Feidhlim Woods, MBBCh, BAO, MRCP(UK) Fresenius Medical Care Asia Pacific, Hong Kong, SAR (China)

Nick Woodward, MBBS, MRCP, FRCR Department of radiology, Royal Free London NHS Foundation Trust, London, UK

Dominic Yu, MBBS, MRCPI, FRCR Department of radiology, Royal Free London NHS Foundation Trust, London, UK

Liam Plant Department of radiology, Cork University Hospital, University College Cork, Ireland

1 Assessment of the Renal Patient

Maryam Khosravi, Edward Kingdon, and Ben Caplin

Nephrologists encounter a spectrum of renal disease, from asymptomatic incidental findings to newly diagnosed renal impairment to life-threatening metabolic disturbance in a critically ill patient. Many of these patients will have significant comorbidity, often alongside previously diagnosed chronic renal disease. These factors mean the assessment of the 'renal patient' can be a challenging proposition. There are numerous approaches to the assessment of patients with kidney disease, and practitioners will develop their own style with time. The 'practical' strategy we outline here is only one of many but one that we find successful in day-to-day practice.

In this chapter we approach the assessment of the renal patient with a series of such questions. This strategy is outlined in Fig. 1.1. Unsurprisingly, as with any area of acute medicine, the first priority will be to ask if the patient is safe. This question provides the starting point of this chapter.

After addressing any life-threatening emergency, the usual next question in any renal patient will be to ask: What is this patient's intravascular volume status? An accurate assessment of this is absolutely central to both the diagnosis and management of patients with kidney disease. Assessment of fluid balance is usually based on multiple sources of clinical information, and we discuss the utility of these in the second section of this chapter. However assessing fluid balance is primarily a practical skill, so although tips and guidance can be provided in a textbook, this can be no substitute for repeated practice.

Alongside the assessment of intravascular volume status, the other critical step will be to clarify is this patient already being managed for an underlying kidney condition. The approach to the patient with established kidney disease, for example, a patient receiving dialysis or being treated for an inflammatory glomerulonephritis, will be completely different from the approach to the patient who presents with a renal disorder for the first time. In these cases where the patient is known to a renal service, the assessment will be focused on optimising the management of the underlying condition and addressing associated complications. This aspect of the assessment of the kidney patient is addressed in the last section of the chapter.

If the current presentation is the patient's first consultation with a renal specialist, the primary purpose of the assessment will be to establish the underlying cause of the renal disorder. This is a clinical scenario in which there is often diagnostic uncertainty, representing some of the most interesting and sometimes challenging areas of the nephrology practice. This aspect of the clinical assessment comprises the majority of this chapter. In this section the approach to different renal syndromes is outlined.

M. Khosravi, BSc, MRCP (✉)
UCL Centre for Nephrology, Royal Free Hospital, Rowland Hill Street, Lodnon NW3 2PF, UK
e-mail: m.khosravi@ucl.ac.uk

E. Kingdon, FRCP
Sussex Kidney Unit, Royal Sussex County Hospital, Eastern Road, Brighton BN2 5BE, UK
e-mail: edward.kingdon@bsuh.nhs.uk

B. Caplin, BSc (Hons), MBChB, PhD
Centre for Nephrology, UCL Medical School, Royal Free Campus, Rowland Hill Street, London NW3 2PF, UK
e-mail: b.caplin@ucl.ac.uk

Urgent Assessment for Renal Emergencies

As with any acutely unwell patient, the first priority must be to assess and correct potentially life-threatening physiological dysfunction. Alongside the maintenance of an adequate airway, ventilation and circulation, urgent renal-specific issues are likely to relate to assessment and treatment of either metabolic disturbance, most often hyperkalaemia, acidaemia, or fluid overload. Any of these scenarios may be and indication for urgent renal replacement therapy (RRT) if

M. Harber (ed.), *Practical Nephrology*,
DOI 10.1007/978-1-4471-5547-8_1, © Springer-Verlag London 2014

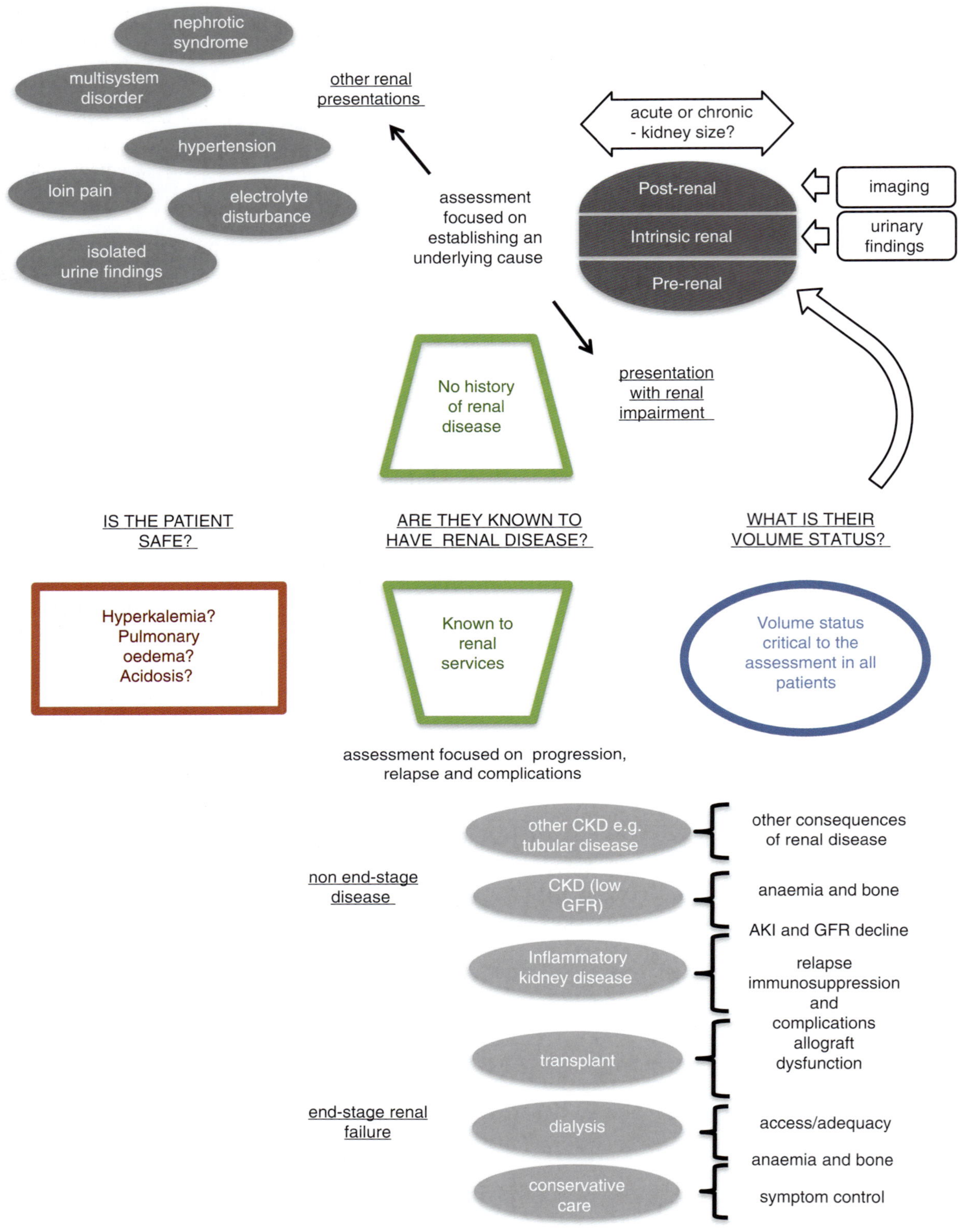

Fig. 1.1 An approach to the assessment of the 'renal patient'. Our approach is initially based on asking three questions. The first priority is always to ensure any life-threatening clinical situation is addressed. Establishing whether a patient is known to renal services is always important. The assessment of a patient with a known renal problem will be focused on progression and complications of their condition. Conversely the work-up will be will be concentrated on making a diagnosis if the patient has no known renal history. Classification of a new presentation into one of the many 'renal syndromes' e.g. acute pre-renal impairment or nephrotic syndrome, will mean further assessment can be appropriately targeted. In parallel, the patient's intravascular volume status will likely be relevant to almost every 'renal patient' whether in the evaluation of potential pre-renal acute kidney injury, management of oedema and hypertension in a patient with nephrotic syndrome or to establish the cause of intradialytic hypotension in a patient receiving outpatient haemodialysis

not responsive to medical manoeuvres. Furthermore uraemic encepholapathy, pericarditis are likely to be absolute indications for instituting dialysis (see Chaps. 7, 9 and 10 on acute renal replacement, acid-base and electrolyte disturbances, respectively).

When there is an indication for urgent renal replacement therapy (RRT) attention must be given to the most appropriate form of dialysis or haemofiltration. Requirements will depend on the need for other organ support, but the use of an extracorporeal circuit, even with the low blood flows used in continuous therapies such as haemofiltration, risks haemodynamic instability. Therefore adequate, usually invasive, monitoring and access to vasopressors or inotropes are mandatory in cardiovascularly unstable patients receiving RRT. Critically, immediate management often depends on whether the acidaemic or hyperkalaemic patient has a remediable medical condition; a patient with urinary retention and potassium of 7.2 mmol/L may respond rapidly to medical therapy following relief of obstruction, whereas a septic oliguric hypotensive patient with a potassium of 5.8 mmol/L is much more likely to need renal replacement in the coming hours.

Assessment of Intravascular Volume Status

The evaluation of fluid status is critical in the assessment and management of all renal patients.

Table 1.1 Clinical assessment of fluid status

History	Paroxysmal nocturnal dyspnoea, orthopnoea, increased weight and worsening oedema are relatively sensitive and fairly specific symptoms of fluid overload. Thirst is a relatively sensitive marker of dehydration or salt overload. A history of significant fluid loss or reduced fluid intake may contribute to the overall assessment of fluid balance
Examination	
Pulse	Tachycardia is a non-specific marker of intravascular volume depletion and may be associated with excessive intravascular volume in the context of heart failure
Blood pressure	Relative hypotension (in comparison with historical blood pressure) and episodes of documented hypotension (intraoperative, hospital or community based) are always significant findings in patients with renal dysfunction. Although trends may be informative, hypotension alone is a non-specific marker of intravascular volume depletion
Orthostatic changes	Changes in blood pressure with changes in posture are useful findings. Changes of 20 mmHg in systolic and 10 mmHg in diastolic blood pressure upon change in posture are widely used as significant thresholds. Reflex tachycardia (increase in 30 beats per minute or more) is non-specific and sensitive for acute large blood loss but insensitive for smaller bleeds or other causes of hypovolaemia
Peripheral temperature	Cool nose, hands or feet at room temperature imply either decreased intravascular volume (low JVP) or cardiac failure (raised JVP). These are not sensitive but easy and reproducible. Unhelpful in patients with peripheral vascular disease or vasodilated patients (sepsis, cirrhosis, thyrotoxicosis)
Jugular venous pressure (JVP)	Operator dependent and sensitivity highly influenced by body habitus. Raised JVP may represent either increased intravascular volume or high right ventricular filling pressure (cardiac failure, pulmonary hypertension, tricuspid regurgitation or stenosis, restrictive defects, tamponade). Common for ESRD patients with previous central venous catheters to have internal jugular stenosis or occlusion (including secondary to current line) or superior vena cava obstruction
Oedema	Diurnal variation (feet swollen in the evening, face in the morning) usually rules out any anatomical cause. A bed-bound patient may have normal ankles but retain substantial salt and water in the sacral or flank oedema. Oedema will also be influenced by drugs and plasma oncotic pressure
Third heart sound (S3 gallop rhythm)	Insensitive indicator of ventricular failure/overload
Ascites and pleural effusions	Non-specific and poorly sensitive
Weight	Extremely useful serial measurement for general nephrology patients as well as those on dialysis with a 'dry weight'. Serial measurements for inpatients are extremely valuable measures of total body water (but not necessarily intravascular volume)
Urine output	Non-specific but important part of AKI classification and relatively a sensitive marker of intravascular volume. Unhelpful as a marker of intravascular volume if coexistent AKI or concentrating defect from an alternative cause, e.g. post-obstructive diuresis
Documentation of inputs and outputs	Anaesthetic charts, ward charts including drain losses and stool charts can be invaluable if accurate
Urine specific gravity	Can be useful but acutely or chronically injured kidneys lose the ability to concentrate urine normally and therefore has limited value in patients with renal disease
Urinary sodium	A low spot urinary sodium or fractional excretion of sodium is indicative of reduced renal perfusion and can be helpful in identifying intravascular volume depletion or hepatorenal syndrome but is invalid in the face of acute tubular injury, diuretics or dopamine

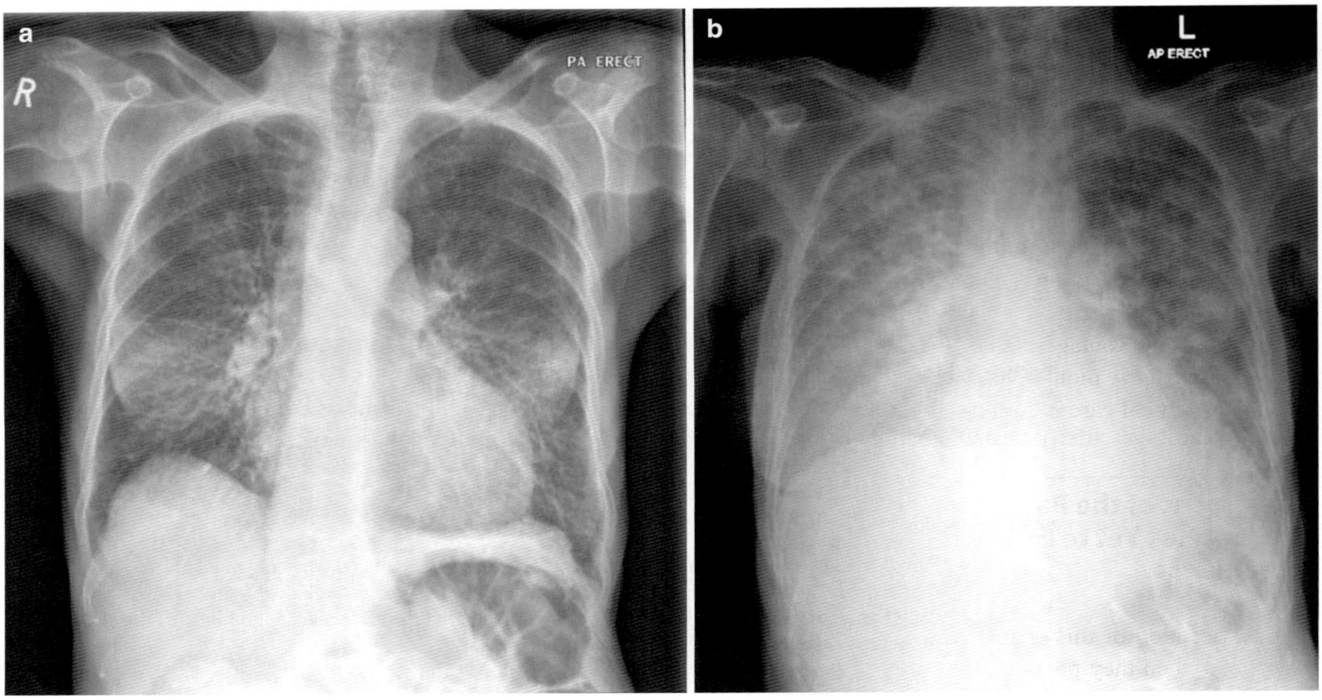

Fig. 1.2 (**a**) CXR of a patient with raised left ventricular end-diastolic pressure (LVEDP) showing upper lobe blood diversion, fluid in the fissure and Kerley B lines. This approximately equates to an LVEDP of 18 mmHg or above. (**b**) Frank pulmonary oedema in the same patient within 24 h in the absence of any filling or cardiac event but in the presence of sepsis. This demonstrates that pulmonary oedema on a CXR is not necessarily indicative of excessive filling pressures per se

Table 1.1 shows some of the clinical parameters that have merit in assessing fluid balance. Some such as serial measurement of weight and orthostatic blood pressure should be incorporated into routine ward observations even on non-renal wards. Where appropriate patients such as those discharged home with recovering AKI or nephrotic syndrome may also benefit from monitoring their own weight and postural blood pressure to help inform changes in fluid status. Other signs such as peripheral temperature and observation of central veins are often useful, whereas skin turgor and dryness of mucous membranes are on the whole poor, insensitive and non-specific clinical tools.

Investigations may also be helpful in assessment of intravascular volume status. The chest radiograph can confirm fluid overload, but is not particularly sensitive for mild/moderate overload, and acute lung injury can occur without an increase of right sided filling pressure (see Fig. 1.2a, b). In one study using pulmonary artery measurements, where fluid overload was defined as a pulmonary artery occlusion pressure ≥18 mmHg, radiologists achieved a diagnostic sensitivity of 55–65 %. This improved to 70 % by including cardiothoracic ratio (CTR) >0.55 and a vascular pedicle width (VPW) (the horizontal distance between the point where the superior vena cava crosses the right main bronchus and the origin of the left subclavian artery) measurement of >70 mm [1]. Therefore in practical terms a single chest-x-ray is unlikely to be useful, it may be a valuable tool when serial measurements are used.

In addition, there are also near-patient tests that may become more commonly utilised. Bioimpedance is one such technique and is an inexpensive and non-invasive technique to estimate body water. Given the difficulties with the clinical assessment of fluid status, the possibility of an easily usable objective measure is attractive. Unfortunately as with many of the clinical parameters guiding assessment of fluid balance, a single measurement in an individual patient does appear to add significant value to clinical assessment. Serial measures may again be more useful, so this technique may be most appropriate in patients regularly attending dialysis or the outpatient department rather than in the acute situation [2].

Biochemical measures that have been advocated as indices of fluid status such as a disproportionately high urea:creatinine ratio, raised serum urate or elevated serum lactate also lack sensitivity and specificity but may be helpful as part of a constellation of features associated with intravascular volume depletion.

A number of methods using continuous monitoring and aimed at detecting changes in cardiac output in response to altered venous return (e.g. using respiratory cycle variation, passive leg raising or a fluid challenge) are useful in experienced hands. Importantly however, measures of fluid-responsiveness are likely to reflect a number of variables rather than just intravascular volume, so should always be considered as part of a more comprehensive assessment. Finally a variety of invasive cardiovascular measurements can be used to more accurately assess fluid status where sophisticated monitoring is available and are reviewed comprehensively elsewhere [3]. There remains significant debate as to the advantages and disadvantages of the various methods of invasive monitoring, and the knowledge base in this area of critical care is continuously evolving.

Assessment of the Patient When the Renal Disorder Has Yet to Be Identified and/or Characterised

This next section of this chapter discusses the approach to the patient when they present for the first time with a renal disorder to the reviewing nephrologist. In these cases a diagnosis needs to be established. Although renal physicians are faced with an enviable variety of clinical scenarios, these can usually be grouped into a number of renal 'syndromes'. These renal syndromes although not diagnoses in themselves are useful descriptions to help direct further investigation and to facilitate communication between physicians. An initial approach to these renal syndromes is outlined below. Following this the more general aspects of the history and the clinical examination, which might be helpful in establishing the cause of a renal disorder in patients presenting with any one of these renal syndromes is presented.

Presentation with Renal Impairment

An impaired kidney function, as identified by an increase in the serum creatinine, is the commonest reason for referral to a nephrologist. Patients may first present with symptoms directly related to renal dysfunction (Table 1.2). Often however, the presence of renal impairment will be identified by blood tests performed following a clinical presentation unrelated to the kidney.

Does the Patient Have Acute or Chronic Renal Injury?

The urgency of further investigation in a patient with renal impairment is critically dependent on whether the identified kidney dysfunction is acute (occurring over days to weeks) or chronic (occurring over months to years). Differentiation of these clinical scenarios is straightforward if the patient has been historically diagnosed with CKD, if previous blood tests are available or if the patient is aware of previous episodes of AKI or CKD. The distinction can be all the more difficult in cases of acute on chronic renal dysfunction where only knowledge of baseline creatinine figures will uncover whether there is an element of acute deterioration in GFR. Suggestive evidence may come from a likely acute precipitating event, the long-standing presence of a risk factor or a childhood history raising the possibility of previously undiagnosed renal dysplasia. Often, however, these clues are not immediately to hand, so other evidence may needed to judge the likely time course of the presenting renal dysfunction.

The duration of symptoms can be a useful indicator of chronicity; however, the high prevalence of subclinical advanced renal impairment means that in many cases the underlying disorder may have been present for some time before the patient reports the onset of illness. Furthermore the presence of risk factors or a systemic disorder known to put the patient at risk of chronic kidney disease (see below) does not provide definite evidence for pre-existing renal dysfunction. The single best markers of long-standing (and consequently irreversible) renal impairment are radiological measurements. Bipolar kidney length <10 cm in combination with an increase in cortical echogenicity (defined as a higher pixel density in the renal cortex than the liver) are the best predictors of advanced chronic kidney disease [4]. Exceptions to this rule occur where the size of chronically diseased kidneys is preserved, most typically in diabetes but also cystic diseases such as APCKD, protein deposition diseases such as amyloid, chronic obstruction, xanthomatous pyelonephritis and HIV nephropathy.

Table 1.2 Symptoms attributable to renal dysfunction

Uraemia	Anorexia, nausea, pruritus, malaise and sleep disturbance are all common symptoms in ESRD. Patients may also complain of headaches, reduced mental agility, chest pain (pericarditis), prolonged bleeding or bruising
Anaemia	Lethargy, palpitations, shortness of breath
Electrolyte disturbance	Palpitations, musculoskeletal pain, cramps, restless limbs, seizures, confusion
Fluid maldistribution or excess	Facial or peripheral swelling, shortness of breath or reduced exercise tolerance, orthopnoea, paroxysmal nocturnal dyspnoea
Urinary symptoms	Oliguria, nocturia (a common symptom in CKD)

Biochemical markers such as potassium, calcium, phosphate, parathyroid hormone and haemoglobin have been described in textbooks as indicators of chronicity of renal dysfunction. However, these parameters have limited utility in practice since all can also change rapidly in the context of AKI.

Diagnostic Breakdown of Acute or Chronic Renal Dysfunction

Assessment of a patient with AKI is described in detail in Chap. 5; however, the classical subdivision into prerenal, intrinsic and postrenal causes of impairment is a useful approach in any patient presenting with either acute or chronic renal impairment, so it will also be outlined here.

Prerenal

A 'prerenal' aetiology suggests hypoperfusion of the kidney. This is a critical component of the assessment of patients with AKI as this form of insult is usually associated with an acute presentation. However, renal artery stenosis and chronic hypovolaemia in patients with high output gastrointestinal stomas may develop more insidiously and present as CKD. Therefore, potential precipitants of prerenal injury should be sought in all patients with renal dysfunction.

Circulatory shock, whether vasodilatory, cardiogenic or hypovolaemic, will invariably lead to an acute prerenal injury (even if it is subclinical) and should be straightforward to identify. Other more subtle forms of prerenal kidney injury (such as those due to a less clinically apparent degree of intravascular volume depletion) may be less obvious initially but remain important considerations. The potential precipitants of prerenal injury are outlined in Table 1.3.

Postrenal Causes

Postrenal causes of renal impairment are particularly important to detect since the associated renal injury often reversible with relief of the obstruction. Furthermore, obstruction is a common cause for unexpected deterioration in patients with established kidney disease.

Although the clinical history or examination (Table 1.4) may suggest an obstructive cause of kidney injury, the exclusion of a postrenal cause of renal impairment cannot be made without radiological investigation. A renal ultrasound is often the first-line investigation. There are important limitations which should be considered when interpreting evidence of obstruction on renal ultrasound:

- 'False positives' can occur in cases of chronic dilation of the pelvi-calyceal system. Functional imaging should be pursued in attempting to establish the significance of morphological abnormality where kidney function is adequate for these tests to be useful. Renograms with the addition of diuretics using nuclear medicine tracers can be helpful in this context (discussed in Chap. 38).
- 'False negatives' can occur in anuric patients who may not have pelvi-calyceal dilatation. If the history is suggestive, more detailed anatomical imaging such as MRI or CT may be helpful. Occasionally in these cases a diagnostic trial of relief of obstruction should be considered.

Symptomatic changes in urine volume are not usually diagnostically helpful. Patients with significant obstruction usually notice no change in their urine volume. Clinical presentations and past history that might suggest a postrenal cause of kidney dysfunction are shown in Table 1.4.

Table 1.3 Assessment of potential precipitants of prerenal kidney injury

Relative hypotension, i.e. drop in BP for whatever cause in normally hypertensive patient	
Cardiogenic shock	
Intravascular volume depletion	
Blood loss	
Poor oral intake	Consider the confused patient or the patient without access to fluids
Fever, sweating	
Vomiting, diarrhoea	Patients with short bowel syndrome or high output stomas are at particular risk of volume depletion
Polyuria	Prescribed or non-prescribed diuretics, mannitol Central polyuria – salt-losing nephropathy, diabetes insipidus Tubular dysfunction – Addison's disease, nephrogenic DI, lithium toxicity, salt-losing nephropathies, hyperglycaemia, diuresis associated with recovery of kidney function
Fluid redistribution with reduced arterial perfusion	
Ascites	Liver disease
Fluid accumulation in the GI tract	Bowel obstruction, post-op ileus
Oedema secondary to nephrotic syndrome	
Septic/anaphylactic shock	
Local hypoperfusion	
Arterial occlusion	Emboli, most commonly following endovascular intervention; arterial dissection; malignant infiltration
Renal artery stenosis	May be suggested by 'crash' pulmonary oedema, profound reduction in GFR post-renin-angiotensin blockade
Venous obstruction	Renal vein thrombosis, consider in association with a procoagulant state (nephrotic syndrome); Page kidney following kidney biopsy or trauma

NB Patient notes (including anaesthetic records) are invaluable for identifying episodes of relative hypotension, poor IV or oral intake, excessive losses or weight changes. The better the documentation, the more accurate the interpretation is likely to be

Table 1.4 Symptoms, findings and clinical history suggestive of urinary tract obstruction or conditions associated with obstruction

Anuria	Suggests bilateral ureteric or bladder outlet obstruction. Beware of nonobstructive causes
Symptoms of bladder outlet obstruction	Urinary frequency, dysuria, poor flow, nocturia, urgency, double micturition, hesitancy, post-micturition dribbling, incontinence (overflow obstruction), sensation of incomplete emptying
NB Acute urinary retention can be painless with a neuropathic bladder	
Spraying on micturition	Urethral stricture, phimosis or paraphimosis
Loin pain	Any cause of obstruction On micturition (suggestive of vesicoureteric reflux) On excessive drinking (suggestive of PUJ obstruction)
Visible haematuria	Nephrolithiasis, malignancy, papillary necrosis
Medications	Anticholinergics, withdrawal of alpha blockers
Disseminated or pelvic malignancy	
Iatrogenic obstruction	Pelvic surgery or radiation therapy
Nephrolithiasis	
Pregnancy	Collecting systems can be dilated without functional obstruction
Childhood UTI or enuresis	May suggest congenital abnormalities of the urinary tract
Schistosomiasis infection	

Table 1.5 Simple classification and diagnostic clues to intrinsic renal causes of renal dysfunction

Toxins: endogenous	Any history to suggest rhabdomyolysis, intravascular haemolysis, tumour lysis syndrome, multiple myeloma, enteric hyperoxalosis, cholesterol emboli, hypercalcaemia
Toxins: exogenous	Drugs prescribed or illicit, herbal remedies, poisons Sepsis, snake bite, IV contrast
Glomerular injury	Features to suggest nephritic (or nephrotic) syndrome, haematuria or cola-coloured urine, recent or current infections, constitutional symptoms consistent with systemic inflammatory or autoimmune disease or malignancy, e.g. fevers, weight loss, ENT symptoms, red eyes, alopecia, rashes, haemoptysis, pleurisy, arthralgia, oedema. Bruising or bleeding in TMA such as HUS
Primary tubulointerstitial disease	Autoimmune, infiltrative, e.g. lymphoma, or inflammatory, e.g. TB or sarcoid
Any cause of unresolved prerenal injury	

Intrinsic Renal

Intrinsic renal causes of AKI and CKD are numerous but can be grouped into broad categories for the purpose of initial assessment (Table 1.5). Other chapters in the rest of this textbook are devoted to the assessment and management of each of these conditions.

Examination of the urine is absolutely critical in establishing the diagnosis of intrinsic renal injury, and the role of urinalysis and urine microscopy is discussed in detail in Chap. 2.

Presentations Other than with Biochemical Evidence of Change in Renal Function

Although the majority of patients referred for the first time to nephrologists will have a degree of kidney dysfunction, not all patients will present with renal failure. Patients with isolated urinary abnormalities are often sent for expert review, and the assessment of isolated haematuria and proteinuria is discussed in detail in the following chapter. In addition to urinary abnormalities, nephrologists will find themselves faced with a diverse range of clinical syndromes secondary to disorders of the kidney. Similarly these syndromes and the logical diagnostic approaches are discussed in detail in the chapters devoted to the presenting syndrome or the underlying diagnoses. However an introduction to these presentations alongside important diagnostic clues is discussed briefly below.

Haematuria

Haematuria can originate from anywhere along the urinary tract, so it is important to identify coexistent lower urinary tract symptoms in any patient with visible blood in the urine. Intermittent visible haematuria can be temporarily associated with an upper respiratory tract infection (suggestive of IgA nephropathy) or related to exercise. Periodic haematuria can be seen in patients with endometriosis. Finally myoglobinuria will often lead to a false-positive dipstick urinalysis for haematuria.

Proteinuria

Proteinuria is identified either on dipstick testing, during routine medical, as part of a surveillance programme (e.g. for diabetes), or for the investigation of associated oedema, but patients with nephrotic range proteinuria can on occasion present having noticed frothy urine. History of past episodes of dipstick-positive proteinuria is helpful but is rarely recalled by patients.

Nephrotic Syndrome

The presentation of nephrotic syndrome is usually unambiguous. Diagnostic difficulties can occur in the presence of anuria, advanced renal failure or in the context of other causes for hypoalbuminaemia. For patients with nephrotic syndrome, swelling of the face or 'puffy eyes' in the morning can be an early symptom, pedal oedema and frothy urine may be noted, and fatigue or tiredness are also common complaints. For some individuals nephrotic syndrome may be precipitated by vaccinations, insect bites or non-specific infections. The definition, investigation and initial management of nephrotic syndrome are covered in Chap. 12.

Hypertension

Uncontrolled or unexpected hypertension is a fairly common referral to the nephrologist. Beyond emergency care, and determining duration, severity and compliance, the main consideration is the degree to which an underlying cause should be sought (Table 1.6). A secondary cause is more likely if hypertension occurs before the age of 40 years (the younger the patient, the greater the likelihood of a secondary cause), there is a history of severe end-organ damage, it presents as accelerated hypertension or there is a family history of early hypertension/stroke. It is important to recognise that the commonest cause of secondary hypertension relates to underlying CKD.

Loin Pain

Although kidney stones are a common and potentially serious cause of loin pain, pain arising from the kidneys can occur in numerous conditions (Table 1.7).

Nephrolithiasis is usually accompanied by severe symptoms although it may only be on direct questioning that patients mention passing 'gravel', i.e. small sand-like material. Working or living in hot, dehydrating environments, multiple long flights and salt intake as well as any dietary precipitants such as betel nut are all associated with stones in epidemiological studies. Any history of obstruction, lithotripsy or stone removal is also clearly important. Identifying if and where any stones have been analysed is very helpful and can expedite appropriate preventative therapy if reports can be obtained.

Electrolyte Disorders

The renal physician is often asked to provide assistance in the diagnosis and management of patients with electrolyte abnormalities. Renal tubular syndromes are discussed in detail later in this book, although differentiation of renal tubular abnormalities from endocrine, metabolic or gastroenterological aetiologies can be difficult.

Table 1.6 Evaluation of the patient with hypertension

Age of onset	Early onset <40 years more suggestive of secondary cause
Adherence	Agents tried, evidence of concordance
Severity/end-organ damage	Number of agents, retinopathy, left ventricular hypertrophy/failure, cerebrovascular disease
History of renal disease	
Family history	Examples include Liddle's or Gordon's syndrome but more usually a family history without diagnosis
Abnormalities of great vessels	Congenital heart disease, murmurs or abnormal pulses
Renal artery stenosis	Flash pulmonary oedema is rare. A history of macrovascular disease, deterioration in renal function with ACEI/ARB, absent peripheral pulses are more common
Phaeochromocytoma	*Episodic* headache, palpitations (64 %), sweating (70 %), pallor, hypotension, tremor, flushing, dyspnoea and epigastric pain
Obstructive sleep apnoea	Usually typical history and body habitus
Other endocrine causes	Cushingoid features, signs of acromegaly, etc.

Table 1.7 Pain associated with renal disease

Pyelonephritis	Acute and chronic such as xanthogranulomatous pyelonephritis
Renal stones	Typically severe, sudden onset and radiating (loin to groin)
Acute obstruction	Stone, sloughed papillae, blood clot, intermittent PUJ obstruction (particularly after fluid challenge)
Reflux	Occasionally patients describe loin pain on micturition
Wunderlich syndrome	Spontaneous renal haemorrhage from renal carcinoma, angiomyolipoma (renal AML) or arteriovenous malformation
Abdominal pain	Polyarteritis nodosa, infiltration with tumour
Infarction	Arterial or venous occlusion
Loin pain haematuria	Nutcracker *syndrome*

Where an abnormal finding is unexpected or sudden, the possibility of an aberrant value should be considered. For example, the recognition of the abnormal lab finding as being the result of blood sampling from a drip arm or patient misidentification can save significant anxiety. Symptomatology can be non-specific, such as muscle weakness with hyperkalaemia, or classic such as perioral paraesthesia and latent tetany in hypocalcaemia. The urgency of investigation and treatment will typically depend on both the severity and the chronicity of any abnormality.

Changes in Urinary Volume

Urinary volumes in the absence of disease can vary at least tenfold, so aside from anuria patients may find it difficult to recognise clinically important changes in urinary volume. Oliguria is a manifestation of advanced renal impairment of any cause; however, acute absolute anuria is rare and the causes are listed in Table 1.8.

Conversely, patients may find polyuria difficult to distinguish from urinary frequency, but this is important to differentiate. One approach to assessment is shown in Table 1.9.

Renal Manifestation of Multisystem Disorders

Abnormalities of the kidney occur in a large number and diverse range of systemic disorders with vascular, inflammatory, malignant or infective aetiologies (Table 1.10). Indeed, where the kidney represents the first clinical manifestation of these disorders, the renal physician may be best placed to establish diagnosis with predominantly extrarenal involvement. In these cases it is often attention to a comprehensive clinical history and examination that will reveal an underlying disorder.

General Aspects of the Clinical History Relevant to Establishing a Renal Diagnosis

In patients first presenting to a nephrologist once the presenting renal syndrome (e.g. new renal impairment nephrotic syndrome or an electrolyte disorder) has been determined, a further clinical history and examination can be pursued. A clear understanding of what brought the patient to seek medical attention at this time alongside a past medical and surgical history is likely to provide further valuable information.

Table 1.8 Causes of acute anuria

Vascular 1. Arterial catastrophe	Aortic dissection or thromboembolic event to single functioning kidney
Vascular 2. Venous thrombosis	Bilateral venous thrombosis (e.g. nephrotic syndrome or IVC occlusion)
Urinary leak	Usually traumatic rupture, occasionally after instrumentation or surgery
Anti-GBM disease	Probably the only intrinsic renal disease that can result in abrupt anuria
Profound shock	In patient with underlying CKD
Obstruction	Bilateral obstruction or obstruction of single functioning kidney, bladder outlet obstruction, surgical obstruction
Page kidney	Single functioning kidney
Urinary leak	For example, bladder rupture, leaking transplant ureter

Table 1.9 Assessment of polyuria

Polyuria associated with thirst	
Due to increased urine output:	
Renal tubular disorders, congenital	
Nephrogenic diabetes insipidus	Patients may give a childhood history of drinking from puddles or any available water
Bartter syndrome	
Medullary cystic kidney disease	Nephronophthisis, childhood thirst and polyuria
Renal tubular disorders acquired	
Recovery from AKI	
Medication	Lithium, diuretics, etc.
Acquired medullary pathology	Pyelonephritis, obstructive uropathy, HbSS, analgesic nephropathy, light chains
Hypercalcaemia, hypokalaemia	
Osmotic diuresis	Glucose, mannitol, contrast
Endocrine causes	Cranial diabetes insipidus, Addison's disease, hyporeninemic hypoaldosteronism
Due to increased intake:	Xerostoma (Sicca syndrome) anticholinergic medication
Polyuria without thirst	
Psychogenic polydipsia	
Following fluid loading	Beer drinking, IV fluids

Table 1.10 Common multisystem disorders with renal involvement

Diabetes	Diabetic nephropathy or atherosclerosis
Atherosclerosis	Large vessel or small vessel renal involvement
Connective tissue disorders	Scleroderma renal crisis Interstitial disease: sarcoidosis, treatment related (calcineurin inhibitors) Glomerulonephritis: systemic lupus erythematosus, systemic vasculitis, treatment related (gold penicillamine) AA amyloidosis: rheumatoid arthritis
Malignancy (primary or metastatic disease)	Obstruction, hypercalcaemia, tumour lysis syndrome, AL amyloid (paraproteinaemia) Direct infiltration Thrombotic microangiopathy Glomerulonephritis: membranous (breast, lung, GI), minimal change (lymphoma) Treatment related
Infections	
Tuberculosis	Sterile pyuria, haematuria, cystitis, nephrolithiasis Interstitial disease Glomerular – MCGN type 2, focal proliferative, amyloid Treatment-associated nephropathy
Enterohaemorrhagic bacteria	Thrombotic microangiopathy
Other bacterial infections	Postinfectious glomerulonephritis
Schistosomiasis	Chronic cystitis, bladder fibrosis, malignancy, ureteric obstruction and vesicoureteric reflux Interstitial fibrosis Glomerulopathy
Blood-borne viruses, e.g. hepatitis B and C, HIV	Disease associated. Glomerular, thrombotic microangiopathy, cryoglobulin Treatment-related nephropathy
Chronic suppurative infection	AA amyloidosis
Gout	Urate nephropathy, uromodulin disorder
Chronic pain	Analgesia use – nephropathy/TIN
Chronic neurological disorder	Bladder dysfunction
Inflammatory bowel disease	Short bowel syndrome/ileostomy losses, treatment associated, oxalate nephropathy, AA amyloidosis
Hepatic failure	Hepatorenal syndrome
Ear, nose and throat disorders	Deafness – Alport's syndrome, Anderson-Fabry's disease Epistaxis – cocaine or systemic vasculitis
Pulmonary renal syndromes	Haemoptysis: systemic vasculitis, lupus, anti-GBM syndrome Asthmatic: eosinophilic granulomatosis with polyangiitis

Age

The age at presentation can be a clue to diagnosis in a patient with renal impairment. A patient presenting with ESRD in his or her 20s may well have an inherited or congenital cause, and it is important to determine if symptoms started in childhood or adolescence. Age may make some diagnoses much less likely. For example, it is very unusual for lupus nephritis to present late in life, whereas primary vasculitides may well present in a patient's eighth or ninth decade. In addition, the significant age-associated decline in GFR and increase in the prevalence of CKD mean that the elderly are more vulnerable to acute kidney injury (AKI).

Gender

Some renal diseases show a significant gender bias and patterns of inheritance may give a significant clue to the diagnosis when a clear family history is available. For example, X-linked conditions like Alport's syndrome and Anderson-Fabry's disease have a male bias, whereas conditions such as Takayasu's arteritis, fibromuscular dysplasia and systemic lupus erythematosus have a very strong female preponderance.

Ethnicity and Country of Origin

Ethnicity and country of origin may be pointers to increased exposure to risk factors for some renal diseases and comorbid conditions that may affect the kidneys. There are many examples of this and some examples are given in Table 1.11.

Family History

In a new patient it is important to ask about a family history of any kidney problems such as dialysis, renal transplantation or familial renal disease (Table 1.12). If there is evidence of a family history and the diagnosis is not obvious, then age of onset, severity and phenotypic characteristics are helpful. Efforts should be made to obtain (with consent) medical diagnoses of the relatives; information from another renal

Table 1.11 Ethnicities and countries of origin associated with increased risk of kidney disease

Examples of populations at increased risk of CKD in the West	
UK	South Asian and Black populations have higher rates of diabetic nephropathy and hypertension
	Sickle cell nephropathy, systemic lupus erythematosus (SLE), focal segmental glomerulosclerosis in the Black population. Possibly chronic TIN in Asian population
United States	Increased CKD in the Black and Native American population
Australasia	Aborigines, Maoris and Pacific Islanders at increased risk of diabetic nephropathy and hypertension
Examples of geographically prevalent nephropathy	
Danube river	Balkan nephropathy is chronic tubulointerstitial nephropathy. A familial predisposition also exists. There is also a higher prevalence of renal tract tumours in this population
Tunisia and France	Ochratoxin associated with chronic interstitial nephritis
China and Indian subcontinent	Aristolochic acid causing 'Chinese herb nephropathy'
	Takayasu's arteritis
	Heavy metal poisoning
Italy	Hepatitis C-associated kidney disease
Cyprus	CFHR5 nephropathy
Africa and Indian subcontinent	Genitourinary tuberculosis in distribution of TB prevalence
Sub-Saharan Africa	Schistosoma haematobium – lower urinary tract disease and glomerulopathy
	HIV-associated nephropathy
Africa and South/Central Asia	Schistosoma mansoni – glomerulopathy
Africa, Australasia and Indian subcontinent	Post-streptococcal glomerulonephritis
East Asia	IgA nephropathy, SLE, hepatitis B-associated glomerulonephritis
Middle East	Nephrolithiasis
	Familial Mediterranean fever
Central American Pacific Coast	Tubulointerstitial disease

Table 1.12 Family history in renal disease

CKD or ESRD (dialysis or transplantation)	Cause as identified by renal unit, age of onset, pattern of inheritance
Hypertension and diabetes	Polygenic influence, RCAD syndrome
Stones	Calcium nephrolithiasis
Reflux nephropathy	Dysplastic kidneys, PUV or any other congenital abnormality of the urogenital tract
Renal tumours	Age of onset, numbers, other non-renal malignancies (including phaeochromocytoma), epilepsy, learning disabilities, pneumothorax, fibroids, skin lesions – may indicate VHL, BHD, HLRCC or TSC
Subarachnoid haemorrhage	May indicate PKD or the need for screening if known PKD; in haematuria may suggest hereditary angiopathy with nephropathy, aneurysms and cramps (HANAC) syndrome
Deafness	Alport's syndrome, female family members may have history of isolated haematuria suggesting X-linked Alport's syndrome, Fabry's disease, autosomal dominant history suggestive of branchio-oto-renal syndromes, MYH9 mutations, mitochondrial disorders, ciliopathies
Microscopic haematuria	X-linked or autosomal recessive Alport's syndrome; thin basement membrane nephropathy; CFHR5 nephropathy; HANAC syndrome; MYH9-associated nephropathies (Epstein/Fechtner's syndromes)
Retinitis pigmentosa	Bardet-Biedl syndrome and other ciliopathies; mitochondrial disorders
Liver fibrosis and cysts	Autosomal recessive polycystic kidney disease
Heart disease	Anderson-Fabry's disease; hereditary amyloidosis
Gout	Uromodulin-associated disease (MCKD2)
Electrolyte disorders	Hyper- or hyponatraemia, kalaemia, calcaemia, magnesaemia or phosphataemia or a history of polyuria, periodic paralysis

unit may expedite a diagnosis and prevent an unnecessary further investigation. The pattern of inheritance is crucial: affected siblings with unaffected parents suggest recessive disease, especially if there is endogamy or consanguinity. Affected individuals in consecutive generations are consistent with autosomal dominant, mitochondrial and X-linked inheritance; male-to-male transmission of a trait excludes X-linked disease or mitochondrially encoded disorder.

Obstetric History

An abnormal obstetric history can be a pointer to chronic underlying renal disease. Moreover, dipstick urinalysis and blood pressure measurement are recorded regularly from booking until delivery as part of routine maternity care. These findings may unveil both pregnancy-associated and pre-existing renal disease. If the patient is not clear about the details, it is often worthwhile pursuing via her family practitioner or obstetric unit.

The number of pregnancies, including miscarriages, stage of pregnancy reached and any reason for early delivery can be highly relevant as outlined in Table 1.13.

Occupation

Occupation may be a factor in the risk of developing some renal conditions (Table 1.14). Sometimes the exposure is not immediately apparent, and a detailed history of both occupation and hobbies is important to avoid continued risk of deterioration.

Travel and Hobbies

In addition to considering the patient's geographical origins, a travel history should be sought. This is particularly important in the context of AKI. Relevant questions are shown in Table 1.15. Relevant hobbies include water sports (leptospirosis), pets (hantavirus) and endurance sports (haematuria, rhabdomyolysis).

Psychosocial History

There are several aspects of the psychosocial history that are germane to the care of the renal patient. There remains a significant bias to CKD in lower socio-economic groups. Lower educational attainment, mental health problems, substance misuse and unstable home circumstances can pose barriers to engagement with medical professionals, delay recognition of ill health and diagnosis, limit adherence and influence suitability for home therapies. Getting a clear understanding of a patient's psychosocial history is therefore fundamental to the delivery of full and effective care. In addition, there are certain abused substances that have associations with renal disease shown in Table 1.16.

Medication and Allergy

The kidneys are susceptible to a wide range of adverse effects from medications and their active metabolites. Different medications may cause toxicity in a variety of sites within the kidney. It is essential to obtain a history of (1) prescribed and (2) non-prescription drugs and (3) recreational or illicit drugs. Ward prescription charts and inpatient procedural records such as anaesthetic charts, as well as redundant

Table 1.13 Obstetric history and renal disease

Multiple miscarriages	May suggest anti-cardiolipin antibody syndrome. Occurs in advanced CKD of any cause
Hypertension	Stage of pregnancy, severity and number of agents required to treat. Hypertension early in pregnancy, e.g. at booking, is highly suggestive of a non-pregnancy-related cause
Proteinuria	Proteinuria (or haematuria) at booking or heavy proteinuria early in pregnancy is very suggestive of underlying renal disease. Prolonged proteinuria post-partum may also suggest that pre-eclampsia was not the only cause for proteinuria
Pre-eclampsia	Early (<20/40) PET is suggestive of underlying renal disease (20 % have underlying CKD). An underlying renal cause is more likely if hypertension worsens in second pregnancy (with same partner)
UTIs (lower tract or pyelonephritis)	Pyelonephritis is more common in pregnancy and may result in renal scarring
Obstetric sepsis/severe haemorrhage	AKI following either may rarely result in cortical necrosis

Table 1.14 Occupations predisposing or exacerbating renal disease

Occupation/exposure	Pathology
Solvents	Glomerular and tubular pathology
Aniline dye	Urothelial tumours
Sewage workers	Leptospirosis
Outdoor workers in endemic areas	Hantavirus, leptospirosis
Old paint work/plumbing	Lead nephropathy
Cooks	Renal stones
Heavy metal workers/exposure/soldering	Heavy metal nephropathy

Table 1.15 Key travel questions

Details of travel, particularly in the previous 12 months
Pretravel vaccinations and malaria prophylaxis
Rural vs. urban destinations
Unwell contacts
Time period between return and onset of symptoms
Accommodation and food/drink exposures
Fresh water swimming
Animal contacts or bites – tick, animal, bird or bat bites and scratches
Occupation and hobbies – e.g. water sports or agricultural employment
Recent dental work, surgical procedures
Sexual history

Table 1.16 Substance misuse

Smoking	Hastens the progression of renal disease associated with both diabetes and hypertension Increased microalbuminuria Increased likelihood of pulmonary haemorrhage in anti-GBM disease
Alcohol	IgA nephropathy in alcoholic liver cirrhosis Cirrhosis and hepatorenal syndrome
Solvent	Toluene in 'glue sniffing' has been associated with numerous tubular and glomerular lesions
Cocaine	Renal ischaemia, vasculitis or rhabdomyolysis
Heroin	FSGS
Intravenous drug injection	Blood-borne viruses Infective endocarditis AA amyloid
Ketamine	Inflammatory cystitis and obstructive uropathy
Ecstasy/MDMA	Increased risk of rhabdomyolysis and acute hyponatraemia

completed drug charts, should be reviewed to identify potential toxins in use at the onset of renal dysfunction. Accurately identifying a complete drug history may be time-consuming, but confirming prior use of aminoglycosides, exposure to a common cause of tubulointerstitial nephritis or that a patient is taking a product containing aristolochic acid may be critically important to establishing the cause of renal dysfunction. Key elements of the drug history are shown in Table 1.17.

Table 1.17 Key elements of medication history

Prescribed medication Start and stop dates Route of administration Previous exposure and timeline
Non-prescribed, over-the-counter or commercially purchased medication Particularly analgesic and NSAID use which may not be volunteered Include use of creams and gels with consideration to systemic absorption
Drug interactions Anticipated/dose adjustment/drug level monitoring
Drug reactions Fever, rash, arthralgia may occur in suspected AIN Reversibility of effect Concomitant administration of prophylaxis for side effects IV radiocontrast
Dietary supplements Creatine-based sports supplements Dieting supplements Nutritional additives Laxatives and diuretics
Herbal preparations Whenever possible ascertain the origin and obtain a sample for analysis since it may contain heavy metals or NSAIDs Consider interactions with prescription medication, for example, via cytochrome P450
Illicit drug abuse Modality – frequency of needle use and sharing between individuals or participation in needle exchange Route – intravenous or subcutaneous (increased risk of amyloid) associated with thrombophlebitis or cellulitis Risk factors for infective endocarditis

Clues on Clinical Examination to Help Establish the Cause of a Renal Disorder

A thorough clinical examination is an essential part of the approach to any patient presenting either acutely or to the outpatient department. Accurate fluid assessment will be critical to most presentations to the renal physician and is discussed in detail above. Alongside intravascular volume assessment, other findings on clinical examination can provide important clues to the aetiology of a renal presentation. These examination findings are summarised in Table 1.18.

Assessment of the Patient with Known Renal Disease

Many renal conditions are chronic, and it is common to encounter patients who have previously been investigated or treated either locally or in another centre. When a patient is known to suffer from a renal disorder, the aim of the assessment will usually be focused on the management of the underlying condition or associated complications rather than the underlying cause of the renal disease (which may or may not have already been diagnosed). Those in contact with renal services frequently have complex and chronic histories, and the importance of handling the transfer of care cannot be overstated (see Chap. 49). Fortunately patients are increasingly involved in their own care, have a good understanding of their disease and have access to their clinical records. When they do not, it is important to make the effort to trace historical imaging, blood and urine results. In all patients known to have renal disease, the nature and duration of the condition, as well as histological details if available, are an essential starting point of any assessment. Patients with known renal disease will broadly fall into the following groups allowing the clinician to focus their clinical assessment on relevant issues.

Table 1.18 Examination tips and renal disease

Habitus	Obesity (OSA), Bardet-Biedl syndrome (renal cysts) (short stature), Noonan syndrome (short and webbed neck – renal dysplasia), Turner's syndrome (short stature, webbed neck – horseshoe kidney), Down's syndrome (renal dysplasia), Jeune's syndrome (short limbs, narrow rib cage). Lipodystrophy (MPGN). Limb abnormalities VACTERL association. *Any form of CKD in childhood can result in short stature*
Hair	Scaring alopecia (SLE), diffuse alopecia (heavy metal poisoning, tacrolimus, steroids), hirsutism (cyclosporine)
Ears	Otitis, inflammation of the pinna with granulomatosis with polyangiitis (GPA), preauricular pit, sensorineural deafness (branchio-oto-renal syndrome (BOR), Alport's syndrome, Anderson-Fabry's disease (AFD), CHARGE syndrome (ear abnormalities))
Nose	Crusting, nasal bridge collapse, GPA; cocaine
Mouth	Dentition (infective endocarditis (IE)), mouth ulcers (vasculitis SLE, herpes viral infections), fungal infections, macroglossia (useful sign of amyloid)
Polydactyly	Jeune's, Bardet-Biedl, Meckel-Gruber syndromes
Nails	Periungual fibromas (tuberous-sclerosis complex (TSC), dysplastic nails (nail patella syndrome), splinter haemorrhages (infective endocarditis), Muehrcke's bands (episodes of nephrotic syndrome))
Skin	*Signs of renal disease*: vasculitic rashes, palpable purpura (Henoch-Schönlein purpura (HSP)), palpable subcutaneous nodules/ulcers (polyarteritis nodosa), malar flush (systemic lupus erythematosus (SLE)), cutaneous lupus erythematosus, alopecia (SLE, tacrolimus), neurofibroma, viral exanthem, erythema nodosum, tracheostomy scar (previous ICU admission), xanthelasma, nicotine stains (atherosclerotic disease), Janeway lesions (IE), bruising (amyloid), livedo reticularis (cholesterol emboli, SLE, anti-cardiolipin syndrome), angiokeratoma (AFD), Raynaud's disease (SLE, scleroderma, anti-cardiolipin syndrome), facial angiofibromas, ash-leaf macule and shagreen patch (TSC) *Signs of immunosuppression*: purpura, thin skin, gum hypertrophy (cyclosporine), sebaceous gland hyperplasia, actinic keratosis, Kaposi's sarcoma, squamous cell carcinoma, basal cell carcinoma, hypertrichosis (cyclosporine), cushingoid features and striae (steroids) *Signs of advanced CKD*: xerosis, acquired perforating dermatosis, porphyria cutanea tarda, calciphylaxis
Eyes	Retinopathy (hypertensive, diabetic); retinitis pigmentosa/dysplasia (Bardet-Biedl; Senior-Loken syndrome, nephronophthisis; Jeune's syndrome; Kearns-Sayre mitochondrial cytopathy); uveitis (tubulointerstitial nephritis with uveitis); band keratopathy, sicca (Sjögren's syndrome); corneal clouding (cystinosis); lenticonus (Anderson-Fabry's disease); proptosis (GPA, IgG-4-related disease); angiomatosis retinae (VHL); coloboma (renal coloboma syndrome CHARGE and COACH syndromes), periorbital bruising (amyloid), iritis, scleritis, retinal vasculitis (vasculitis), drusen (dense deposit disease)
Lymphoproliferative	Lymphadenopathy (tuberculosis, lymphoma); splenomegaly (IE, sarcoid, lymphoproliferative disorder)
CVS	Atrial fibrillation (emboli), pericardial rub (SLE, infections, uraemic pericarditis), murmur/pacing wire (endocarditis), radiofemoral delay/missing pulses (aortic coarctation/mid-aortic syndrome, Takayasu's arteritis), bruits (renovascular disease, fibromuscular dysplasia), ventricular failure (right or left sided)
Chest	Pneumothorax (tuberosclerosis); pleural rub (SLE, vasculitis, infection); asthma (eosinophilic granulomatosis with polyangiitis); pulmonary fibrosis (systemic vasculitis, scleroderma, SLE, Sjogren's syndrome, drugs); signs of bronchiectasis (amyloid)
Abdominal	Signs of chronic liver disease (hepatorenal syndrome, viral hepatitis), stoma (high output), absent abdominal musculature (prune-belly syndrome)
Neurological	Asterixis/tremor (uraemic encephalopathy, calcineurin inhibitor toxicity), hemiparesis (bladder dysfunction, infection-associated amyloid), spina bifida (occulta)
Musculoskeletal	Polyarthropathy (rheumatoid arthritis, SLE, ankylosing spondylitis), monoarthritis (hyperuricaemia), infection including IE, Charcot joint, absent patellae (nail patella syndrome)

Patients with ESRD Treated with Dialysis

Patients with ESRD may have been receiving renal replacement therapy for many years and have been treated with several treatment modalities. Renal physicians will often be integral to the holistic care of patients on dialysis programmes. Therefore, alongside dialysis-related issues the renal specialist increasingly needs at least a basic understanding of a broad range of medical, surgical and psychiatric problems so that appropriate further expertise can be sought when necessary. When thinking about dialysis-related problems, presentations will commonly be related to dialysis access (including infection) and intradialytic issues (instability, adequacy or complications). Important considerations for the assessment of the patient on dialysis are outlined in Table 1.19.

Table 1.19 Clinical assessment specific to the dialysis patient

Underlying cause of ESRF	
Duration of ESRF and different treatment modalities	
Most recent dialysis session and intradialytic problems	Date/duration of last session, problems with treatment, loss of circuit
Dialysis access PD catheter Temporary vascular access for HD AVF or AV grafts	Date of formation/insertion, signs of infection, adequate function, position (temporary HD catheters or PD catheters)
Fluid status	
Dialysis adequacy	URR or KT/V, serum potassium, residual native kidney function, ultrafiltration volumes, intradialytic weight gains (HD), constipation (PD)
Blood pressure control	Antihypertensive medication, sodium intake, intradialytic hypotension
Traditional cardiovascular risk factors	Smoking, dyslipidaemia and treatment
Complications of CKD and treatment	Anaemia, bone-mineral disorder
Transplant listing status	May impact on decisions regarding transfusion, imminent recipient of live donor transplant, etc.
Nutritional status	Changes in 'dry weight' may indicate occult chronic infection or malignancy

Table 1.20 Clinical assessment specific to the transplant patient

Underlying cause of ESRF	
Duration of ESRF and different treatment modalities	
Previous transplantation	Date, duration, reason for graft loss
Current transplant	
Donor details	Age, donor type, donor comorbidity/COD
Immunological details	Overall sensitisation (% CRF) (donor-specific and non-specific antibodies), mismatch, cross-match details, posttransplant donor-specific antibodies
Surgical details	Cold and warm ischaemic times, arterial and venous anatomy, ureteric anastomosis
Post-operative course	Delayed graft function, infection, rejection, thrombosis, obstruction (stent removal)
Allograft biopsies	Tubular injury, rejection, recurrence of primary disease, degree of fibrosis
Immunosuppressive treatment	Induction, maintenance, treatment for rejection, steroid withdrawal, drug levels
Infection risk and prophylaxis	Donor and recipient viral immunity, prophylaxis, infection history, BK virus
Recent allograft imaging	Ultrasound, MRA/angiography, nuclear medicine
Baseline function	Look out for slow declines over many months
Non-allograft issues	
Fluid status	
Evidence of infection	Urine, chest, GI, neurological, atypical organisms
Evidence of malignancy	Weight loss, breast/cervical screening
Blood pressure control	Antihypertensive medication, sodium intake
CV risk	Smoking, dyslipidaemia (posttransplant), diabetes
Osteoporosis	Fractures, prophylaxis
Complications of CKD and treatment	Anaemia, bone-mineral disorder

Patients with ESRD with Functioning Kidney Transplants

The management of graft dysfunction will represent a substantial workload for any transplant unit, so the nephrologist needs to be fluent in the further management of a transplant patient with a rise in the serum creatinine. Once again assessment of intravascular volume status is a critical element. In addition, the management of immunosuppression-related complications such as infection and malignancy will need specific attention in transplant patients. Finally, patients with kidney transplants will often present to their 'home' transplant unit with transplant-related issues and problems not immediately associated with the allograft or associated complications. Table 1.20 outlines aspects of clinical assessment important in the patient with a functioning renal allograft.

Table 1.21 Clinical assessment specific to the patient with inflammatory renal disease

Underlying diagnosis	
Duration of disease, relapses, multisystem involvement	
Baseline kidney function	
Renal biopsies	Active disease, chronic fibrosis
Immunosuppressive treatment	Induction, maintenance, steroid withdrawal, drug levels
Evidence of relapse	Including extrarenal symptoms and signs
Fluid status	
Infection risk and prophylaxis	Infection history, viral immunity, prophylaxis
Evidence of infection	Urine, chest, GI, neurological, atypical organisms
Evidence of malignancy	Weight loss, breast/cervical screening
Blood pressure control	Antihypertensive medication, sodium intake
CV risk	Smoking, statins, diabetes
Osteoporosis	Fractures, prophylaxis
Complications of CKD	Anaemia, bone-mineral disorder

Patients with ESRD on Conservative Care Programmes

Increasingly renal units have large and successful conservative care programmes. One of the reasons patients may have decided that they do not wish to receive active care for ESRF is to reduce time spent in a medical environment. Although these patients may have decided not to undergo dialysis or transplantation, the assessment and prompt management of fluid status, anaemia, bone-mineral disorders, nausea and pain can have a significant impact on quality of life and should be pursued as a priority.

When patients are clearly close to death the renal physician may need to play an active part in ensuring that the appropriate end-of-life care can be effectively delivered and in the most appropriate environment.

Patients with CKD and a Reduced GFR

Some form of chronic kidney disease is thought to affect between 5 and 10 % of the population in Western countries. Nephrologists will often be asked to help manage this group of patients who may often suffer with multiple comorbidities. The increasing recognition of the increased risk of AKI in those with CKD as well as the contribution of AKI to the future progression of CKD means that a key focus of the assessment of this group of patients surrounds the management, and prevention, of a further decline in kidney function. The approach to this clinical situation should be similar to that set out in the section on establishing the cause of previously undiagnosed renal impairment set-out in detail above.

Patients with CKD also commonly present with fluid overload, and the nephrologist will often be asked for advice, again underlying the importance of thorough assessment of intravascular volume status.

In this group of patients particular attention should also be focused on the prescription of medication at the dose appropriate for the patients GFR. Failure to dose-reduce medications can lead to acute-on-chronic kidney injury or alternatively significant adverse effects due to drug or metabolite accumulation (see Chap. 56).

The management of patients with stable CKD also needs to address the complications of decreased renal function, specifically anaemia, bone-mineral disorder and cardiovascular risk. These are addressed in the chapters on chronic kidney disease management.

Patients with Inflammatory Renal Diseases and/or Requiring Immunosuppression

Patients suffering from systemic vasculitis, SLE, nephrotic syndrome or other inflammatory renal conditions will often be taking immunosuppressive drugs. In addition to the issues related to CKD or dialysis, the possibility of disease relapse and the consequences of immunosuppression needs to be considered when these patients present to renal services. An approach to this group of patients is outlined in Table 1.21.

Summary

Patients attending renal specialists present with an enormous diversity of clinical problems. An approach to the review of patients using a system similar to the one outlined in this chapter allows for comprehensive and organised recognition of both the background and current problems. In this group of often extremely complex patients, it is by focusing the assessment on answering the relevant questions at hand that clinical problems will be appropriately prioritised and timely and safe treatment instigated. The critical importance of accurate assessment of intravascular volume status in almost all areas of renal medicine cannot be overemphasised, and this is a skill that can only be learned with repeated practice. Although as experience is gained each clinician will develop their own unique approach to clinical assessment, it is only with a systematic approach that nephrologists can be confident of providing safe, efficient and high-quality care to their patients.

References

1. Ely EW. Radiologic determination of intravascular volume status using portable, digital chest radiography: a prospective investigation in 100 patients. Crit Care Med. 2001;29(8):1502–12.
2. Olde Rikkert MG, et al. Validation of multi-frequency bioelectrical impedance analysis in detecting changes in fluid balance of geriatric patients. J Am Geriatr Soc. 1997;45(11):1345–51.
3. Kalantai K, et al. Assessment of intravascular volume status and volume responsiveness in critically ill patients. Kidney Int. 2013;83:1017–28.
4. Moghazi S, et al. Correlation of renal histopathology with sonographic findings. Kidney Int. 2005;67:1515–20.

2 Urine Analysis

Scott R. Henderson and Mark Harber

Introduction

Formation of urine allows a cheap, noninvasive and novel insight into the pathological processes affecting the kidneys and urinary tract and has been shown to be an essential tool to the practising nephrologist [1, 2]. Urine analysis has evolved from 'the art of uroscopy', practised in medieval times [3], to detailed chemical analysis and microscopy, allowing early detection and differentiation of renal disease.

This chapter outlines the practical aspects of urine analysis and routine urine dipstick and aims to guide the interpretation of pathognomic features of urinary abnormalities on microscopy to relevant clinical situations.

Sample Collection

At the outset, it is important to optimise sample collection: poorly procured samples have little value and may result in inappropriate management (see Table 2.1 for guidance on sample collection). It is also important to ensure that samples are delivered without delay for processing; microscopy or cytology samples dispatched at the end of the day and left overnight are likely to be useless and waste lab resources. As a guideline, samples for cytology should ideally reach the laboratory within 2 h, whereas samples for culture may be refrigerated, if required, for 24 h at 4 °C. It is therefore worth ensuring that a system is in place for prompt sample delivery and that nursing staff routinely educate patients on how to reliably provide 'clean-catch' midstream urine (MSU) samples.

A variety of clean-catch systems are commercially available to reduce contamination, although to date there is very limited evidence of benefit. For those patients unable to cooperate, and in whom urine analysis is important, then alternatives include 'in-out' catheterisation or suprapubic aspiration (common in paediatrics) both of which may be contaminated by erythrocytes, but worth considering when urine analysis is critical.

Indwelling catheter specimens are invariably contaminated by blood and low-level proteinuria. Ileal conduits, urostomies and indwelling catheters are also very frequently (*universally*) colonised with bacteria, and there is little point obtaining samples in the asymptomatic patient except to exclude gross proteinuria or for analysis of electrolytes.

Physical Appearance

Prior to any testing of a urine sample, physical appearance should be assessed, particularly *colour*, *odour* and *turbidity* as certain circumstances result in specific appearances, as outlined in Table 2.2. Normal urine is clear when analysed in a transparent container against a white background, and colour ranges from light yellow to dark amber depending on the amount of urochromes present and solute concentration.

Urine Dipstick

Urine dipstick abnormalities are widely prevalent in both community and hospital practice and is most often the

S.R. Henderson, MBChB, BScMedSci (Hons), MRCP (✉)
UCL Department of Nephrology, Royal Free Hospital,
Pond Street, London NW3 2QG, UK
e-mail: scotthenderson@nhs.net

M. Harber, MBBS, PhD, FRCP
UCL Department of Nephrology,
Royal Free London NHS Foundation Trust,
Pond Street, Hampstead, London NW3 2QG, UK
e-mail: mark.harber@nhs.net

M. Harber (ed.), *Practical Nephrology*,
DOI 10.1007/978-1-4471-5547-8_2, © Springer-Verlag London 2014

Table 2.1 Health Protection Agency standard method of MSU sample collection in men and women [4]

Midstream sample of urine is always preferential
Quality of urine sample determines accuracy of analysis
Clear instructions should be provided prior to voiding to avoid contamination
Males: retract foreskin and clean glans
Females: clean labia and urethral meatus
Place container midstream in the flow of urine
Analysis should be performed as soon as possible to avoid decomposition of cellular elements
As a general rule, samples should be exposed to minimal light and not be stored at room temperature for longer than 2 h
First morning urine provides a concentrated urine sample most likely to contain clinically important elements
Quick link: http://www.hpa-standardmethods.org.uk/documents/bsop/pdf/bsop41.pdf

Table 2.2 Physical characteristics of urine [5]

Colour	*Yellow/brown* – hyperbilirubinaemia, chloroquine, nitrofurantoin
	Orange – rifampacin, senna
	Red/brown – blood, myoglobin, phenytoin, beetroot (anthocyanins), blackberries, rhubarb, chronic lead or mercury poisoning
	Pink – propofol (especially in alcoholics)
	Blue – methylene blue, *Pseudomonas* infection, indicanuria
	Green – propofol, amitriptyline, indomethacin, phenergen
	White/milky – chyluria
	Black – ochronosis, porphyria (on standing, pink under UV light), melanomatosis, copper poisoning, chloroquine, primaquine, metronidazole, phenol poisoning, alkaptonuria, tyrosinosis
	Causes of urine darkening on standing – alkaptonuria, typically when left exposed to open air caused by oxidation and polymerisation of excess homogentisic acid, enhanced with alkaline pH
Odour	*Offensive* – consider bacterial infection
	'*Maple syrup*' – maple syrup urine disease
	Acetone – diabetic ketoacidosis
	'*Sweaty feet*' – isovaleric acidaemia
Turbidity	'*Cloudy*' – high concentration of either/or leucocytes, erythrocytes, epithelial cells, bacteria or crystals. Consider genital tract contamination (females), white cloudy can occur with phosphaturia (disappears with acetic acid)
	'*Milky*' – lipid-rich material (chyluria); consider abnormal connection between lymphatic and urinary systems
	'*Gas*' – termed pneumaturia, an important symptom that occurs in the presence of colovesical fistula or emphysematous pyelonephritis
	'*Frothy*' – indicative of nephrotic range proteinuria

first clue to the presence of renal disease. Careful interpretation of dipstick abnormalities is therefore important and should guide further appropriate investigations and specialist referral. Sample collection is an undervalued yet essential component of urinary examination and should be performed by standard methods as outlined in Table 2.1.

A variety of dipstick testing kits are available, but standard combination strips routinely include five or seven of the following tests: *protein*, *blood*, *glucose*, *ketones*, *pH*, *bilirubin* and *urobilinogen*. Other characteristics detected on urine dipstick are *specific gravity* and the presence of *leucocytes* and *nitrites*. Table 2.3 outlines common abnormalities, possible causes and important false positive situations to consider. Specific urine dipstick tests are also available in specialist practice with the most widely available tests including Micral-Test II® or Microbumintest® (microalbuminuria), Ictotest® (bilirubin), Acetest® (ketones) and Clinistix® (glycosuria only).

Urine Microscopy

> Urine...... can provide us day by day, month by month and year by year with a serial story of the major events going on within the kidney.
>
> Thomas Addis (1948) [6]

Urine microscopy performed by a nephrologist is a cheap, noninvasive and educational test that, in the right setting, can substantially aid the diagnosis. Before investing in resources, it is worth approaching local laboratories for used centrifuges and microscopes. The requirements are:

1. A centrifuge capable of taking 10 ml samples at 1,500 rpm
2. Centrifuge tubes
3. Disposable pipettes
4. Microscope slides
5. Cover slips
6. Microscope (with phase contrast)
7. Appropriate bench space (usually dirty utility room)
8. Individual with responsibility for maintaining equipment

   (*Draconian penalties for leaving the microscope on or in a mess – optional*)

Suitably preparing urine for microscopy is essential to obtaining informative results. A midstream sample should be obtained by the method outlined (Table 2.1) and at least 10 ml of urine should be collected and analysed *within 2 h*. Table 2.4 shows how to prepare a urine sample for light microscopy, and Table 2.5 shows technical information on analysing the urine sediment.

The urine sediment may contain a vast number of cellular elements. This section is not an exhaustive atlas, but rather a summary of the important components which should be recognised on examination in association with the relevant clinical syndromes, helping guide the practising nephrologist in the pursuit of diagnosis.

Table 2.3 Urinary dipstick abnormalities (*for haematuria and proteinuria see below*)

Specific gravity	Polyuria associated with low SG <1.010
Normal range 1.002–1.035	Low with polydipsia (psychogenic, beer drinking) and diabetes insipidus
NB: varies according to urine concentration	Tends to be fixed (c.1.010) in acute tubular injury or CKD
	High levels (≥1.035) seen in shock and dehydration (appropriately concentrated)
	Artificially high with glycosuria, proteinuria and following IV contrast
	Useful cheap measure of fluid intake for patients with recurrent UTI or stone disease if renal function is normal
pH	Low pH in acidosis and high-protein diet and promotes uric acid and cysteine stone formation
Normal range 5–8, Western diet pH=~6	High pH in (1) renal tubular acidosis (inappropriately alkaline urine (>5.5) in face of acidosis) (pH <5.4 excludes distal RTA), (2) low-protein/low-vegetarian diet and (3) urinary tract infection, particularly from urease-producing organisms such as *Proteus mirabilis*
	High pH promotes calcium-phosphate deposition
Glucose	Freely filtered at glomerulus, but almost completely reabsorbed at the proximal tubule
In normal homeostasis, glucose is not present in urine	Causes of glycosuria
	Pregnancy (normal physiological response)
	Hyperglycaemia (diabetes mellitus)
	Impaired proximal tubular reabsorption in isolation (SGLT2 defect)
Ketones	Ketones are produced following increased metabolism of fat. Ketone bodies (acetoacetic acid, acetone and 3-hydroxybutyrate *not detected*) are freely filtered in the glomerulus
In normal homeostasis, ketones are not present in the urine	Causes of ketonuria
	Type 1 diabetes mellitus (diabetic ketoacidosis)
	Starvation states (prolonged fasting, anorexia nervosa)
Bilirubin	Bilirubin is normally conjugated and excreted into the gastrointestinal tract as a water-soluble molecule. Small bowel bacterial metabolism converts bilirubin to urobilinogen which is then reabsorbed at the distal small bowel lumen and partially excreted in the urine
Urobilinogen gives urine its 'normal' physical appearance	*Positive bilirubin dipstick test* – suggests failure of hepatic conjugation of bilirubin preventing excretion and conversion of urobilinogen
	Negative urobilinogen dipstick test – indicates failure of hepatic excretion of conjugated bilirubin (biliary obstruction)
Nitrites	Most bacteria convert nitrates to nitrites during growth and replication. Positive nitrite test is suggestive of infection, but a negative test is not exclusive. A minimum time period is required for bacterial transformation
In health, nitrites are excreted in variable amounts, although are undetectable in the majority	Bacteria that do not reduce nitrate compounds include
	Enterococcus
	Pseudomonas species
	Streptococcus faecalis
	Staphylococcus albus
	Neisseria gonorrhoea
Leucocytes	Urine dipstick detects the enzymatic reduction of a synthetic ester substrate by urinary neutrophil esterase to a blue derivative in the presence of air
The presence of leucocytes in the urine suggests inflammation or infection NB: *may be absent in neutropenia*	Leucocyte esterase reaction has a reported better sensitivity than nitrite testing for the diagnosis of urinary tract infection, but false negatives can occur in the presence of tetracyclines, cephalosporins, glucose, albumin and ketones

Isolated Haematuria

Haematuria on dipstick should *always* be confirmed by microscopy to exclude false positives (pigment nephropathy, hypochlorite solutions, oxidising agents, bacterial peroxidase) and false negative results (vitamin C, gentisic acid).

New patients over 40 years of age (or younger for those with risk factors for urinary tract malignancy, e.g. previous cyclophosphamide or aristolic acid exposure) with proven micro- or macroscopic haematuria should be screened for urinary tract malignancy [7] or another cause of lower urinary tract bleeding. There is a strong argument for an integrated uro-nephrology approach to haematuria in this

Table 2.4 Preparation of urine for microscopy

Collect 10 ml midstream urine sample in sterile universal container
Centrifuge 10 ml at 1,500 rpm
Discard supernatant (9.5 ml)
Resuspend 500 µl sediment using *Pasteur* pipette
Transfer 50 µl of urinary sediment to slide
Apply cover slip (24 × 32 mm)

Table 2.5 Technical aspects of urine microscopy

Microscope	Indications
Phase contrast	Allows best identification of cellular elements, less need for special stains
Light	Poor visualisation of contents with low refractive index
Polarised light	Positive birefringence allows detection of crystalluria
Stains	
Wright's	Lymphocytes
Papanicolaou's	'Decoy cells' pathognomic of Bk viruria
May-Grünwald-Giemsa	Eosinophils
Hansel's	Haemosiderin
Prussian blue	

group of patients (Table 2.6). Perhaps the most patient-orientated approach is a '*haematuria one-stop shop*' where patients are seen and assessed by urologists with urine microscopy, renal blood tests, same-day ultrasound of kidneys and bladder and cystoscopy when appropriate. Those deemed not to have a urological cause for haematuria can then be assessed by a nephrologist in reserved slots on the same day. This takes a bit of organising, but the dividends for the patient and the clinician are obvious in terms of providing an efficient and joined-up approach.

Lower urinary tract bleeding is indicated by erythrocytes (RBC) with essentially normal and homogenous morphology. In haematuria due to glomerular disease, RBC presumably become distorted as they pass through the glomerular basement membrane and down the tubule resulting in heterogenous and dysmorphic shapes including acanthocytes, best seen with phase-contrast microscopy (Fig. 2.1a). A large quantity of dysmorphic red blood cells is suggestive of an aggressive glomerular lesion, whereas scanty dysmorphic RBC are more indicative of a subacute GN. The presence of a red blood cell cast is highly suggestive of an aggressive glomerulonephritis and, to paraphrase the old adage, '*one RBC cast makes a Summer*'. As this is one of the most important and specific findings in urine microscopy, it is extremely helpful to train the nephrologist's eye with the urine of patients known to have acute renal vasculitis/lupus.

Isolated Proteinuria

The detection of protein on urine dipstick is affected by (1) concentration (consider specific gravity), (2) macroscopic haematuria and (3) urine pH >8.0. Urine dipstick testing does, however, provide a semi-quantitative measurement of proteinuria as outlined in Table 2.7, but whilst dipstick reagent testing is sensitive to albumin, it has low sensitivity to other proteins, such as tubular proteins and light chain immunoglobulins. Proteinuria should therefore be confirmed by additional testing, and for the vast majority of patients, a random urine protein:creatinine ratio (uPCR) or urine albumin:creatinine ratio (uACR) (monitoring of choice in diabetes) is sufficient for diagnosis and monitoring. Table 2.8 outlines different types of proteinuria with important clinical considerations.

Although largely superseded by simpler tests, occasionally 24 h collections may be helpful for the assessment of proteinuria particularly if combined with other diagnostic tests such as 24 h sodium, urine volume, creatinine clearance and Bence-Jones proteinuria. It is noteworthy that the value of such tests is diminished if incomplete collection is performed. For 24 h collections, patients should be given clear guidance and a pre-labelled large volume container and instructed to empty their bladder first thing in the morning (ideally a nonworking day with no heavy exercise) and then collect all urine until the following morning including finishing with an empty bladder on rising.

Acute Kidney Injury

Urine analysis is absolutely critical in guiding the diagnosis and initial management of patients with AKI, and although the clinical picture is often complex, there are several scenarios when urine analysis can substantially guide or cleverly make the diagnosis. It is important that your referring wards and emergency departments try, where possible, to obtain a fresh urine prior to catheterisation (and reliably record residual urine volume on catheterisation):

1. *Acute tubular injury*: The majority of AKI is secondary to hypoperfusion-induced acute tubular injury, and, in the absence of an intrinsic renal disease, the urine is likely to have minimal haematuria or proteinuria, and urine microscopy therefore reveals large numbers of renal epithelial cells (Fig. 2.1b) and granular casts (not specific) and limited numbers of erythrocytes with no red cell casts. Urine festooned with tubular cells is highly suggestive of acute tubular injury, but more often it is the exclusion of an active glomerular lesion that is critical.

Table 2.6 Decision algorithm for the investigation and referral of haematuria

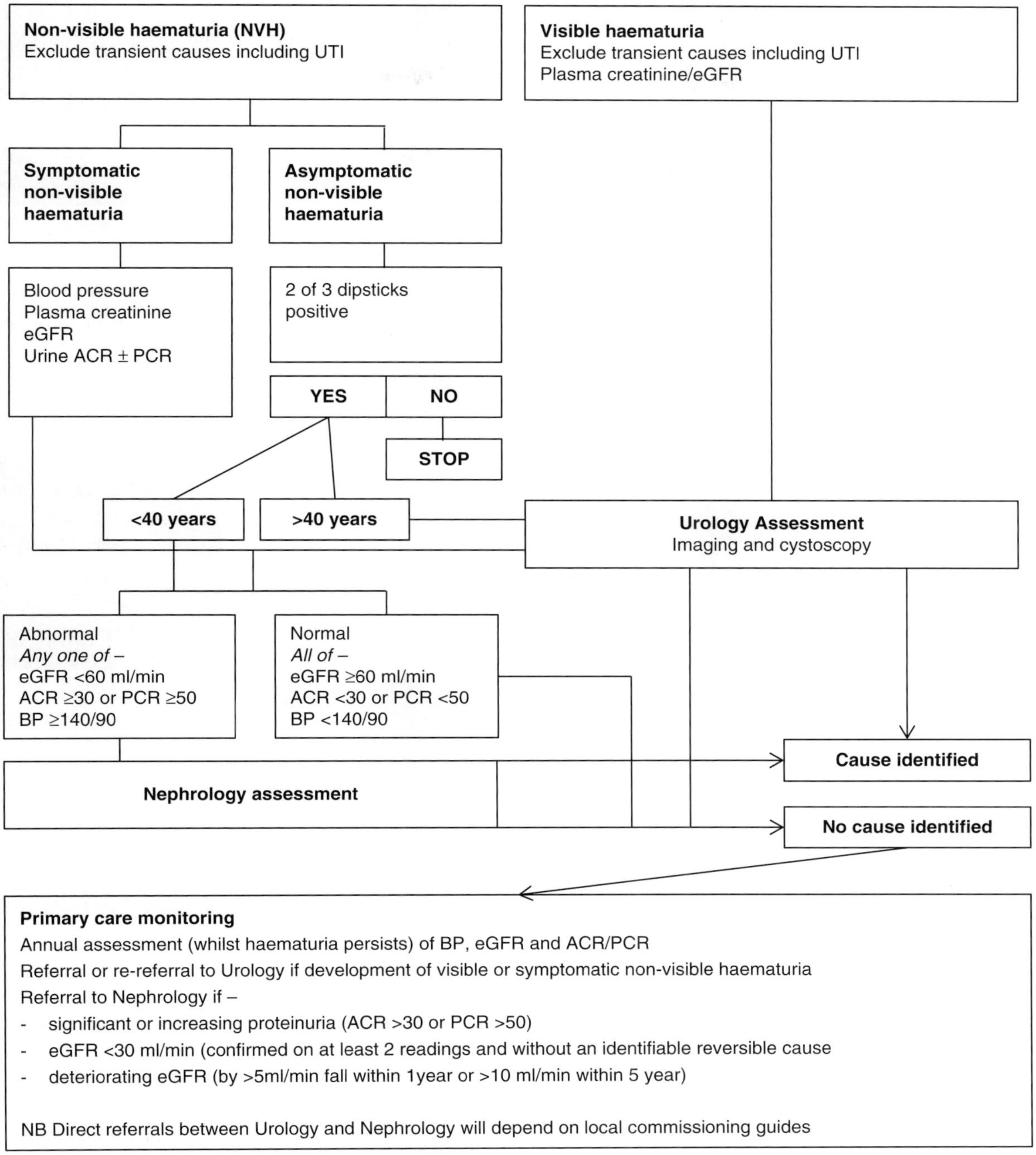

Adapted from the UK Renal Association Clinical Guidelines [7]

2. *Pigment nephropathy*: This is a great opportunity to make a rapid diagnosis in that myoglobinuria and haemglobinuria both result in a dark urine and positive haemstix test, but microscopy will show an absence of RBC. Thus, +++ haematuria but no RBC on microscopy is highly suggestive of a pigment nephropathy. If sent rapidly enough, rhabdomyolysis may be confirmed by the presence of myoglobin in the urine, but this is evanescent. Although not strictly urine analysis, intravascular haemolysis can then be cunningly distinguished from rhabdomyolysis by spinning the

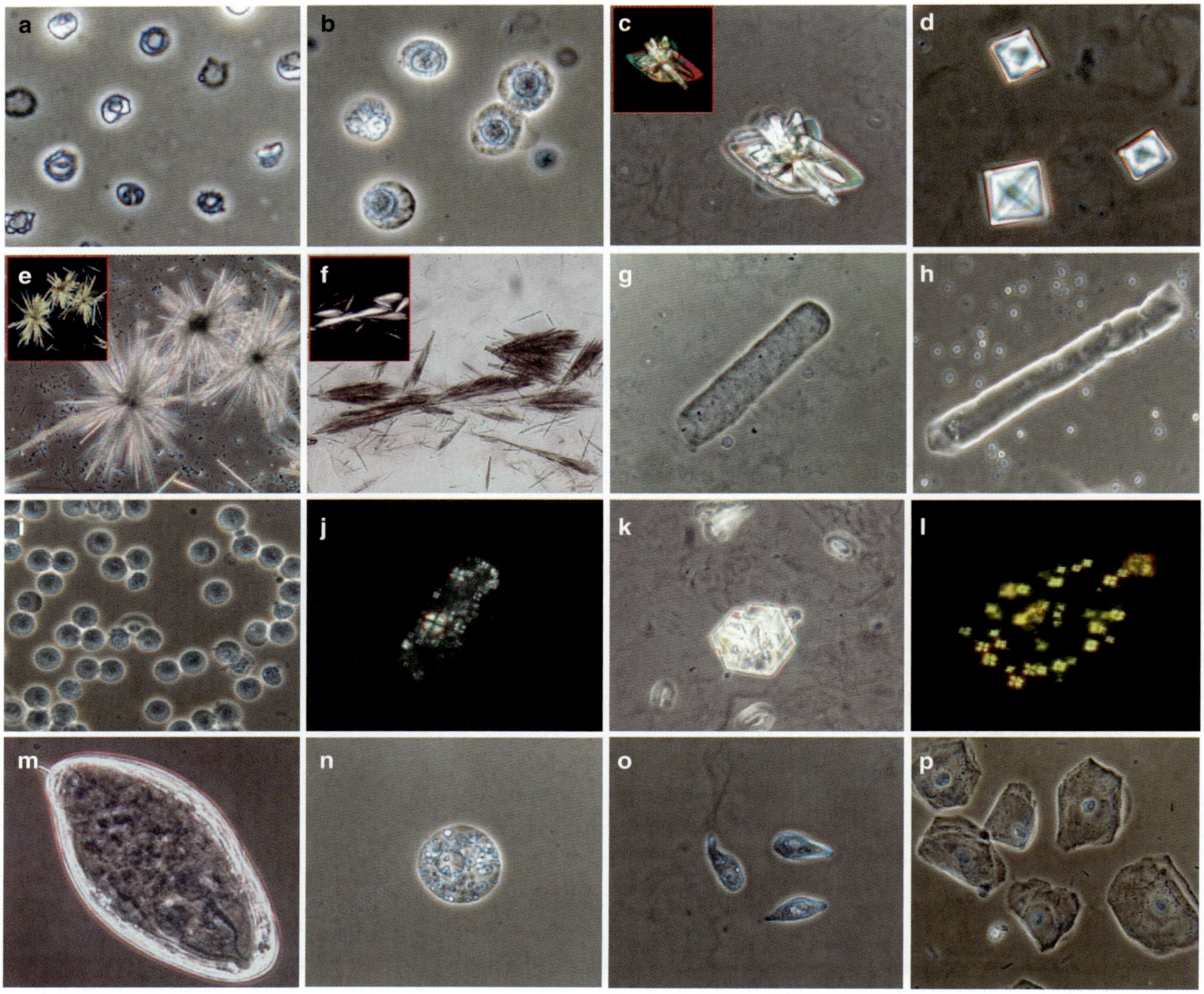

Fig. 2.1 Magnification ×400. (**a**) Dysmorphic erythrocytes; (**b**) proximal renal tubular epithelial cells – round shape, large nucleus and granular cytoplasm; (**c**) rhomboidal uric acid crystal with polychromatic birefringence under polarised light; (**d**) bipyramidal appearance of bihydrated calcium oxalate crystals; (**e**) ciprofloxacin crystals with birefringent star-like shape; (**f**) amoxicillin crystals appearing as needles, strong birefringence; (**g**) hyaline granular cast; (**h**) waxy cast; (**i**) leucocyturia; (**j**) 'Maltese cross' crystals on polarised light; (**k**) hexagonal crystals of cysteine; (**l**) 2,8-dihydroxyadenine crystals; (**m**) *Schistosoma haematobium* eggs; (**n**) granular macrophage; (**o**) deep urothelial cells; (**p**) squamous cells [8, 9] (Reprinted with permission from Fogazzi et al. [8] and Bouzidi et al. [9])

patient's blood and demonstrating pink serum. Myoglobin and haemoglobin can stain granular and epithelial casts orange/brown, and this can be a late useful clue.

3. *Rapidly progressive glomerulonephritis* (*RPGN*): The presence of a classical 'active urine', i.e. significant blood and protein and dysmorphic RBC in large numbers (and ideally a RBC cast), is extremely helpful contributory evidence for RPGN. Similarly, the absence of any dysmorphic RBC may be very reassuring in a complex patient with AKI.
4. *Acute interstitial nephritis* (*AIN*): There are no truly discriminatory findings in the urine of patients with AIN, but patients often have low to moderate levels of haematuria/proteinuria but can occur with neither, emphasising the importance of urine microscopy for white blood cells; large amounts of either blood or protein tending to make the diagnosis less likely (e.g. urine PCR >200). Classically AIN is associated with a sterile pyuria and eosinophiluria* is common, but neither particularly specific nor sensitive (**visible on Giemsa staining*). Of note, simultaneous measurement of urinary albumin and protein to creatinine ratio allows determination of urinary albumin to total protein ratio, and it has been shown that a measurement of <0.40 is highly sensitive and specific for the diagnosis of AIN [10].
5. *Crystal nephropathy*: The rhomboid shapes of uric acid crystals in otherwise 'quiet' urine may be indicative of

tumour lysis syndrome (Fig. 2.1c). Bipyramidal crystals of calcium oxalate may be extensive in acute oxalosis secondary to ethylene glycol ingestion or hyperoxalosis of any cause, although they can occur in normal urine (Fig. 2.1d). Occasionally it may be possible to heroically make the diagnosis of drug-induced crystal nephropathy relating to aciclovir, antiretroviral therapy or antibiotics, such as ciprofloxacin and amoxicillin (Fig. 2.1e, f).

In summary whilst many cases of AKI result from multiple insults, sometimes, careful assessment of the urine can cheaply and noninvasively hone the differential diagnosis that significantly or reassuringly excludes some important disease groups.

Chronic Kidney Disease (CKD)

The kidney loses the ability to substantially regulate urine concentration (beyond 1.010) or control pH in CKD. The concentration of creatinine in the urine tends to remain stable with worsening renal function as GFR falls but plasma creatinine rises. Low levels of proteinuria are very common in CKD, but substantial proteinuria (3+), especially if combined with haematuria, suggests a primary glomerular lesion. Microscopy of urine in CKD is usually dominated by signs of progressive tubular damage including tubular cell casts, waxy casts, coarse granular casts and leucocytes (Fig. 2.1g–i).

Table 2.7 Semi-quantitative correlation of dipstick proteinuria

	Protein concentration (mg/dl)	Estimated daily protein excretion (g/day)
Trace	5–20	
1+	30	<0.5
2+	100	0.5–1
3+	300	1–2

Is There Any Value in Urine Analysis in Suspected CKD?

The role of urine analysis in chronically damaged kidneys is rather more limited than in AKI. However, when faced with a new patient who has marked renal impairment, it is critical to distinguish between AKI and CKD. This is often resolved by detailed clinical history, historical creatinine results or renal ultrasound; however, urine microscopy demonstrating granular and tubular cell casts with an *absence* of acute cellular casts, dysmorphic red cells or features of an 'active urine deposit' may be helpful confirmatory evidence of CKD and exclusion of a rapidly progressive glomerulonephritis or urinary tract infection.

A significant proportion of patients with ESRF have no definite renal diagnosis, and occasionally thoughtful urine analysis in CKD can narrow down the differential diagnosis and sometimes achieve a diagnostic coup and is worth considering in new patients, for example:

- The identification of '*Maltese cross*' on polarised light microscopy (Fig. 2.1j) in a patient with CKD and low-level proteinuria is highly suggestive of Anderson-Fabry disease, although it can occur in any heavily nephrotic state. In Anderson-Fabry's disease, these represent myelin bodies free within the urine or within hyaline casts and can be definitively distinguished by electron microscopy.
- Extremely broad *hyaline casts* are said to be indicative of medullary cystic disease or reflux nephropathy and maybe helpful in early CKD but can occur in any advanced CKD.
- The oval or bipyramidal crystals of *calcium oxalate* (Fig. 2.1d) may indicate either acute or chronic hyperoxalaemia, although oxalate crystals are a fairly nonspecific finding.

Table 2.8 Types of proteinuria with important clinical considerations

Glomerular proteinuria Predominantly albumin and an early, important indicator of glomerular injury. Standard dipsticks sensitive	*Physiological* – ACR <30 mg/24 h (but raised acutely if febrile, see below) *Microalbuminuria* – ACR >30–300 mg/24 h (not detectable with standard dipstick) *Overt proteinuria* – ACR > PCR *Nephrotic range proteinuria* – ACR > PCR>
Tubular proteinuria Suspect with low-level proteinuria especially if uPCR out of proportion to dipstick/uACR or accompanied by other features of tubular injury/inflammation such as sterile pyuria or features of Fanconi syndrome	Rarely greater than 100 mg/mmol or 1 g/l Indicated by normal ACR but raised PCR Specific tests for tubular proteins include retinol binding protein (RBP), α-1 microglobulin and N-acetyl β glucosamine (NAG) Causes include drug toxicity (eg. cisplatin, tenofovir etc.), causes of acquired tubulointerstitial nephritis, heavy metal poisoning and Dent's disease
Overflow proteinuria	Overproduction of proteins, most commonly light chains Not detected by standard urine dipsticks Negative or low-level dipstick with disproportionate urine PCR may suggest overflow or tubular proteinuria
Benign proteinuria	'Physiological': febrile proteinuria, post-exercise proteinuria Orthostatic proteinuria: isolated low-level proteinuria, often in young males, possibly associated with 'nutcracker kidney' (arterial compression of renal veins occasionally with loin pain). Proteinuria is absent on rising sample, present after being ambulant so easily diagnosed with paired rising and ambulant uPCRs

- Hexagonal crystals of *cysteine* (Fig. 2.1k) are always pathological and thus indicate cystinosis if not already identified or isolated cystinuria as a cause of stones.
- *2,8-Dihydroxyadenine crystals* (Fig. 2.1l) are indicative of the rare adenine phosphoribosyltransferase deficiency – an important diagnosis to make in terms of treatment and risk of recurrence.
- Urine microscopy (of early morning sample) is a cheap and widely used method for diagnosis of *Schistosoma haematobium* (Fig. 2.1m) in endemic areas and may give the diagnosis in CKD secondary to obstructive uropathy.
- In the setting of CKD, significant blood and glomerular range proteinuria is suggestive of a *subacute glomerular disorder* (such as IgA or Alport's syndrome).

Figure 2.1 also shows additional frequent findings on urine microscopy which are important to recognise including granular macrophage (Fig. 2.1n), deep urothelial cell (Fig. 2.1o) and squamous cells (Fig. 2.1p).

Tubular Disorders

The causes of tubular and interstitial disease are numerous, but there are less pathognomic signs on urine microscopy than that found in the context of glomerular injury. Nevertheless, the presence of isolated mild proteinuria should always raise the possibility of a tubular disorder and may be supported by the detection of granular or 'waxy' casts on urine microscopy. In addition, the diagnosis of tubular clinical syndromes is often heralded by urinary abnormalities. Tubular syndromes result from abnormal handling of waste products, electrolytes and hydrogen ions and bicarbonate compounds without a necessary change in GFR:

1. *Renal tubular acidosis* may be associated with either a consistently elevated urine pH (distal RTA, type 4) or may be variable (proximal RTA, type 1) according to changes in bicarbonate reabsorption.
2. *Fanconi syndrome* is associated with reduced urine pH, but rather than an isolated bicarbonate reabsorption defect being present, additional proximal tubular function is impaired. Characteristic urinary abnormalities are phosphaturia, glycosuria (normoglycaemia), uricosuria and aminoaciduria. These abnormalities may be found in association with 'tubular' proteinuria.
3. *Tubular proteinuria* is a term used interchangeably with low molecular weight proteinuria and usually implies chronic proximal tubular dysfunction with the abnormal presence of β2-microglobuin, α-microglobulin, retinol binding protein and Clara cell protein within the urine. It is rarely more than 1 g/l and may be indicated by minimal protein on dipstick (detecting albumin) or normal ACR with a raised PCR.
4. *Acute and chronic tubulointerstitial nephritis* as mentioned above tend to be associated with low levels (<1.5 g/l) of proteinuria (PCR ≫ ACR), pyuria (more common in AIN than chronic TIN), occasionally eosinophiluria (nice to see but very low sensitivity and uncertain specificity) and sometimes microscopic haematuria.

Urinary Tract Infection (UTI)

The initial appearance of cloudy, offensive urine (especially in a symptomatic patient) may convincingly make a rapid diagnosis of UTI. It is often helpful to see urine at presentation, and it is important to get fresh samples to the laboratory swiftly for culture in order to confirm the diagnosis and guide antimicrobial chemotherapy. Urine analysis findings both in favour and against of a significant/clinically relevant UTI in a MSU specimen are shown in Table 2.9. Sterile pyuria has to be considered in the differential diagnosis prior to confirmation of bacterial culture as the hallmark 'nonspecific' features on initial urine analysis may also be

Table 2.9 Considerations in the diagnosis of a significant/clinically relevant UTI

	Features suggestive of UTI	Features against clinically relevant UTI
Appearance	Cloudy/turbid/offensive	Clear urine in asymptomatic patient
Urine dipstick	*Leucocyte esterase* positive (sensitive and very specific for pyuria) *Nitrites* (helpful if present but low sensitivity) *Low-level proteinuria/haematuria* (sometimes macroscopic), particularly if not previously present	Negative *leucocyte esterase* and *nitrite* dipstick have a strong negative predictive value (caveats above)
Microscopy	*White cell casts* (rare but important finding, very strong evidence of pyelonephritis) *Pyuria* (for other causes of sterile pyuria see Table 2.10) *Bacteruria* (if present on high-power field in clean catch, unspun urine, correlates with 10^5 or more bacteria/ml). Two clean-catch specimens in asymptomatic woman with 10^5 or more bacteria/ml represent a 95 % probability of true bacteruria	Absence of pyuria (NB: pyuria may be absent in neutropenic patients)
Culture	Pure growth of single organism with >10^5 cfu/ml	Bacteruria in the absence of pyuria and or multiple squamous cells contaminating sample Mixed growth of organisms (bona fide in 5 % of UTIs)

explained by the causes of sterile pyuria as outlined in Table 2.10.

Considerable thought also needs to be applied to the interpretation of urine from patients with indwelling catheters, ileal conduits and urostomies in that these frequently demonstrate all the features of a urinary tract infection as a result of chronic colonisation, and these samples frequently do not represent clinically relevant UTI.

Table 2.10 Causes of sterile pyuria

Urinary tract infection during or immediately post-antibiotics
Children with pyrexia of non-urinary tract origin
Urinary tract infection with fastidious organism
Symptomatic patient but no bacteria: *Neisseria gonorrhoeae*, *Chlamydia trachomatis*, *Mycoplasma genitalium*
Asymptomatic tuberculosis, fungal infections
Interstitial nephritis
Chronic prostatitis
Papillary necrosis
Radiation or chemical cystitis
Renal stones
Solvent abuse

Urinary Electrolytes

Measurement of urinary electrolytes and osmolality is often performed in clinical practice in an attempt to guide diagnosis. However, interpretation is complex, compounded by the intricate mechanisms regulating solute excretion and osmolality. It is useful to remember that urinary electrolytes and osmolalities do not have fixed 'normal' values but rather parameters, based on the clinical setting.

From a practical perspective, testing is now routinely performed on a 'random' 10 ml clean-catch MSU sample, although certain circumstances require 24-h collection. Common indications and clinical scenarios when testing of urinary electrolytes and osmolality is appropriate are outlined in Table 2.11. However, the physiological principles underpinning water and solute excretion need to be continually considered; for example, urine osmolality assesses the action of ADH in the collecting ducts and hence water excretion, whilst urinary sodium is a measure of tubular function with the majority of freely filtered sodium being reabsorbed by the renal tubules. Table 2.11 is intended to be a helpful guide to interpreting urinary electrolytes, rather than an exhaustive atlas.

Table 2.11 Guide to interpretation of urine electrolytes [11]

	Urinary abnormalities	Considerations
Acute kidney injury		
'Prerenal' volume-depleted AKI	UNa^+ <20 mmol/l, $UOsm$ ↑, FE_{Na^+} <1 %, FE_{urea} <35 %	Abnormalities in urinary electrolytes in AKI reflect disease/damage to renal tubules with concentrating ability usually preserved in 'prerenal' volume-depleted AKI
Acute tubular necrosis (ATN)	UNa^+ >20 mmol/l, $UOsm$ ↔, FE_{Na^+} >3 %, FE_{urea} <35 % (*Hepatorenal syndrome* – UNa^+ *<20 mmol/l*, FE_{urea} ↓)	UNa^+ in post-obstructive uropathy is *not* reliable despite volume depletion
Contrast nephropathy Pigment nephropathy	FE_{Na^+} typically <1 % (*Also seen in cardiac failure*)	In any post-operative patient, vasopressin release alters urine concentration ability
Interstitial nephritis	Usually 'salt-wasting' state – UNa^+ >20 mmol/l, FE_{Na^+} >3 %	
Chronic kidney disease		
Crystal nephropathy	24-h urine collection most useful. Need to measure:	Risk factors for calcium stone formation:
Renal stone disease	Volume, calcium (acid preservative), phosphate, oxalate (acid preservative), uric acid (alkaline preservative), sodium, citrate, creatinine (ensure adequate collection), pH	Hypercalciuria, hypocitraturia, hyperoxaluria, hyperuricosuria, RTA (*see also* Chap. 36)
Nephrocalcinosis	In addition, random urine sample to measure:	
Fanconi syndrome	Amino acids, β2-microglobulin, glucose	
	Phosphaturia, glycosuria (normoglycaemia), uricosuria and aminoaciduria	

UNa^+ urine sodium, $UOsm$ urine osmolality, FE_{Na^+} fractional excretion of sodium, FE_{Urea} fractional excretion of urea

$$FE_{Na^+} = \frac{\text{urine Na}^+ \times \text{plasma creatinine}}{\text{plasma Na}^+ \times \text{urine creatinine}} \times 100, \quad FE_{Na^+} = \frac{\text{urine urea} \times \text{plasma creatinine}}{\text{plasma urea} \times \text{urine creatinine}} \times 100$$

Summary

Urine analysis remains an important tool available to all clinicians and offers particularly useful information to the practising nephrologist. From initially inspecting the urine to performing routine urine dipstick and microscopy, clinical information is available at each stage and should therefore always be considered as an extension of the physical examination.

References

1. Bagshaw SM, Haase M, Haase-Fielitz A, Bennett M, Devarajan P, Bellomo R. A prospective evaluation of urine microscopy in septic and non-septic acute kidney injury. Nephrol Dial Transplant. 2012; 27(2):582–8.
2. Kanbay M, Kasapoglu B, Perazella MA. Acute tubular necrosis and pre-renal acute kidney injury: utility of urine microscopy in their evaluation – a systematic review. Int Urol Nephrol. 2010;42(2): 425–33.
3. Connor H. Medieval uroscopy and its representation on misericords – part 1: uroscopy. Clin Med. 2001;1(6):507–9.
4. HPA. Investigation of Urine. Health Protection Agency. National Standard Method BSOP41. 2009. http://www.hpa-standardmethods.org.uk/documents/bsop/pdf/bsop41.pdf. Accessed 1 Feb 2012.
5. Berman LB. Urine in technicolor. JAMA. 1974;228(6):753.
6. Addis T. Glomerular nephritis. Diagnosis and treatment. New York: Macmillan; 1948. p. 2.
7. BAUS/RA Guidelines. Joint Consensus Statement on the Initial Assessment of Haematuria. Renal Association. 2008. http://www.renal.org/Libraries/Other_Guidlines/Haematuria_-_RA-BAUS_consensus_guideline_2008.sflb.ashx.
8. Fogazzi GB, Verdesca S, Garigali G. Urinalysis: core curriculum 2008. Am J Kidney Dis. 2008;51(6):1052–67.
9. Bouzidi H, Lacour B, Daudon M. 2,8-dihydroxyadenine nephrolithiasis: from diagnosis to therapy. Ann Biol Clin (Paris). 2007;65(6): 585–92.
10. Smith ER, Cai MMX, McMahon LP, Wright DA, Holt SG. The value of simultaneous measurements of urinary albumin and total protein in proteinuric patients. Nephrol Dial Transplant. 2012;27(4): 1534–41.
11. Winter SD, Gabow PA. Measurement of urine electrolytes: clinical significance and methods. Clin Rev Clin Lab Sci. 1981;14(3): 163–87.

3 Imaging in Nephrology

Benjamin Salt and Antony Goode

Imaging is fundamental to the management of patients with renal disease, and access to increasingly sophisticated techniques is growing. As a consequence of this, renal disease is being identified coincidentally by other specialities, and patients with chronic renal problems can easily clock up large doses of radiation, gadolinium and radio-contrast. A close working relationship with radiology and nuclear medicine specialists is vital as is a thoughtful assessment of the most appropriate form of imaging and/or intervention, and a structured process is necessary for this.

The Multidisciplinary Team Meeting

The clinico-radiological meeting, or 'X-ray meeting', is a long-standing tradition in hospital medicine and provides an opportunity to meet with a radiologist to discuss the diagnosis and management of that patient along with relevant imaging and for any further imaging strategies to be decided. In modern practice, the meeting may well involve other professionals who have a role in management of specialty patients, for example, a pathologist, specialist nurse or physiotherapist, and is now known as the multidisciplinary team meeting (MDTM). Renal cancer MDTMs have become an integral part of the management of patients with renal cancer, and attendance includes a surgeon, oncologist, radiologist and pathologist, together with specialist nurses. The organisation of a cancer MDTM is tightly defined and subject to peer review for quality assurance, and there are published guidelines on the conduct of a cancer MDTM for radiologists [1].

Non-cancer MDTMs, such as the nephrology MDTM, are not subject to such tight regulation; however, the standards may still be used to guide the organisation of such an MDTM. The nephrology MDTM should be attended by both junior and consultant nephrologists and specialist nurses and be taken by a radiologist with an appropriate interest. Local practices will vary, but in a unit where vascular access for dialysis is performed, a surgeon who performs these procedures should attend and likewise if the centre performs renal transplants. Some units may run separate MDTMs for vascular access or transplant issues.

The Royal College of Radiologists recommend that all imaging to be presented at the MTDM should be reviewed by the radiologist beforehand, and where resources allow, an MDTM coordinator may be employed to prepare a list of patients beforehand. Decisions taken during an MDTM should be recorded in the patient's notes, and the MDTM coordinator may assist with this – where possible this should be done electronically with the record made visible to all members of the MDTM. The appointment of a nominated chairperson for the MDTM will allow the meeting to progress efficiently.

Radiation

Much of imaging involves the use of ionising radiation (in the form of X-rays for plain radiography, CT or fluoroscopy and gamma rays in the case of nuclear medicine) to form diagnostic images. As such, it is prudent to consider the risks and damages this poses to patients and staff. When radiation is absorbed by the tissues, the biological effects can then manifest over a much longer period of time. Doses from certain examinations can be orders of magnitude greater than the yearly average background dose for an individual, which is 2.7 mSv [2], and with serial examinations or multiphase CT, this can constitute significant risk.

B. Salt, MBBS, MA
Department of Radiology, Royal Free Hospital,
Pond Street, London, UK
e-mail: bcsalt@doctors.org.uk

A. Goode, BSc (Hons), MBBS, MRCP, FRCR (✉)
Radiology Department, Royal Free London NHS Foundation
Trust, Pond St, London NW3 2QG, UK
e-mail: antonygoode1@nhs.net

M. Harber (ed.), *Practical Nephrology*,
DOI 10.1007/978-1-4471-5547-8_3, © Springer-Verlag London 2014

Table 3.1 Radiation dose for common imaging protocols

Examination	Effective dose (mSv)
1 day of background radiation	0.006
Chest X-ray	0.02
Abdomen X-ray	0.7
CT chest	7
CT pulmonary angiogram	15
CT KUB (low dose)	5
CT abdomen and pelvis	14
CT IVU	28
Nuclear medicine MAG3	2.6
Nuclear medicine DMSA	3.3
Whole body PET-CT	25

Adverse outcomes related to radiation risk can be divided into deterministic events and stochastic effects. Deterministic effects are those which will not happen below a certain threshold dose. Once this dose is achieved, the likelihood of the event occurring increases to a level where it is inevitable. Examples of this are cataracts and skin erythema. These events occur at relatively high doses for patients and are therefore only really of consideration in certain circumstances, for example, complex interventional procedures where there may be a long period of screening over one part of the body. This effect is not cumulative – the skin repairs itself so if the patient undergoes a further procedure in the future, skin erythema would require the same dose of radiation again. Pregnancy is a special case in that there is a threshold dose of radiation above which foetal abnormalities, such as growth retardation, Down's syndrome or spontaneous abortion, occur. The risk of this is greatest in the third to eighth week of pregnancy, and it is essential to minimise the radiation risk to any patients who are pregnant.

Stochastic effects of radiation relate to the risk of cancer or genetic abnormalities. This is manifested as a risk that increases linearly with the dose of radiation. For stochastic effects, the most useful measurement of radiation exposure is the effective dose of radiation. This is a theoretically calculated value that gives a weighted view of the radiation dose to the entire body. It cannot be measured directly; rather the values given are calculated from the known radiation output and exposure of different body parts, and the dose is measured in sieverts. The effective doses for different examinations are shown in Table 3.1. These doses are the average expected doses for each examination and will vary depending upon how modern the equipment is, the size of the patient, etc.

The risk of developing a fatal cancer is 5 % per sievert (Sv) effective dose or 1:20,000 per millisievert (mSv). This is a cumulative risk – i.e. the risk increases with subsequent exposures even if there has been a significant time period between them.

CT

Computed tomography (CT) uses X-rays to generate an image based on the density of the tissues being examined and is responsible for a large proportion (40 %) of the annual dose of ionising radiation due to medical exposures, despite representing a smaller proportion of the number of examinations performed annually. The use of CT is therefore largely dictated by concerns over radiation dose a patient may receive and IV contrast if required.

Intravenous Contrast

Most soft tissues within the body attenuate X-rays by the same amount and therefore appear as the same density or same shade of grey on an unenhanced CT scan. Intravenous contrast agents concentrate in different organs to different degrees and so improve the distinction between tissues and organs. IV contrast agents contain iodine which, due to its high atomic number relative to soft tissues within the body, appears as a denser medium. This improves visualisation of blood vessels or tissues which have a higher blood flow.

Patients requiring contrast need to be assessed for factors increasing their risk of an adverse reaction (see below). In addition, they need a cannula in situ, the size and position of which is dependent upon the type of procedure being performed (examinations such as CT pulmonary angiography for pulmonary emboli require a higher rate of contrast injection and as such a larger cannula is required). In addition there are different types of contrast media with differing toxicities, and the decision of which to use will depend upon the clinical scenario and risk factors as discussed below.

Adverse Reactions

Incidence of severe reactions is about 0.04 % with modern contrast media.

Patients at increased risk:

1. Previous reaction.
2. Asthma – increases risk of a severe reaction by 6–10 times.
3. Renal impairment (up to date eGFR or creatinine is essential).
4. Multiple allergies – patients with multiple allergies or a single severe allergy are at increased risk. Contrary to popular belief, there is no specific link with reactions to shellfish or topical iodine in acute contrast reactions. There is no evidence to support the use of prophylactic steroids.
5. Diabetes.

Metformin – as this is exclusively excreted by the kidneys, there is a theoretical risk of accumulation and subsequent lactic acidosis if a patient has a fall in eGFR secondary to IV contrast. However, there is no evidence that this is a risk in patients with a normal function. The current advice is that patients with normal renal function should continue metformin; however, in cases where eGFR < 60 ml/min or creatinine is abnormally raised, a consideration to stop metformin for 48 h after contrast should be made by the referring clinic.

Reactions

Anaphylactoid

The guidelines for treatment of acute contrast anaphylaxis are the same as for any other acute anaphylactic reaction.

Skin Reactions

Delayed reactions can occur up to 1 week after IV contrast. The significance of these is unclear and symptomatic treatment only is required.

Thyroid

Due to the high iodine content of IV contrast, patients with uncontrolled hyperthyroidism should not be administered contrast material due to a high risk of thyrotoxicosis. Prophylactic treatment can be arranged after discussion with endocrinology team.

Contrast-Induced Acute Kidney Injury (CI-AKI)

This is an uncommon consequence (incidence 1–2 %) of intravenous contrast that is due to a combination of afferent arteriolar vasoconstriction and direct toxicity of the contrast media on epithelial cells of the renal tubules, and creatinine usually peaks 72 h post-contrast.

Risk Factors Increasing Chance of CI-AKI

(a) Chronic kidney disease – eGFR <60 ml/min/1.73 m^2
(b) Age >75 years
(c) Cardiac failure
(d) Nephrotoxic drugs
(e) Hypovolaemia
(f) Sepsis
(g) High dose of contrast
(h) Multiple doses

In cases where there is an increased risk, the first consideration is whether a different imaging modality such as MRI or ultrasound will answer the clinical question or whether the CT can be performed without IV contrast. If contrast must be administered, the management focusses on prevention as there is no specific treatment after the event.

For patients with eGFR <60 ml/min, preventative measures should be used (with the use of *low-osmolality* contrast agents). For eGFR <30, iodinated contrast media should be avoided if possible with the caveat that making the correct diagnosis may take precedence over the risk of AKI (if the patient is already on haemodialysis, then the risk of AKI is less important but even then due consideration should be given to preserving renal function where possible).

If IV contrast needs to be administered, the following preventative measures are currently recommended by the renal association:

Volume expansion – IV 0.9 % sodium chloride at a rate of 1 ml/kg/h for 12 h pre- and post-contrast and intravenous isotonic sodium bicarbonate have both been shown to significantly reduce the risk of CI-AKI [3].

No reliable data have yet been produced to support the use of one versus the other [4]. The most important issue is dose reduction and having a robust system for ensuring the patient is well hydrated. There is currently no compelling evidence to support the use of *N*-acetylcysteine (NAC) in preventing CI-AKI; although there is conflicting evidence, a large randomised controlled trial showed NAC to have no effect in reducing CI-AKI [5].

Nephrotoxic Drugs: Withhold Any Potentially Nephrotoxic Drugs

Minimise the volume of contrast media – by selecting the appropriate examination depending upon the clinical question, the need for repeat examinations can be minimised and therefore only a single bolus of contrast needs to be administered.

Measure renal function – in stable patients, eGFR is the preferred measurement; however, in patients with AKI, this should not be used. eGFR should be measured pre-examination in those at risk and 48–72 h post-IV contrast to ensure it has remained stable.

Advantages

1. Multiplanar – CT builds the images using data about the body as a volume; therefore, the area of interest can be examined in different planes, and its relationship to other structures can be studied.
2. Speed – modern CT scanners can cover the whole body in a matter of a few seconds, making rapid examination possible which can be vital for unstable patients.
3. Availability.

Disadvantages

The major disadvantage of CT as described above is the use of radiation and associated increased risk of cancer. However, certain other factors need to be considered.

Table 3.2 Sensitivity and role of CT scanning protocols for renal pathologies

Parenchyma	Mass lesions	76 % Sensitivity for lesions <1 cm, 95 % sensitivity 1–2 cm. Allows assessment of fat, calcium and soft tissue content and enhancement pattern with IV contrast
	Vascularity	Renal perfusion can be assessed as can the renal vasculature. Anatomical delineation for pre-transplant assessment
Collecting system	Calculi	>90 % Sensitivity. Also allows assessment of other causes of flank pain
	Tumour	89–100 % Sensitivity for TCC on CT IVU
	Obstruction	Sensitive for obstruction and helps demonstrate cause; however ,US is better first-line test
Ureters	Calculi	98 % Sensitive for ureteric calculi. Also allows demonstration of inflammatory change which may indicate recent stone passage
	Tumour	CT IVU is 96 % sensitive and 99 % specific for TCC of the ureter. Also allows staging
Bladder	Wall lesions	CT IVU 79 % sensitive for bladder wall tumours
	Emptying	No role

Movement and breathing during the scan can produce blurred images obscuring pathology. As such, patients who are hyperventilating or unable to lie still due to pain or confusion can produce non-diagnostic imaging. Patients therefore need to be prepared for their scan with adequate analgesia +/– sedation if appropriate.

As most soft tissues within the body attenuate X-rays by a similar amount, it is often not possible to distinguish between normal and abnormal soft tissues on a plain CT, although this is improved by the use of IV contrast, this carries its own risks.

Protocols

The need for IV contrast and the timings of the scan after injection of contrast need to be guided by the clinical picture and question to be answered. The scan can be timed so that IV contrast is within the arteries or the venous system or delayed, so it is within the ureters or bladder depending upon what organ needs to be assessed or which pathological process is suspected – Table 3.2 describes the sensitivity of CT for different aspects of the renal system. The protocol of the CT examination is therefore tailored by the clinical details. Examples of some commonly used protocols are below:

CT KUB

This is a lower-dose procedure which does not involve the use of intravenous contrast for the detection of renal tract calculi. The decreased dose reduces the sharpness of the scan slightly and the lack of IV contrast reduces soft tissue contrast, so this is not optimal for looking at the parenchyma of the kidneys or other solid organs.

Contrast-Enhanced Abdomen

The 'standard' abdominal/pelvic CT involves IV contrast and is timed so the majority of the contrast is within the venous system. This is good for distinguishing lesions from normal soft tissue.

CT IVU

This is a multiphase protocol. It involves an unenhanced phase to detect calculi, followed by a venous/nephrogenic phase to study the renal parenchyma and finally a delayed phase that displays the collecting system and ureters. There is a relatively high radiation dose, so patient selection is important.

CT Angiogram

This involves timing the scan so the IV contrast is within the arterial system. One of the main uses is for delineating arterial anatomy for assessment prior to live renal transplant donation.

MRI

Because it does not rely upon the differential absorption of X-rays by tissues, rather giving images more dependent upon the chemical makeup of the tissue, MRI gives excellent contrast between soft tissue structures. As such, it is very useful for imaging and assessing tumours and soft tissue masses. The addition of gadolinium contrast can show enhancement patterns of lesions as well as visualising vessels to assess for anatomy and stenosis.

Contraindications

Due to the high magnetic field used, there are risks with MR imaging and metallic objects. There is variability in what orthopaedic and cardiac implants can safely be imaged with MRI (Table 3.3), and as such it is vital to obtain accurate records of any medical, cosmetic or other implants.

MRI Contrast

Incidence of anaphylactoid reactions with gadolinium is <0.01 % with an increased risk in patients with previous

Table 3.3 Contraindications for MRI scanning with implants

Absolute contraindication	Pacemaker
	Otic implant
	Metal in the eye or orbit
	Implanted cardiac defibrillator
Likely contraindication	Heart valve or aneurysm clip installed before 1996
Possible contraindication	Heart valve or aneurysm clip installed after 1996
	Any type of prosthesis
Usually allowable 6–8 weeks after implantation	Passive implants, weakly ferromagnetic (e.g. coils, filters and stents; metal sutures or staples)
Usually allowable immediately after implantation	Passive implants, non-ferromagnetic (e.g. bone/joint pins, screws or rods; coils, filters and stents; metal sutures or staples)
	Rigidly fixed passive implants, weakly ferromagnetic (e.g. bone/joint pins, screws or rods)

reactions – the second reaction often being more severe. Asthma or atopy also confer a 3.7x adverse reaction rate.

Nephrogenic Systemic Fibrosis (NSF)

There is a well-documented link between exposure to gadolinium-based contrast agents (GBCAs) and development of NSF. Patients with end-stage renal failure (eGFR <15 ml/min) have a 1–7 % chance of developing NSF. Increased frequency is seen with repeated exposure. NSF has not been reported in patients with eGFR >60.

Gadolinium is toxic, and so GBCAs are formed of chelates which bind gadolinium ions. The hypothesis is that gadolinium ions are released from chelates in GBCAs due to the prolonged clearance time in patients with renal failure, as a result of displacement of the gadolinium ion by another metallic ion such as calcium or zinc, in a process known as transmetallation. The gadolinium ion binds with free anions and precipitates out in various tissues resulting in fibrosis.

Clinical features include initial pain, pruritus, swelling and erythema, usually starting in the legs. This progresses to thickening and fibrosis of the skin and subcutaneous tissues and fibrosis of internal organs. Time of onset ranges from the day of exposure to several months. Patients with eGFR <60 who are not on dialysis or patients with chronic renal failure on dialysis are considered high risk. In these patients, alternative imaging tests or MRI without gadolinium should first be considered. If there are no alternatives, dose should be limited to 0.1 mmol/kg with a low-toxicity agent – some GBCAs are based on a chelate with a cyclical structure rather than a linear structure, and these so-called cyclical agents appear to be less susceptible to transmetallation. In patients already on dialysis, post-examination dialysis within a few hours is recommended; however, this will not clear gadolinium completely (approximately 9 h of dialysis is required to completely clear the gadolinium dose). In patients not already on dialysis, post-examination dialysis has not been shown to have any effect on the incidence of NSF.

Pros and Cons

Advantages

1. Good soft tissue contrast.
2. No ionising radiation – for younger patient or patients undergoing serial scans for follow-up purposes, MRI is preferable to minimise the radiation exposure.

Disadvantages

1. Time – whereas a CT scan takes a matter of seconds to perform, MRI takes many minutes to obtain the different sequences and planes necessary. As such, patients are required to lie still, making it unsuitable for patients in pain who are unable to lie flat or confused/agitated patients.
2. Availability – due to the high cost of MRI scanners combined with the time taken for each examination, availability is much less readily available than for other imaging modalities.
3. Claustrophobia – the bore of the scanner, inside which the patient is placed for imaging, is about 60 cm, smaller and longer than a CT. This can be very disconcerting for claustrophobic patients, and sedation may therefore be required. In addition, the narrow bore makes it unsuitable or obese patients. Wide-bore or open MRI scanners are available at specialist institutes however to address these factors, although image quality is usually poorer with these types of magnets.

Generally MRI is used for assessing soft tissue lesions and the vascular system in renal imaging. Table 3.4 demonstrates the sensitivity of MRI for different renal pathologies.

Nuclear Medicine

Nuclear medicine examinations also involves the use of radiation; however, instead of projecting a beam of X-rays through the patient as in plain radiography or CT, an unstable isotope (often technetium-99 m) is chemically bound to a pharmaceutical with affinity for the relevant target organ. This is then ingested or injected, and as the radioisotope decays, it releases gamma rays. These gamma rays are detected by a gamma camera, and the image is constructed over time. As the pharmaceutical can be selected specifically for the area of interest, this allows either static or dynamic imaging (as in the case of MAG3) and places a greater

Table 3.4 Sensitivity and role of MRI for specific renal pathologies

Parenchyma	Mass lesions	100 % Sensitivity and 94 % specificity for solid mass detection
	Scarring	
Collecting system	Calculi	No role
	Tumour	No role
	Obstruction	MRU increasingly used for anatomical and functional assessment of obstruction
Ureters	Calculi	
	Tumour	
	Obstruction	
Bladder	Wall lesions	Excellent for assessing invasion of tumour beyond bladder and involvement of local structures
	Emptying	No role
Vasculature		87 % Sensitive and 69 % specific for RAS. Often overestimates the degree of stenosis
		MR venography is useful for demonstrating venous anomalies but also for assessing the central thoracic veins when considering fistulas or long-term IV access for haemodialysis
		MRA and MRV are also used to assess the pelvic vasculature when planning renal transplantation, in conjunction with unenhanced CT (MR does not show calcification in vessels well)

emphasis on function rather than anatomical detail. Table 3.5 describes the different applications of nuclear medicine examinations to various aspects of the renal system.

Pros and Cons

Advantages

Functional data is obtained – the uptake and excretion of the radiopharmaceutical is dependent upon the function of the organ, giving an indication of the physiological process within that organ.

Disadvantages

1. Radiation – the use of ionising radiation has risks as described above. In addition, the added risk with nuclear medicine is that the radiopharmaceutical and subsequently the patient's bodily fluids are radioactive, increasing risk to other patients, carers and staff members.
2. Anatomical resolution – whilst it does give good dynamic data regarding organ function, the spatial resolution is quite poor giving low anatomical detail. As such, some investigations are combined with CT (e.g. PET-CT) to enable spatial localisation of the physiological data shown by the nuclear medicine component.

Table 3.5 Role of nuclear medicine in renal imaging

Parenchyma	Mass lesions	PET-CT useful for staging metastatic disease or recurrent disease
	Scarring	DMSA is gold standard for assessment of focal renal scarring
	Vascularity	
	Function	MAG3 for assessment of function and excretion. DMSA shows relative function
Collecting system	Calculi	No role
	Tumour	No role
	Obstruction	
Ureters	Calculi	No role
	Tumour	
	Obstruction	MAG3 for assessing drainage and function of the kidney. Will demonstrate obstruction
Bladder	Wall lesions	
	Emptying	

3. Time – many of the scans require a large amount of time to acquire the necessary data.
4. Renal impairment – the sensitivity of all radionuclide imaging techniques is diminished in moderate to severe renal dysfunction.

MAG3

MAG3 (mercaptoacetyltriglycine) is chelated with radioactive technetium-99m to form the radiopharmaceutical. It is cleared from the body by the kidneys via both glomerular filtration and tubular secretion.

This type of scan is useful as a dynamic renal study to assess renal perfusion, divided function, drainage and ureteric clearance. The patient is initially asked to empty their bladder and then the radiopharmaceutical is administered whilst they are on the gamma camera. The whole examination takes about 20–40 min after administration of the radiopharmaceutical during which time acquisitions are taken to show curves of activity related to time within the kidneys, known as a renogram. This is supplemented with static images of the kidneys, ureter and bladder. A diuretic (furosemide 0.5 mg/kg maximum dose 40 mg given 20 min prior to scanning in a well-hydrated patient) is used if clinical suspicion of obstruction or if a kidney is seen to not have drained satisfactorily during the scan, as this will diurese the radiopharmaceutical into the collecting system. If it still does not clear, this demonstrates an obstruction to drainage of the collecting system.

The dynamic nature of the scan allows gross assessment of the parenchymal perfusion and morphology and good dynamic visualisation of the parenchymal clearance and collecting system drainage.

DMSA

In this examination, dimercaptosuccinic acid is chelated with technetium-99 m to form the radiopharmaceutical. After injection, this concentrates within the renal parenchyma and becomes bound to proximal tubular cells. It is then slowly excreted within the urine.

Unlike the dynamic nature of MAG3, DMSA is used to assess the renal parenchyma for anatomy or scarring. As such, it is useful in cases of horseshoe or solitary kidneys or for localisation of an ectopic kidney. It is also used to assess renal scarring and parenchymal damage in acute pyelonephritis and later postinfection. The relative function of the two kidneys is also calculated.

Once the radiopharmaceutical is injected, the patient waits approximately 3 h for it to accumulate within the kidneys. Images are then acquired with a gamma camera.

Ultrasound

Medical sonography uses high-frequency sound waves (>20 kHz). Fluid (e.g. bladder or cystic structures) does not reflect any sound allowing it to pass through, and this therefore appears as black. Bone or calcification reflects the sound, and this appears as a white area.

Doppler sonography uses the Doppler effect to detect flow and is thus a highly useful non-invasive way to examine gross effects in arterial supply and venous drainage.

Because of its versatile nature, ultrasound can supply a myriad of information concerning pathological lesions (Table 3.6). As it does not use ionising radiation, it displays different properties of tissues than CT does, relying on their reflectivity rather than their X-ray absorbance. It is therefore excellent at distinguishing between solid and cystic lesions, studying the kidneys for evidence of hydronephrosis and giving information on the size and parenchymal thickness of the kidneys with any structural abnormalities.

Table 3.6 Role of ultrasound in renal imaging

Parenchyma	Mass lesions	20 % Sensitivity for lesions <1 cm, 70 % 1–2 cm. Allows Bosniak characterisation of cystic lesions superior to CT
	Scarring	37–100 % Sensitivity when compared to DMSA
	Vascularity	Good for demonstrating general vascularity of the kidney and patency of main renal artery and vein. RAS – 0–70 % sensitivity in experienced operators, increasing to >90 for transplant kidneys. Ultrasound does have a role in looking for asymmetry in renal sizes to suggest RAS
Collecting system	Calculi	30–90 % Sensitive for collecting system calculi. Sensitivity poor for small calculi
	Tumour	TCC appears as solid hypoechoic mass. Can be mistaken for hydronephrosis
	Obstruction	First-line test for diagnosis and grading of hydronephrosis. Excellent visualisation of the pelvicalyceal system when dilated
Ureters	Calculi	Poor visualisation of ureters with USS makes detection of calculi difficult. Will show if there is obstruction, hydronephrosis
	Tumour	No role
Bladder	Wall lesions	63 % Sensitivity for bladder tumours, direct visualisation is therefore needed in macroscopic haematuria to exclude. Endoscopic ultrasound is more sensitive but invasive
	Emptying	Volumetric measurement of bladder pre- and post-micturition is simple and fast. Can also show bladder wall trabeculation or diverticula, which suggest chronic outflow obstruction

Pros and Cons

Pros

1. Cheap – compared to CT and MRI scanners, ultrasound machines are orders of magnitude less expensive.
2. No radiation.
3. Bedside – many small portable ultrasound machines are currently available which are versatile enough to be used as a bedside scanner for patients who are too unstable to be transferred.

Cons

1. Small field of view – with ultrasound only a single plane is seen at one time: the view directly in front of the probe. As such, it can be difficult to fully assess larger structures or properly ascertain the anatomical relationships between different objects.
2. Operator dependent – the images produced in ultrasound are very dependent upon the skill and experience of the person performing the ultrasound.
3. Image review – due to the factors above, an ultrasound can only really be interpreted by the person who has performed it. Unlike CT where the whole scan is available for review at a later point, ultrasound only allows a few selected images to be reviewed at a later date, usually attempting to demonstrate the salient pathology.

4. Patient dependent – many patient factors can degrade the ability of ultrasound to demonstrate pathology. Movement and breathing mean that it can be difficult to obtain good views of the area of interest. In addition, the subcutaneous fat within obese patients causes significant attenuation of the sound waves, meaning that visualisation of deeper structures is challenging. This can be partly compensated; however, this again depends upon operator expertise.

Special Imaging Considerations

Renal artery stenosis – ultrasound is not commonly used to image native renal artery stenosis as visualisation of the whole renal artery is technically very difficult with ultrasound. However, initial screening ultrasound can often detect a discrepancy in the size of kidneys which may indicate stenosis of the afferent artery of the smaller kidney. This can then be assessed with MR angiography. The exception to this is with transplanted kidneys as the whole artery can often easily be visualised to the point of anastomosis.

Pyelonephritis – ultrasound is not diagnostic for pyelonephritis. The kidneys do show changes under ultrasound; however, these rarely manifest early, and if the kidneys appear normal, this does not rule out a pyelonephritis. The role of ultrasound is better for detecting obstruction or renal/perirenal abscess or collection secondary to the infection.

Intravenous pyelography – this is rarely performed now, as CT is superior for most applications. The IVP is however superior to CT in the diagnosis of medullary sponge kidney and papillary necrosis, as the superior spatial resolution of film radiography over CT better demonstrates the typical findings of both these conditions.

Interventional Radiology

Many nephrology and dialysis patients will undergo a procedure in interventional radiology (IR) during their diagnosis and treatment, and the planning and work-up of these patients are important in order to maximise the benefit and reduce the risk from the IR procedure. When a patient is referred to the IR department, clinical information should be comprehensive and relevant so that the radiologist can decide whether or not the proposed treatment is indicated or indeed feasible. Often the case of the patient will have been discussed at a nephrology or vascular access MDTM, but for those that are not, a discussion with a radiologist prior to referral will assist in requesting the correct procedure and will also allow any specific steps in patient preparation that are necessary.

Some general points on clinical information and preparation are listed in Table 3.7. It is worth noting that many departments will have their own guidelines which may vary from these. There are also specific notes about common procedures, including complications, that may be encountered.

Table 3.7 General preparations for interventional radiology

Clinical information:	Relevant history and indications, diagnostic question or therapeutic aim. Significant patient history, e.g. confusion, high levels of patient anxiety, previous procedures, bleeding diathesis, allergies
Need for interpreter	Important and frequently forgotten issue
Infection risk	Hepatitis C and B and HIV, MRSA, VRE, ESBL
Requirements	For example, oxygen, monitoring
Preparation	
IV access	Of sufficient size for contrast need
Nil by mouth	If having IV sedation
Coagulation	Haemoglobin, platelets, clotting screen, whether on low molecular weight or other prophylactic heparin
Urea and electrolytes	For example, degree of hyperkalaemia
Patient information	Patient information leaflet (ideally in first language), reasons for procedure discussed and explained

Patients attending the interventional radiology department should have their case notes, observation chart, drug prescription chart and any other relevant charts such as glucose monitoring chart and blood transfusion forms. Consent forms (see below) may be completed on the ward prior to attendance or in the IR department.

Consent

Patient consent is a legal requirement for non-emergency medical care, and the nature of interventional radiological procedures is such that written consent is required prior to all elective and planned urgent procedures. The act of signing the consent form usually occurs when the patient arrives in the interventional radiology department; however, the process of consent begins when the proposed treatment is initially discussed with the patient and will include an assessment of capacity of the patient to give consent, a description of the treatment proposed and the benefits and risks of that treatment. Sometimes the patient will have met the interventional radiologist during an outpatient attendance; however, in most cases the process of consent will begin with the clinical team who have referred the patient to interventional radiology; it is therefore essential that any clinician referring a patient for an interventional procedure has a good understanding of what the procedure entails. The provision of patient information leaflets is a valuable aid to the consent process. Further resources are available about the process of consent as follows:

http://www.gmc-uk.org/guidance/ethical_guidance/consent_guidance_index.asp

Standards for patient consent, particular to radiology, 2nd edition. RCR 2012
http://www.medicalprotection.org/uk/wales-factsheets/consent-the-basics

Fistuloplasty and Venoplasty

This involves accessing a stenotic or occluded segment of a native or prosthetic AV fistula and placing a guidewire across the abnormal segment to allow passage of an angioplasty balloon for venous dilatation. Access sheaths may be placed into the fistula vein, into the prosthetic graft or into an internal jugular vein or common femoral vein.

The procedure is often performed with the use of intravenous sedation and analgesia, as venous dilatation is often very painful. For a native AV fistula, no antibiotics are given as premedication; however, for an AV fistula with a prosthetic graft, antibiotic prophylaxis with gram-positive, gram-negative and anaerobic cover is commonly given.

Complications

Haemorrhage – this is not usually clinically significant at the puncture site, even when an arterialised segment of fistula vein has been punctured, as manual compression is sufficient to obtain haemostasis.

Infection – prosthetic grafts at risk; see above for antibiotic prophylaxis.

Rupture of fistula – risk greatest if there has been very recent surgical revision of the fistula or if there is infection present.

Central venous perforation – this may occur due to perforation by a guidewire or during angioplasty of a central vein and may be serious due to the potential for significant intrathoracic haemorrhage.

Nephrostomy and Antegrade Stent

Antegrade renal drainage may be used to established drainage of an obstructed kidney when retrograde drainage has been unsuccessful or cannot be attempted. No data exists which demonstrates whether antegrade or retrograde drainage is safer; however, there are specific situations when retrograde drainage may not be possible. These include extensive distal tumour, ureteric injury and reimplantation of the ureter, e.g. the transplant kidney. Urgent drainage should be considered in an obstructed infected PC system or obstructed single kidney (including transplant) with acute derangement or renal function.

The procedure requires IV analgesia, sedation and antibiotic prophylaxis.

Complications

1. Haemorrhage – may be sufficient to threaten kidney or life. Bleeding may occur from the kidney or from the abdominal wall.
2. Infection – puncture of an obstructed and infected PC system may result in septic shower and rapid instability of the patient.
3. Deterioration in renal function – haemorrhage may lead to loss of the kidney or renal compression and reduced function. Renal damage may also occur due to secondary infection.

Permacath (See Video on Line Insertion)

Vascular access for haemodialysis may be performed by radiologists, nephrologists, surgeons or other paramedical staff groups, such as nurses, who have had appropriate training. Patients who have had multiple lines however eventually lose the common sites for line insertion, such as the jugular veins, and there may also be stenoses or occlusions of the brachiocephalic veins, SVC, IVC or iliac veins. These patients may need associated venoplasty to facilitate line insertion, or an unusual access site such as a translumbar IVC line, and some may require insertion of a line surgically, for example, directly into an iliac vein.

Antibiotic prophylaxis is not usually given for line insertion.

Mesenteric, Coeliac, Splenic, Renal, Iliac and Femoral Angiography, Angioplasty and Stent Insertion

Renal angiography is used for diagnosis of conditions such as renal vasculitis, fibromusculodysplasia and renal artery stenosis and is usually done with a transfemoral approach. It is safe, with a complication rate of 1 % for femoral arterial injury and <1 % for renal arterial damage. Mesenteric angiography is often performed at the same time when investigating vasculitis.

Renal angioplasty is indicated for the treatment of fibromuscular dysplasia; however, stent insertion is not performed for this indication due to the potential provocation of neointimal hyperplasia within the stent leading to in-stent restenosis.

The finding of the Angioplasty and STenting for Renal Artery Lesions (ASTRAL) trial resulted in a large reduction in the number of patients with atherosclerotic renal artery stenosis being treated with angioplasty and stent insertion. The trial showed no benefit of intervention over medical therapy in both preventing deterioration of renal function and treating hypertension. Despite this, there are still situations in which angioplasty with/without stent insertion may be appropriate:

- Transplant renal artery stenosis – intervention may lead to stabilisation of renal function. Stent insertion is not usually performed due to the difficulty in treating in-stent restenosis should this occur.
- Renal artery stenosis with flash pulmonary oedema – stent insertion may reduce episodes of pulmonary oedema.
- New deterioration of renal function in established renovascular disease.
- Severe stenosis and singe kidney with significant impairment of renal function.

Many patients with renal disease require peripheral arterial revascularisation. The preparation is the same as for renal angiography, although the complication rate is higher, at 4 %.

Complications include arterial damage or haemorrhage at the puncture site and distal embolisation following angioplasty, which at worst may be limb threatening (<1 %). Antibiotic prophylaxis is not usually necessary.

Summary

Renal imaging and intervention just gets better and better and increasingly cross-sectional imaging will be combined with functional imagining, further aiding diagnosis and management.

Governance issues in terms of consent, total burden of radiation or gadolinium, MDT working and documentation all need to be considered by nephrologists and renal departments. Radiologists and nephrologists should consider ways of prospectively documenting cummulative doses of radiation and gadolinium for renal patients.

References

1. Board of the Faculty of Clinical Radiology. The Royal College of Radiology. Cancer multidisciplinary team meeting-standards for clinical radiologists. 2005. www.rcr.ac.uk/docs/radiology/pdf/MDTM2005Webprint.pdf.
2. Health protection agency. The risk of solid cancers following radiation exposure: report of the independent advisory group on ionising radiation. 2011. www.hpa.org.uk/webc/HPAwebFile/HPAweb_C/1313155169469.
3. Mertgen GJ, Burgess WP, Gray LV, et al. Prevention of contrast induced nephropathy with sodium bicarbonate: a randomised controlled trial. JAMA. 2004;291:2328–34.
4. Hoste EA, De Waele JJ, Gevaert SA, Uchino S, Kellum JA. Sodium bicarbonate for prevention of contrast-induced acute kidney injury: a systematic review & meta-analysis. Nephrol Dial Transplant. 2010;25(3):747–58.
5. ACT Investigators. Acetylcysteine for prevention of renal outcomes in patients undergoing coronary and peripheral vascular angiography: main results from the randomised Acetylcysteine for Contrast induced nephropathy trial. Circulation. 2011;124(11):1250–9.

4 Kidney Biopsy

Nick Woodward and Mark Harber

The percutaneous renal biopsy (PRB) is a little over 60 years old, and despite the advances in other diagnostic tests, it remains critical to the diagnosis, management and prognosis of the renal transplant and many nephrological conditions [1].

In experienced hands using real-time ultrasound and spring-loaded biopsy guns, the procedure has become routine, often performed as a day case, and should have a diagnostic yield of 95 % with a significant complication rate of <5 % [2]. This chapter will discuss the indications and practical aspects of nondirected renal biopsy.

Indications and Contraindications for Renal Biopsy

However prosaic biopsies have become, obtaining a suitable diagnostic core safely is a skilled procedure; thus, for those providing a renal biopsy service and those requesting a biopsy, the risk:benefit ratio for the patient remains an important consideration. If the operators are relatively inexperienced and doing infrequent biopsies, then the risk for the patient is likely to be significantly higher.

Indications (See Table 4.1)

This will very much be determined by individual circumstances; whether the likely diagnosis can be established without a biopsy, how high risk the treatment for the presumed diagnosis is and how safely a biopsy could be done. In essence, what is the question being asked in terms of diagnosis, prognosis, response to treatment, and can it be reliably answered without a biopsy? A unit with a fairly inexperienced biopsy service should have a higher threshold for PRB and may benefit from developing skilled urine microscopy.

Acute Kidney Injury: In the majority of cases of AKI, the diagnosis is not in doubt and the acute tubular injury is explained by preceding hypotension, sepsis or medication especially in the setting of pre-existing CKD; in these circumstances a biopsy is likely to contribute little but hazard. However, there are times when a biopsy can add substantially to the management of AKI (see Table 4.1):

1. Rapidly progressive glomerular nephritis AKI. In the setting of an active urine deposit, a biopsy may be critical to exclude a rapidly progressive glomerular nephritis for which getting the *correct* treatment urgently has very significant consequences (e.g. anti-GBM disease or infective endocarditis).
2. A proportion of patients will present with AKI in the absence of any obvious hypotension or sufficient co-morbidity to fit with the degree of renal impairment, and in these individuals a biopsy may diagnose either a chronic underlying renal disease or an active unanticipated renal disease such as acute interstitial nephritis.
3. Occasionally AKI occurs in the setting of unexplained constitutional illness, and assuming there is convincing evidence of direct renal involvement (haematuria, proteinuria or pyuria), then a renal biopsy may be the most direct approach to a diagnosis (e.g. sarcoid, tuberculosis, systemic vasculitis, cryoglobulinaemia, endocarditis).
4. Finally, in a patient who would be expected to recover renal function within days or a few weeks of a limited renal insult. When this is not the case and the persistence of

N. Woodward, MBBS, MRCP, FRCR
Department of Radiology, Royal Free London NHS Foundation Trust, Pond Street, London NW3 2QG, UK
e-mail: nick.woodward@nhs.net

M. Harber, MBBS, PhD, FRCP (✉)
UCL Department of Nephrology,
Royal Free London NHS Foundation Trust,
Pond Street, Hampstead, London NW3 2QG, UK
e-mail: mark.harber@nhs.net

Electronic supplementary material The online version of this chapter (doi: 10.1007/978-1-4471-5547-8_4) contains supplementary material, which is available to authorized users. Videos can also be accessed at http://www.springerimages.com/videos/978-1-4471-5546-1.

M. Harber (ed.), *Practical Nephrology*,
DOI 10.1007/978-1-4471-5547-8_4, © Springer-Verlag London 2014

Table 4.1 Indications for nondirected renal biopsy

AKI	1. Rapidly progressive AKI 2. AKI without obvious explanation 3. AKI in the setting of undiagnosed systemic illness 4. Failure to recover from AKI
Proteinuria	Nephrotic syndrome in adults Steroid-resistant nephrotic syndrome in children Moderate unexplained proteinuria with renal impairment or haematuria
Microscopic haematuria	Non-lower urinary tract haematuria with renal impairment, hypertension or in potential live donor
Pyuria	Unexplained pyuria in the context of renal impairment
Tubular dysfunction	Unexplained tubular abnormalities without an obvious aetiology
CKD	Unexplained CKD in the setting of relatively preserved renal size/cortex
Diagnosis and monitoring of systemic disease	Response to treatment and prognosis in, e.g. vasculitis, SLE, myeloma, sarcoid
Transplantation	Graft dysfunction (exclusion of rejection, recurrent disease, BKV and other infections, quantification of IFTA) Protocol biopsy

oliguria is unexpected, then a biopsy may be helpful in determining prognosis of recovery or establishing renal disease such as acute TIN or renal infection. As a rule of thumb if the patient is still oliguric 6 weeks post-AKI then a biopsy may be helpful; however, the timing for this would be sooner if the primary insult was mild or the threshold would be higher if there have been multiple significant insults.

Nephrotic syndrome is a common indication for renal biopsy; however, in paediatric practice, it is unusual to biopsy a patient at first presentation as the real issue is whether the nephrotic syndrome is steroid responsive. Thus, patients are only offered a biopsy if they fail to respond to a course of steroids. In adults the equation is very different; for example, a significant proportion of nephrotic adults will have membranous glomerulonephritis, amyloid or mesangiocapillary glomerulonephritis for which there is no evidence that steroid monotherapy has any benefit. Committing all nephrotic adults to a prolonged course of steroids on spec would inflict serious side effects with no benefit for a significant proportion, and thus most units have a low threshold for biopsy in adults with nephrotic syndrome.

In patients with isolated sub-nephrotic range proteinuria, the indications are more controversial; significant proteinuria in any renal disease is an adverse prognostic factor, and reduction of proteinuria by any means such as control of blood pressure and blockade of the renin angiotensin system improves the prognosis. Therefore, the majority of patients are going to receive this treatment whatever the underlying condition; however, it is common to biopsy nondiabetic patients with isolated proteinuria >1 g/day or a consistent PCR >100 to exclude other potentially treatable conditions particularly if there is evidence of declining renal function.

With *isolated microscopic haematuria*, it is usual, in patients over 40, to exclude lower urinary tract disease/malignancy before assuming a renal lesion. The underlying renal pathology is usually either IgA glomerulonephritis, hereditary abnormalities of the GBM (e.g. Alport syndrome) or thin basement membrane disease. In this setting there is very little in the way of specific treatments and thus benefits of a biopsy predominantly relate to prognosis for the patient (particularly for insurance purposes), especially in the context of potential live donation, and family if excluding a heritable GBM abnormality. In practical terms and in the absence of the indications above, most units will merely recommend observation unless hypertension or renal impairment intervenes.

It is conventional wisdom to avoid a renal biopsy in the context of a UTI for fear of generating an abscess; however, it is not unheard of to make a diagnosis of pyelonephritis on a biopsy with a culture-negative MSU, and there is little or no data indicating the degree of risk for abscess formation following a biopsy. Similarly, the diagnosis of renal TB or sarcoid may only be made following a biopsy in a patient with sterile pyuria and renal impairment.

It is rare that a biopsy is necessary for the diagnosis of tubular disorders, but very occasionally electron microscopy can reveal the underlying cause, for example, in Fanconi syndrome an underlying mitochondrial cytopathy, dysproteinuria and heavy metal poisoning are worth considering if the primary diagnosis is not obvious.

Patients with CKD 4–5 with small kidneys are at very high risk from a biopsy, and it is much less common that the risk:benefit ratio justifies the investigation.

There is a stronger imperative if the primary disease cannot be diagnosed by less invasive tests, and there is a high likelihood of clinically relevant recurrence post-transplant. In practice this is rare; diseases with significant impact if not identified such as Goodpasture's syndrome, atypical HUS, systemic vasculitis and SLE can usually be diagnosed without recourse to a biopsy, and conditions such as IgA which require a biopsy for diagnosis have limited impact post-transplant and would not alter management. However, very rarely conditions with significant impact on a future transplant such as membranoproliferative GN and primary hyperoxalosis may only be diagnosed via renal biopsy.

Finally, renal biopsy can be critical in establishing a more systemic disease, and occasionally repeat biopsy can act as a barometer of disease control in the absence of other less invasive markers. Most commonly this is in the context of connective tissue diseases such as vasculitis and SLE with an active urine deposit. However, a biopsy may demonstrate deposition of light chains in myeloma or evidence of HIV-related nephropathy which might provoke treatment for either condition. Similarly biopsy of enlarged kidneys with dysfunction can diagnose infiltration and escalation of treatment in lymphoproliferative disorders.

Table 4.2 Contraindications to nontargeted native renal biopsy

Renal mass	Risk of neoplastic spread
Polycystic kidneys	High-risk and low diagnostic yield
Small end-stage kidneys	Very-high-risk and low diagnostic yield
Acute bacterial pyelonephritis	Risk of perinephric abscess formation, lower UTI is a relative contraindication
Solitary kidney, horseshoe kidney	Increased risk of dialysis dependence but relatively safe in experienced hands, open or laparoscopic biopsy alternatives
Obstructed kidneys	Increased risk of urinary leak
Bleeding diathesis	Absolute contraindication if uncontrolled, relative if correctable (see coagulation in renal disease chapter 52)
Uraemia	Relative contra-indication, due to platelet dysfunction; where possible correct prior to biopsy
Severe hypertension	Kidney vasculature poorly able to autoregulate even if blood pressure is acutely controlled
Severe obesity	Biopsy becomes technically more difficult and dangerous with increasing obesity. Transjugular, laparoscopic and open biopsy may offer significant advantage
Uncooperative patient	Absolute contraindication if unable or unwilling to cooperate with breath holding. If lacking capacity and biopsy essential, consider biopsy under a general anaesthetic
Third trimester pregnancy	Relatively contraindicated, dilated system, sitting, risk of foetal loss, but very rarely necessary after second trimester and before delivery
Vascular abnormalities	Aneurysms (e.g. PAN), arteriovenous malformations

Contraindications

In the majority of patients with contraindications to renal biopsy, it is possible to make a diagnosis and management plan based on urine microscopy and other clinical features. However, it is important to note that most of the contraindications to renal biopsy (Table 4.2) are relative in that if a biopsy is *really* critical to patient management, it is often possible to reduce the risk of a PRB or to use alternative approaches. The coagulopathy of renal failure is covered in chapter 52, but a uraemic patient is likely to have significant platelet dysfunction and in practical terms there is no routinely available test that can predict this accurately (including bleeding time). In uraemic patients there is a correlation with risk of bleeding at haemoglobins below 10 g/dl; thus, in high-risk patients it is common to optimise the risk by dialysis (if dialysis dependent) and transfusion the day before a biopsy. Amyloidosis was said to increase the risk of PRB, but a recent retrospective study has demonstrated no apparent excess in complications.

It is important for the unit to have a robust system in place to ensure that low molecular weight heparins (which will not be detectable with PT and PTT assays) are crossed off 24 h prior to biopsy.

Finally, an increasing proportion of renal patients are on anti-platelet agents. Conventionally aspirin is stopped a week before an elective biopsy; however, when given for secondary prevention, there seems to be an increased risk of acute coronary events [3] and cerebrovascular events [4] on stopping aspirin. A recent review suggests stopping clopidogrel 3–5 days prior to surgical procedures and continuing aspirin in general patients [5]. Clearly the risk:benefit ratio needs to be decided on an individual basis with the caveat that a patient with significant cardiovascular morbidity is unlikely to tolerate a substantial bleed well.

Desmopressin (DDAVP) V2 antagonist results in a release of stored ultra-large von Willebrand factor multimers and factor VIII. The effect lasts from 1 to 24 h and can be used in uraemic high-risk patients to promote platelet aggregation. One randomised trial demonstrated a reduction in bleeding and haematoma size with prophylactic DDAVP in PRB [6]. However, it can induce coronary vasospasm in patients with ischaemic heart disease, and our practice is to ensure that it is given slowly (>1 h).

Procedure PRB

Renal biopsies are now generally obtained using spring-loaded biopsy guns using 14–18 gauge needles (typically 16G for native and 18G for transplants); increasingly the guns are also disposable, but if using a non-disposable gun, a robust process for post-procedure sterilisation is mandatory. Biopsies should be performed under real-time ultrasound (curvilinear ultrasound probes are preferred as lower-frequency range gives a larger field of view and greater depth than linear probes). The probe should be covered by a sterile, disposable probe cover procedure performed with full aseptic technique.

The technique for native biopsies is beautifully illustrated in the video produced by Dr Peter Topham and Dr Sue Carr at Leicester Royal Infirmary (see Video 4.1). The technique for transplant biopsies is slightly different and again nicely illustrated on the video produced by Mr Peter Veitch and Arundhati M. UCL Centre for Nephrology (see Video 4.2).

Skewing things in your favour by ensuring a good- and high-resolution US scanner, properly darkened room and good positioning of a relaxed patient is fundamental to success.

It is important to note that patients are often, understandably, nervous about the procedure, and it is also very important to ensure that the patient is thoughtfully talked through the procedure and reassured.

It is rarely necessary to biopsy a patient in the third trimester, but sometimes a biopsy is required in the second trimester, and if not possible to do this prone, the patient can be sat upright on the bed with arms and head resting on a table. Obese patients can sometimes be biopsied lying laterally with pillows supporting their middle.

Anatomy and Complications and Consent

See Figs. 4.1, 4.2, 4.3 and 4.4.

Complication rates in the literature vary significantly depending on definition, how studiously they were looked for and how high risk the biopsy. There is almost certainly a significant publication bias in favour of low rates. What follows is a rough and hopefully reasonable summation of the risks; ultimately complications will depend on local practice and experience, but individuals and units should be audited against these outcomes on a regular basis [7–9].

Temporary local pain and discomfort on administration of local anaesthetic is universal but should subside rapidly and patients should be prewarned of this. Native renal biopsies tend to be more uncomfortable than biopsy of a superficial denervated renal transplant kidney.

1. Failure of technique or diagnostic inadequacy of 5 %.
2. Percutaneous infection with aseptic technique seems extremely rare and the risk of a renal/perirenal abscess following a biopsy in the presence of urosepsis is difficult to define and neither tends to be consented for.
3. Biopsy of non-renal tissue should be rare; however, it is not unheard of to obtain small bowel with native PRB; anecdotal evidence seems to suggest this is of little consequence. Biopsy of large bowel or pancreas is rarer but potentially more serious, and patients should be carefully reassessed if this occurs.
4. Macroscopic haematuria (1–2 %).
5. Arteriovenous fistulae (AVF) on the other hand appear to be very common with an incidence of roughly 10 % on screening. As 95 % of AVF appear to resolve

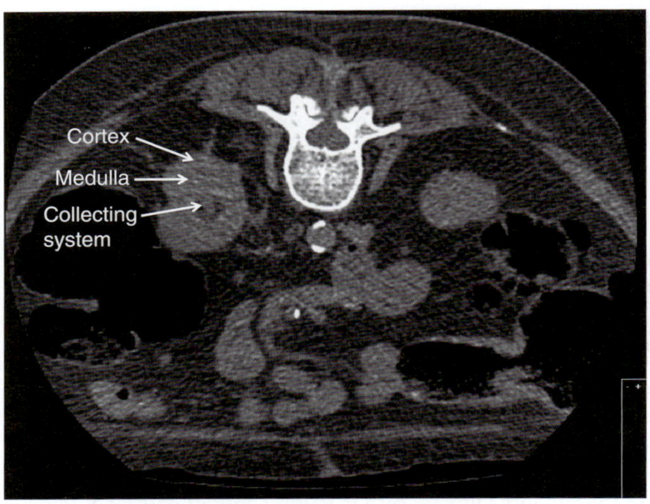

Fig. 4.1 Prone unenhanced CT at the level of the lower pole of the left kidney

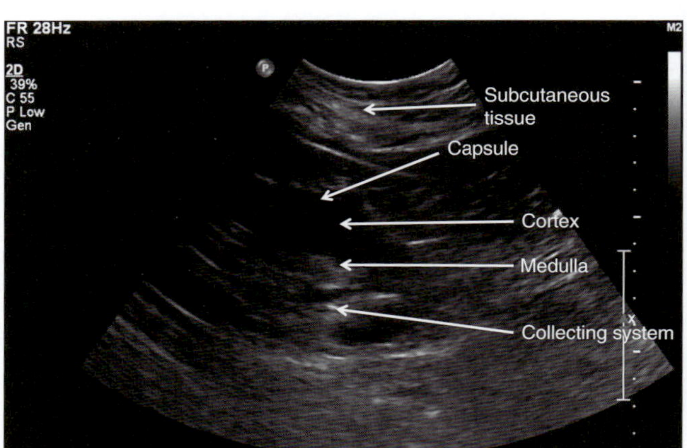

Fig. 4.2 Prone ultrasound, same patient

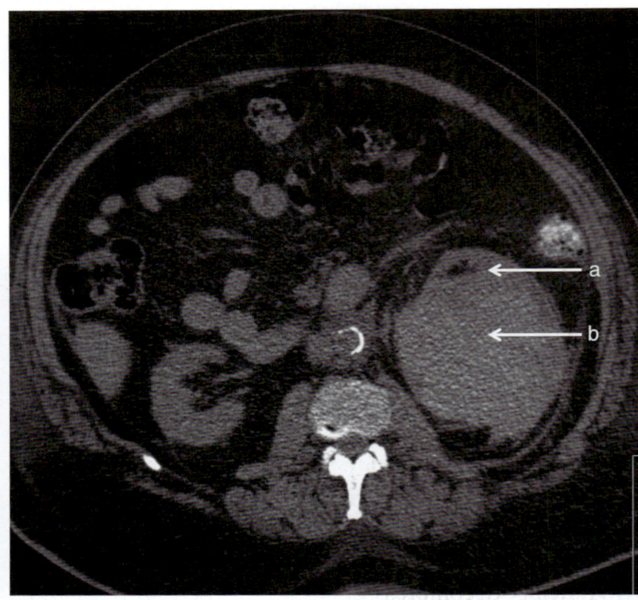

Fig. 4.3 CT scan of subcapsular haematoma following biopsy of the left kidney. The left kidney (*a*) is displaced anteriorly, secondary to a high-density collection (*b*)

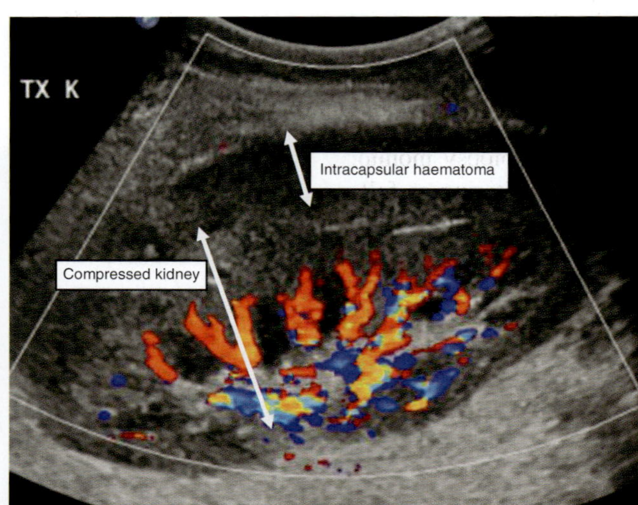

Fig. 4.4 Intracapsular haematoma causing gross compression of the kidney (Page kidney) and anuria in a transplant recipient. Urine flow was restored instantly with surgical decompression

spontaneously, this complication tends not to be quoted for consent. However, AVF that do not resolve pose a potential hazard for future biopsies (a bruit over the kidney and fall in GFR should raise suspicion) or significant steal from the kidney.

6. Perirenal haematoma appears to be a very common complication with rates of 57–85 %, although this data comes from studies done 30 years ago, and for the majority of patients, haematoma in itself appears to have had little consequence. However, rarely a subcapsular haematoma may cause a 'Page kidney' (see Figs. 4.3 and 4.4) and, in a single kidney, acute oliguria requiring urgent surgical decompression.
7. Bleeding requiring transfusion, 1 % if standard risk and >2 % if high risk.
8. Embolisation rate post-PRB is rather dependent on access to this, but we quote rates of 1:400.
9. The data on loss of kidney or nephrectomy is scant but usually quoted at less than 1 in 1,000 and is important to discuss for transplant and solitary kidney biopsy.
10. Mortality is associated with PRB and the literature suggests this to be 1 in 2,000–5,000 biopsies.

Acute oligoanuria post-transplant is likely due to the following:

(a) Shock: this is usually pretty obvious.
(b) Clot retention: easily diagnosed by US or catheterisation.
(c) Page kidney: this may cause complete anuria in a transplant, but often missed in native biopsies once identified urgent surgical decompression can instantly restore perfusion to a transplant kidney but risks further bleeding by removing any tamponade; the optimum option is to surgically decompress the kidney and perform selective radiological embolisation immediately if haemostasis cannot be achieved.
(d) Urinary leak: this may be identifiable on delayed film MAG-3.

Post-biopsy Monitoring

Typical post-biopsy monitoring would be pulse and blood pressure monitoring as follows: every 15 min for an hour, then if stable; every 30 min for 2 h, then if stable; every hour for 4 h, and then if stable and passed urine (without haematuria), mobilise and discharge; if an inpatient (high-risk patient), then continue four-hourly monitoring.

The most critical aspect of post-biopsy monitoring is that nursing and medical staff are familiar with the procedure and are comfortable escalating monitoring and requesting medical review at the first sign of a complication.

The timing of complications is important and somewhat controversial; one large study detected 42 % of complications within 4 h, 67 % by 8 h, 85 % by 12 h and 89 % by 24 h [6]. This data would imply that day case biopsies would not be safe, yet a third of complications occurring after 8 h does not seem to be general experience, and day case biopsies in standard-risk patients seem to have a high safety record.

Day Case vs Inpatient Procedure

In the last two decades, standard-risk PRBs have been increasingly performed as day case procedures. The published audits seem to have a good safety record, benefits to patients and significant cost savings [10, 11].

There are no standard guidelines for who is suitable for day case biopsy but the criteria below seem to have been arrived at independently by several units and represent a reasonable starting place.

Suggested criteria for day case renal biopsy:

1. Two kidneys ≥10 cm
2. Blood pressure ≤150/90
3. eGFR ≥30
4. Hb ≥10 g/dl
5. Platelets ≥100
6. INR ≤1.2 PTT ≤1.2
7. Off aspirin or clopidogrel for 7 days
8. Lack of significant cardiovascular co-morbidity
9. BMI ≤30 (not significant centripetal obesity)
10. A responsible adult to transport home and at home to provide care and support for 24 h post-transplant
11. Experienced operator and day ward staff

The good outcome data presumably, in part, reflects that patients suitable for a day case biopsy are carefully selected; thus, if the above criteria are breached, then the decision to proceed as a day case biopsy must be discussed with the patient and should be made at a senior level.

Example of day case and inpatient renal biopsy pro formas are attached and can be modified for local practice.

For inpatient biopsies it is less easy to be absolutist because there may be compelling reasons to perform a biopsy despite the increased risk, and depending on local expertise, options such as open, laparoscopic or transjugular biopsy might be employed.

Alternatives to PRB in High-Risk Patients (Table 4.3)

As levels of obesity and co-morbidity increase, we will be increasingly faced with high-risk patients. There are a variety of alternatives to stand PRB nicely summarised in a review by Stiles et al. [12].

Open Renal Biopsy (ORB)

The definitive series of ORB was of 934 patients and had 100 % tissue adequacy and apparently no significant complications [13]. Open (and laparoscopic) approaches

Table 4.3 Alternatives to PRB in high-risk patients

Technique	Advantages	Disadvantages	Possible indications
Open biopsy	Direct vision, very high diagnostic yield, direct haemostasis, suitable for ventilated patient	General anaesthetic, long recovery and hospitalisation, cost	Single kidney, kidney with multiple cysts, obese patient, patient unable to cooperate with breath holding
Laparoscopic biopsy	Direct vision, very high diagnostic yield, direct haemostasis, less invasive than open biopsy, suitable for ventilated patient	General anaesthetic, long recovery, hospitalisation, cost	Single kidney, kidney with multiple cysts, obese patient, patient unable to cooperate with breath holding
Transvenous biopsy	Suitable for grossly obese, contractures preventing PRB, abnormal clotting, diagnostic yield 78–97 % Suitable for ventilated patient	Contrast load, smaller sample size predominance of medulla	Simultaneous liver kidney biopsy, concomitant with dialysis line placement, obese patient, bleeding diathesis, patient unable to cooperate with breath holding

offer the distinct advantage of direct vision and direct haemostasis and thus can be helpful in patients with cysts or other focal abnormalities as well as other high-risk patients and those already ventilated. The need for general anaesthetic and significant recovery time however are not justified in standard-risk patients.

Laparoscopic Renal Biopsy (LRB)

There are several case series of LRB usually in the setting of high-risk patients. As with ORB direct vision means the diagnostic yield approaches 100 % and immediate haemostasis can be performed. This offers a significant advantage in patients with a body habitus preventing PRB, mild bleeding disorders or focal abnormalities of the kidney. As with ORB this technique obligates a general anaesthetic but is less invasive and the recovery time is likely to be less than for an ORB and again can be considered in patients already ventilated on ITU.

Transvenous Renal Biopsy (TVRB)

Transvenous renal biopsy (TVRB) (usually transjugular) has been reported in the setting of bleeding diathesis [14–17] or obesity [18] (mean BMI 44). The theoretical advantages are that (a) the capsule is less likely to be punctured, (b) any bleeding should be back into the vein, (c) any acute extracapsular bleeds demonstrated at the time can be embolised if significant and (d) tissue can be obtained in patients in whom the percutaneous approach is not feasible, e.g. grossly obese. Diagnostic yields of 78–97 % have been reported and, in the largest study to date, major complications of only 1 % [14], but other smaller studies have had significantly higher rates and it is easy to inadvertently perforate the capsule. In short TVRB is a useful technique for high-risk patients if there is sufficient local expertise; however, it is not without risk and remains extremely important to correct coagulopathies as much as possible prior to biopsy.

Standards for Renal Biopsy

In 2010 the British Association for Paediatric Nephrology published suggested standards for renal biopsy [2] which are also a useful benchmark for adult patients with some amendments to consider added in italics:

1. All patients should receive an appropriate patient information leaflet (PIL) about the biopsy procedure[1] (*in advance and, ideally, in their first language*) (*the patient or guardian should have a clear understanding of the indication for the biopsy*).
2. *Complication rates for macroscopic haematuria, transfusion, embolisation and loss of kidney (if single or transplant) should be quoted as part of consent.*
3. For both native and transplant biopsies, ≤3 passes should be achieved in 80 % of occasions.
4. There should be adequate tissue for diagnosis on 95 % of occasions.[2]
5. Major complications (defined as delay in discharge as a result in post-biopsy complications or requirements for further investigations or monitoring) should be <5 %.
6. *There should be on site access to interventional radiology and surgeons experienced in dealing with a major renal bleed.*

[1]The renal association has produced a PIL available on the website (www.renal.org), and there is a similar PIL available on MedlinePlus and includes Spanish translation.

[2]Adequacy: the general consensus is that for native renal biopsies, 10–15 glomeruli are an optimal number to exclude a focal glomerulonephritis (>20 ideal), but this definition of adequacy may be a little rigid as sometimes it is possible to make the diagnosis on a single glomerulus. Conversely, a sample of less than 10–15 may miss focal disease and therefore be unable to rule out other disease (such interstitial nephritis or rejection in transplantation). For transplant biopsies, the Banff classification requires >10 glomeruli and two arteries with a minimum of seven glomeruli and one artery. A more pragmatic definition of adequacy is that if the cause of the renal dysfunction is identified, then the sample was adequate, if not, then adequate only if containing ≥10–15 glomeruli.

7. *Operators should maintain a prospective audit of adequacy and complications.*

Informative, detailed request forms greatly assist the pathologist, uninformative ones do not; it is thus good practice to ensure that the indication and clinical details are of a high standard.

The workup of a renal biopsy is reviewed in more detail elsewhere [19]; however, assessment requires light microscopy always, immunohistochemistry frequently and electron microscopy occasionally. Although there are many different approaches to technical aspects of these, the most important factor is the competence of the pathologist who is giving a report on the specimen. Different pathologists have their own preferences for the number of sections, whether serial sections are cut, which stains are used, whether immunofluorescence usually on frozen sections or an enzyme method such as immunoperoxidase on paraffin sections is used for immunohistological studies and whether electron microscopy, if available, is necessary on a particular specimen. Importantly if your laboratory processes biopsies for immunoperoxidase, then it is often possible to retrospectively obtain tissue for electron microscopy (see Howie [20]). Renal pathology is a highly specialised field, and it is important to have close liaison between clinicians and pathologists as well as consider presenting difficult cases between renal teams and pathologists.

Finally pathology MDT meetings are an invaluable liaison between clinicians and pathologists, and it is important to document, in real time (ideally electronically), conclusions of these discussions and consequent treatment plans.

References

1. Richards NT, Darby S, Howie AJ, Adu D, Michael J. Knowledge of renal histology alters patient management in over 40 % of cases. Nephrol Dial Transplant. 1994;9(9):1255–9.
2. Hussain F, Mallik M, Marks SD, Watson AR. Nephrology on behalf of the BA of P. Renal biopsies in children: current practice and audit of outcomes. Nephrol Dial Transplant. 2010;25(2): 485–9.
3. Ferrari E, Benhamou M, Cerboni P, Marcel B. Coronary syndromes following aspirin withdrawal: a special risk for late stent thrombosis. J Am Coll Cardiol. 2005;45(3):456–9.
4. Sibon I, Orgogozo JM. Antiplatelet drug discontinuation is a risk factor for ischemic stroke. Neurology. 2004;62(7):1187.
5. O'Connor SD, Taylor AJ, Williams EC, Winter TC. Coagulation concepts update. Am J Roentgenol. 2009;193(6):1656–64.
6. Manno C. Desmopressin acetate in percutaneous ultrasound-guided kidney biopsy: a randomized controlled trial. Am J Kidney Dis. 2010;57(6):850–5.
7. Whittier WL, Korbet SM. Timing of complications in percutaneous renal biopsy. J Am Soc Nephrol. 2004;15(1):142–7.
8. Preda A, Van Dijk L, Van Oostaijen J, Pattynama P. Complication rate and diagnostic yield of 515 consecutive ultrasound-guided biopsies of renal allografts and native kidneys using a 14-gauge Biopty gun. Eur Radiol. 2003;13(3):527–30.
9. Hergesell O, Felten H, Andrassy K, Kühn K, Ritz E. Safety of ultrasound-guided percutaneous renal biopsy-retrospective analysis of 1090 consecutive cases. Nephrol Dial Transplant. 1998;13(4): 975–7.
10. Khajehdehi P, Junaid SMA, Salinas-Madrigal L, Schmitz PG, Bastani B. Percutaneous renal biopsy in the 1990s: safety, value, and implications for early hospital discharge. Am J Kidney Dis. 1999;34(1):92–7.
11. Hussain F, Watson A, Hayes J, Evans J. Standards for renal biopsies: comparison of inpatient and day care procedures. Pediatr Nephrol. 2003;18(1):53–6.
12. Stiles KP, Yuan CM, Chung EM, Lyon RD, Lane JD, Abbott KC. Renal biopsy in high-risk patients with medical diseases of the kidney. Am J Kidney Dis. 2000;36(2):419–33.
13. Nomoto Y, Tomino Y, Endoh M, Suga T, Miura M, Nomoto H, Sakai H. Modified open renal biopsy: results in 934 patients. Nephron. 1987;45(3):224–8.
14. See T, Thompson B, Howie A, Karamshi M, Papadopoulou A, Davies N, Tibballs J. Transjugular renal biopsy: our experience and technical considerations. Cardiovasc Intervent Radiol. 2008;31(5): 906–18.
15. Cluzel P, Martinez F, Bellin MF, Michalik Y, Beaufils H, Jouanneau C, Lucidarme O, Deray G, Grenier PA. Transjugular versus percutaneous renal biopsy for the diagnosis of parenchymal disease: comparison of sampling effectiveness and complications1. Radiology. 2000;215(3):689–93.
16. Misra S, Gyamlani G, Swaminathan S, Buehrig CK, Bjarnason H, McKusick MA, Andrews JC, Johnson CM, Fervenza FC, Leung N. Safety and diagnostic yield of transjugular renal biopsy. J Vasc Interv Radiol. 2008;19(4):546–51.
17. Sarabu N, Maddukuri G, Munikrishnappa D, Martin KJ, Qazi RA, Alvarez A, Schmitz PG. Safety and efficacy of transjugular renal biopsy performed by interventional nephrologists. Semin Dial. 2011;24(3):343–8.
18. Fine DM, Arepally A, Hofmann LV, Mankowitz SG, Atta MG. Diagnostic utility and safety of transjugular kidney biopsy in the obese patient. Nephrol Dial Transplant. 2004;19(7):1798–802.
19. Amann K, Haas CS. What you should know about the work-up of a renal biopsy. NDT. 2006;21:1157–61.
20. Howie AJ. Handbook of renal biopsy pathology. 2nd ed. New York: Springer; 2008.

5 Acute Kidney Injury: Epidemiology and Assessment

Rachel M. Hilton

Acute renal failure, now called acute kidney injury (AKI), is common and costly and carries a very high morbidity and mortality. As it is often preventable, identification of at-risk patients and institution of appropriate preventive measures are crucial; rapid recognition and treatment may prevent irreversible nephron loss, even death. Most cases of AKI are initially managed by non-specialist clinicians, often comparatively junior ones; therefore, all clinicians need to be au fait with the initial assessment and management of AKI. Nephrologists need to ensure that referring teams are supported in recognising the symptoms and signs of AKI, requesting and interpreting initial investigations, initiating appropriate treatment and knowing when to refer on to the renal team. This chapter covers the common causes of AKI, defines at-risk populations, outlines the clinical diagnostic approach and highlights ways of predicting risk of AKI.

Definitions and Classifications

The clinical syndrome of AKI is characterised by a sudden decline in glomerular filtration rate (GFR) over a period of hours to days and manifest as retention of creatinine, urea and other metabolic waste products. This traditional description lacks precise definition and fails to highlight the importance of early recognition of this life-threatening condition. Consequently, in 2000, a group of experts from critical care and nephrology came together as the Acute Dialysis Quality Initiative (ADQI) to develop a consensus definition whereby AKI is stratified based on the severity and duration of injury into stages of Risk, Injury, Failure, Loss and End-Stage disease (RIFLE) [1]. The Acute Kidney Injury Network (AKIN) comprising the ADQI group and others later modified this definition [2] based on the recognition that even small changes in serum creatinine are associated with increased mortality. At the same time, the term acute kidney injury (AKI) was introduced to encompass the entire spectrum of renal injury from minor changes in kidney function to dialysis dependency. Most recently, the international guideline group Kidney Disease: Improving Global Outcomes (KDIGO) has agreed a definition and staging system that harmonises the previous systems proposed by both ADQI and AKIN [3]. It is anticipated that this definition and staging system will be adopted globally and will validate future comparisons of the incidence, outcomes and efficacy of therapeutic interventions for AKI. Under the KDIGO classification scheme, AKI is defined as an abrupt (within 48 h to one week) rise in serum creatinine or as a sustained (more than 6 h) reduction in urine output and can be further classified into three stages based on the absolute or relative increase in serum creatinine or duration of reduction in urine output (Table 5.1).

These classifications help define the degree of kidney dysfunction at diagnosis, aid tracking of the clinical course, are widely validated and have been shown to predict outcomes in diverse patient populations and in large international databases. Under all classification schemes, loss of kidney function requiring dialysis for more than 3 months constitutes end-stage kidney disease. For audit, education and prevention consider implementing routine, prospective AKI scoring for hospital inpatients.

Epidemiology

The worldwide incidence of AKI is poorly known because of under-reporting, regional disparities and differences in definition and case mix. Most epidemiological studies have focused on hospital or critical care inpatients, and relatively few have addressed the incidence in the general population. In one large population-based study in Scotland [4], the

R.M. Hilton, MA, PhD, FRCP
Department of Nephrology and Transplantation,
Guy's and St Thomas' NHS Foundation Trust,
Great Maze Pond, London SE1 9RT, UK
e-mail: rachel.hilton@gstt.nhs.uk

M. Harber (ed.), *Practical Nephrology*,
DOI 10.1007/978-1-4471-5547-8_5, © Springer-Verlag London 2014

Table 5.1 KDIGO classification of acute kidney injury [3]

AKI stage	Serum creatinine criteria	Urine output criteria
1	Increase in serum creatinine of ≥26 μmol/L (0.3 mg/dL) within 48 h or increase to ≥1.5–1.9 × baseline serum creatinine within 1 week	<0.5 mL/kg/h for >6 consecutive hours
2	Increase in serum creatinine to >2.0–2.9 × baseline serum creatinine	<0.5 mL/kg/h for >12 consecutive hours
3	Increase in serum creatinine to >3-fold from baseline or serum creatinine of ≥354 μmol/L [≥4.0 mg/dL] or commenced on renal replacement therapy irrespective of stage	<0.3 mL/kg/h for >24 consecutive hours OR anuria for 12 h

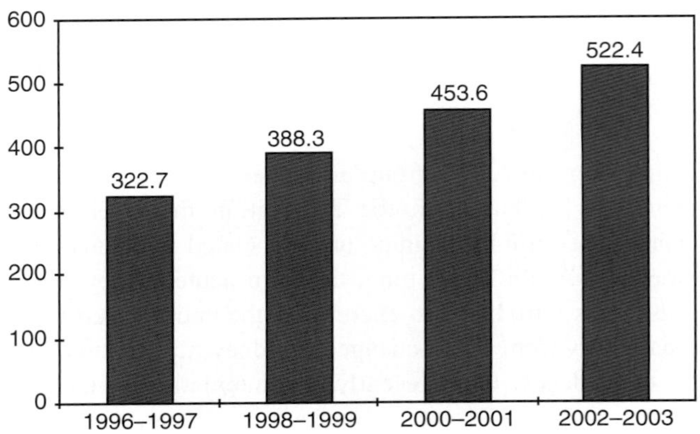

Fig. 5.1 Community-based incidence rates (per 100,000 person-years) of non-dialysis-requiring ARF by calendar year (Reproduced with permission from Hsu et al. [5])

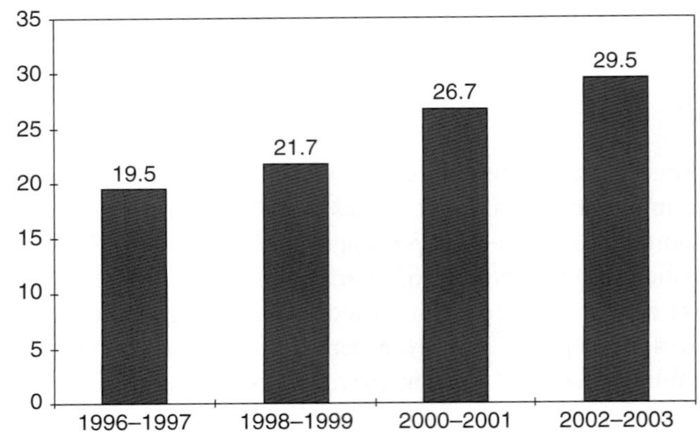

Fig. 5.2 Community-based incidence rates (per 100,000 person-years) of dialysis-requiring ARF by calendar year (Reproduced with permission from Hsu et al. [5])

annual incidence of AKI according to RIFLE criteria was 2,147 per million population, with sepsis as the leading cause. The community-based incidence of AKI is increasing over time. In a different study in Northern California, among members of one of the largest integrated healthcare systems in the USA and using different diagnostic criteria, the annual incidence of AKI was 4,085 per million population [5], more commonly occurring in men and among the elderly (Figs. 5.1 and 5.2).

AKI is an increasingly common cause of acute hospitalisation [6], particularly when superimposed on chronic kidney disease (CKD) (Fig. 5.3). Retrospective studies suggest that the incidence of hospital-acquired AKI varies between 3.2 % if defined by AKIN criteria [7] and 18 % if defined by RIFLE criteria [8] and can be as high as 60 % in patients with severe sepsis [9]. A number of large prospective and retrospective studies have been undertaken which analyse the incidence of AKI in critical care units in various centres. In a large study of more than 120,000 patients admitted to intensive care units across Australia [10], AKI according to RIFLE criteria occurred in 36 % of patients and was associated with a threefold increase in hospital mortality. An even larger study reported on more than 300,000 patients admitted to intensive care in the USA and found the overall AKI incidence using AKIN criteria to be 22 %, mostly AKI stage 1 [11].

Whereas in developed countries AKI occurs predominantly in urban intensive care units in older patients in association with multi-organ failure and sepsis, in rural regions of the developing world, AKI more commonly develops in response to infection (e.g. gastroenteritis or severe infection such as malaria or leptospirosis), obstetric complications or toxins, such as snake bite, and in younger otherwise healthy individuals [12].

For both the community and hospital setting, there are several features that predict a significantly increased risk of AKI (Table 5.2). Given the substantial increased mortality associated with AKI, it is clearly important to have systems in place to identify who is at risk. The awareness, for example, among general medical and surgical teams that an elderly patient with cardiac impairment on an angiotensin-converting enzyme inhibitor (ACEI) undergoing surgery is at significant risk of AKI, is an important first step in prevention of this serious complication.

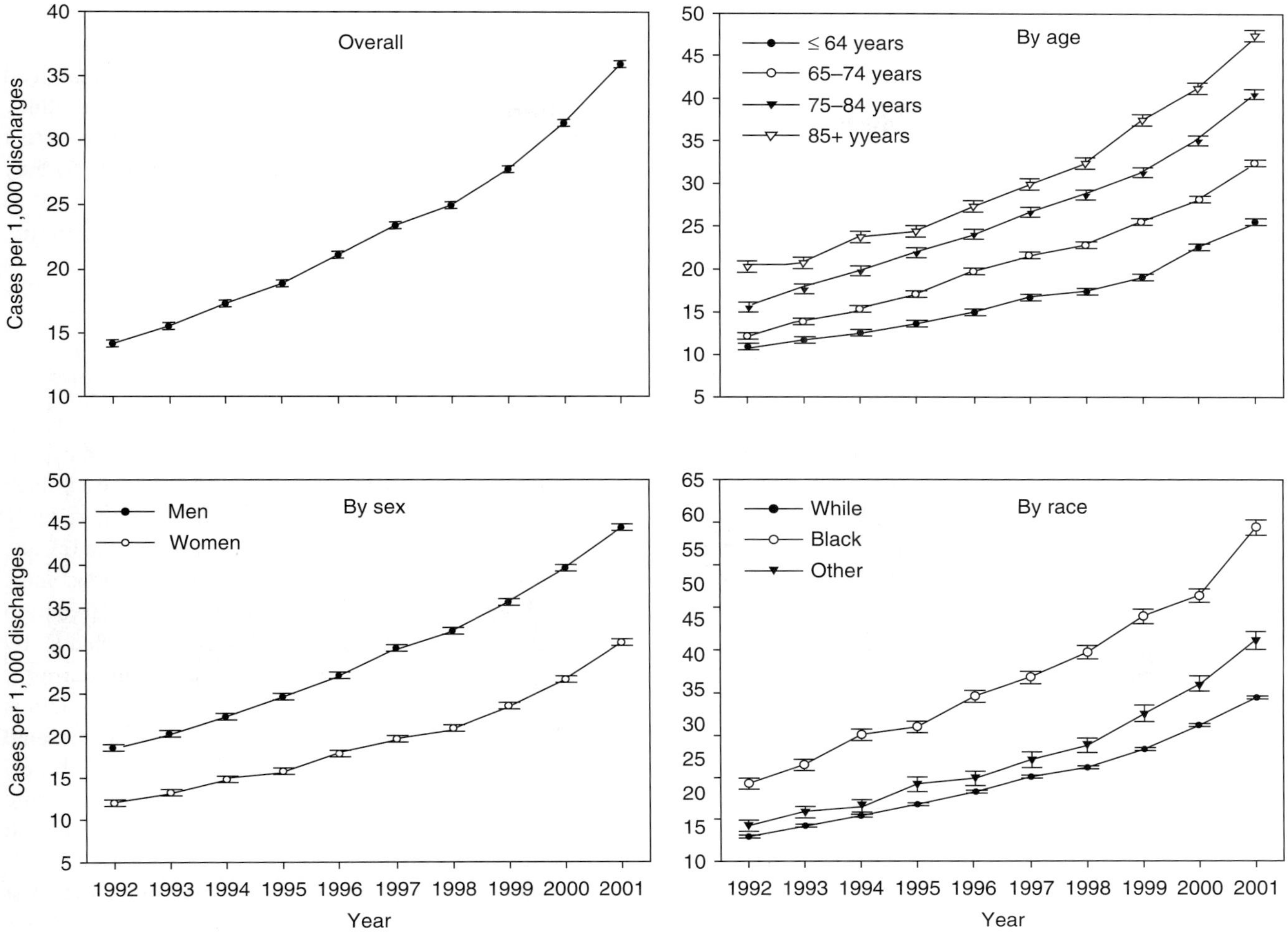

Fig. 5.3 Number of cases of AKI per 1,000 hospital discharges of US Medicare beneficiaries, 1992–2001. I-bars represent Standard Error (Reproduced with permission from Xue et al. [6])

Table 5.2 Risk factors for AKI

1. Pre-existing CKD (especially diabetes, myeloma)
2. Reduced intravascular volume (reduced renal perfusion): (a) Hypovolaemia (impaired oral intake, haemorrhage, GI losses, renal losses, skin losses) (b) Reduced effective arterial blood volume (cirrhosis, nephrotic syndrome, third-spacing, e.g. pancreatitis, complex fractures, acute lung injury, peritonitis)
3. Impaired cardiac output (reduced renal perfusion)
4. Old age (reduced GFR, reduced renal reserve, co-morbidity)
5. Sepsis (reduced renal perfusion)
6. Prolonged surgery (any, but especially if involving cross-clamping of the aorta or renal arteries)
7. Jaundice
8. Exposure to toxins: (a) Endogenous (sepsis), rhabdomyolysis (myoglobin), tumour lysis syndrome (urate), intravascular haemolysis (free haemoglobin), multiple myeloma (light chains) (b) Exogenous (intravenous contrast and other nephrotoxic agents/drugs; drugs preventing normal renal autoregulation, e.g. ACEI, angiotensin II receptor antagonists, nonsteroidal anti-inflammatory drugs)

Pathophysiology

The susceptibility of the kidney to injury from ischaemia and toxins derives partly from the vulnerability of tubular cells in the outer medulla to ischaemia and hypoxia and partly from the role of the nephron in filtering, concentrating and potentially reabsorbing substances from the tubular lumen that may cause local epithelial cell injury, typically drugs and contrast media.

There are two components that contribute to the acute decrease in GFR in AKI: a "vascular" component and a "tubular" component. Ischaemic injury to the kidney is the most common cause of AKI, but it must be remembered that contributory factors include not only diminished renal blood flow and oxygen and substrate delivery but also a relative increase in oxygen demand by the tubular cells. Acute ischaemia has been shown experimentally to be associated with a loss of renal autoregulation, and in addition, rather than the usual autoregulatory renal vasodilatation that occurs in response to decreased renal perfusion, there is evidence for renal vasoconstriction. Outer medullary congestion is another prominent feature that may worsen the relative hypoxia in the outer medulla and thus potentiate hypoxic injury. As well as intrarenal vasoconstriction, vascular congestion in the outer medulla and activation of tubuloglomerular feedback (the "vascular" component), there is also tubular obstruction, transtubular backleak of filtrate and interstitial inflammation (the "tubular" component). Injured epithelial cells generate and recruit inflammatory and vasoactive mediators that can further compound renal vasoconstriction and inflammation. So tubular injury may be a direct consequence of metabolic pathways activated by ischaemia but is potentiated by inflammation [13].

Key Causes

The causes of AKI can be grouped into those that lead to decreased renal blood flow (prerenal acute kidney injury, 40–70 % of patients), those that lead to direct renal parenchymal damage (intrinsic acute kidney injury, 10–50 % of patients) and those that lead to obstructed flow of urine (postrenal acute kidney injury, 10 % of patients).

Prerenal Acute Kidney Injury

Prerenal causes are the most common and include any condition that leads to under-perfusion of the kidney (Table 5.3). Renal blood flow and GFR remain roughly constant across a wide range of mean arterial pressures due to changes in pre- and post-glomerular arteriolar resistance. This renal autoregulation mainly depends on a combination of pre-glomerular arteriolar vasodilatation, mediated by prostaglandins and nitric oxide, and post-glomerular arteriolar vasoconstriction, mediated by angiotensin II. Drugs that interfere with these mediators may provoke prerenal acute kidney injury in particular clinical settings. The at-risk population includes older people with atherosclerotic cardiovascular disease, those with pre-existing CKD and those with chronic renal hypoperfusion (e.g. cardiac failure, hepatorenal syndrome). In critical care units, the most common cause of AKI is sepsis. In tropical and developing countries, prerenal AKI commonly occurs secondary to dehydration due to diarrhoeal diseases or shock secondary to trauma, affecting a relatively younger population, often children.

Table 5.3 Main causes of prerenal AKI

Causes	Examples
Hypovolaemia	Severe bleeding
	Volume depletion, for example, gastrointestinal fluid losses, burns, polyuria (post-obstructive, over-diuresis, salt-wasting nephropathy, hyperglycaemia, diabetes insipidus)
Hypotension (NB: this may be relative in previously hypertensive patient)	Cardiogenic shock
	Distributive shock ("3rd spacing"), for example, sepsis, anaphylaxis, severe pancreatitis
Reduced renal blood flow	Drugs:
	Nonsteroidal anti-inflammatory drugs (NSAIDs)
	Selective cyclo-oxygenase 2 inhibitors
	Angiotensin-converting enzyme (ACE) inhibitors
	Angiotensin II receptor antagonists
	Renal artery stenosis, occlusion or embolisation
	Hepatorenal syndrome
Decreased effective arterial blood volume	Heart failure
	Liver cirrhosis
	Nephrotic syndrome

Table 5.4 Main causes of intrinsic AKI

Causes	Examples
Glomerular disease	
(a) Inflammatory	Postinfectious glomerulonephritis
	Henoch-Schönlein purpura
	Systemic lupus erythematosus
	Anti-neutrophil cytoplasmic antibody glomerulonephritis
	Anti-glomerular basement membrane disease
	Cryoglobulinaemia
(b) Thrombotic	Disseminated intravascular coagulopathy
	Thrombotic microangiopathy, for example, haemolytic uraemic syndrome
Tubular injury	Ischaemia secondary to prolonged renal hypoperfusion
	Toxins:
	Drugs, for example, aminoglycosides
	Radio contrast
	Snake bite
	Pigments, myoglobin and haemoglobin
	Heavy metals, for example, cisplatinum
	Metabolic, for example, hypercalcaemia and immunoglobulin light chains
	Crystals, for example, urate, oxalate and some medications
Interstitial injury	Drug induced, for example, NSAIDs and antibiotics
	Infiltrative, for example, lymphoma
	Granulomatous, for example, sarcoidosis and tuberculosis
	Infection related, for example, postinfective and pyelonephritis
Vascular injury	Vasculitis, usually ANCA associated
	Cryoglobulinaemia
	Polyarteritis nodosa
	Thrombotic microangiopathy
	Cholesterol emboli
	Renal artery or renal vein thrombosis

Intrinsic Acute Kidney Injury

Intrinsic acute kidney injury may be caused by conditions affecting the glomeruli, renal tubules, interstitium or vasculature (Table 5.4). The most important causes are listed here.

Postrenal Acute Kidney Injury

It is important to recognise obstructive nephropathy because rapid diagnosis and prompt intervention can result in improvement or even complete recovery of kidney function (Table 5.5).

Table 5.5 Main causes of postrenal AKI (see Chap. 37)

Causes	Examples
Intrinsic	Intraluminal, for example, stone, blood clot and papillary necrosis
	Intramural, for example, urethral stricture and bladder tumour
Extrinsic	Prostatic hypertrophy or malignancy
	Autonomic bladder
	Anticholinergics
	Constipation, immobility, pain
	Pelvic malignancy
	Retroperitoneal fibrosis
	Radiation fibrosis
	Abdominal compartment syndrome[a]

[a]Abdominal compartment syndrome is an under-recognised contributor to AKI when the peritoneal cavity pressure is high. The mechanism for causing a fall in GFR is not known but is likely to be due to a combination of renal hypoperfusion and renal vein congestion [14]

Clinical Approach to Diagnosis

The diagnostic approach to a patient with AKI requires a careful history, scrutiny of the medical notes, drug charts, observations charts and anaesthetic records, thorough physical examination and interpretation of appropriate investigations including laboratory tests and imaging. It is vital to obtain historical blood tests, urine analysis and recent drug history where possible.

For each patient with apparent AKI, the following questions need to be considered:

1. Is this acute kidney injury or chronic kidney disease?
2. What is the intravascular volume status of the patient?
3. Has obstruction been excluded?
4. Is there evidence of intrinsic AKI other than acute tubular injury?

History and Examination

Although there may be nonspecific symptoms, renal impairment is often asymptomatic and may only be diagnosed by laboratory tests. However, patients with chronic kidney disease may have a long history of symptoms such as fatigue, nausea, nocturia or itch (Table 5.6). A history of underlying chronic disease such as diabetes, hypertension or peripheral vascular disease may be present, whereas patients with AKI

Table 5.6 Some specific conditions associated with AKI

Diabetes	Hypovolaemia, renal losses HONK and DKA; urosepsis, acute sepsis and pyelonephritis; obstruction, secondary to sloughed papilla (papillary necrosis), and secondary to autonomic bladder Underlying (often subclinical) diabetic nephropathy is a significant contributing risk factor for AKI. NB: pyelonephritis may be subacute and asymptomatic
Gastrointestinal	Acute diarrhoeal illnesses (hypovolaemia +/− sepsis), diarrhoea-associated HUS, hypovolaemia secondary to high output ileostomy, obstruction secondary to stones in short bowel Acute oxalate nephropathy (pancreatic insufficiency or short bowel), interstitial nephritis secondary to sulphasalazines in inflammatory bowel disease (IBD) Chronic diarrhoea often associated with malnutrition and a low creatinine belies a poor GFR secondary to multiple AKI events IBD may have underlying amyloid (proteinuria); acute oxalate nephropathy can cause rapid AKI and is important to diagnose (check plasma oxalate levels or oxalate on phase contrast microscopy of biopsy)
Liver disease	Reduced effective arterial blood volume: 1. Hepatorenal syndrome 2. Variceal haemorrhage 3. Hypovolaemia post-paracentesis 4. Over-diuresis 5. Hypoalbuminaemia 6. Fulminant hepatitic failure any cause Abdominal compartment syndrome Infections: Sepsis, e.g. spontaneous bacterial peritonitis Leptospirosis, Legionnaire's disease, Hantavirus, Hepatitis B and C, etc. Drugs Paracetamol, rifampicin, isoniazid, azathioprine, tetracycline, etc. Toxins Amanita phalloides (mushroom poisoning), hydrotetracarbon inhalation, etc. Jaundice and reduced effective arterial blood volume make patients with chronic liver disease exquisitely sensitive to AKI from other insults such as hypovolaemia, sepsis or nephrotoxic drugs. Abdominal compartment syndrome is an under-recognised contribution to AKI and should be suspected in anyone with a tense abdomen
Cardiovascular	Acute coronary syndrome: 1. Myocardial stunning/decreased cardiac output 2. Contrast nephropathy 3. Acute cholesterol emboli syndrome 4. Renal arterial embolism Chronic heart failure: Hypoperfusion due to reduced cardiac output Over-diuresis Atherosclerotic renal artery stenosis Takayasu's aortitis and middle aorta syndrome Surgery involving cross-clamping suprarenal aorta or renal arteries Infective endocarditis IVC thrombosis extending to renal vein Renal vein thrombosis and pulmonary emboli AKI common in the setting of large myocardial infarction, chronic heart failure is often associated with underlying CKD, and these patients are very sensitive to hypovolaemia particularly in the context of renin:angiotensin blockade. An abrupt deterioration in renal function may be due to renal artery or vein thrombosis, often silent and only detectable by MAG-3 scan

Table 5.6 (continued)

Cancer	Endogenous toxins: 1. Hypercalcaemia 2. Tumour lysis syndrome (hyeruricaemia) 3. Light-chain nephropathy (myeloma) Exogenous toxins: Cisplatin, methotrexate, ifosfamide, etc. Radiation (fibrosis and TMA) Reduced renal perfusion, e.g. hypovolaemia nausea/vomiting/anorexia Drug-induced cardiomyopathy Direct infiltration: Lymphoma (and PTLD), chronic lymphocytic leukaemia, acute lymphoblastic leukaemia Obstruction Glomerular lesions Rapid progressive glomerulonephritis Minimal change GN (lymphoma) Membranous GN (solid organ malignancy) TMA
Pulmonary-renal syndrome (AKI and acute pulmonary impairment)	1. Heart failure or fluid overload (AKI and pulmonary oedema) 2. Infective endocarditis 3. Pulmonary emboli secondary to renal vein thrombosis 4. Vasculitis: Goodpasture's syndrome GCA Microscopic polyangiitis Churg-Strauss syndrome Crescentic IgA and Henoch-Schönlein purpura Cryoglobulinaemia Systemic lupus erythematosus 5. Infections: Bacterial: Legionnaire's disease, pneumococcal pneumonia, hantavirus, HIV, tuberculosis 6. Sarcoidosis 7. Any cause multi-organ failure (ARDS) The commonest presentation of pulmonary and renal failure is pulmonary oedema in the context of CKD or ESRF, and this can mimic many lung pathologies Diagnosing the much rarer vasculitic pulmonary-renal syndrome requires a high index of suspicion especially if active urine deposit. Urine microscopy and *urgent* immunology are critical
Blood-borne viruses	Hepatitis C: Cryoglobulinaemia (+/– MCGN), interstitial nephritis Hepatitis B: Cryoglobulinaemia (+/– MCGN), membranous nephropathy, interstitial nephritis, polyarteritis nodosa HIV Thrombotic microangiopathy, HIVAN, immune complex GN, vasculitis, MCGN, membranous GN Tubular toxicity: foscarnet, tenofovir, iv pentamidine, cidofovir, amphotericin, aminoglycosides. Crystal nephropathy : acyclovir, indinavir, sulphadiazine
Pregnancy	TMA: (a) eclampsia, (b) HUS, (c) HELLP, (d) acute fatty liver of pregnancy Septic shock (following septic abortion) Hypovolaemia (hyperemesis gravidarum) Obstruction Pyelonephritis Exacerbation of autoimmune disease

(continued)

Table 5.6 (continued)

Tropical AKI	Diarrhoeal diseases Haemolytic uraemic syndrome (has replaced diarrhoeal diseases as the commonest cause of AKI in children in several tropical countries) Intravascular haemolysis and G6PD deficiency (acute haemolysis in individuals deficient in G-6-PD is a frequent cause of AKI in some ethnic populations in tropical countries and is the usual cause of AKI in typhoid as ciprofloxacin is widely used for this condition) Infection, e.g. malaria, leptospirosis, typhoid Plant, animal and chemical toxins: Snake bite (common cause of AKI, e.g. in Southern India) Bee, wasp and hornet stings and spider bites Mushroom poisoning Heat stroke Obstetric AKI (remains a major preventable cause of AKI)
Haematological disease	AL amyloidosis Myeloma: 1. Dehydration 2. Hypercalcaemia 3. Infection 4. NSAIDs 5. Myeloma cast nephropathy Sickle-cell disease (AKI can occur in conjunction with any other complication in sickle-cell disease, most notably sepsis): 1. Prolonged painful crises 2. Acute chest syndrome 3. NSAIDs 4. Rhabdomyolysis 5. Papillary cell necrosis Paroxysmal nocturnal haemoglobinuria Acute and chronic leukaemias Tumour lysis syndrome Bone marrow transplantation (AKI is one of the most frequent complications of bone marrow transplantation, usually occurring within the first month): 1. Sepsis 2. Hypovolaemia 3. Nephrotoxic drugs 4. Obstructive uropathy (tumour, calculi) 5. Tumour lysis syndrome 6. Haemolytic uraemic syndrome

are more likely to have an acute illness. The most useful and important clue comes from previous creatinine measurements. It is therefore critical to retrieve historical results and imaging from other sources if possible, as this indicates whether the kidney impairment is new or pre-existing and gives an idea of the rate of decline in kidney function. There may be a history of excessive fluid loss from haemorrhage, diarrhoea, vomiting or sweating, coupled with insufficient fluid replacement, especially in patients who are unable to take oral fluids. On direct questioning, there may be constitutional symptoms indicative of a systemic autoimmune disease, infection or malignancy. Current and new medication use maybe relevant, particularly antibiotics, nonsteroidal anti-inflammatory drugs and proton pump inhibitors, because these can cause acute interstitial nephritis. Almost any drug may cause an idiosyncratic reaction, sometimes many months after initiation. A history of illicit drug use and herbal remedies may also be pertinent. It is important to enquire about previous kidney stones or symptoms of bladder outflow obstruction such as hesitancy, frequency and nocturia as well as abnormalities in the urine such as haematuria, dark or offensive urine. Complete anuria is unusual in early AKI and suggests (1) urinary tract obstruction, (2) renal infarction/profound shock, (3) urinary leak or (4) Goodpasture's syndrome.

The focus of clinical examination should be to:

(a) Assess the effective arterial blood volume
(b) Identify any systemic disease
(c) Exclude lower urinary tract obstruction (i.e. palpable bladder or ballotable kidney)
(d) Identify any intrinsic renal disease (i.e. urine dipstick)

A careful assessment of the patient's fluid status, in particular intravascular volume, is essential. Pulse rate and volume, *relative* blood pressure, postural blood pressure, JVP and peripheral perfusion are important and useful clinical signs (reduced skin turgor and dry mucous membranes may be unhelpful signs in older people). Response to fluid challenges, i.e. sustained or transient rise in blood pressure or central venous pressure following a bolus of fluid, is very helpful in determining whether a patient is intravascularly replete. Examination may reveal features of underlying systemic disease, such as skin rashes, scleritis, episcleritis, nasal bridge collapse, alopecia, mouth ulcers, arthritis or stigmata of endocarditis. You should consider cholesterol embolism in the differential diagnosis of AKI in older patients following interventions such as angiography, vascular surgery, thrombolysis or anticoagulation. This is characterised by the triad of livedo reticularis, AKI and eosinophilia, frequently accompanied by signs of peripheral ischaemia in a patient with signs of macrovascular disease such as vascular bruits [15]. The onset is typically 1–4 weeks after the procedure, and patients may have forgotten about the procedure by the time they present.

Investigation

Tailor investigations to individual circumstances. It is not necessary to request a full battery of immunological tests in a patient with postoperative acute tubular injury or urinary tract obstruction, but this would be appropriate if uncertain about the diagnosis or if there was suspicion of an inflammatory condition. However, it is critical to ensure that a urine dipstick test and microscopy is done on all patients with AKI to avoid missing an inflammatory process (see Chap. 2 Henderson/Harber) (Table 5.7). Blood or protein on dipstick or dysmorphic red cells or red cell casts strongly suggests glomerulonephritis. Eosinophils on microscopy suggest acute interstitial nephritis; both situations require prompt

Table 5.7 Key investigations in acute kidney injury (italic for essential initial tests in patient with unexplained AKI)

	Test	Comment
Urinalysis	*Dipstick for blood and/or protein*	Suggestive of a renal inflammatory process
	Microscopy for cells, casts, crystals	Red cell casts diagnostic in glomerulonephritis
Biochemistry	*Serial urea, creatinine, sodium, potassium, calcium, phosphate, urate, serum bicarbonate*	Important metabolic consequences of acute renal failure include hyperkalaemia, metabolic acidosis, hypocalcaemia, hyperphosphataemia
	(If sick) blood gas analysis and lactate	Markedly elevated creatine kinase and myoglobinuria suggestive of rhabdomyolysis
	Creatine kinase, myoglobinuria	Non-specific marker of infection or inflammation
	C-reactive protein	Immune paresis, monoclonal band on serum protein electrophoresis and Bence Jones proteinuria suggestive of myeloma
	Serum immunoglobulins, serum protein electrophoresis, Bence Jones proteinuria	
Haematology	*Full blood count, blood film*	Eosinophilia may be present in acute interstitial nephritis, cholesterol embolisation or vasculitis
	Coagulation studies	Thrombocytopenia and red cell fragments suggestive of thrombotic microangiopathy
		Disseminated intravascular coagulation associated with sepsis
Immunology (if haematuria/proteinuria)	Antinuclear antibody (ANA)	ANA positive in systemic lupus erythematosus (SLE) and other autoimmune disorders; anti-double-stranded DNA antibodies more specific for SLE
	Anti-double-stranded DNA antibodies	Associated with systemic vasculitis
	Anti-neutrophil cytoplasmic antibody (ANCA)	c-ANCA and anti-PR3 antibodies associated with GPA granulomatosis; p-ANCA and anti-MPO antibodies present in microscopic polyangiitis
	Antiproteinase 3 (PR3) antibodies	Low in SLE, acute postinfectious glomerulonephritis, cryoglobulinaemia
	Antimyeloperoxidase (MPO) antibodies	Present in Goodpasture's disease
	Complement levels	Elevated following streptococcal infection
	Anti-glomerular basement membrane antibodies	
	Antistreptolysin O and anti-DNAse B titres	
Virology	*Hepatitis B and C; HIV*	Important implications for infection control within the dialysis area
Radiology	*Renal ultrasound*	Renal size, symmetry, evidence of obstruction
	Chest X-ray	May reveal pulmonary oedema or cardiomegaly
Histopathology	Renal biopsy	May be performed if clinical and laboratory assessment suggests systemic disease or if the diagnosis is unclear

specialist referral. Positive haematuria on dipstick in the absence of RBC on microscopy strongly suggests a pigment nephropathy, i.e. either rhabdomyolysis or significant intravascular haemolysis.

Renal ultrasound is non-invasive, cheap and absolutely critical for (1) excluding obstruction (upper or lower urinary tract), (2) differentiating between acute (normal size) and chronic kidney disease (small) (with the caveat that CKD secondary to diabetes or amyloid may be associated with normal or large kidneys), (3) cortico-medullary differentiation (CMD) (bright kidneys with loss of CMD and thinning of cortex imply CKD and (4) Doppler confirmation of arterial and venous flow. Ultrasound may also identify other causes: multiple cysts of APKD, heterogeneity consistent with pyelonephritis, and scarring or very bright kidneys in acute crystal nephropathy. It is recommended [16] that all cases of apparent AKI should have a renal ultrasound within 24 h, and this should be within 12 h in the setting of urosepsis.

Special Areas

Children

In developing countries, AKI is a disease of the young and children, in whom volume-responsive "prerenal" mechanisms are common [17] and AKI-related mortality is very high despite commonly being due to reversible conditions such as post-streptococcal glomerulonephritis, malaria and diarrhoeal illnesses [18]. In developed countries, AKI is approximately 20-fold less common in children than in adults. Special considerations in children include a higher likelihood of acute obstructive uropathy due to congenital malformations such as imperforate prepuce, urethral stricture, prune belly syndrome, and posterior urethral valves. Other causes of AKI that are relatively more common in children include microangiopathies due to underlying damage to kidney endothelial cells, particularly diarrhoea-associated haemolytic uraemic syndrome (HUS) arising from endothelial damage by bacterial endotoxin such as the toxin expressed by *Escherichia coli* 0157 [19].

Pregnancy (See Chapter on "Pregnancy and Renal Disease")

AKI in pregnancy may be due to any disorder that can cause AKI in the general population, but there are additional complications characteristic of each trimester of pregnancy that can result in AKI. During the first trimester, the most common causes are hypovolaemia due to hyperemesis gravidarum or acute tubular injury following a septic abortion. Later in pregnancy a variety of less common disorders can cause AKI. These include acute pyelonephritis, which occurs in 1–2 % of pregnancies and can be associated with hypovolaemia and septic shock. The gravid uterus may cause ureteric obstruction, particularly if the pregnancy is multiple or if there is polyhydramnios. Endothelial changes in pregnancy may contribute to a number of conditions including a predisposition to thrombotic microangiopathies (TMA) such as haemolytic uraemic syndrome and thrombotic thrombocytopenic purpura [20]. During the third trimester, catastrophic hypotensive events such as placental abruption or severe post-partum haemorrhage may result in acute cortical necrosis from severe ischaemic injury, and globally, this remains an important cause of AKI. Acute fatty liver of pregnancy is an extremely rare variant of pre-eclampsia and may be associated with AKI or multi-organ failure. In developing countries, AKI remains a common and potentially preventable cause of maternal mortality, which varies between 6 and 30 % in reported series [21].

The Elderly

The incidence of AKI is highest in elderly patients [5], who make up an ever-growing proportion of the general population. Pre-existing CKD is a powerful risk factor although few studies have focused on this area [22]. In older people, the commonly used signs to gauge volume depletion can be misleading. Severely ill patients may have gross oedema while at the same time being intravascularly depleted. Reduced skin turgor and a dry mouth are increasingly common in older people and cannot be relied upon to indicate dehydration. More useful signs include postural hypotension and a low jugular venous pressure. The limitations of serum creatinine to estimate GFR are much more pronounced in the elderly, including its dependence on muscle mass and the presence of multiple drug use and co-morbidities [23]. Older age is also associated with a greater risk of non-recovery of renal function back to baseline, which, given the increasing incidence of AKI, raises significant public health concerns about the absolute number of elderly people developing incident CKD.

Rhabdomyolysis

Rhabdomyolysis was first described in the victims of crush injury during the 1940–1941 World War II bombing raids in London, and its complications remain significant problems for those injured in disasters such as earthquakes and bombings. Rhabdomyolysis is characterised by the leakage of muscle-cell contents, including electrolytes, myoglobin, creatine kinase and other proteins, into the circulation. High circulating plasma myoglobin levels (lasting for only 1–6 h) can cause acute tubular injury and AKI. The cause of rhabdomyolysis is often self-apparent (Table 5.8), but if not it may occasionally be due to an inherited muscle enzyme deficit [24]. AKI complicates up to 50 % of cases of severe rhabdomyolysis and substantially worsens the prognosis [25]. Rhabdomyolysis is a relatively common cause of AKI, accounting for 8–15 % of cases in the USA [26]. The classic presentation is with myalgia, limb weakness, pigmenturia due to myoglobinuria (very transient) with positive dipstick for blood but without haematuria on microscopy and a markedly raised CK (in tens of thousands, starting 2–12 h post insult and peaking between 1 and 3 days). Serum potassium is usually raised (in the presence of renal impairment often dangerously so), phosphate levels are disproportionately high for the degree of renal impairment and calcium levels are low (in part due to sequestration by damaged muscle). Occasionally, patients will present with AKI several days after the event with an unremarkable CK level: (1) subsequent hypercalcaemia (2) calcification in the affected muscles on X-ray or (3) a bone scan showing uptake in the muscles may make the diagnosis (Fig. 5.4).

Table 5.8 Causes of rhabdomyolysis

Direct injury or hypoxia	Direct trauma, crush injury, burns, frost-bite, electrocution Ischaemia secondary to immobility-falls, coma (medical or drug induced), prolonged surgery Ischaemia secondary to acute vascular insufficiency or compartment syndrome	
Excessive muscle activity	Grand mal fit, status epilepticus, acute psychosis, prolonged myoclonus, dystonia, status asthmaticus Excessive exercise e.g. marathon running, military training of new recruits	NB clinically relevant rhabdomyolysis secondary to excessive exercise *usually* only occurs in the presence of dehydration (or heat stroke) unless underlying medical predisposition or drug exposure
Muscle enzyme defects	Deficiency of glycol(geno)lytic enzymes 1. Myophosphorylase deficiency (McArdle's) 2. Phosphorylase kinase deficiency 3. Phosphorylase mutase deficiency 4. Lactate dehydrogenase deficiency Abnormal lipid 1. Carnitine palmitoyltransferase deficiency 2. Carnitine deficiency Miscellaneous 1. Neuroleptic malignant syndrome 2. Malignant hyperthermia 3. Myoadenylate deamine deficiency 4. Idiopathic rhabdomyolysis syndrome	Rare causes, usually presenting before the age of 20. Look out for history of 1. Exercise intolerance 2. Cramps 3. Intermittent dark urine 4. Family history (most autosomal recessive) 5. More than one episode of rhabdomyolysis with minor exercise or no obvious precipitant If suspicious refer for muscle biopsy Hyperthermia or hypothermia
Metabolic	1. Hypokalaemia 2. Hypophosphataemia 3. Hyponatraemia 4. Hypothyroidism 5. Diabetic ketoacidosis 6. Hyperosmolar non-ketotic diabetic coma	Hypokalaemia, hypophosphataemia and hyponatraemia important predisposing risk factors
Infectious	1. Viral (Influenza, adenovirus, echovirus, HIV, EBV, Coxsackie, enterovirus) 2. Bacterial (staphylococcus aureus, streptococcus pneumoniae, salmonella) all can cause direct bacterial myositis (thyphoid, shigella, *E. coli*, leptospirosis, legionella, chlostridium perfinges)	

(continued)

Table 5.8 (continued)

Drugs	1. Statins and fibrates 2. Chronic and acute alcohol abuse 3. Cocaine 4. Heroin 5. Amphetamines 6. Theophylline 7. Antibiotics 8. Barbiturates 9. Abrupt withdrawal of L-dopa in Parkinson's syndrome	Risk of lipid lowering myositis increased with dual fibrate/statin therapy, dose, concomitant renal or liver disease, hypothyroidism Also inhibitors of cytochrome p450 macrolide antibiotics, warfarin, cyclosporine, azoles, digoxin (Fluvastatin, pravastatin and atorvastatin are metabolised independently of cytochrome p450 and therefore lower risk)
Toxins	1. Snake bite 2. Hornet stings 3. Spider bite 4. Scorpion 5. Hemlock 6. Not forgetting quail fed on hemlock or hellebore	Alcohol is a significant risk factor in part because of associated electrolyte abnormalities and risk of hypothermia and crush injury
Autoimmune myositis	1. Polymyositis 2. Dermatomyositis	Check autoimmune screen including Anti-JO-1

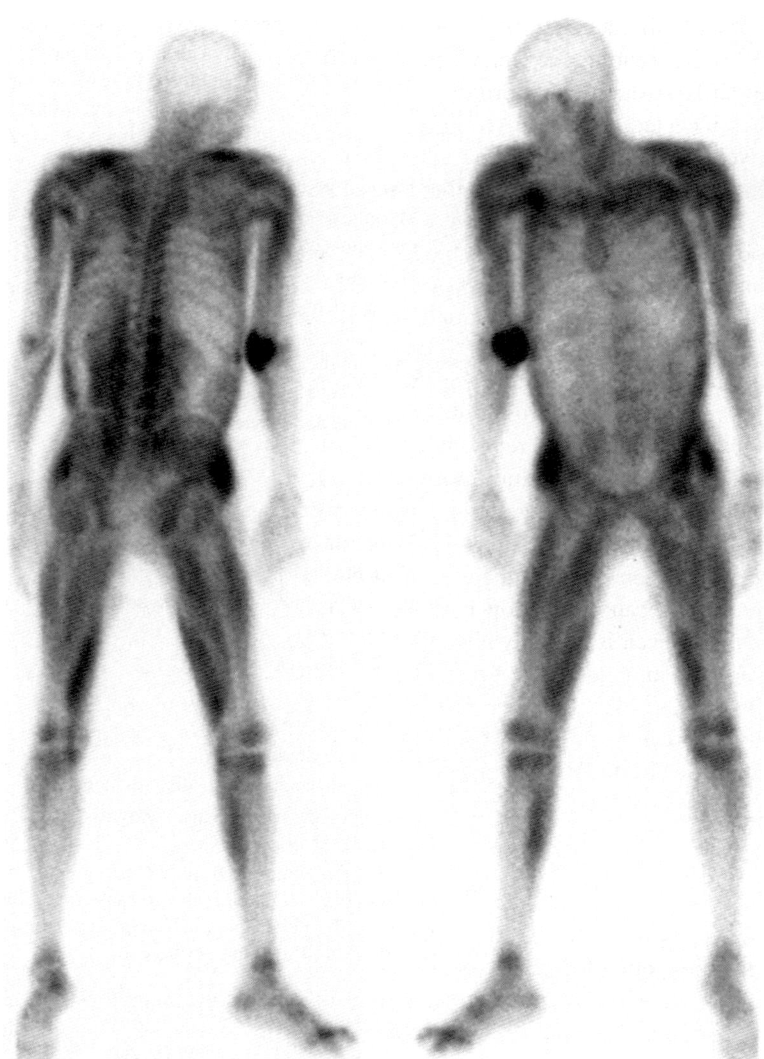

Fig. 5.4 Rhabdomyolysis visualised with a Tc99-labelled diphosphonate bone scan. Posterior (*left*) and anterior (*right*) views (Reproduced with permission from Walsh and Fan [27])

Contrast Nephropathy

Contrast-induced AKI is an important complication in the use of iodinated contrast media and is the third commonest cause of hospital-acquired AKI [28]. Patients at particular risk include those with (1) pre-existing renal impairment, (2) diabetes mellitus, (3) volume depletion, (4) haemodynamic instability, (5) those receiving other nephrotoxic medications or (6) multiple doses of contrast and (7) large volumes of contrast (8) use of hyperosmolar contrast. These risk factors have an additive effect [29]. In high-risk patients, alternative imaging should be considered where possible, but otherwise, the patient should be pre-hydrated, and the lowest volume necessary of nonionic iso-osmolar contrast medium should be used.

Nephrotoxic Drugs

Administration of nephrotoxic drugs has been implicated as a causative factor in up to 25 % of all cases of severe AKI in critically ill patients [30]. There are many drugs with nephrotoxic potential (see Chap. 55), and it is very important to ascertain exactly what drugs, prescribed or illicit, a patient has received and when. Aminoglycoside treatment is relatively commonly associated with nephrotoxicity, occurring in 10–20 % of cases. Aminoglycosides are non-protein bound, primarily cleared by glomerular filtration, then transported into proximal tubular cells where they accumulate and induce cell death. Risk factors for nephrotoxicity include high peak serum levels, cumulative dose and duration and frequency of administration. Proximal tubular cell uptake of aminoglycosides is saturable; therefore, single large doses permit more of the drug to be excreted without undergoing tubular resorption, so reducing cell injury. Numerous meta-analyses have shown similar clinical efficacy with once-daily aminoglycoside dosing, though none has shown a significant reduction in nephrotoxicity [30]. Amphotericin B has for decades been the antifungal drug of choice for critically ill patients because of its low cost and broad spectrum of activity. However, it is highly nephrotoxic with renal dysfunction reported in up to 80 % of patients, the risk relating to cumulative dose [31]. Over the last few years, randomised trials have shown that lipid-based formulations of amphotericin B are significantly less nephrotoxic.

Cancer

AKI is a common complication in patients with cancer. The development of AKI is associated with poor prognosis, although early recognition and treatment are associated with better outcomes [32]. It is difficult to assess the overall prevalence, but studies carried out in specific diseases such as multiple myeloma have shown that 15–30 % of patients have evidence of renal impairment [33]. Important risk factors are dehydration, use of nephrotoxic drugs, pre-existing renal impairment and large tumour burden. Common causes include those resulting from the malignancy itself (e.g. obstruction or infiltration, cast nephropathy in multiple myeloma, paraneoplastic syndromes such as hypercalcaemia), those resulting from treatment (e.g. nephrotoxic drugs, tumour lysis syndrome) and general causes (e.g. volume depletion, sepsis, radiocontrast). Tumour lysis syndrome (TLS) deserves special mention as an oncological emergency most often seen in patients with bulky, rapidly proliferating and treatment-responsive lymphoproliferative malignancies (e.g. acute leukaemias and high-grade non-Hodgkin lymphomas such as Burkitt's lymphoma) after chemotherapy, radiation or corticosteroids. TLS may occur spontaneously in the absence of any treatment but is rare in patients with solid tumours. It is particularly important to identify those at risk, especially so in those with pre-existing renal impairment and monitor their potassium and renal function closely. Risk factors and clinical markers of TLS are shown in Table 5.9 and reviewed in reference [34].

Table 5.9 Risk factors and clinical features of tumour lysis syndrome

Risk Factors for tumour lysis syndrome:
1. High tumour burden (bulky tumour or extensive metastases)
2. High cell lysis potential (rapidly proliferating tumour – LDH is a surrogate marker for this; high cancer-cell sensitivity to therapy; intensity of therapy)
3. Pre-existing patient factors (older age; renal impairment; dehydration; acidic urine; hypotension; nephrotoxic drugs)
4. Inadequate supportive care (inadequate hydration; lack of allopurinol or rasburicase prophylaxis)
Clinical markers of tumour lysis syndrome:
1. Hyperuricaemia (uric acid >0.4 mmol/L)
2. Hyperphosphataemia (serum phosphate >1.5 mmol/L in adults; >2.1 mmol/L in children)
3. Rapid (sometimes life-threatening) rise in potassium (serum potassium >6.0 mmol/L)
4. Hypocalcaemia (corrected calcium <1.75 mmol/L; ionised calcium <0.3 mmol/L)
5. Raised lactate dehydrogenase
6. Acute kidney injury

Outcomes

AKI is a powerful predictor of important clinical outcomes such as hospital mortality, need for renal replacement therapy and prolonged hospital stay in critically ill patients [35]. In uncomplicated AKI, reported mortality rates can be as high as 10 % [36, 37]. In contrast, patients presenting with AKI and multi-organ failure have reported mortality rates of over 50 %. If renal replacement therapy is required, the mortality rate rises further to as high as 80 % [38, 39]. Even

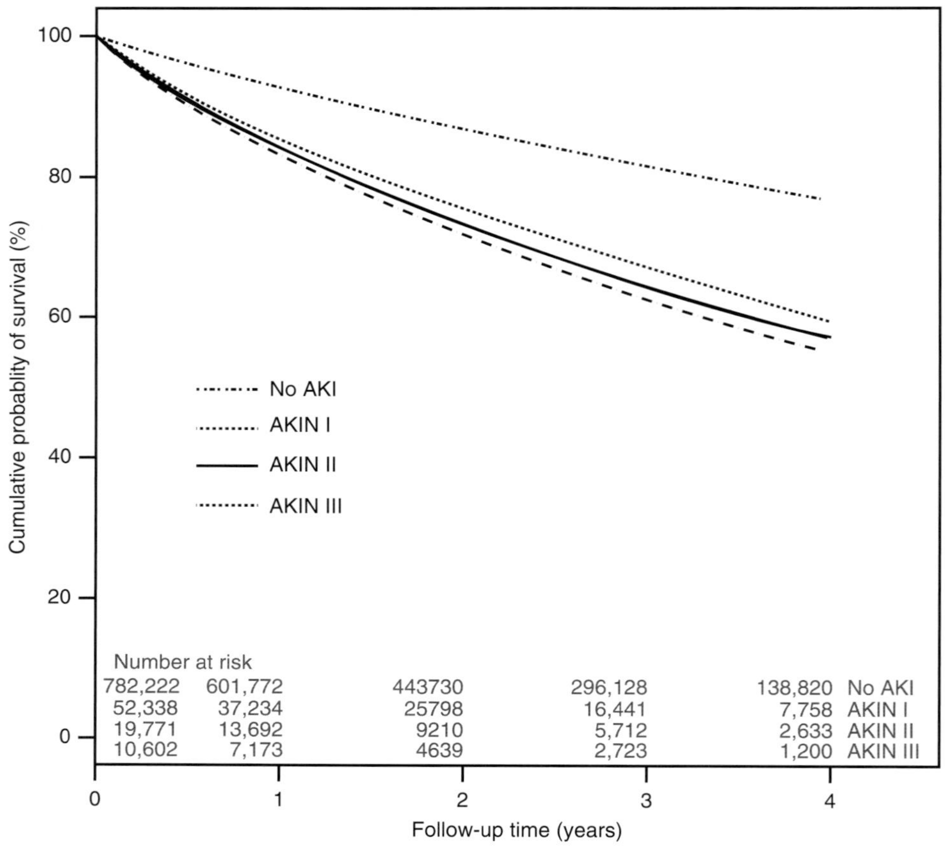

Fig. 5.5 Severity of AKI is associated with increasing risk for death (Reproduced with permission from Lafrance and Miller [40])

milder forms of AKI, not just dialysis-dependent acute renal failure, are associated with excess mortality (Ref. [4] and Fig. 5.5), so recognition and treatment of even very early AKI is likely to improve outcomes. Although long considered a completely reversible syndrome, a wealth of data from experimental and clinical studies indicates that AKI may result in permanent kidney damage (i.e. CKD) (Ref. [41] and Fig. 5.6) and may also result in damage to non-renal organs. A recent meta-analysis identifies AKI as an independent risk factor for CKD, end-stage kidney disease, death and other important non-renal outcomes such as congestive heart failure [42]. There remain considerable challenges in the optimal management of AKI to reduce mortality and improve outcomes, and more research is urgently needed. Tools to predict prognosis in AKI are also much needed, and key advances in this area are likely to come from the rapidly developing field of AKI biomarkers.

Summary

With an ageing population and an increasing prevalence of CKD, heart failure and other morbidities, it seems likely that the incidence of AKI will continue to rise. Although often reversible, AKI has very significant short- and medium-term implications for the individual, and for those where dialysis is not available or tolerated, it may be fatal. Given that many of the multiple risk factors for AKI are predictable, it is beholden on clinicians (and the nephrologists supporting them) to have robust systems in place to prevent, identify early and treat AKI.

Information Resources for Patients

National Kidney and Urologic Diseases Information Clearinghouse (kidney.niddk.nih.gov/index.htm)—US website with information about diseases of the kidneys and urological system for patients, families, healthcare professionals and the general public.

Patient.co.uk (www.patient.co.uk) – an online medical resource supplying evidence based information on a wide range of medical and health topics to patients and health professionals.

Renalinfo (www.renalinfo.com/uk/en/)—Offers help, advice, and support to people being treated for kidney failure.

Royal Infirmary of Edinburgh Renal Unit (http://www.edren.org/pages/edreninfo.php)—Source of information about kidney diseases for patients and non-specialist doctors.

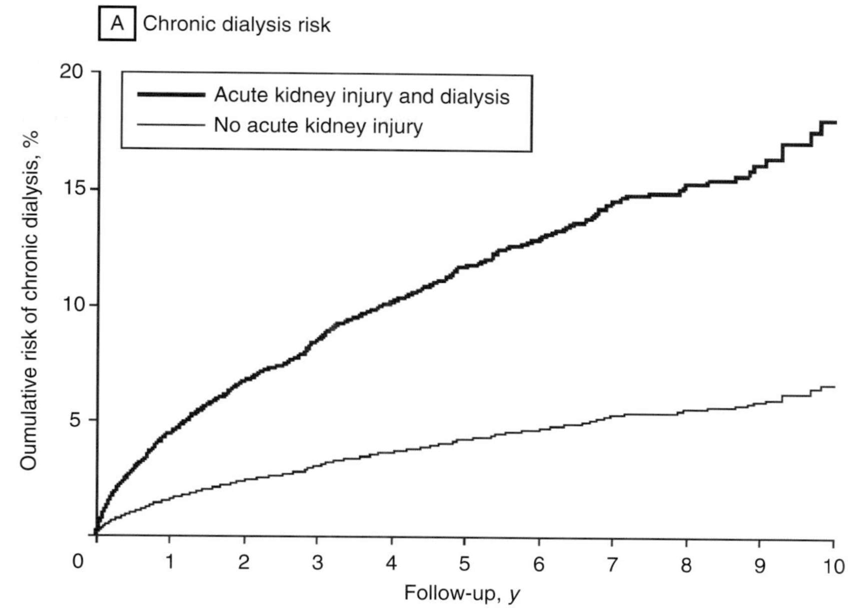

No. at risk

Acute kidney injury and dialysis	3,769	2,761	2,118	1,683	1,305	964	676	462	294	158	58
No acute kidney injury	13,598	10,224	7,850	6,080	4,639	3,383	2,342	1,555	905	473	169

Fig. 5.6 Risk of chronic dialysis in association with acute kidney injury and dialysis during index hospitalisation (Reproduced with permission from Wald et al. [41])

References

1. Bellomo R, Ronco C, Kellum JA, Mehta RL, Palevsky P, Acute Dialysis Quality Initiative workgroup. Acute renal failure – definition, outcome measures, animal models, fluid therapy and information technology needs: the Second International Consensus Conference of the Acute Dialysis Quality Initiative (ADQI) Group. Crit Care. 2004;8(4):R204–12.
2. Mehta RL, Kellum JA, Shah SV, Molitoris BA, Ronco C, Warnock DG, Levin A, Acute Kidney Injury Network. Acute Kidney Injury Network: report of an initiative to improve outcomes in acute kidney injury. Crit Care. 2007;11(2):R31.
3. Kidney disease: improving global outcomes. Clinical practice guideline on acute kidney injury. 2011. www.kdigo.org.
4. Ali T, Khan I, Simpson W, et al. Incidence and outcomes in acute kidney injury: a comprehensive population-based study. J Am Soc Nephrol. 2007;18:1292–8.
5. Hsu CY, McCulloch CE, Fan D, Ordoñez JD, Chertow GM, Go AS. Community-based incidence of acute renal failure. Kidney Int. 2007;72:208–12.
6. Xue JL, Daniels F, Star RA, et al. Incidence and mortality of acute renal failure in Medicare beneficiaries, 1992 to 2001. J Am Soc Nephrol. 2006;17:1135–42.
7. Fang Y, Ding X, Zhong Y, et al. Acute kidney injury in a Chinese hospitalized population. Blood Purif. 2010;30:120–6.
8. Uchino S, Bellomo R, Goldsmith D, et al. An assessment of the RIFLE criteria for acute renal failure in hospitalized patients. Crit Care Med. 2006;34:1913–7.
9. Murugan R, Karajala-Subramanyam V, Lee M, et al. Acute kidney injury in nonsevere pneumonia is associated with an increased immune response and lower survival. Kidney Int. 2010;77:527–35.
10. Bagshaw SM, George C, Bellomo R. A comparison of the RIFLE and AKIN criteria for acute kidney injury in critically ill patients. Nephrol Dial Transplant. 2008;23:1569–74.
11. Thakar CV, Christianson A, Freyberg R, et al. Incidence and outcomes of acute kidney injury in intensive care units: a Veterans Administration study. Crit Care Med. 2009;37:2552–8.
12. Cerdá J, Bagga A, Kher V, Chakravarthi RM. The contrasting characteristics of acute kidney injury in developed and developing countries. Nat Clin Pract Nephrol. 2008;4:138–53.
13. Schrier RW, Wang W, Poole B, Mitra A. Acute renal failure: definitions, diagnosis, pathogenesis, and therapy. J Clin Invest. 2004; 114(1):5–14.
14. World Society of Abdominal Compartment Syndrome. http://wsacs.org/. Accessed 13 Mar 2012.
15. Dupont PJ, Lightstone L, Clutterbuck EJ, Gaskin G, Pusey CD, Cook T, Warrens AN. Lesson of the week: cholesterol emboli syndrome. BMJ. 2000;321(7268):1065–7.
16. UK renal association clinical practice guideline on acute kidney injury. 2011. http://www.renal.org/guidelines/modules/acute-kidney-injury#sthash.MHcUy3ia.dpbs. Accessed 13 Jan 2014.
17. Cerdá J, Lameire N, Eggers P, Pannu N, Uchino S, Wang H, Bagga A, Levin A. Epidemiology of acute kidney injury. CJASN. 2008; 3(3):881–6.
18. Pereira BJ, Narang A, Pereira S, Gupta A, Sakhuja V, Chugh KS. Acute renal failure in infants in the tropics. Nephrol Dial Transplant. 1989;4(6):535–8.
19. Askenazi D. Evaluation and management of critically ill children with acute kidney injury. Curr Opin Pediatr. 2011;23(2):201–7.
20. Ganesan C, Maynard SE. Acute kidney injury in pregnancy: the thrombotic microangiopathies. J Nephrol. 2011;24(5):554–63. doi:10.5301/JN.2011.6250.
21. Bentata Y, Housni B, Mimouni A, Azzouzi A, Abouqal R. Acute kidney injury related to pregnancy in developing countries: etiology and risk factors in an intensive care unit. J Nephrol. 2012;25(5): 764–75. doi:10.5301/jn.5000058.
22. Coca SG, Cho KC, Hsu CY. Acute kidney injury in the elderly: predisposition to chronic kidney disease and vice versa. Nephron Clin Pract. 2011;119 Suppl 1:c19–24. Epub 2011 Aug 10.

23. Haase M, Story DA, Haase-Fielitz A. Renal injury in the elderly: diagnosis, biomarkers and prevention. Best Pract Res Clin Anaesthesiol. 2011;25(3):401–12.
24. Bosch X, Poch E, Grau JM. Rhabdomyolysis and acute kidney injury. N Engl J Med. 2009;361:62–72.
25. Melli G, Chaudhry V, Cornblath DR. Rhabdomyolysis: an evaluation of 475 hospitalized patients. Medicine (Baltimore). 2005; 84(6):377–85.
26. Bagley WH, Yang H, Shah KH. Rhabdomyolysis. Intern Emerg Med. 2007;2(3):210–8.
27. Walsh S, Fan SL. Visualising rhabdomyolysis. Lancet. 2009;373(9658):154.
28. Nash K, Hafeez A, Hou S. Hospital-acquired renal insufficiency. Am J Kidney Dis. 2002;39(5):930–6.
29. McCullough PA. Contrast-induced acute kidney injury. J Am Coll Cardiol. 2008;51(15):1419–28.
30. Pannu N, Nadim MK. An overview of drug-induced acute kidney injury. Crit Care Med. 2008;36(4 Suppl):S216–23.
31. Costa S, Nucci M. Can we decrease amphotericin nephrotoxicity? Curr Opin Crit Care. 2001;7(6):379–83.
32. Denker B, Robles-Osorio ML, Sabath E. Recent advances in diagnosis and treatment of acute kidney injury in patients with cancer. Eur J Intern Med. 2011;22(4):348–54.
33. Humphreys BD, Soiffer RJ, Magee CC. Renal failure associated with cancer and its treatment: an update. J Am Soc Nephrol. 2005; 16:151–6.
34. Howard SC, Jones DP, Pui C-H. The tumor lysis syndrome. N Engl J Med. 2011;364:1844–54.
35. Barrantes F, Tian J, Vazquez R, et al. Acute kidney injury criteria predict outcomes of critically ill patients. Crit Care Med. 2008;36(5):1397–403.
36. Hou SH, Bushinsky DA, Wish JB, Cohen JJ, Harrington JT. Hospital-acquired renal insufficiency: a prospective study. Am J Med. 1983;74:243–8.
37. Shusterman N, Strom BL, Murray TG, Morrison G, West SL, Maislin G. Risk factors and outcome of hospital-acquired acute renal failure. Clinical epidemiologic study. Am J Med. 1987;83: 65–71.
38. Liaño F, Junco E, Pascual J, Madero R, Verde E. The spectrum of acute renal failure in the intensive care unit compared with that seen in other settings. The Madrid Acute Renal Failure Study Group. Kidney Int. 1998;53:S16–24.
39. Cosentino F, Chaff C, Piedmonte M. Risk factors influencing survival in ICU acute renal failure. Nephrol Dial Transplant. 1994;9:179–82.
40. Lafrance J-P, Miller DR. Acute kidney injury associates with increased long-term mortality. J Am Soc Nephrol. 2010;21(2): 345–52.
41. Wald R, Quinn RR, Luo J, et al. Chronic dialysis and death among survivors of acute kidney injury requiring dialysis. JAMA. 2009;302(11):1179–85.
42. Coca SG, Singanamala S, Parikh CR. Chronic kidney disease after acute kidney injury: a systematic review and meta-analysis. Kidney Int. 2012;81(5):442–8. doi:10.1038/ki.2011.379.

Acute Kidney Injury: Management and Prevention

6

Yogita Aggarwal, Mark Harber, and Christopher M. Laing

Until relatively recently, and somewhat to the discredit of nephrology, the management of AKI has been rather a Cinderella subject breeding a nihilistic approach to both the treatment and importance of this common phenomenon. However, overwhelming data demonstrating the high mortality associated with developing AKI, and that AKI predisposes to CKD, have spawned intense interest in AKI and approaches to safely manage patients who develop it. To this end there are now a welter of very good clinical guidelines including 2012 KDIGO [1] NICE [2], intensive care society (www.ics.ac.uk) and the National Confidential Enquiry into patient outcome and death 'Adding Insult to Injury' [3]. The London AKI Network has produced pragmatic and practical guidelines covering the care bundle for the management of patients with AKI which can be modified to suit local practice [4] (http://londonaki.net/clinical/index.html and London AKI app). Imaginative, novel and inspirational approaches are being developed to foster AKI networks harmonising protocols, audit and overall patient care. The challenge for nephrologists is to raise the profile of AKI and implement systems and training that support the prevention and rapid treatment of all patients with AKI.

Y. Aggarwal, MBCh.B, MRCP, Pg.Cert.Med.Edn., MA
Renal Department, Royal Free Hospital,
Hampstead, London NW3 2QG, UK
e-mail: dr_y_aggarwal@hotmail.com

M. Harber, MBBS, PhD, FRCP
UCL Department of Nephrology,
Royal Free London NHS Foundation Trust,
Pond Street, Hampstead, London NW3 2QG, UK
e-mail: mark.harber@nhs.net

C.M. Laing, MBChB, MRCP, Md (Res) (✉)
UCL Centre for Nephrology,
Royal Free London NHS Foundation Trust
and University College London Hospitals, Pond Street,
London NW3 2QG, UK
e-mail: chris.laing@nhs.net

M. Harber (ed.), *Practical Nephrology*,
DOI 10.1007/978-1-4471-5547-8_6, © Springer-Verlag London 2014

Prevention of AKI

Given that there is a notable dearth of effective 'cures' for established AKI, prevention is profoundly important and there is a lot of potential for improvement on current practice. There are three aspects to prevention: (1) identifying patients at increased risk, (2) avoidance of renal insults and (3) prophylactic treatments.

Identifying Patients at Increased Risk of AKI

In terms of identification, it is clear that some patients are at much greater risk. Alerting surgeons, anaesthetists, general practitioners and other specialists to this heightened risk is critical to reducing the incidence of AKI. Some established predisposing risk factors for AKI are shown in Table 6.1.

The trick is having a systematic and robust mechanism for ensuring that all such patients are identified. Some risk factors are more quantifiable than others; nutritional state and vascular disease are not simple metrics, and cardiac and liver disease can be broadly categorised by severity, but perhaps the most accessible risk factors are (a) age, (b) eGFR, (c) proteinuria and (d) previous AKI (KDIGO Group. KDIGO 2012 clinical practice guideline for the evaluation and management of chronic kidney disease). Heat maps have been generated showing the risk of AKI based on proteinuria and degree of CKD [5]. A representation of this data is shown in Fig. 6.1 illustrating the profound risk of AKI associated with proteinuria or CKD or both.

Others have developed a more elaborate scoring system to predict AKI following surgery (mostly cardiothoracic surgery) [6]. Easy to use and electronically generated scoring systems need to be developed to flag patients as high, medium or normal risk of AKI. Simple yes/no versions of this can be used in surgical pre-assessment clinic and in emergency rooms.

The UK National Confidential Enquiry into Patient Outcome and Death (NCEPOD) [3] reviewing deaths of

Acute Renal Replacement Therapy

7

Andrew Davenport

Initiation of Dialysis

The decision when to initiate renal replacement therapy (RRT) in patients with acute kidney injury (AKI) is extremely variable and tends to be based on empiricism, depending upon the immediate and projected trajectory of the clinical situation, clinician experience and local institutional practices and resources. For example, RRT is typically initiated for oliguria, acidosis and correction of volume overload in the intensive care unit (ICU), whereas in the renal ward azotaemia and hyperkalaemia are more common triggers to initiate RRT.

The indications for RRT depend on both or either the clinical scenario or biochemical abnormalities and also on whether the situation is expected to improve following appropriate resuscitation or supportive or interventional management, and as such indications may be relative or absolute (Table 7.1). Current clinical practice is to consider initiating RRT in patients with AKI, defined by an abrupt fall of glomerular filtration rate, who are at risk of clinically significant solute imbalance, toxicity or volume overload.

Does the Timing of RRT Influence Outcome in AKI?

Historic data suggests that 'early' initiation of RRT in AKI was associated with improved survival when RRT was started with BUN levels of 100 mg/dl (35.7 mmol/l) or less.

More recently several retrospective studies reported improved clinical outcomes with earlier institution of dialysis at urea levels <21.5 mmol/l or initiation of CRRT in post-cardiac-surgery patients with a urine output of <100 ml/8 h, and an observational study reported a twofold increased mortality starting RRT at higher urea concentrations. However, a prospective randomised study did not show any survival advantage with early initiation, although this study was somewhat underpowered.

Although early introduction of RRT as soon as a patient enters RIFLE-F or AKI stage 3 [2], may be of potential benefit, so that the patient is not exposed to the potential deleterious effects of metabolic abnormalities or volume overload. However, early initiation of RRT could equally cause some patients to suffer complications of RRT, including hypotension, access catheter-associated bacteraemia and anticoagulant-induced haemorrhage. In addition some patients with AKI, especially those with single organ failure, may recover renal function without ever requiring RRT. Indeed one study from Pittsburgh which followed over 5,000 patients admitted to ICU reported that <1 % of 2,273 who developed RIFLE-I required RRT and only 14 % of 1,511 who developed RIFLE-F [3].

Although retrospective and observational studies suggest that 'early' initiation of RRT in AKI is associated with improved patient survival, this remains to be confirmed by appropriately powered, prospective multicentre randomised trials. In everyday clinical practice, clinicians typically start RRT earlier in critically ill patients with multiple organ failure than in those with single organ AKI alone. 'It is important to ensure that the sick oliguric patient who is unlikely to recover function with filling identify alone, is identified early and RRT anticipated rather than precipitated as an emergency'.

When Should RRT Be Withdrawn in AKI?

There have been no formal studies performed as to when to switch patients from CRRT to intermittent dialytic therapies or withdraw RRT. Typically withdrawal of RRT is an empiric decision made by clinicians based on a falling predialysis urea or creatinine concentrations, increasing urine output and general improvement in the clinical condition of the

A. Davenport, MD
UCL Centre for Nephrology, Royal Free Hospital, Pond Street, London NW4 1AH, UK
e-mail: andrewdavenport@nhs.net

M. Harber (ed.), *Practical Nephrology*,
DOI 10.1007/978-1-4471-5547-8_7, © Springer-Verlag London 2014

Table 7.1 Clinical and biochemical indications to consider initiation of renal replacement therapy in the patient with acute kidney injury

Indication	Characteristics	Absolute/relative	Trigger to initiate RRT
Azotaemia	Blood urea nitrogen (serum urea)	Relative	>76 mg/dl (27 mmol/l)
		Absolute	>100 mg/dl (35.7 mmol/l)
			Pericarditis
			Uraemic encephalopathy
Metabolic acidosis	pH	Relative	<7.25 and >7.15
	pH	Absolute	<7.15
	Lactic acidosis	Absolute	Secondary to metformin
Anuria/oliguria	RIFLE Class R	Relative	
	RIFLE Class I	Relative	
	RIFLE Class F	Relative	
Volume overload	Diuretic sensitive	Relative	Need to create space for blood, plasma products, nutrition
	Diuretic resistant	Absolute	Refractory pulmonary oedema
Severe hyperkalaemia	<6.5	Relative	ECG – tenting of T waves
	6.5	Absolute	ECG-additional ECG abnormalities to T wave changes
Electrolyte abnormalities	Hypo/hypernatraemia	Relative	Correction of hyponatraemia prior to liver transplantation
	Hypo/hypercalcaemia	Absolute	Coma, refractory to medical management
Tumour lysis syndrome	Hyperuricaemia	Relative	Urate >1.0 mmol/l, phosphate >4.0 mmol/l
	Hyperphosphataemia	Absolute	Failure to respond to medical therapy
Metabolic coma	Urea cycle defects	Relative	Acidaemia
	Organic acidaemia, hyperammonaemia	Absolute	Coma, failure to respond to conservative management
Poisoning, drug overdosage	Water-soluble drugs/poisons, relative small volume of distribution	Relative	e.g. Alcohols, lithium depending upon serum concentrations
		Absolute	Coma, failure to respond to supportive management
Thermal regulation	Hyperpyrexia	Relative	Temperature >40° and <32 °C
	Hypothermia	Relative	Coma, unresponsive to other therapies

RIFLE criteria relate to changes in baseline serum creatinine [1], discussed in Chap. 5

patient. As such, some clinicians favour abrupt cessation, whereas others reduce the dose of CRRT or intermittent dialytic therapies, and then if no deterioration in chemistries stop RRT. For those undergoing continuous RRT there may be an advantage transitioning the recovering patient to IHD to permit greater mobility and physiotherapy. Either way it is important to establish close liaison between ITU and the renal unit who may inherit patients with multiple medical problems.

Treatment Options for RRT

Whereas in the early 1980s the options for RRT therapy were limited to intermittent haemodialysis (IHD) and peritoneal dialysis (PD), the currently available therapies in the developed world now include various forms of continuous renal replacement therapy (CRRT) (Fig. 7.1 shows the difference between convective (haemofiltration) and diffusive (haemodialysis) blood purification techniques) and newer 'hybrid' therapies variously termed extended duration dialysis (EDD) (Table 7.2), sustained low-efficiency dialysis (SLED) and prolonged intermittent renal replacement therapy (PIRRT) and the single batch dialysate Genius® system (Fresenius, Bad Homburg, Germany) [4] (Table 7.3) offer a variety of alternative approaches. In the intensive care setting, a variety of additional therapies are currently being trialled as add-on therapies for treating septic patients including dialysers designed to enhance endotoxin clearance, endotoxin filters and plasma separators with adsorption cartridges.

The significant difference in urea clearance between modalities is emphasized in Fig. 7.2.

Does Modality of Renal Replacement Therapy Affect Outcomes?

Mortality

Although it is widely perceived that CRRT is superior to IHD in haemodynamically unstable critically ill adult patients, prospective randomised clinical trials have failed to confirm this supposition. In many of the earlier trials, the more critically ill patients received CRRT rather than IHD, and as such mortality was greater for patients treated with CVVH [Swartz]. Correcting for illness severity mortality was similar for both modalities.

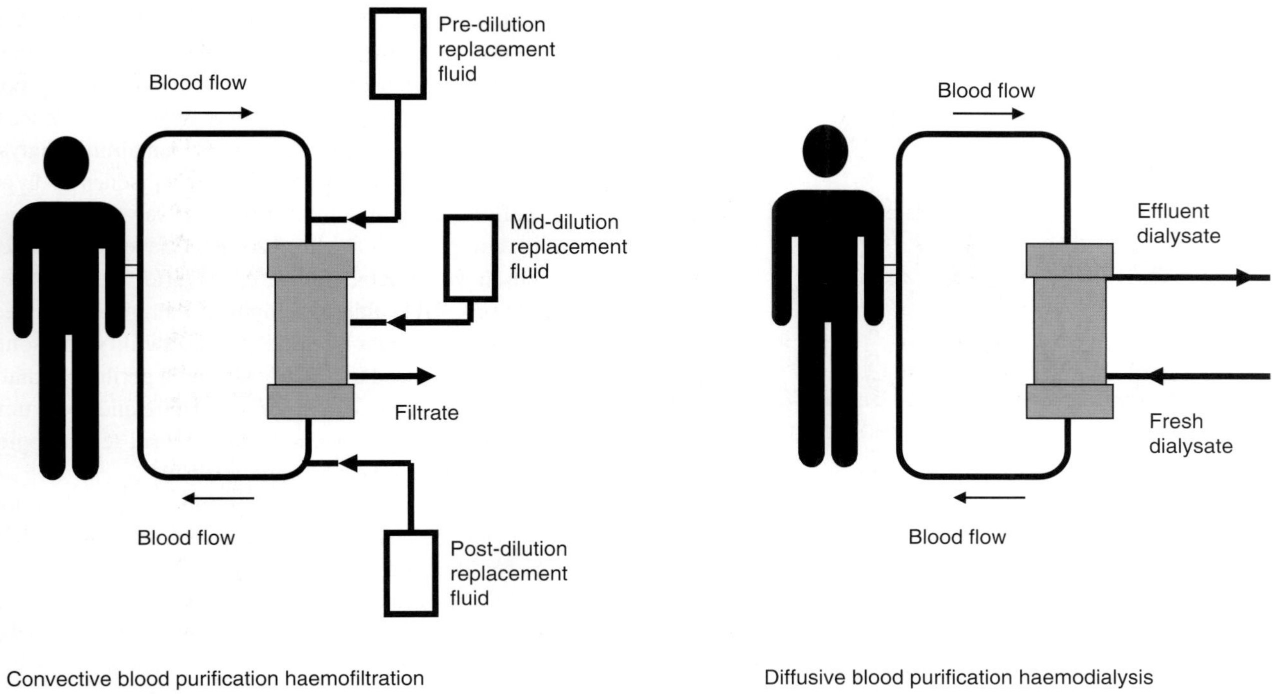

Fig. 7.1 Comparison of haemodialysis and haemofiltration modalities for acute renal replacement

Table 7.2 Comparison of renal replacement modalities: equipment and costs

Modality	Machine technology	Machine costs	Special requirements	Nurse time training	Therapy cost
Peritoneal dialysis	Yes/no	None/++	PD fluid	++	+/++
Intermittent haemodialysis	Yes	+++	Water supply	++++	+
Intermittent haemofiltration	Yes	+++	HF fluids/OL-F ultrapure water	++++	++++
Intermittent HDF	Yes	+++	Water supply ultrapure water	++++	+
Hybrid techniques PIRRT	Yes	+++	Water supply	+++++	++
CVVH	Yes	++++	HF fluids	++++++	++++
CVVHD	Yes	++++	HF fluids	++++++	++++
CVVHDF	Yes	++++	HF fluids/OL-F ultrapure water	++++++	++++++

Costs – assuming no online fluids for CRRT and intermittent haemofiltration
HF haemofiltration, *OL-F* online fluid production

Table 7.3 Different modalities of renal replacement therapy

Modality	CVVH	CVVHD	CVHDF	PD	PIRRT	IHD
Qb ml/min	100–250	100–250	100–250	None	100–300	200–350
Qd ml/min	none	25–50	25–50	32–50	200–300	300–800
Therapy time h	24	24	24	24	6–12	4–6
Primary solute transport	Convection	Diffusion	Diffusion convection	Diffusion	Diffusion	Diffusion
Ultrafiltrate l/h	1.5–3.0	Variable	1.5–3.0	Variable	Variable	Variable
Effluent volume l/day	36–72	36–72	36–72	20–25	Variable	Variable
Replacement fluid l/h	1.5–3.0	None	1.5–3.0	None	None	None
Urea clearance ml/min	20–40	25–45	25–45	15–35	90–140	150–180

Continuous veno-venous haemofiltration (*CVVH*), haemodialysis (*CVVHD*), haemodiafiltration (*CVVHDF*), peritoneal dialysis (*PD*), prolonged intermittent renal replacement therapy (*PIRRT*) and intermittent haemodialysis (*IHD*)

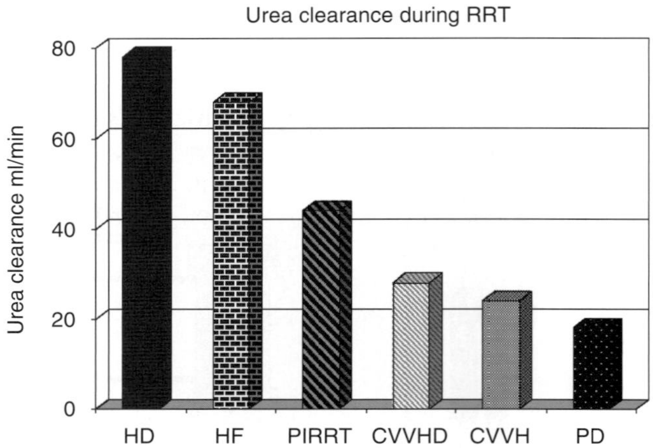

Fig. 7.2 Comparison of clearance between acute renal replacement dialysis modalities

Several randomised prospective controlled trials comparing CRRT and IHD from Europe and the USA have been reported in recent years. These trials excluded very seriously ill patients with limited life expectancy, and also some of the trials had a high crossover of patients, typically CCRT switching to IHD due to recurrent problems with circuit clotting and IHD to CRRT due to hypotension. No trial showed that modality impacted on overall survival. Several trials observed greater cardiovascular stability with CRRT. However, the largest of these studies, the Hemodiafe study, a multicentre randomised controlled trial of 359 patients, successfully delivered IHD to patients despite marked haemodynamic instability with very little crossover between treatment groups [5]. Is this trial IHD used cooled dialysate combined with a very high dialysate sodium concentration and extended session time to minimise cardiovascular instability during IHD and compared to other studies delivered the highest Kt/V dose in the IHD group.

Although there have been few comparisons of PIRRT and CRRT, those which have been reported have not shown any effect of modality on patient survival [4].

Recovery of Residual Renal Function

Although there was no obvious difference in overall survival, two large prospective observational studies reported greater recovery of residual renal function and dialysis independence in survivors treated by CRRT compared to IHD. One study from the Cleveland Clinic reported that intradialytic hypotension during the first IHD session predicted dialysis dependence in survivors [6], and as many ICU patients have haemodynamic instability and intradialytic hypotension during IHD is more likely in hypotensive patients requiring vasopressors, this has led to the suggestion that CRRT may be associated with an increased likelihood for recovery of renal function. Interestingly in the Hemodiafe study, there were a similar number of hypotensive episodes during both IHD and CRRT and no difference in dialysis dependence in the survivors [5]. As such the risk of remaining dialysis dependent would appear to be related to episodes of hypotension rather than treatment modality per se.

Studies comparing other forms of RRT have been limited. No studies have directly compared 'hybrid' treatments to either IHD or CRRT, although 'hybrid' therapies have been shown to provide similar haemodynamic stability and solute control when compared to CRRT. Although peritoneal dialysis is widely used in paediatric practice, more and more units are using various forms of CRRT and hybrid technologies, but as of yet there is no comparative data.

As such, analysis of the currently published studies does not allow evidence-based guidelines for the selection of RRT modality for the treatment of AKI. The modality chosen should therefore be guided by the individual patient's clinical status, local medical and nursing expertise and availability of equipment.

Tailoring Intermittent Therapies for Patients with Acute Kidney Injury

Haemodialysis

In the 1980s, IHD in the ICU was typically delivered thrice weekly, using bio-incompatible low-flux cellulosic dialysers and low sodium acetate-based dialysate at body temperature and with machines that did not have accurate volume regulation. However, just as CRRT has developed, so has IHD with the introduction of volumetric machines, fitted with relative blood volume monitoring, temperature control modules and biofeedback control, along with synthetic high-flux biocompatible membranes and bicarbonate dialysate. In addition the importance of daily or at least alternate-day extended treatments designed to reduce ultrafiltration requirements coupled with higher sodium and lower dialysate temperatures to reduce the frequency of intradialytic hypotension is now recognised, such that the introduction of this so-called bundle effect has been shown to have had a marked impact on reducing IHD-associated hypotension, reducing the frequency of intradialytic hypotension to that of CRRT.

However, the limitation of these technological advances has to be appreciated. For intermittent haemodialysis/haemodiafiltration, relative blood volume measurements which are the cornerstone of biofeedback systems, which then regulate ultrafiltration rates, coupled with changing dialysate sodium or temperature depend upon the concept that if the rate of ultrafiltration exceeds plasma volume refill, then haematocrit and whole blood viscosity increase. However, there

Table 7.4 Theoretical advantages and disadvantages of different renal replacement modalities

Modality	Potential role	Advantages	Disadvantages
PD	Paediatrics	Technically simple	Low clearances in patients with reduced mesenteric blood flow
			Unpredictable fluid removal
	Single organ failure	No anticoagulation	Intact peritoneum required
	Haemodynamically unstable	Gradual removal of azotaemic toxins	
		Usually haemodynamically stable	Risk of peritonitis hyperglycaemia and hypostatic pneumonia

are a number of errors that need to be appreciated. The main error is determining the starting point; then as ultrafiltration proceeds, the normal physiological response is to close down small capillaries, but as the haematocrit in these small vessels is less than that in the inferior vena cava, blood returning to the central vessels is relatively dilute, minimising changes recorded by the blood volume monitoring modules. In addition, there is a marked intra-patient variation to ultrafiltration, which is more marked in the ICU patient, particularly those with sepsis and liver failure by affecting endothelial function and integrity. As such the changes recorded by these modules lag behind what is actually occurring in the body, and although these devices can reduce the frequency and severity of intradialytic hypotension, they cannot prevent hypotension [7].

Haemofiltration

Intermittent haemofiltration (IHF) which was introduced in the late 1970s has mainly been superseded by intermittent haemodiafiltration (IHDF). IHF was reported to reduce the frequency of hypotensive episodes compared to IHD. Initially this was thought to be due to the convective loss of cardiodepressant factors, but was more likely to be due to the cooling effect of IHF, as subsequent studies showed that the frequency of intra-treatment hypotension was similar between modalities provided the same degree of cooling was achieved. Typically cooling is greater with predilutional rather than postdilutional fluid replacement (Fig. 7.1).

IHF as with CRRT requires a sterile replacement solution. IHDF in the outpatient dialysis clinic uses ultrapure water to reduce costs. Many ICUs only have access to a domestic water supply, rather than the specialised water treatment plant in the chronic haemodialysis unit. However, with the addition of simple particle filters, in combination with carbon filters and portable reverse osmosis machines, some units can provide water of ultrapure quality, when using dialysis machines fitted with ultrafilters.

Continuous Renal Replacement Therapies (CRRT)

CRRT initially started with continuous arteriovenous haemofiltration (CAVH), but as the clearances were often low, many patients required additional intermittent haemodialysis sessions to control biochemistries. To improve efficiency, countercurrent dialysate was added, continuous arteriovenous haemodialysis (CAVHD), and then a blood pump to allow veno-venous systems. Initially there were no specialised replacement solutions or dialysates, so peritoneal dialysates were often used. Over time replacement fluids and dialysates based on extracellular fluid composition became commercially available.

Although CRRT machines are volumetrically controlled, as the fluid management systems are often based on 24 h periods, then volume errors can occur with reprogramming following repeatedly overriding error messages and replacing circuits due to clotting.

Hybrid Therapies

Hybrid therapies encompass a group of treatments which are essentially based on extending the duration and slowing down the rate of diffusion of IHD. Most regimens use standard IHD machines with slower blood and dialysate flow rates (Table 7.1). There is in addition a batch IHD machine (Genius®, Fresenius, Bad Homburg, Germany) in which the blood and dialysate flows are linked by a single pump so that the flow rates are of similar magnitude, and this treatment can be extended for more than 12 h by slowing the flow rates down to 100 ml/min, although 150–200 ml/min is more common in clinical practice.

Depending on the design, hybrid therapies can provide diffusive clearances of small solutes such as urea of around 36 ml/min and greater solute clearances of vitamin B12 or beta-2 microglobulin, some 50–66 % of that with CRRT. In addition hybrid therapies can also be set up to provide haemodiafiltration, so then achieving comparable larger solute clearances to CRRT.

Whereas circuit thrombus formation has been reported in 20–25 % of hybrid therapies using standard haemodialysis machines using heparin, clotting is much less frequent with the batch dialysate therapies, such as the Genius®. This may be due to the difference in blood pump technology between the systems, with much greater leukocyte and platelet activation with standard occlusive roller pump.

Peritoneal Dialysis

Although the role of peritoneal dialysis for adult AKI is declining in Europe and North America, it is still used in developing countries and also for paediatric AKI, particularly post cardiac surgery and in patients with single organ failure. Peritoneal dialysis machines are useful but not obligatory. Clearances achieved in paediatric AKI are certainly comparable to those targeted for chronic kidney disease.

However, there have been debates as to whether peritoneal dialysis can provide adequate clearances for treating adult AKI. Traditionally acute peritoneal dialysis was practised by using rapid small volume cycling designed to

Dose of Renal Replacement Therapy for AKI

In patients with chronic kidney disease stage 5, treated by regular dialysis, the term 'dose' describes urea clearance achieved during RRT. The evidence from chronic kidney disease suggests that although urea per se is not a major azotaemic toxin, failure to achieve a minimum urea clearance target results in increased patient morbidity and mortality. However, the question arises as to whether patients with AKI, who often have increased catabolism, require a greater dose of dialysis, and due to the lack of prospective studies addressing the minimum 'dose' of RRT required in AKI, the multinational Acute Dialysis Quality Initiative (ADQI) consensus panel recommended that patients with AKI receive at least the minimum dose considered appropriate for patients with end-stage renal disease. However, due to the difficulty in assessing the true volume of distribution of urea in patients with AKI, several studies have shown that the delivered dose of IHD can be markedly lower than that prescribed.

There are very few haemodialysis studies, but one prospective study reported improved survival and more rapid recovery of AKI with daily haemodialysis rather than alternate-day treatments. However, the increased dose associated with more frequent dialysis was also accompanied by lower ultrafiltration rates and less intradialytic hypotension. Whereas there have been a number of studies investigating the effect of dose in CRRT. Some of which suggested a benefit, particularly for septic AKI patients with greater delivered dose of RRT. For example, Ronco and colleagues randomised 425 patients to one of three CVVH doses, defined by achieved daily ultrafiltration rates of 20, 35 and 45 ml/kg/h [10]. Mortality was markedly lower in the intermediate- and high-dose arms (43 and 42 %, respectively) compared to the low-dose arm (59 %, $p<0.001$). Although these findings were supported by some smaller studies, not all studies showed an effect of dose on outcomes.

Two major trials each with more than 1,000 patients were devised to try and answer whether the dose of RRT was important in determining outcomes in AKI. The NIH/VA ATN trial stratified patients according to illness severity and randomised the less critically ill patient to standard thrice-weekly haemodialysis to achieve a sessional Kt/V of 1.2 or to six-times-weekly dialysis [11]. This study showed no differences in outcomes, and paradoxically intradialytic hypotension was greater in the more frequent dialysis group, but this transpired to be due to increased fluid administration and higher ultrafiltration requirements in the more frequent dialysis group. The more critically ill patients were randomised to CRRT prescribed to achieve ultrafiltration rates of 35 vs 20 ml/kg/h, respectively, and again there were no differences in outcomes between the groups. The RENAL trial compared two doses of haemofiltration, 25 vs 40 ml/kg/h, and again showed no differences in outcomes [12]. Whereas the Ronco study compared delivered CRRT dosages, these latter trials compared prescribed and not delivered doses. Both of these trials reported increased CRRT clotting with the more intensive regimes, and as such the delivered dose of RRT was most likely somewhat lower than that prescribed. Even so taken together, it is unlikely that above a critical threshold of a sessional Kt/V for intermittent treatments and 20 ml/kg/h for CRRT additional treatments do not appear to offer benefit. As it takes time for azotaemic toxins to accumulate, then in AKI, probably correction of volume overload and electrolyte and acid–base disturbances are more important than removing azotaemic solutes above a critical threshold.

In terms of other treatment modalities, there are no studies looking at the optimum dose of peritoneal dialysis required for patients with single organ and/or multiple organ failure, and there is a similar paucity of data on the recently introduced PIRRT (Genius®, EDD and SLED). Preliminary studies suggest that EDD systems have comparable small solute clearances to conventional CRRT but are less effective in terms of middle molecule clearances.

Pulsed High-Volume CRRT or Haemodiafiltration

Although there appears to be no benefit from continued increased dosage of RRT, several single-centre reports suggested a benefit of an initial high pulse of RRT, in keeping with ICU policies of initial active fluid resuscitation, as part of early goal-directed therapy and early administration of antibiotics for sepsis.

It has been suggested that high-volume treatments can help reduce the inflammatory milieu, but equally the improved cardiovascular stability reported could be attributable to increased sympathetic drive secondly to additional cooling, accompanied by positive sodium and calcium balance. The positive outcomes reported with this treatment come from single centres, and the one randomised prospective dual-centre trial of high-dose CRRT was abandoned as there was no observed patient benefit for high-dose therapy.

Choice of Dialysate and Substitution Replacement Fluid

Studies from both chronic haemodialysis patients and patients with AKI have shown an increased incidence of supraventricular arrhythmias, typically precipitated by a relative reduction in effective plasma volume. These arrhythmias and intradialytic hypertension can be ameliorated by using higher sodium dialysate, of around 5 mmol/l above the serum concentration, up to 145 mmol/l, with

not be able to control chemistries in patients with hypercatabolic AKI, and this has led to the development of novel techniques, such as continuous flow through peritoneal dialysis, with recycling of the peritoneal dialysate effluent.

However, the number of patients suitable for peritoneal dialysis may be limited by surgical procedures, and complications include mechanical leaks and peritonitis.

as such smaller solute clearances tend to be lower with predilutional fluid replacement compared to postdilutional fluid replacement. In addition, as some of the fresh predilutional fluid is removed during its first passage through the haemofilter, more fluid is required to achieve solute clearances, increasing costs.

some reports using even higher gradients, coupled with higher potassium dialysates, minimising the serum to dialysate potassium gradient to 2 mmol/l or less, and higher dialysate calcium concentrations between 1.35 and 1.5 mol/l, although there is a suggestion that a further increase in dialysate calcium concentrations may actually cause cardiovascular instability. In addition bicarbonate-based dialysates provide greater cardiovascular stability than acetate. Cooling of the dialysate also reduces the risk of intradialytic hypotension. Dialysis machines may have dialysate temperature modules, which can reduce the dialysate temperature to prevent patient warming or an increase in heat energy, as during dialysis blood skin flow falls, reducing thermal energy dissipation and increasing core temperature, which if it reaches a critical threshold can cause reflex vasodilatation. Recent studies have shown that greater cardiovascular stability can be achieved by simply cooling the dialysate to 35 °C. One of the differences between haemodiafiltration compared to haemodialysis is the additional cooling achieved with haemodiafiltration, which is greatest with predilutional mode.

Lactate and acetate have been used as the primary buffers for both replacement fluids and dialysates for CRRT, due to ease of sterility and prolonged storage life. Lactate and acetate are indirectly metabolised, in the liver and skeletal muscle, through to bicarbonate. The blood lactate level can increase during lactate-based CRRT, if the rate of administration exceeds the rate of metabolism, particularly in patients with pre-existent lactic acidosis and/or impaired hepatic function, potentially contributing to increased protein catabolism and impaired myocardial contractility. Relatively recently, commercially available bicarbonate-buffered fluids have been introduced for CRRT, and although there has been no study showing a significant effect on patient survival, some studies have reported improved cardiovascular stability and control of metabolic acidosis with bicarbonate-based fluids.

There is a wide range of commercially available dialysates and replacement fluids for CRRT. As the amount of lactate and chloride is balanced to the sodium and other cations, if a fluid has a high chloride concentration, then the lactate concentration will be lower and vice versa. The spectrum of fluids available varies from 95 mmol/l chloride and 46 mmol/l lactate to 115 mmol/l chloride and 30 mmol/l lactate. As such, after a few days, and more noticeably with higher volume exchanges, patients typically develop a hypochloraemic alkalosis with the first fluid and conversely a hyperchloraemic acidosis with the second fluid composition.

In addition during purely convective therapies, as the dialyser membrane is charged, the ratio of a small cation in the ultrafiltrate will be less than that of plasma water and conversely anions greater. This effect also depends upon whether fluids are replaced in predilutional or postdilutional mode. As such sodium and calcium balances are most positive with postdilutional fluid replacement, whereas chloride gains are greatest with predilutional fluid replacement. Again as sodium and calcium content of fluids also varies, the actual electrolyte balances will vary between fluid compositions.

Choice of Anticoagulation During IHD/Hybrid and CRRT

AKI is often associated with systemic inflammation, and as such these patients are more likely to have clotting problems with extracorporeal circuits than chronic kidney disease patients attending for routine haemodialysis. On the other hand, systemic anticoagulants may be contraindicated as patients with AKI may have recently undergone surgery or be at increased risk of haemorrhage.

Clotting in the extracorporeal circuit typically occurs in the dialyser, venous air detector chamber and catheter access. The risk of clotting can be reduced by careful priming to remove air from the circuit, reducing air-blood interfaces, and using tubing within minimum changes in lumen diameter and joins, minimising turbulence.

Anticoagulation-Free Options

Although prefilter normal saline flushes can be used to avoid anticoagulation during intermittent haemodialysis, particularly for short sessions by reducing haemoconcentration during passage through the dialyser, other options include heparin adsorption to the dialyser and citrate dialysate. Unfractionated heparin (UFH) is very negatively charged and as such can adsorb to dialyser membranes. This has led to a number of centres devising their own protocols, recirculating 10–20,000 IU UFH for 30–60 min and then rinsing out the circuit to avoid systemic anticoagulation. Taking this one step further, the polyacrylonitrile membrane has been specially modified to increase UFH adsorption and is now commercially available (AN 69ST®) [13]. Citrate is an effective anticoagulant by binding calcium. Formal citrate anticoagulation adds a degree of cost and complexity to haemodialysis circuits (see Fig. 7.3), and an alternative is to replace acetate in the dialysate with citrate. As such the patient is exposed to a low concentration of citrate (Citrasate®), which may permit short session systemic anticoagulant-free dialysis [14].

It is usually possible to perform anticoagulant-free CRRT by prediluting fluid replacement, minimising haemoconcentration and circuitry as well as careful priming to exclude all air.

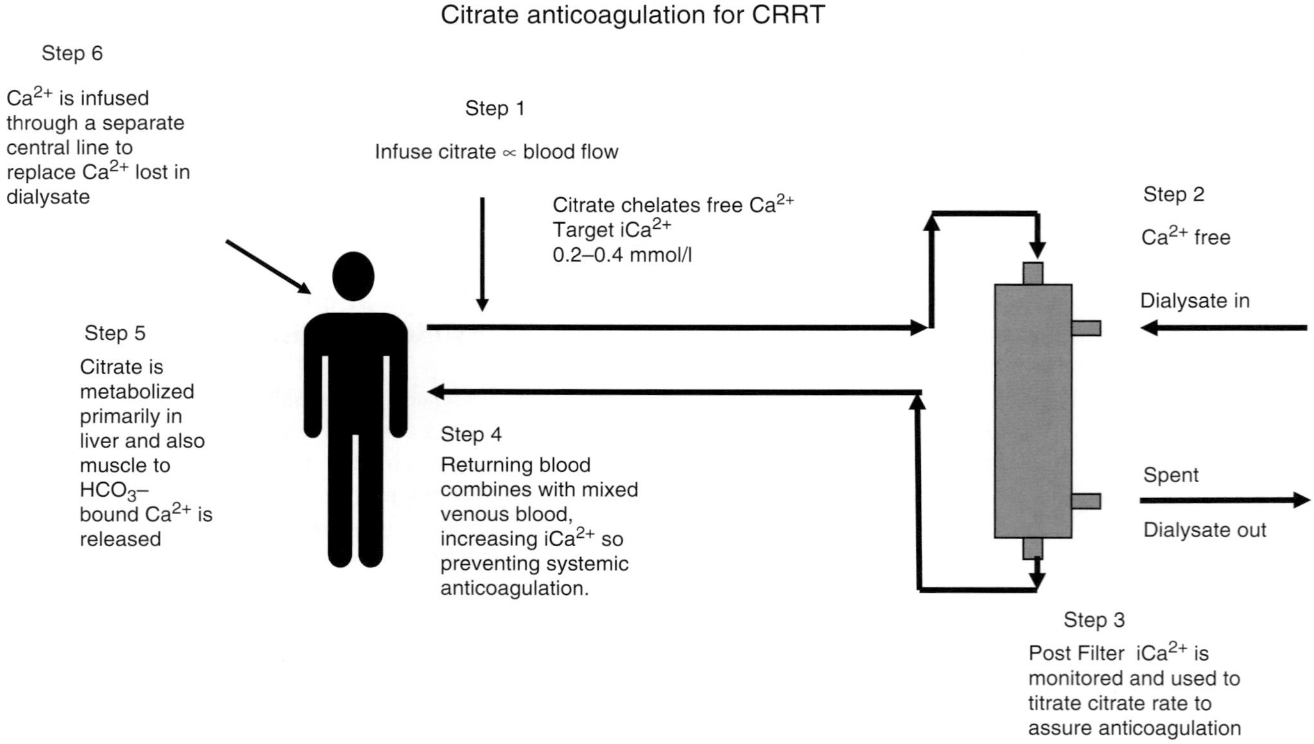

Fig. 7.3 Shows circuit for continuous citrate anticoagulation with calcium replacement

Systemic Anticoagulants

UFH is typically administered as a bolus (500–1,000 IU depending on the risk of haemorrhage), and as it has a relatively short half-life then infused (500–1,000 IU/h) until 30–60 min prior to the end of the session. Low molecular weight heparins (LMWHs) have a more prolonged half-life and as such typically are administered as a single bolus (tinzaparin 1,500–2,500 IU, enoxaparin 0.4–0.8 mg/kg depending upon duration of session and risk of haemorrhage). UFH is a series of large molecules, but LMWHs are smaller molecules, and as such there can be loss if administered as a single bolus prior to a high-flux or high-permeability dialyser, before it has become protein coated.

UFH remains the most widely used anticoagulant for CRRT. Although an effective anticoagulant for IHD in patients with chronic kidney disease, UFH may be less effective in AKI, as many critically ill patients have reduced levels of antithrombin, especially during CRRT. In addition, heparin is associated with a risk of bleeding and with the development of heparin-induced thrombocytopenia (HIT). LMWHs can equally be used for CRRT, with either an initial bolus followed by an infusion or simply starting with a greater infusion rate, and then titrated according to anti-Xa activity, aiming for a target of around 0.4 anti-Xa IU/ml. Regional heparinisation protocols, with reversal of heparin by infusion of protamine into the return line, have been developed to prevent systemic anticoagulation and minimise bleeding risk. Unfortunately, these protocols are cumbersome, may be associated with paradoxical increased risk of bleeding if excess protamine is infused and do not alter the risk of HIT. Protamine may cause anaphylaxis, particularly in patients allergic to salmon.

If patients with HIT develop thrombosis, or other major complications, then systemic anticoagulation with either the heparinoids, danaparoid, fondaparinux or the direct thrombin inhibitors, hirudin and argatroban, is required. If, however, patients have HIT antibodies, but no symptoms or signs of thrombosis, then other anticoagulants, including prostacyclin (prostaglandin I_2), nafamostat and citrate are safe in patients with a history of HIT, provided all exposure to heparin has ceased. In the laboratory there may be cross reaction between the heparinoids and HIT antibodies, although only occasionally has this led to clinical cross reactivity. Heparinoids, such as danaparoid, have an increased half-life in AKI and require anti-factor Xa monitoring. For CRRT an initial bolus dose of 1,500 IU is followed by an infusion of 150 IU/h adjusted to maintain anti-Xa levels between 0.2 and 0.4 IU/ml. Hirudin irreversibly binds to thrombin, and although some hirudin is removed during convective techniques, particularly with polysulphone membranes, the half-life can be markedly extended by the development of anti-hirudin antibodies. As such there is a major risk of bleeding with hirudin, and

Table 7.5 Citrate dose for varying blood flows (Qb)

Qb ml/min	4 % TCA ml/h	ACD-A ml/h
100	175	210
150	262	315
200	350	420
250	438	525
300	525	630

Trisodium citrate (*TCA*) and acid citrate dextrose (*ACD-A*)

many centres use a small bolus of 5–10 mg and then monitor the activated partial thromboplastin ratio (aPTTr) and simply give a second bolus when the aPTTr falls to <1.5. The relationship between plasma hirudin concentration and aPTTr is not linear, and as such aPTTr of 1.9 or greater may reflect a dangerously high hirudin concentration, as such direct measurement of plasma hirudin is recommended in patients with an aPTTR >1.7. Anaphylaxis may rarely occur with hirudin, and further exposure should be avoided.

Argatroban requires a continuous infusion, starting at 0.8 ug/kg/min followed by dose adjustment to maintain an aPTTr of 1.8–2.0 and additional dose reduction in liver disease (starting at 0.02 ug/kg/min). The major metabolite of argatroban has biological activity and accumulates with time. In addition argatroban also prolongs the prothrombin time. Although available in North America, argatroban has only recently been introduced into Europe.

Regional Anticoagulants

Over the last decade citrate has emerged as a very effective regional anticoagulant for CRRT. Citrate is infused into the prefilter line and works by chelating calcium, aiming for a prefilter ionised calcium of 0.2–0.4 mmol/l. As such the amount of citrate to be infused depends upon blood flow (Table 7.5). Calcium is then reinfused separately, or into the return line, to maintain a normal systemic ionised calcium [15]. Citrate comes as a sodium salt, either trisodium citrate or acid citrate dextrose, and each citrate molecule is indirectly converted to three bicarbonates, so there can potentially be changes in sodium balance and acid–base status depending upon the citrate load and the ability of the patient to adequately metabolise citrate. Thus, most centres that used citrate developed their own in-house calcium-free dialysates and reinfusion fluids. It is only recently that pharmaceutical and dialysis companies have marketed specialised dialysates and reinfusion fluids designed for citrate systems. The advent of these commercially available fluids for citrate-based anticoagulation has increased the usage in both adult and particularly paediatric practice, where circuit clotting has been a greater clinical problem. There have been few prospective comparative studies of UFH and citrate anticoagulation; in two such CRRT studies, the median circuit survival time was significantly prolonged with citrate (70 h vs. 40 h and 124 vs. 38 h) with reduced blood transfusion requirement and/or haemorrhage in the citrate groups.

In AKI citrate is primarily metabolised in the liver and muscle, so patients with acute liver failure and cardiogenic shock may not be able to adequately metabolise citrate, leading to an increase in total serum calcium, with a lowered ionised calcium, due to increasing calcium-citrate complexes, termed the calcium gap, and a metabolic acidosis. Citrate accumulation or toxicity is likely when the ratio of total serum calcium to ionised calcium exceeds 2.5 [16]. Treatment includes increasing dialysate flow to increase circuit citrate losses, stopping or reducing the rate of citrate infusion and increasing blood flow. On the other hand, excess citrate delivery, which is metabolised through to bicarbonate, can lead to a metabolic alkalosis.

Other regional anticoagulants include prostacyclin (5–10 ng/kg/min), which is a potent vasodilator. As such patients should be made volume-replete prior to administration and infusions started at 0.5 ng/kg/min and titrated upwards prior to starting CRRT. In Japan, nafamostat maleate is used as a regional anticoagulant and appears to have similar efficacy and safety profile to citrate.

Acute Brain Injury

During a standard intermittent outpatient haemodialysis session, the brain swells. This is due to a combination of a relatively faster fall in serum urea compared to that in brain extracellular fluid and astrocytes, which regulate the blood–brain barrier. As water moves some 20 times faster than urea, water passes back into the brain along a concentration gradient. In addition as the effective plasma volume decreases, then middle cerebral artery blood flow falls. In patients with acute traumatic brain injury or acute cerebral oedema, then autoregulation may not be intact, and as such intradialytic hypotension may lead to a fall in cerebral perfusion pressure with increased local cerebral oedema in areas of ischaemia.

As such the two key objectives for RRT in patients with acute brain injury are to maintain cardiovascular stability and avoid a rapid reduction in serum urea. Patients with intracranial monitoring devices, particularly intraventricular drains and subdural catheters, are at increased risk of local bleeding around these devices if given systemic anticoagulants.

In clinical practice acute brain injury requiring RRT is encountered in two main scenarios, firstly chronic dialysis patients who have sustained an intracranial haemorrhage or ischaemic stroke and secondly acute traumatic brain injury or cerebral oedema and AKI. As the brain typically takes

10–14 days to adapt to injury, RRT should be modified during this period. In patients with compromised cerebral perfusion pressure (<60 mmHg) or major midline shift on brain scanning, standard intermittent haemodialysis should be avoided. Peritoneal dialysis is an option, as changes in serum urea are slower than those during intermittent haemodialysis, but dialysates are hyponatraemic, and patients may require additional hypertonic saline. Large volume cycles, particularly using hypertonic glucose dialysates, can alter cardiac filling by sudden changes in intraperitoneal pressure and compression of the inferior vena cava and so may lead to sudden falls in cerebral perfusion pressure. As such, tidal exchanges or smaller fill cycle fill volumes are to be preferred. CRRT provides the greatest cardiovascular stability, and haemofiltration is less effective at clearing urea than dialysis, so it causes a slower reduction in plasma osmolality. In addition by performing predilutional CVVH, patients achieve greater cooling, so they are less likely to suffer hypotension, and predilution reduces urea clearance compared to postdilution. In cases of raised intracranial hypertension, with lower or borderline cerebral perfusion, hypertonic saline infusions can be given during CRRT, to raise serum sodium or 20 % mannitol.

Typically in cases of AKI following acute traumatic brain injury, or acute cerebral oedema with liver failure, urea and creatinine concentrations are not high, and RRT is initiated for oliguria and metabolic acidosis, so disequilibrium due to too rapid urea shifts is less likely, but maintaining cerebral perfusion pressure and cardiac output is key to patient management, and so dialysis machines equipped with relative blood volume monitoring are preferred. Whereas in acute intracranial haemorrhage in established dialysis patients, urea levels are often raised, and the major management decision is to balance the risks of early RRT to deferring treatment but then starting with a higher urea and risking greater disequilibrium. Although there have been no randomised trials, most centres aim to maintain the serum urea <15 mmol/l. If haemodialysis is the only modality available, then the rate of change in plasma osmolality can be reduced by using a smaller surface area dialyser (0.6–0.8 m^2), slowing blood flow to 200 ml/min with a slower dialysate flow of 300 ml/min and using a dialysate sodium of +5 mmol/l up to 145 mmol/l. To maintain cardiovascular stability, the ultrafiltration rate needs to be slowed by extending dialysis session time in combination with higher dialysate sodium, potassium and calcium concentrations, with the dialysate cooled to 35 °C. So in essence haemodialysis becomes PIRRT. Predilutional haemodiafiltration would provide additional cooling. Daily treatments would lower ultrafiltration requirements and also help prevent rises in serum urea, leading to a lower time averaged urea concentration. If there are contraindications to systemic anticoagulation, then predilutional fluid replacement, with either citrate in the dialysate or citrate anticoagulation, would be preferable. Both hypertonic saline and mannitol can be administered during haemodialysis as short infusions.

To minimise the risk of hypotension when first connecting the patient to the extracorporeal circuit, then priming with isotonic bicarbonate, by reducing negative charge, reduces the risk of anaphylatoxin- and bradykinin-induced vasodilatation. Similarly if a bolus of UFH or LMWH is administered into the venous limb of the circuit, this reduces the charge effect from anticoagulants. Some centres prime the circuit with albumin to precoat the dialyser with proteins prior to directly connecting the patient to the RRT circuit.

Cardiorenal Syndrome

Increasingly nephrologists are encountering patients with cardiac failure who have developed AKI following an additional insult.

Although cardiorenal syndromes can occur with both acute cardiac and renal dysfunction following drugs or toxins, and acute myocardial infarction, most patients developing a cardiorenal syndrome do so, on a background of both chronic heart and kidney disease [17]. Patients with acute multi-organ dysfunction should preferably be managed in the ICU setting by CRRT. As although peritoneal dialysis is technically possible, low blood pressure in cases of cardiogenic shock will limit mesenteric blood flows, reducing solute clearances and water removal.

Most patients with heart failure have a normal or increased cardiac output and only a minority around 10 % with cardiogenic shock and reduced cardiac output [18] (taken from European Heart Society guidelines on heart failure). As such peritoneal dialysis may be an effective therapy. Increased right-sided cardiac filling pressures contribute to renal dysfunction, and as such fluid removal by peritoneal dialysis using smaller fill volumes may help restore renal function. As these patients may behave as fast peritoneal transporters, 7.5 % icodextrin exchanges may be required to achieve ultrafiltration without exposing the patient to hypertonic glucose dialysates. After stabilisation some patients can be discharged home on one overnight icodextrin exchange. However, for some patients peritoneal dialysis is not initially effective in correcting volume overload, due to increased peritoneal permeability and loss of glucose gradients, and for these patients CRRT or daily intermittent dialysis or PIRRT is required. Later, when stabilised, these patients may well return to peritoneal dialysis. As outlined above for dialysing patients with brain injury, dialysis needs to be tailored to improve cardiovascular stability and minimise ultrafiltration rates, utilising machines capable of relative blood volume monitoring. Angiotensin-converting enzyme inhibitors also block bradykinin degradation and as such may increase the risk of hypotensive reactions when starting RRT.

For patients with acute cardiorenal syndromes treated by haemodialysis, there is an increased risk of intra-treatment hypotension, which may then convert a potentially reversible acute episode into one of established dialysis-dependent kidney failure. The main risk of hypotension is due to an ultrafiltration rate which removes plasma water at a rate faster than tissue fluid can refill the plasma water. Even for a healthy dialysis outpatient, once the ultrafiltration rate exceeds 7 ml/kg/h, the risk of intradialytic hypotension rises exponentially. Thus, to minimise ultrafiltration rates, patients should be dialysed more frequently, ideally daily if possible. The risk of arrhythmias on dialysis depends upon both relative intravascular hypovolaemia and also electrolyte shifts. To minimise electrolyte shifts patients should be dialysed against a dialysate potassium of at least 2 or 3 mmol/l, to reduce the gradient between serum and dialysate potassium concentration. Dialysate calcium concentrations also affect cardiovascular stability, and although higher dialysate calcium concentrations confer cardiovascular stability over lower concentrations (1.5 vs 1.0 mmol/l), too high a calcium (>1.5 mmol/l) also increases the risk on cardiac instability. Dialysate bicarbonate also affects the flux of ions between the plasma water and cells, and although bicarbonate-based dialysate confers cardiovascular stability compared to acetate-based dialysate, the higher bicarbonate concentrations (>32 mmol/l) increase the risk of electrolyte fluxes. Cooling the dialysate also reduces the risk of intradialytic hypotension. Some dialysis machines can be programmed to provide isothermic dialysis, so as the patient starts to warm up during dialysis due to the relative increase in core blood flow and reduced skin blood flows, the dialysis machine automatically cools the dialysate to prevent any increase in body temperature. If this technology is available, then simply setting the dialysate temperature to 35 °C will be equally, if not be more effective. During dialysis the plasma urea concentration falls exponentially, and so reduces plasma osmolality, and this may reduce plasma water refilling rate and so risk intradialytic hypotension. Thus, using a higher dialysate sodium can reduce this fall in osmolality and so better maintain blood pressure. Most studies have advocated a dialysate sodium set at 5 mmol/l above serum sodium up to a maximum dialysate sodium of 147 mmol/l. Advances in haemodialysis machine technology have brought a new generation of dialysis machines that can monitor relative blood volume, based on changes in haematocrit or blood viscosity, and can therefore sense if the ultrafiltration rate exceeds plasma refilling. This can be visually displayed allowing the supervising dialysis nurse or technician to respond to sudden changes. The more sophisticated machines have feedback loops which automatically adjust ultrafiltration rate and/or dialysate sodium to these changes, reducing the risk of intradialytic hypotension. When dialysis first starts, the passage of blood across the dialyser leads to activation of platelets and leukocytes, with pulmonary sequestration and fall in arterial oxygen tension, typically during the first 20 min, and this then tends to resolve after 1 h. In cases of patients who have recently suffered myocardial ischaemia, then supplemental oxygen should be considered to prevent any reduction in arterial oxygen tension. Several reports have advocated haemodiafiltration over haemodialysis due to the additional cooling effect in maintaining cardiovascular stability, whilst achieving required ultrafiltration. As fluid volume control is achieved, then cardiac biomarkers such as NTproBNP fall.

Chronic Cardiorenal Syndromes

Patients who have recovered from a major myocardial infarction or patients with other cardiac pathology, such as cardiac amyloid infiltration, may be left with chronic hypotension and symptomatic dyspnoea. As such quality of life may be poor, and the decision whether to offer such patients dialysis to help control fluid volume should not be taken lightly. However, if patients can tolerate chronic hypotension and wish to have palliative dialysis, then peritoneal dialysis using a single overnight 2 l exchange of 7.5 % icodextrin may help to contain volume overload without significantly reducing systemic blood pressure. As patients are often incapacitated, then exchanges may have to be performed by a family member or assistant. However over time, the underlying cardiac pathology will typically progress, and patients may lose residual renal function, requiring standard peritoneal dialysis. At this stage the role of palliative peritoneal dialysis should be reassessed, as ultrafiltration volumes are often unpredictable with peritoneal dialysis, leading to periods of volume overload interspersed with hypotensive episodes, as typically patients require higher glucose exchanges to sustain adequate ultrafiltration.

Some patients may opt for haemodialysis, but this needs to be viewed as a palliative therapy. As haemodialysis risks exacerbation of hypotension, then patients typically require more frequent dialysis sessions (four to six times a week) to allow adequate volume control. Patients should be dialysed with cooled dialysate and higher potassium and calcium dialysates (Table 7.6), but continuous exposure to high dialysate sodium will lead to increased thirst and weight gains, and as such dialysate sodium should be set to around 140 mmol/l. For patients with excessively low systemic blood pressures (<80 mmHg), then vasoconstrictive agents such as midodrine or terlipressin may prevent intradialytic hypotension but risk ischaemia to the heart, gastrointestinal tract and other organs, and these risks have to be considered on an individual basis.

Table 7.6 Dialysis prescription for patient with acute cardiorenal syndrome secondary to myocardial infarction

Modality	Haemodiafiltration preferred to haemodialysis
Frequency	Preferably daily
Duration	3–4 h
Dialyser	Small surface area biocompatible dialyser
Dialysate	Sodium +5 mmol/l above serum sodium Potassium 3 mmol/l Calcium 1.35–1.5 mmol/l Bicarbonate 32 mmol/l Isothermic or cooled dialysate to 35 °C Dialysate flow 500 ml/min
Blood pump speed	250–300 ml/min
Ultrafiltration rate	<5 ml/kg/h
Anticoagulation	Depends on whether patient systemically anticoagulated with bivalirudin, low molecular weight heparin or antiplatelet agents

Severe Electrolyte Imbalances

Hyponatraemia in AKI

When asked to provide RRT in a patient with severe hyponatraemia, then first establish volume status, and if the patient has hypovolaemic hyponatraemia, this should be corrected before initiating RRT, to avoid hypotension during RRT. Peritoneal dialysis uses fixed hyponatraemic dialysates (Na 132/133 mmol/l), and haemodialysis machines are typically designed to deliver dialysates of 136–145 mmol/l, and outside this range, machines would have to recalibrated to provide more hyponatraemic dialysates. Even so this would be prone to errors, and accurate concentrations could not be guaranteed.

Depending upon the clinical situation, dialysis would be designed to increase the serum sodium to 125 mmol/l over the first 12–24 h. As such only CRRT would allow a slow rise in serum sodium from 110 mmol/l or so compared to peritoneal or intermittent therapies, especially as the risk to pontine demyelination also depends on cerebral oxygen delivery and perfusion [19]. Although the replacement fluids and dialysates for CRRT come with a fixed sodium (typically 138–144 mmol/l), it is possible to tailor the composition of the dialysate/replacement fluid by using a combination of commercial fluids and Hartmann's, dextrose and either 0.9 % saline or dextrose saline, to achieve an initial dialysate 5 mmol/l above the serum dialysate (e.g. 5 l. of commercial fluid Na 143 mmol/l and 4.0 l Hartmann's with a sodium of 132 mmol/l and 1.0 l of 5 % dextrose provide a sodium of 124 mmol/l). Reducing exchange volumes to 1.0 l/h and using postdilutional CVVH to slow the rate of rise in serum sodium. Regular monitoring of the serum sodium allows a controlled rise in serum sodium and determines changes in replacement fluid/dialysate sodium composition so that a serum sodium of 125 mmol/l is achieved over 24 h. Thereafter serum sodium can be steadily increased.

Hypernatraemia

As with hyponatraemia volume status needs to be assessed, as if the patient has hypovolaemic hypernatraemia, this should be corrected before initiating RRT due to the risks of hypotension with RRT. Similarly serum sodium concentration should be reduced slowly. Whereas peritoneal dialysis and haemodialysis machines have relatively fixed dialysate sodium concentrations, CRRT allows the possibility of tailoring the dialysate/replacement solution sodium concentration, by adding hypertonic saline to achieve the desired composition.

Hypercalcaemia

In cases of severe hypercalcaemia (>4.0 mmol/l) in moribund patients not responding to standard medical practices, then RRT can be used to reduce the serum calcium and prevent soft tissue calcification. Standard peritoneal dialysates have a fixed calcium concentration of 1.25–1.75 mmol/l, and as this is equivalent to ionised calcium concentrations, these fluids are not hypocalcaemic. Similarly standard dialysates for haemodialysis start at 1.0 mmol/l and thus will allow calcium clearance with haemodialysis, down to an ionised calcium of 1.0 mmol/l. To increase calcium losses, then a large surface area dialyser should be coupled with a prolonged session time, moving from intermittent haemodialysis to PIRRT. The standard dialysates and fluid replacement fluids designed for CRRT are typically hypercalcaemic, as they were designed for critically ill patients who are often hypocalcaemic. However, following the introduction of citrate as an anticoagulant for CRRT, there are now commercially available fluids designed for citrate which contain no calcium. As such these fluids will correct hypercalcaemia, and a greater calcium loss is achieved with predilutional rather than postdilutional mode, with 3 l hourly cycles. If these fluids are not available, then CRRT could be performed using 0.9 % saline with potassium and phosphate supplements as appropriate.

Poisoning

RRT should be considered in severe cases of poisoning or drug intoxication that have not responded to standard supportive medical treatment, and patients have serum levels of drugs and/or poisons which are known to result in significant risk of patient mortality and/or organ failure, and also if the

Table 7.7 Serum drug/poison concentrations at which extracorporeal removal may be beneficial

Drug	Serum (mg/l)	Concentration (mmol/l)
Phenobarbital	100	0.43
Glutethimide	40	0.18
Methaqualone	40	0.16
Salicylates	800	4.4
Theophylline	40	0.22
Paraquat	0.1	0.5
Methanol	500	16
Ethylene glycol	500	8.1
Meprobamate	100	0.46
Lithium acute	4.0	4.0
Lithium chronic	>2.5	>2.5
Phenytoin	30	120
Valproate	1,000	7.0

Table 7.8 Drugs and toxins preferentially removed by HD and HP

HD effective	HP effective
Lithium	Lipid soluble
Bromide	Barbiturates
Ethanol	Sedatives
Methanol	Tranquilizers
Ethylene glycol	Theophylline
Salicylates	Paraquat
Antimicrobials	Mushroom
Antivirals	Phenytoin
Valproate	Trichloroethanol
Carbamazepine	Disopyramide
Metformin	

rate of extracorporeal clearance exceeds that of endogenous hepatic and/or renal clearance (Table 7.7).

Volume of Distribution

Although RRT is most effective when treating drugs/toxins with a small volume of distribution, there may be a role in treating tissue/protein-bound compounds, if a temporary reduction in plasma concentration results in reversal of life-threatening toxic effects.

Haemodialysis and Haemodiafiltration

HD provides rapid clearance for water-soluble drugs/toxins, particularly those of a low molecular weight with a small volume of distribution, including alcohols, organic acids (which accumulate in urea cycle defects of metabolism), aminoglycosides, atenolol and lithium (Table 7.8). Larger drugs such as amphotericin (9241 D) can be cleared using high-flux dialysers and by adding in predilutional HDF. As such HDF is the preferred option for clearing valproate, vancomycin and hirudin. In cases of cardiovascular instability, then CRRT with high-volume exchanges should be considered, but clearances will not be as effective as intermittent HD or HDF.

In cases of drugs which have substantial tissue binding and haemoperfusion is not available, then HD and HDF may still be effective in reducing drug toxicity, provided that session times are prolonged to PIRRT. For example, methotrexate can be effectively cleared by extending dialysis times to 6 h and performing two dialysis sessions with only a short break between.

Haemoperfusion

Haemoperfusion (HP) uses a sorbent cartridge, typically carbon, or an exchange resin to bind protein-bound drugs or poisons, including arsenic, calcium channel blockers, benzodiazepines, phenytoin and tricyclic antidepressants (Table 7.7). HP will also remove lipophilic drugs/toxins more effectively than HD [20]. Depending upon the column, there may be an increased risk of hypotension due to bradykinin and nitric oxide generation and increased risk of clotting due to the combination of platelet activation and also the adsorption of the natural anticoagulant protein C, particularly to anionic exchange resins. As such anticoagulants with a predominately antiplatelet effect (prostacyclin, prostanoids, and citrate) are more potent anticoagulants than heparins for haemoperfusion.

The key difference between haemoperfusion and HD is that the haemoperfusion cartridge will become saturated depending upon the plasma concentration of the substance to be adsorbed, with a typical cartridge becoming saturated in 4–6 h. Thus, in cases of severe poisoning, two HP treatments should be performed in series, with a short break in between, rather than waiting to perform the second haemoperfusion on the following day. Is there a website on how to do haemoperfusion, that is, would it be helpful to have a how-to-do-it guide? Of course not.

Useful Websites

Acute Dialysis Quality Initiative. www.adqi.net.

Acute Kidney Injury Network. www.akinet.org.

Continuous Renal Replacement Therapies. www.crrtonline.com.

International Society for Peritoneal Dialysis. www.ispd.org/lang-en/treatmentguidelines/guidelines.

Kidney Disease Improving Global Outcomes. www.kdoqi.org.

National Institute for Clinical Excellence acute kidney injury. www.nice.org.uk/nicemedia/live/12959/54435/54435.pdf.

National Confidential Enquiry into Patient Outcomes and Deaths – AKI: Adding Insult to Injury Report (2009). www.ncepod.org.uk.

References

1. Bellomo R, Ronco C, Kellum JA, Mehta RL, Palevsky P, Acute Dialysis Quality Initiative workgroup. Acute renal failure – definition, outcome measures, animal models, fluid therapy and information technology needs: the Second International Consensus Conference of the Acute Dialysis Quality Initiative (ADQI) Group. Crit Care. 2004;8:R204–12.
2. Molitoris BA, Levin A, Warnock DG, Joannidis M, Mehta RL, Kellum JA, Ronco C, Shah S, Acute Kidney Injury Network. Improving outcomes from acute kidney injury. J Am Soc Nephrol. 2007;18:1992–4.
3. Hoste EA, Hoste EA, Clermont G, Kersten A, Venkataraman R, Angus DC, De Bacquer D, Kellum JA. RIFLE criteria for acute kidney injury are associated with hospital mortality in critically ill patients: a cohort analysis. Crit Care. 2006;10:R73.
4. Kielstein J, Kretschmer U, Ernst T, Hafer C, Bahr M, Haller H, Fliser D. Efficacy and cardiovascular tolerability of extended daily dialysis in critically ill patients: a randomized controlled study. Am J Kidney Dis. 2004;43:342–9.
5. Vinsonneau DCC, Combes A, Costa de Beauregard MA, Klouche K, Boulain T, Pallot JL, Chiche JD, Taupin P, Landais P, Dhainaut JF. A prospective, multicentre, randomized clinical trial comparing continuous venovenous hemodiafiltration to intermittent hemodialysis for the treatment of acute renal failure in intensive care unit patients with multiple organ dysfunction syndrome. Lancet. 2006;368:379–85.
6. Augustine JJ, Sandy D, Seifert TH, Paganini EP. A randomized controlled trial comparing intermittent with continuous dialysis in patients with ARF. Am J Kidney Dis. 2004;44:1000–7.
7. Davenport A. Can advances in hemodialysis machine technology prevent intradialytic hypotension? Semin Dial. 2009;22:231–9.
8. Phu NH, Hien TT, Mai NT, Chau TT, Chuong LV, Loc PP, Winearls C, Farrar J, White N, Day N. Haemofiltration and peritoneal dialysis in infection-associated acute renal failure in Vietnam. N Engl J Med. 2002;347:895–902.
9. Gabriel DP, Nascimento GV, Caramori JT, Martim LC, Barretti P, Balbi AL. High volume peritoneal dialysis for acute renal failure. Perit Dial Int. 2007;27:277–82.
10. Ronco C, Bellomo R, Homel P, Brendolan A, Dan M, Piccinni P, La Greca G. Effects of different doses in continuous veno-venous haemofiltration on outcomes of acute renal failure: a prospective randomised trial. Lancet. 2000;356:26–30.
11. VA/NIH Acute Renal Failure Trial Network, Palevsky PM, Zhang JH, O'Connor TZ, Chertow GM, Crowley ST, Choudhury D, Finkel K, Kellum JA, Paganini E, Schein RM, Smith MW, Swanson KM, Thompson BT, Vijayan A, Watnick S, Star RA, Peduzzi P. Intensity of renal support in critically ill patients with acute kidney injury. N Engl J Med. 2008;359:7–20.
12. RENAL Replacement Therapy Study Investigators, Bellomo R, Cass A, Cole L, Finfer S, Gallagher M, Lo S, McArthur C, McGuinness S, Myburgh J, Norton R, Scheinkestel C, Su S. Intensity of continuous renal-replacement therapy in critically ill patients. N Engl J Med. 2009;361:1627–38.
13. Brunet P, Frances J, Vacher-Coponat H, Jaubert D, Lebrun G, Gondouin B, Duval A, Berland Y. Hemodialysis without heparin: a randomized, controlled, crossover study of two dialysis membranes (AN69ST and polysulfone F60). Int J Artif Organs. 2011;34: 1165–71.
14. Hanevold C, Lu S, Yonekawa K. Utility of citrate dialysate in management of acute kidney injury in children. Hemodial Int. 2010;14 Suppl 1:S2–6.
15. Davenport A, Tolwani A. Citrate anticoagulation for continuous renal replacement therapy (CRRT) in patients with acute kidney injury admitted to the intensive care unit. Nephrol Dial Transplant Plus. 2009;2:439–47.
16. Meier-Kriesche HU, Gitomer J, Kinkel K, DuBose T. Increased total to ionised calcium ratio during continuous venovenous haemodialysis with regional citrate anticoagulation. Crit Care Med. 2001;29:748–52.
17. House AA, Anand I, Bellomo R, Cruz D, Bobek I, Anker SD, Aspromonte N, Bagshaw S, Berl T, Daliento L, Davenport A, Haapio M, Hillege H, McCullough P, Katz N, Maisel A, Mankad S, Zanco P, Mebazaa A, Palazzuoli A, Ronco F, Shaw A, Sheinfeld G, Soni S, Vescovo G, Zamperetti N, Ponikowski P, Ronco C, Acute Dialysis Quality Initiative Consensus Group. Definition and classification of Cardio-Renal Syndromes: workgroup statements from the 7th ADQI Consensus Conference. Nephrol Dial Transplant. 2010;25:1416–20.
18. Bagshaw SM, Cruz DN, Aspromonte N, Daliento L, Ronco F, Sheinfeld G, Anker SD, Anand I, Bellomo R, Berl T, Bobek I, Davenport A, Haapio M, Hillege H, House A, Katz N, Maisel A, Mankad S, McCullough P, Mebazaa A, Palazzuoli A, Ponikowski P, Shaw A, Soni S, Vescovo G, Zamperetti N, Zanco P, Ronco C, Acute Dialysis Quality Initiative Consensus Group. Epidemiology of cardio-renal syndromes: workgroup statements from the 7th ADQI Consensus Conference. Nephrol Dial Transplant. 2010;25: 1406–16.
19. Wszolek ZK, McComb RD, Pfeiffer RF, Steg RE, Wood RP, Shaw Jr BW, Markin RS. Pontine and extrapontine myelinolysis following liver transplantation. Relationship to serum sodium. Transplantation. 1989;48:1006–12.
20. Winchester JF, Harbord NB, Rosen H. Management of poisonings: core curriculum 2010. Am J Kidney Dis. 2010;56:788–800.

Hepatorenal Syndrome

8

Aisling O'Riordan

Renal dysfunction, particularly acute kidney injury (AKI), is relatively common in patients with cirrhotic liver disease. Both prerenal and intrinsic renal causes predominate. Hepatorenal syndrome (HRS) is a specific form of prerenal failure characterised by systemic vasodilatation with renal vasoconstriction in patients with portal hypertension and cirrhotic liver disease. It can also occur with acute liver failure such as alcoholic hepatitis. Hepatorenal syndrome is often a diagnostic challenge with a complex underlying pathophysiology, but greater understanding has led to therapeutic advances over recent decades. However, it remains a serious complication signifying a poor prognosis for some, particularly those not suitable for liver transplantation (LT) [1, 2].

Definition and Classification

Diagnostic criteria published in 2007 build upon a 1996 definition and are outlined in Table 8.1. Hepatorenal syndrome is subdivided into two categories with HRS type 1 being an acute, rapidly progressive illness with a very poor prognosis without a LT and HRS type 2, a less severe condition with a more gradual onset that is more amenable to pharmacological interventions. The classification and clinical characteristics are summarised in Table 8.2 [2, 3]. A further consensus conference was held in 2010 where the term "hepatorenal disorders" in the setting of advanced liver disease was introduced. This is not meant to replace the 2007 definition of HRS, but instead aims to improve the classification and early detection of all types of renal dysfunction in patients with liver failure. It builds upon the definitions of the Acute Kidney Injury Network with the proposed definition for AKI in cirrhosis being a rise in serum creatinine by >26.4 μmol/L or >50 % from baseline in <48 h, with HRS type 1 being one possible cause of this. The coexistence of HRS and chronic kidney disease (CKD) was also explored. Currently the presence of significant proteinuria and/or structural renal damage preclude the diagnosis of HRS, but allowance for this has been made in the new definition of acute on CKD in cirrhosis where the baseline is GFR <60 mL/min [4–7].

Incidence

Hepatorenal syndrome is a relatively common complication in cirrhotic patients. Using the 1996 definition of HRS, two studies identified HRS type 1 to be the cause for a serum creatinine >133 μmol/L in between 8.2 and 16.7 % of patients. Hepatorenal syndrome type 2 was identified in another 4.8–6.6 %. If the 2007 diagnostic criteria were applied to the larger of these patient cohorts, then HRS would actually have been the principle diagnosis in 43 % of those with renal dysfunction, thereby making it the most common cause of renal dysfunction in hospitalised cirrhotic patients [8, 9].

Table 8.1 Diagnostic criteria for hepatorenal syndrome

1. Presence of cirrhosis with portal hypertension and ascites
2. A serum creatinine over 133 μmol/L (1.5 mg/dL)
3. No improvement in serum creatinine below the described threshold following 2 days of fluid resuscitation with albumin (1 g/kg/day to a maximum of 100 g/day) and withdrawal of diuretic therapy
4. Absence of shock
5. No treatment with nephrotoxic drugs
6. No evidence of parenchymal damage, i.e. a normal renal ultrasound, urinary protein <500 mg/day or haematuria (<50 red cells/high-power field on microscopy)

Adapted from Salerno et al. [2] with permission

A. O'Riordan, MBBCh, BAO, MRCPI, MD
Renal Department, Royal Free NHS Foundation Trust, Pond Street, London NW3 2QG, UK
e-mail: aisling.o'riordan@nhs.net

M. Harber (ed.), *Practical Nephrology*,
DOI 10.1007/978-1-4471-5547-8_8, © Springer-Verlag London 2014

Investigations

The first step in diagnosing HRS is to detect a falling estimated glomerular filtration rate (eGFR) or a rising creatinine, and both should be monitored regularly in this patient population to facilitate early diagnosis. This is particularly true for those with diuretic-resistant ascites, hyponatraemia, peritonitis or gastrointestinal haemorrhage. However, these biomarkers are problematic as creatinine is a notoriously poor indicator of renal function in patients with cirrhotic liver failure due to poor nutrition, reduced hepatic creatinine production and muscle mass. Estimated GFR equations overestimate true GFR, when compared to radioisotopic methods potentially leading to a delay in diagnosing and treating HRS. However, despite these reservations, creatinine and eGFR are the easiest and most widely available tools for assessment of renal function [4, 7].

One of the most notable biochemical features of HRS is hyponatraemia. Water retention can exceed that of sodium, and so a dilutional hyponatraemia develops in about two thirds of patients. This parameter can be useful in differentiating HRS from other aetiologies of renal impairment such as acute tubular necrosis. Natriuresis is impaired so one of the other classical findings in HRS is a urinary sodium <10 mmol/L in the context of a serum sodium <135 mmol/L and a urine osmolality that is greater than that of serum.

To help distinguish HRS from other parenchymal causes of renal impairment in cirrhotics, a urinary protein-creatinine ratio is useful along with examination of urinary sediment for casts. If the proteinuria is found to be >500 mg/dL, there is microscopic haematuria (>50 urinary red cells per high-powered field) or any other clinical features to suggest parenchymal renal disease, then consider an alternative diagnosis. A renal biopsy may be useful in this scenario to help determine the underlying aetiology. This is particularly so if a combined liver and kidney transplant is being considered, as the degree of renal fibrosis will help predict renal prognosis post LT and avoid unnecessary renal transplantation in those with HRS. The latter is characterised by a lack of significant parenchymal histological changes and typically recovers with LT alone. The platelet count and INR will need to be corrected sufficiently to allow a biopsy to proceed safely as complications can occur in approximately 30 % of cirrhotic patients. As with all other causes of renal impairment, performing a renal ultrasound scan should be a priority to evaluate for evidence of parenchymal disease and to exclude obstruction. A summary of the renal investigations is outlined in Table 8.3.

Differential Diagnosis

Hepatorenal syndrome is a diagnosis of exclusion. When dealing with a patient with cirrhotic liver disease and renal impairment, the differential diagnosis is broad: AKI and CKD due to other causes are very common as illustrated in Table 8.4. Getting the diagnosis of renal dysfunction correct may have critical implications for patient management and prognosis.

Prerenal

Complications such as sepsis, gastrointestinal haemorrhage or diarrhoea and vomiting are common and can cause renal hypoperfusion and consequently AKI. Patients are frequently exposed to relatively high doses of diuretics with the potential to precipitate volume depletion. Nonsteroidal anti-inflammatory agents inhibit prostaglandin synthesis and in turn renal perfusion and so should be avoided. For similar reasons, ACE inhibitors can precipitate renal dysfunction in this patient population.

Renal

If hypoperfusion is prolonged, it can lead to renal ischaemia, tubular damage and even necrosis. Acute tubular injury is the principal differential to consider in cirrhotics with prolonged AKI, and the presence of muddy brown urinary casts supports this diagnosis. Contrast administered during radiological investigations or aminoglycosides are other potential tubular hazards. Tubulointerstitial nephritis from drugs such as antibiotics or proton pump inhibitors should always be considered, particularly in those with an eosinophilia. Glomerular pathology, such as IgA nephropathy, has been described in chronic liver disease, particularly those with alcoholic liver disease. This diagnosis is suggested by the presence of proteinuria and microscopic haematuria and is easily diagnosed by renal biopsy. In addition to IgA nephropathy, there are numerous reports of conditions such as

Table 8.3 Typical results of renal investigations in hepatorenal syndrome

Laboratory (serum)	Laboratory (urine)	Radiology	Histology
Creatinine >133 µmol/L (type 2) and >226 µmol/L (type 1)	Proteinuria <500 mg/day	Normal renal ultrasound	Normal renal histopathology
Sodium <130 mmol/L	Sodium <10 mEq/L		
	Red blood cells <50 per high-powered field		

(afterload) are common findings in HRS as is a hyperdynamic with or at risk of developing HRS. This is not isolated to the

Table 8.4 Differential diagnosis

Prerenal	Excessive diuretics Gastrointestinal haemorrhage Inadequate fluid resuscitation Diarrhoea from excessive laxative use Septic shock Drugs, e.g. nonsteroidal anti-inflammatory agents
Renal	Acute tubular injury from persistent hypoperfusion or nephrotoxins, e.g. contrast, aminoglycosides Drug-induced interstitial nephritis from, e.g. antibiotics Glomerular disease can be related to the cause of the underlying cirrhosis, e.g. alcohol, hepatitis B or C virus infection: IgA, membranous or membranoproliferative glomerulonephritis Other causes of renal failure should be considered in cirrhotics with proteinuria/haematuria including: Diabetes, myeloma, vasculitis
Postrenal	Obstruction (rare cause)

membranoproliferative or membranous glomerulonephritis in those with hepatitis B and C viral infection. Again, dipstick urinalysis will give a clue to this diagnosis. Complement levels may also be depleted. Other infective causes of both liver and renal failure should also be taken into consideration such as leptospirosis. Clearly, if the patient has a long-standing condition such as diabetes with retinopathy, then diabetic nephropathy must be part of the differential diagnosis in chronically impaired renal function. Other conditions such as myeloma, vasculitis or lupus are rare but should always be considered in all patients with unexplained AKI or CKD with a positive dipstick urinalysis [1, 2, 10, 17].

Precipitating Factors, Prevention and Initial Therapy

Hepatorenal syndrome can occur spontaneously but is frequently triggered by complications such as peritonitis, acute alcoholic hepatitis and gastrointestinal haemorrhage. Hence, prompt diagnosis and effective treatment is imperative to prevent the development of HRS.

As previously alluded to, nonsteroidal anti-inflammatory drugs inhibit renal perfusion and so should not be used in those with cirrhosis. Other drugs such as aminoglycosides and angiotensin-converting enzyme inhibitors should also be avoided. Radiological contrast should be administered with caution in those at risk of developing HRS. Overzealous diuresis can have a negative impact on renal perfusion and hence precipitate HRS. Typically ascites is initially treated with fluid and sodium restriction, but diuretics such as spironolactone, an aldosterone antagonist, are frequently required. However, this agent can precipitate dangerous hyperkalaemia and so should not be used in those with type 1 HRS. Preventative strategies include regular monitoring of renal function in all those on diuretics. If renal function does deteriorate, then the first step is to correct intravascular volume depletion and diuretic doses should be reduced or even stopped. In this scenario the optimum treatment is paracentesis, with appropriate albumin support for those who require removal of large volumes of over 5 L (8 g/L of ascites drained). Without albumin, approximately 20 % will develop HRS. Paracentesis may also relieve raised intra-abdominal pressure impeding renal venous return.

There needs to be a low threshold for hospital admission in patients with deteriorating renal function aiming to restore renal perfusion. Some may even require high dependency or intensive care unit support to facilitate close monitoring of vital signs and urine output. Continuous central venous pressure monitoring can be utilised to guide and optimise fluid resuscitation, preferably with 20 % albumin. Adrenal insufficiency may be an exacerbating factor in some, and so hydrocortisone administration may also have a role.

Hepatorenal syndrome is triggered by bacterial peritonitis in about a third of patients and is associated with increased cytokine levels including tumour necrosis factor α and interleukin 6. Tumour necrosis α is linked to cardiomyopathy in bacterial peritonitis and triggers an inability to compensate for the disturbed systemic circulation seen in HRS. Prompt treatment of any sepsis, including peritonitis, is imperative. Along with antibiotic therapy, albumin administration has also been shown to decrease the risk of HRS by 66 % in those with peritonitis if it is given on day 1 and 3. This is felt to be due to an improvement in haemodynamics and renal perfusion along with antioxidant effects. For high-risk patients, the use of antibiotic prophylaxis with norfloxacin or ceftriaxone helps to reduce the risk of spontaneous bacterial peritonitis and HRS and improves survival. Finally, pentoxifylline (a tumour necrosis factor inhibitor) use has been shown to reduce the risk of HRS in those suffering from alcoholic hepatitis [1, 10, 18–22].

Treatment

If preventative strategies fail and HRS develops, then a number of therapies are available. The key treatment options in the management of HRS are outlined in Tables 8.5 and 8.6.

Table 9.1 Epidemiology of hyponatraemia: some associations with high incidence [2]

Cirrhosis	~35–50 %, depending on severity of disease
Heart failure	~20 %, depending on severity of disease
Elderly	Significantly increased risk with age, especially in institutionalized, with feeding or fluids (up to 30 %)
Thiazides	~15 % in the elderly and low body weight significant risk factors (apparent within 2 weeks)
Serotonic uptake inhibitors	~10–20 % (apparent within 2 weeks)
Hospital admissions	Variable depending on environment 5–40 % common when associated with diarrhoeal illnesses
Emergency department	~3 % (hypovolaemia common)
Hospital acquired	~15 %
Post-operative	(<130 mmol/L) 4–5 %
ICU	10–15 %
Endurance athletes	Marathon runners 10–20 %, severe hyponatraemia ~0.5 %
Pneumonia	~10 %
HIV	Untreated HIV high incidence but also pseudohyponatraemia
Anorexia nervosa	20 %
3,4-Methylenedioxymethylamphetamine	Ecstasy

brain is normally protected from osmotic injury by the regulation of intracellular electrolytes and intraneural osmotic osmolytes. Electrolytes such as potassium can be transferred out of the neural cells rapidly to reduce intracellular osmolality in hyponatraemia, but as reduction in organic intraneural osmolytes takes longer, it explains why sudden drops in sodium (<48 h) are more dangerous than worse hyponatraemia that develops over a longer period. While mild hyponatraemia is often tolerated by physicians and felt to be harmless, one study of 'asymptomatic' hyponatraemia (mean sodium 128 mmol/L) demonstrated significantly delayed response to audiovisual stimuli, a significant increase in errors and a very significantly increased risk of falls [3] as well as osteoporosis (RR 2–3×) [4].

Causes of Hyponatraemia and Differential Diagnosis of Hyponatraemia

Although relatively rare, it is important to exclude pseudohyponatraemia; when the laboratory plasma sodium is lower than the real plasma sodium. This can occur in hyperlipidaemia (especially triglycerides or high protein levels, e.g. myeloma or polyclonal gammopathy in HIV), in which case plasma osmolality will be normal. Measuring sodium with an ion-specific electrode can overcome this and thus arterial or venous blood gases will give a more accurate sodium. Mannitol and maltose (with IVIg infusions) can also cause pseudohyponatraemia but with a raised plasma osmolality.

There are many causes of hyponatraemia, and in any one patient it is not unusual for two or more causes to contribute (see Table 9.2). Hyponatraemia is due to either decrease in the content of sodium or retention of water, and three common pathophysiologies of hyponatraemia are: (a) pure increase in total body water (euvolaemia), (b) increase in total body sodium and water (hypervolaemia) and (c) genuine reduction in total body sodium (hypovolaemia); this is the most practical way of dividing very different potential causes and is important for directing management.

Assessment and Investigations of Hyponatraemia

Assuming that pseudohyponatraemia and factitious hyponatraemia (diluted sample) have been excluded and hyperosmolar states are also excluded; then assessment of hyponatraemia requires a careful history of fluid balance – losses and gains, significant comorbidities as cranial lesions, cardiac, hepatic, adrenal, thyroid or renal disease. For hospitalized patients, careful review of fluid balance and weights can be diagnostic. The physical assessment, apart from excluding obvious causes, needs to ascertain whether the patient has a raised, normal or low effective arterial blood volume; that is whether they have gained total body sodium and water, gained total body water or lost total body sodium (Table 9.3).

In theory this should be straightforward, but in complex patients with multiple co-morbidities it can be tricky. Not all the tests shown in Table 9.3 are required in all patients, but even with these there may remain diagnostic uncertainty.

Some Specific Causes of Hyponatraemia

Psychogenic polydipsia and beer potomania: the kidneys are so efficient at free water clearance that you have to be a determined drinker of 12–15 L a day to become hyponatraemic (urine should be maximally dilute) and a diagnosis of psychogenic polydipsia needs to be one of exclusion (beer potomania is usually obvious). However, some patients may be more predisposed (those with a low body mass or malnourished), and secondary causes of hyponatraemia (e.g. the use of antidepressants or renal impairment) may lower the fluid threshold required; moreover with dedicated polydipsia

Table 9.2 Causes of hyponatraemia

		Disease
Increased EABV (hypervolaemia)	*Increase in total body sodium < increase in water*	
	Increased renin:angiotensin system activity	Cirrhosis (low urinary sodium)
		Congestive cardiac failure (low urinary sodium)
		Nephrotic syndrome (low urinary sodium)
		Renal failure (high urinary sodium)
Normal EABV (euvolaemia)	*Increased total body water*	Water intoxication, psychogenic polydipsia, excessive beer drinking, ecstasy
		Syndrome of inappropriate ADH (high urinary sodium)
		Medication (thiazides, SSRIs, opiates)
		Hypothyroidism (thyroxin required for maximal free water clearance; high urinary sodium)
		Hypoadrenalism (cortisol required for maximal free water clearance; high urinary sodium)
		Pregnancy
Reduced EABV (hypovolaemia)	Reduction in total body sodium > reduction in body water	
	(a) *Renal losses* (high urinary sodium)	Diuretics
		Hypoadrenalism
		Salt-losing nephropathies
		Cerebral salt-wasting (excessive BNP)
	(b) *Extra-renal losses* (low urinary sodium)	Sweating (and water intake, endurance exercise, vomiting, diarrhoea)
	(c) *Low solute intake*	
Hyperosmolar and iso-osmolar hyponatraemia	*Hyperosmolar states*	Hyperglycaemia, Mannitol
	Iso-osmolar state	Absorption of irrigation fluid
Pseudohyponatraemia		Hyperlipidaemia, high protein (immunoglobulin levels),
Factitious hyponatraemia		diluted sample, e.g. from drip arm or Munchausen syndrome

EABV effective arterial blood volume
BNP brain naturetic peptide

Table 9.3 Investigations of hyponatraemia

Serum electrolytes and glucose plus osmolality to exclude hyperosmolar hyponatraemia
Triglycerides albumin and total protein to exclude pseudohyponatraemia
Renal function tests, urate and if appropriate liver function tests and brain natriuretic peptide
Urine and plasma osmolality
Urinary potassium
Urinary sodium (low urinary sodium (<20 mmol/L) associated with cirrhosis, heart failure, nephrotic syndrome, hypovolaemia of any cause and water intoxication) (urinary sodium >20 mmol/L associated with renal loss, SIADH and renal impairment) assuming no diuretics
Thyroid function tests, Adrenal function tests (both hormones required for maximal free water clearance)

the counter-current multiplier will get washed out and the ability to generate free water clearance is reduced.

Endurance sports are becoming increasingly popular and hyponatraemia is common in this setting. Risk factors seem to relate to body size, duration of exercise (e.g. marathons over 4 h), fluid intake (failure to lose weight or actually gaining weight) during a marathon is an adverse risk factor) and the use of NSAIDs. Most legitimate sports drinks are hypotonic and likely to contribute; illegitimate supplements could contain almost anything.

Some medication has a particular association; thiazide diuretics and selective serotonine uptake inhibitors both have a high incidence. Again, it is the elderly and those having low body weight who are at the highest risk. For thiazides, those gaining weight within 48 h of starting have increased risk. Fortunately, for both classes of medication, hyponatraemia usually becomes apparent within 2 weeks, and testing at this time in high risk patients is likely to identify most.

Post-operative hyponatraemia is common and is related to SIADH secondary stress, opiates, pain and nausea, resulting in the non-osmotic release of ADH, often in the setting of hypotonic fluid administration. This can have very severe consequences. In one landmark study among 15 women undergoing elective surgery and incurring hyponatraemia (mean 108 mmol/L), 27 % died and 60 % suffered persistent vegetative state [5].

Table 9.4 Causes of SIADH

Malignancy	Predominantly lung but reported with many tumour types
Pulmonary	Infections, asthma, cystic fibrosis, respiratory failure associated with positive pressure ventilation
Central nervous system disease	CNS tumours, encephalitis, meningitis, demyelination, acute intermittent porphyria
Medication	SSRIs, thiazide diuretics, chlorpropamide, tricyclic antidepressants, NSAIDs, carbamazepine, opiates, nicotine, DDAVP, oxytocin, vincristine, cyclophosphamide, ifosfamide, ecstasy
Miscellaneous	Stress, pain, nausea, endurance sports, gain of function mutations in the V2 receptor (nephrogenic syndrome of inappropriate anti-diuresis)

Ecstasy induced hyponatraemia has caused deaths in otherwise healthy young adults and appears to be a combination of polydipsia and inappropriate ADH; advice to drink copious quantities of water is probably inappropriate.

The incidence of hyponatraemia in institutionalized elderly patients is very high and causes multifactorial, including polypharmacy, low body weight and low solute intake. In this setting even moderate hyponatraemia can have a profound effect, decompensating patients with co-morbidity. Those patients receiving IV fluids or medical feeding are particularly at risk. Dissecting the principal cause of hyponatraemia may be very difficult and identifying the patient at risk is critical.

Syndrome of inappropriate ADH is a relatively common cause of hyponatraemia, particularly in the setting of surgery; some common causes are shown in Table 9.4.

The diagnosis is one of exclusion and needs to be in the absence of hypothyroidism or hypoadrenalism or renal impairment and in the absence of a pre-renal element. Assuming all these are satisfied, the diagnosis is suggested by the clinical circumstances, hypo-osmolar serum (<275 mmol/L) in a euvolaemic patients, a high urine osmolality (low serum urea and urate also suggestive, urine sodium often >40 mmol/L), a relatively concentrated urine osmolarity (>100 mmol/L) and a urinary sodium of >20 mmol/L. The precipitating cause may be obvious such as pneumonia, but if not, suspending any potentially culpable medication may need to be followed by a search for malignancy.

Treatment of Hyponatraemia

This depends on the clinical state of the patient, the acuteness of the hyponatraemia and the underlying cause. The main concern with treating hyponatraemia is the risk of central pontine myelinolysis (CPM). Rapid correction of serum osmolality causes osmotic dehydration of neural cells; classically at risk is the central pons but basal ganglia and cerebellum can also be involved. Having shed organic osmolytes and electrolytes, neurons are particularly vulnerable to an increase in plasma osmolality. Reaccumulation of osmolytes such as the major osmolyte myoinositol is slower than their loss, although reuptake of myoinositol is faster in patients with uraemia, therefore protecting them somewhat from CPM – yet another reason, if any more were needed, in the merit of renal disease.

Treatment relies on identifying and treating the cause, and specific management of the low sodium depends on whether there is a sodium deficit, SIADH or sodium and water excess. The fundamental rules, however, are for the patient to be in a place of safety and for very frequent monitoring; to avoid CPM the aim is to correct but slowly. In a seminal study looking at patients with severe hyponatraemia (<105 mmol/L), no patients, who had increments of ≤12 mmol/L in 24 h or 18 mmol/L in 48 h suffered neurological injury [6]. As these are maximum increments, the aim is no greater correction than 8–10 mmol/L in 24 h if hyponatraemia is likely to have been present for ≥48 h. In those with hyponatraemic encephalopathy (seizures, neurological signs and neurogenic pulmonary oedema), the initial correction should be with 100 mL of 3 % (hypertonic) saline plus or minus an infusion of the same at 1–2 mL/kg/h, ensuring that correction is no greater than 8–10 mmol/L/24 h. This can be given in conjunction with loop-diuretic but again the concern is that correction may be too rapid if not monitored extremely closely. Oxygenation is important for anyone at risk of hyponatraemic encephalopathy.

Non-peptide vasopressin receptor antagonists (vaptans) conivaptan (IV) and tolvaptan (oral) offer an elegant way of promoting free water clearance acting on V1a and V2 receptors (tolvaptan more selectively on the latter). They are effective at increasing sodium in euvolaemic and hypervolaemic states and appear safe, but are contraindicated in hypovolaemic states and not the treatment of choice in hyponatraemic emergencies. Patients can become polyuric and over-correct, so close monitoring on initiation is important and fluid restriction may need to be limited or reversed (caution with patients who do not have free access to fluids, and do not use simultaneously with hypertonic saline and diuretics). There is a danger that vaptans will be used willy-nilly but concerns over liver toxicity, extortionate cost and lack of long-term outcome benefits mean the role of these drugs for long-term conditions is not yet established: It seems likely in the right setting, and if carefully handled they are a welcome addition to the therapeutic armamentarium [7].

1. For patients who are hypovolaemic and sodium deplete, the treatment is usually with saline replacement and treating the underlying cause such as GI losses, correcting adrenal or thyroid insufficiency or sodium supplementation

Table 9.5 Causes of hypernatraemia

Increased EABV (hypervolaemia)	*Excessive mineralocorticoid activity*	For example, Cushing's syndrome, Conn's usually associated with hypokalaemia and hypertension and low urinary sodium
	Excessive salt intake	Hypertonic feed, hypertonic saline, normal saline and colloid have a sodium of 155 mmol/L, high salt load medication (e.g. some antibiotics, sodium bicarbonate, glucocorticoids and mineralocorticoids), associated with high urinary sodium
Normal EABV (Euvolaemia)	*Renal water loss*	Nephrogenic diabetes insipidus Central diabetes insipidus (with inadequate water intake)
	Extra renal water loss	Insensible losses e.g. hyperventilation
Reduced EABV (hypovolaemia)	*Renal water losses*	Diuretics, especially osmotic diuretics, vaptan therapy
	Extra renal water loss	Vomiting, diarrhoea, sweating, NG suction

in patients with salt-losing nephropathies; potassium deficits if present should be corrected. Vaptans are contraindicated.

2. Euvolaemic patients, i.e. those who are water overloaded, require treatment of the underlying condition and fluid restriction. Demeclocycline (300–600 mg bid) (which inhibits cAMP in the collecting duct, inducing nephrogenic diabetes insipidus and AVP resistance) can be used in SIADH but is slow acting and potentially nephrotoxic. Urea can also be used but is not well tolerated. Vaptans achieve free water clearance without natriuresis or kaliuresis and are well suited for the treatment of euvolaemic hyponatraemia if progress is not made with simpler measures. In hyponatraemic emergencies hypertonic saline and/or loop-diuretic is the treatment of choice and should be used as a temporary measure to make a gentle increment in serum sodium while correcting the underlying cause.
3. Patients with salt and water overload require fluid restriction, usually with loop diuretics and treatment of the underlying condition, in combination with salt restriction chronically. ADH is often inappropriately high in these conditions and vaptans have been used to promote free water clearance.

Prevention of hyponatraemia is probably under-practised given that the consequences of hyponatraemia can be so severe. It is important to ensure that hypotonic solutions are not used routinely as post-operative fluid replacement. Identification and close monitoring of high risk patients such as the elderly, institutionalized or malnourished is also sensible including checking of plasma sodium within 2 weeks of starting a thiazide or SSRI. Similarly, advising endurance athletes to avoid NSAIDs anddrink no more than 800 mL/h are all relatively straight-forward and practical approaches to consider.

Outcomes of Hyponatraemia

Hospital associated hyponatraemia is a universal and independent risk factor for worse outcome, be it worsening ascites in liver disease, readmission with heart failure, admission to ICU and ventilation, length of stay or death. In many cases this may simply be a reflection of illness but even so low sodium becomes an important biomarker for risk [8].

Hypernatraemia

Defined as a plasma, sodium of >145 mmol/L is also relatively common in the hospital setting, affecting between 1 and 5 % of hospitalized patients, and associated with very high mortality (40–75 %) when severe. It is caused by either loss of body water or, less commonly, a gain in total body sodium. Powerful protective mechanisms usually prevent hypernatraemia, and in the former scenario it is usually related to impaired thirst, reduced access to water, impaired AVP release or impaired AVP responsiveness. Consequently, the elderly, confused, debilitated, ventilated and infants are at greatest risk. A list of causes are shown in Table 9.5 and can be categorized in the same way as hyponatraemia based on EABV, but more than one cause may be in play.

Clinical Features

As with hyponatraemia, symptoms depend on the extent of the abnormality and the rate of change, and as with hyponatraemia, the brain compensates for hypernatraemia by manipulating intracellular osmolality (increasing intracellular osmolytes in this case). Again the symptoms and signs are relatively non-specific, including lethargy, muscle weakness, impaired mental ability, confusion, coma and death. Acute hypernatraemia results in osmotic shrinkage of the brain and can result in subarachnoid haemorrhage.

Assessment and Investigation of Hypernatraemia

As with hyponatraemia, hypernatraemia is usually either detected incidentally or in the investigation of a patient who has impaired mental state (Table 9.6). A carefully obtained history including changes in weights and fluid balance with emphasis on water intake, GI losses and polyuria is key. As

Table 9.6 Initial investigation of hypernatraemia

Careful history and examination	GI losses, skin losses or polyuria, history of poor water intake, excessive thirst. Is the patient hypovolaemic?
Plasma urea and electrolytes including calcium	
Plasma osmolality	
Glucose	To exclude non-ketotic hyperosmolar diabetic coma
Urine osmolality	If >600 mosmol/kg this suggests unreplaced gastrointestinal, renal or insensible water losses, sodium overload or a primary defect in thirst. If 300–600 mosmol/kg, consider the presence of an osmotic diuretic. If <300 mosmol/kg this suggests diabetes insipidus
Urine Na^+	Low urinary sodium (<20 mmol/L) suggestive of extra renal water losses/volume depletion or excessive mineralocorticoid activity, raised urinary sodium (>20 mmol/L) suggesting salt poisoning or iatrogenic sodium loading
Water deprivation test	If suspicious of diabetes insipidus (DI)
ADH levels	If suspicious of DI (low in cranial DI, normal or high in renal DI)

with hyponatraemia it is critical to determine the patient's EABV both in terms cause and management.

Water Deprivation Test

The water deprivation test is a test to distinguish diabetes insipidus from primary (psychogenic) polydipsia, and furthermore to differentiate central diabetes insipidus (CDI) vs. nephrogenic diabetes insipidus (NDI).

Water deprivation would normally cause a rise in plasma osmolality (P_{osm}), which stimulates ADH secretion from the posterior pituitary. ADH then leads to increased renal water reabsorption via aquaporin-2 water channel insertion in the distal tubule and the collecting duct. Subsequently, the urine osmolality (U_{osm}) will rise to a maximum value of 800–1,400 mosm/kg and U_{Volume} will fall to <0.5 mL/min, reflecting the maximum ADH effect on the kidney. This is reached when P_{osm} is 285–295 mosm/kg.

In individuals with defects in either ADH release (CDI) or ADH effect (NDI), their U_{osm} remains inappropriately low despite a rise in P_{osm} to levels ≥295 mosm/kg.

Test Instructions

- Patient should stop drinking 2–3 h before starting the test. Avoid overnight fluid depletion as severe hypernatreamia and dehydration may occur. Keep nil by mouth during the test.
- Measure baseline U_{osm}, P_{osm}, P_{Sodium} and body weight
- Measure U_{osm}, U_{Volume} and body weight every hour
- Measure P_{Sodium} and P_{osm} every 2 h

Stop the test once any of the following endpoints are reached:

1. U_{osm} reaches a value above 600 mosmol/kg (appropriate response).
2. Inappropriate response:
    - U_{osm} is stable on two to three successive hourly measurements despite a rising P_{osm}.
    - P_{osm} exceeds 295–300 mosmol/kg.
    - P_{Sodium} is 145 meq/L or higher.
    - Body weight falls below 97 % from baseline.

- dDAVP (desmopressin) can then be administered for further differentiation (10 mcg by nasal insufflation or 1–2 mcg intravenously), and U_{osm} and U_{Volume} are monitored every 30 min over the next 2 h. Desmopressin administration should lead to an increase in U_{osm} of at least 50 % or a significant fall in Urine Output in CDI, but will have no or only little effect in NDI.

Test Interpretation [9–11]

Condition	Urine osmolality in mosm/kg, after water deprivation	U_{osm} rise in response to dDAVP administration
Normal response	>800	No response
Primary polydipsia	>600[a]	No response
CDI	<300	>100% (complete CDI) 15–50 % (partial CDI)
NDI	<300	≤45 % (partial NDI) No response (complete NDI)

[a]Primary polydipsia will be associated with a rise in urine osmolality, usually to above 500–600 mosmol/kg, but maximum concentrating ability is frequently impaired in this disorder. This defect may be due to downregulation of the release of AVP in response to hypertonicity in those patients [12]

Test Limitations and Errors

The water restriction test has proven to establish the correct diagnosis in 80 %; however, the main limitation seems to be the differentiation between partial CDI and primary polydipsia, as some patients with partial CDI have an upregulation of ADH receptors. Those patients are polyuric at normal P_{osm}, but will be able to concentrate their urine normally when P_{osm} rises to 295. They will not respond to dDAVP administration. Hence, they may be mistakenly diagnosed with primary polydipsia.

In equivocal cases, a trial of desmopressin may be helpful as patients with partial CDI will get quick relief of polyuria, whereas patients with primary polydipsia may have some fall in urine output, but if they continue to have excessive water intake, they may develop severe hyponatraemia. Careful monitoring of P_{Sodium} is therefore advisable.

Treatment of Hypernatraemia

For the majority of patients, treatment of hypernatraemia involves defining and treating the underlying cause and then supplying adequate water. The overall water deficit can be calculated from the following formula and will give an idea of the amount of water replacement to achieve normal hydration:

$$\text{Overall water deficit} = \left(\frac{[\text{plasma Na}^+] - [\text{desired plasma Na}^+]}{[\text{desired plasma Na}^+]}\right) \times \text{TBW}$$

$$\text{TBW} = 0.6 \times \text{weight (assuming 60\% of body weight is water)}$$

where TBW total body weight.

For some, correction merely involves providing ready access to water, for the infirm it may be via NG water, 5 % dextrose or 0.45 % normal saline. Hypovolaemia should be corrected with colloid or isotonic saline. In the elderly a calculation factor of 0.5 may be used. This water deficit is not a prescription for replacement, as it does not account for on-going renal or other losses. Titration with regular measurement and clinical assessment is critical. As with hyponatraemia, rapid correction of acute (≤48 h) hypernatraemia is relatively safe but with chronic hypernatraemia rapid correction risks cerebral oedema. Correction must therefore be cautious and a maximum of 1 mmol/L/h is recommended for very acute hypernatraemia, 0.4 mmol/L/h for anything remotely chronic, with a total maximum decrease of 10 mmol/L in 24 h. In hypervolaemic hypernatraemia, diuretics (which promote salt and water excretion) may aid normalization of plasma sodium (usually requiring concomitant water and salt restriction).

Diabetes Insipidus (DI)

DI is relatively rare but can result in severe and recurrent hypernatraemia. Causes of DI are shown in Table 9.7 and can be divided into cranial (central) and nephrogenic DI. Congenital causes of cranial or pure nephrogenic DI usually present in infancy with dehydration, failure to thrive and hypernatraemia; children may give a history of drinking water from any source including puddles; polyuria typically manifests as frequency, nocturia and enuresis. Urine outputs of up to 20 L can occur (although more commonly less than this) and an important secondary feature is chronic bladder distension causing bladder dysfunction. Other genetically acquired renal diseases can also result in predominantly collecting tubule damage and usually a milder version of NDI as the disease progresses. Urine osmolality is low in the face of high plasma osmolality whereas urinary sodium is variable.

Table 9.7 Causes of diabetes insipidus

Cranial diabetes insipidus (CDI)	
Inherited/congenital	Inherited AD, very rare and resulting from mutations of AVP-NPII, carrier protein neurophysin II and its co-peptide, Wolfam syndrome (DI, DM, Optic atrophy and deafness), birth trauma
Acquired	Trauma and vascular (head injury (especially basal skull fracture), subarachnoid haemorrhage, aneurysm), surgery, especially hypophysectomy, pituitary apoplexy (Sheehan's syndrome: post-partum pituitary necrosis)
	Idiopathic
	Tumour-related: craniopharyngioma, hypothalamic lesions, metastases, lymphoma, pineal gland tumours, optic gliomas
	Granulomatous and autoimmune conditions: Sarcoidoisis, Histiocytosis-X
	Infection related: meningitis, encephalitis, cerebral abscess
Nephrogenic diabetes insipidus (NDI)	
Inherited	X-linked defect of vasopressin receptor (AVPR2 gene) (90 %), rarer still (10 %) AR mutation of aquaporin 2 gene (AQP2)
	Medullary cystic disease, juvenile nephronophthesis, ADPKD, Bartter syndrome, renal dysplasia
Acquired	Drug-induced: Lithium commonest drug cause can result in acute or chronic NDI, amphotericin-B, cidofovir, ifosfomide, demeclocycline and by definition vaptans
	Chronic hypercalcaemia, chronic hypokalaemia
	Amyloidosis, light chain disease, sickle cell disease, recurrent pyelonephritis, any cause of papillary necrosis, post-obstruction, Sjogren's syndrome
'Mixed central and nephrogenic' diabetes insipidus	Placental secretion of enzyme vasopressinase metabolizing ADH, resulting in a very rare (and spontaneously resolving) complication of third trimester with polyuria

Treatment of Diabetes Insipidus

Cranial diabetes insipidus is treatable with nasal or oral desmopressin (DDAVP). NDI is more tricky to treat, but resolving any secondary causes is important (treating hypercalcaemia and avoiding culpable medication). If it is possible to stop lithium or reduce the dose then this should be done; if not possible then amiloride may compete for lithium uptake and potentially reduce acute toxicity. A high water intake (with planning for this and toilets), low salt and modest protein diet are first line. If symptoms cannot be controlled with this then thiazide or amiloride diuretics may help induce a mild contraction of the EABV. Non-steroidal anti-inflammatory drugs can be useful for NDI and lithium induced DI.

Patients need to have a clear understanding of the condition (www.patient.co.uk/health/diabetes-insipidus), ensure that they do not take excessive amounts of fluid with DDAVP and keep a close eye on daily weights especially if unwell; a Medical alert bracelet or equivalent is very sensible.

Patients with chronic profound polyuria should have surveillance ultrasound to check for 'functional' high-pressure obstruction as well as to perform checks of renal function.

Potassium Disorders

Ninety-eight percent of total body potassium is within cells and potassium is the main intracellular cation at *~100 mmol/L*, which is why tissue necrosis can be associated with fulminant hyperkalaemia. The large gradient between intra- and extracellular compartments is actively maintained by the Na^+-K^+-ATPase. It is via the Na^+-K^+-ATPase that β_2-adrenoreceptor agonists and insulin act to shift potassium into cells, acidosis and α_1-adrenoreceptor stimulation (increased in CKD) having the opposite effect. The concentration of extracellular potassium is critical as it influences the voltage difference across cell membranes [13].

The proximal tubule is the site of reabsorption of the majority (55 %) of filtered potassium via paracellular diffusion and further reabsorption occurs via the Na^+-K^+-$2Cl^-$ co-transporter in the thick ascending limb of the loop of Henle. Potassium is also actively secreted via the ROM-K transporter. Only 10 % of filtered potassium reaches the distal convoluted tubule and cortical collecting duct where critical control of potassium secretion occurs.

Hypokalaemia

Oral intake is approximately 100 mmol/day and 95 % of potassium is excreted via the kidney, with 5 % from the colon. Hypokalaemia is relatively uncommon in healthy individuals as the kidney is able to avidly retain potassium (excreting less than 15 mmol/day). Thus, hypokalaemia, defined as serum potassium less than 3.5 mmol/L (moderate 2.5–3.0 mmol/L, severe <2.5 mmol/L), is normally the consequence of significant underlying pathology or drug use and is extremely common in hospital with up to 20 % of patients developing hypokalaemia. Mostly this relates to medication, fluid losses, fevers, malnutrition, eating disorders and potassium-lite fluid replacement [13]. Gastrointestinal losses are a common cause of hypokalaemia (and hypomagnesaemia) globally and can be fatal in severe diarrhoea, particularly in countries with limited health care. Causes of hypokalaemia are shown in Table 9.8 and are often multifactorial such as a patient with poor nutritional state on loop or thiazide diuretics who develops GI losses.

Clinically hypokalaemia (usually below 3.0 mmol/L except in those predisposed to cardiac dysrhythmias) causes mainly cardiac dysrhythmias including atrial or ventricular dysrhythmias due to increased myocardial excitability, but muscle weakness may also occur (see Appendix 1). Hypokalaemia increases renal ammonia production, predisposing to decompensation of hepatic encephalopathy. Acute and chronic hypokalaemia may cause polyuria, and previously chronic hypokalaemia was thought to cause tubulointerstitial damage, but this is somewhat controversial and may merely be an association with the primary causes of hypokalaemia.

Investigation of hypokalaemia (Table 9.9) should determine if the cause is related to redistribution secondary to intracellular uptake or to renal or extra-renal losses of potassium. Baseline tests include urea and electrolytes, magnesium and glucose, blood pH (bicarbonate), plasma and urine osmolality and urine potassium. Excessive non-renal losses from any cause (usually the GI tract) will be associated with reduced urinary excretion of potassium (<15 mmol/24 h) (or urine K^+: urine creatinine <1.5, whereas an inappropriately high urinary potassium excretion of >15 mmol/24 h) (or urine K^+: urine creatinine ratio of >1.5) suggests renal losses and is most commonly the result of kaliuretic medication or toxicity to the proximal convoluted tubule.

Urinary potassium is a useful test to discriminate between renal and non-renal losses: a level of <15 mmol/day is suggestive of extra-renal losses, the fractional excretion of potassium (FE_{K+}) or transtubular potassium gradient (TTKG) should both be <2 % in the presence of hypokalaemia of extra-renal origin.

In the context of a renal cause of hypokalaemia, hypertension suggests either hyperaldosteronism or mineralocorticoid excess such as accelerated phase hypertension, renal artery stenosis, Conn's, glucocorticoid remediable aldosteronism (GRA) or causes of mineralocorticoid excess such as Cushing's syndrome. Urinary chloride will be useful with

Table 9.8 Causes of hypokalaemia

Reduced total body potassium	
Deficient intake	Rare on Western diet but seen in alcoholics, elderly and those with wasting disease such as cancer, may predispose to re-feeding hypokalaemia
Extrarenal losses (low urine potassium (<15 mmol/day))	Chronic or severe acute diarrhoea, laxatives, gastrointestinal and biliary drains, sweating, vomiting[a] (NB secondary hyperaldosteronism and alkalosis in this setting cause predominantly renal losses of potassium)
Renal losses (high urine potassium)	*Drugs*: Diuretics (loop and thiazide (hypokalaemia more common in women on thiazide)) (potent synergistic effect of loop and thiazide in combination), mineralocorticoid and glucocorticoids, medication causing proximal tubular injury, e.g. aminoglycosides, amphotericin-B, cisplatin. Excess licorice *Primary hyper-reninaemia* (high renin and aldosterone) Malignant hypertension, renal artery stenosis, coarctation, renin secreting tumour, Page kidney *Primary hyperaldosteronism* (low renin, high aldosterone) Conn syndrome, adrenal hyperplasia, glucocorticoid remediable aldosteronism (GRA) *Excess mineralocorticoid activity* Cushing's syndrome, congenital adrenal hyperplasia, apparent mineralocorticoid excess, exogenous mineralocorticoid, licorice *Increased delivery of sodium or non-reabsorbable ions to distal nephron* Diuretics proximal to connecting tubule and cortical collecting duct (see above), magnesium deficiency, Bartter and Gitelman syndrome, Liddle syndrome, chronic metabolic acidosis including proximal and distal RTA, Fanconi syndrome, ketoacidosis, starvation
Redistributive hypokalaemia	Hyperinsulinaemia, alkalosis, increased beta-adrenergic receptor, alkalosis activation (stress response or the use of beta agonists for chronic airwasy disease)
Miscellaneous	Rapid uptake with correction of B12 deficiency, hypokalaemic periodic paralysis, hypothermia, thyrotoxicosis. Overdose of chloroquine, respiridone, quetiapine, barium and caesium
Pseudohypokalaemia	Massive leucocytosis (usually chronic leukaemias) (can be avoided by rapid separation of cells from plasma), artifactual hypokalaemia from drip-arm or poorly flushed central line.

[a]Vomiting can be associated with high urinary potassium because of secondary hyperaldosteronism

Table 9.9 Investigations of hypokalaemia

History	GI losses, laxatives, diuretics, medication
Examination	EABV, blood pressure, evidence of Cushing's syndrome or macrovascular disease suggestive of RAS, nutritional state
Urea, electrolytes, bicarbonate, osmolality, magnesium	
Urine potassium	*Extra-renal* <15 mmol/day or urine K^+:urine creatinine <1.5 *Renal* >15 mmol/day or urine K^+:urine creatinine >1.5
Fractional excretion of potassium: FE_{K+} = (Urine K^+ × Plasma Creatinine/Plasma K^+ × Urine Creatinine) × 100	
Transtubular potassium gradient (TTKG) = (Urine K^+ × Plasma osmol)/(Plasma K^+ × Urine osmol)	
Urinary chloride	*Low* gastric losses, non-resorbable anions, *High* diuretics, Gitelman, Bartter syndrome, magnesium deficiency
Urinary pH	Alkaline urine with acidosis; RTA
Renin:Aldosterone	See Table 9.8
Specialist endocrine tests	
Urine laxative and diuretic screen	If suspicion of illicit use

gastric losses and non-reabsorbable anions, high with diuretics, magnesium deficiency, Bartter and Gitelman syndromes. Urine diuretic screen and laxative screen can also be useful particularly if hypokalaemia is intermittent.

Non-specific tubular interstitial damage may cause hypokalaemia usually in association with hypovolaemia and secondary (appropriate) hyperaldosteronism. Distal renal tubular acidosis is covered in this chapter, but hypokalaemia is then associated with hyperchloraemic acidosis (measure serum bicarbonate and urine pH). Some rare renal conditions causing hypokalaemia are discussed here.

Some Specific Conditions Causing Hypokalaemia

Bartter and Gitelman syndromes (BS and GS) are rare, inherited tubulopathies characterized by hypokalaemic metabolic alkalosis and hyper-reninaemic hyperaldosteronism.

Bartter Syndrome

BS results from mutations of one of a number of transporters necessary for the proper functioning of the sodium potassium chloride co-transporter (NKCC2) in the thick ascending limb of the loop of Henle. This results in disruption of the normal water reabsorbing function of the loop, and severe salt and water loss. Due to volume depletion they have aggressive activation of their renin–angotensin–aldosterone system (RAAS) and thus hyperaldosteronism. This results in a metabolic alkalosis and hypokalaemia, which may be severe and usually has a more severe phenotype with lower potassium levels than GS. NKCC2 is the pharmacologic target of loop diuretics and the biochemical features of Bartter are the same as those found with loop diuretic administration.

Given the variety of different genes that can be involved, the phenotype is quite variable, but patients usually present in infancy with failure to thrive and dehydration but unlike GS polyhydramnios may be present on antenatal screening. Muscle cramps, polydipsia, polyuria, enuresis and salt craving are typical.

There is no curative treatment, and treatment is oral replacement of electrolyte losses with oral potassium and magnesium supplementation, as required. Angiotensin converting enzyme inhibition, angiotensin receptor blockade, aldosterone antagonists and potassium sparing diuretics can be helpful in maintaining safe potassium levels. Non-steroidal anti-inflammatory drugs may also help to increase serum potassium and reduce salt and water loss, via prostaglandin inhibition and reduction of the GFR. In practical terms, management of BS (and GS) can be challenging, as it involves titrating large quantities of tablets in children and adults for an indefinite period. Periods of non-compliance and intercurrent illness are not uncommon.

Gitelman Syndrome

Gitelman syndrome is an autosomal recessive condition, with a prevalence of 25 per million population, making it one of the commonest inherited tubular disorders. Gitelman syndrome results from inactivating mutations (of which there are many reported) of the SLC12A3 gene encoding for the thiazide-sensitive sodium chloride cotransporter (NCC) in the distal convoluted tubule. As this is distal to the loop, it leaves the free water absorbing mechanism of the loop functional, and the salt and water loss in Gitelman is much less pronounced than in Bartter and hypokalaemia is typically milder. Again, there is activation of the RAAS and subsequent hyperaldosteronism, causing a metabolic alkalosis and hypokalaemia. Hypomagnesaemia is frequently present and may also be severe.

Patients usually present in late childhood or early adulthood with a coincident illness during which routine blood tests reveal hypokalaemia but the clinical manifestations are highly variable between families. Clinical features relate to the metabolic upset and include muscle weakness, cramps (often exercise intolerance), tetany, paraesthesia, nocturia, thirst, salt craving, abdominal pain, chondrocalcinosis and growth retardation may also occur. Blood pressure is often normal or low.

Gitelman patients are often referred to nephrologists with marked hypokalaemia but also have hypomagnesaemia and hypocalciuria, unlike Bartter patients. Thiazide diuretics mimic exactly the effect of the mutation, and therefore thiazide abuse (as well as laxative abuse) mimics the condition (easily excluded by toxicology screens *if* done at the right time). Joint X-rays may show chondrocalcinosis.

There is no specific treatment and therapy relies on oral salt replacement, with oral potassium and magnesium supplementation; this is often a considerable burden of tablets, and gastrointestinal disturbance can rapidly cause hypokalaemia, so patients need to be counselled on this and the importance of seeking medical aid early.

Liddle Syndrome

Liddle syndrome is an extremely rare autosomal dominant condition caused by mutations of the epithelial sodium channel (ENaC) causing it to be overactive. ENaC is normally activated by aldosterone, so Liddle mimics hyperaldosteronism, causing hypertension (which may be severe), metabolic alkalosis, low renin, hypokalaemia and unlike Conn syndrome characteristically normal or low aldosterone levels. Presentation is usually in childhood. Treatment is with a low salt diet and amiloride, which is a specific inhibitor of ENaC. Spironolactone is ineffective as aldosterone is suppressed.

Fanconi Syndromes

The Fanconi syndromes (FS) are inherited or acquired syndromes of generalized proximal tubular dysfunction, causing low molecular weight proteinuria, aminoaciduria, phosphaturia, uricosuria, glycosuria and bicarbonaturia. Bicarbonate is usually reabsorbed by the proximal tubular cells, but can be less efficiently absorbed in the loop. This means that, as bicarbonate is freely filtered, when bicarbonate falls below approximately 14 mmol/L, it will all be absorbed from the filtrate and disappear from the urine. Bicarbonate is not reabsorbed in the collecting duct, and remains in the lumen. As it is an anion, this makes the lumen more electronegative, favouring the secretion of positive potassium ions into the lumen. Thus, Fanconi will cause hypokalaemia only when there is bicarbonate in the urine, e.g. when it first develops, or when the Fanconi is treated with enough bicarbonate supplements to increase the serum bicarbonate enough to cause bicarbonaturia.

Clinical features relate to the metabolic impact and include polyuria, polydipsia, muscle weakness, hypophospataemic rickets (in children) or osteomalacia (in adults) due to phosphate depletion. Severely affected children fail to thrive but lesser involvement may be clinically silent.

Table 9.10 Causes of Fanconi syndrome

Genetic	*Cystinosis, Wilson's disease, Lowe's (X-linked) (oculocerebral syndrome), Dent's disease (X-linked), tyrosinaemia (type 1), galactosaemia, glycogen storage diseases, hereditary fructose intolerance, mitochondrial disorders*
Acquired	*Heavy metals*: arsenic, lead, mercury and cadmium poisoning/toxicity
	Drugs: tenofovir, adefovir, aminoglycosides, ifosfamide
	Light chain diseases: amyloid, multiple myeloma, light chain deposition disease
	Interstitial Nephritis: Sjogren's syndrome, other causes of interstitial nephritis

The causes of inherited and acquired FS are shown in Table 9.10. The diagnosis of FS is usually made by demonstrating a combination of hyperchloraemic metabolic acidosis, hypokalaemia, hypophosphataemia and hypouricaemia with evidence of inappropriate urine losses of phosphate, potassium, bicarbonate and aminoaciduria. Glycosuria in the face of normal serum glucose is suggestive and a cheap screening test but may be negative. Depending on the cause there is often low molecular weight tubular proteinuria (retinol binding protein, β2 microglobulin, α1 macroglobulin). The cause of FS needs to be established and treatable secondary causes excluded.

The treatment of FS is to treat the underlying condition where possible (for example remove potential drug causes, and treatment of plasma cell dyscrasia). Otherwise treatment is to replace bicarbonate, phosphate, vitamin D and if necessary potassium, aiming for a bicarbonate above 20 mmol/L and a potassium >3 mmol/L.

Dent's Disease

It comprises a heterogenous group of rare X-linked proximal tubulopathies associated with nephrolithiasis, nephrocalcinosis (75 %), hypercalciuria (95 %), hypophosphataemia and low molecular weight proteinuria. It results from mutations in CLCNS (encoding for the Chloride/Hydrogen exchanger) in Dent's disease-1 or mutations in OCRL-1 encoding for phosphatidylinositol bisphosphate 5-phosphatase in Dent's disease-2. As yet there is no clear genotype:phenotype correlation, and there is considerable variation between families; some patients presenting with incomplete FS and low molecular weight proteinuria may be the only clue.

Clinical features are proximal tubular dysfunction, Fanconi syndrome, hypercalciuria, nephrocalcinosis and low molecular weight proteinuria (beta 2 microglobulin, retinol binding protein). Detection of low molecular weight proteinuria can be a useful screening test in female carriers. Dent's disease is one of the few causes of nephrocalcinosis associated with end-stage renal disease, and 30–80 % of affected males require renal replacement therapy between the third and fifth decades of life; thus, it is an important (albeit rare) cause of unexplained renal failure. Renal transplantation is curative.

Lowe Syndrome

It is a very rare (estimated at roughly one in a million) X-linked oculocerebrorenal syndrome with a similar renal phenotype to Dent's disease, also resulting from mutations of the OCRL gene encoding the PIP phosphatase involved in endosomal trafficking. Aside from a relatively mild FS and metabolic acidosis, male patients develop severe cataracts antenatally, glaucoma is common and visual deficit almost universal. Hypotonia results in severe motor developmental delay, and scoliosis is common, often resulting in chest infections. Severe hypophosphataemia may result in rickets. Although rare, this condition is relevant to adult nephrologists as patients may live to middle age, often have complex needs and patients have been successfully transplanted [14].

Glucocorticoid Remedial Hyperaldosteronism

Glucocorticoid remedial hyperaldosteronism (or type 1 familial hyperaldosteronism) is a rare autosomal dominant disease caused by a mutation resulting in a chimeric CYP11B1/CYP11B2 gene. This causes aldosterone synthetase (in the zona glomerulosa of the adrenal cortex) to become sensitive to ACTH and inappropriately upregulated. A happy consequence of this is that it also becomes suppressible by physiological doses of glucocorticoid. As this is a condition of hyperaldosteronism, there is hypertension, metabolic alkalosis and hypokalaemia. Clinical features include fatigue, headaches, muscle cramps, polyuria and consequent polydipsia. The condition is usually diagnosed in childhood or adolescence as part of the investigation of secondary hypertension.

Apparent Mineralocorticoid Excess

This is a rare autosomal recessive syndrome of juvenile hypertension associated with metabolic alkalosis and hypokalaemia but with a low serum aldosterone. It is caused by mutations in the HSD11B2 gene encoding for 11β-hydroxysteroid dehydrogenase type 2. This enzyme normally converts cortisol to cortisone (temporary inhibition of 11β-hydroxysteroid dehydrogenase type 2 is how excessive liquorice is thought to cause hypertension). This conversion is important as cortisol activates the mineralocorticoid receptor as powerfully as aldosterone, and the plasma cortisol

Table 9.11 Causes of pseudohyperkalaemia

Sample taking and processing:	Traumatic venesection with red blood cell lysis or sample squirted through needle into bottle
	Contamination with anticoagulant from another sample (potassium EDTA)
	Increased release from muscles during venesection (excessive hand clenching, prolonged tourniquet time)
	Cell death during long delay/storage prior to analysis (more common with out-of-hospital samples)
Predisposing medical conditions:	Marked leucocytosis such as chronic leukaemias
	Thrombocytosis
	Hereditary and acquired red cell disorders predisposing to cell lysis including familial pseudohyperkalaemia

concentration is orders of magnitude higher than aldosterone. AME is also glucocorticoid responsive and may be treated with dexamethasone, which suppresses endogenous cortisol production without stimulating the mineralocorticoid receptor, or by inhibiting ENaC using amiloride, or the receptor itself with eplenerone or spironolactone. AME, secondary to excess liquorice ingestion, just requires a little more restraint in the confectionary department.

Treatment of Hypokalaemia

As most potassium is intracellular, low serum potassium often represents a profound deficit in total body potassium, potassium levels of <3.0 and <2.0 representing deficits of ~200 and 300 mmol of potassium, respectively [13], and thus it may take several days to become replete.

In hypokalaemic emergencies (such as arrhythmia), IV potassium is helpful, especially when depletion is severe or when oral intake is insufficient or unreliable. Intravenous potassium chloride may be given peripherally in normal saline or 5 % dextrose at a rate of up to 10 mmol/h. The risk of phlebitis limits the peripheral route for faster rates than this, whereas rates of up to 40 mmol/h are felt to be safe via a central line with high dependency cardiac (and potassium) monitoring [15].

Potassium may be given orally as potassium chloride and potassium citrate, titrated against response with the caveat that effervescent potassium is poorly tolerated in large amounts (dose should be split) and slow-release potassium has the nasty habit of accumulating before absorption and causing oesophageal ulcers if taken before bed. Treating the underlying causes, be they extrarenal or renal in origin, is obviously important as is correcting any concomitant hypomagnesaemia. In chronic potassium wasting conditions (such as Gitelman, Bartter and renal Fanconi syndrome, syndromes of mineralocorticoid excess or diuretic dependence), other strategies including the use of ACE inhibitors and the potassium sparing diuretics amiloride and spironolactone may need to be considered.

Hyperkalaemia

Hyperkalaemia (>5 mmol/L) is relatively uncommon in the general population, but relatively common in patients with renal disease or who are taking drugs which limit renal excretion. The efficacy of renin:angiotensin blockade in proteinuric renal disease and cardiac failure has resulted in 'clinic hyperkalaemia' being a frequent occurrence. Values of more than 6.0 mmol/L are viewed as medical emergencies while values greater than 6.5 mmol/L are genuinely life threatening, although patients with CKD and chronically high total potassium seem to tolerate higher levels.

Pseudohyperkalaemia is where there is a red cell leak of potassium in extracted blood. This can be due to direct haemolysis (from the collection process) or red cell leakage (haematological disease, infectious mononucleosis or inherited red cell membrane abnormalities); see Table 9.11.

Causes of Hyperkalaemia

Causes of hyperkalaemia are shown in Table 9.12, but reduced GFR is a key risk factor as are drugs that reduce renal potassium excretion, and dietary excess only really comes into play if a patient is predisposed by reduced renal excretion. Less common are endocrine causes of reduced urinary potassium loss such as mineralocorticoid deficiency (Addison's disease) (resulting in aldosterone deficiency) or pseudohypoaldosteronism (aldosterone resistance), and as with hypokalaemia, redistributive shifts between ECF and ICF can result in significant changes in serum levels.

Assessment and Investigation of Hyperkalaemia

As always, a thorough clinical assessment, including drug (ideally seeing the medication) and dietary history as well as volume status, is essential, but an ECG takes precedence in the setting of severe hyperkalaemia as this will establish whether the patient is at imminent risk of life-threatening bradycardia, asystole and death (see Appendix 1). Pseudohyperkalaemia should be excluded in unexpectedly hyperkalaemic patients, particularly in the absence of ECG changes (see Table 9.11). Here a fresh sample should be rapidly spun and separated (avoiding haemolysis or ongoing red cell potassium leakage).

Initial investigations should include: urea, creatnine and electrolytes, glucose, bicarbonate (acid–base status) and urinary potassium (see below) lactate dehydrogenase if

Table 9.12 Causes of hyperkalaemia

Reduced renal loss (low urinary potassium)	*Drugs*: Angiotensin converting enzyme inhibitors (ACEi), angiotensin receptor antagonists (ARBs), beta-blockers, aldosterone receptor antagonists (spironolactone, eplerone), potassium sparing diuretics (amiloride, triamterene), calcineurin inhibitors (CNIs), trimethoprim, non-steroidal anti-inflammatory drugs (NSAIDs), heparin *Endocrine*: Addison's disease (aldosterone/mineralocorticoid deficiency), some forms of congenital adrenal hyperplasia *Renal*: Most causes of reduced GFR, Type I renal tubular acidosis and Type IV renal tubular acidosis, Gordon's syndrome (pseudohypoaldosteronism type II)
Excessive production	Rhabdomyolysis, intravascular haemolysis, massive transfusion (especially incompatible transfusion), tumour lysis syndrome, significant tissue infarction (especially in case of impaired renal function), severe exercise
Redistributive	Acidosis, beta-blockade, insulin deficiency, digoxin toxicity, suxamethonium muscle relaxant, hyperkalaemic periodic paralysis
Reduced non-renal losses	Rarely clinically relevant but constipation can worsen hyperkalaemia in patients with reduced GFR
Excessive intake	Only usually relevant in context of reduced renal excretion (but becomes a common, and avoidable cause in patients with ESRD or supplemented patients with AKI), the notable exception being lethal injection. Lo-salt condiment has high levels of potassium and is not suitable for patients with reduced GFR
Pseudohyperkalaemia	See Table 9.11

haemolysis or infarction are a possibility, cortisol, renin and aldosterone where the cause is not otherwise clear.

Twenty-four hours urinary potassium excretion is the gold standard and will differentiate renal from non-renal hyperkalaemia; <20 mmol/24 h, in the face of hyperkalaemia suggests a problem with renal excretion. Alternatively, and more conveniently, potassium excretion can be assessed using the transtubular potassium gradient (TTKG) from a spot urinary potassium, while correcting for variations in urine concentration due to water reclamation.

$$\text{TTKG} = \left(\frac{\text{urine potassium} \times \text{serum osmolarity}}{\text{serum potassium} \times \text{urine osmolarity}} \right).$$

A value of less than five in the face of hyperkalaemia is abnormal, while a value of >7 is considered appropriate (unreliable with a very dilute urine or urinary sodium >25 meq/L) [16]. If renal potassium excretion is reduced, in the face of a normal GFR, the patient must then be investigated for hypoaldosteronism or aldosterone resistance.

Gordon's syndrome pseudohypoaldosteronism (type II) is a rare inherited mutation of WNK1, WNK4, CUL3 or KLHL3 genes resulting in gain of function of the thiazide-sensitive sodium-chloride co-transporter (NCC) which is inhibited in Gitelman syndrome. This results in excess sodium and chloride retention, hyperkalaemia, hyperchloraemic metabolic acidosis and low renin, low aldosterone hypertension which can become severe by the third decade. The diagnosis is usually difficult, and patients are often investigated for difficult hypertension or hyperkalaemia for a long time before this is made. Urinary potassium excretion is inappropriately low (fractional excretion or TTKG); renin and aldosterone will also tend to be low. Genotyping may be available at specialist centres. Treatment is with thiazide diuretic (which often totally resolves the hypertension and hyperkalaemia) and a low salt diet.

Management of Hyperkalaemia

The management of hyperkalaemia (Table 9.13) is dependent on the degree of hyperkalaemia and the presence or absence of ECG changes.

It is critical to emphasize to junior medical staff the reducing plasma potassium by redistribution is just a temporary measure. It is essential to initiate treatment that will reduce total body potassium to avoid recurrent hyperkalaemia. Moreover, it needs to be made clear that in an oliguric, hyperkalaemic patient with AKI or ESRD, early plans need to be made for renal replacement therapy unless there is a rapidly reversible element.

Calcium Disorders

The most abundant mineral in the body, the majority of total body calcium is stored in the skeleton with the remainder overwhelmingly intracellular, where its effects are regulated by calmodulin. Extracellular calcium is either protein bound, ionized (the active form) or complexed with phosphate, citrate, bicarbonate or sulphate. Total body calcium is closely regulated and determined by the balance of gut uptake and renal excretion with the skeleton being a large reservoir (see Chap. 50) [17].

Table 9.13 Treatment of hyperkalaemia

Cardiac stabilization	If ECG changes present, then IV *calcium gluconate* 10 mL of 10 % instant effect, can be repeated
Redistribution (combination treatment more effective)	*Insulin and dextrose*: 50 mL of 50 % dextrose with 10 units of insulin IV effect with 15 min, effect lasting for about 4 h *Beta$_2$-agonists*: Nebulized but high dose required, e.g. salbutamol 10–20 mg (drop in K^+ by 0.6 and 0.85 mmol/L) *Correction of acidosis*: with bicarbonate both redistributes potassium and can lead to sustained reduction in the setting of CKD with chronic acidosis
Reduce/stop intake	Stop supplements and dietary excess (consider dietary review)
Stop/suspend/reduce potassium sparing medication	ACEI, ARB, aldosterone antagonists, NSAID, trimethoprim, heparin, CNIs
Lowering total body potassium:	
1. Renal losses	*Diuresis*: Loop diuretics (plus or minus thiazides in case of poor renal function), thiazides for CNI-induced hyperkalaemia *Mineralocorticoid*: Fludrocortisone, for patients with adrenal insufficiency supplementing hydrocortisone and fludrocortisone
2. Gastrointestinal losses	*Binders*: For example, calcium resonium, very limited evidence (should be given with laxatives which may be more effective than resins) *Laxatives*: An important and under-used method of reducing total body potassium in a tight corner (NB: ensure the laxative does not contain potassium)
3. Renal replacement therapy	*Haemofiltration, haemodialysis or acute peritoneal dialysis* highly effective at reducing total body potassium

Most calcium assays measure total (bound and unbound) calcium correcting for albumin levels using the following formula:

$$\text{Adjcalmmol} / \text{L} = \text{mscmmol} / \text{L} + 0.02 \times 40 - \text{sag} / \text{L}$$

This becomes inaccurate if the patient is very acidotic, with paraproteinaemia and at extremes of albumin. It is changes in ionized calcium that are most clinically significant and this can be obtained via blood gas analyzers, although in practical terms most of the diagnosis and decisions are made on the corrected calcium.

Hypercalcaemia

Hypercalcaemia (corrected calcium of >2.6 mmol/L) is a relatively common disorder, affecting around 1 % of the population, often with chronically, mildly elevated levels but occasionally presenting with severe hypercalcaemia (≥3.5 mmol/L) and life threateningly high levels, sometimes involving nephrology intervention, or at levels precipitating AKI.

Causes of Hypercalcaemia

The causes of hypercalcaemia are shown in Table 9.14, with malignancy and primary hyperparathyroidism being the causes in over 90 % of cases. Malignancy can cause hypercalcaemia in a variety of ways in part through the production of PTH-related protein (PTHrP) (typically through solid malignancies with metastases, classically breast and squamous cell carcinoma). Alternative mechanisms include malignancy associated cytokine release (IL-6, IL-1, TGF-β), direct bone involvement, prolonged immobility and increased macrophage production of 1,25 $(OH)_2$ vitamin D with some haematological malignancies.

Clinical Features of Hypercalcaemia

Non-specific symptoms such as malaise, anorexia, nausea and vomiting, depression and lethargy often predominate and may be subtle if the hypercalcaemia is not severe and particularly if chronic as with primary hyperparathyroidism. Renal effects include polyuria, thirst, renal failure, nephrocalcinosis and kidney stones (most commonly associated with primary hyperparathyroidism as chronic). Bone pain is common but often non-specific; however, worsening bone pain in known malignancy should provoke a calcium check. Pruritis and conjunctivitis may also occur. Neurological complications include depression, inability to concentrate, confusion, reduced neural excitability resulting in neurological depression, ataxia, upper motor neurone signs and (in severe cases) coma as well as reduced smooth and striated muscle movement. Constipation is a common feature in part due to reduced smooth muscle activity, hypercalcaemia induces increased gastrin secretion and peptic ulcers can occur as can pancreatitis. Cardiotoxicity may occur in severe hypercalcaemia with ECG changes including short QT interval and ST changes mimicking acute coronary syndrome (see Appendix 1).

Table 9.14 Causes of hypercalcaemia

Malignancy	PTHrP (squamous cell carcinoma, breast malignancy), pro-inflammatory cytokine release, immobilization, direct bone involvement (multiple myeloma), increased synthesis of 1,25 $(OH)_2$ vitamin D (lymphoma)
Hyperparathyroidism	
Primary	85 % single adenoma > primary hyperplasia, MEN, parathyroid carcinoma
Tertiary	Exacerbated by high doses of vitamin D, aluminium intoxication and adynamic bone disease
Granulomatous diseases	Classically TB and sarcoidosis but potentially any chronic inflammatory process involving accumulation of macrophages (sometimes unmasked by vitamin D supplementation)
Vitamin D intoxication	Hypervitaminosis D, food faddists but not uncommon iatrogenic cause in patients with CKD on large doses of supplements
Vitamin A intoxication	
Aluminium intoxication	
Medication	Thiazides, lithium, excess antacid ingestions (milk-alkali syndrome)
Endocrine causes	Addison's disease, acromegaly, hyperthyroidism, phaechromocytoma
Familial hypocalciuric hypercalcaemia	Secondary to calcium sensing receptor mutations
Prolonged immobilization	Unusual as a sole cause; Paget's disease only causes hypercalcaemia in the immobile patients
Recovery phase of Rhabdomyolysis	Hypercalcaemia 1–2 weeks post AKI may be the only clue as to the aetiology of missed rhabdomyolysis

MEN multiple endocrine neoplasia

Assessment and Investigation of Hypercalcaemia

A history of long-standing symptoms, especially stones, is suggestive of primary hyperparathyroidism, whereas constitutional symptoms of malignancy may suggest this as a primary cause (although symptoms of hypercalcaemia may mimic neoplasia). Rarely there may be a family history of MEN or familial hypocalciuric hypercalcaemia. Examination may reveal signs of malignancy, granulomatous conditions, an underlying endocrine cause or very rarely (but very satisfyingly) corneal calcification. As with all electrolyte disorders, volume status needs to be assessed. Blood tests should include PTH level, alkaline phosphatase, phosphate, albumin, total proteins and renal function (magnesium and potassium will be important for subsequent management). In general, hyperparathyroid patients have inappropriately high PTH and a low phosphate. In such cases parathyroid ultrasound and radioisotope scanning may be performed. If the PTH is not suppressed in the face of hypercalcaemia, then the patient has primary or tertiary hyperparathyroidism (the caveat being that some patients have this *and* a secondary cause such as malignancy). If the PTH is suppressed then a more detailed assessment of secondary causes is warranted, e.g. serum ACE (unhelpful if on ACEI), 25 (OH) vitamin D and 1,25 (OH) vitamin D levels, paraproteins, Bence Jones proteinuria, protein electrophoresis and immunofixation, chest X-ray and, where appropriate, further imaging with mammogram, CT scanning or gallium. An ECG is necessary to exclude any electrophysiological changes.

Treatment of Hypercalcaemia

The treatment of hypercalcaemia is directed at restoring intravascular volume and treating the underlying cause; see NICE guidance [18]. Severe and symptomatic hypercalcaemia requires urgent corrective therapy with most agreeing that a calcium above 3.0 mmol/L requires admission and urgent correction. Cessation of contributing medication (antacids, thiazides, lithium, vitamin D supplements) is appropriate. Volume expansion with normal saline promotes a diuresis and is calciuric; in fact anything promoting a natriuresis promotes calciuresis. Once euvolaemia has been achieved, saline may be given in tandem with intravenous or oral loop diuretics, promoting renal losses further. In hypercalcaemia due to sarcoidosis, other granulomatous disease, vitamin D intoxication and some malignancies, prednisolone therapy is effective and of course is part of the treatment of adrenal insufficiency. Bisphosphonates can be given to inhibit bone resorption, although they are relatively contraindicated in patients with GFR <30, and a judgement call needs to be made on the risk benefit in patients with severe hypercalcaemia and low GFR. Subcutaneous calcitonin also blocks bone resorption and increases urinary calcium excretion by inhibiting calcium reabsorption and can be useful in severe acute hypercalcaemia.

The calcimimetic agent cinacalcet has been shown to lower calcium in hyperparathyroidism related to reduced GFR, although surgical parathyroidectomy remains the standard UK approach in the absence of contraindications to surgery and occasionally should be considered as an urgent procedure. Finally severe hypercalcaemia around 4 mmol/L or above (lower if ECG changes) may be better treated by acute renal replacement therapy (highly effective at acutely reducing calcium) especially if the patient has significant AKI or CKD.

Table 9.15 Causes of hypocalcaemia

High PTH	*Renal failure* (falling 1α (OH) vitamin D and rising phosphate) *25 (OH) Vitamin D deficiency* (reduced ultra violet exposure, short-bowel syndromes, malabsorption, liver disease) *Pseudohypoparathyroidism* Resistance to PTH (Albright hereditary osteodystrophy (type 1a) short fourth and fifth metacarpals and round facies)
Low/normal PTH	*Magnesium deficiency (severe)* (lowers PTH secretion and end-organ resistance) *Hypoparathyroidism*: Post-operative parathyroidectomy (acute 'Hungry bones') (chronic PTH deficiency with removal of all four glands), post-operative (thyroidectomy/neck trauma), infiltrative malignancy, autoimmune (including part of polyglandular syndrome-1), haemochromatosis, Di George syndrome (thymic aplasia and absent parathyroid glands), Barakat (HDR) syndrome (hypoparathyroidism, sensorineural deafness and renal disease (dysplasia, reflux, cystic)), idiopathic hypoparathyroidism
Hyperphosphataemia	Rhabdomyolysis (acutely), tumour lysis syndrome, phosphate supplements (including phosphate enemas in patients with advanced renal impairment)
Medication	Cinacalcet, bisphosphonates, loop diuretics, proton pump inhibitors, cisplatin, phenobarbitone, phenytoin
Miscellaneous	Acute pancreatitis, burns, sepsis, massive transfusion
Artifactual	Low albumin (correction for serum albumin or ionized calcium give true status)
Redistributive	Alkalosis (e.g. hyperventilation)

Hypocalcaemia

Hypocalcaemia (corrected calcium <2.1 mmol/L) is less common than hypercalcaemia but familiar to nephrologists in the setting of CKD and nutritional deficiency and very common among hospital inpatients. Severe hypocalcaemia (<1.75 mmol/L) can have life-threatening consequences in terms of seizures and cardiac arrhythmias.

Causes of Hypocalcaemia

The commonest cause of hypocalcaemia is artifactual and relates to a low serum albumin, the corrected calcium and ionized calcium should be normal if no deficiency. Parathyroid hormone level (PTH) can be useful in dividing possible aetiologies, especially if chronic, but may be less discriminatory in acute illness such as burns or pancreatitis. Beyond renal disease as a cause of hypocalcaemia, vitamin D deficiency is epidemic and may be a contributing factor with other causes of hypocalcaemia (see Table 9.15). 'Hungry bone syndrome' is worth special mention as it occurs in renal practice following parathyroidectomy in patients with tertiary hyperparathyroidism and can result in life-threatening hypocalcaemia. It results from reduced bone resorption, a marked influx of calcium into calcium depleted bones, and reduced calcium absorption from the gut secondary to a fall in PTH. Advanced age, hypomagnesaemia, vitamin D deficiency and size of the gland removed are risk factors, but it is largely dependent on how severe the parathyroid bone disease is [19] and occurs in 25–90 % of those patients with radiological evidence of hyperparathyroidism compared to only 0–6 % of those without radiological change.

Clinical Features of Hypocalcaemia

Perioral paraesthesia and numbness, dystonia, bronchospasm, laryngospasm, seizures, tetany, and respiratory arrest are well known neuromuscular features of severe hypocalcaemia. Prolonged QTc, heart block and flat T waves, reduced PR interval and U waves, Torsades de pointes and ventricular fibrillation are cardiovascular sequelae (see Appendix 1). Chronic hypocalcaemia may be associated with rickets and/or osteodystrophy, basal ganglia calcification, poor dentition and cataracts. More moderate hypocalcaemia may also be associated with more subtle symptoms chronically such as depression, irritability, muscle cramps and dementia. Chvostek's sign (ipsilateral facial muscle contraction on tapping of the facial nerve) and Trousseau's sign (hand and wrist flexion on inflating a blood pressure cuff above systolic blood pressure) may confirm a clinical suspicion of significant hypocalcaemia.

Investigation of Hypocalcaemia

Albumin, total protein and bicarbonate help confirm genuine hypocalcaemia. PTH, vitamin D, phosphate, renal function and magnesium are useful first line tests. Checking serum amylase, creatine kinase and exclusion of malabsorption and liver disease may be helpful if there is no obvious cause. Osteomalacia may be apparent on X-rays. The presence of a low PTH in the absence of surgical removal requires further investigation (see Table 9.15).

Treatment of Hypocalcaemia

Treatment depends largely on the underlying cause, but acute symptomatic hypocalcaemia should be treated with intravenous calcium (e.g. 10 % calcium gluconate) which may need repeat doses or an infusion, for example in the setting of 'hungry bone syndrome'. Hungry bone syndrome tends to cause a nadir of calcium at 2–4 days post-operatively but may continue for a significantly longer period. IV calcium supplements are often necessary initially before transferring to oral calcium (often calcium carbonate but taken *after* meals to avoid reducing phosphate) at doses of 6–12 g/day may be required. Correction of magnesium is important, and large doses of 1,25 (OH) vitamin D are necessary. Pre-treatment with high doses of vitamin D pre-surgery

Table 9.16 Causes of hypophosphataemia

Renal	
Inherited phosphate wasting disorders	Autosomal dominant hypophosphataemic rickets (via impaired metabolism of FGF-23), (variable age of presentation, may appear in early adulthood), autosomal recessive hypophosphataemic rickets (dentin matrix protein-1 (DMP1) via impaired inhibition of FGF-23), X-linked hypophosphataemic rickets (phosphate regulating endopeptidase (PHEX) mutation via FGF-23), childhood rickets and inappropriately low or normal vitamin D
	Hereditary hypophosphataemic rickets with hypercalciuria (defect of NaPi2 co-transporter, increased vitamin D levels and risk of stones)
Proximal tubular disorders	Fanconi syndrome (see Table 9.10), Dent's disease, cystinosis
Medication/drugs	Diuretics (acetazolamide, loop and thiazide diuretics), cisplatin, ifosfamide, tetracyclines, aminoglycosides, tenofovir, adefovir, imatinib, streptozocin, toluene, mannitol (pseudohypophosphataemia), IV iron maltose
Post-transplant	FGF-23 mediated, usually short term
Tumour-induced osteomalacia (TIO)	Mostly benign mesenchymal tumours via FGF-23
Fibrodysplasia	May be associated with endocrine abnormalities and café au lait spots in McCune–Albright syndrome (facial or long bone asymmetry)
Hyperparathyroidism/vitamin D deficiency	Reduced sodium:phosphate co-transporter expression
Gastrointestinal	Malnutrition from any cause, chronic alcoholism (common), eating disorders, short-bowel syndrome, chronic use of phosphate binders (especially in context of improving renal function)
Redistributive	Refeeding syndrome, insulin and/or glucose infusion, respiratory alkalosis, salicylate poisoning, catecholamines, diabetic ketoacidosis, postpartial hepatic resection
Miscellaneous	Post-dialysis (especially in malnourished patients) with continuous renal replacement therapy (HDU/ITU), bisphosphonates

for several days and bisphosphonate pre-op if high PTH is present, appears to significantly reduce the severity of postoperative hypocalcaemia, although the evidence base for the use of bisphosphonates is limited.

Stopping causative drugs, correcting magnesium deficiency and treatment with calcium and vitamin D are helpful with any cause of hypocalcaemia. Thereafter, maintenance is with calcium and vitamin D (calcitriol if significant CKD, colecalciferol if 25 (OH) vitamin D deficient). Deficiencies in diet, sun exposure, and malabsorption should be addressed where possible. Severe hyperphosphataemia and hypocalcaemia may be corrected with dialysis in, for example, rhabdomyolysis or tumour lysis syndrome. Getting the dose of IV and/or oral calcium supplements right can be tricky as the requirements alter, and close monitoring is essential in severe hypocalcaemia.

Phosphate Disorders

Over 99 % of total body phosphate is intracellular (muscles and visceral) as well as bone (where it forms a key structural component). It is the most abundant intracellular anion and essential for normal cell structure and membrane integrity, nucleic acid synthesis and metabolism, buffering, energy metabolism via ATP synthesis and is crucially involved in activation of intracellular molecules involved in signalling and metabolism. Phosphate is abundant in most diets and absorbed predominantly in the duodenum and upper jejunum via passive transcellular uptake as well as active sodium:phosphate coupled transport. Gut absorption is increased by hypophosphataemia and 1,25 (OH) vitamin D via up-regulation of the sodium:phosphate cotransporter.

Total body phosphate balance is in part regulated by gut uptake but largely maintained by the kidney. Phosphate is freely filtered, but the vast majority (>75 %) is actively resorbed in the proximal convoluted tubule via a sodium: phosphate co-transporter. Some additional phosphate reabsorption occurs in the distal convoluted tubule. Renal excretion of phosphate is influenced by several factors including dietary intake, 1,25 (OH) vitamin D, PTH and phosphatonins such as fibroblast growth factors 23 and 7 (FGF-23, FGF-7) and secreted frizzled-related protein-4 (sFRP-4) [20]. Rather critically, phosphate excretion is also dependent on GFR in that secretion is impaired once the kidney reaches CKD3b and progressively so with further decline.

The skeleton is critical as a store of phosphate but also highly dependent on adequate supplies for healthy mineralization and remodelling of bone.

Like potassium, phosphate can translocate between the intracellular and extracellular compartments under the influence of insulin.

Hypophosphataemia

Hypophosphataemia (0.65–0.81 mmol/L mild, 0.32–0.64 mmol/L moderate and <0.32 mmol/L severe) is common in hospitalized patients (up to 5 %), particularly so in

Table 9.17 Investigation of hypophosphataemia

Urea, creatinine and electrolytes	Phosphate, magnesium, calcium, potassium, glucose
Acid:Base	Venous bicarbonate or arterial blood gases (may reflect proximal tubular acidosis, respiratory alkalosis)
Liver function	Evidence of liver disease, GGT for alcoholism, ALP for osteomalacia
PTH and vitamin D	Hyperparathyroidism, vitamin D deficiency
Urine phosphate	*Extra-renal* loss <10 mmol/day
	Renal loss >20 mmol/day
Fractional excretion of phosphate:	$FE_{phosphate}$ = (Urine Phosphate × Plasma Creatinine/Plasma Phosphate × Urine Creatinine) × 100
	$FE_{Phosphate}$ >20 % renal wasting
	$FE_{Phosphate}$ <20 % Deficiency, gastrointestinal wasting or redistribution
Nutritional status/gastrointestinal disease	Overall nutritional state and evidence of malabsorption (low BMI or recent poor intake increases risk of refeeding syndrome), vitamin and trace elements
Imaging of the skeletal system	Focused X rays or bone densitometry as appropriate in chronic hypophosphataemia
Imaging for tumours	In otherwise unexplained renal phosphate wasting to exclude TIO

malnourished patients particularly in the setting of refeeding syndrome, alcoholism, malabsorption, acute sepsis, ITU admission (especially with continuous filtration) and in patients with diabetic ketoacidosis.

Causes of Hypophosphataemia

Causes of hypophosphataemia are shown in Table 9.16 and can broadly be separated into renal causes (increased excretion), gastrointestinal causes (decreased absorption) and redistributive. Renal causes can be further subdivided into those secondary to FGF-23 and those not; this is not a very practical division as clinical assays for FGF-23 are not readily available in most health settings but do add a certain something. Medication is thought to be a contributing factor in a significant proportion of cases, and malnourished patients are substantially predisposed.

The majority of inherited renal causes causing phosphate wasting are diagnosed in childhood, but autosomal dominant hypophosphataemic rickets can present in adulthood with bone pain and osteomalacia. Presentation of acquired renal wasting depends on the cause or insult resulting in either a selective or, more commonly, diffuse proximal convoluted tubular dysfunction. Not infrequently a combination of factors is present in patients with malabsorption, malnutrition or alcoholism, and such patients with depleted total body phosphate levels are at very high and predictable risk of refeeding syndrome.

Clinical Features of Hypophosphataemia

The majority of patients with hypophosphataemia is asymptomatic with perhaps non-specific weakness, paresthesia and fatigue; however, severe hypophosphataemia can result in a proximal myopathy resulting in rhabdomyolysis and respiratory failure as well as acute cardiomyopathy. Intravascular haemolysis and depressed white cell function occur with severely low levels, and neurotoxicity in the form of neuropathy, metabolic encephalopathy and seizures are also consequences of severe deficiency. More chronically in adults hypophosphataemia results in osteomalacia with diffuse bone pain and fracture risk; in children with inherited forms of hypophosphataemia, rickets and growth retardation are common.

Assessment and Investigation of Hypophosphataemia

Hypophosphataemia is often a surrogate marker for malnutrition or renal proximal tubular disease, and investigations should include an overall assessment of the patient's nutritional status and clinical features of tubular disorders as well as signs of osteomalacia and rickets and proximal myopathy (Table 9.17).

Unless the cause of hypophosphataemia is obvious, renal excretion of phosphate is helpful in distinguishing between renal and extra-renal causes. If the cause is renal then further tests for diffuse proximal tubular disease such as Fanconi syndrome are warranted. Family history is essential in children and young adults with isolated phosphate wasting who should be offered genetic screening.

Treatment of Hypophosphataemia

The underlying cause of hypophosphataemia should be established and where possible, it should be treated (e.g. vitamin D supplementation, cessation of tubular toxins such as tenofovir if possible, resolution of malabsorption). Acute mild to moderate hypophosphataemia can usually be managed with high phosphate foods with or without oral phosphate supplements (although diarrhoea is a common and frequently limiting side effect of phosphate supplements). The evidence base for dosing in acute moderate to severe hypophosphataemia is somewhat limited [21]; anticipation, close monitoring and common sense are probably the best guides. IV phosphate should be considered in patients with severe (<0.32 mmol/L) acute hypophosphataemia particularly if they already have cardiorespiratory compromise (e.g. ventilated patients), those with a predisposition to seizures or those unable to take enteral feed. As always, with electrolyte abnormalities the response depends on the stability of the deficit and the

Table 9.18 Causes of hyperphosphataemia

Reduced renal excretion[a]	AKI and CKD, hypoparathyroidism, pseudohypoparathyroidism (PTH promotes phosphate excretion).
Increased renal absorption	Acromegaly, familial tumoral calcinosis.
Cell lysis	Tumour lysis syndrome (TLS), rhabdomyolysis, significant infarction, intravascular haemolysis and extravascular haemolysis (e.g. extensive haematoma), high LDH, lactate, urate, potassium and creatine kinase may rise, depending on cause.
Excess intake	Inappropriate supplementation (especially IV phosphate); phosphate enemas can cause an acute rise in phosphate and thus can be hazardous in patients with significant renal impairment, especially those with pre-existing vascular calcification. Intake of phosphate-rich foods (see Chap. 55) is rarely an issue in patients with normal renal function but common place in patients with advanced CKD.
Vitamin D intoxication	Rare cause of hyperphosphataemia in the general population but contributory in patients with CKD (vitamin D 25 (OH) and 1,25 (OH) levels may be helpful).
Redistributive	Acidosis promotes shift from intracellular to extracellular location.

[a]Reduced GFR-significant predisposition to all other causes

direction of travel. For example, those with hypophosphataemia with ongoing losses such as continuous renal replacement therapy or anticipated re-feeding syndrome in a sick patient are likely to need IV supplements whereas a healthy post-transplant patient with a level of 0.30 mmol/L, who is able to take a high phosphate diet, vitamin D and oral supplements may not need to be given IV phosphate, if it is clear that the level has reached a nadir and is no longer falling. An important caveat with supplementation, especially intravenous, is that it can worsen hypocalcaemia and hypomagnesaemia, both of which must be corrected and monitored, and over-aggressive poorly monitored supplementation may result in phosphate-induced AKI (which does not look good for a nephrologist).

If there is associated vitamin D deficiency, then supplementation is essential (patients with malabsorption, starvation or alcoholism sufficient to cause hypophosphataemia are likely to have multiple vitamin and other nutritional deficiencies as well). Resection of the causative tumour is curative in tumour-induced osteomalacia (TIO)-induced hypophosphataemia [22].

Hyperphosphataemia

Hyperphosphataemia, serum phosphate >1.5 mmol/L, is uncommon in the general population but omnipresent in advanced CKD (in the absence of phosphate lowering measures) (see Chap. 50). Acute hyperphosphataemia can occur, usually in the setting of significant cell death or inappropriate supplementation; in both scenarios this is much more likely to occur with impaired renal function (Table 9.18).

Clinical Features of Hyperphosphataemia

The major clinical consequence of hyperphosphataemia is calcium-phosphate deposition in multiple tissues and particularly arterial vessels which may manifest as conjunctivitis or tenosynovitis. It is usually asymptomatic but if chronic will lead to calcium-phosphate deposition in multiple tissues, the most significant being vascular and with important cardiovascular consequences including calciphylaxis (see Chap. 52). Occasionally and particularly in dialysis patients, a large hard mass may develop in soft tissue (Teutschlander's disease), sometimes secondary to calcification of a haematoma. These are often painful and may ulcerate but X-ray imaging usually makes the diagnosis fairly evident and rules out more sinister causes. Sudden acute hyperphosphataemia may lead to acute tissue calcification, hypocalcaemia and acute kidney injury.

Treatment of hyperphosphataemia

The treatment of hyperphosphataemia needs to be directed at the underlying cause and in the case of CKD is covered in Chaps. 50 and 54. Management of acute and severe hyperphosphataemia involves prevention in the setting of tumor lysis syndrome (TLS) (see Chap. 31), volume expansion to promote renal excretion (in case of good renal function), with the possible addition of a loop diuretic to promote renal excretion (with monitoring of calcium). Although the evidence base is weak, there is at least a good theoretical argument for acute haemodialysis or haemofiltration in the setting of tumour lysis syndrome, or rhabdomyolysis associated with hyperphosphataemia in the context of AKI and is worth considering, especially if potassiums are becoming bothersome.

In patients with CKD, management relies on patient engagement with the issue, excellent and clear education on how to have a good and culturally relevant low phosphate diet and the purpose and importance of phosphate binders.

Magnesium Disorders

Magnesium is critical for cellular and metabolic processes, mitochondrial function, inflammation, neuromuscular function, cardiac electrical activity and blood pressure regulation. It is the most abundant intracellular cation after potassium, 99 % of total body magnesium is intracellular and is stored in muscle, liver and bone. Of the 1 % that is extracellular 20 %

abnormalities (importantly hypokalaemia) take precedence over correction of the acidosis.

Evidence for benefit for bicarbonate replacement in DKA is lacking [18, 19]; however, no randomised trials have been performed on DKA patients with severe acidosis (pH<6.9). There are concerns about using bicarbonate therapy in DKA:

- There is some evidence that giving bicarbonate may delay the recovery from the ketosis; this was suggested by one small study of seven patients in which bicarbonate administration delayed recovery form ketosis by 6 h [20], although this was not the case in a randomised study of bicarbonate treatment in DKA with less severe acidosis [19].
- Insulin treatment will cause the ketoacids to eventually be metabolised to bicarbonate, and thus bicarbonate administration during treatment may lead to eventual metabolic alkalosis.

However, there are potential benefits for bicarbonate therapy in DKA:

Patients have impaired cardiac contractility and vasodilatation with a serum pH of less than 7.0; therefore, alkali therapy in this cohort may improve tissue perfusion; this effect is unlikely to be significant above a pH of 7, as insulin therapy will rapidly improve pH in any case.

If the serum potassium is dangerously high, then intravenous bicarbonate will act to shunt some of the extracellular potassium intracellularly, lowering the serum potassium concentration.

The ketoacidosis seen in alcoholic patients can be severe, whilst that seen in fasting patients rarely is (bicarbonate levels rarely fall below 14 mmol/L).

This reflects the additional burden of pathophysiology present in the alcoholic ketoacidotic patient; a lack of carbohydrates reduces insulin secretion and raises glucagon, whilst alcohol inhibits liver gluconeogenesis and stimulates lipolysis contributing to increased ketoacid formation. Ethanol metabolism to acetaldehyde and then acetic acid will also contribute to the acidosis.

It may be difficult in the alcoholic patient with a high anion gap metabolic acidosis to distinguish between alcoholic ketoacidosis, diabetic ketoacidosis and methanol or ethylene glycol poisoning. It is therefore essential to take a careful history, demonstrate ketoacidosis, perform urinalysis (for oxalate crystals) and measure serum levels of possible toxins, if the assays are available.

In fasting and alcoholic ketoacidosis, as in DKA, correction of the underlying metabolic defect will lead to metabolism of the ketoacids and resolution of the acidosis. In both cases this is achieved by infusion of dextrose to increase insulin and decrease glucagon secretion and saline to volume expand the patient. In alcoholics it is important to give intravenous (or intramuscular) thiamine before IV dextrose to prevent precipitating Wernicke encephalopathy or Korsakoff psychosis.

Lactic Acidosis

Acute Metabolic Acidosis AG: High

Like ketoacidosis, in lactic acidosis, the lactate replaces bicarbonate. Once the stimulus for lactic acid production is removed, lactate is metabolised to bicarbonate, ending the acidaemia.

This means that the role of alkali therapy in lactic acidosis is limited to control of the acute acidosis. There is some evidence [21, 22] that acidosis impairs cardiac contractility, and in severe acidosis, acute therapy with intravenous bicarbonate may improve tissue perfusion.

However, there are a number of reasons to be cautious with bicarbonate replacement in lactic acidosis:

- Fluid overload and posttreatment metabolic alkalosis when the excess lactate is converted to bicarbonate, as with ketoacidosis.
- CO_2 retention may be a problem in patients with compromised cardiac and pulmonary function; as bicarbonate buffers excess hydrogen ions, CO_2 is formed, and normally this would be eliminated via the lungs; if the pulmonary circulation is inadequate to vent the CO_2, it will be retained [23], adding an additional acid burden.
- It has been proposed that intravenous bicarbonate could cause a paradoxical drop in intracellular pH [24], worsening hepatic lactate metabolism and cardiac contractility [22]. This was based on isolated cell experiments and several lines of evidence show that this is probably not the case in vivo [25].
- Bicarbonate therapy may cause a fall in serum ionised calcium by increasing calcium binding to albumin [26]; this could potentially worsen cardiac contractility.

Thus, much like in ketoacidosis, the role for bicarbonate therapy is probably only for the acute control of severe acidaemia (~pH 7.1).

Ingestion of Methanol or Ethylene Glycol

Acute Metabolic Acidosis AG: High

Both methanol and ethylene glycol poisoning tend to occur in the setting of ethanol substitution, either deliberate (i.e. drinking methylated spirits or deliberate self-harm) or accidental (i.e. methanol contamination of domestically distilled alcohol or occult ethylene glycol substitution in illegally produced spirits).

Unlike ketoacidosis and lactic acidosis, the inorganic anions generated in methanol or ethylene glycol poisoning are not metabolised to bicarbonate; they are toxic and must be removed. Therefore, treatment is much more active in these cases.

Both methanol and ethylene glycol are both relatively harmless alcohols (both can cause sedation), but they both form very toxic metabolites when oxidised by alcohol dehydrogenase and (to a lesser extent) aldehyde dehydrogenase.

Methanol is metabolised to *formate*. Formate toxicity causes visual impairment from optic disc oedema and direct retinal damage, leading eventually to permanent *blindness*, as well as *injury to the basal ganglia*, probably via mitochondrial toxicity [27].

Ethylene glycol is metabolised to *glycolate*, glyoxylate and *oxalate*. These metabolites cause *acute kidney injury*, mainly from tubular injury caused by glycolate, but also via oxalate precipitation in the kidney. The kidney injury will further delay the elimination of the ethylene glycol. Hypocalcaemia may occur due to calcium oxalate precipitation.

Inhibition of alcohol dehydrogenase is an important strategy, to prevent metabolism of the parent alcohols to their toxic metabolites. *Fomepizole* is an alcohol dehydrogenase inhibitor, which is superior to ethanol therapy, is safe and easy to administer. Alternatively, alcohol dehydrogenase can be competitively inhibited by *ethanol* which has a higher affinity for alcohol dehydrogenase than either methanol or ethylene glycol. However, it is vastly inferior to fomepizole, as it is difficult to administer, monitor and adjust; it is irritant to veins and most importantly causes central sedation, possibly leading to obtundation and airway compromise. Although this is only effective if done early, co-ingestion with ethanol is very common and will delay the appearance of the toxic metabolites, so it is worth attempting inhibition even hours after ingestion.

Alkalinisation: Both formate and glycolate and/or oxalate are more likely to penetrate their target tissues when they are protonated (and therefore uncharged), and this is more likely to occur when the patient is acidaemic. There is thus a clear rationale for alkalinisation with bicarbonate in these patients, especially as the metabolic acidosis in these cases is often severe (bicarbonate often as low as 8 mmol/L). Intravenous bicarbonate should be given with an aim for an arterial pH of 7.35.

Haemodialysis is the best way to rapidly clear both the parent alcohols and their toxic metabolites. It should be started rapidly in a case of suspected methanol or ethylene glycol poisoning, and the patient has evidence of acidaemia and/or end organ damage (renal failure or visual impairment); confirmatory levels of methanol or ethylene glycol should not delay treatment. Repeated courses of haemodialysis may be necessary in massive overdoses or in those whom renal failure results from ethylene glycol poisoning. Haemodialysis may also shorten the course of alcohol dehydrogenase inhibitor therapy. Haemodialysis may not be necessary in ethylene glycol ingestion if fomepizole has been given, there is no acidaemia (i.e. there is little or no glycolate circulating) and renal function remains normal.

Aspirin Overdose

Acute (Rarely Chronic) Respiratory Alkalosis/ Metabolic Acidosis AG: High

Aspirin (and other salicylates, such as salicyclic acid and methyl salicylate) is common and can cause multiple toxic effects (tinnitus, nausea and vomiting, altered mental state and seizures, tachyarrhythmias, acute lung and liver injury), including a complex acid-base disturbance.

Salicylates directly stimulate the respiratory centre causing hyperventilation and *respiratory alkalosis*. This is followed by a high anion gap *metabolic acidosis*, caused by accumulation of organic anions, including lactate and ketoacids. Approximately a third of salicylate overdoses are a part of mixed overdoses, often with respiratory depressants, so the respiratory alkalosis may be ameliorated or a respiratory acidosis may be present in these cases.

Salicylate is also uncharged when protonated and able to cross cell membranes; thus, acidaemia will increase its delivery to target tissues.

Alkalinisation of serum and urine is therefore desirable, not just to reduce tissue penetration but also to enhance the renal elimination of the salicylate. Intravenous bicarbonate should be given, even if there is a mild respiratory alkalosis.

Haemodialysis removes salicylate and should be considered in patients with cerebral or pulmonary oedema, renal failure, depressed level of consciousness, a very high salicylate level (>700 mg/dL) and clinical deterioration despite good supportive treatment.

Chronic Renal Failure

Chronic Metabolic Acidosis AG: N

Excess acid consumed in the diet is excreted renally, mainly as ammonium. In chronic kidney disease, as the GFR falls, the ammonium production per nephron increases to maintain normal acid excretion; however, this compensation starts to fail at about a GFR of 40–50 ml/min. After this there will be a net retention of acid, which may progress to a significant metabolic acidaemia.

Even in salt and water retaining patients with advanced chronic renal failure, oral sodium bicarbonate is well tolerated [28], and treatment of the acidosis has three main aims:

Retardation of the progression of renal impairment. Oral bicarbonate supplementation has been shown to retard the progression of CKD in acidotic CKD patients compared to patients receiving no bicarbonate supplementation [29]. The mechanism for this effect is not clear.

Bone protection. As a chronic acidosis, the acidosis of CKD causes calcium and phosphate leeching from bone in order to buffer the extra hydrogen ions. Preventing this by bicarbonate supplementation may delay the onset of osteopenia, in dialysis patients at least [30].

Improved nutritional status. Acidosis in CKD can cause muscle wasting and weakness, probably by a direct effect of the acidaemia in stimulating genes that promote muscle proteolysis, an effect ameliorated by bicarbonate [31]. Bicarbonate is also beneficial in preventing the growth retardation caused by chronic acidosis in children with CKD.

Surreptitious Vomiting

Chronic Metabolic Alkalosis AG: N

The urinary sodium concentration is often used as an indicator of volume status. However, it should be borne in mind that in acute metabolic alkalosis, the urine concentrations of both sodium and potassium are high, even if there is volume depletion. In fact, the urinary losses of potassium are the main cause of hypokalaemia in vomiting; the potassium loss in vomitus itself is minimal.

In this setting a much better indicator of volume depletion is the urinary chloride concentration, which will be low as the kidney appropriately retains chloride, both for volume expansion and due to the hypochloraemia due to chloride loss in the vomitus.

In protracted vomiting, the reabsorbative capacity of the nephron is increased in order to deal with the increased filtered load of bicarbonate; at this point the urinary concentrations of sodium and potassium will become very low and the urine pH will fall.

Surreptitious Diuretic Abuse

Chronic Metabolic Alkalosis AG: N/High

As mentioned above, the biochemical profile of a patient taking a loop diuretic is identical to that of Bartter syndrome, and the profile of someone taking a thiazide is the same as that of Gitelman syndrome. If a patient is taking either of these drugs surreptitiously, they may present as either of these conditions.

The only biochemical clue may come from the urine; patients with either Bartter or Gitelman have constant inappropriate urinary losses of chloride. Patients on loop or thiazide diuretics will also have inappropriately high urinary chloride losses, but only during the duration of action of the diuretic (~6 h), during which time, the diuretic should be detectable in the urine. After this time, the urinary chloride will fall precipitously, as the kidney tries to conserve chloride, and the diuretic will be undetectable.

Sudden Relief of Hypercapnia

Acute Metabolic Alkalosis AG: N

Chronic hypercapnia will cause an appropriate compensatory metabolic increase in renal hydrogen ion secretion. Sudden correction of the hypercapnia (e.g. by mechanical ventilation) can cause a metabolic alkalosis due to the sustained high serum concentration of HCO_3^-. This may be enough to increase cerebral pH and cause a neurological deficit or even death [32]. As chloride is exchanged for bicarbonate in the cortical collecting duct and hypercapnic patients may have a chloride deficit [33], it is often necessary to administer IV sodium chloride to allow the excess bicarbonate to be excreted.

References

1. Schwartz WB, Relman AS. A critique of the parameters used in the evaluation of acid-base disorders. "Whole-blood buffer base" and "standard bicarbonate" compared with blood pH and plasma bicarbonate concentration. N Engl J Med. 1963;268:1382–8.
2. Madias NE, Adrogue HJ, Horowitz GL, Cohen JJ, Schwartz WB. A redefinition of normal acid-base equilibrium in man: carbon dioxide tension as a key determinant of normal plasma bicarbonate concentration. Kidney Int. 1979;16(5):612–8.
3. Balasubramanyan N, Havens PL, Hoffman GM. Unmeasured anions identified by the Fencl-Stewart method predict mortality better than base excess, anion gap, and lactate in patients in the pediatric intensive care unit. Crit Care Med. 1999;27(8):1577–81.
4. Kaplan LJ, Kellum JA. Initial pH, base deficit, lactate, anion gap, strong ion difference, and strong ion gap predict outcome from major vascular injury. Crit Care Med. 2004;32(5):1120–4.
5. Cusack RJ, Rhodes A, Lochhead P, Jordan B, Perry S, Ball JA, et al. The strong ion gap does not have prognostic value in critically ill patients in a mixed medical/surgical adult ICU. Intensive Care Med. 2002;28(7):864–9.
6. Dubin A, Menises MM, Masevicius FD, Moseinco MC, Kutscherauer DO, Ventrice E, et al. Comparison of three different methods of evaluation of metabolic acid-base disorders. Crit Care Med. 2007;35(5):1264–70.
7. Siggaard-Andersen O, Fogh-Andersen N. Base excess or buffer base (strong ion difference) as measure of a non-respiratory acid-base disturbance. Acta Anaesthesiol Scand Suppl. 1995;107:123–8.
8. Kurtz I, Kraut J, Ornekian V, Nguyen MK. Acid-base analysis: a critique of the Stewart and bicarbonate-centered approaches. Am J Physiol Renal Physiol. 2008;294(5):F1009–31.
9. Adrogue HJ, Madias NE. Changes in plasma potassium concentration during acute acid-base disturbances. Am J Med. 1981;71(3):456–67.
10. Oberleithner H, Greger R, Lang F. The effect of respiratory and metabolic acid-base changes on ionized calcium concentration: in vivo and in vitro experiments in man and rat. Eur J Clin Invest. 1982;12(6):451–5.
11. Perez GO, Oster JR, Rogers A. Acid-base disturbances in gastrointestinal disease. Dig Dis Sci. 1987;32(9):1033–43.
12. Khositseth S, Bruce LJ, Walsh SB, Bawazir WM, Ogle GD, Unwin RJ, et al. Tropical distal renal tubular acidosis: clinical and epidemiological studies in 78 patients. QJM. 2012;105(9):861–77.

13. Poux JM, Peyronnet P, Le Meur Y, Favereau JP, Charmes JP, Leroux-Robert C. Hypokalemic quadriplegia and respiratory arrest revealing primary Sjogren's syndrome. Clin Nephrol. 1992;37(4):189–91.
14. Walsh SB, Shirley DG, Wrong OM, Unwin RJ. Urinary acidification assessed by simultaneous furosemide and fludrocortisone treatment: an alternative to ammonium chloride. Kidney Int. 2007;71(12):1310–6.
15. Wrong O, Davies HE. The excretion of acid in renal disease. Q J Med. 1959;28(110):259–313.
16. Mundy AR. Metabolic complications of urinary diversion. Lancet. 1999;353(9167):1813–4.
17. McDougal WS. Metabolic complications of urinary intestinal diversion. J Urol. 1992;147(5):1199–208.
18. Lever E, Jaspan JB. Sodium bicarbonate therapy in severe diabetic ketoacidosis. Am J Med. 1983;75(2):263–8.
19. Morris LR, Murphy MB, Kitabchi AE. Bicarbonate therapy in severe diabetic ketoacidosis. Ann Intern Med. 1986;105(6):836–40.
20. Okuda Y, Adrogue HJ, Field JB, Nohara H, Yamashita K. Counterproductive effects of sodium bicarbonate in diabetic ketoacidosis. J Clin Endocrinol Metab. 1996;81(1):314–20.
21. Narins RG, Cohen JJ. Bicarbonate therapy for organic acidosis: the case for its continued use. Ann Intern Med. 1987;106(4):615–8.
22. Orchard CH, Kentish JC. Effects of changes of pH on the contractile function of cardiac muscle. Am J Physiol. 1990;258(6 Pt 1):C967–81.
23. Adrogue HJ, Rashad MN, Gorin AB, Yacoub J, Madias NE. Assessing acid-base status in circulatory failure. Differences between arterial and central venous blood. N Engl J Med. 1989;320(20):1312–6.
24. Adrogue HJ, Madias NE. Management of life-threatening acid-base disorders. First of two parts. N Engl J Med. 1998;338(1):26–34.
25. Goldsmith DJ, Forni LG, Hilton PJ. Bicarbonate therapy and intracellular acidosis. Clin Sci (Lond). 1997;93(6):593–8.
26. Cooper DJ, Walley KR, Wiggs BR, Russell JA. Bicarbonate does not improve hemodynamics in critically ill patients who have lactic acidosis. A prospective, controlled clinical study. Ann Intern Med. 1990;112(7):492–8.
27. Wallace KB, Eells JT, Madeira VM, Cortopassi G, Jones DP. Mitochondria-mediated cell injury. Symposium overview. Fundam Appl Toxicol. 1997;38(1):23–37.
28. Husted FC, Nolph KD, Maher JF. NaHCO3 and NaC1 tolerance in chronic renal failure. J Clin Invest. 1975;56(2):414–9.
29. de Brito-Ashurst I, Varagunam M, Raftery MJ, Yaqoob MM. Bicarbonate supplementation slows progression of CKD and improves nutritional status. J Am Soc Nephrol. 2009;20(9):2075–84.
30. Lefebvre A, de Vernejoul MC, Gueris J, Goldfarb B, Graulet AM, Morieux C. Optimal correction of acidosis changes progression of dialysis osteodystrophy. Kidney Int. 1989;36(6):1112–8.
31. Bailey JL, Wang X, England BK, Price SR, Ding X, Mitch WE. The acidosis of chronic renal failure activates muscle proteolysis in rats by augmenting transcription of genes encoding proteins of the ATP-dependent ubiquitin-proteasome pathway. J Clin Invest. 1996;97(6):1447–53.
32. Rotheram Jr EB, Safar P, Robin E. CNS disorder during mechanical ventilation in chronic pulmonary disease. JAMA. 1964;189:993–6.
33. Schwartz WB, Hays RM, Polak A, Haynie GD. Effects of chronic hypercapnia on electrolyte and acid-base equilibrium. II. Recovery, with special reference to the influence of chloride intake. J Clin Invest. 1961;40:1238–49.

Diagnosis and Investigation of the Hypertensive Patient

11

Marc Jonathan George, Reecha Sofat,
Aroon D. Hingorani, and Raymond MacAllister

Hypertension is the most prevalent, modifiable risk factor for cardiovascular disease (CVD), stroke, chronic kidney disease (CKD), heart failure and peripheral arterial disease [1].

The risk of death, myocardial infarction (MI) and stroke has a continuous relationship on a log scale with both systolic and diastolic blood pressure (BP), though the relationship is steeper for stroke than MI. As an indication of the strength of the relationship, at ages of 40–69 years for every 20/10 mmHg rise in BP above 115/70 mmHg, these risks roughly double [2] (Fig. 11.1). The converse is also true, so that reduction of blood pressure by 20/10 mmHg will approximately halve the risk of cardiovascular events. In addition, BP also shows a continuous, independent relationship with CKD, heart failure and peripheral artery disease.

According to the Global Burden of Disease 2000 study, approximately 50 % of strokes and MIs and an estimated 7.6 million deaths per year (13.5 % of all deaths worldwide) can be attributed to hypertension [3].

M.J. George, MBChB (Hons), BSc (Hons) • R. Sofat
Department of Clinical Pharmacology and Therapeutics,
University College London Hospital,
235 Euston Road, London NW1 2BU, UK
e-mail: marc.george@uclh.nhs.uk

A.D. Hingorani, MA, FRCP, PhD
Department of genetic epidemiology,
Institute of Cardiovascular Science,
University College London and University College London
Hospitals NHS Foundation Trust, 1-19 Torrinton Place,
London WC1E 6BT, UK
e-mail: a.hingorani@ucl.ac.uk

R. MacAllister, FRCP, MD (✉)
Division of Medicine,
Centre for Clinical Pharmacology,
University College London,
Rayne Building, 5 University Street,
London WC1E 6JF, UK
e-mail: r.macallister@ucl.ac.uk

The relationship between CKD and hypertension is complex, given the kidney's role in regulation of body fluid volumes and BP homeostasis. More than 80 % of CKD patients are hypertensive and teasing out whether the hypertension is primary and the cause of the CKD can be a challenge. However, data from cohort studies in patients with hypertension and no baseline renal disease demonstrate the graded relationship between increasing BP and the development of CKD [4].

Given the importance of hypertension as a risk factor for cardiovascular and renal disease, this chapter will discuss the approach to defining and diagnosing hypertension before discussing the approach to investigation of patients with suspected resistant and secondary hypertension.

Defining Hypertension and Setting Treatment Thresholds

BP has a well-recognised skewed normal distribution in the population, and given the continuous log-linear relationship with cardiovascular and renal disease, down to at least a level of 115/70 mmHg [2], the BP cut-off that defines 'hypertension' is arbitrary.

Definitions of hypertension and treatment thresholds and targets have been issued by more than 100 organisations worldwide including the National Institute of Clinical Excellence (NICE) in the UK [5], the American Heart Association (AHA) [6], European Societies of Hypertension (ESH) and Cardiology (ESC) [7, 8], Japanese Society of Hypertension (JSH) [9] and the World Health Association (WHO) [10].

Table 11.1 summarises the definitions of hypertension used in these particular guidelines. All of these sample guidelines agree that the term hypertension be applied to a patient with a clinic BP of ≥140/90 mmHg. However, BP is further subdivided using a variety of terms such as optimal, normal, high-normal, pre-hypertension and grades (or stages) 1–3.

M. Harber (ed.), *Practical Nephrology*,
DOI 10.1007/978-1-4471-5547-8_11, © Springer-Verlag London 2014

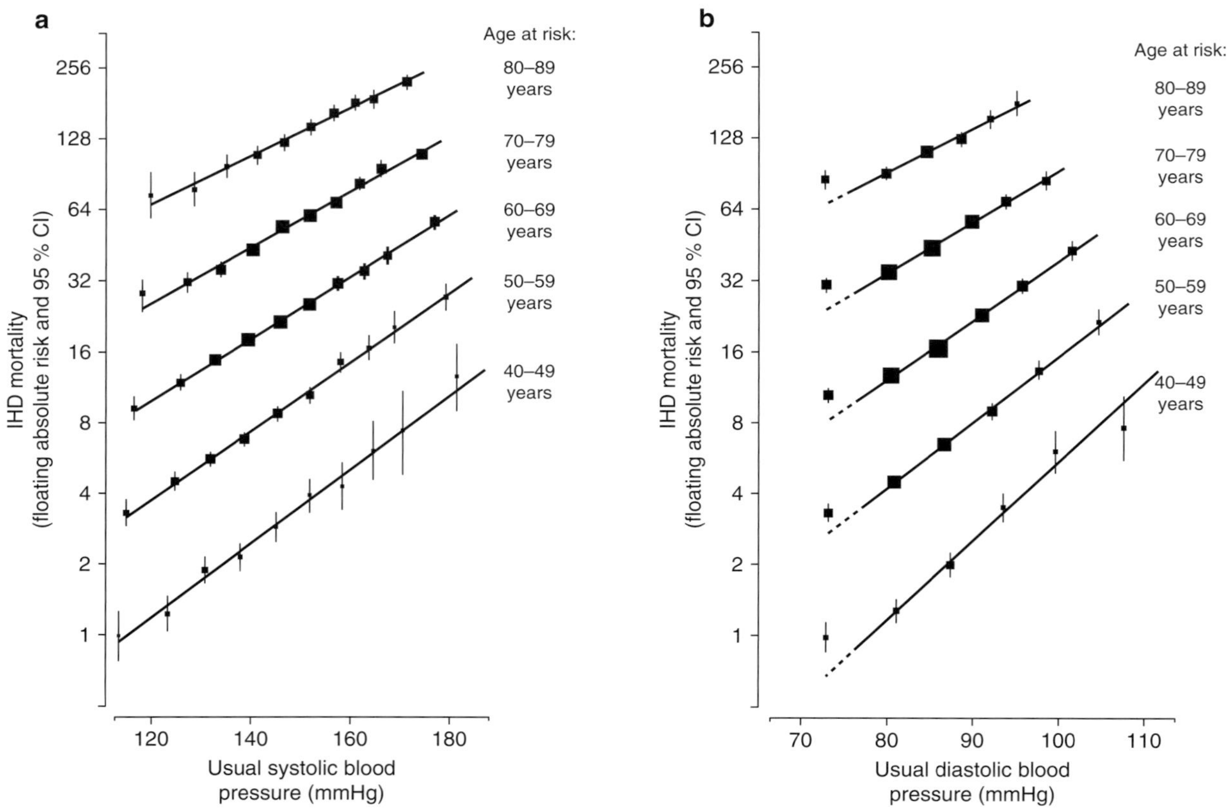

Fig. 11.1 Association between blood pressure and ischaemic heart disease. (**a**) Systolic blood pressure. (**b**) Diastolic blood pressure (Reproduced with permission from Lewington et al. [2])

Table 11.1 Definitions of hypertension in international guidelines

Term	Clinic sBP	Clinic dBP
NICE 2011 [5]		
Stage 1 hypertension	140–159	90–99
Stage 2 hypertension	160–179	100–109
Severe hypertension	≥180	≥110
JSH 2009 [9], *ESH 2007* [7], *WHO 2007* [10]		
Optimal BP	<120	<80
Normal BP	120–129	80–84
High-normal BP	130–139	85–89
Grade 1 hypertension	140–159	90–99
Grade 2 hypertension	160–179	100–109
Grade 3 hypertension	≥180	≥110
AHA 2007 [6]		
Pre-hypertension	130–139	80–89
Hypertension	≥140	≥90

Treatment thresholds and targets differ between guidelines. However, in general, there is a clear delineation in all guidelines between lower- and higher-risk groups. High-risk groups are those with additional cardiovascular risk factors, including diabetes mellitus (DM), established CKD, pre-existing cardiovascular disease (including cerebrovascular, heart disease and peripheral arterial disease), subclinical end-organ damage (Table 11.2) or a '10-year cardiovascular risk' of a predefined level (Table 11.3). The summary of the baseline investigations required to make a reasonable assessment of cardiovascular risk for a patient with hypertension is listed in Box 11.1.

Treatment Thresholds in Low-Risk Patients

As described, a low-risk patient is one with no history of DM or vascular disease in any territory, with no evidence of subclinical end-organ damage and a low calculated 10-year cardiovascular risk. In general, such patients are under represented in clinical trials, as the selection of high-risk patients maximises the number of events collected and thus the power of trials. Furthermore, most trials are of a short duration (4–5 years), whereas the additional life expectancy for middle-aged hypertensives is 20–30 years. Consequently, there is a lack of quality evidence and therefore consensus regarding treatment thresholds in this cohort.

Nevertheless, in the largest overview of blood pressure treatment trials conducted by Law et al. [14], it is shown that in all patients, a sustained reduction over 5 years of 5–6 mmHg in sBP reduces coronary events by approximately

Table 11.2 Investigation of subclinical end-organ damage

Abnormality	Investigations[a]	Suggested threshold[b]
Heart		
Left ventricular hypertrophy	*ECG*	Sokolow-Lyon >38 mm
	Echocardiogram	LVMI M $\geq$125 g/m^2, W $\geq$110 g/m^2
Arteries		
Carotid intima-media thickening (IMT)	Ultrasound Doppler carotid	IMT >0.9 mm
Renal		
Low estimated glomerular filtration rate (eGFR) (MDRD formula)	*Serum eGFR*	<60 ml/min/1.73 m^2
Microalbuminuria	*Urine dip*	1+ Protein (proceed to measure of quantity)
	Random urine: albumin/creatinine ratio	M >22 W >31 mg/g creatinine
	24 h urine collection	30–300 mg/24 h
Cerebrovascular		
Small vessel ischaemia	MRI	Presence of cerebrovascular lesions
Retinal		
Hypertensive retinopathy	*Fundoscopy*	≥Grade 2 changes

[a]Investigations in bold are first-line and should be performed in all patients, and others may have a role in selected patients
[b]Thresholds (other than fundoscopy) taken from 2007 ESH guidelines [7]

Table 11.3 10-Year cardiovascular risk calculators

Calculator	Notes	Data fields	URL
Framingham	Based on the long-standing prospective Framingham cohort studies	BP	http://www.framinghamheartstudy.org/risk/coronary.html
	Included in AHA guidelines	Age	
	Risk calculated after cumulative points total (based on series of charts)	Sex	
		Diabetes	
		Smoking	
		LDL cholesterol	
		Total cholesterol	
		HDL cholesterol	
QRisk	Based on data collected by general practitioners in NHS	BP	http://www.qrisk.org/
	Online risk calculator	Age	
		Sex	
		Ethnicity	
		Smoking	
		Diabetes	
		Family history	
		Renal function	
		AF	
		On BP Rx	
		Rheumatoid arthritis	
		Cholesterol/HDL ratio	
		BMI	
WHO	Included in WHO/ISH guidelines	BP	http://www.who.int/cardiovascular_diseases/guidelines/PocketGL.ENGLISH.AFR-D-E.rev1.pdf
	A series of region-specific prediction charts	Sex	
	Less number of fields required	Age	
		Diabetes	
		Smoking	
		Total cholesterol	
		Region	

Box 11.1: Initial Investigations in a Patient with Hypertension

- Blood electrolytes, creatinine and eGFR
- Fundoscopy
- Random blood glucose
- Serum total and HDL cholesterol
- Urine strip for protein (and blood)
- Weight and height for BMI
- 12 lead ECG

20 % and strokes by 40 % [14]. The percentage reductions in CVD events and stroke were similar in people *with or without* cardiovascular disease and *regardless* of blood pressure before treatment (down to 110 mmHg systolic). This is in keeping with evidence from overviews of prospective observational studies that predict lowering BP by this degree confers the same magnitude of protection [2]. The authors of this review suggested that their results indicated the importance of lowering blood pressure in *everyone* over a certain age (55 years old), rather than in just those with higher-risk profile.

Despite this data, guidelines differ in their recommendations for low-risk individuals.

The guidelines produced by NICE, WHO and JSH do not recommend treatment in this group when BP is between 140 and 160 mmHg [5, 9, 10]. However, the ESH and the AHA [6, 7] do recommend treatment if BP is uncontrolled by lifestyle measures. All guidelines agree that treatment should be commenced when the clinic BP is >160/100 mmHg.

Treatment Thresholds in High-Risk Patients

As described above, the majority of hypertension trial data relates to higher-risk patients. In all cited guidelines, blood pressure thresholds for treating these higher-risk groups are lower; however, there is also a lack of consensus in this group. Suggested treatment thresholds in these high-risk patients range from a clinic BP of 130/80 mmHg in the AHA guidance [14] to 140/90 mmHg in the recent NICE guidelines [5]. However, it must be noted that the evidence suggests that all patients considered high risk would benefit from blood pressure lowering, *regardless* of their initial BP [14].

Recent trials have illustrated the benefits of aggressive BP lowering in higher-risk cohorts. For example, in the ADVANCE trial [12], sBP lowering to <110 mmHg in patients with DM was associated with progressively lower rates of renal events such as development of microalbuminuria and progression to end-stage renal disease [12]. Similarly in the PROGRESS trial [22] of patients who had previously had a stroke, analyses of follow-up BP showed that the lowest risk of recurrence was among the one-quarter of participants with the lowest follow-up BP levels (median 112/72 mmHg).

Thus, treatment should be aggressive in high-risk individuals with the aim of achieving blood pressure lowering without causing symptomatic hypotension. Aiming for an sBP of 130 mmHg as suggested by many guidelines is pragmatic, but cardiovascular and renal risks continue to fall beyond this target.

Measuring Blood Pressure and Diagnosing Hypertension

The extremely large evidence base on which the treatment for hypertension is founded, including cohort studies with approximately one million participants and randomised studies in over 500,000 individuals [14], is based on using clinic BP measurements. Such measurements are cheap, readily available and require no specialised training or equipment over and above what is usually available in a clinic setting, and treatment based on these measurements is cost effective, worldwide.

However, BP can be highly variable and is influenced by multiple factors including the time of day, posture, stress, pain and room temperature. Indeed, even with serial back-to-back measurement, BP reproducibly falls. Thus, one-off clinic readings, even performed under ideal conditions, may give limited information about a patient's BP and thus cardiovascular risk. In order to overcome this limitation, multiple measurements over time are required to make a diagnosis, and this is advocated in multiple guidelines. However, increasing emphasis is being put on the value of ambulatory blood pressure measurement (ABPM) in diagnosing hypertension.

Ambulatory Blood Pressure Measurement (ABPM) in the Diagnosis of Hypertension

ABPM requires a patient wearing a cuff and bladder connected to electronic sensors which measures BP by the oscillometric technique. Serial BP measurements are performed (usually every 30–60 min), whilst going about their daily routine, over a period of time (usually 24 h). This allows their diastolic and systolic blood pressures to be plotted over time and allows calculation of various measures, including mean ambulatory BP over 24 h, diurnal variation (by comparing mean BP at night- with the daytime mean) and the overall range and variability of BP.

Cohort studies, performed in the last 10 years, have examined whether utilising ABPM-derived values, rather than clinic values to measure BP, is more accurate at predicting adverse cardiovascular outcomes. Of nine such studies identified by the NICE 2011 clinical guideline, eight (including over 25,000 patients) found that mean 24 h blood pressure values derived from ABPM were more strongly associated with cardiovascular events than clinic measurements [5].

The authors of the NICE guideline were persuaded to recommend (somewhat contentiously) that ABPM be used in all patients with a clinic BP greater than 140/90 mmHg to confirm the diagnosis of hypertension [5], but not to use ABPM in monitoring the response to treatment. At present, of the major hypertension guidelines, only NICE have recommended using ABPM to make the diagnosis of hypertension in all patients. Other international guidelines recommend its use in a more targeted fashion. Other indications for its use include investigating patients with suspected resistant, white coat or masked hypertension and monitoring response to treatment, particularly when there is a concern regarding iatrogenic hypotension.

Although the predictive value of ABPM is well established, there is no randomised evidence to guide the selection of an average BP threshold at which treatment would be indicated. In an effort to address this, Head et al. [13] compared mean 24 h BP and mean daytime BP (n=8,575) with clinic BP in a different cohort (n=1,693) and, using least product regression analysis, established that clinic BP was 6/3 mmHg higher than daytime mean ambulatory BP and 10/5 mmHg higher than 24 h mean ambulatory BP. The differences were more marked at higher BPs. On the basis of this data, the ABPM daytime equivalent to 140/90 mmHg in guidelines is 135/85 [10, 11].

The ultimate impact of utilising ABPM more frequently in clinical practice is yet to be fully appreciated, and further prospective research is required to address whether it is of benefit to patients and how to use it most appropriately.

Home Blood Pressure Monitors

An alternative to ABPM is home monitoring. Patients have their own home BP monitoring device which allows for similar benefits to ABPM as well as other potential benefits, such as allowing patients to assess their response to antihypertensive medications and providing frequent measurements over longer periods of time. However, concerns have been raised that such monitors may cause anxiety and obsessive behaviours and that the readings may be subject to observer prejudice and may produce unreliable readings.

Resistant Hypertension

Resistant hypertension is defined as hypertension (clinic BP >140/90 mmHg) despite treatment with a rational combination of at least 3 antihypertensive agents or controlled hypertension on 4 agents. Cohort studies suggest a prevalence of 10–15 % among those diagnosed with hypertension [15]. Apparent resistant hypertension may be due white coat hypertension (WCH), due to poor adherence with prescribed medication or due to a secondary cause.

Careful clinical evaluation of patients with suspected resistant or secondary hypertension is critical as the diagnosis may significantly alter treatment. A list of suggested first-line investigations in patients with resistant hypertension is presented in Table 11.4.

Table 11.4 Suggested first-line investigations in resistant hypertension

Cause	First-line investigation(s)
White coat hypertension	24 h ABPM
Poor adherence	Directly observed therapy OR measurement of serum/urinary levels of antihypertensives
Renal parenchymal disease	Blood electrolytes, creatinine and eGFR Urine strip for protein and blood
Renal artery stenosis	CT or MR renal angiogram
Primary aldosteronism	Plasma renin (+/− aldosterone) Cross-sectional imaging of adrenal gland (can be done concurrently with CT/MR renal angiogram)
Cushing's syndrome	24 h urinary cortisol, single-dose dexamethasone suppression test
Phaeochromocytoma	Plasma free metanephrines/catecholamines OR Urine free metanephrines/catecholamines

White Coat Hypertension

WCH or 'isolated clinic hypertension' is a condition in which BP measured in clinic is hypertensive, but that measured out of the clinic is normal (measured by ABPM or home monitors). This phenomenon is observed in approximately 30 % of patients with a clinic BP >140/90 mmHg [16], and the prognosis of these patients is good compared with those with sustained hypertension. However, whether or not the patients with WCH should be treated with antihypertensives is controversial.

Several studies have linked WCH with subclinical end-organ damage including left ventricular hypertrophy [17] and proteinuria [19]; however, these findings have not been reproduced across all studies. Multiple longitudinal studies suggest that WCH increases the long-term risk of stroke [20], cardiovascular events [21] and all-cause mortality [16], but to a significantly lesser degree than sustained hypertension. The relative risk of WCH versus sustained hypertension is nicely demonstrated in the Kaplan-Meier curves derived from the PAMELA study (Fig. 11.2) [18].

Thus, patients with WCH appear to have an intermediately increased risk of cardiovascular events, compared with normotensives and hypertensives. Several reasons for this increased risk have been proposed, most notably that BP variation (inherently higher in those with white coat hypertension) is itself an independent risk factor for cardiovascular events and that over time, a significant proportion of patients with WCH develop sustained hypertension.

ABPM is the investigation of choice to investigate whether a patient has WCH. Although, as mentioned, some guidelines advocate all patients undergoing ABPM, others

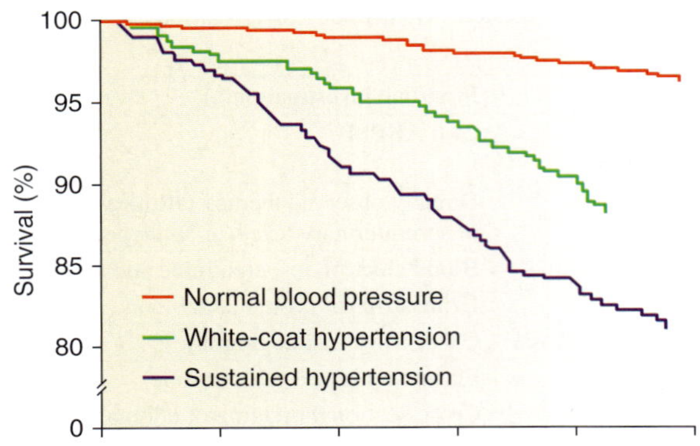

Fig. 11.2 Kaplan-Meier curves depicting the survival of patients with normal BP (*red*), WCH (*blue*) and sustained hypertension (*purple*) (Reprinted with permission from Sega et al. [18])

suggest its use when there is a high index of suspicion. This may be the case if patients have home readings that are significantly lower than those in the clinic, in patients that show signs of over treatment (such as postural symptoms) and in patients with high office BP with no target organ damage [6].

There is no trial evidence to guide whether or not patients with WCH would benefit from treatment, and some guidelines, including NICE, do not advocate treatment in patients with clinic sBP 140–160 mmHg and mean daytime sBP <135 mmHg [5]. However, the ESC guidelines suggest starting treatment if there is evidence of end-organ damage [7], and overall, a decision to treat should be taken after consideration of multiple factors, including the ABPM, clinic BP measurements and the 10-year cardiovascular risk in addition to assessment of end-organ damage.

Masked Hypertension

Masked hypertension or isolated ambulatory hypertension is the inverse of WCH, in which clinic BP measurements are <140/90 mmHg, whereas the mean BP on ABPM is elevated (>135/85 mmHg). This occurs in approximately 15 % of the population [23], and since the associated cardiovascular risk is similar to that of sustained hypertension, it represents a significant diagnostic challenge. A high index of suspicion is warranted in patients with a normal clinic BP who have multiple cardiovascular risk factors and evidence of organ damage.

Poor Adherence

Poor adherence is a major cause of lack of blood pressure control and, along with WCH, accounts for the majority of patients who appear to have resistant hypertension. Retrospective analyses indicate that up to 40 % of patients with newly diagnosed hypertension will discontinue their medication within the first year of treatment [24], and over 5–10 years this figure may rise to over 60 % [25]. Assessing whether or not this is the case can be challenging, as patients may not be forthright about their adherence. Several strategies have been developed to overcome this, including directly observed therapy and measurement of urinary or serum antihypertensive levels. Directly observed therapy may necessitate an admission to a day ward or overnight inpatient stay and should be conducted with caution – giving multiple antihypertensives to a non-compliant patient at once may cause profound and life-threatening hypotension, and thus giving only 1–2 agents initially is advised.

Once this diagnosis is established, management can be a challenge, but focusing on patients' motivations and considering side-effect profiles of available antihypertensives should both form part of the strategy.

Secondary Hypertension

Secondary hypertension is hypertension in which there is an identifiable cause. It is thought to account for up to 10 % of patients with hypertension although this figure is likely to increase with the increasing prevalence of hypertension and obesity. In addition to patients with apparently resistant hypertension, secondary causes should be considered in those who present:

1. Young (<40 years)
2. With accelerated hypertension/hypertensive emergencies
3. Have suddenly worsening hypertension
4. Severe end-organ damage
5. Family history of early onset hypertension/stroke

Secondary causes of hypertension may be split into four broad groups: renal, endocrine, drugs (see Table 11.5 and Box 11.2) and 'other causes'. A comprehensive summary of these is presented in Table 11.6. The most important of these will now be discussed.

Renal Causes of Secondary Hypertension

Renal Parenchymal Disease

Renal parenchymal disease is the most common cause (50–75 %) of secondary hypertension, with cohort studies suggesting a prevalence of approximately 6 % in patients with hypertension [26]. Given this, and that cardiovascular risks increase significantly once hypertensive nephropathy is established, all patients with newly diagnosed hypertension should have serum urea, creatinine, electrolytes measured and an estimation of glomerular filtration rate

Table 11.5 Effect of antihypertensives on serum renin and aldosterone levels

Drug group	Examples	Effect on renin	Effect on aldosterone	Comments
Beta-blockers	Atenolol, bisoprolol, metoprolol	↓	↓	Generally consistent effect
Potassium-sparing diuretics	Amiloride, spironolactone	↑	↑	Very large increases in renin
ACE inhibitors	Enalapril, perindopril, ramipril	↑	↓	Large increases in renin. Effect on aldosterone less consistent
Thiazide (and thiazide-like) diuretics	Bendroflumethiazide, chlortalidone, metolazone	↑	↑	Consistent effect with renin, more variable with aldosterone
Loop diuretics	Bumetanide, Furosemide	↑	↔/↓	Only small changes seen
Calcium channel antagonists	Amlodipine, felodipine, nifedipine	↔/↓/↑	↔/↓/↑	Variable, unpredictable effects
Alpha channel antagonists	Doxazosin, indoramin, tamsulosin	None significant	None significant	Best when measuring renin and aldosterone

Box 11.2: Drugs Which Increase BP

- Oestrogens (e.g. in contraceptives)
- Non-steroidal anti-inflammatory drugs
- COX-2 inhibitors
- Weight-loss agents (amphetamine related)
- Stimulants (e.g. cocaine)
- Mineral and glucocorticoids
- Antiparkinsonian agents (serotoninergic)
- Monoamine oxidase inhibitors (serotoninergic)
- Anabolic steroids
- Sympathomimetics including decongestants
- Migraine treatments (triptans – serotoninergic)

Table 11.6 An evidence-based guide to treating high blood pressure

Who to treat	Anyone older than 55 will benefit from BP lowering[a]
	Anyone with a prior cardiovascular event
	Anyone with evidence of end-organ damage, irrespective of BP level
	Anyone with extreme elevation of BP[b]
What to treat with	Diet and lifestyle for all
	BP lowering medication; once contraindications are checked, use any as a first-line agent and when adding any combination so long as tolerated
What treatment target	The lower the BP achieved without producing symptoms of hypotension, the better
	Address all other risk factors

[a]Lifestyle advice first – reduce salt and alcohol intake, weight loss, increase aerobic exercise and fruit/vegetable and oily fish consumption

[b]Investigate for secondary causes of raised BP, particularly in the young, if all negative, proceed to directly observed therapy to ensure non-adherence as a cause of persistently elevated BP despite presumed adequate therapy

(eGFR) as well as a urine dip for protein, erythrocytes and leucocytes. There should be a robust referral pathway for patients with renal impairment or an abnormal urine sediment.

Renal Artery Stenosis (See Chap. 34)

Renal artery stenosis (RAS) is a common cause of secondary hypertension. Its prevalence in the general hypertension population is approximately 2–5 % [27] and is more than 30 % in patients undergoing cardiac catheterisation [28] and may account for up to 14 % of patients with end-stage renal failure [28]. The culprit stenoses are of the extra-renal arteries and are most commonly caused by atherosclerotic plaques or by fibromuscular dysplasia, which is more common in younger female patients, but may also be the result of vasculitis, neurofibromatosis, congenital bands and extrinsic compression.

Classically, RAS is suggested by the presence of an abdominal bruit, progressively worsening renal function, acutely worsening renal function after the introduction of an angiotensin-converting enzyme (ACE) inhibitor (poor sensitivity and specificity) and episodes of unexplained flash pulmonary oedema or angina.

The gold standard diagnostic test is intravenous contrast-enhanced digital subtraction angiography. However, non-invasive tests are often sufficient in confirming the diagnosis. Due to its wide availability and low cost, ultrasonography and colour Doppler studies are often the first imaging study used to investigate RAS; however, results are operator dependent and stenotic lesions are often missed. Preferable imaging modalities are computed tomography (CT) and magnetic resonance (MR) angiography. Both have sensitivities over 90 % and the choice of modality may be guided by factors such as renal function and the presence of implanted devices.

Rarer causes of renovascular hypertension include middle-aortic syndrome, Takayasu's aortitis, Page kidney and suprarenal coarctation of the aorta.

Distal Tubular Disorders

Rare, inherited dysfunctions of the distal renal tubule can cause increased sodium absorption and hypertension. The most important of these is Liddle's syndrome.

Liddle's syndrome is the result of mutations in the genes which encode the amiloride-sensitive epithelial sodium channel (ENaC) in the distal nephron which increases both the numbers and activity of the channels. This results in increased sodium and water retention and therefore hypertension. It is inherited in an autosomal dominant fashion and is probably the most common type of monogenic hypertension [29]. It usually presents in childhood or early adulthood with hypertension and hypokalaemia. A key diagnostic feature is that plasma renin and aldosterone levels are markedly suppressed. Treatment includes dietary salt restriction and inhibitors of the ENaC such as amiloride.

Another familial autosomal disease of the distal nephron is Gordon's syndrome (pseudohypoaldosteronism type II). Gain-of-function mutations in the thiazide-sensitive sodium chloride co-transporter result in excessive sodium and chloride reabsorption, hypertension and hyperkalaemia.

Endocrine Causes of Secondary Hypertension

There are multiple endocrine causes of secondary hypertension which should be considered in any secondary work-up. In addition to mineralocorticoid excess, Cushing's syndrome and phaeochromocytoma which are all detailed below, hypertension may also be a feature of the following endocrine disorders:

1. Hyper- and hypothyroidism
2. Hyperparathyroidism
3. Acromegaly
4. Carcinoid syndrome

Mineralocorticoid Excess

Mineralocorticoid excess results in increased renal sodium reabsorption and hypertension. It is most often the result of primary aldosteronism (see below) but rarer causes include the following:

1. Congenital adrenal hyperplasia – defects in 11-hydroxylase and 17-hydroxylase (key enzymes in the production of adrenal steroids) result in excessive accumulation of intermediate products with mineralocorticoid activity. In addition to hypertension, patients have genital ambiguity.
2. Glucocorticoid-remediable aldosteronism – a rare autosomal dominant disorder in which a fusion of 2 genes results in aldosterone production being stimulated by adrenocorticotropic hormone (ACTH).
3. Apparent mineralocorticoid excess – a rare autosomal recessive disorder in which an inactivating mutation of the 11 B-hydroxysteroid dehydrogenase type 2 enzyme allows cortisol to activate the mineralocorticoid receptor.
4. Exogenous mineralocorticoid excess – may be the result of fludrocortisone administration or excess liquorice ingestion.

Primary aldosteronism is characterised by overproduction of the mineralocorticoid aldosterone. Approximately 30 % are due to adenomas, with the majority being due to bilateral hyperplasia. Rarely it may be due to unilateral adrenal hyperplasia.

The incidence of primary aldosteronism may be as high as 20 % in patients with resistant hypertension [30], and primary aldosteronism is the most common curable cause of secondary hypertension. Hypokalaemia is not a reliable indicator as less than 15 % may present with this finding [31], and thus previous studies which were reliant on this finding to make the diagnosis grossly underestimated its prevalence.

A good initial screening test is measurement of plasma renin levels, with or without the addition of plasma aldosterone levels and calculation of a renin:aldosterone (R:A) ratio. A suppressed renin and elevated aldosterone – resulting in an elevated ratio (>800) – is suggestive of primary aldosteronism; a ratio >2,000 with aldosterone >250pmol/l makes the diagnosis almost certain.

However, this test must be interpreted with caution in the elderly or black patients who may have low renin and those on drugs which interfere with the renin-angiotensin-aldosterone pathway (Table 11.5). This is clearly a common problem in patients with resistant hypertension that may be on several of these agents. Ideally, the antihypertensives are stopped 2 weeks prior to the measurement of serum renin and aldosterone levels. Alpha-blockers, slow-release verapamil or hydralazine can be used to treat the hypertension during this period. Calcium channel blockers have unpredictable effects on renin and aldosterone but are nonetheless commonly used to control blood pressure in such patients. Time of day, posture and serum potassium levels are other important factors which may affect renin. Ideally potassium should be corrected into the normal range, and R:A ratio following normal saline infusion is said to be more specific.

Confirmatory functional tests involve aldosterone suppression utilising oral or intravenous salt loading, fludrocortisone or captopril, although these are seldom used in practice. CT or MR imaging is required to identify the presence of an adenoma. Subsequently, adrenal vein sampling allows for confirmation and localisation of the primary aldosteronism to one, or both, of the adrenals. This is a technically challenging procedure that should be carried out by an experienced practitioner. However, this is particularly important as identified adenomas may be non-functioning or may in fact be the result of nodular hyperplasia. More recently, positron emission tomography (PET) CT, utilising the radiotracer (11)C-metomidate, a potent inhibitor of adrenal steroidogenic enzymes, has been developed as a non-invasive alternative to adrenal vein sampling [32].

Cushing's Syndrome

Cushing's syndrome is caused by excess glucocorticoids, which is most commonly iatrogenic. It may also be due to overproduction of ACTH by the pituitary gland (Cushing's disease) or by production of cortisol by a tumour of the adrenal gland or rarely by ectopic release from another organ or gland. The syndrome affects <0.1 % of the total population but causes hypertension in approximately 80 % of those affected [33].

Screening tests include 24 h urinary cortisol excretion, late night salivary cortisol or the single-dose (1 mg) dexamethasone suppression test. Positive results should be confirmed by performing at least 1 other tests or midnight cortisol. Subsequent localising tests include plasma ACTH, long dexamethasone suppression tests and the corticotrophin-releasing hormone stimulation test.

Phaeochromocytoma

Phaeochromocytoma is a rare cause of secondary hypertension accounting for <0.5 % of patients with hypertension [34] (M:F 2:1), but some case series have reported an incidence of 4 % in patients with resistant hypertension [35]. Approximately 85 % arise from the adrenal glands, with the remainder termed 'paragangliomas' arising from extra-adrenal chromaffin tissue, typically in the abdomen, urinary bladder or mediastinum. They can be inherited, often as part of a multiple endocrine neoplasia syndrome, or acquired.

The diagnosis should be suspected in patients if episodic headaches, palpitations (64 %) and sweating (70 %) are features in addition to hypertension. Episodic pallor, tremor, flushing, epigastric pain, dyspnea, syncope and hypotension are also important findings. Of note, previous cohort studies have suggested that up to 70 % of such patients are hypertensives, but since many are now picked up incidentally, hypertension is only a feature in approximately half. Screening tests (in order of sensitivity) include plasma free metanephrines (99 %), urinary fractionated metanephrines (97 %), urinary and plasma catecholamines (85 %), urinary total metanephrines (77 %) and vanillylmandelic acid (VMA) (64 %) [36].

Confirmatory tests include glucagon stimulation and clonidine suppression tests, and cross-sectional imaging is required to localise the tumour. In the case of extra-adrenal tumours, isotopic scanning with meta-iodobenzylguanidine (MIBG) can be of use.

Other Causes of Secondary Hypertension

There are several other secondary causes of hypertension which are listed in Table 11.6. Coarctation of the aorta and obstructive sleep apnoea are reversible causes and therefore particularly significant.

Coarctation of the Aorta

Coarctation is a rare but important cause, representing about 6–8 % of all congenital heart disease and 1 in 2,500 births [37]. It is seven times more common in white than Asian children. Patients may present as children or adolescents with symptoms of dyspnea, leg cramps on exercise, chest pain, fainting and shortness of breath but are increasingly identified earlier because of other congenital heart disease or as investigation of mid-systolic murmur (radiating to the back). Making the diagnosis is critical as untreated there is a 80 % mortality by 50 years and diagnosis before 14 results in a significantly reduced mortality compared to diagnosis after this. Cool feet and poor lower limb pulses are a strong clue; radiofemoral delay and unequal blood pressure in limbs are non-invasive and simple clinical examinations. Treatment is either surgical correction or angioplasty with currently no evidence to recommend one over the other.

Obstructive Sleep Apnoea

There is a strong association between obstructive sleep apnoea (OSA) and hypertension (present in 50–90 % of patients with OSA [38]), and with increasing severity, the associated hypertension is more difficult to control. The proposed mechanism to explain this association is that intermittent hypoxemia induces a sustained increase in sympathetic nervous system activity, which in turn raises blood pressure by well-described mechanisms. The cardiovascular risk of OSA is significant and an important cause of hypertension is not to miss. Loss or reversal of nocturnal dipping (the usual 10 % drop in BP at night) may be prominent and a clue, but history or body habitus of OSA should prompt exclusion of OSA as a contributor to hypertension as correction can sometimes have a marked effect on hypertension and cardiovascular risk.

Obesity

Although not strictly considered a secondary cause of hypertension, obesity is a strong independent risk factor for hypertension. Furthermore, the observation that there are an increasing number of children and adolescents with hypertension is likely attributed to the rising prevalence of obesity. In 2010 16.9 % of children and adolescents in the USA were obese, which was significantly higher than a decade before [39] and has been driven by diet and lifestyle changes. If this trend continues, there will be an epidemic of hypertension and other obesity-related co-morbidities in western countries.

Summary

As hypertension is the most important modifiable risk factor for cardiovascular and renal disease, an understanding of its diagnosis and thresholds for treatment is crucial. National and international published guidelines provide a useful framework for the diagnosis of hypertension, but differences in approach exist. When measuring blood pressure and making decisions to treat, considerations not only include the measured clinic blood pressure but an overall assessment of cardiovascular risk, end-organ damage (clinical or subclinical) and the need for 24 h ABPM. Further considerations and investigations of secondary causes are required in those that present young, with accelerated hypertension or apparent resistant hypertension.

References

1. Lloyd-Jones D, Adams R, Carnethon M, et al. Heart disease and stroke statistics—2009 update a report from the American Heart Association Statistics Committee and Stroke Statistics Subcommittee. Circulation. 2009;119:480–6.
2. Lewington S, Clarke R, Qizilbash N, et al. Age-specific relevance of usual blood pressure to vascular mortality: a meta-analysis of individual data for one million adults in 61 prospective studies. Lancet. 2002;360:1903–13.
3. Lawes CMM, Vander Hoorn S, Rodgers A. Global burden of blood-pressure-related disease, 2001. Lancet. 2008;371:1513–8.
4. Hsu C, McCulloch CE, Darbinian J, et al. Elevated blood pressure and risk of end-stage renal disease in subjects without baseline kidney disease. Arch Intern Med. 2005;165:923–8.
5. NICE. CG127 Hypertension: NICE guideline. http://publications.nice.org.uk/hypertension-cg127. Accessed 24 Aug 2012.
6. Rosendorff C, Black HR, Cannon CP, et al. Treatment of hypertension in the prevention and management of ischemic heart disease a scientific statement from the American Heart Association Council for high blood pressure research and the councils on clinical cardiology and epidemiology and prevention. Circulation. 2007;115:2761–88.
7. Mancia G, De Backer G, Dominiczak A, et al. 2007 Guidelines for the management of arterial hypertension: the task force for the management of arterial hypertension of the European Society of Hypertension (ESH) and of the European Society of Cardiology (ESC). Eur Heart J. 2007;28:1462–536.
8. Mancia G, Laurent S, Agabiti-Rosei E, et al. Reappraisal of European guidelines on hypertension management: a European Society of Hypertension Task Force document. J Hypertens. 2009;27:2121–58.
9. Chapter 2. Measurement and clinical evaluation of blood pressure. Hypertens Res. 2009;32:11–23.
10. World Health Organisation. Prevention of cardiovascular disease. Guidelines for assessment and management of cardiovascular risk. WHO Press, Geneva, Switzerland. 2007;1–85. http://whqlibdoc.who.int/publications/2007/9789241547178_eng.pdf?ua=1.
11. Verberk WJ, Kroon AA, Kessels AGH, et al. The optimal scheme of self blood pressure measurement as determined from ambulatory blood pressure recordings. J Hypertens. 2006;24:1541–8.
12. De Galan BE, Perkovic V, Ninomiya T, et al. Lowering blood pressure reduces renal events in type 2 diabetes. J Am Soc Nephrol. 2009;20:883–92.
13. Head GA, Mihailidou AS, Duggan KA, et al. Definition of ambulatory blood pressure targets for diagnosis and treatment of hypertension in relation to clinic blood pressure: prospective cohort study. BMJ. 2010;340:c1104.
14. Law MR, Morris JK, Wald NJ. Use of blood pressure lowering drugs in the prevention of cardiovascular disease: meta-analysis of 147 randomised trials in the context of expectations from prospective epidemiological studies. [Review] [60 refs]. BMJ. 2009;338:b1665. doi:10.1136/bmj.b1665.
15. De la Sierra A, Segura J, Banegas JR, et al. Clinical features of 8295 patients with resistant hypertension classified on the basis of ambulatory blood pressure monitoring. Hypertension. 2011;57:898–902.
16. Mancia G, Facchetti R, Bombelli M, et al. Long-term risk of mortality associated with selective and combined elevation in office, home, and ambulatory blood pressure. Hypertension. 2006;47:846–53.
17. Páll D, Juhász M, Lengyel S, et al. Assessment of target-organ damage in adolescent white-coat and sustained hypertensives. J Hypertens. 2010;28:2139–44.
18. Sega R, Trocino G, Lanzarotti A, et al. Alterations of cardiac structure in patients with isolated office, ambulatory, or home hypertension: data from the general population (Pressione Arteriose Monitorate E Loro Associazioni [PAMELA] Study). Circulation. 2001;104:1385–92.
19. Palatini P, Mormino P, Santonastaso M, et al. Target-organ damage in stage I hypertensive subjects with white coat and sustained hypertension: results from the HARVEST study. Hypertension. 1998;31:57–63.
20. Verdecchia P, Reboldi GP, Angeli F, et al. Short- and long-term incidence of stroke in white-coat hypertension. Hypertension. 2005;45:203–8.
21. Gustavsen PH, Høegholm A, Bang LE, et al. White coat hypertension is a cardiovascular risk factor: a 10-year follow-up study. J Hum Hypertens. 2003;17:811–7.
22. Arima H, Chalmers J, Woodward M, et al. Lower target blood pressures are safe and effective for the prevention of recurrent stroke: the PROGRESS trial. J Hypertens. 2006;24:1201–8.
23. Hansen TW, Jeppesen J, Rasmussen S, et al. Ambulatory blood pressure monitoring and risk of cardiovascular disease: a population based study. Am J Hypertens. 2006;19:243–50.
24. Caro JJ, Speckman JL, Salas M, et al. Effect of initial drug choice on persistence with antihypertensive therapy: the importance of actual practice data. CMAJ. 1999;160:41–6.
25. Van Wijk BL, Klungel OH, Heerdink ER, et al. Rate and determinants of 10-year persistence with antihypertensive drugs. J Hypertens. 2005;23:2101–7.
26. Sinclair AM, Isles CG, Brown I, et al. Secondary hypertension in a blood pressure clinic. Arch Intern Med. 1987;147:1289–93.

27. Lao D, Parasher PS, Cho KC, et al. Atherosclerotic renal artery stenosis–diagnosis and treatment. Mayo Clin Proc. 2011;86: 649–57.
28. Harding MB, Smith LR, Himmelstein SI, et al. Renal artery stenosis: prevalence and associated risk factors in patients undergoing routine cardiac catheterization. J Am Soc Nephrol. 1992;2:1608–16.
29. Vehaskari VM. Heritable forms of hypertension. Pediatr Nephrol. 2009;24:1929–37.
30. Calhoun DA, Nishizaka MK, Zaman MA, et al. Hyperaldosteronism among black and white subjects with resistant hypertension. Hypertension. 2002;40:892–6.
31. Stowasser M, Gordon RD, Gunasekera TG, et al. High rate of detection of primary aldosteronism, including surgically treatable forms, after 'non-selective' screening of hypertensive patients. J Hypertens. 2003;21:2149–57.
32. Burton TJ, Mackenzie IS, Balan K, et al. Evaluation of the sensitivity and specificity of (11)C-metomidate positron emission tomography (PET)-CT for lateralizing aldosterone secretion by Conn's adenomas. J Clin Endocrinol Metab. 2012;97:100–9.
33. Newell-Price J, Bertagna X, Grossman AB, et al. Cushing's syndrome. Lancet. 2006;367:1605–17.
34. Reisch N, Peczkowska M, Januszewicz A, et al. Pheochromocytoma: presentation, diagnosis and treatment. J Hypertens. 2006;24:2331–9.
35. Martell N, Rodriguez-Cerrillo M, Grobbee DE, et al. High prevalence of secondary hypertension and insulin resistance in patients with refractory hypertension. Blood Press. 2003;12:149–54.
36. Lenders JWM, Pacak K, Walther MM, et al. Biochemical diagnosis of pheochromocytoma: which test is best? JAMA. 2002;287: 1427–34.
37. Kenny D, Hijazi ZM. Coarctation of the aorta: from fetal life to adulthood. Cardiol J. 2011;18:487–95.
38. Nieto FJ, Young TB, Lind BK, et al. Association of sleep-disordered breathing, sleep apnea, and hypertension in a large community-based study. Sleep Heart Health Study. JAMA. 2000;283:1829–36.
39. Ogden CL, Carroll MD, Kit BK, et al. Prevalence of obesity and trends in body mass index among US children and adolescents, 1999–2010. JAMA. 2012;307:483–90.

Management of High Blood Pressure

12

Reecha Sofat, Marc Jonathan George, Aroon D. Hingorani, and Raymond MacAllister

Treatment of blood pressure in the context of renal disease is important for three reasons. First, high BP can cause ESRD; second, high BP is a consequence of renal disease; and third, high BP is a major modifiable risk factor for CVD which in turn is the main cause of mortality and morbidity in individuals with ESRD. The approach to treatment of BP should be similar in those with and without established renal disease. This approach reflects the totality of the evidence base.

Randomised controlled trials (RCTs) demonstrate BP reductions, whether by diet, lifestyle or drug therapy, reducing the risk of CHD, stroke and ESRD. Overviews of RCTs of drugs that lower BP show that a sustained reduction over 5 years of 5–6 mmHg in BP reduces coronary events by approximately 20 % and strokes by 40 % [1]. This is in keeping with evidence from overviews of prospective observational studies that predict lowering BP by this degree confers the same magnitude of protection [2]. Therefore, the overarching aim should be reduction of blood pressure rather than the drug used to achieve this.

R. Sofat • M.J. George, MBChB (Hons), BSc (Hons)
Department of Clinical Pharmacology and Therapeutics, University College London Hospital, 235 Euston Road, London NW1 2BU, UK
e-mail: marc.george@uclh.nhs.uk

A.D. Hingorani, MA, FRCP, PhD
Department of Genetic Epidemiology, Institute of Cardiovascular Science, University College London and University College London Hospitals NHS Foundation Trust, 1-19 Torrinton Place, London WC1E 6BT, UK
e-mail: a.hingorani@ucl.ac.uk

R. MacAllister, FRCP, MD (✉)
Division of Medicine, Centre for Clinical Pharmacology, University College London, Rayne Building, 5 University Street, London WC1E 6JF, UK
e-mail: r.macallister@ucl.ac.uk

M. Harber (ed.), *Practical Nephrology*,
DOI 10.1007/978-1-4471-5547-8_12, © Springer-Verlag London 2014

Non-pharmacological Management of Hypertension

A number of non-pharmacological interventions have been shown to be effective in randomised controlled trials, at producing sustained reductions in blood pressure. These measures can therefore be a useful first strategy for lowering BP in individuals, particularly where no end-organ damage has been identified. Such measures include:

- Salt (reducing sodium intake from 10 to 5 g/day leads to a ~5/3 mmHg reduction in BP) [3, 4]
- Alcohol (change depends on amount consumed) [5]
- Weight (expect 1–2 mmHg BP reduction for every kg lost) [6]
- Aerobic exercise (thrice weekly aerobic exercise leads to a ~4/3 mmHg reduction) [7]
- Diet rich in fresh fruit and vegetables (increased dietary potassium) [8]
- Oily fish [9–11]

Drugs Used to Lower Blood Pressure

The British National Formulary lists ~50 BP-lowering drugs drawn from 7 drug classes. Four drug classes dominate prescribing in England and Wales: angiotensin-converting enzyme (ACEi) inhibitors and angiotensin receptor blockers (ARB) (A-class drugs), β-blockers (B-class drugs), calcium channel blockers (CCB) (C-class drugs) and diuretics (D-class drugs). Each class has a differing mechanism of action [12], but all classes have been shown in RCTs to be effective in reducing the risk of cardiovascular and renal outcomes.

Evidence from an overview of short-term trials (with blood pressure as the outcome) indicate that all classes of blood pressure-lowering drugs at either standard, half or quarter standard doses result in broadly comparable reductions in BP [13] (Fig. 12.1). Moreover, combinations of drugs from different classes at low dose may provide a way of achieving additive reductions in blood pressure with a

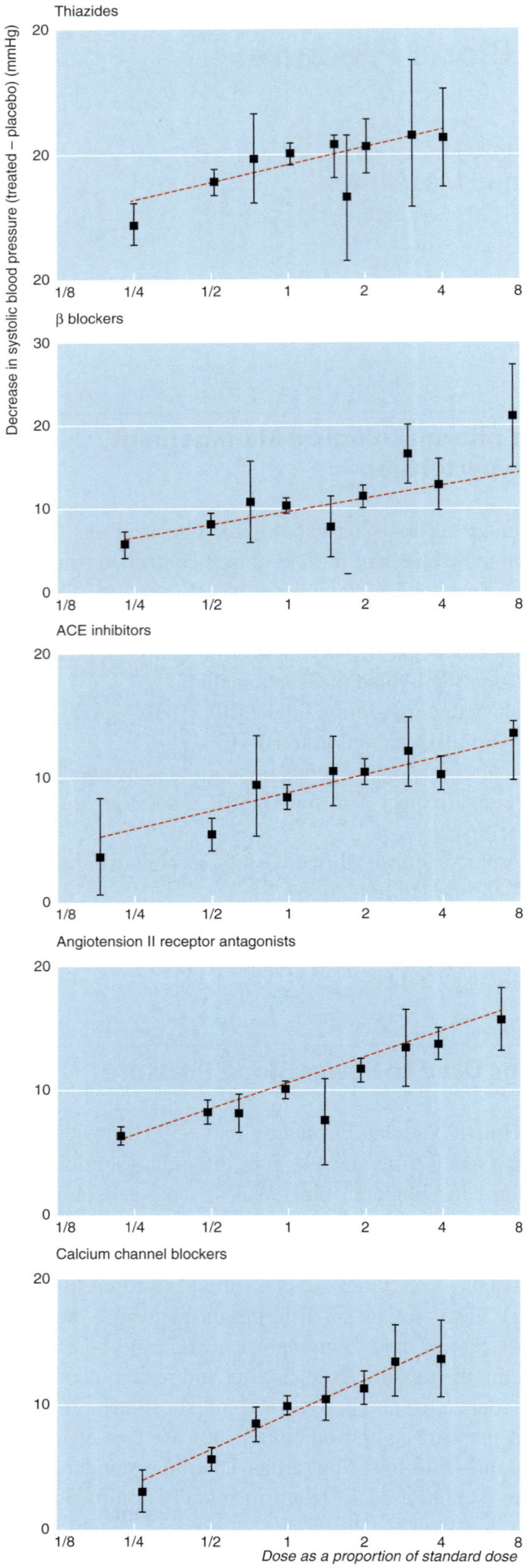

possible advantage of a reduction of dose-related mechanism-based adverse effects, which are important causes of discontinuation of therapy [13].

Generic drugs are available for all the major drug classes. Reduced acquisition costs of drugs translate into cost savings to health providers, provided branded medications are avoided (from within these major classes). Newer agents available currently (e.g. aliskiren) or in the future can only be rationally prescribed if there are persuasive reasons to think that they are superior to existing generic drugs.

The evidence base on the efficacy of BP-lowering drugs from all the major classes is large, encompassing ~150 RCTs over four decades. Three types of trial that have been conducted are as follows: first, those that test active treatments versus placebo (long-term trials are no longer ethical because of the established benefits of BP lowering); second, those that test a more intensive versus a less intensive BP lowering; and third, trials of one active drug versus another. The first two categories of trial answer questions about the efficacy of BP lowering on outcome. However, differences between classes might be inferred by exploring evidence for heterogeneity in effect sizes across trials of different agents. The third category of trial investigates class- or drug-specific differences in efficacy. To ensure a fair test in a head-to-head trial of this type, the achieved BP in the two arms of such a trial *must* be similar, to confirm that differences in outcome event rates are not simply due to BP differences between the two arms. Two recent overviews [1, 14] have both interpreted the evidence in the context of achieved BP reductions and emphasised the similarity in effectiveness of different BP-lowering drugs in the prevention of cardiovascular outcomes with two possible exceptions: beta-blockers may have a class-specific advantage in reducing recurrent CHD events in patients who have suffered an MI, and dihydropyridine calcium channel blockers may have an advantage over other classes in the prevention of stroke. The number of patients with kidney disease in these trials is small, but is reasonable to extrapolate the findings from these studies to patients with kidney disease.

Controversies in Blood Pressure Management

Despite this evidence there continue to be controversies in the pharmacological management of BP. Up to 2006, international guidance on BP management was largely uniform. The

Fig. 12.1 Average reductions in systolic blood pressure according to drug class and dose as a proportion of a given standard dose (here shown as 1). Results are adjusted for SBP change in the placebo group, and data are based on analysis form 354 randomised controlled trials (Reproduced with permission from Law et al. [13])

message was clear, and the recommendation was that the overarching benefit of antihypertensive medication is lowering of BP rather than the drug used to achieve it. Subsequent to the publication of influential trials and meta-analysis [15, 16], guidance in England and Wales has evolved. As a consequence, pharmacological updates of joint guidance issued by NICE and the British Hypertension Society (BHS) guidance since 2006 have led to recommendation of A-class drugs as initial treatment in those <55 years and C-class drugs in those >55 years of age, while B-class drugs have been relegated to being a third- or fourth-line option. In the most recent NICE/BHS guidelines (http://www.nice.org.uk/CG127), D-class drugs were relegated to a third-line option because they were considered to be less effective in reducing BP variability than C-class drugs. The *proposed* reasons for the emphasis of updated guidelines on drug choice rather than BP reduction can be summarised as follows:

1. BP-lowering drugs differ in their BP-lowering efficacy in younger and older patients: drugs that target the renin-angiotensin system (A-class/B-class drugs) are considered to be more effective in lowering BP in younger patients (age <55 years) than in older patients where renin concentration is low and C/D class drugs are considered more effective.
2. Differences exist in the efficacy and safety of different BP-lowering drug classes. Specifically:
    - B-class (β-blockers) and D-class (thiazide diuretics) increase the risk of type 2 diabetes.
    - B-class (β-blockers) in general and atenolol in particular confer less protection from stroke than other drug classes.
    - A-class drugs have a class-specific advantage, over and above BP lowering, in protection from renal disease.
3. Apparent differences in cardiovascular outcomes between the different drug classes might arise because of differences in their effect on diabetes risk, their effect on central (aortic) compared to peripheral (brachial artery) BP and their effect on BP variability.

However, the extent to which these proposals are supported by the evidence is debated, and indeed European and US guidelines on the treatment of hypertension remain largely similar to the pre-2006 UK guidance. The arguments are discussed below.

Age as a Determinant of BP-Lowering Response to Different Drug Classes

Recommendations that BP is best lowered with A-class drugs in patients aged under 55 years (in whom an activated renin-angiotensin system may be an important mechanism) and D-class diuretics or C-class calcium channel blockers in older patients (because sodium retention, with suppression of the renin-angiotensin system, may be more important) were based primarily on the findings of a mechanistic study ($n=36$) that rotated young patients through monthly treatment with each of four main classes of BP-lowering drugs and assessed the effect on BP [17]. Since renin declines with age [18], and the major drug classes differ in their effect on the renin-angiotensin system [19], age has been suggested as a proxy for stratifying the response of BP medications on cardiovascular outcomes. However, on the few occasions when potential effect modification by age of the effect of BP treatment on cardiovascular outcomes has been evaluated, no major differences have been observed [14]. Similar analyses using renin concentrations (now possible with a rapid, cheap assay [20]) have yet to be conducted, and this therefore remains a hypothesis.

β-Blockers and Stroke Prevention

Two sources of evidence were influential in the relegation of B-class β-blockers from first-line treatment of the NICE guidance: the 2005 Anglo-Scandinavian Cardiovascular Outcomes Trial (ASCOT) [15] and three meta-analyses examining the efficacy of β-blockers in prevention of cardiovascular events, published in 2005–2006 [16, 21, 22]. ASCOT was a randomised trial comparing a C-class drug (amlodipine)–based treatment regimen (with addition of perindopril and then doxazosin if required) with a B-class drug (atenolol)–based treatment regimen (with the addition of bendroflumethiazide and then doxazosin if required) to achieve a BP <140/90 mmHg. The trial was terminated early on the advice of the data safety monitoring committee because of a significant treatment difference in favour of patients randomised to the C-class-based regimen for two secondary end points (stroke and total cardiovascular events). There was no evidence of a difference in the primary end point of nonfatal myocardial infarction or fatal coronary heart disease. BP after intervention was lower in the group randomised to amlodipine compared to atenolol by around 2.7/1.9 mmHg on average throughout the trial. The trialists' analysis suggested the BP difference was insufficient to explain the disparity in event rates, but others have reached the opposite conclusion [23].

A subsequent meta-analysis examined trials comparing B-class drugs with any other BP-lowering drugs [16]. Stroke risk was 16 % higher (95 % CI 4–30 %) among patients randomised to B-class drugs than among those taking other drugs. Other meta-analyses reached similar conclusions [21, 22]. However, these meta-analyses were sensitive to the criteria for including RCTs and did not take full account of differences in achieved BP between treatment arms. These limitations were confirmed by a recent reanalysis of such

...analysis suggested ...mparator drug over B-class ...hich may explain the apparent ben- ... drugs over β-blockers. The BP disparity is ... to be because β-blockers are inherently less effec-tive at lowering BP than other drugs but rather because achieving a precisely equivalent BP reduction in two arms of a comparator trial is extremely challenging.

The pairwise meta-analyses conducted by Law et al. [1] and that by the Blood Pressure Lowering Treatment Trialists Collaboration [14] now supersede these studies. These examined the efficacy of all major BP drug classes (not just B-class drugs) in the context of the achieved reductions in BP. The Blood Pressure Lowering Treatment Trialists Collaboration' Collaboration, which incorporated information from 190 to 606 participants across 31 treatment trials, concluded that all classes of drug were broadly equivalent with respect to protection from major cardiovascular events. The investigators found a log-linear association between BP reduction and the relative risk of cardiovascular events, in keeping with predictions from observational studies. A second analysis by Law and colleagues, which included information from 147 published trials among 464,000 participants, concluded that the protective effect of lowering BP on coronary heart disease was the same for all drug classes in primary prevention, with the possible exception of the effect of C-class drugs on stroke [1]. The authors considered that this probably accounted for most of the apparent disadvantage of B-class drugs in stroke protection, because C-class calcium channel blockers had been the most common comparator drug in trials of B-class drugs.

BP-Lowering Drugs and the Risk of Type 2 Diabetes

Patients receiving B- or D-class drugs rather than A-class drugs are at higher risk of diabetes. But what is the magnitude of the blood glucose increase, by how much is the absolute risk of diabetes increased and, importantly, how does this affect the risk of cardiovascular events?

In the ASCOT trial, diabetes risk was increased among people randomised to the B-class arm (atenolol-bendroflumethiazide) (the hazard ratio comparing C-class (amlodipine) with B-class (atenolol) was 0.70, 95 % CI 0.63–0.78, equating to a risk difference of 11 per 1,000 people over 5 years). However, the average absolute difference in blood glucose concentration was only 0.2 mmol/L (SD 2.08 mmol/L, $P<0.0001$). The substantial increase in the risk of diabetes arises because an average increase in glucose of as little as 0.2 mmol/L leads to an increase in the proportion of people marginally exceeding the diagnostic fasting blood glucose threshold of 7 mmol/L and therefore being classified as diabetic (Fig. 12.2 [10]).

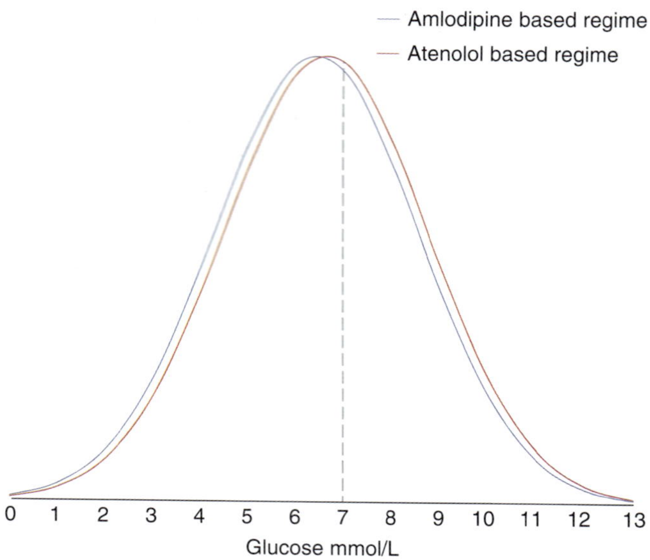

Fig. 12.2 Estimated distribution of on treatment blood glucose in individuals randomised to amlodipine compared to those randomised to atenolol in the ASCOT-BPLA trial. Curves are constructed using the reported mean and SD in the trial. The diagnosis of diabetes is made at an arbitrary level of 7 mmol/L, indicated below. A greater number of individuals may just cross this threshold if on atenolol compared to amlodipine and therefore labelled as diabetic, although their overall vascular risk may not change based on the absolute measurement of glucose (Reproduced with permission from Sofat et al. [24])

The evidence is not compelling that this small average increase in glucose translates into a shortfall in protection from stroke or coronary heart disease. Recent overviews of prospective observational studies [25, 26] indicate that although the risk of coronary heart disease is linearly and modestly increased above a fasting glucose value of 5 mmol/L, the risk of stroke is substantially raised only at fasting glucose values well above 7 mmol/L [26].

In the ALLHAT trial (in which 33,357 patients were randomised to A-class (lisinopril), C-class (amlodipine), or D-class (chlortalidone)), there was a difference in blood glucose of 0.16 mmol/L in the amlodipine group compared with the chlortalidone group with an odds ratio for diabetes of 0.73 (0.58–0.91) [27]. Yet the hazard ratio for stroke after 4.9 years of follow-up was 0.93 (0.82–1.06). There was only a small BP disparity between the chlortalidone arm and amlodipine arms (mean difference for amlodipine versus chlortalidone 0.8 mmHg systolic ($P=0.03$)). This suggests that observed differences in the risk of stroke in these trials are more likely to be explained by between-arm differences in BP, rather than glucose. The relevance of the small average increase in glucose is further questioned by results of recent trials that indicate that, after 5 years follow-up, tight glucose control does not necessarily lead to a reduction in cardiovascular event rates [28].

A-Class Drugs and Protection from Renal Disease

UK guidance [29, 30] has encouraged the use of drugs that specifically block the renin-angiotensin system (including ACEi and ARBs) as first-line treatment to reduce proteinuria and slow the progression of renal disease. The recommendation, initially for those with diabetes and evidence of renal impairment, is now more generally applied even to those without diabetes. These recommendations evolved following randomised studies of A-class ACEi and subsequently ARBs that showed a reno-protective effect. Implicit in the interpretation of the guidance is that inhibition of the renin-angiotensin system with ACEi/ARBs has specific reno-protective effects beyond lowering BP alone. However, the RCTs on which this guidance was based compared ACEi and ARBs against placebo rather than another BP-lowering agent. Given that systemic BP is a major determinant of the progression of renal disease [31], and that BP differences are inevitable when comparing placebo with BP-lowering drugs, the between-treatment-arm BP differences must confound effects on renal outcomes in placebo-controlled trials of ACEi/ARBs.

A previous systematic review and meta-analysis of RCTs investigated the effect of different classes of antihypertensive drugs in the progression of renal disease [32]. ACEi/ARBs, when compared to other BP-lowering drugs, stratified by degree of BP lowering, yielded a relative risk of 0.74 (95 % CI 0.59–0.92) in the group with greatest degree of BP lowering (–6.9 mmHg) and an RR of 0.9 (95 % CI 0.72–1.12) in the group with the smallest degree of BP lowering (1.5 mmHg), reinforcing the major role of BP differences as the mechanism to explain the proposed advantages of A-class drugs over other BP-lowering drugs in renal outcomes. Moreover, smaller studies showed a smaller overall benefit in renal end points. There was little evidence of an advantage in the diabetic subgroup, in which the relative risk for end-stage renal failure was 0.89 (95 % CI 0.74–1.07). Despite these findings and a lack of large trials, UK (and in this instance other international) guidelines recommend the use of A-Class drugs first line to treat hypertension and retard progression of renal disease [29, 33]. While a good example of drug policy that overreached its evidence base, it is an academic point given that most patients with kidney disease will require combination antihypertensive treatment.

Effectiveness of Thiazides in Prevention of Cardiovascular Events

The 2011 NICE guidance relegated diuretics (D-class drugs) from first to third choice. Diuretics as a class are among the most widely studied of all BP-lowering drugs and remain the preferred first-line agent for high BP treatment in the USA [34]. The prominence given to C-class calcium channel blockers over D-class diuretics was based on recent analysis of observational studies that BP variability might be more predictive of adverse cardiovascular outcomes than usual BP and that C-class drugs reduce BP variability to a greater extent than D-class drugs [35]. However, the evidence base on the relationship between usual BP and cardiovascular outcomes far exceeds that for BP variability, and no randomised trial has tested the influence of a reduction in BP variability on cardiovascular outcomes. The recommendation to use D-class thiazide-like diuretics rather than D-class thiazide diuretics was based on the interaction of these agents with carbonic anhydrase, which is no longer the major therapeutic target of these drugs.

Management of Hypertensive Crises

A hypertensive crisis or emergency is defined as an acute elevation of blood pressure in the presence of acute, ongoing or rapidly deteriorating end-organ damage and is shown in Table 12.1. It is very important to distinguish hypertensive emergencies from severe hypertension without *acute* end-organ damage. While the latter does involve intensive treatment, it does not require immediate parenteral treatment. It is also important to note that although most hypertensive emergencies are associated with a systolic blood pressure (SBP) of greater than 180 mmHg or a diastolic blood pressure (DBP) of greater than 110 mmHg, they rarely present with normal or high normal blood pressures. Hypertensive crises require rapid but careful reduction in blood pressure in a high dependency setting (e.g. intensive care) whereone-to-one nursing, arterial blood pressure and cardiac monitoring are available. This is critical as significant harm can be done by over-rapid correction of blood pressure resulting in end-organ ischaemia or infarction.

In contrast to the management of BP, where there is a mature evidence base, there are no large randomised trials in the setting of hypertensive emergencies. This is likely to be due to the small numbers of individuals presenting in this way (1 % of all those with hypertension) and the heterogeneity of the presentation (Table 12.1). Management is therefore based on consensus rather than evidence.

Pathophysiology

Pathophysiology of hypertensive crises is not well understood. A crisis can develop de novo or can complicate an underlying primary or secondary cause of hypertension. The vast majority of hypertensive crises appear to occur in patients with background hypertension the exceptions being eclampsia and de novo nephritic syndrome. A key first step is thought to be a rapid increase in systemic vascular resistance (SVR) precipitated by vasoconstrictor substances (e.g. noradrenalin,

Table 12.1 Summary of hypertensive crises, signs and symptoms associated with their presentation and pharmacological approach for each

Hypertensive emergency	Important signs/symptoms	Key investigations	Preferred agent
Hypertensive encephalopathy	Headache, altered conscious level, seizures, focal neurological signs, haemorrhage/exudates and papilloedema on fundoscopy	MRI brain	Labetalol
Dissecting aortic aneurysm	Chest and back pain, BP in both arms, palpation of all peripheral pulses	CT or MRI aorta	Labetalol, GTN (only after labetalol to counter reflex tachycardia)
Acute ventricular failure with pulmonary oedema	Breathlessness, gallop rhythm, raised JVP, third heart sound, inspiratory crackles on auscultation	CXR, echo may be useful	GTN
Acute myocardial ischaemia/ infarction	Chest pain, diaphoresis, breathlessness	ECG, cardiac enzymes	GTN, labetalol, esmolol
Eclampsia	Visual fields, headaches, altered mental state, acute stroke, abdominal pain, heart failure, oliguria		Labetalol (and delivery)
Acute kidney injury	Oliguria, uraemia, electrolyte-associated arrhythmias	Urea, creatinine, electrolytes, urinalysis	Labetalol, nicardipine
Sympathetic crisis (cocaine induced)	Labile blood pressure	Toxicology screen	Verapamil/diltiazem/ nicardipine
Catecholamine-associated crisis	Labile blood pressure with associated flushing	Urine catecholamines	Phentolamine

angiotensin II) or relative hypovolaemia. Like many other biological systems, the endothelium attempts to compensate by release of vasodilators to counter increases in SVR. However, sustained hypertension overwhelms compensatory mechanisms, leading to further endothelial dysfunction, increase in vascular permeability, fibrinoid necrosis of the vessel wall, activation of platelet aggregation and the coagulation cascade. Activation of these systems can promote further inflammation of the endothelium, thrombosis and vasoconstriction.

Assessment and Clinical Evaluation

A targeted history and examination supported by key laboratory and imaging investigations is essential. Salient features in any evaluation should establish preexisting hypertension, its treatment, control and adherence to medication, concurrent clinical conditions that could precipitate a hypertensive crises and drugs including prescribed, over the counter or illicit such as cocaine. Examination should focus on identifying syndromes where rapid intervention can be life-saving (aortic dissection, eclampsia, hypertensive encephalopathy) as a priority but should not preclude a full examination as other complications may also be present. Assessment should be made of BP in both arms, in the supine, seated and standing position if possible, to determine volume status. Cardiac compromise in particular left ventricular failure can be assessed by examination of the jugular venous pressure, the presence of a gallop rhythm and/or fourth heart sound and presence of inspiratory crackles on auscultation of the lungs. Hypertensive encephalopathy can be detected by assessment of the conscious level, assessment of focal neurology and grades III or IV hypertensive retinopathy. Assessment and symmetry of all pulses should also be made and is particularly important where aortic dissection is suspected.

Investigations

Bedside tests should include urine analysis to identify glomerulonephritis, an electrocardiogram to assess ischaemic changes, and in particular ST segment elevation which can be present in both acute myocardial infarction and aortic dissection. A chest radiograph in the presence of clinical signs and symptoms of left ventricular failure or aortic dissection can indicate a widened mediastinum (computed tomography (CT) aortogram or a magnetic resonance image (MRI) being the investigation of choice). In individuals presenting with hypertensive encephalopathy, CT brain imaging may be helpful to rule out intracranial haemorrhage or large infarcts although magnetic resonance imaging (MRI) is more sensitive to changes associated with hypertensive encephalopathy with typical findings of cerebral oedema and white matter changes. These can be extensive or more localised to the posterior part of the brain (occipital and parietal lobes), when it is known as posterior reversible encephalopathy syndrome (PRES) (see Fig. 12.3). PRES can however also be due to other causes such as calcineurin inhibitors, thrombotic microangiopathies and HIV. Changes associated with PRES

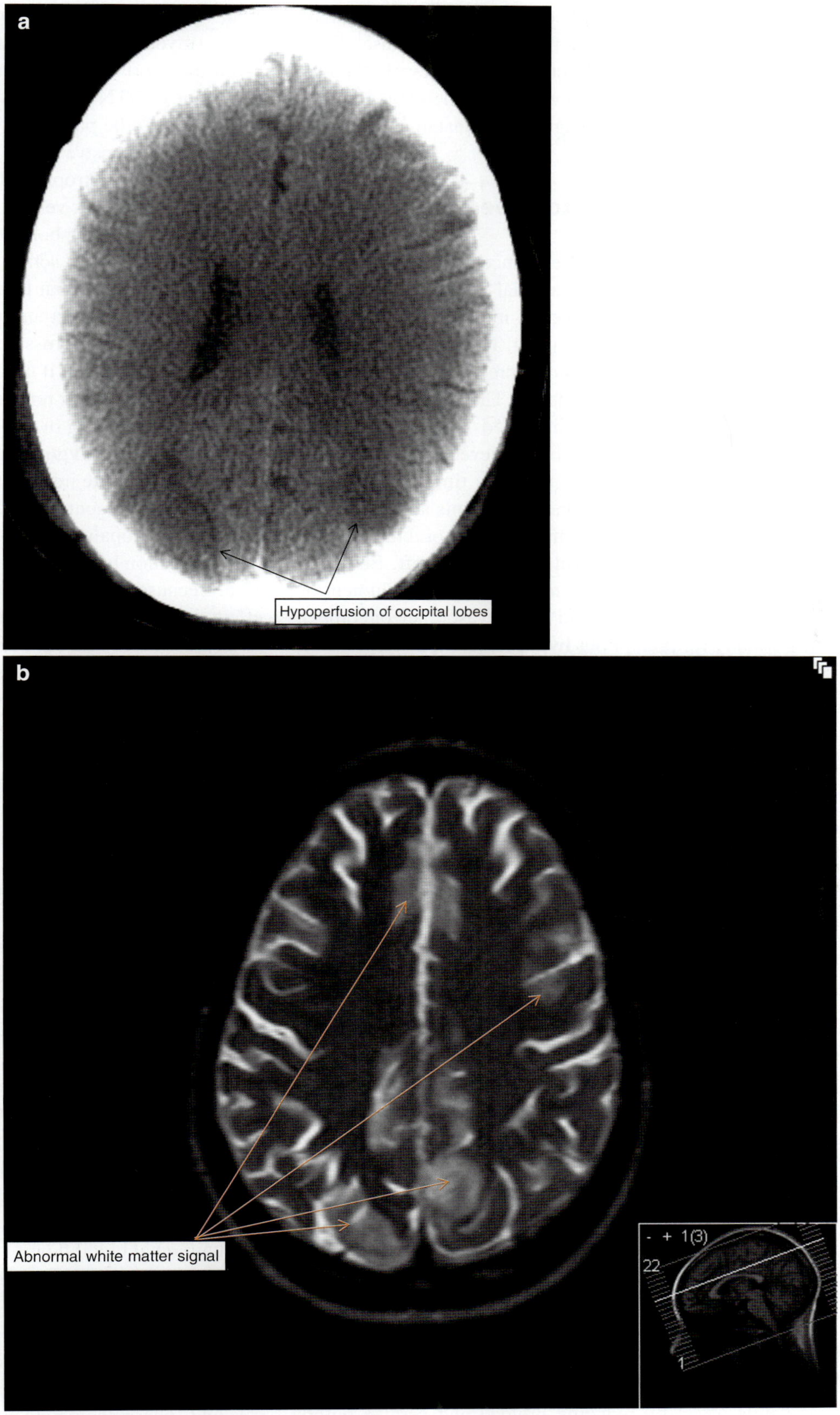

Fig. 12.3 (**a**) CT scan of a patient with CKD who developed bilateral cortical blindness with a blood pressure of 165/105 mmHg. The scan shows bilateral hypoperfusion consistent with posterior reversible leucoencephalopathy syndrome (PRES), and patient went on to recover her vision. (**b**) MRI scan showing extensive white matter changes in a 21-year-old with systemic lupus erythematosus and a blood pressure of 230/140 mmHg

as well as hypertensive encephalopathy are potentially reversible with treatment of the underlying cause. Blood tests should include renal function, electrolytes, LDH and a full blood count/platelet count with a peripheral blood film to exclude a thrombotic microangiopathic anaemia.

Therapeutic Approach to Hypertensive Crisis

In the absence of randomised evidence, consensus guidance recommends lowering mean arterial pressure by no more than 20–25 % within a period of minutes up to 2 h or a decrease in DPB to 100–110 mmHg. This is best achieved by parenteral administration of blood-pressure-lowering agents that are short acting and titratable. The one instance when more rapid BP reduction is indicated is aortic dissection, where BP lowering should be achieved within 10 min, whereas in all other crises an arbitrary time to achieve BP control of 1 h is often used. Once end points are reached and maintained, patients can be commenced on oral maintenance therapy while parenteral agents are weaned off. End-organ vessels are often grossly abnormal with narrowed lumens but also unable to autoregulate and cannot vasodilate or compensate normally for precipitous hypoperfusion; therefore, overzealous or poorly monitored blood pressure reduction carries a significant risk.

Pharmacological Agents

Agents for the management of hypertensive crises need to be fast acting, rapidly reversible and titratable with minimal adverse effects. In the absence of one ideal agent, knowledge of the pharmacological properties of agents that are available can be used to tailor treatments for a given clinical situation. Parenteral preparations of most drug classes are available with preferred options in UK-based practice being beta-blockers (labetalol and esmolol) and nitric oxide donors (glyceryl trinitrate).

Beta-blockers (esmolol and labetalol) are often the preferred drug, as they are rapidly acting (esmolol within 60 s and labetalol within 5 min) and are the drug of choice where cardiac output, heart rate and blood pressure are all increased. They achieve control of systemic vascular resistance, lowering this without reduction in total peripheral blood flow. They are the agents of choice in aortic dissection, eclampsia (labetalol does not cross the placenta) and myocardial ischaemia (in the absence of left ventricular failure).

Glyceryl trinitrate (GTN) is the nitric oxide donor commonly used in the UK. It acts by venodilation with effects on arterial tone only at higher doses. It therefore achieves its therapeutic effect by reducing preload and cardiac output, but can cause a reflex tachycardia and significant hypotension, which may be disadvantageous in certain hypertensive crises (myocardial ischaemia, aortic dissection). However, given the short duration of action and plasma half-life, the advantage of GTN is that unwanted effects are rapidly reversible. GTN can be particularly useful in individuals presenting with hypertensive crises associated with left ventricular failure. Sodium nitroprusside, another nitric oxide donor, also acts by reducing venous tone, with more of an effect on arterial tone, reducing both preload and after load. Like GTN it has a rapid onset of action, with a short duration of action and plasma half-life, but like GTN it also can be associated with reflex tachycardia and precipitous BP falls. The other disadvantage of nitroprusside is the association with cyanate or thiocyanate toxicity if used over days, particularly in individuals with hepatic or renal dysfunction. This should be offset by use of the drug over a short period of time and a dose not exceeding 2 μg/kg/min. If needed at higher doses, concurrent thiosulphate infusions can be considered.

Other useful agents include hydralazine, calcium channel blockers and dopamine-1 receptor agonists. Hydralazine acts by vasodilation but can cause precipitous BP falls which last 12 h. Because of this prolonged and somewhat unpredictable effect on blood pressure lowering and inability to titrate dose to BP, it is no longer used first line, but can be reserved for more complex refractory cases with careful administration and monitoring. Parenteral preparations of calcium channel blockers are available (nicardipine), which act by vasodilation. These are more water soluble than nifedipine, whose use in the setting of hypertensive emergencies or urgencies can cause sharp falls in BP when chewed and swallowed, an effect which can last up to 8 h, and therefore not recommended. In contrast nicardipine given as an intravenous infusion has a rapid onset of action (5–15 min) with a duration of 4–6 h. It can therefore be titrated to BP, although the shorter-acting beta-blockers and nitric oxide donors are of greater use for rapid titration.

The dopamine receptor agonist fenoldopam has been approved by the Food and Drug Administration (FDA) for hypertensive emergencies. Although similar to dopamine in mechanism, fenoldopam is a much more specific agonist at peripheral dopamine-1 receptors. Like dopamine it increases renal blood flow and promotes natriuresis. It can be given by the intravenous route and has a rapid onset of action (5 min), with a duration of action of 30–60 min. It may therefore be useful in hypertensive crises with a renal cause, in order to maintain renal blood flow.

Prostacyclin has a very short half-life and often used in the treatment of scleroderma renal crisis.

Hypertensive emergencies require rapid diagnosis and immediate treatment in a place of safety. Recognition of the underlying clinical syndrome is essential to guide both clinical and pharmacological management. BP lowering in hypertensive emergencies should be carried out in a high dependency setting where close nursing, cardiac and arterial monitoring are available. Drugs that are short acting with a short half-life are preferable so that doses can be titrated to BP.

Summary

A simple approach to BP management is therefore summarised below. The evidence for the approaches described in this table has been discussed throughout this chapter. The key concepts are to encourage non-pharmacological strategies for lowering BP and overall cardiovascular risk in all; however, in the presence of end-organ damage, individuals will require pharmacological intervention. The overarching goal of BP management should be reduction of BP regardless of the agent used to achieve this.

An evidence-based guide to treating high blood pressure	
Who to treat	Anyone older than 55 will benefit from BP lowering[a]
	Anyone with a prior cardiovascular event
	Anyone with evidence of end-organ damage, irrespective of BP level
	Anyone with extreme elevation of BP[b]
What to treat with	Diet and lifestyle for all
	BP-lowering medication; once contraindications are checked, use any as a first-line agent, and when adding any combination so long as tolerated
What treatment target	The lower the BP achieved without producing symptoms of hypotension, the better
	Address all other risk factors

[a]Lifestyle advice: reduce salt and alcohol intake, lose weight and increase aerobic exercise and fruit/vegetable and oily fish consumption
[b]Investigate for secondary causes of raised BP, particularly in the young; if all negative, proceed to directly observed therapy to ensure non-adherence as a cause of persistently elevated BP despite presumed adequate therapy

Tips and Tricks

Poor compliance is a common cause of poor blood pressure control; therefore consider urine medication levels, and observe dosing of medication in patients on multiple agents but poor control (with the caveat that a completely noncompliant patient given several prescribed anti-hypertensives may have a profound drop in blood pressure).

It is critical for medical teams to distinguish between a hypertensive crisis (requiring urgent parenteral treatment and high dependency monitoring) and severe hypertension without acute end-organ damage (which requires immediate attention but not parenteral anti-hypertensives).

Overzealous correction of blood pressure in patients with a thrombotic microangiopathy may result in worse renal function and prolonged dialysis dependence.

Generally we are poor at achieving blood pressure targets in the CKD and transplant populations; electronic alerts, setting a target blood pressure with the patient and regular audits are all helpful strategies for focusing effort.

References

1. Law MR, Morris JK, Wald NJ. Use of blood pressure lowering drugs in the prevention of cardiovascular disease: meta-analysis of 147 randomised trials in the context of expectations from prospective epidemiological studies. BMJ. 2009;338:b1665.
2. Lewington S, Clarke R, Qizilbash N, Peto R, Collins R. Age-specific relevance of usual blood pressure to vascular mortality: a meta-analysis of individual data for one million adults in 61 prospective studies. Lancet. 2002;360(9349):1903–13.
3. He FJ, MacGregor GA. Effect of longer-term modest salt reduction on blood pressure. Cochrane Database Syst Rev. 2004;(3):CD004937.
4. Hooper L, Bartlett C, Davey SG, Ebrahim S. Advice to reduce dietary salt for prevention of cardiovascular disease. Cochrane Database Syst Rev. 2004;(1):CD003656.
5. Xin X, He J, Frontini MG, Ogden LG, Motsamai OI, Whelton PK. Effects of alcohol reduction on blood pressure: a meta-analysis of randomized controlled trials. Hypertension. 2001;38(5):1112–7.
6. Horvath K, Jeitler K, Siering U, Stich AK, Skipka G, Gratzer TW, Siebenhofer A. Long-term effects of weight-reducing interventions in hypertensive patients: systematic review and meta-analysis. Arch Intern Med. 2008;168(6):571–80.
7. Fagard RH, Cornelissen VA. Effect of exercise on blood pressure control in hypertensive patients. Eur J Cardiovasc Prev Rehabil. 2007;14(1):12–7.
8. Sacks FM, Svetkey LP, Vollmer WM, Appel LJ, Bray GA, Harsha D, Obarzanek E, Conlin PR, Miller 3rd ER, Simons-Morton DG, Karanja N, Lin PH. Effects on blood pressure of reduced dietary sodium and the dietary approaches to stop hypertension (DASH) diet. DASH-Sodium Collaborative Research Group. N Engl J Med. 2001;344(1):3–10.
9. Appel LJ, Miller 3rd ER, Seidler AJ, Whelton PK. Does supplementation of diet with 'fish oil' reduce blood pressure? A meta-analysis of controlled clinical trials. Arch Intern Med. 1993;153(12):1429–38.
10. Geleijnse JM, Giltay EJ, Grobbee DE, Donders AR, Kok FJ. Blood pressure response to fish oil supplementation: metaregression analysis of randomized trials. J Hypertens. 2002;20(8):1493–9.
11. Morris MC, Sacks F, Rosner B. Does fish oil lower blood pressure? A meta-analysis of controlled trials. Circulation. 1993;88(2):523–33.
12. Rang HP, Dale MM. Rang and Dale's pharmacology. 7th ed. Edinburgh: Elsevier Churchill Livingstone; 2012.
13. Law MR, Wald NJ, Morris JK, Jordan RE. Value of low dose combination treatment with blood pressure lowering drugs: analysis of 354 randomised trials. BMJ. 2003;326(7404):1427.
14. Turnbull F, Neal B, Ninomiya T, Algert C, Arima H, Barzi F, Bulpitt C, Chalmers J, Fagard R, Gleason A, Heritier S, Li N, Perkovic V, Woodward M, MacMahon S. Effects of different regimens to lower blood pressure on major cardiovascular events in older and younger adults: meta-analysis of randomised trials. BMJ. 2008;336(7653):1121–3.

15. Dahlof B, Sever PS, Poulter NR, Wedel H, Beevers DG, Caulfield M, Collins R, Kjeldsen SE, Kristinsson A, McInnes GT, Mehlsen J, Nieminen M, O'Brien E, Ostergren J. Prevention of cardiovascular events with an antihypertensive regimen of amlodipine adding perindopril as required versus atenolol adding bendroflumethiazide as required, in the Anglo-Scandinavian Cardiac Outcomes Trial-Blood Pressure Lowering Arm (ASCOT-BPLA): a multicentre randomised controlled trial. Lancet. 2005;366(9489):895–906.
16. Lindholm LH, Carlberg B, Samuelsson O. Should beta blockers remain first choice in the treatment of primary hypertension? A meta-analysis. Lancet. 2005;366(9496):1545–53.
17. Dickerson JE, Hingorani AD, Ashby MJ, Palmer CR, Brown MJ. Optimisation of antihypertensive treatment by crossover rotation of four major classes. Lancet. 1999;353(9169):2008–13.
18. Belmin J, Levy BI, Michel JB. Changes in the renin-angiotensin-aldosterone axis in later life. Drugs Aging. 1994;5(5):391–400.
19. Seifarth C, Trenkel S, Schobel H, Hahn EG, Hensen J. Influence of antihypertensive medication on aldosterone and renin concentration in the differential diagnosis of essential hypertension and primary aldosteronism. Clin Endocrinol. 2002;57(4):457–65.
20. de Bruin RA, Bouhuizen A, Diederich S, Perschel FH, Boomsma F, Deinum J. Validation of a new automated renin assay. Clin Chem. 2004;50(11):2111–6.
21. Bradley HA, Wiysonge CS, Volmink JA, Mayosi BM, Opie LH. How strong is the evidence for use of beta-blockers as first-line therapy for hypertension? Systematic review and meta-analysis. J Hypertens. 2006;24(11):2131–41.
22. Khan N, McAlister FA. Re-examining the efficacy of beta-blockers for the treatment of hypertension: a meta-analysis. CMAJ. 2006;174(12):1737–42.
23. Staessen JA, Birkenhager WH. Evidence that new antihypertensives are superior to older drugs. Lancet. 2005;366(9489):869–71.
24. Sofat R, Casas JP, Grosso AM, Prichard BN, Smeeth L, MacAllister R, Hingorani AD. Could NICE guidance on the choice of blood pressure lowering drugs be simplified? BMJ. 2012;344:d8078.
25. Lawlor DA, Fraser A, Ebrahim S, Smith GD. Independent associations of fasting insulin, glucose, and glycated haemoglobin with stroke and coronary heart disease in older women. PLoS Med. 2007;4(8):e263.
26. Sarwar N, Gao P, Seshasai SR, Gobin R, Kaptoge S, Di Angelantonio E, Ingelsson E, Lawlor DA, Selvin E, Stampfer M, Stehouwer CD, Lewington S, Pennells L, Thompson A, Sattar N, White IR, Ray KK, Danesh J. Diabetes mellitus, fasting blood glucose concentration, and risk of vascular disease: a collaborative meta-analysis of 102 prospective studies. Lancet. 2010;375(9733):2215–22.
27. Barzilay JI, Davis BR, Cutler JA, Pressel SL, Whelton PK, Basile J, Margolis KL, Ong ST, Sadler LS, Summerson J. Fasting glucose levels and incident diabetes mellitus in older nondiabetic adults randomized to receive 3 different classes of antihypertensive treatment: a report from the Antihypertensive and Lipid-Lowering Treatment to Prevent Heart Attack Trial (ALLHAT). Arch Intern Med. 2006;166(20):2191–201.
28. Patel A, MacMahon S, Chalmers J, Neal B, Woodward M, Billot L, Harrap S, Poulter N, Marre M, Cooper M, Glasziou P, Grobbee DE, Hamet P, Heller S, Liu LS, Mancia G, Mogensen CE, Pan CY, Rodgers A, Williams B. Effects of a fixed combination of perindopril and indapamide on macrovascular and microvascular outcomes in patients with type 2 diabetes mellitus (the ADVANCE trial): a randomised controlled trial. Lancet. 2007;370(9590):829–40.
29. National Collaborating Centre for Chronic Conditions. Type 2 diabetes: national clinical guideline for management in primary and secondary care (update). London: Royal College of Physicians; 2008.
30. NICE. CG73 Early identification and management of chronic kidney disease in adults in primary and secondary care. Chronic kidney disease.2008:1–29.guidance. http://guidance.nice.org.uk/CG73/NICE Guidance/pdf/English.
31. Hsu CY, McCulloch CE, Darbinian J, Go AS, Iribarren C. Elevated blood pressure and risk of end-stage renal disease in subjects without baseline kidney disease. Arch Intern Med. 2005;165(8):923–8.
32. Casas JP, Chua W, Loukogeorgakis S, Vallance P, Smeeth L, Hingorani AD, MacAllister RJ. Effect of inhibitors of the renin-angiotensin system and other antihypertensive drugs on renal outcomes: systematic review and meta-analysis. Lancet. 2005; 366(9502):2026–33.
33. Consensus statement on management of early CKD. Royal college of Physicians of Edinburgh and Renal Association. 2007. http://www.renal.org/docs/default-source/clinical-service/clinical-service/RA_RCP_Edinburgh_Consensus_Statement_on_Management_of_Early_CKD_February_2007.pdf?sfvrsn=0. http://www.renal.org/CKDguide/consensus.html.
34. Chobanian AV, Bakris GL, Black HR, Cushman WC, Green LA, Izzo Jr JL, Jones DW, Materson BJ, Oparil S, Wright Jr JT, Roccella EJ. Seventh report of the Joint National Committee on Prevention, Detection, Evaluation, and Treatment of High Blood Pressure. Hypertension. 2003;42(6):1206–52.
35. Rothwell PM, Howard SC, Dolan E, O'Brien E, Dobson JE, Dahlof B, Sever PS, Poulter NR. Prognostic significance of visit-to-visit variability, maximum systolic blood pressure, and episodic hypertension. Lancet. 2010;375(9718):895–905.

Podocytopathies

13

Peter W. Mathieson

Podocytes are the cells located on the outer (urinary) aspect of the glomerular capillary wall and are also known as visceral glomerular epithelial cells. Podocytopathies are diseases where the cell that is primarily injured/dysfunctional is the podocyte. The term is most literally applied to a group of genetically mediated conditions where a mutation in a podocyte-specific gene leads to a clinical phenotype including proteinuria. These relatively rare genetic conditions have been enormously important in helping us to understand podocyte biology, structure and function [reviewed in 1]. The knowledge thus acquired has accelerated our ability to study podocytes in other disease situations, including some of the most common forms of acquired kidney disease such as diabetic nephropathy. Minimal change nephropathy (MCN) and focal segmental glomerulosclerosis (FSGS) are the two forms of acquired glomerular disease that are most widely accepted to be podocytopathies: both are covered in separate chapters so that only the general concepts of podocytopathies illustrated by these diseases will be covered here. There is evidence of podocyte injury, plus good reasons for believing that the extent thereof is an important prognostic factor, in a variety of other renal diseases including diabetic nephropathy, membranous glomerulonephritis, IgA nephropathy and even renal transplant glomerulopathy, so that some degree of podocytopathy could be said to be a very widespread phenomenon. For the sake of brevity, I will focus on the issues raised by the genetic podocytopathies and by MCN and FSGS.

P.W. Mathieson, PhD, FRCP, FMedSci
Academic Renal Unit,
University of Bristol and Southmead Hospital,
Bristol BS10 5NB, UK
e-mail: p.mathieson@bristol.ac.uk

M. Harber (ed.), *Practical Nephrology*,
DOI 10.1007/978-1-4471-5547-8_13, © Springer-Verlag London 2014

Manifestations of Podocyte Injury/Dysfunction

In health, the glomerular capillary wall is relatively impermeable to protein and its selective sieving action is maintained via a complex tripartite structure involving podocytes on the outside, glomerular endothelial cells on the inside and the glomerular basement membrane in between the two cellular layers. Podocytes have a specialised structure comprising a cell body and primary and secondary processes (Fig. 13.1). The secondary processes interdigitate together and the slits they form, analogous to the teeth of a zipper, are the filtration slits through which glomerular filtration occurs. Each is bridged by a slit diaphragm (Fig. 13.2a). The complex architecture of the podocyte is maintained by actin fibres arranged throughout the cytoplasm of the cell and when there is foot process effacement, the distribution of

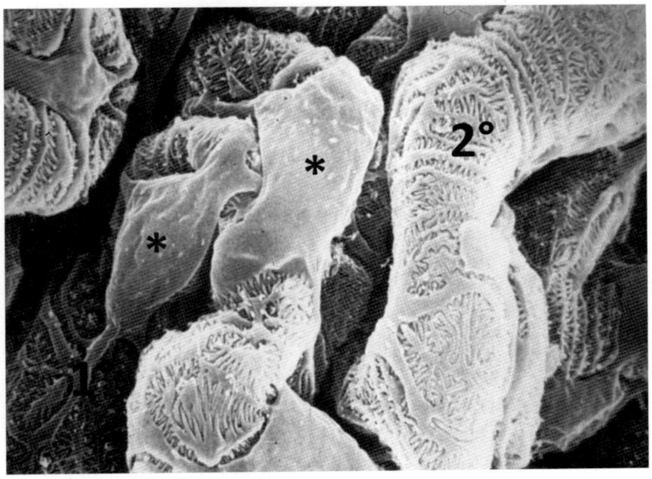

Fig. 13.1 Scanning electron micrograph of external (urinary) aspect of normal human glomerular capillary showing podocyte cell bodies (*) and primary (1°) and secondary (2°) processes

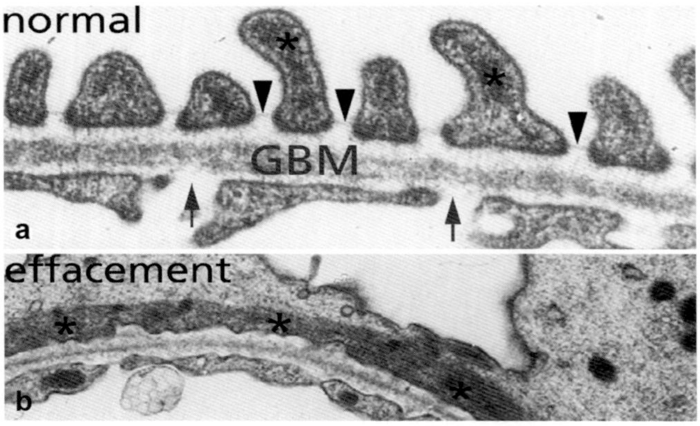

Fig. 13.2 (**a**) Transmission electron micrograph of glomerular capillary wall showing podocyte foot processes with dense actin fibres (*), slit diaphragms (*arrowheads*) and glomerular endothelial cells with fenestrations (*arrows*). (**b**) Podocyte foot process effacement (as in minimal change nephropathy). Note flattening of actin filaments (*)

actin fibres is markedly deranged (Fig. 13.2b). The selective filtration function of the glomerular capillary wall is then disrupted and proteinuria results. Podocytes have a very limited capacity for repair or regeneration [2], so that when podocytes are irreversibly damaged or lost they are not adequately replaced, proteinuria continues and progressive loss of kidney function can supervene.

Podocyte-Specific Gene Mutations

In truth, few genes are absolutely cell specific, and this applies to podocytes as it does to most other cell types. However, relative cell specificity and/or cell specificity in a particular organ or location certainly do occur and the podocyte is a good example of a cell that relies on a particular set of relatively specific gene products to maintain its structure and function. The first podocyte-specific gene mutation to be discovered was identified by a positional cloning approach in families with one or more individual affected by the autosomal recessive condition known as congenital nephrotic syndrome of the Finnish type. This gene locus, denoted NPHS1 and encoding a protein called nephrin, was identified by Tryggvason's group in 1999 [3]. Nephrin is a signalling molecule: it is predominantly located at the slit diaphragm, but its natural ligands and precise function remain uncertain. Its identification was swiftly followed by that of NPHS2, encoding podocin [4], which when mutated leads to steroid-resistant nephrotic syndrome. Subsequently, numerous other podocyte-specific gene mutations have been described, each leading to proteinuria [5]. The unifying factor in most genetically mediated podocyte disorders seems to be disruption of the actin cytoskeleton: even mutations in the cation channel TRPC6, leading to constitutive activity of the channel and unregulated calcium entry into the cell, seem to exert some or all of their effects via alterations in the actin cytoskeleton and therefore in the cell shape [5, 6].

There have been two major spin-offs from the study of these genetic disorders: the first is that a series of key proteins and protein functions have been identified that are essential for the health of the podocyte. These form logical therapeutic targets for novel treatments aimed at preserving podocyte health or inducing podocyte repair. The second is that the availability of cell-specific gene promoters has allowed podocyte-specific gene manipulation in experimental systems [7]. For clinical nephrologists, the tantalising question is whether these advances are helpful in the management of patients with the more common, apparently sporadic, forms of proteinuric disease. The answer seems to be a tentative yes: as many as 20 % of children with early onset nephrotic syndrome will have one or more mutation in the podocin gene [8], and it is possible that heterozygous mutations in this and other genes could act as susceptibility loci for later-onset nephrotic syndrome. The importance of finding a gene mutation is that this means that the patient is most likely to be steroid resistant (and therefore shouldn't be exposed to prolonged steroid therapy in the vain hope that they will respond) and also that recurrence after a renal transplant is much less likely when the original disease was genetic in origin and the transplant comes from a genetically distinct donor.

Podocyte Injury in MCN and FSGS

The clinical presentation, and sometimes the initial renal biopsy, may be indistinguishable in these two conditions. Steroid responsiveness is typical in MCN and less so in FSGS, although 20–50 % of patients with the latter condition will also respond to steroids and have a good prognosis [9]. Both conditions are characterised by podocyte injury: in MCN this is the only discernible morphological correlate of disease (Fig. 13.3) and in FSGS this is the earliest feature. Experimental models in which podocytes are selectively targeted invariably lead to FSGS [10]. So what is it that separates the two conditions? In the author's opinion it is the reversibility of the podocyte injury: in MCN, proteinuria may be acute and very severe yet complete remission can be achieved with steroids or other therapies. Thus, the injury must be reversible. This seems to also be true in a subset of patients with FSGS, but we do not yet have any means of

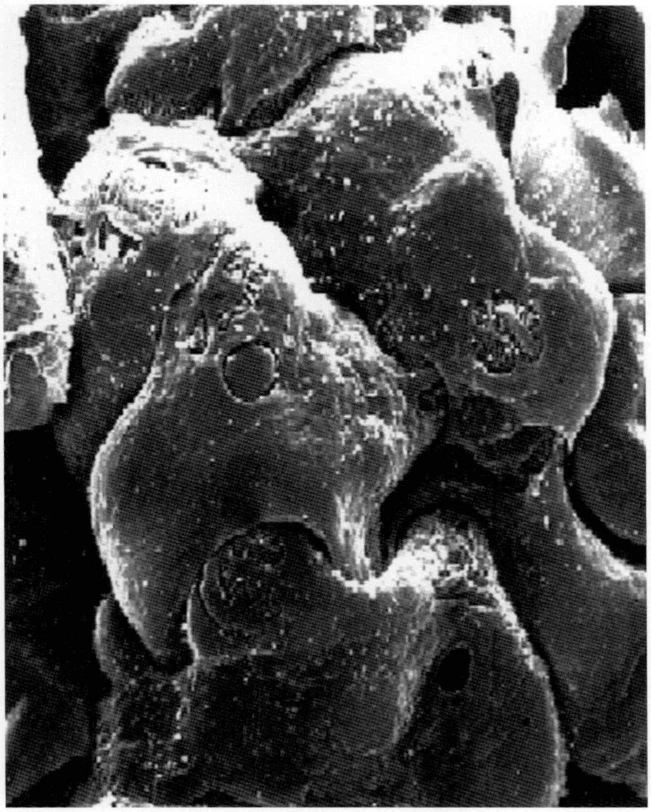

Fig. 13.3 Scanning electron micrograph of podocytes showing foot process effacement

prospectively identifying this subset. In the remainder of patients with FSGS, podocyte injury is either more severe or more sustained and leads to podocyte detachment and loss such that permanent injury is caused. We need better ways of identifying and quantifying podocyte injury: detection of detached podocytes in the urine shows some promise [11] but has not proved widely reproducible. Existing therapies including steroids, cyclosporin and even rituximab have direct effects on podocytes [12]: new therapeutic approaches need to be more specifically targeted toward podocyte repair/regeneration.

References

1. Patrakka J, Tryggvason K. New insights into the role of podocytes in proteinuria. Nat Rev Nephrol. 2009;5:463–8.
2. Mathieson PW. Update on the podocyte. Curr Opin Nephrol Hypertens. 2009;18:206–11.
3. Kestila M, Lenkkeri U, Mannikko M, et al. Positionally cloned gene for a novel glomerular protein–nephrin–is mutated in congenital nephrotic syndrome. Mol Cell. 1998;1:575–82.
4. Boute N, Gribouval O, Roselli S, et al. NPHS2, encoding the glomerular protein podocin, is mutated in autosomal recessive steroid-resistant nephrotic syndrome. Nat Genet. 2000;24:349–54.
5. McCarthy HJ, Saleem MA. Genetics in clinical practice: nephrotic and proteinuric syndromes. Nephron Exp Nephrol. 2011;118: e1–8.
6. Tian D, Jacobo SM, Billing D, et al. Antagonistic regulation of actin dynamics and cell motility by TRPC5 and TRPC6 channels. Sci Signal. 2010;3:ra77.
7. Quaggin SE. A "molecular toolbox" for the nephrologist. J Am Soc Nephrol. 2002;13:1682–5.
8. Hinkes B, Vlangos C, Heeringa S, et al. Specific podocin mutations correlate with age of onset in steroid-resistant nephrotic syndrome. J Am Soc Nephrol. 2008;19:365–71.
9. Mathieson PW. Minimal change nephropathy and focal segmental glomerulosclerosis. Semin Immunopathol. 2007;29:415–26.
10. D'Agati VD. Pathobiology of focal segmental glomerulosclerosis: new developments. Curr Opin Nephrol Hypertens. 2012;21: 243–50.
11. Sun D, Zhao X, Meng L. Relationship between urinary podocytes and kidney diseases. Ren Fail. 2012;34:403–7.
12. Mathieson PW. The podocyte as a target for therapies, old and new. Nat Rev Nephrol. 2011;8:52–6.

Management of the Nephrotic Patient: The Overall Approach to the Patient with Nephrotic Syndrome (NS)

14

Mark Harber

NS has a significant associated morbidity and mortality, and although there are several complications of NS, three are particularly life-threatening: thromboembolism, infection and AKI. Systems need to be firmly established and adequately implemented to protect patients from these risks. For some patients NS is a chronic or relapsing condition with implications for quality of life and work, and nephrologists need to ensure joined up, patient-centred care.

Diagnosis

An accurate diagnosis is important; while it is much more common (rather depressingly) to be eventually referred a patient who has been investigated for heart failure or cirrhosis before NS has been identified, occasionally these conditions, tamponade and IVC thrombosis, can exacerbate oedema in a patient with mild to moderate proteinuria. While in children the practical issue is whether the lesion is steroid responsive, in adults the proportion of patients with a steroid-responsive element is much less, and the risk:benefit ratio much more in favour of a biopsy.

It is critical in NS to ascertain if the glomerular lesion is 'primary' or 'secondary' to another disease (for example malignancy or infection), as almost universally treatment of secondary NS should focus on treating the underlying condition. The specific treatments for different causes of NS are covered within those chapters, but the more generic clinical aspects of NS are discussed here.

M. Harber, MBBS, PhD, FRCP
UCL Department of Nephrology,
Royal Free London NHS Foundation Trust,
Pond Street, Hampstead, London NW3 2QG, UK
e-mail: mark.harber@nhs.net

Hypertension and Proteinuria

NS may or may not be associated with hypertension (some patients, e.g. those with amyloid or severe NS, may be significantly hypotensive), but for those that are hypertensive, tight control of blood pressure results in cardiovascular protection and delays progression. The KDIGO guidelines recommend a target blood pressure of 130/80 or even 125/75 if proteinuria >1 g [1]. There is good evidence in support of renin-angiotensin blockade (RAS) as the optimum treatment, and ACEI/ARBs are recommended as first line to reduce cardiovascular risk and progression. Aldosterone antagonists (such as spironolactone) reduce proteinuria and are worth considering as an add-on particularly in patients intolerance of ACEI. Reduction in proteinuria should be a parallel aim to BP control; proteinuria is toxic to the tubule-interstitium, and the quantity of protein correlates very strongly with cardiovascular risk and progression of renal disease. Almost any reduction in proteinuria either partial remission or reduction through blood pressure control and RAS blockade is associated with improved outcome, and this should be maximised in all patients with chronic proteinuria >1 g. Beyond BP control, ACEI/ARB and spironolactone, non-dihydropyridine calcium channel antagonists also have an anti-proteinuric effect and probably preferable to dihydropyridine agents. Calcineurin inhibitors (CNIs) can also be useful in nonspecifically reducing proteinuria through a haemodynamic effect but risking deterioration in renal function and need to be monitored closely. Occasionally proteinuria is so torrential that the native kidneys are sacrificed by medical (usually high-dose NSAIDs, CNIs and RAS blockade) or surgical nephrectomy. Although rare this may be the only practical treatment for the grossly hypotensive, hypoalbuminaemic patient with a poor renal prognosis and is sometimes done in children prior to a planned live donor transplantation.

M. Harber (ed.), *Practical Nephrology*,
DOI 10.1007/978-1-4471-5547-8_14,

Management of the Nephrotic Patient: Treatment of ECF Volume Expansion Due to Nephrotic Syndrome in Adults

15

Liam Plant

How Comparable Are the Different Salt-Retaining States?

Salt-retaining states are common medical problems, particularly as clinical manifestations of chronic heart failure (CHF) and chronic kidney disease (CKD). Nephrotic syndrome (NS) in adults is a relatively less common manifestation of kidney disease, with an estimated annual incidence of three new cases per 100,000 [1]. In childhood it is most commonly due to minimal change disease. Most cases of NS in adults are due to primary glomerular diseases, but some are due to secondary glomerular diseases such as diabetes mellitus, systemic lupus erythematosus and amyloidosis [1]. Cardinal features are proteinuria, hypoalbuminaemia and oedema.

Expansion of extracellular fluid (ECF) volume can be very disabling, with peripheral oedema, pulmonary oedema, gut oedema and ascites. If disease-specific therapies do not rapidly induce a remission, it is often difficult to bring these symptoms under control with generic therapies. Patients with NS may then seem to be 'diuretic resistant', in much the same way as some patients with CHF or CKD are considered to so be [2]. However, it may be a mistake to view all oedematous patients who are 'slow' to respond to initial therapies as being 'the same' just because the general principles of therapy are similar. It is important to recognise that the pathophysiological basis of oedema differs between different underlying conditions and this may have implications for choices in therapy. Furthermore, differences in drug pharmacokinetics and pharmacodynamics influence response to treatment [2–5].

An example of the increasing interest in more precise characterisation and treatment of oedematous states has been that focused on acute decompensated heart failure (ADHF) and associated cardio-renal syndromes (CRS) [6]. This acknowledges pathophysiological interactions between the heart and the kidney as well as the effects of neurohumeral activation [7]. Salt restriction, use of diuretics and use of other agents are demonstrated to exhibit a complex interplay in such cases. Some of these factors will overlap with the pathophysiology/treatment of ECF expansion in NS, some will not. Important trials on how to use diuretics in ADHF have been published [8]. The findings of these studies may not translate directly to strategies for treating oedematous NS patients.

Why Do Nephrotic Patients Become Oedematous?

The traditional explanation has been that proteinuria leads to hypoalbuminaemia, which causes a decrease in plasma oncotic pressure. The consequent imbalance in Starling forces across the capillary wall causes fluid to 'leak' into the interstitium. Effective hypovolaemia follows and this triggers activation of the renin-angiotensin-aldosterone system, sympathetic nervous system and arginine vasopressin system, with inhibition of the release of atrial natriuretic peptide. All of this leads to secondary renal salt and water retention. However, observations in clinical cases and in experimental models have called this 'underfill' hypothesis into question, and whilst it may play some role, contemporary opinion favours a greater role for a specific renal salt retention process coupled with an alteration in capillary permeability independent of changes in oncotic gradients [9, 10].

No compelling and consistent explanation for the dysregulation in sodium balance in NS has yet been universally accepted, but it is notable that many studies indicate an upregulation of epithelial sodium channel (ENaC) expression in the distal nephron, independent of aldosterone and other systemic hormones [10]. Recent studies postulate a role for plasminogen and plasmin, both of which appear in nephrotic urine. It is postulated that, in NS, plasminogen enters the

L. Plant
Cork University Hospital, University College Cork, Ireland

M. Harber (ed.), *Practical Nephrology*,
DOI 10.1007/978-1-4471-5547-8_15, © Springer-Verlag London 2014

urine through more permeable glomerular capillaries; that it is then activated to plasmin by urokinase; and that plasmin activates distal nephron ENaC channels [11]. Thus, a prominent aspect of NS is a particular salt avidity in the distal nephron, mediated through ENaC and occurring in concert with other mechanisms (possibly reflecting the 'underfill' hypothesis) enhancing salt retention at other sites.

What Are the Clinical Goals of Specific Management of NS?

These are dealt with elsewhere in this book and relate to inducing a remission of proteinuria and preserving glomerular filtration rate. There are extensive reviews and guidelines on potential therapies to induce remission/reduce proteinuria [12]. All make reference to the necessity for salt restriction and use of diuretics, but there is heterogeneity in clinical practice strategies, with a need to individualise such treatments. Consensus on how to achieve this is not prominent in the literature; in one very extensive guideline [12], the word 'diuretic' appears only 13 times in a 15-page document!

What Are the Clinical Goals of Generic Management of NS?

The objective of generic therapy is to initiate and sustain an increased natriuresis until the patient has returned to clinical euvolaemia. It should then be easier to maintain homeostasis at the new desired steady state, particularly if dietary salt restriction is appropriately introduced.

Total body salt and water will not decrease unless excretion exceeds intake. Dietary salt intake frequently exceeds 100 mmol/day (~6 g salt/day). Thus, for example, a patient will need to excrete 300 mmol of sodium *over and above* that needed to balance daily intake if he/she is to lose 2 kg of excess ECF volume.

Whilst salt avidity persists, this requires the use of (various) natriuretic agents – usually referred to as 'diuretics' – with specific pharmacokinetic and pharmacodynamic properties, in different doses and combinations.

Dietary salt intake also needs to be restricted, ideally to <80 mmol/day, but this may be difficult to achieve. Most salt intake is not 'elective', but occurs because of addition in food processing. Furthermore, many patients find diets containing less than 80 mmol/day to be bland and unpalatable.

Unexpected failure to lose weight/ECF volume in a patient on a seemingly appropriate diuretic dose should prompt enquiry into salt intake. Measurement of 24-h sodium excretion may help. A patient passing 150 mmol/day or more but not losing weight is likely to have an excess intake.

What Are the Different Classes of Diuretics and How Do They Work?

Diuretics are different classes of drugs that inhibit sodium reabsorption at different sites along the nephron and by increasing natriuresis achieve clinical benefit [2–5]. However, clinical goals may not always be easily achieved.

Site of action classifies the commonly used agents (Table 15.1). Although most (60–70 %) filtered sodium is reabsorbed in the proximal tubule, agents acting at this site (e.g. acetazolamide) are of relatively little clinical use in oedematous states because the increased sodium loss is offset by increased reabsorption further down the nephron in the thick ascending loop of Henle. The same principle applies to the proximal tubular effect of some thiazide diuretics.

Loop diuretics (e.g. furosemide, bumetanide, torasemide) are organic anions, secreted into the tubular lumen by the organic anion transporter (OAT1) in the proximal tubule (Table 15.2). They act on the luminal aspect of the thick ascending loop of Henle where they exhibit high affinity for the chloride-binding site of the sodium-potassium-2 chloride (NKCC2) transporter – a member of the solute carrier family 12 group of proteins [2, 4]. This directly inhibits sodium and chloride reabsorption and indirectly leads to decreased reabsorption of calcium and magnesium. Up to 20 % of filtered sodium can be excreted using these agents.

Thiazides and related compounds (e.g. bendroflumethiazide, hydrochlorothiazide, chlorthalidone, indapamide, metolazone) are organic anions also secreted by OAT1 in the proximal tubule. They act on the distal tubule and connecting segment where they bind to a number of transporters, principally the sodium-chloride cotransporter (NCC) – another member of the solute carrier family 12 protein group – directly inhibiting sodium reabsorption (Table 15.2). This indirectly increases calcium reabsorption. The maximum natriuresis is less than that achieved with loop diuretics, but a combination of these classes can be especially potent [13].

The potassium-sparing diuretics include amiloride, triamterene and spironolactone [2–5]. These have slightly different modes of action. Amiloride and triamterene are organic cations secreted into the lumen of the proximal tubule, but acting on the luminal aspect of the epithelial sodium channel (ENaC) in the cortical collecting duct. Spironolactone and eplerenone, by contrast, enter the principal cells of the cortical collecting duct from the plasma and interfere with the activation of the intracellular aldosterone receptor. This leads to a reduction in the activity of the baso-lateral sodium-potassium ATPase and a reduction in luminal expression of ENaC.

Table 15.1 Classes of diuretic agents

Class	Examples	Site of action
Loop diuretics	Furosemide Bumetanide Torasemide	Thick ascending loop of Henle (TALH)
Thiazide/thiazide-like diuretics	Hydrochlorothiazide Bendroflumethiazide Chlorthalidone Metolazone Indapamide	Distal convoluted tubule (DCT)
Potassium-sparing diuretics	Amiloride Triamterene Spironolactone Eplerenone	Cortical collecting duct (CCD)

Table 15.2 Ion transporters

Transporter	Role	Location
Organic anion transporter (OAT-1)	Secretion of loop diuretics and thiazide/thiazide-like diuretics into tubular lumen	Proximal convoluted tubule
Sodium-potassium-2 chloride transporter (NKCC-2)	Site of action of loop diuretics	Thick ascending loop of Henle
Sodium-chloride cotransporter (NCC)	Site of action of thiazide/thiazide-like diuretics	Distal convoluted tubule
Epithelial sodium channel (ENaC)	Site of action of amiloride and triamterene Expression influenced by activation of aldosterone receptor	Cortical collecting duct (principal cells)

What Are the Pharmacokinetic Barriers to Achieving Therapeutic Objectives?

The primary driver of natriuresis is the rate of excretion of diuretic in the tubular fluid. This relationship exhibits a threshold phenomenon, following which the rate of sodium excretion reflects diuretic excretion in a linear dose-dependent pattern [3, 4]. Failure to deliver a sufficient dose of diuretic to exceed the natriuretic threshold may be described as 'diuretic resistance', but more usually reflects a failure to appreciate pharmacokinetic principles (Table 15.3).

Most prescribing choices to address pharmacokinetic issues involve administering larger doses of diuretic or enhancing bioavailability.

The first step is to ensure that an adequate dose of diuretic enters the bloodstream and is delivered to the kidney for excretion into the tubular lumen. Diuretics differ in their oral bioavailability. The oral bioavailability of furosemide ranges from 20 to 70 %, decreasing with increased gut oedema. On the other hand, bumetanide has an oral bioavailability approaching 80 %. When faced with a very oedematous patient, administering a higher dose of oral furosemide and switching to bumetanide or administering the agent intravenously are all rational therapeutic choices.

Loop and thiazide diuretics are transported bound to albumin and other plasma proteins. In NS, levels of albumin and other plasma proteins are often extremely low, and the consequent increased volume of distribution decreases the amount delivered to the kidney [14]. Increasing the dose administered is the appropriate response to this; coadministration of albumin with diuretic has not been consistently demonstrated as being of additional benefit [15, 16].

Diuretics compete with other anions for excretion by OAT1 into the proximal tubule [3–5]. Such anions accumulate particularly in the presence of renal failure and hepatic failure. In such circumstances the expected dose–response to loop and thiazide diuretics may be less than anticipated. Certain drugs (such as cimetidine) also compete for excretion. This problem does not occur with spironolactone, which does not require to be excreted into the tubular lumen, and its diuretic effect is less affected by liver failure.

A fall in GFR, particularly when combined with a low cardiac output, will decrease diurectic delivery and also initial filtered sodium load making a substantial naturiesis even more difficult to achieve. It was previously postulated that urinary protein bound to diuretic in the tubular lumen decreased its effectiveness. This view has not been substantiated by experimental studies [17].

Therefore, there are many factors active in NS that act as additional pharmacokinetic 'hurdles' to achieving a degree of diuretic excretion sufficient to initiate a natriuresis. In most circumstances, increasing the prescribed dose or otherwise enhancing the bioavailability of that dose is the appropriate strategy. An illogical, but common, error is to repeat the same ineffective dose more frequently. If there is doubt as to whether or not a natriuresis has been initiated, measurement of 24-h sodium excretion (or even 6-h excretion following the dose) is a rational choice.

What Are the Pharmacodynamic Barriers to Achieving Therapeutic Objectives?

Once a natriuresis is initiated, it needs to be sustained until the patient has been restored to the desired steady state. Once diuretics are administered and natriuresis achieved, there is a rapid functional and structural response in the nephron that acts to reduce the degree of enhanced natriuresis [2–5]. This can be viewed as 'diuretic blunting' and reflects pharmacodynamic principles.

Most of the adaptation occurs downstream from the site of action of the initially deployed diuretic. Changes in the expression and activity of transporters in the distal tubule

Minimal Change Disease and Focal Segmental Glomerulosclerosis

16

Philip David Mason

Minimal change disease (MCD) and focal segmental glomerulosclerosis (FSGS) are considered together since, although their aetiology may be different, they share clinical features and are, at least initially, managed in a similar way.

MCD is the cause of the nephrotic syndrome in~90 % of children aged under 10 years (most common age 2–7 years), about 50–70 % of older children and 20–35 % of adults. The incidence in boys is twice that in girls although there is no gender difference in adolescents or adults. The reported incidence varies geographically. In the UK it has been reported to be as low as 1 per million but up to 27 per million in the USA. It is commoner in Indo-Asians and Native Americans but is rarer in Black Africans (who are much more likely to have FSGS with steroid-resistant nephrotic syndrome). Since children with nephrotic syndrome are very likely to have MCN, they are not usually biopsied and the term steroid-responsive nephrotic syndrome is used if they respond to steroids.

Primary FSGS is the cause of nephrotic syndrome in <10 % of children, the middle aged and the elderly but is the diagnosis in up to 20 % of nephrotic adolescents and young adults. It has an incidence of about two per million in a white European population [1] but is commonest cause in adult African Americans and the incidence appears to be rising [2]. Overall, it is the cause of renal failure in about 2.5 % of patients on renal replacement therapy in the USA, but this is more than 10 % in younger patients [3].

It is important to remember that both MCD and FSGS are defined by histopathology and the clinical presentation with nephrotic syndrome. Similar histopathologic appearances are seen in patients with non-nephrotic proteinuria who have other conditions with different prognoses and are, therefore, managed differently.

P.D. Mason, BSc, PhD, MBBS, FRCP
Oxford Kidney Unit, The Churchill Hospital,
Headington, Oxford OX3 7LE, UK

M. Harber (ed.), *Practical Nephrology*,
DOI 10.1007/978-1-4471-5547-8_16, © Springer-Verlag London 2014

Aetiology and Pathogenesis

In a minority of patients, nephrotic syndrome with MCD is associated with a secondary factor (Table 16.1). FSGS may also be found in association with a wide range of other conditions and genetic mutations (Table 16.2). These include a variety of infections, non-renal conditions and pre-existing renal diseases. These secondary forms of FSGS are more likely if the proteinuria is not in the nephrotic range. Nephrotic FSGS may also be a consequence of genetic mutations, mostly in podocyte proteins involved with the actin cytoskeleton and integrity of the slit diaphragm [4].

In normal glomeruli, the filtration barrier to protein is provided by a combination of size barriers and charge selectivity so that neutral molecules larger than 4–4.5 nm are excluded. Albumin molecules are smaller but are excluded because as anionic molecules they are repelled by the normal negative charge on the epithelial cells and glomerular basement membrane (GBM) (predominantly heparan sulphate). In MCD and FSGS the clearance of small neutral molecules is actually less than normal, suggesting that the large albumin

Table 16.1 Factors associated with the onset of nephrotic syndrome in minimal change disease

Drugs
Nonsteroidal anti-inflammatory drugs
Lithium: rare (usually causes chronic interstitial nephritis)
Interferon-α
Gold: rare (usually associated with membranous nephropathy)
Allergies
Pollens
House dust
Insect stings
Immunizations
Malignancies
Hodgkin's disease
Mycosis fungoides
Chronic lymphocytic leukaemia: uncommon (usually associated with MPGN)

Table 16.2 Secondary FSGS

Genetic
Autosomal recessive:
NPHS1 (nephrin)[a], NPHS2 (podocin)[b], NPHS3 (phospholipase Cε1), CD2-associated protein, MYO1E (non-muscle myosin)
Autosomal dominant:
TRPC6 (Ca channel), ACTN4 (a-actinin-4), INF2 (formin)[c]
Uncertain:
APOL1[d]
Viral infections
HIV (collapsing FSGS, HIV-associated nephropathy [HIVAN])
Rarely CMV and parvovirus
Drugs
Heroin (sometimes also with HIV)
Lithium
Pamidronate
γ-Interferon
Sulphasalazine
Anabolic steroids (possibly by hyperfiltration)
'Adaptive' in response to hyperfiltration
Obesity
Reduced nephron mass (e.g. subtotal nephrectomy)
Renal dysplasia
Reflux nephropathy
Congenital heart disease (cyanotic)
Sickle cell anaemia
Chronic allograft (transplant) nephropathy

[a]Most common cause of Finnish congenital nephrotic syndrome
[b]Most common genetic cause of SRNS in children
[c]Most common cause of adult familial FSGS—usually non-nephrotic
[d]Mutations confer resistance to *Trypanosoma brucei* but predispose (uncertain aetiology) to FSGS

filtration is primarily the result of loss of GBM surface charge. The cause of this is uncertain, and the presence of circulating cationic factors (which may result in a generalised increased capillary permeability) remains controversial. The characteristic podocyte foot process fusion is seen in other patients with heavy proteinuria (e.g. due to FSGS), suggesting that these changes may be secondary. Finding foot process fusion in children dying of kwashiorkor with severe hypoalbuminaemia, but no proteinuria, and the absence of foot process fusion in patients with heavy proteinuria with early recurrent FSGS following transplantation would support this.

Minimal Change Disease

Various data have implicated an immune aetiology of MCD, which seems likely to be a systemic condition rather than an intrinsic disease of the kidney. Before corticosteroids were found to be effective, the nephrotic syndrome often remitted in children who contracted measles, which is known to have potent inhibitory effects on cell-mediated immunity. MCD is associated with lymphomas (especially Hodgkin's disease) and atopy (in some series in up to 30 % of children) and responds to immunosuppressive drugs. There are also many reports of abnormal humoral and cellular immunity in patients with MCD during relapse and sometimes in remission as well, but not in those with other causes of nephrotic syndrome. Finally, there is an association (in some ethnic groups) with HLA-DR7 in steroid-responsive individuals. There are many anecdotal reports of MCD relapse following exposure to an allergen in sensitive individuals. As a result, patients with identified food allergies have been managed with exclusion diets with reported complete or partial remissions and relapse following reintroduction of the offending food. However, even if the relationship is real, it is possible that the allergic events merely trigger relapse, as may infections.

Some data suggest that a primary podocyte abnormality may be involved. Podocyte expression of CD80 (B7.1) has been reported in patients with MCD and the soluble molecule found in their urine [5], and experimentally, CD80 expression by podocytes results in shape change and the development of proteinuria.

There is circumstantial evidence that a circulating factor is involved in the pathogenesis. Lymphocyte-derived cytokines have been proposed but remain elusive, and T regulatory cells have been reported to be abnormal in MCD and that there is generalised activation of T cells during active disease. In one small study, plasma haemopexin (an acute phase reactant found in human plasma) was increased in MCD patients in relapse with some evidence of an altered isoform [6]. It is unclear how this relates to clinical disease although the authors suggest that protease inhibitors might normally mask its activity. Reduced levels of dystroglycans (adhesion molecules believed to anchor podocytes to the GBM) have also been reported in MCD but not in FSGS, with normalisation following corticosteroid treatment. Evidence of a circulating factor in humans is also supported by the observation that proteinuria resolved within days following transplantation from a cadaveric donor with MCD [7].

Experimental studies have implicated T lymphocyte-derived IL-13 in causing the proteinuria by a mechanism involving induction of CD80 in the podocyte and this cytokine is associated with allergic states, and MCD may be triggered by vaccination or exposure to an allergen in sensitive individuals [8]. Exciting recent experimental studies have implicated an overproduction of angiopoietin-like 4 by podocytes which binds to the GBM causing proteinuria, foot process effacement and loss of GBM charge [9], but clinical correlates are needed.

Primary Focal Segmental Glomerulosclerosis

Evidence for a circulating factor in FSGS is more substantial, mainly based on the high incidence of recurrence following transplantation, with heavy proteinuria developing sometimes within hours (with resolution reported in one case report of an affected transplant after re-transplantation into a second recipient [10]). In another case report, transmission of heavy proteinuria to the foetus of a mother with FSGS resolved rapidly after delivery [11]. Following transplantation the histologic picture is initially MCD later developing into FSGS. Plasma exchange and elution with protein A or anti-IgG columns can lead to temporary remission in transplant recurrence of FSGS, and eluates from the columns may induce proteinuria [12]. A soluble factor that causes increased protein permeability in cultured human glomeruli has also been described [13]. This has not been definitively characterised although cardiotrophin-like cytokine-1 (structurally similar to interleukin-16) is a potential candidate and upregulated receptors have been demonstrated on the podocytes of patients with recurrent disease [14]. Upregulated expression of transforming growth factor-β (TGF-β), a pro-fibrotic cytokine, has been described in patients with FSGS, but it is unclear whether this is a primary or secondary phenomenon.

A number of genetic abnormalities of podocyte proteins are known to be associated with FSGS (Table 16.2), and many other aetiological factors have also been identified. More recently soluble urokinase-type plasminogen activator receptors (suPAR) have been demonstrated to be present in two-thirds of patients with FSGS and high levels seem to be predictive of recurrence following transplantation [15]. It is believed that the suPAR activate β3 integrin, which plays a major role in anchoring the podocyte to the GBM, resulting in dysregulation.

There are a large number of secondary (non-genetic) causes of FSGS (Table 16.2). These are often associated with podocyte injury or result from adaptive changes in response to glomerular loss from scarring resulting in hyperfiltration [16].

The close clinical relationship between MCD and FSGS has led some to suggest a shared pathogenesis. The non-sclerotic regions of glomeruli in FSGS are indistinguishable from MCD. Patients with FSGS sometimes have a diagnosis of MCD in initial biopsy. This may merely be a reflection of early disease and sampling error, but there are well-documented cases of patients with steroid-sensitive MCD developing into FSGS after many years of relapses.

Natural History and Complications

MCD

- A relapsing–remitting course is common and more frequent in children.
- Those presenting at an earlier age are more likely to have a longer disease course before long-term remission occurs (see Fig. 16.1).
- Relapse occurs in >2/3 of children and ~50 % relapse more than four times, usually following steroid cessation or reduction. If relapse occurs during steroid reduction, the patient is described as steroid dependent.
- <5 % of children with MCD enter adulthood still relapsing, although the younger the onset of the first attack, the longer the child is likely to continue having relapses [17].

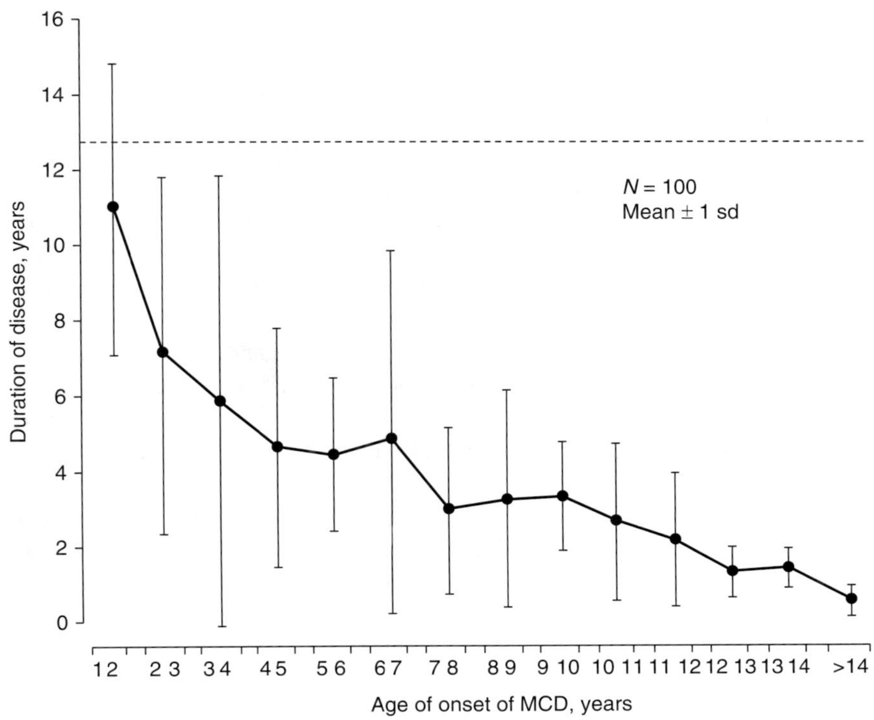

Fig. 16.1 Long-term outcome in childhood-onset minimal change disease. The duration of disease is inversely related to the age of presentation (Reproduced with permission from Trompeter et al. [17])

Fig. 16.2 Prognosis in primary focal segmental glomerulosclerosis. The risk of developing renal failure is related to the extent of proteinuria. Those with nephrotic-range proteinuria are much more likely to develop renal failure than those with low-grade proteinuria. The figures indicate the number of at-risk patients at different time points. (Reproduced with permission from Rydel et al. [18])

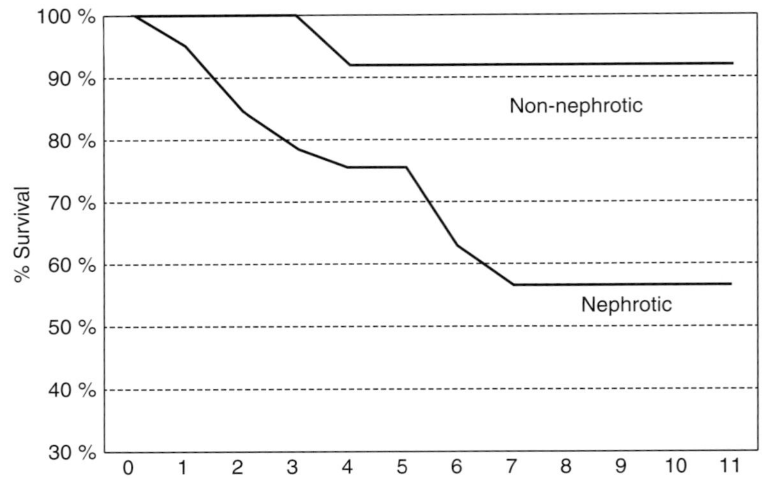

	0	1	2	3	4	5	6	7	8	9	10	11
Non-nephrotic	21	20	16	16	13	12	10	9	8	8	8	6
Nephrotic	60	46	32	26	21	19	13	11	11	11	11	9

- In general, increasing time since last relapse reduces the risk of further relapse, but occasionally adults relapse after an interval of >10 years.
- MCD does not progress to renal failure, although a number of patients with this diagnosis are found to have FSGS on subsequent biopsies. It is unclear whether the focal nature of the disease resulted in the correct diagnosis being missed on the initial biopsy or whether evolution from MCD to FSGS occurs.

FSGS

- The incidence of progressive renal failure in primary FSGS is often quoted as around 50 %, although there may be variation in the exact diagnostic criteria.
- The prognosis is clearly related to the level of proteinuria and the response to treatment [18] (Figs. 16.2 and 16.8).
- Non-nephrotic patients with normal plasma albumin and proteinuria of <3 g/day have a 10-year incidence of renal failure of just 10–15 %, but many of these will have secondary FSGS.

The complications of MCD and FSGS are generally the same as for any cause of nephrotic syndrome and include infection (especially with encapsulated bacteria and including spontaneous bacterial peritonitis particularly in children), life-threatening venous or arterial thrombosis, AKI (especially adults) (as discussed in Chap 14). Before the introduction of corticosteroids, the morbidity and mortality of patients with MCD were high because of complications, particularly infection. This is still a serious problem for children and adults whilst they are nephrotic that must not be forgotten. Peritonitis is mainly seen in children and is still a major cause of death in the Third World.

Clinical Features

The symptoms and clinical signs are the same as those for the nephrotic syndrome from any cause, but it is worth noting:

- In MCD, a fairly rapid onset of oedema is common with increased risks of hypovolaemia (especially in children).
- Severe fluid retention exceeding 3 % of the body weight and often much more.
- 60 % of presentations and relapses follow an infection (most often upper respiratory tract); however, minor infections are common in children and following remission most infections do not trigger a relapse, so it is uncertain whether or not these are of causative significance.
- Children commonly present with pleural effusions, ascites and hepatomegaly and may present with abdominal pain.
- Pericardial effusions may occur, but pulmonary oedema is uncommon except following treatment with albumin or with coexisting cardiac disease.
- Oedema is gravitational, but a puffy face is common and genital swelling may be very uncomfortable, especially in men. Gross oedema may result in ulceration and infection of dependent skin and lacerations and needlestick punctures may weep fluid profusely.
- Striae commonly appear even without steroids.
- Bowel oedema may cause diarrhoea and increased capillary leak has been suggested as a mechanism for losing protein via the gut.
- Other clinical features include white nails, sometimes in bands (Muehrcke's bands) correlating with periods of clinical relapse. Rarely xanthomata are associated with gross hyperlipidaemia.
- Microscopic haematuria is rare in MCD but is more common in FSGS.

- In MCD hypertension is present in 30–43 % of adults [19] and in 14–21 % of children, when compared with age- and sex-matched blood pressure reference ranges [20]. This usually resolves during remission, especially in children. Hypertension is sometimes associated with expansion of the intravascular volume but may paradoxically be secondary to hypovolaemia and activation of the renin–angiotensin axis.
- Hypertension is more common in FSGS, especially with impaired function [20].
- AKI is present or develops in ~18 % of patients with MCD.
- Other complications, as for any cause of nephrotic syndrome, include thromboembolism, infection and hyperlipidaemia.

Diagnosis and Differential Diagnosis

The clinical diagnosis of nephrotic syndrome is usually obvious, with oedema and heavy proteinuria, usually without microscopic haematuria on urine dipstick testing. The differential diagnosis is that of nephrotic syndrome and requires a renal biopsy to make a definitive diagnosis. In patients with conditions that may be associated with the nephrotic syndrome (e.g. diabetes or amyloidosis), the decision to biopsy needs to be carefully considered.

Investigations

Routine Investigations

Hyaline and sometimes lipid casts may be seen on urine microscopy. There is nephrotic-range proteinuria (>3.5 g/24 h in adults or >40 mg/h per m^2 in children or a protein/creatinine ratio >350 mg/mmol).

Routine blood biochemistry confirms hypoalbuminaemia and hyperlipidaemia. Hyponatraemia may be present even before treatment, and elevated urea and creatinine are more common in adults.

Usually IgG levels are low and IgM is normal or raised. Serum complement levels are normal. In children, steroid-responsive MCD is usually associated with 'selective' proteinuria of smaller molecules including albumin and transferrin but not of larger molecules such as immunoglobulins and ferritin. A selectivity index can be derived from the ratio of IgG to albumin clearance:

$$\text{Selectivity index (SI)} = \frac{[\text{IgG}]_U\,[\text{Albumin}]_S}{[\text{IgG}]_S\,[\text{Albumin}]_U}$$

where U and S are the concentrations in urine and serum. A SI of <0.1 % indicates 'highly selective' proteinuria, and an SI of >0.2 % is 'non-selective'. This is of limited clinical value since highly selective proteinuria is less common in adult MCD and does not influence a decision to treat with steroids. However, highly selective proteinuria, when present, does indicate that MCD is more likely to be the diagnosis, and some argue that such patients should be given a trial of steroids without a renal biopsy.

Renal Biopsy

In children (especially <12 years), renal biopsy is unnecessary unless the patient does not respond to corticosteroid treatment. In adults, since steroid-responsive disease is less likely (<30 %) and a wide differential diagnosis for nephrotic syndrome exists, a renal biopsy is recommended to establish the diagnosis. In the absence of a specific contraindication to steroid therapy, some argue that a therapeutic trial of steroids should be given, reserving renal biopsy for nonresponders. However, adults with steroid-responsive nephrotic syndrome may take up to 12 weeks before induction of remission and so the morbidity from steroids does become significant outweighing the small risks of a renal biopsy. Even when there is a typical biopsy appearance, it is always important to consider whether the patient may have a secondary cause of MCD or FSGS.

Histopathology

Minimal Change Disease

- Classically completely normal glomeruli on light microscopy and immunohistology with podocyte foot process effacement on electron microscopy (Fig. 16.3) as the only (but nonspecific finding) abnormality.

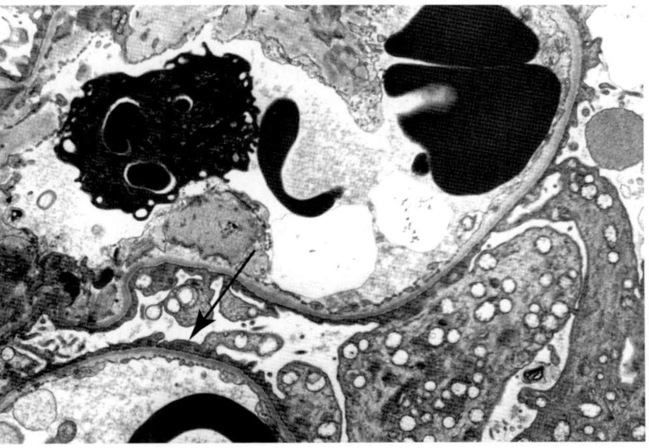

Fig. 16.3 Podocyte foot process fusion in minimal change disease. The epithelial cells (*arrows*) are completely effaced along the glomerular basement membranes (electron micrograph ×6,000). (Courtesy of Prof Ian Roberts, Oxford University Hospitals NHS Trust)

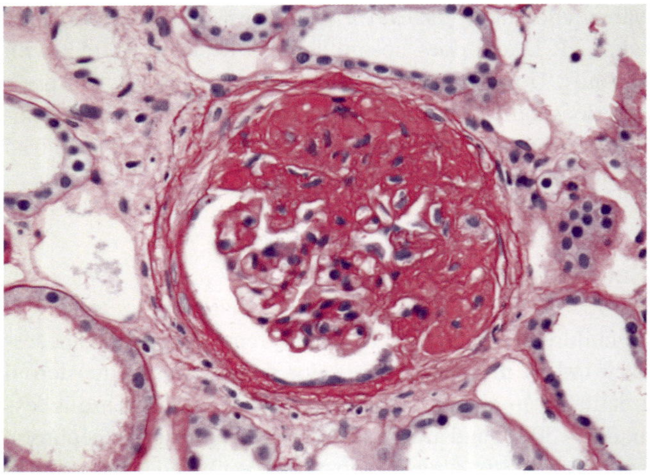

Fig. 16.4 Light microscopic appearances in focal segmental glomerulosclerosis. Segmental scars with capsular adhesions in otherwise normal glomeruli [periodic acid–Schiff, ×300] (Courtesy of Prof Ian Roberts, Oxford University Hospitals NHS Trust)

- Mild mesangial hypercellularity is now accepted as an infrequent finding, as are small amounts of mesangial IgG, complement C3 and occasionally IgA (partly based on patients whose clinical course is indistinguishable from classical MCD). Mesangial hypercellularity may be a predictor of steroid resistance, a poorer prognosis.
- The presence of mesangial IgM is considered by some to define a separate entity (see below).
- Hyaline casts obstructing tubules, foam cells and appearances consistent with acute tubular injury may be seen, especially if AKI is present at the time of biopsy.

Focal Segmental Glomerulosclerosis

Light Microscopy

- As the name implies, there is focal segmental glomerular scarring (Fig. 16.4). Typically juxta-medullary glomeruli are affected first, and so it is possible to miss the diagnosis if there are only a few glomeruli in the biopsy sample and a glomerulus containing a sclerotic segment may be missed on a single section (examination of serial sections increase the incidence of lesions [21]).
- Glomerular capillaries in affected segments are obliterated by acellular matrix and hyaline deposits, sometimes with adhesions to Bowman's capsule.
- As more glomeruli are affected as the disease progresses, there is more global sclerosis with tubular atrophy with the development of interstitial fibrosis. A diagnosis of FSGS in a nephrotic patient might be suggested by focal tubular atrophy and interstitial fibrosis with normal looking glomeruli (especially with a small biopsy specimen), in which case serial sections may reveal the typical glomerular changes.

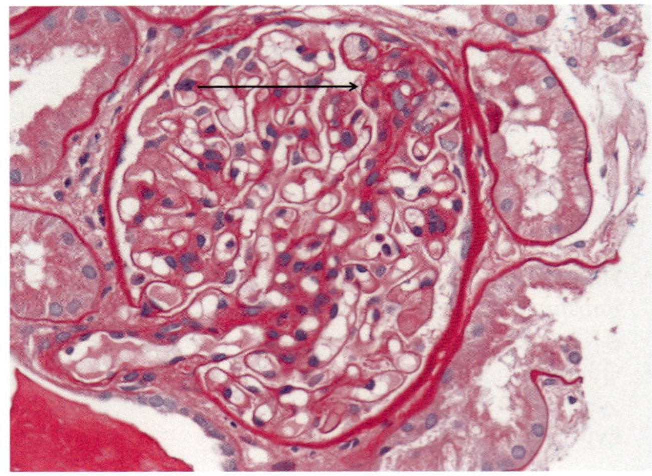

Fig. 16.5 The glomerular 'tip' lesion. A glomerulus in a renal biopsy from an adult with steroid-responsive nephrotic syndrome. The glomerular tuft is normal away from the tubular origin, but at the tubular origin, there is adhesion to Bowman's capsule with protrusion into the tubular lumen (methenamine silver stain ×300) (Courtesy of Prof Ian Roberts, Oxford University Hospitals NHS Trust)

Immunofluorescence

- Sclerotic segments are often positive for IgM and C3 complement (thought to be a nonspecific consequence of the injury, possibly caused by passive trapping of large molecules in damaged capillary loops).

Electron Microscopy

- Foot process fusion of non-sclerotic segments and unaffected glomeruli may be indistinguishable from that seen in MCD, but diffuse foot process fusion predominates in the sclerotic segments, with partial effacement in surrounding apparently normal lobules.

Histologic Variants of Primary FSGS

There is considerable overlap in the descriptions of histologic variants of FSGS and uncertainty as to whether they should be regarded as distinct entities.

- *Collapsing variant* (best defined histologically variant): segmental sclerotic lesions are associated with glomerular tuft collapse and clinically associated with nephrotic syndrome and rapidly progressive AKI similar to HIV-associated FSGS.
- *Glomerular 'tip' lesion*: segmental scars are described as 'hilar' when related to the vascular pole, 'peripheral' when opposite the tubular pole or 'intermediate'. The 'tip' lesion refers to peripheral segmental sclerosis adjacent to the tubular pole of Bowman's capsule, often with adhesions or synechiae to Bowman's capsule and may prolapse into the proximal tubular lumen (Fig. 16.5). The glomerular capillary loops adjacent to the proximal

tubule may be dilated, with accumulation of foamy cells. 'Tip' lesions are seen in other proteinuric conditions including normal glomeruli consistent with MCD (more often in adults than children) which may explain why they have been reported to be more likely to be steroid responsive with a better long-term prognosis. However, most series do not support an association with a better prognosis, possibly reflecting a more widespread use of the term 'tip' lesion when glomerular changes at the tubular origin occur in other glomerular disorders with proteinuria, including membranoproliferative glomerulonephritis and IgA nephropathy (and renal transplants).

The most important reason to recognise the lesion is to prevent a misdiagnosis of a proliferative glomerulonephritis.

- *The cellular variant*: characterised by podocyte hyperplasia and proliferation, often overlying segmental scars or areas of collapsed capillary loops, sometimes with endocapillary hypercellularity, foam cells, leukocytes and nuclear debris, mimicking proliferative glomerulonephritis. Clinicopathologic correlates of this variant are variable.
- *Mesangial hypercellular variant*: there are contradictory data regarding the significance of this [22], but many consider mesangial hypercellularity to be an intermediate step in the evolution (progression) of MCD to FSGS.
- *IgM nephropathy*: Patients with mesangial deposits of IgM, usually with minor mesangial hypercellularity, are more likely to be associated with haematuria (usually microscopic) and less likely to respond to steroids (50 % compared with 90 % for MCD). However, since IgM deposits are seen in MCD, FSGS and mesangial proliferative glomerulonephritis in a similar proportion of patients, it may not be a specific entity in its own right. Similar arguments apply to the rarer finding of mesangial complement C1q deposition, sometimes labelled as C1q nephropathy.

Management

As described in the chapter on the general management of nephrotic syndrome, all patients should receive general management of the nephrotic syndrome to control oedema with fluid and salt restriction and diuretics (used less often in children because of the greater risk of hypovolaemia). Consideration should be given to prophylaxis against thrombosis and infection and, in nonresponders, control of hyperlipidaemia.

More than 90 % of patients with MCD and about 40 % of those with FSGS respond to steroids, although there is considerable variation in the recommended doses and duration and when to introduce second-line treatments, reflecting the dearth of adequate controlled trials. Therefore, the recommendations here are pragmatic and justified, where possible, by evidence from clinical trials.

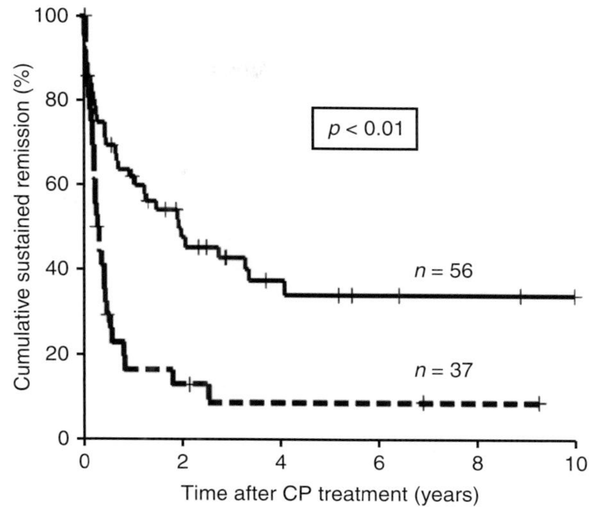

Fig. 16.6 Older children are more likely to respond to cyclophosphamide than younger children. Sustained remission in older (*solid line*) and younger (<5.5 years, *dotted line*) children following cyclophosphamide treatment (Reproduced with permission from Vester et al. [45])

Childhood Minimal Change Disease

The ISKDC recommends that the first episode should be treated with oral prednisolone 60 mg/m^2/day or 2 mg/kg to a maximum of 60 mg/day (calculated on estimated 'dry' weight). Response rates are 75 % within 2 weeks, 80–85 % within 4 weeks and over 90 % within 8 weeks (Fig. 16.7). Assuming urinary remission, steroids should be continued at the initial dose for 6 weeks followed by a switch to alternate-day dosing at 1.5 mg/kg (maximum 40 mg per day) for 6 weeks, but subsequent tapering is no longer recommended [23, 24]. Children remain on steroids for 3–4 months, which is associated with a lower 1-year relapse rate compared with those receiving steroids ≤2 months (19 % v. 64 %, respectively) based on several studies and a meta-analysis [25, 26]. The 2-year sustained remission rate is 49 % with a 29 % frequent relapse rate although this is higher in younger children.

For children still proteinuric after 4 weeks on steroids, there is anecdotal evidence that either increasing the steroid dose or giving an intravenous pulse of methylprednisolone (1 g/1.73 m^2) improves the probability of inducing a remission. However, it is important to consider reasons for treatment failure including noncompliance and poor absorption from an oedematous bowel, especially in the presence of diarrhoea, both of which would make intravenous steroids logical. Even in the absence of diarrhoea, prescription of non-enteric-coated steroid formulations is recommended,

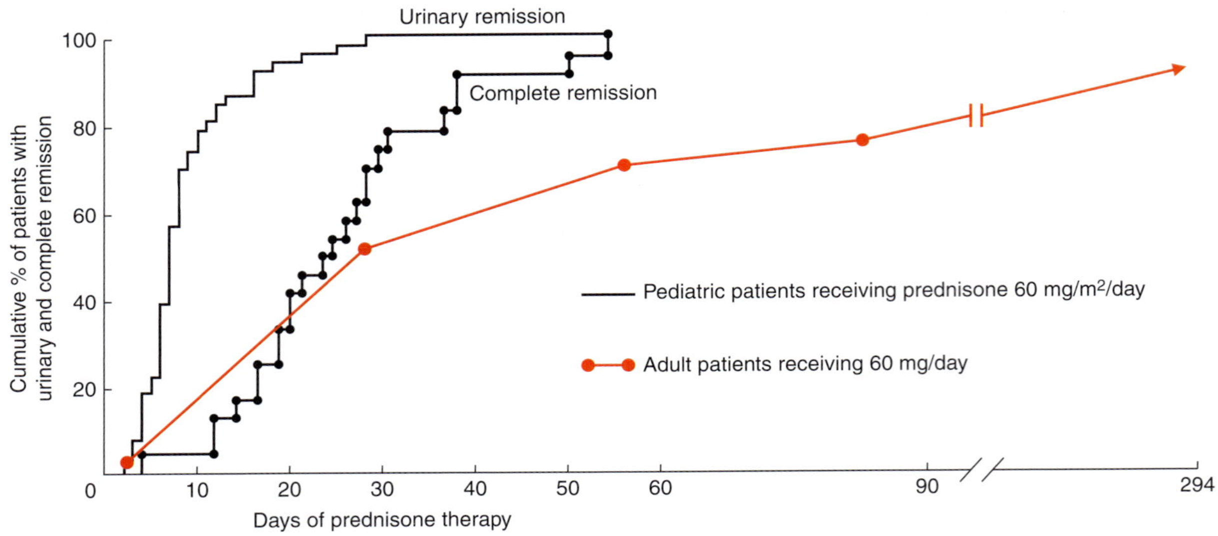

Fig. 16.7 Corticosteroid responses in children and adults (Adapted from [25, 32])

since occasionally enteric-coated tablets are poorly or not absorbed.

Diagnosis and Treatment of Initial and Infrequent Relapses

Daily urine testing should continue after remission in order to detect and treat relapses early. Relapse should be diagnosed on the basis of dipstick 3+ proteinuria for 3 consecutive days. The first relapse is treated with a 2nd induction course of steroids but of shorter duration, for instance, halving the dose after 3 consecutive days of a dipstick-negative/1+ urine for 4 weeks and then stopping is probably as effective as a more prolonged course.

Subsequent relapses may be treated similarly or by tapering the prednisolone to 15 mg/m^2 on alternate days and continuing for 12–18 months (assuming this is above the 'steroid threshold' at which relapse occurs in that individual). Clearly the acceptability of this approach depends on the 'steroid threshold'.

Frequent Relapsers

There is wide variation in the management of frequent relapsers, with a paucity of controlled data, but generally 'second-line' drugs are used to avoid steroid toxicity, most commonly alkylating agents (cyclophosphamide and chlorambucil), levamisole, ciclosporin or tacrolimus and, more recently, rituximab.

Alkylating agents were originally first line, although increasingly other agents are now being tried first, mainly because of the potential side effects of alkylating agents (immediately infection and alopecia, and subsequently sterility [27], haemorrhagic cystitis and longer-term risks of hematologic malignancy). Although these are small for a 3-month course, they need to be balanced against the fact that MCD is usually self-limiting and the permanent remission rate is not very high. On the basis of one but not all studies, cyclophosphamide (2–2.5 mg/kg daily) for 12 weeks is more effective than an 8-week course, giving a 2-year remission rate of 60 % versus 30 % [28]. Younger children are less likely to have a sustained response to cyclophosphamide (Fig. 16.6). Chlorambucil (0.2 mg/kg daily) for 2 months appears to have a similar effect to cyclophosphamide and, apart from not provoking haemorrhagic cystitis, has similar adverse effects. Frequent relapsers are more likely to have a long-term remission following an 8-week course of cyclophosphamide or chlorambucil than steroid-dependent children (75 % versus 35 %). Second courses are not recommended as they are less effective and the cumulative dose of 150–250 mg/kg [27] is likely to be exceeded.

During treatment with cyclophosphamide or chlorambucil, blood counts should be checked weekly and dose reductions made to avoid cytopenias. Herpes zoster infection is potentially catastrophic, serostatus must be checked on starting treatment, and in case of unavoidable contact with active zoster, children should be given hyperimmune immunoglobulin and antivirals.

Azathioprine has no proven role in the management of children with MCD and was ineffective in a randomised trial. It may perhaps have a place as a 'steroid-sparing' agent in steroid-dependent children who have failed second-line treatments and have to be maintained on long-term steroids.

Ciclosporin (up to 150 mg/m^2 or 4 mg/kg per day with initial target trough levels of 50–150 ng/ml) is generally effective in children with both steroid-dependent and frequently relapsing nephrotic syndrome [29]. Unfortunately relapse within 3 months of stopping treatment is very common, and there is a risk of nephrotoxicity, even with careful monitoring of blood levels, renal function and blood pressure control. The aim of therapy is that ciclosporin will maintain steroid-free remission until the underlying disease remits. The optimum duration of therapy is not established, but treatment for 1–2 years followed by its slow withdrawal is recommended. Limited reports suggest that tacrolimus is as effective as ciclosporin and may be used if hypertrichosis or gingival hypertrophy is a problem, but diabetes may be more common.

The choice between a calcineurin inhibitor and cyclophosphamide needs to be individualised and may be influenced by the frequency of relapses and how quickly the child responds to steroids, and often the relative side effects are discussed with the parents. Also relevant is that younger children are less likely to have a sustained remission after cyclophosphamide (Fig. 16.6).

The antihelminthic drug levamisole (2.5 mg/kg on alternate days for 3 months) has been shown to be effective [30]. However, relapse within 3 months of stopping the drug is very common although, as with ciclosporin, it may provide a relatively nontoxic alternative to steroids until spontaneous remission of the condition occurs.

Newer Agents

There have been recent positive reports of the use of mycophenolate and the B-cell depleting anti-CD40 monoclonal antibody, rituximab, in difficult-to-treat patients with MCD. These have been mostly small uncontrolled series, and others have failed to demonstrate efficacy and adequately powered randomised controlled trials are needed. A recent open randomised controlled trial in children with steroid- and calcineurin inhibitor-dependent MCD demonstrated that rituximab with lower dose of steroid and calcineurin inhibitor was non-inferior to standard management [31].

Although there continue to be many unresolved issues, the clinical setting may suggest an obvious approach to frequent relapsers. For instance, a child who presents at a very young age (and is, therefore, statistically likely to continue to relapse for many years) and who is a frequent relapser but not steroid dependent may stand to benefit more from an alkylating agent than an older, steroid-dependent patient.

Adult Minimal Change Disease

With few adequate controlled studies in adults, treatment recommendations are extrapolated from the paediatric experience, but lower doses of oral prednisolone (1 mg/kg daily up to 80 mg/day) are traditionally prescribed. The response rate is lower and up to 25 % do not respond despite 3–4 months treatment [32] (Fig. 16.7). The reasons for this are likely to include lower relative doses of steroids given to children and higher chance of underlying FSGS, missed on the original biopsy, which is more often steroid resistant. After 1 week of urinary remission, the prednisolone dose is halved for 4–6 weeks, followed by further tapering to stop after a further 4–6 weeks aiming, as in children, for a total steroid course of 3–4 months (not evidence-based in adults). Steroid treatment should be combined with gastric protection (an H2 blocker or proton pump inhibitor) and bone protection with a bisphosphonate.

Relapse

The relapse rate is slightly lower than in children (30–50 %), and older adults have fewer relapses and are less likely to require second-line agents [33]. It is important to remember that transient non-nephrotic relapses may occur, so treatment should await confirmation of relapse with 3–5 consecutive days of proteinuria >2+ on urine dipstick and weight gain, the development of oedema or a fall in plasma albumin. Initial relapses are treated with prednisolone (1 mg/kg up to 80 mg/day) but with a much more rapid tapering after urinary remission is achieved (e.g. halving dose every 5 days until 10–15 mg/day, then reduce by 5 mg/day every 5 days until stopped).

Second-line treatments are given to frequently relapsing patients and those who are steroid dependent (who relapse as the steroid dose is reduced but remain in remission as long as a 'threshold' dose is maintained). As in children, cyclophosphamide or calcineurin inhibitors are used. A permanent remission is achieved with cyclophosphamide more often than in children (75 and 66 % at 2 and 5 years, respectively) [32], and based on the paediatric data, a 12-week course may be more effective than 8 weeks. Adults may be less susceptible to gonadal damage, and men can be given the opportunity to bank sperm prior to treatment.

Ciclosporin (4–6 mg/kg/day, aiming for 50–150 ng/ml) is an alternative (and may be preferred in younger adults) or can be used if cyclophosphamide fails. Relapse usually follows dose reduction or withdrawal, but since immunosuppression-free remission eventually occurs in up to 75 % of patients, it is an effective strategy to maintain patients non-nephrotic. There are no controlled studies to inform the best length of time on ciclosporin. My practice is to treat for 1 year and then taper the dose gradually to stop over 4–6 months. Relapse would indicate a longer course of treatment. Since nephrotoxicity is more common after >1-year treatment [34], careful monitoring of renal function and ciclosporin levels is essential, and if the GFR falls, a biopsy is indicated to distinguish between calcineurin inhibitor toxicity or the development of FSGS. Tacrolimus is similarly effective and useful for patients with side effects from ciclosporin.

Reports of the use of mycophenolate and rituximab are, as for children, anecdotal and need to await further studies. The largest published study of rituximab in adult steroid-dependent

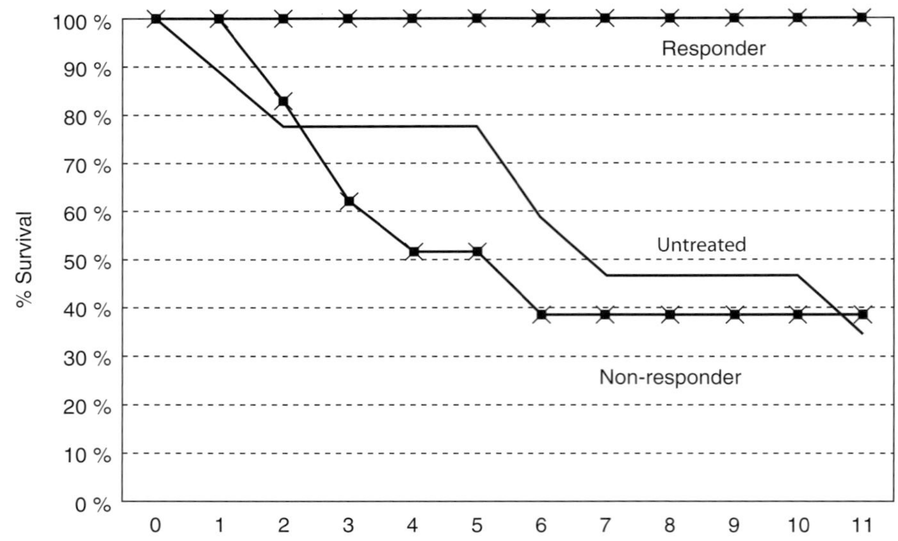

Responder	15	14	10	9	7	7	5	5	5	5	5	5
Non-responder	15	13	10	7	5	5	3	3	3	3	3	2
Untreated	30	21	14	12	11	9	8	5	5	5	5	4

Years

Fig. 16.8 Renal survival is good in patients with FSGS who respond to steroids (Reproduced with permission from Rydel et al. [18])

or frequently relapsing MCN suggests that a significant proportion of patients (65 %) maintained a remission for >2 years, and it appeared to be more effective when given in remission [44]. However, the study was retrospective, and although patients were adults, 12/17 had developed NS as children. Controlled prospective trials are needed.

'Minimal Change' Appearance with Non-nephrotic Proteinuria and Normal Albumin

Steroid treatment is not indicated, but hypertension should be treated with an ACE inhibitor or angiotensin II receptor antagonist. Proteinuria and renal function should be monitored with re-biopsy in case of increased proteinuria of reduced renal function.

Focal Segmental Glomerulosclerosis

Traditionally, FSGS has been thought to have a poor prognosis, with a low rate of response to steroid treatment and about 50 % of patients progressing to ESRD in 10 years [35] although only those who are nephrotic seem to be at particular risk (Fig. 16.2). However, since up to 40 % of nephrotic patients (adults and children alike) respond to steroids with complete remission and, in those who respond, the 5-year actuarial renal survival exceeds 95 % [18], treatment is definitely indicated (Fig. 16.8).

Currently there is no way of identifying those patients who will respond although if the recently described suPAR is confirmed as a reliable marker, this may change. The only (retrospective) factor identified in published studies seems to be the duration of steroid treatment, but recommended protocols vary widely. For example, one study showed that 87 % of responders received 60 mg prednisolone for 1 month and 67 % for 2 months and that the median response time was 3.7 ± 2 months [36].

A pragmatic approach is to treat nephrotic adults with FSGS with prednisolone 1 mg/kg daily for at least 3 months (2 months in children) after considering patient comorbidities and possible contraindications and after discussion with the patient. Responders, in whom the proteinuria reduces or remits, are treated with reducing doses for about 6 months, whilst the steroids are tapered and stopped within 4 weeks in nonresponders. Patients should be monitored for steroid side effects and decisions to abandon treatment need to be made on an individual basis.

Frequent relapsers and those who become steroid dependent may benefit from a 3-month course of cyclophosphamide [37], but steroid-unresponsive patients rarely, if ever, obtain a sustained remission [37, 38] and so the risks outweigh the benefits.

Ciclosporin is sometimes effective, especially in the steroid-dependent patients and although, as in the MCD patients, relapse usually follows withdrawal of the drug [35], it may have a role in those patients with refractory nephrotic syndrome. There are several randomised controlled trials of ciclosporin, including patients with steroid-resistant FSGS [35]. Treated patients received ciclosporin for 6 months, followed by gradual withdrawal. Only 20 % of patients achieved complete remission, but a further 60 % had a partial remission, although there were many relapses following dose reduction. There have been anecdotal reports that patients kept in remission for 12 months can then have ciclosporin successfully withdrawn without relapse [39]. Currently the largest randomised trial of ciclosporin includes only 49 adults: all patients were steroid resistant (and 40 % had also received cyclophosphamide) and received prednisolone (0.15 mg/kg/day) and 6 months of either ciclosporin (3.5 mg/kg/day adjusted to trough levels 125–225 ng/ml) or placebo. Complete (12 %) or partial (58 %) remission followed in the ciclosporin arm compared with 4 % (combined) in the placebo group. Although the relapse rate was high (4 and 35 % respectively still in remission at 1 and 4 years), the treated cohort had a significantly lower rate of progression of renal failure [40]. Based on these limited data, I treat steroid non-responders with ciclosporin (aiming for trough levels of 150–200 ng/ml) for 6 months if remission is not achieved but continue for 1 year with tapering over 3–6 months if remission does occur. This takes advantage of the proven long-term beneficial effects of 6 months of ciclosporin with control of nephrotic syndrome. Ciclosporin is restarted in patients who subsequently relapse again but with careful monitoring of renal function.

Other approaches that have been tried include tacrolimus and very aggressive regimens such as prolonged courses of daily cyclophosphamide (up to 2 years), extended therapy with pulse steroids and intravenous cyclophosphamide or cyclical treatments with corticosteroids and chlorambucil, similar to that introduced by Ponticelli for the treatment of membranous nephropathy. More recently mycophenolate has been reported by several groups to be effective, but no controlled trials are available and the risks of potentially toxic treatments need to be carefully weighed against likelihood of success and alternatives, even if these include progression to ESRD with medical or surgical nephrectomy for intractable and debilitating nephrotic syndrome. All patients, whilst proteinuric, especially those who are steroid resistant should receive angiotensin-converting enzyme (ACE) inhibitors or ARBs to reduce proteinuria and treatment for hyperlipidaemia.

Focal Segmental Glomerulosclerosis with Non-nephrotic Proteinuria

Careful evaluation is required to exclude secondary FSGS in those with non-nephrotic proteinuria. There is no convincing evidence that these patients are steroid responsive, and the risks of treatment outweigh the benefits.

Transplant Recurrence

Recurrence is common after transplantation, but because the label FSGS may often include non-nephrotic native renal disease, an accurate proportion is difficult to assess. It is often reported to be 20 % but is probably higher (~40 %) for patients with true nephrotic FSGS. Recurrence is more likely with rapid progression in native kidneys, previous recurrence following transplantation (up to 80 %) and paediatric recipients [41]. In the future it is possible that assays for suPAR (see above) may prove useful to predict recurrence and direct treatment.

Recurrence may be evident early, even within hours, although the median time to appearance is 14 days and acute renal failure and acute rejection are common. Because of the evidence that a circulating agent is pathogenic in FSGS, patients with recurrent disease following transplantation have been managed with plasma exchange. There is no doubt that plasma exchange can reduce proteinuria, although the response is not absolutely reliable [42]. The best chance of a lasting response occurs when plasma exchange is initiated as soon as possible after the appearance of proteinuria and in those whose recurrence is in the first few weeks after transplantation. The effect can be dramatic and long lasting, but unfortunately the nephrotic syndrome frequently recurs within a few months of discontinuing plasma exchange, and there is much less evidence that a further course of plasma exchange is useful. Some have suggested that pre-emptive plasma exchange is logical, especially for those with a rapid course in native kidneys, but others have found no benefit [43].

High-dose ciclosporin and rituximab [44] have both been tried anecdotally with mixed results. I generally treat with daily plasma exchange for 7 days if this occurs, with reducing frequency depending on response, but sometimes treatments are continued for weeks with plasma exchange associated with reduction in proteinuria and improvement or preservation of renal function.

References

1. Schena FP. Survey of the Italian Registry of Renal Biopsies. Frequency of the renal diseases for 7 consecutive years. The Italian Group of Renal Immunopathology. Nephrol Dial Transplant. 1997;12(3):418–26.
2. Haas M, Meehan SM, Karrison TG, Spargo BH. Changing etiologies of unexplained adult nephrotic syndrome: a comparison of renal biopsy findings from 1976–1979 and 1995–1997. Am J Kidney Dis. 1997;30(5):621–31.
3. Kitiyakara C, Eggers P, Kopp JB. Twenty-one-year trend in ESRD due to focal segmental glomerulosclerosis in the United States. Am J Kidney Dis. 2004;44(5):815–25.
4. Rood IM, Deegens JK, Wetzels JF. Genetic causes of focal segmental glomerulosclerosis: implications for clinical practice. Nephrol Dial Transplant. 2012;27(3):882–90.
5. Garin EH, Diaz LN, Mu W, Wasserfall C, Araya C, Segal M, et al. Urinary CD80 excretion increases in idiopathic minimal-change disease. J Am Soc Nephrol. 2009;20(2):260–6.
6. Bakker WW, van Dael CM, Pierik LJ, van Wijk JA, Nauta J, Borghuis T, et al. Altered activity of plasma hemopexin in patients with minimal change disease in relapse. Pediatr Nephrol. 2005;20(10):1410–5.
7. Ali AA, Wilson E, Moorhead JF, Amlot P, Abdulla A, Fernando ON, et al. Minimal-change glomerular nephritis. Normal kidneys in an abnormal environment? Transplantation. 1994;58(7):849–52.
8. Abdel-Hafez M, Shimada M, Lee PY, Johnson RJ, Garin EH. Idiopathic nephrotic syndrome and atopy: is there a common link? Am J Kidney Dis. 2009;54(5):945–53.
9. Clement LC, Avila-Casado C, Mace C, Soria E, Bakker WW, Kersten S, et al. Podocyte-secreted angiopoietin-like-4 mediates proteinuria in glucocorticoid-sensitive nephrotic syndrome. Nat Med. 2011;17(1):117–22.

10. Gallon L, Leventhal J, Skaro A, Kanwar Y, Alvarado A. Resolution of recurrent focal segmental glomerulosclerosis after retransplantation. N Engl J Med. 2012;366(17):1648–9.
11. Kemper MJ, Wolf G, Muller-Wiefel DE. Transmission of glomerular permeability factor from a mother to her child. N Engl J Med. 2001;344(5):386–7.
12. Dantal J, Godfrin Y, Koll R, Perretto S, Naulet J, Bouhours JF, et al. Antihuman immunoglobulin affinity immunoadsorption strongly decreases proteinuria in patients with relapsing nephrotic syndrome. J Am Soc Nephrol. 1998;9(9):1709–15.
13. Savin VJ, Sharma R, Sharma M, McCarthy ET, Swan SK, Ellis E, et al. Circulating factor associated with increased glomerular permeability to albumin in recurrent focal segmental glomerulosclerosis. N Engl J Med. 1996;334(14):878–83.
14. McCarthy ET, Sharma M, Savin VJ. Circulating permeability factors in idiopathic nephrotic syndrome and focal segmental glomerulosclerosis. Clin J Am Soc Nephrol. 2010;5(11):2115–21.
15. Wei C, El Hindi S, Li J, Fornoni A, Goes N, Sageshima J, et al. Circulating urokinase receptor as a cause of focal segmental glomerulosclerosis. Nat Med. 2011;17(8):952–60.
16. D'Agati VD. Pathobiology of focal segmental glomerulosclerosis: new developments. Curr Opin Nephrol Hypertens. 2012;21(3):243–50.
17. Trompeter RS, Lloyd BW, Hicks J, White RH, Cameron JS. Long-term outcome for children with minimal-change nephrotic syndrome. Lancet. 1985;1(8425):368–70.
18. Rydel JJ, Korbet SM, Borok RZ, Schwartz MM. Focal segmental glomerular sclerosis in adults: presentation, course, and response to treatment. Am J Kidney Dis. 1995;25(4):534–42.
19. Waldman M, Crew RJ, Valeri A, Busch J, Stokes B, Markowitz G, et al. Adult minimal-change disease: clinical characteristics, treatment, and outcomes. Clin J Am Soc Nephrol. 2007;2(3):445–53.
20. Nephrotic syndrome in children: prediction of histopathology from clinical and laboratory characteristics at time of diagnosis. A report of the International Study of Kidney Disease in Children. Kidney Int. 1978;13(2):159–65.
21. Fuiano G, Comi N, Magri P, Sepe V, Balletta MM, Esposito C, et al. Serial morphometric analysis of sclerotic lesions in primary "focal" segmental glomerulosclerosis. J Am Soc Nephrol. 1996;7(1):49–55.
22. Border WA. Distinguishing minimal-change disease from mesangial disorders. Kidney Int. 1988;34(3):419–34.
23. Ehrich JH, Brodehl J. Long versus standard prednisone therapy for initial treatment of idiopathic nephrotic syndrome in children. Arbeitsgemeinschaft fur Padiatrische Nephrologie. Eur J Pediatr. 1993;152(4):357–61.
24. Gipson DS, Massengill SF, Yao L, Nagaraj S, Smoyer WE, Mahan JD, et al. Management of childhood onset nephrotic syndrome. Pediatrics. 2009;124(2):747–57.
25. Short versus standard prednisone therapy for initial treatment of idiopathic nephrotic syndrome in children. Arbeitsgemeinschaft fur Padiatrische Nephrologie. Lancet. 1988;1(8582):380–3.
26. Hodson EM, Willis NS, Craig JC. Corticosteroid therapy for nephrotic syndrome in children. Cochrane Database Syst Rev. 2007(4):CD001533.
27. Trompeter RS, Evans PR, Barratt TM. Gonadal function in boys with steroid-responsive nephrotic syndrome treated with cyclophosphamide for short periods. Lancet. 1981;1(8231):1177–9.
28. Cyclophosphamide treatment of steroid dependent nephrotic syndrome: comparison of eight week with 12 week course. Report of Arbeitsgemeinschaft fur Padiatrische Nephrologie. Arch Dis Child. 1987;62(11):1102–6.
29. Niaudet P, Broyer M, Habib R. Treatment of idiopathic nephrotic syndrome with cyclosporin A in children. Clin Nephrol. 1991;35 Suppl 1:S31–6.
30. Levamisole for corticosteroid-dependent nephrotic syndrome in childhood. British Association for Paediatric Nephrology. Lancet. 1991;337(8757):1555–7.
31. Ravani P, Magnasco A, Edefonti A, Murer L, Rossi R, Ghio L, et al. Short-term effects of rituximab in children with steroid- and calcineurin-dependent nephrotic syndrome: a randomized controlled trial. Clin J Am Soc Nephrol. 2011;6(6):1308–15.
32. Nolasco F, Cameron JS, Heywood EF, Hicks J, Ogg C, Williams DG. Adult-onset minimal change nephrotic syndrome: a long-term follow-up. Kidney Int. 1986;29(6):1215–23.
33. Tse KC, Lam MF, Yip PS, Li FK, Choy BY, Lai KN, et al. Idiopathic minimal change nephrotic syndrome in older adults: steroid responsiveness and pattern of relapses. Nephrol Dial Transplant. 2003;18(7):1316–20.
34. Melocoton TL, Kamil ES, Cohen AH, Fine RN. Long-term cyclosporine A treatment of steroid-resistant and steroid-dependent nephrotic syndrome. Am J Kidney Dis. 1991;18(5):583–8.
35. Korbet SM. Primary focal segmental glomerulosclerosis. J Am Soc Nephrol. 1998;9(7):1333–40.
36. Banfi G, Moriggi M, Sabadini E, Fellin G, D'Amico G, Ponticelli C. The impact of prolonged immunosuppression on the outcome of idiopathic focal-segmental glomerulosclerosis with nephrotic syndrome in adults. A collaborative retrospective study. Clin Nephrol. 1991;36(2):53–9.
37. Siegel NJ, Gaudio KM, Krassner LS, McDonald BM, Anderson FP, Kashgarian M. Steroid-dependent nephrotic syndrome in children: histopathology and relapses after cyclophosphamide treatment. Kidney Int. 1981;19(3):454–9.
38. Tarshish P, Tobin JN, Bernstein J, Edelmann Jr CM. Cyclophosphamide does not benefit patients with focal segmental glomerulosclerosis. A report of the International Study of Kidney Disease in Children. Pediatr Nephrol. 1996;10(5):590–3.
39. Meyrier A, Noel LH, Auriche P, Callard P. Long-term renal tolerance of cyclosporin A treatment in adult idiopathic nephrotic syndrome. Collaborative Group of the Societe de Nephrologie. Kidney Int. 1994;45(5):1446–56.
40. Cattran DC, Appel GB, Hebert LA, Hunsicker LG, Pohl MA, Hoy WE, et al. A randomized trial of cyclosporine in patients with steroid-resistant focal segmental glomerulosclerosis. North America Nephrotic Syndrome Study Group. Kidney Int. 1999;56(6):2220–6.
41. Keith DS. Therapeutic apheresis rescue mission: recurrent focal segmental glomerulosclerosis in renal allografts. Semin Dial. 2012;25(2):190–2.
42. Artero ML, Sharma R, Savin VJ, Vincenti F. Plasmapheresis reduces proteinuria and serum capacity to injure glomeruli in patients with recurrent focal glomerulosclerosis. Am J Kidney Dis. 1994;23(4):574–81.
43. Gonzalez E, Ettenger R, Rianthavorn P, Tsai E, Malekzadeh M. Preemptive plasmapheresis and recurrence of focal segmental glomerulosclerosis in pediatric renal transplantation. Pediatr Transplant. 2011;15(5):495–501.
44. Munyentwali H, Bouachi K, Audard V, Remy P, Lang P, Mojaat R, et al. Rituximab is an efficient and safe treatment in adults with steroid-dependent minimal change disease. Kidney Int. 2013;83(3):511–6.
45. Vester U, Kranz B, Zimmermann S, Hoyer PF. Cyclophosphamide in steroid-sensitive nephrotic syndrome: outcome and outlook. Pediatr Nephrol. 2003;18(7):661–4.

Membranous Nephropathy

17

Peter W. Mathieson

Membranous nephropathy (MN) is the most common cause of primary nephrotic syndrome in adults: recent figures from the Netherlands show an incidence of around ten per million population per year [1]. Identical clinical presentation and histological appearances can occur whether the condition is primary or 'idiopathic' (IMN) or when it is secondary to various drugs, infections or tumours (see Table 17.1), so that careful consideration to exclude an underlying cause is needed when assessing each new patient. When such a cause can be identified, the prognosis is that of the underlying condition and management should be directed towards that condition: causative drugs should be stopped and infections or tumours treated and eradicated if possible. If successful the secondary MN can be expected to resolve.

Epidemiology

IMN has a slight male preponderance (1.3–2.2:1) and is increasingly common with advancing years, being relatively rare in children (<5 %). Consequently MN becomes increasingly high on the differential diagnosis of an elderly patient presenting with frank or subacute nephrotic syndrome. There is very little global variation in incidence of IMN which represents roughly 70–80 % of all membranous glomerulonephritis; however, the incidence of secondary MN relates to the prevalence of the underlying conditions, in particular infections such as hepatitis B. Consequently, and in contrast to IMN, secondary causes of MN are a significant cause of nephrotic syndrome in children in developing countries [2]. Although familial cases have been reported, these are perhaps surprisingly rare given the role immunogenetics is now thought to play in the aetiology of the disease.

Several forms of glomerulonephritis are associated with malignancy and are covered in an excellent recent review [3]. However, MN has the strongest association with approximately 10 % of patients with MN having malignancy, and 70 % of patients with carcinoma and nephrotic syndrome having MN as the cause of their nephrotic syndrome. The common tumours are shown in Table 17.1, but lung and gastrointestinal carcinomas predominate with age over 65 and >20 pack year history of smoking being substantial risk factors [4].

There is a caveat in attributing a secondary cause; MN is a common cause of nephrotic syndrome with increasing age, malignancies, autoimmune diseases and medication are also very common and for an individual the combination does not prove causality. However, there are very clear associations with some infections such as hepatitis B, and potentially any malignancy or chronic infection could be associated with neoantigens that might precipitate MN. Identifying and treating potential secondary causes makes absolute sense.

Pathogenesis

There have been several significant recent advances in the understanding of the pathogenesis and treatment of MN, and I will focus on these rather than the older history of the condition which has been extensively reviewed elsewhere [5, 6]. Suffice to say MN is a discrete pathological entity (Fig. 17.1) which can only be identified by renal biopsy including examination of the tissue by electron microscopy. The glomerular capillary wall is expanded but the cellularity of the glomerulus is not typically increased (Fig. 17.1a). Immune deposits typically including IgG and complement are found in a granular distribution along the glomerular capillary wall (Fig. 17.1b), and electron microscopy shows electron dense deposits in the sub-epithelial space adjacent to the foot processes of the glomerular epithelial cells or podocytes (Fig. 17.1c, see also separate Chap. 13).

P.W. Mathieson, PhD, FRCP, FMedSci
Academic Renal Unit,
University of Bristol and Southmead Hospital,
Bristol BS10 5NB, UK
e-mail: p.mathieson@bristol.ac.uk

M. Harber (ed.), *Practical Nephrology*,
DOI 10.1007/978-1-4471-5547-8_17, © Springer-Verlag London 2014

Table 17.1

Causes of MN	Comments and investigations
Idiopathic (primary) MN 70–80 %	Anti-PLA2R antibody Exclusion of secondary causes
Secondary MN	
Malignancy associated: 1. Carcinomas Lung Gastric Oesophageal Renal Prostate Breast Colon Ovary Oropharyngeal 2. Malignancy associated: others Lymphoproliferative: lymphomas and CLL Melanoma Mesothelioma Wilm's tumour Schwannoma Neuroblastoma Hepatic adenoma	Thorough clinical assessment in all patients for symptoms or signs of neoplasia. Consider clinically appropriate investigations to exclude malignancy on the basis of assessment Consider staining for IgG_1 and IgG_2 on biopsy especially in patients with inflammatory infiltrate
Secondary MN	
Infection associated: Hepatitis B Hepatitis C HIV Syphilis Malaria Schistosomiasis Filariasis Leprosy Hydatid	Hepatitis B by far the commonest cause worldwide Hepatitis B sAg, eAg, delta, HIV, hepatitis C, syphilis serology, blood film, schistosomiasis, hydatid and microfilaria serology
Secondary MN	
Autoimmune associated: Systemic lupus erythematosus Rheumatoid arthritis Grave's disease Hashimoto's thyroiditis Sjogren's syndrome Mixed connective tissue disorder Ankylosing spondylitis Scleroderma Myasthenia gravis Bullous pemphigoid Dermatomyositis Primary biliary cirrhosis Guillain-Barre syndrome	Autoimmune disease usually clinically apparent but following tests appropriate on all patients with MN, anti-nuclear antibody, complement (C_3/C_4), ENA screen, dsDNA, rheumatoid factor, thyroid function tests and antithyroid antibodies
Alloimmune associated: Transplant glomerulopathy/de novo MN Graft vs. host disease	Donor-specific antibodies

Table 17.1 (continued)

Causes of MN	Comments and investigations
Secondary MN	
Medication associated: Penicillamine Gold NSAIDs and COX-2 inhibitors Lithium Captopril Clopidogrel Probenecid Toxin associated: Mercury Hydrocarbons Formaldehyde	Accurate drug and exposure history critical, not least as many rheumatological conditions can be associated with MN in their own right
Secondary MN	
Miscellaneous: Diabetes Sarcoidosis Sickle-cell disease α-1 Antitrypsin deficiency Mastocytosis Urticarial vasculitis Myelodysplasia Dermatitis herpetiformis IgG4-related disease	Serum ACE, haemoglobin electrophoresis, α-1 antitrypsin deficiency: Haemoglobin electrophoresis, IgG subtypes

Much of the early understanding of MN was based on analysis of animal models, especially Heymann nephritis in rats [7]; it is clear from more recent work that the pathogenesis of IMN in humans is likely a conventional autoimmune one in genetically predisposed individuals, with the podocyte being the major target of injury. Therapeutic advances, as is so often the case, have lagged behind the basic science progress, but there are very good reasons for optimism that our ability to manage IMN will improve rapidly in the next few years.

An autoimmune pathogenesis has long been assumed in IMN because of the immune deposits in the glomerulus and the analogies with Heymann nephritis. The first major advance in recent years was the elegant description by Pierre Ronco and colleagues of MN due to alloimmunisation against neutral endopeptidase (NEP). Babies born to NEP-deficient mothers developed transient neonatal MN due to transplacental transfer of IgG anti-NEP induced in the mother by an immune response to NEP in a previous foetus [8]. This was a beautiful demonstration of the induction of human MN by an IgG antibody; unfortunately it soon became clear that NEP was not the auto-antigenic target in sporadic IMN. In 2009, Larry Beck and colleagues reported [9] that around 70 % of patients with IMN have autoantibodies directed against the phospholipase A2 receptor PLA2R1. This has been confirmed by others [10] and in different populations

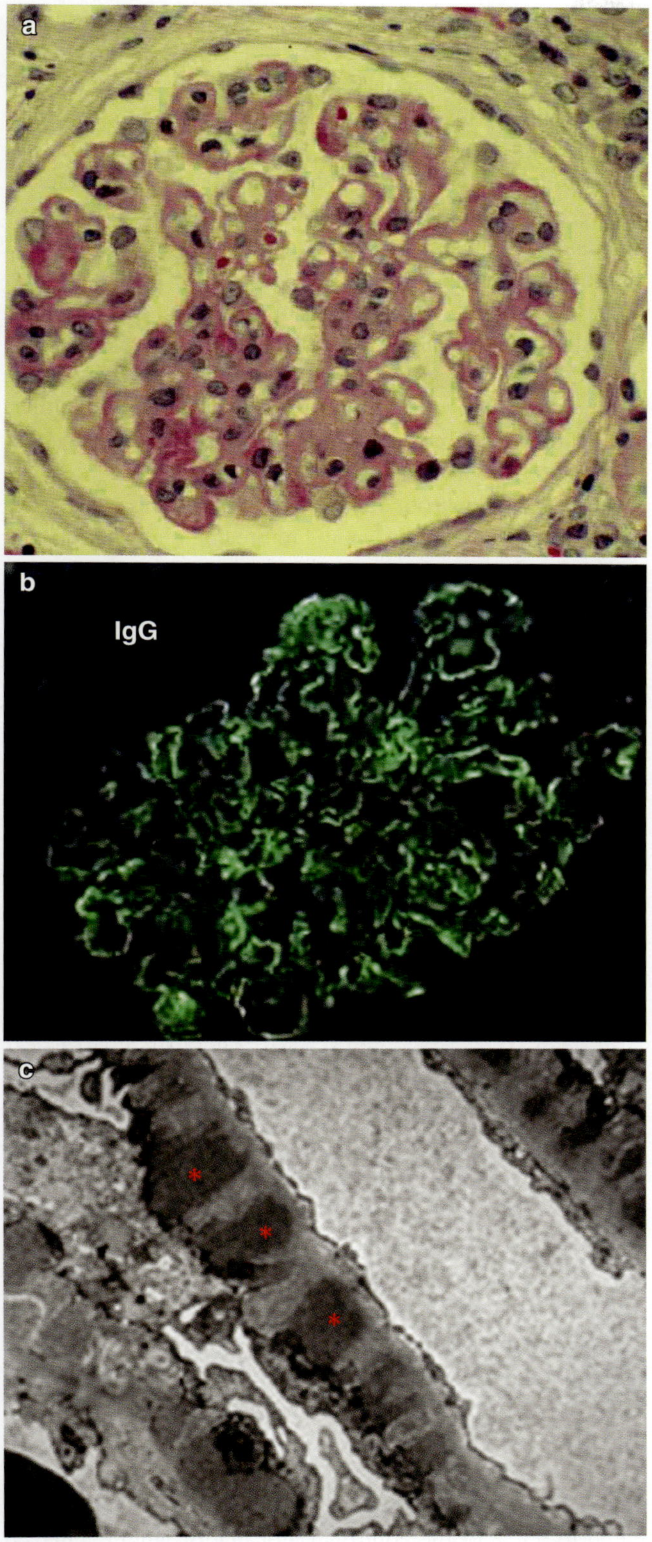

Fig. 17.1 Renal biopsy appearances of membranous nephropathy. (**a**) Light microscopy (haematoxylin and eosin stain). (**b**) Immunofluorescence, in this case for IgG, but similar appearances typically seen for C3. (**c**) Electron microscopy: electron dense deposits are shown by *asterisks*

[11]. There is a suggestion that anti-PLA2R1 antibody levels correlate with disease activity and/or with response to treatment [12], so testing for this autoantibody shows promise not only in diagnosis of IMN but also in monitoring and commercial assays for anti-PLA2R1 are now available. PLA2R1 is expressed by podocytes [13], but it is not yet clear whether the immune response is primarily directed against podocyte PLA2R1 or whether the podocyte is an innocent bystander that is injured by the anti-PLA2R1 antibody response. Either way, podocytes are the target of injury, presumably mediated by complement: the predominant autoantibodies in IMN are of IgG4 subclass and although this is not regarded as a complement-activating subclass of IgG, recent data, also from Beck et al. [presented at 9th International Podocyte conference, Miami, March 2012], show that anti-PLA2R1 autoantibodies do activate complement, mainly via the lectin pathway. Novel approaches to therapy could therefore be directed against the anti-PLA2R1 autoimmune response or towards measures to protect, repair and/or regenerate the podocytes that have been injured.

The other recent major advance in IMN has been the elucidation of the genetics of the condition. Stanescu et al. [14] reported genome-wide association studies in three European populations and showed that two genetic regions are closely involved in predisposition to IMN. One is on chromosome 6 in the major histocompatibility complex, with the strongest association being with HLA-DQA1 and the other is on chromosome 2, most likely the gene encoding PLA2R1 itself. That the condition should result from predisposing genes in the MHC, an immune response gene, and in the autoantigen itself is intriguing although curiously few familial cases of IMN are reported. The MHC association was the strongest, and this together with the fact that 20–30 % of patients with IMN do not apparently have autoantibodies to PLA2R1 suggests that other autoantigens must be involved. Other candidates include aldose reductase and manganese superoxide dismutase [15].

Clinical Features

Roughly ¾ of adults with IMN present frankly nephrotic, often with very heavy and sustained proteinuria (sometimes life-threateningly severe). The remaining ¼ present with sub-nephrotic (but still significant) proteinuria with or without overt renal impairment. Microscopic haematuria is not unusual (40–50 %) even in patients who are grossly nephrotic, but red cell casts are rare unless associated with other renal pathology such as lupus nephritis. Renal impairment and hypertension are said to be unusual at presentation but does not exclude the diagnosis, and AKI in the setting of severe nephrotic syndrome is common requiring rapid identification and correction of prerenal elements.

Patients may have features suggestive of a secondary cause such as symptoms and signs of underlying malignancy, SLE/rheumatoid arthritis or an infective cause, which may be obvious but if not should be searched for (see Table 17.1). For MN associated with malignancy, the two conditions are usually identified within 12 months of each other with 80 % of malignancies being present before or at time of the diagnosis of nephrotic syndrome.

The reported incidence of thromboembolism in MN varies hugely in the literature (3–48 %) but is undoubtedly a significant risk. A summary of studies suggests 11 % of patients having a DVT, 11 % of patients a clinically significant pulmonary embolus and 35 % (5–60 %) of patients having a renal vein thrombosis [16]. A recent retrospective study demonstrated a hazard ratio for VTE of 22 compared to patients with IgA nephropathy, and even after correction for age, cancer history and degree of proteinuria, the HR was roughly ten times that of IgA and twice as high as FSGS [17]. The frequency of RVT is surprising for most clinicians and clearly depends on how aggressively the diagnosis is pursued, but RVT does genuinely seem to be more common in MN and if it occurs carries an adverse renal prognosis. The reasons for this difference thromboembolism and renal vein thrombosis in patients with different pathologies who are equally nephrotic remain unclear.

IMN has a variable natural history, with around a third of patients undergoing spontaneous remission and having an excellent long-term prognosis and a third remaining stable, but the final third experiencing progressive deterioration of excretory renal function and developing chronic kidney disease (CKD) with all its attendant morbidity and mortality. It is important to note that spontaneous remission can be complete or partial, but critically can take up to 2 years to occur with a mean of about a year [18].

Treatment

KDIGO guidelines have recently been published for the treatment of IMN with graded recommendations on the limited evidence available and offer excellent guidance [19]. As in all proteinuric conditions, patients with IMN should be treated with dietary salt restriction, angiotensin system blockade (even if not hypertensive, but if they are hypertensive, strict blood pressure control is of course essential), modification of cardiovascular risk by smoking avoidance/lifestyle modification/cholesterol lowering therapy and diuretics as required for oedema control.

There is evidence in favour of prophylactic anticoagulation in patients with severe hypoalbuminaemia due to IMN (at or below 2.5 g/dl or 25 g/l) [20]. Secondary causes of MN should be screened for and the underlying condition, e.g. infection or malignancy, should be treated. It is also important to consider vaccination against encapsulated bacteria and consideration of antibiotic prophylaxis in those with persistent hypogammaglobulinaemia.

The more controversial question is whether patients with IMN should be given immunosuppressive therapy and if so how patients should be selected for treatment, when it should be given and which agent(s) should be used. As mentioned earlier, the variable natural history of the condition means that data from uncontrolled trials should be treated with great caution; sadly there is a shortage of controlled trials in IMN. In part because of spontaneous remission and in part because the risk: benefit studies of immunosuppression in IMN are so limited, KDIGO guidelines only recommend initiating immunosuppressive medication in those patients with either:

(a) Severe, disabling or life-threatening symptoms related to nephrotic syndrome or
(b) Persistent nephrotic range (>4 g/l) proteinuria unresponsive to antihypertensive and renin: angiotensin blockade over at least 6 months or
(c) Progressive rise in creatinine (>30 %) over 6–12 months unexplained by other renal insults

It is NOT recommended to initiate immunosuppressive therapy for IMN in patients with small kidneys (e.g. <8 cm in adults) or if eGFR <30 ml/min/1.73 m^2 or in the presence of severe/life-threatening infection.

To prescribe immunosuppressive therapy outside these parameters exposes patients to potentially toxic medication in the absence of any supportive data. Furthermore, there is no evidence that steroids alone, or mycophenolate mofetil, have any role in the initial treatment of IMN.

A Cochrane review [21] and more recently the KDIGO guidelines [19] have concluded that the treatment for which there is the best evidence is the combination of prednisolone with an alkylating agent (chlorambucil or cyclophosphamide with the latter recommended as first choice as it has similar remission rates but fewer severe adverse effects), originally popularised from Italy by Claudio Ponticelli [22, 23]. The safe administration of the Ponticelli regimen is covered with other immunosuppressive regimens in this chapter, but in summary, it consists of a 6-month course of treatment with alternating 30-day cycles starting with 1 g methylprednisolone daily for 3 days followed by oral methylprednisolone 0.5 mg/kg/day for the rest of the month. For the second month patients either receive oral cyclophosphamide (2 mg/kg/day) OR chlorambucil (0.15–2 mg/kg/day) for the month, then repeating the cycle by returning to the steroid regimen. The 10-year follow-up of this impressive RCT demonstrated complete or partial remission in 61 % of the treated compared to 33 % of the controls (very few of whom achieved complete remission). The treatment group also had better patient and renal survival [22]. In the recently reported UK randomised controlled trial focusing on the subset of patients with deteriorating renal function, prednisolone plus chlorambucil has been shown to provide significant protection of renal function compared to cyclosporine or supportive treatment alone [24]. Adverse events with this approach are very frequent and for this reason plus the fact that in the UK trial the deterioration was slowed rather than prevented, better treatments are still needed. Perhaps the two most promising are rituximab [25] and adrenocorticotropic hormone, ACTH [26]. Rituximab targets B lymphocytes and since we now know that the disease is associated with an auto-antibody, at least in the majority of cases, a drug that prevents synthesis of this antibody does seem logical. This drug has not yet been tested in randomised controlled trials (RCTs), the responses are mostly in terms of reductions in proteinuria rather than long-term protection of excretory renal function, and there are important concerns about the cost of rituximab and also its long-term safety [27]. ACTH has only been studied in small series but does show promise. It is probably working not by stimulating adrenal steroid production but by direct effects on podocytes, which express the appropriate receptor and show responsiveness to ACTH in vitro [28].

Calcineurin inhibitors (cyclosporine or tacrolimus) are undoubtedly capable of reducing proteinuria although there is a very high risk of relapse when they are stopped. They should be reserved for patients who are not suitable for, or fail, 6 months of steroids plus an alkylating agent; should be used with great caution in patients with impaired renal function; should be reduced to as low a dose as possible in those that respond; and should be stopped promptly in those that don't.

Recurrent and De Novo MN Following Transplantation

Recurrent IMN is common and occurs in roughly a third of patients (7–44 %) by 3years and resulting in 50 % ESRD by 10 years [29]. Recurrent disease presents earlier than de novo MN typically within 2 years (15 months vs. 4 years for de novo). As yet there seem to be no markers to identify patients at risk of recurrence, but it may be that titres of anti-PLAR1 will be predictive.

De novo MN seems to be very common and apparent on as many as 2 % of all transplants, and again the reason for this is not clear but may be associated with donor-specific antibodies (HLA or non-HLA). As with native IMN some success has been claimed for the use of rituximab in small series [30], but the numbers are small and the area is crying out for a large RCT before this agent slips into routine use.

Prognosis

The prognosis of secondary MN is very dependent on the underlying cause and its response to therapy, but there are many examples of remission following treatment of malignancy or the associated infectious disease. The prognostic indicators for IMN are really little different from most other kidney diseases; adverse factors include *severity and duration of proteinuria*, hypertension, *reduced and progressively declining GFR, glomerulosclerosis and tubulointerstitial fibrosis/atrophy* in addition to being male and progressive age (children seem to fare well); the severity of the membranous changes on biopsy has no correlation to outcome [31]. Duration and severity of proteinuria is of practical use: 32 % of patients with nephrotic range proteinuria developing a decline in GFR compared to 12 % of those with sub-nephrotic proteinuria. 66 % of those patients having >8 g/day of proteinuria for >6 months progress to ESRD, however even a significant proportion of patients in this category do not share this fate and approximately 20 % of those with very heavy proteinuria undergo spontaneous remission. Conversely a female patient presenting with no tubulointerstitial fibrosis/glomerulosclerosis and sub-nephrotic proteinuria has a good prognosis. In common with all nephrotic disease, any reduction in proteinuria, in the absence of reduced GFR, is associated with a very significantly better outcome. 10-year renal survival is 100, 90 and 50 % in complete, partial and no remission, respectively.

Summary

MN is a common cause of nephrotic syndrome in adults and associated with significant morbidity. Distinguishing IMN from secondary MN is critical and anti-PLA2 receptor antibodies may help identify IMN. Furthermore, genuinely remarkable developments in the understanding of IMN are afoot which will hopefully result in better treatments, and well-designed RCTs of newer agents are urgently needed.

The National Kidney Federation has a good website providing patient information, and the membranous page is a good first stop for newly diagnosed patients: www.Kidney.org.uk/Medical-Info/Kidney-disease/memb-neph.html

References

1. Hofstra JM, Wetzels JFM. Introduction of a cyclophosphamide-based strategy and the risk of ESRD in patients with idiopathic membranous nephropathy: a nationwide survey in the Netherlands. Nephrol Dial Transplant. 2008;23:3534–8.
2. Ponticelli C. Membranous nephropathy. J Nephrol. 2007;20(3):268–87.
3. Lien YH, Lai LW. Pathogenesis, diagnosis and management of paraneoplastic glomerulonephritis. Nat Rev Nephrol. 2011;7(2):85–95.
4. Beck LH Jr. Membranous nephropathy and malignancy. Semin Nephrol. 2010;30(6):635–44.
5. Mathieson PW. Membranous nephropathy. Br J Ren Med. 2002;7:17–20.
6. Glassock RJ. The pathogenesis of idiopathic membranous nephropathy: a 50-year odyssey. Am J Kidney Dis. 2010;56:157–67.
7. Cybulsky AV. Membranous nephropathy. Contrib Nephrol. 2011;169:107–25.

8. Debiec H, Nauta J, Coulet F, et al. Role of truncating mutations in MME gene in fetomaternal alloimmunisation and antenatal glomerulopathies. Lancet. 2004;364:1252–9.
9. Beck Jr LH, Bonegio RG, Lambeau G, et al. M-type phospholipase A2 receptor as target antigen in idiopathic membranous nephropathy. N Engl J Med. 2009;361:11–21.
10. Debiec H, Ronco P. PLA2R autoantibodies and PLA2R glomerular deposits in membranous nephropathy. N Engl J Med. 2011;364:689–90.
11. Qin W, Beck Jr LH, Zeng C, et al. Anti-phospholipase A2 receptor antibody in membranous nephropathy. J Am Soc Nephrol. 2011;22:1137–43.
12. Cravedi P, Ruggenenti P, Remuzzi G. Circulating anti-PLA2R autoantibodies to monitor immunological activity in membranous nephropathy. J Am Soc Nephrol. 2011;22:1400–2.
13. Beck Jr LH, Salant DJ. Membranous nephropathy: recent travels and new roads ahead. Kidney Int. 2010;77:765–70.
14. Stanescu HC, Arcos-Burgos M, Medlar A, et al. Risk HLA-DQA1 and PLA(2)R1 alleles in idiopathic membranous nephropathy. N Engl J Med. 2011;364:616–26.
15. Makker SP, Tramontano A. Idiopathic membranous nephropathy: an autoimmune disease. Semin Nephrol. 2011;31:333–40.
16. Nickolas TL, Radhakrishnan J, Appel GB. Hyperlipidemia and thrombotic complications in patients with membranous nephropathy. Semin Nephrol. 2003;23(4):406–11.
17. Barbour SJ, Greenwald A. Djurdjev O, et al. Disease-specific risk of venous thromboembolic events is increased in idiopathic glomerulonephritis. Kidney Int. 2012;81(2):190–5.
18. Polanco N, Gutierrez E. Covarsi A, et al. Spontaneous remission of nephrotic syndrome in idiopathic membranous nephropathy. J Am Soc Nephrol. 2010;21(4):697–704.
19. KDIGO clinical practice guidelines for glomerulonephritis. Kidney Int Suppl. 2012;2(2):187–97.
20. Glassock RJ. Prophylactic anticoagulation in nephrotic syndrome: a clinical conundrum. J Am Soc Nephrol. 2007;18(8):2221–5.
21. Schieppati A, Perna A, Zamora J, et al. Immunosuppressive treatment for idiopathic membranous nephropathy in adults with nephrotic syndrome. Cochrane Database Syst Rev. 2004;(4):CD004293.
22. Ponticelli C, Zucchelli P, Passerini P, et al. A 10-year follow-up of a randomized study with methylprednisolone and chlorambucil in membranous nephropathy. Kidney Int. 1995;48:1600–4.
23. Ponticelli C, Altieri P, Scolari F, et al. A randomized study comparing methylprednisolone plus chlorambucil versus methylprednisolone plus cyclophosphamide in idiopathic membranous nephropathy. J Am Soc Nephrol. 1998;9:444–50.
24. Howman A, et al. The UK randomised controlled trial of immunosuppression for progressive membranous nephropathy. Lancet. 2013;381(9868):744–51.
25. Beck Jr LH, Fervenza FC, Beck DM, et al. Rituximab-induced depletion of anti-PLA2R autoantibodies predicts response in membranous nephropathy. J Am Soc Nephrol. 2011;22:1543–50.
26. Ponticelli C, Passerini P, Salvadori M, et al. A randomized pilot trial comparing methylprednisolone plus a cytotoxic agent versus synthetic adrenocorticotropic hormone in idiopathic membranous nephropathy. Am J Kidney Dis. 2006;47:233–40.
27. Molloy ES, Calabrese LH. Progressive multifocal leukoencephalopathy associated with immunosuppressive therapy in rheumatic diseases: evolving role of biologic therapies. Arthritis Rheum. 2012;64:3043–51.
28. Lindskog A, Ebefors K, Johansson ME, et al. Melanocortin 1 receptor agonists reduce proteinuria. J Am Soc Nephrol. 2010;21:1290–8.
29. Ivanyi B. A primer on recurrent and de novo glomerulonephritis in renal allografts. Nat Clin Pract Nephrol. 2008;4(8):446–57.
30. Sprangers B, Lefkowitz GI, Cohen SD, et al. Beneficial effect of rituximab in the treatment of recurrent idiopathic membranous nephropathy after kidney transplantation. Clin J Am Soc Nephrol. 2010;5(5):790–7.
31. Reichert LJ, Koene RA, Wetzels JF. Prognostic factors in idiopathic membranous nephropathy. Am J Kidney Dis. 1998;31(1):1–11.

Membranoproliferative Glomerulonephritis and C3 Glomerulopathy

18

Daniel P. Gale and Mared Owen-Casey

The terms membranoproliferative glomerulonephritis (MPGN) and mesangiocapillary glomerulonephritis (MCGN) are interchangeable and refer to the light microscopic appearances of cellular proliferation in the mesangial regions of the glomeruli, with expansion of both cells and mesangial matrix, accompanied by thickening of the glomerular capillary walls. Rather than being a specific disease, MPGN is a morphological pattern which is associated with a wide range of distinct (and usually systemic) diseases. Recent developments in the understanding of these conditions emphasise the importance of establishing underlying disorder.

Classification: MPGN and C3 Glomerulopathy

The first description of MPGN as a distinct histomorphological entity was only in 1961 [1]. MPGN was at first subdivided purely on the basis of light microscopic morphology, but the introduction of electron microscopy and immunostaining in the 1960s led to the classical subdivision into 'type 1', 'type 2' and 'type 3' MPGN (see Table 18.1). Using this system, a diagnosis of type 2 MPGN prompted the search for complement alternative pathway dysregulation, and a diagnosis of type 1 or type 3 MPGN suggested excessive or aberrant immunoglobulin production. Although this categorisation proved clinically useful, over the last 5 years, improved understanding of the pathophysiology of MPGN has led to the move towards classifying proliferative GN according to the underlying clinicopathological process, rather than relying entirely on the morphological features seen in the kidney biopsy. This has been driven by three crucial observations. Firstly, while the degree of inflammatory change (e.g. mesangial hypercellularity and crescent formation) seen on kidney biopsy is correlated with renal prognosis, histomorphological type *per se* is not [2]. Secondly, the morphological changes defining 'type 1' MPGN sometimes occur *without* the deposition of immunoglobulins, and in these cases evidence of dysregulation of the complement alternative pathway is frequently present [3]. The third observation was that dense transformation of the GBM (regarded as pathognomonic of 'type 2 MPGN') is more often seen without the accompanying light microscopic changes of MPGN, leading to the unsatisfactory diagnosis of 'type 2 MPGN without MPGN' in a number of cases [4].

These considerations have led to the introduction of the term 'C3 glomerulopathy' which encompasses the disorders in which complement C3 accumulates in the kidney in the absence of significant immunoglobulin deposition there. This is the hallmark of complement alternative pathway dysregulation and represents pathophysiology, prognosis and underlying aetiology which are distinct from those cases of proliferative GN in which strong immunostaining for immunoglobulin is seen in the glomerulus, whatever the morphology may be by light or electron microscopy. Differential diagnoses suggested by biopsy appearances are summarised in Fig. 18.1, and the patterns associated with specific diseases are shown in Table 18.2.

In addition to immune-mediated proliferative glomerulonephritis and C3 glomerulopathies, light microscopic appearances resembling MPGN are sometimes seen in patients with chronic thrombotic microangiopathies (TMAs). In this situation there is no deposition of immunoglobulin or complement in the glomeruli – rather there is accumulation of electron-lucent, flocculent material (thought to be composed of fibrin and its breakdown products) beneath the endothelial cells. This can result in capillary wall thickening and other light microscopic features of MPGN. Electron microscopy easily distinguishes this from the dense, osmiophilic

D.P. Gale, MA, MBBChir, MRCP(UK) PhD (✉)
UCL Centre for Nephrology, Royal Free Hospital, Rowland Hill Street, London NW3 2PF, UK
e-mail: d.gale@ucl.ac.uk

M. Owen-Casey, MBBCh, FRCPath
Histopathology Department, Betsi Cadwaladar University Health Board, Croesnewydd Road, Wrexham LL13 7TD, UK
e-mail: mared.owencasey@wales.nhs.uk

M. Harber (ed.), *Practical Nephrology*,
DOI 10.1007/978-1-4471-5547-8_18, © Springer-Verlag London 2014

Table 18.1 Traditional classification of membranoproliferative glomerulonephritis (MPGN) by location of electron dense deposits

MPGN type	Electron microscopic appearances	Typical immunostaining	Serum complement	Other
1	Discrete electron dense material in mesangium and *subendothelial* GBM	IgG ± IgA ± IgM + C3 + C1q	Normal ± reduced C4 and C3	Infections, autoimmune disease, cryoglobulinaemia
2	Dense transformation of GBM *lamina densa*	C3 only	Reduced C3, normal C4	C3NeF
3	*Subendothelial* and *subepithelial* GBM electron dense deposits	IgG ± IgA ± IgM + C3 + C1q	Normal ± reduced C4 and C3	Infections, autoimmune disease, cryoglobulinaemia

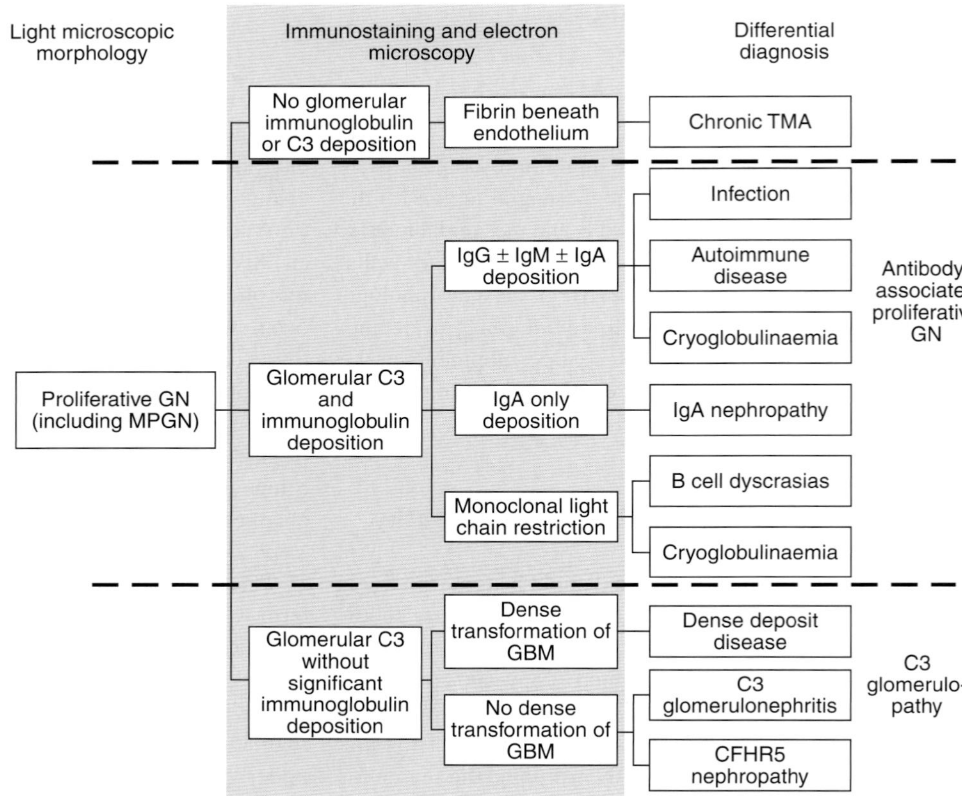

Fig. 18.1 Histological categorisation and commoner causes of proliferative glomerulonephritis (*GN*), *GBM* glomerular basement membrane, *CFHR5* complement-factor-H-related protein 5, *TMA* thrombotic microangiopathy

basement membrane deposits seen in immune complex GN or C3 glomerulopathies. Causes of TMAs which may result in these kidney biopsy appearances are summarised in Table 18.3.

Epidemiology

The incidence of MPGN varies significantly across the world with higher rates in developing countries. MPGN is diagnosed in approximately 2 % patients undergoing renal biopsy in the UK and is the underlying primary glomerulopathy in 5–10 % patients with nephrotic syndrome. However, up to 29 % of biopsies in countries such as Romania or Nigeria show MPGN [5, 6]. Comparisons between different countries are difficult since reporting of, indications for and access to renal biopsy can vary markedly, longitudinal data suggest that rates are falling over time [6–8] probably related to reduction in chronic infection-related MPGN.

Aetiology and Pathophysiology

Excessive or prolonged immunological stimulation and antibody production (whether as a consequence of infection, autoimmunity or blood cell dyscrasias) can result in proliferative glomerulonephritides, including MPGN. In this

Table 18.2 Histological characteristics of different diseases causing MPGN pattern

Diagnosis	LM	IP	EM
Antibody-associated membranoproliferative glomerulonephritis	Global and diffuse mesangial proliferation and glomerular hypercellularity, doubled GBMs with mesangial interposition. The glomerulus may have a distinct lobular/nodular appearance	IgG and C3 +/– IgM on the inside of glomerular capillary walls with occasional mesangial deposits	Subendothelial deposits and occasional mesangial deposits
Acute postinfectious glomerulonephritis	Global and diffuse increase in mesangial matrix and cellularity with an infiltrate of neutrophils within capillary loops	Coarse C3 and IgG on the outside of glomerular capillary loops	Irregular and variably sized electron dense subepithelial deposits that appear as humps
Dense deposit disease	Normal, mild or variable mesangial proliferation with thickened GBMs without spikes. Often the GBM does not stain strongly with silver and has a more characteristically brown colour with no doubling of the GBM. The main differential diagnosis to consider on H&E is membranous nephropathy	Coarse, granular C3 deposition in glomerular capillary walls, without immunoglobulins. Sometimes complement can also be seen within mesangium, Bowman's capsule and within tubular basement membranes	Intramembranous electron dense deposits with ring-like mesangial deposits and corresponding deposits within Bowman's capsule and tubular basement membranes
C3 glomerulopathy	Variable increase in mesangial matrix and cellularity with or without doubling or thickening of the GBM	Isolated complement (C3) deposits in GBMs and mesangium	Subendothelial +/– subepithelial and mesangial electron dense deposits
Cryoglobulinaemic glomerulonephritis	Global and diffuse mesangial proliferation, mesangial hypercellularity, doubled basement membranes with acellular eosinophilic material in capillary loops, possibly representing cryoprecipitate, occasionally vasculitic changes are seen in glomeruli	Intraluminal glomerular capillary IgM +/– IgG, kappa/lambda	Organised subendothelial deposits often with a recognisable substructure
Lupus nephritis	Various glomerular changes including subendothelial membranoproliferative pattern with doubled basement membranes	Mesangial deposition of IgG, IgA, IgM and complement. However, if the disease is inactive there may be no immune deposits	Electron dense subendothelial and mesangial deposits that correspond to immune deposits on IP. Often tubuloreticular bodies are found in glomerular endothelial cells
Thrombotic microangiopathy (small vessel vasculopathy)	Doubled basement membranes with thickened GBMs, increase in mesangial matrix with a subendothelial membranoproliferative type pattern, occasional glomerular capillary thrombi. Fibrinoid necrosis within arterioles and oedematous intimal expansion and vascular thrombi of small arteries are characteristic	Fibrin and fibrinogen +/– IgM within glomerular capillary thrombi. No immune deposits	Electro-lucent expansion of the subendothelial space that may extend into the para-mesangial basement membrane

Diagnosis, light microscopy, immunofluorescence and electron microscopy
LM light microscopy, *IP* immunoperoxidase, *EM* electron microscopy

Table 18.3 Causes of thrombotic microangiopathy

Disease	Investigations
Thrombotic thrombocytopaenic purpura	ADAMTS13 level
Haemolytic uraemic syndrome	Mutation screening: CFH, C3, MCP, FB
Pre-eclampsia/eclampsia	
Antiphospholipid syndrome	Anti-cardiolipin antibodies, lupus anticoagulant
Accelerated hypertension	
Systemic sclerosis	ANAs: anti-Scl-70/RNP
Systemic lupus erythematosus	ANAs: anti-dsDNA; C3/C4
Allograft rejection	Donor-specific antibodies
Drugs (e.g. cyclosporin A, tacrolimus, gemcitabine)	
Radiation exposure	

ANA antinuclear antibodies, *CFH* complement factor H, *MCP* membrane cofactor protein, *FB* factor B

context, immunostaining of the kidney biopsy reveals evidence of activation of the classical complement pathway (i.e. C1q deposition) alongside C3 in the kidney and in addition to the immunoglobulins themselves. The recognition that isolated activation of the alternative pathway (See "The Complement System" below) is sufficient to cause proliferative GN with deposition of complement C3 (in the absence of immunoglobulin or C1q) reinforces the view that renal

Table 18.4 Causes of antibody-associated proliferative glomerulonephritis

Disease category	Examples	Additional investigation(s)
Chronic infections	Viral – hepatitis B, hepatitis C, HIV ± cryoglobulinaemia type 2	Viral serology; RF; cryoglobulins; C3/C4
	Bacterial – endocarditis, infected shunt or prosthesis, abscess	Blood cultures; imaging; transoesophageal echo
	Protozoal – malaria, schistosomiasis	Blood film; serology
	Other – mycoplasma, mycobacterial	Cultures; imaging
Autoimmune diseases	Systemic lupus erythematosus (SLE)	ANAs: anti-dsDNA; C3/C4
	Sjögren syndrome ± cryoglobulinaemia	ANAs: anti-Ro/La
	Rheumatoid arthritis	Rheumatoid factor (RF)
	Scleroderma	ANAs: anti-Scl-70/RNP
	Coeliac disease	Endoscopy; anti-endomysial Abs
Paraprotein deposition diseases	Cryoglobulinaemia type 1	Serum protein electrophoresis; serum free light chain assay/immunofixation; bone marrow biopsy; imaging
	Waldenström's macroglobulinaemia	
	Immunotactoid glomerulopathy	
	Lymphoproliferative disease	
	Leukaemia	
	Malignant neoplasms	
Inherited complement deficiency	C2 deficiency leading to bacterial infections and SLE	CH_{50}, C3/C4
Chronic liver disease	Cirrhosis and alpha1-antitrypsin deficiency	Liver biopsy, A1AT levels
Renal allograft rejection		Donor-specific antibodies
Unknown (formerly 'idiopathic')	Fibrillary glomerulonephritis	

ANA antinuclear antibodies, *RF* rheumatoid factor, CH_{50} complement haemolytic activity

complement activation *per se* is sufficient to cause disease. Furthermore, abnormalities of complement factor H (CFH, a central regulator of complement alternative pathway activity) are sufficient to dysregulate C3 and can result in MPGN.

In this paradigm, the histomorphological changes that define MPGN can be viewed as the downstream consequence of renal complement activation, which may be caused either by increased antibody production (leading to the generation of antibody-antigen complexes) or by defects in the regulation of the complement system itself. In clinical practice, determining which of these processes is driving the renal disease is crucial in determining the appropriate therapy.

Antibody-Associated Proliferative GN

Proliferative and membranoproliferative GN associated with glomerular antibody deposition can occur in a very wide range of diseases, with examples given in Table 18.4. In approximately one third of patients, immune complexes are detectable in the circulation, but it is important to recognise that most people with such circulating complexes do not develop a GN. The extent to which characteristics of the antigen, immune complexes, local glomerular characteristics, variation in complement regulators or other factors determine which patients develop renal inflammation in this context is unknown (Figs. 18.2 and 18.3).

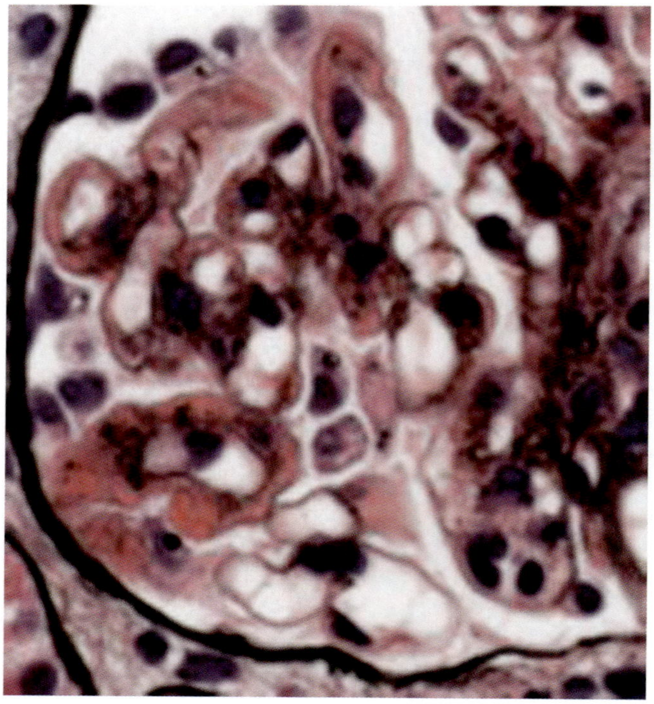

Fig. 18.2 Subendothelial membranoproliferative glomerulonephritis – silver. Part of a glomerulus at high magnification showing doubled basement membranes on silver staining with mesangial interposition, subendothelial immune deposits and increase in mesangial matrix

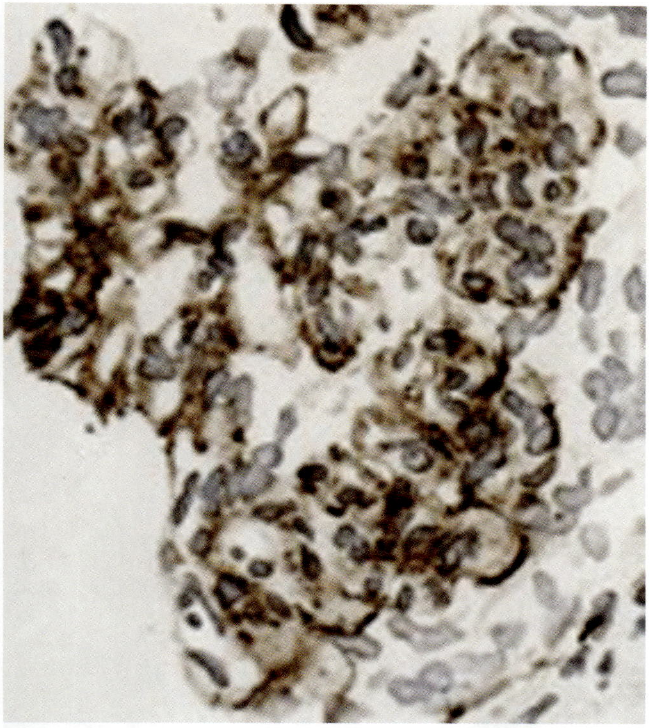

Fig. 18.3 Subendothelial membranoproliferative glomerulonephritis – C9. Immunoperoxidase method to detect C9 (complement component C9 is in the same distribution as C3 but is technically easier to detect than C3 in immunoperoxidase method [15]) shows heavy, granular deposition along the inside of glomerular capillary loops. Similar deposits would be seen with IgG

Clinical Features

The clinical manifestations of MPGN are varied and in part dependent on the underlying disease. However, very approximately one third of patients with MPGN present with the nephrotic syndrome. Another third present with haematuria and sub-nephrotic range proteinuria which is often detected because of symptoms related to primary pathology (such as infection or cryoglobulinaemia, see below). Of the remaining third, patients may present with chronic progressive renal impairment or less commonly with acute kidney injury. Microscopic haematuria is present in the majority of patients, some of whom also report episodes of macroscopic haematuria. High blood pressure in adults with MPGN is common and can be complicated by severe or accelerated phase hypertension. A respiratory tract infection often precedes an acute presentation.

Proliferative GN in Infectious Diseases

Chronic infections are known to be associated with proliferative glomerulonephritis, and, in general, the mechanism is thought to depend on generation of large amounts of antibody-antigen complexes. Although the overall risk of GN is low, some infections, such as endocarditis and viral hepatitis (with or without associated cryoglobulinaemia, see below) seem particularly prone to result in this type of renal injury; infection with *Schistosoma mansoni* is one of the commoner causes of MPGN worldwide, possibly because hepatosplenic disease diverts blood away from the Kupffer cells, allowing increased exposure of the systemic circulation (including the kidney) to the immune complexes that are generated in response to the infection.

Occasionally, glomerular inflammation is seen several days after an acute bacterial (typically streptococcal) infection. In this postinfectious glomerulonephritis, presentation is typically with haematuria, proteinuria (sometimes in the nephrotic range) and renal impairment, with or without oliguria, some 7–14 days following a bacterial infection. The disease is usually self-limiting, although supportive renal replacement therapy may be needed in some cases. Serological tests for antibodies against bacterial antigens such as streptolysin O and DNase B may be positive and hypocomplementaemia is common. However, because some bacterial antigens (or antibodies directed against them) may stabilise the alternative pathway C3 convertase, low serum C3 is not always accompanied by low serum C4 in this condition.

Kidney biopsy typically shows diffuse proliferation of mesangial cells with prominent neutrophil infiltration and large, hump-like deposits on the subepithelial side of the GBM on electron microscopy. Glomerular immunostaining is usually positive for IgG, IgM, C1q and C3 although occasionally immunostain positivity for C3 alone is seen. The pathophysiology of postinfectious glomerulonephritis is not completely understood, but it has been postulated that some bacterial antigens become deposited in the GBM, perhaps as a consequence of their physicochemical properties, and it is the aggressive immunological response to these antigens, including local complement activation, which causes the renal inflammation.

Cryoglobulinaemic GN

Cryoglobulins are immunoglobulins which reversibly precipitate at a temperature of 4 °C. Cryoglobulinaemia is subdivided into three types, based on clonality (see Table 18.5): Type 1 arises as a result of an aberrant, usually IgM-producing, plasma cell clone (e.g. in multiple myeloma or Waldenstrom's macroglobulinaemia). Type 2 comprises monoclonal (usually IgM) bound to polyclonal (usually IgG) immunoglobulins and is most commonly found in people with serological evidence of hepatitis C virus infection. In type 3 cryoglobulinaemia, there is a complex of polyclonal immunoglobulins, and the most common association is with paraneoplastic syndromes.

Table 18.5 Types of cryoglobulinaemia

	Clonality	Associations
Type 1	Monoclonal (usually IgM)	Multiple myeloma, Waldenstrom's macroglobulinaemia
Type 2	Monoclonal IgM bound to polyclonal IgG	RF +ve mixed cryoglobulinaemia and Hepatitis C
Type 3	Polyclonal IgM bound to polyclonal IgG	Hepatitis C, HIV (rarely autoimmune diseases, cancers)

RF rheumatoid factor

In type 2 and type 3 cryoglobulinaemia (collectively referred to as mixed cryoglobulinaemias), tests for rheumatoid factor are positive since the IgM antibody (whether monoclonal or polyclonal) binds to the Fc region of IgG.

The association of cryoglobulins with viral infections is well recognised, with detectable mixed cryoglobulinaemia reported in 15–20 % of people infected with HIV and around 50 % of those infected with hepatitis C [9, 10]. In addition to lymphoproliferative and infectious diseases, cryoglobulinaemia may sometimes occur in the context of autoimmune diseases, with approximately 45 % HCV negative cases of mixed cryoglobulinaemia in one series occurring in patients with Sjögren's syndrome [11]. Clinically significant cryoglobulinaemic disease, however, is only apparent in a proportion of patients in whom a cryoglobulin is detectable serologically.

Cryoglobulins may precipitate anywhere in the body, leading to local complement activation and thrombus formation. Clinically this may manifest as Meltzer's classic triad of palpable purpura, joint pain and muscle weakness, but other manifestations, including neuropathy, may be present. Renal involvement in cryoglobulinaemia usually presents with proteinuria, microscopic haematuria and renal impairment. Nephrotic syndrome is seen in approximately 20 % patients, and around one third of patients have concurrent extrarenal disease at time of presentation. Importantly, over half the patients with HCV-related cryoglobulinaemic MPGN have normal or near normal liver function tests at presentation. Consumption of complement components resulting in reduced plasma levels of C4 and sometimes C3 is frequently seen in active cryoglobulinaemic disease making levels of C3 and C4 excellent screening tests for cryoglobulinaemia. In addition, CH_{50}[1] and C1q levels may also be reduced, again reflecting classical complement pathway activation (Figs. 18.4 and 18.5).

Kidney biopsy in cryoglobulinaemic GN can show typical features of MPGN, but there may also be prominent glomerular hypercellularity with massive infiltration of macrophages or accumulation of eosinophilic material in intraluminal thrombi which probably represent cryoprecipitate within the glomerular capillaries. In approximately one third of patients, there is also associated small- and medium-sized vessel vasculitis [12]. Cryoglobulinaemic MPGN is usually rather indolent, and progression to end-stage renal disease is seen in around 10 % of patients, usually over 10 years or more although often accompanied by severe hypertension. Therapy is usually aimed at treating the underlying cause, for example, by clearing hepatitis C virus infection or suppressing any clonal haematological disorder.

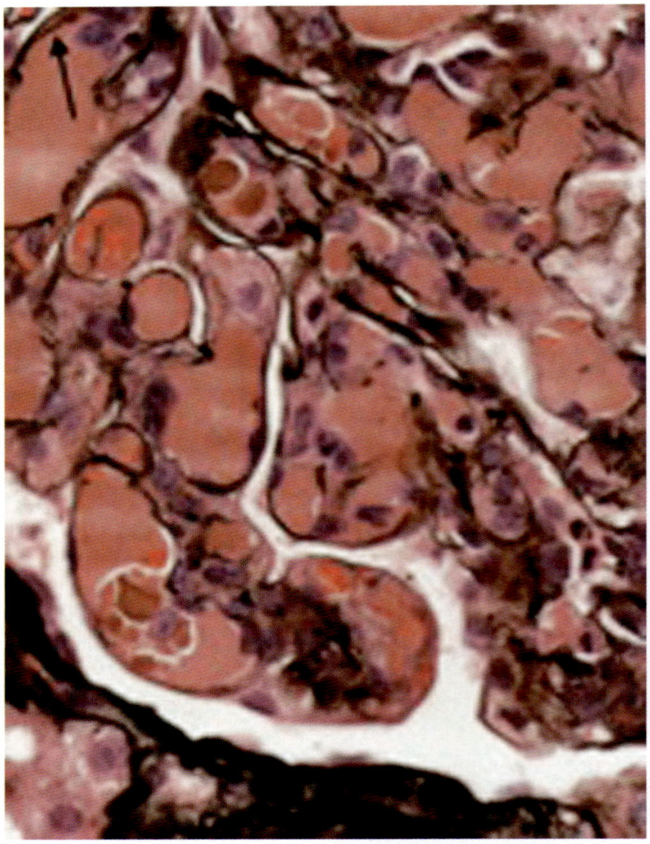

Fig. 18.4 Cryoglobulinaemic glomerulonephritis – silver. Glomerulus from the renal biopsy specimen of a patient with cryoglobulinaemic glomerulonephritis showing eosinophilic, acellular deposits within the majority of capillary loops and occasional doubled basement membranes, *arrowed*

Autoimmune Disease and Proliferative GN

Renal involvement is seen in a variety of systemic autoimmune diseases in which there are circulating antibody-autoantigen complexes. While glomerular changes of MPGN may be present, more commonly proliferation is confined to either the mesangial regions or the capillaries of the glomerular tuft. In this context, positive immunostaining for IgA (but

[1]Complement haemolytic activity: patient serum across a range of dilutions is used to lyse antibody-coated sheep erythrocytes. Lack of haemolysis at a given dilution suggests deficiency of complement component(s).

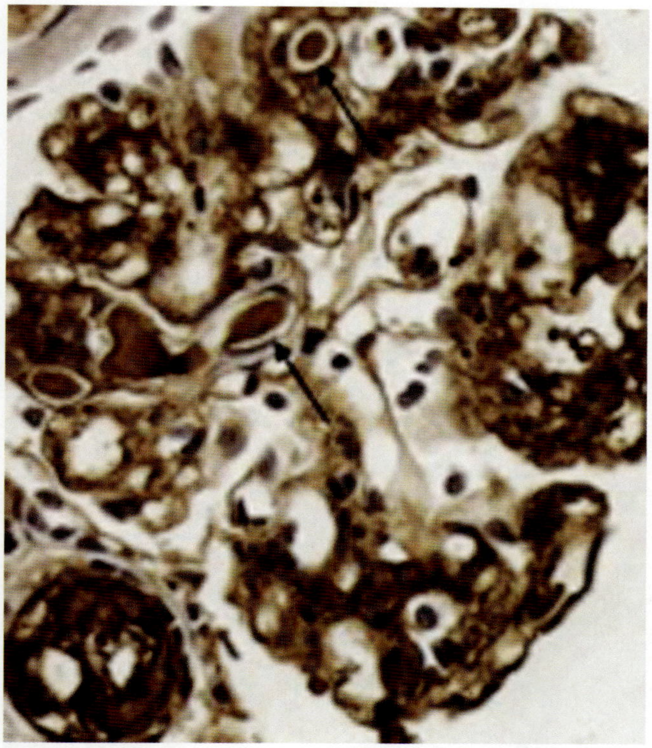

Fig. 18.5 Cryoglobulinaemic glomerulonephritis – IgM. Immunoperoxidase method to detect IgM shows aggregates of IgM in several capillary loops (*arrows*)

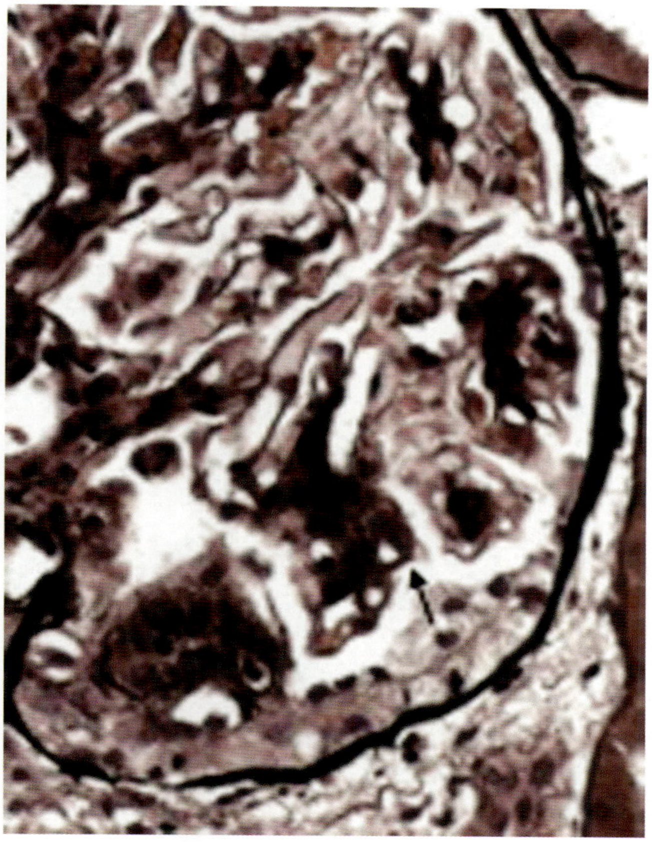

Fig. 18.6 Lupus nephritis – silver. Glomerulus showing features of lupus nephritis seen as a subendothelial membranoproliferative pattern with mesangial increase and occasional doubled basement membranes, *arrowed*

not other immunoglobulins) is diagnostic of IgA nephropathy, and immunostaining for IgA, IgG and IgM is compatible with lupus nephritis (Figs. 18.6 and 18.7). Occasionally, proliferative glomerulonephritis with staining for IgM but not IgA or IgG is seen, and this is sometimes termed IgM nephropathy, although clinical data in this condition are lacking, presumably due to its rarity. In all of these proliferative glomerulonephritides, immunostaining for C1q and C3 is typically positive, reflecting complement activation via the classical pathway.

Treatment of Immune Complex-Associated Glomerulonephritis

Renal prognosis in proliferative GN is ultimately dependent on the course of the underlying disease process responsible. While blood pressure control and angiotensin blockade may delay progressive renal scarring in the presence of hypertension and/or proteinuria from a variety of causes, identification and treatment of any underlying lymphoproliferative, infective or autoimmune process is likely to be the most effective strategy in preventing renal damage in antibody-associated proliferative glomerulonephritis. In patients with MPGN and no identified cause, median time to end-stage renal disease is around 8 years, with 50 % patients needing renal replacement therapy at 10 years. There is some evidence that extent of interstitial fibrosis, glomerular crescent formation and degree of mesangial proliferation provide prognostic information. Importantly, neither age, gender, severity of proteinuria, histomorphological type nor even renal function at presentation seems to predict renal outcomes.

The evidence-base for any treatment in MPGN where a cause is not identified is extremely limited in part because of its rarity and partly because most studies failed to differentiate between the underlying diseases causing the MPGN. Trials were nicely reviewed in 1999 and sadly not much has progressed since then [13]. Alternate-day corticosteroids have been advocated on the basis of small observational studies. One of the best studies was an RCT of steroids in children with MPGN type 1, seeming to show a beneficial effect of alternate-day prednisolone (40 mg/m^2) in those with heavy proteinuria and good function (61 % had stable function vs 12 % of controls) [14] with the recommendation that steroids should be tried in this group; however, there have been no subsequent RCTs. In the 1980s antiplatelet agents in the form of aspirin and dipyramidole were thought to be beneficial, but this has not been supported by clinical trials and has not gained widespread acceptance. Anti-proliferative agents have been reported to have some success in small observational studies with limited

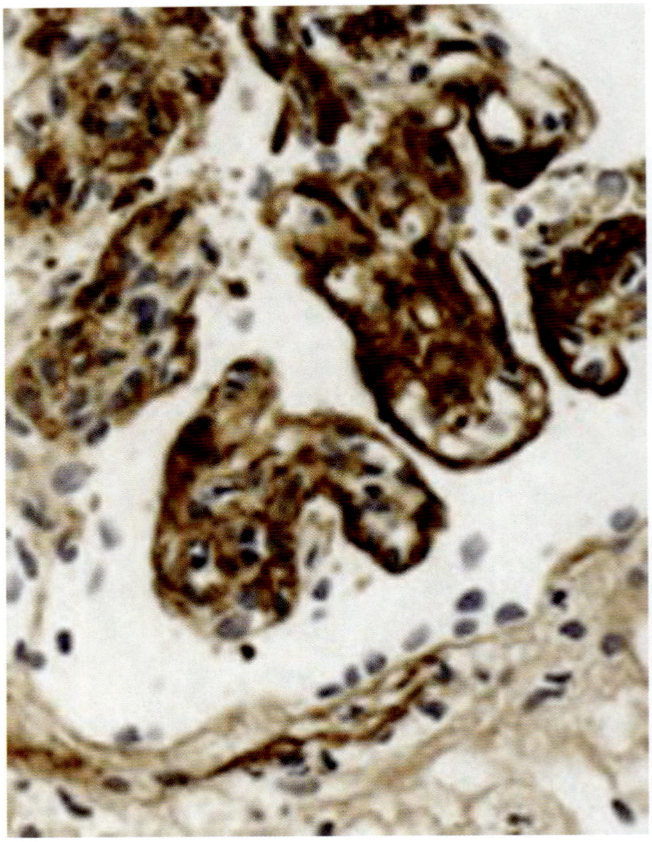

Fig. 18.7 Lupus nephritis – C9. Immunoperoxidase method to detect C9 shows heavy deposition within mesangium and glomerular basement membranes. Similar deposition of IgG, IgM and IgA would also be seen

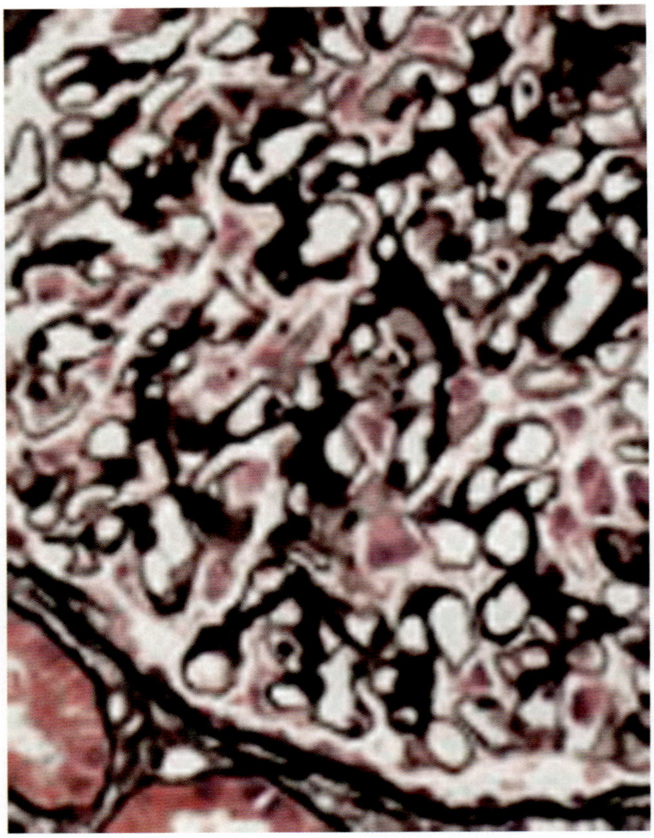

Fig. 18.8 C3 glomerulopathy – silver. Glomerulus at high magnification showing mild increase in mesangial matrix on silver staining and no thickening or doubling of the glomerular basement membrane

follow-up but have never been tested in RCTs. In the face of this paucity of data, the KDIGO guidelines suggest that in idiopathic MPGN in the context of frank nephrotic syndrome and declining function it is reasonable to give a trial of corticosteroids and either cyclophosphamide or mycophenolate mofetil for no more than 6 months initially. It may be that immunosuppressive therapy ameliorates some of the glomerular damage caused by macrophage and neutrophil infiltration in severe disease, and our practice is for a closely monitored trial of immunosuppressive therapy in unexplained MPGN where the kidney biopsy shows substantial glomerular infiltration by immune cells and interstitial fibrosis is not too advanced.

Recurrence Posttransplantation

In view of the systemic nature of these diseases, it is not surprising that they can recur following renal transplantation. Reduction of antibody production is likely to reduce the risk to the allograft, and ability to achieve this will depend on the underlying disease process in each patient. In patients with MPGN and no identified cause, the risk of post-transplantation disease recurrence is greater in younger patients and is correlated with the degree of mesangial proliferation and crescent formation at presentation [2].

C3 Glomerulopathies

It is known that proliferative GN can occur without significant deposition of immunoglobulins or C1q in the glomerulus. While this pattern of immunostaining is characteristic of DDD (formerly known as type 2 MPGN), it is now recognised that it can occur without dense transformation of the GBM (producing appearances which would have formerly been categorised as type 1 or type 3 MPGN). In addition, the degree of inflammatory change and endocapillary proliferation can be subtle (perhaps depending on the timing of the biopsy), so the term C3 glomerulopathy also applies to those cases in which there is not enough proliferative change in the biopsy to be categorised as membranoproliferative GN (Figs. 18.8 and 18.9). This umbrella term is useful because it provides the specific implication that the disease results from complement alternative pathway dysregulation. C3 glomerulopathy can be subdivided into dense deposit disease (DDD), C3 glomerulonephritis (C3GN) and CFHR5 nephropathy.

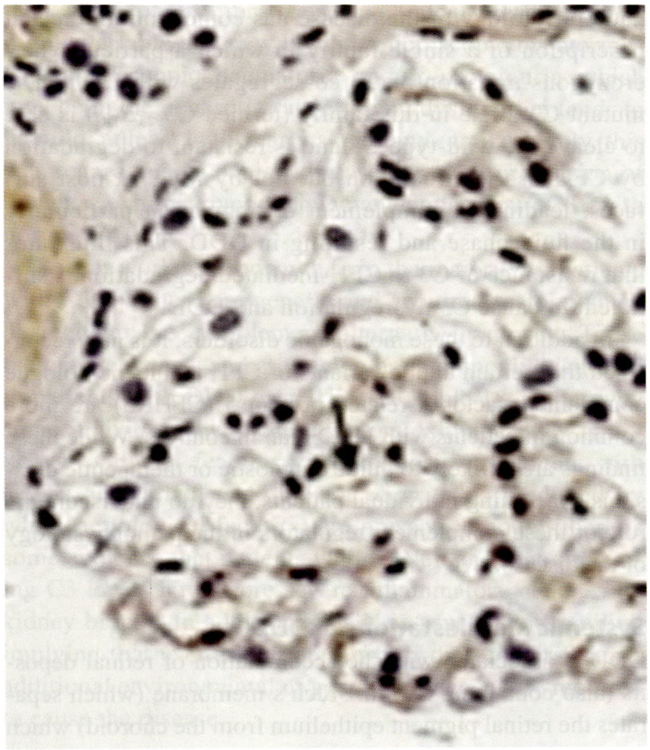

Fig. 18.9 C3 glomerulopathy – C9 IP. Glomerulus at high magnification. An immunoperoxidase method to detect C9 shows irregular, granular deposits within glomerular basement membranes (*arrow*) consistent with the diagnosis of C3 glomerulopathy

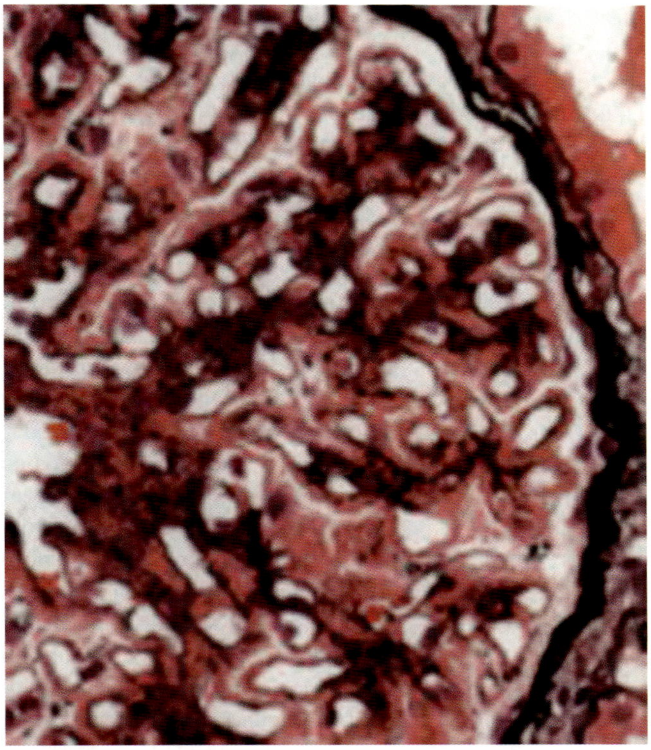

Fig. 18.10 Dense deposit disease – silver. Glomerulus at high magnification showing marked thickening of the majority of glomerular basement membranes. However, unlike membranous nephropathy the thickening is irregular and no spikes are seen. Also, the thickened glomerular basement membranes (GBMs) fail to take the silver stain well, whereas in membranous nephropathy the GBMs appear black

Dense Deposit Disease

Dense deposit disease (DDD, formerly known as type 2 MPGN) is diagnosed by observing the characteristic dense transformation of the *lamina densa* of the GBM (Figs. 18.10 and 18.11). This may be accompanied by the morphological appearances of MPGN, but more often there is more subtle evidence of glomerular inflammation. DDD is a rare disease, affecting around 2–3 per million population. It can occur at any age although is more common in children, accounting for around 15–20 % MPGN in those under 18 years. Clinical presentation is most often with proteinuria, which may be accompanied by the nephrotic syndrome, and microscopic haematuria. There is slowly progressive renal impairment with approximately 50 % patients needing renal replacement therapy within 10 years of diagnosis: poor prognostic features are greater age and greater degree of renal impairment at diagnosis. The disease almost always recurs following kidney transplantation with over 50 % graft loss at 5 years. This reflects the systemic nature of the disease.

Aetiology and Pathophysiology of DDD

DDD is associated with systemic over-activation of the complement alternative pathway and its causes are summarised in Table 18.6. In up to 80 % of patients with DDD, an autoantibody which recognises the C3bBb alternative pathway convertase (called a C3 nephritic factor or C3NeF) is detectable in the circulation. This antibody prevents the normal dissociation and degradation of the C3 convertase, causing runaway activation of the alternative pathway in the circulation and depletion of C3. The presence of a C3NeF is detected by functional assays using, for example, sheep erythrocyte lysis or C3a generation *in vitro* as an indicator for enhanced complement activating ability of patient serum. Circulating C4 levels are typically normal since the classical pathway is not activated. In patients with DDD in whom a C3NeF is not detectable, antibodies which bind to both C3b and factor B have occasionally been identified. In a handful of other C3NeF-negative cases, autoantibodies against complement factor H have been detected. Whether these autoantibodies are causal or contributory is not completely clear at present, and their utility as a diagnostic tool (in DDD) is not known. In addition, DDD sometimes occurs in association with a monoclonal gammopathy, raising the possibility that circulating monoclonal immunoglobulins, in some circumstances, can lead to complement alternative pathway dysregulation.

Rarely, individuals with DDD have been identified who are homozygous (or compound heterozygous) for

with CFHR5 nephropathy is generally very good, the disease recurs following transplantation. While this observation proves that CFHR5 nephropathy results from a systemic factor, extrarenal manifestations of the disease have not been reported, again suggesting that CFHR5 may have a particular role in regulating complement in the kidney.

An important clinical observation which is shared by many disorders of complement alternative pathway regulation (including DDD, C3GN and aHUS) is that otherwise trivial stimulation of the immune system (for instance, by a minor infection) can trigger overt flares of disease and significant kidney damage.

Investigation of C3 Glomerulopathies

Diagnosis of a C3 glomerulopathy (i.e. DDD or C3GN) in a patient should prompt investigation of alternative pathway regulation. Tests for paraproteinaemia, complement C3, complement C4 and C3 nephritic factor are widely available and should be performed in all such patients. In patients with a C3 glomerulopathy who may have Cypriot ancestry, a genetic test for the $CFHR5_{12123\text{-}9}$ mutation should be performed since CFHR5 nephropathy is common in this population (available at the Institute of Child Health in London, http://www.labs.gosh.nhs.uk/laboratory-services/genetics/tests/cfhr5-nephropathy). Additional tests such as serum CFH and CFI levels and tests for autoantibodies against factor B and CFH should be considered if a C3NeF is *not* identified. Where serological tests have not demonstrated the cause of complement dysregulation in a patient, additional genetic testing by mutation screening of the genes for CFH, MCP, CFHR5, factor B and C3 should be considered, especially if there is a family history of kidney disease.

Treatment of C3 Glomerulopathies

Although it is generally presumed that blood pressure control and angiotensin system blockade should be introduced to delay progression of renal damage, there is currently no proven therapy for DDD, C3GN or CFHR5 nephropathy. Since the diseases are rare and rather slowly progressive, robust clinical trial data in humans are lacking. Strategies aimed at suppressing the immune system (e.g. using steroids or anti-proliferative agents such as mycophenolate mofetil) may have some beneficial effects on renal inflammation, but are not expected to control the C3 activation or deposition in the kidney which is driving these diseases. Where a C3NeF is detected, plasma exchange, immunosuppression, cytotoxic therapy or B cell depletion (for instance, using the chimeric anti-CD20 monoclonal antibody Rituximab) may reduce its levels, but trials have not been published showing a clinical benefit of these approaches. It is important to recognise that the C3NeF is playing a different role from that played by circulating antibodies in most autoimmune diseases – only tiny quantities of C3NeF are needed to stabilise the C3 convertase and activate the positive feedback loop of the alternative pathway; thus, strategies to deplete C3NeF must be very efficacious indeed if they are to normalise complement regulation in the circulation.

In patients with genetic defects of complement regulators (e.g. in individuals with deficiency of CFH), plasma infusion or exchange is sometimes beneficial. Where a mutation in a gene for a complement regulator is identified or suspected, removal of the mutant protein (and supplementation of the wild-type protein) using plasma exchange against fresh frozen plasma has been used, sometimes with benefit. Interventions which minimise the frequency of intercurrent infections (such as tonsillectomy in children) have also been reported to provide benefit in CFHR5 nephropathy, which is consistent with the role that infection plays in precipitating acute deterioration of renal function in the disease.

Eculizumab, a humanised monoclonal antibody directed against C5, blocks the terminal complement pathway. The drug is effective in both paroxysmal nocturnal haemoglobinuria and aHUS, but initial reports of its use in DDD and C3GN (in very small numbers of patients) have shown a mixed response.

Summary

Activation of complement can lead to kidney damage with histological appearances ranging from mild proliferative changes to membranoproliferative glomerulonephritis. Complement may be activated via the classical pathway (as a consequence of antibody-antigen complex formation) or by defects in the regulation of the alternative pathway. Excessive complement dysregulation in the circulation is associated with dense deposit disease, whereas complement dysregulation at endothelial surfaces typically leads to atypical haemolytic uraemic syndrome. For reasons which are not completely understood, some defects which result in complement dysregulation either in the circulation or at surfaces result in C3 glomerulonephritis instead.

Treatment of these kidney diseases relies critically on identification and correction of the aetiological factor(s). It is hoped that development of novel drugs which allow the modulation of complement activity directly may provide completely new ways to treat these disorders.

The Complement System

The complement system is a cascade of circulating proteases which plays a pivotal role in defence against infection. In humans, complement has a number of functions, including innate recognition and destruction of invading microorganisms, opsonisation (labelling of foreign material for phagocytosis), activation of cellular immunity and as an effector system for the destruction of antibody-coated microorganisms. Complement therefore bridges innate and adaptive mechanisms of immune defence.

Activation of complement occurs via three pathways, termed the classical, mannose-binding lectin (MBL) and alternative (AP) pathways. All result in the cleavage of the abundant circulating protein C3 to form the active C3b (Fig. 18.12).

The Classical Pathway

Antibody-antigen complexes are recognised by the circulating proteins C1q, r and s to form the C1qrs complex which recruits and cleaves the circulating complement proteins C4 and C2 (releasing the small C4a anaphylatoxin fragment that causes enhanced vascular permeability, histamine release and recruitment of immune cells) to result in the C4b2a complex bound to the cell surface. C4b2a is a C3 convertase which is able to cleave C3 to form C3a (an anaphylatoxin) and the active C3b.

The Mannose-Binding Lectin (MBL) Pathway

Mannose groups on bacterial cell surfaces are recognised by circulating mannose-binding lectin (MBL) proteins which bind to form a complex which, similar to the C1qrs complex, is able to recruit and cleave C4 and C2, producing the C4b2a C3 convertase.

The Alternative Pathway (AP)

C3b is continuously generated by low-grade cleavage of the abundant plasma protein C3 by water hydrolysis – a process known as AP tickover. In the alternative pathway, C3b binds factor B which is cleaved by factor D to result in the non-covalently bound C3bBb complex – a C3 convertase that is able to catalyse the cleavage of C3 to form more C3b. This completes a positive feedback loop which amplifies generation of C3b and which is further amplified by the presence of an appropriate biological surface (such as a cell membrane). In addition to catalysing C3 cleavage, the C3b also acts as an opsonin (labelling the cell to which it is bound for phagocytosis) and forms part of the complex which cleaves circulating C5 to activate the terminal complement pathway.

The Terminal Pathway

The binding of C3b to either of the C3 convertases (C4b2a or C3bBb) produces a C5 convertase which catalyses the cleavage of the circulating protein C5 to release C5a (an

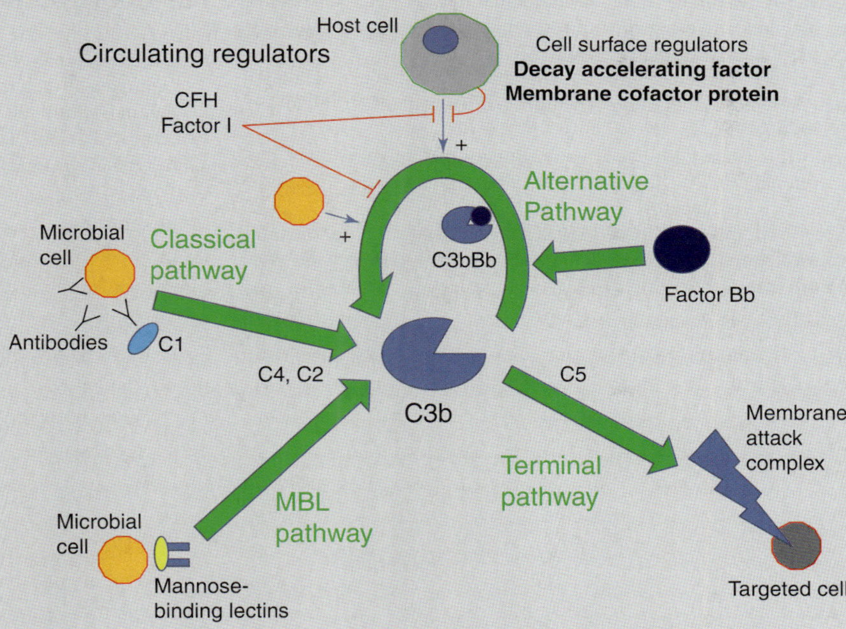

Fig. 18.12 The complement system. *CFH* complement factor H, *CFHR5* CFH-related protein 5

anaphylatoxin) and C5b which initiates the terminal pathway, leading to the recruitment of the tubular membrane attack complex (MAC) which lyses the cell by forming a pore (composed of C6–9) in its surface.

Alternative Pathway Regulation

In order to prevent runaway activation of its positive feedback loop, the AP requires tight regulation. This is achieved by a number of mechanisms, including cleavage of C3b and acceleration of decay of the C3bBb complex and effected by a range of regulators, including factor I and complement factor H (CFH), which prevent over-activation of the pathway both in the circulation and at host surfaces. The *CFH* gene is situated immediately upstream from its five homologues, the *CFH-related* genes 1–5. The proteins encoded by these genes (CFHR1-5) are also present in the circulation (although are much less abundant than CFH) and share some of the complement regulating activities of CFH.

References

1. Habib R, Michielsen P, et al. Clinical, microscopic and electron microscopic data in the nephrotic syndrome of unknown origin. In: Wolstenholme GEW, Cameron MP, editors. Ciba foundation symposium – renal biopsy: clinical and pathological significance. Chichester: Wiley; 1961. p. 70–102.
2. Little MA, Dupont P, et al. Severity of primary MPGN, rather than MPGN type, determines renal survival and post-transplantation recurrence risk. Kidney Int. 2006;69(3):504–11.
3. Servais A, Fremeaux-Bacchi V, et al. Primary glomerulonephritis with isolated C3 deposits: a new entity which shares common genetic risk factors with haemolytic uraemic syndrome. J Med Genet. 2007;44(3):193–9.
4. Walker PD, Ferrario F, et al. Dense deposit disease is not a membranoproliferative glomerulonephritis. Mod Pathol. 2007;20(6):605–16.
5. Abdurrahman MB, Aikhionbare HA, et al. Clinicopathological features of childhood nephrotic syndrome in northern Nigeria. Q J Med. 1990;75(278):563–76.
6. Covic A, Schiller A, et al. Epidemiology of renal disease in Romania: a 10 year review of two regional renal biopsy databases. Nephrol Dial Transplant. 2006;21(2):419–24.
7. Hanko JB, Mullan RN, et al. The changing pattern of adult primary glomerular disease. Nephrol Dial Transplant. 2009;24(10):3050–4.
8. Woo KT, Chan CM, et al. The changing pattern of primary glomerulonephritis in Singapore and other countries over the past 3 decades. Clin Nephrol. 2010;74(5):372–83.
9. Cicardi M, Cesana B, et al. Prevalence and risk factors for the presence of serum cryoglobulins in patients with chronic hepatitis C. J Viral Hepat. 2000;7(2):138–43.
10. Bonnet F, Pineau JJ, et al. Prevalence of cryoglobulinemia and serological markers of autoimmunity in human immunodeficiency virus infected individuals: a cross-sectional study of 97 patients. J Rheumatol. 2003;30(9):2005–10.
11. Matignon M, Cacoub P, et al. Clinical and morphologic spectrum of renal involvement in patients with mixed cryoglobulinemia without evidence of hepatitis C virus infection. Medicine. 2009;88(6):341–8.
12. D'Amico G. Renal involvement in hepatitis C infection: cryoglobulinemic glomerulonephritis. Kidney Int. 1998;54(2):650–71.
13. Levine A. Management of membranoproliferative glomerulonephritis: evidence-based recommendations. Kidney Int Suppl. 1999;70:S41–6.
14. Tarshish P, Bernstein J, et al. Treatment of mesangiocapillary glomerulonephritis with alternate-day prednisone–a report of the International Study of Kidney Disease in Children. Pediatr Nephrol. 1992;6(2):123–30.
15. Howie AJ. Handbook of renal biopsy pathology. 2nd ed. New York: Springer; 2008.

Further Reading

Sethi S, Fervenza FC. Membranoproliferative glomerulonephritis: pathogenetic heterogeneity and proposal for a new classification. Semin Nephrol. 2011;31(4):341–8.

Pickering M, Cook HT. Complement and glomerular disease: new insights. Curr Opin Nephrol Hypertens. 2011;20(3):271–7.

IgA Nephropathy and Henoch-Schönlein Purpura

19

Chee Kay Cheung, Joanna K.F. Boyd, and Jonathan Barratt

Since its initial description by Jean Berger in 1968, immunoglobulin A nephropathy (IgAN) is now recognised as the commonest noninfectious form of glomerulonephritis in the world. Although in many patients it has a benign course, IgAN remains a leading cause of progressive kidney disease, with around 25–30 % of patients progressing to end-stage renal disease within 25 years of diagnosis. IgAN can only be diagnosed by renal biopsy, which is characterised by mesangial deposition of IgA.

Closely related to IgAN is Henoch-Schönlein purpura (HSP). This less commonly seen disease is more frequently found in children. It is a systemic small vessel vasculitis, characterised by IgA deposition in the skin, joints, gut and kidney, leading to a characteristic set of symptoms of rash, arthralgia, abdominal pain and nephritis. The renal biopsy in a patient with HSP nephritis is indistinguishable from IgAN.

IgA Nephropathy

Epidemiology

Reported incidence is highly variable due to national differences in screening policies for asymptomatic urinary abnormalities and biopsy practice between centres [1]. IgAN is most commonly found in Caucasian and Asian populations and is relatively rare in people of African origin. Although patients may present at any age, there is a peak incidence in the second and third decades. There is a 2:1 male to female predominance in North American and Western European populations. This sex difference is not seen in Asian populations. Subclinical IgAN is estimated to occur in up to 16 % of the general population, according to postmortem studies [2].

Aetiology and Pathogenesis

The defining feature of IgAN is mesangial deposition of the immunoglobulin IgA. The IgA molecule in humans exists in two isoforms: IgA1 and IgA2, which can exist as monomers (single molecules) or polymers (most commonly dimeric IgA). It is predominantly polymeric IgA1 that is found in mesangial IgA deposits in IgAN. The major difference between IgA1 and IgA2 is that IgA1 contains a hinge region. Unusual for a serum protein, the IgA1 hinge region carries a variety of *O*-linked oligosaccharides giving rise to a range of IgA1 glucoforms in the serum (Fig. 19.1).

Changes in the composition of the *O*-linked sugars at the IgA1 hinge region is the most consistent finding in patients with IgAN across the world, with identical changes seen in patient cohorts from North America, Europe and Asia [3]. The key change is an increase in the serum of IgA1 *O*-glycoforms that contain less galactose. This increase in undergalactosylated IgA1 *O*-glycoforms is believed to play a central role in the pathogenesis of IgAN. It is believed that undergalactosylated IgA1 *O*-glycoforms form high-molecular-weight circulating immune complexes, either through self-aggregation or through generation of IgG- and IgA-hinge-region-specific autoantibodies. These high-molecular-weight immune complexes are prone to mesangial deposition resulting ultimately in mesangial cell proliferation, release of pro-inflammatory mediators and glomerular injury [4]. Why there should be an increase in the levels of undergalactosylated IgA1 *O*-glycoforms in IgAN is currently not known.

C.K. Cheung, BSc, MBChB
J.K.F. Boyd, MBChB • J. Barratt, PhD, FRCP (✉)
The John Walls Renal Unit, Leicester General Hospital, Gwendolen Road, Leicester LE5 4PW, UK
e-mail: ckc12@le.ac.uk; joannaboyd@nhs.net; jonathan.barratt@uhl-tr.nhs.uk

M. Harber (ed.), *Practical Nephrology*,
DOI 10.1007/978-1-4471-5547-8_19,

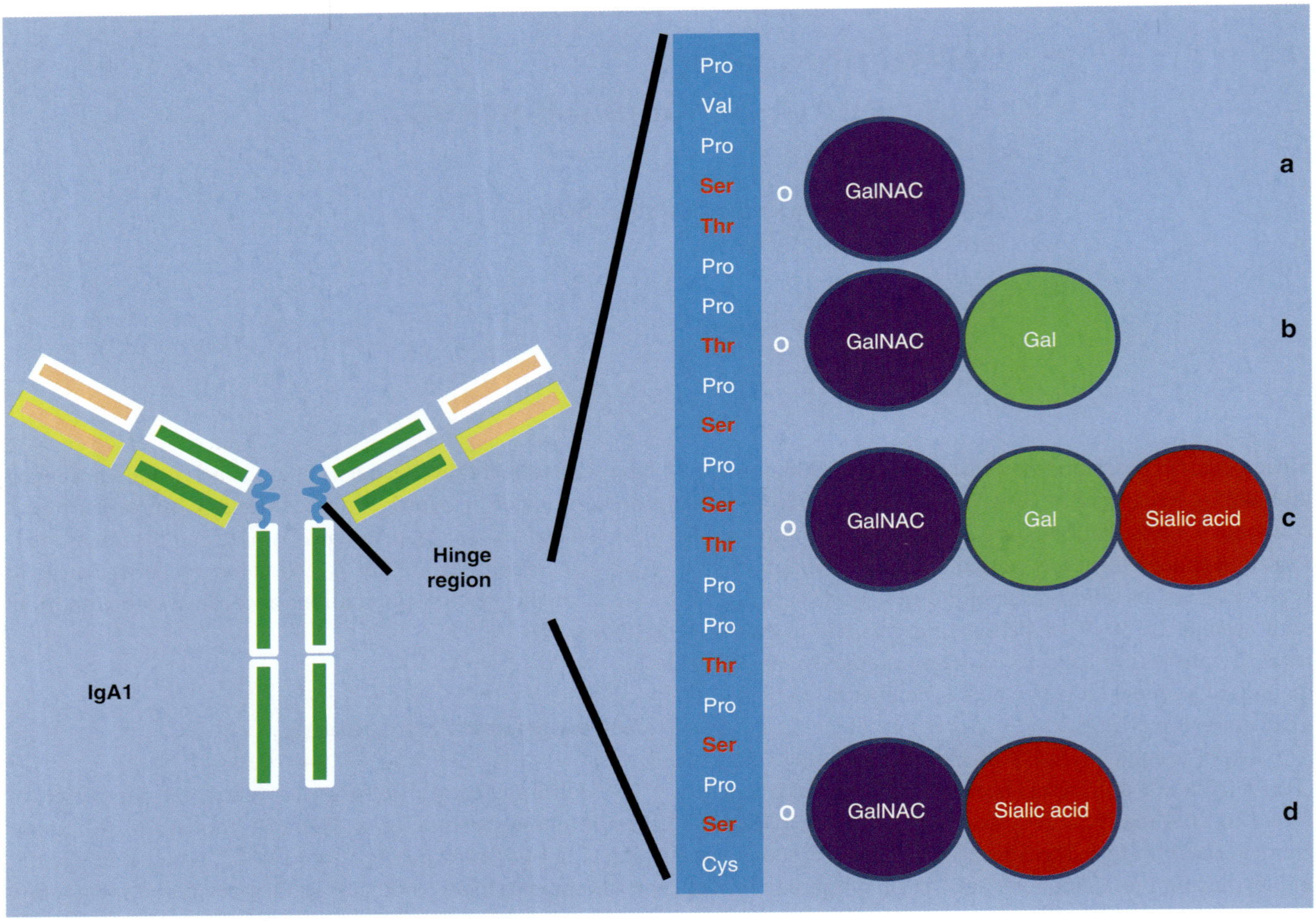

Fig. 19.1 The IgA1 molecule showing the position of the hinge region *O*-glycans. Serine (*Ser*) and threonine (*Thr*) residues in the hinge region provide nine potential *O*-linked glycosylation sites, although to date only six are known to be occupied by *O*-glycans. It is still not known which amino acids are occupied by *O*-glycans and whether it is the same amino acids for all *O*-glycoforms of IgA1. The IgA1 *O*-glycans are all based on *N*-acetylgalactosamine (*GalNAC*) units in *O*-linkage with serine or threonine (*A*). GalNAC may be extended either with galactose (*Gal*) alone (*B*) or with Gal and sialic acid (*C*). Alternatively, the GalNAC may simply carry a sialic acid (*D*)

Natural History

The perceived risk of progressive renal disease in IgAN is heavily influenced by biopsy practice. For example, in centres where there is a low threshold for renal biopsy (e.g. isolated non-visible haematuria), the cohort of patients diagnosed with IgAN will be biased toward those with a lower risk of progressive renal disease.

However, it is generally accepted that:

- Less than 10 % of patients will have complete resolution of urinary abnormalities.
- Episodes of visible haematuria become less frequent with time.
- 25–30 % of patients will progress to end-stage renal disease within 20–25 years of diagnosis.

Clinical Features

Most patients present with either:

- Visible haematuria, typically 12–72 h after an upper respiratory tract infection (less commonly another mucosal infection: gastrointestinal or urinary tract infection)
- Incidental finding of non-visible haematuria ± proteinuria (e.g. on testing for insurance purposes or occupational screening)

  More rarely, patients may present with:

- Acute kidney injury (either due to red cell cast tubular obstruction secondary to massive haematuria or a crescentic glomerulonephritis)
- Overt nephrotic syndrome

- End-stage renal disease
- Malignant hypertension

Differential Diagnosis

Differentiating Between Causes of Isolated Non-visible Haematuria

Urine microscopy in non-visible haematuria due to glomerular disease will typically show dysmorphic red cells and there may also be red cell casts. Non-visible haematuria in glomerulonephritis is often also accompanied by proteinuria and there may also be pre-existing evidence of renal disease with a reduced GFR and development of hypertension.

The three main differential diagnoses of persistent isolated non-visible haematuria due to glomerular disease are:

1. IgA nephropathy
2. Alport syndrome
3. Thin basement nephropathy

Features that may help distinguish between these disorders include:

- Episodes of visible haematuria – this may occur in IgAN or Alport syndrome, but is uncommon in thin basement membrane disease
- Family history
  - Alport syndrome is associated with a family history of end-stage renal disease and deafness. It is most commonly X-linked (80 %) but may be autosomal recessive (15 %) and rarely autosomal dominant (5 %).
  - Thin basement nephropathy is commonly inherited in an autosomal dominant manner.
  - A family history of IgAN is uncommon.

Differentiation between these three disorders does however ultimately require a renal biopsy. However, the likelihood of the biopsy altering the clinical management of a patient with isolated non-visible haematuria is low, so many nephrologists would elect not to biopsy this patient group. The prognosis for most patients with isolated non-visible haematuria is good, although patients with IgAN and Alport syndrome may later develop progressive kidney disease, heralded by the development of proteinuria and renal impairment. Therefore, these patients require long-term follow-up. Thin basement membrane disease typically has a more benign course; however, patients with a COL4A3 or COL4A4 mutation will have a disease course similar to patients with hereditary nephritis.

Other Causes of Recurrent Visible Haematuria

Recurrent visible haematuria in the over 40s should always raise the suspicion of a urinary tract malignancy, and it is essential that initial investigations exclude this as a cause of the haematuria. In terms of glomerulonephritis IgA nephropathy classically occurs around *1–3 days* after an upper respiratory tract infection, whereas *post-streptococcal* glomerulonephritis classically occurs around *2 weeks* after *streptococcal* infection.

Differential Diagnosis of Mesangial IgA Deposition on Renal Biopsy

The three principle differential diagnoses of mesangial IgA deposition are:

1. IgA nephropathy (renal-limited disease).
2. Henoch-Schönlein purpura nephritis (there will be manifestations of an extrarenal vasculitis affecting skin, joints, gut).
3. Lupus nephritis (mesangial deposition of IgA, along with other immunoglobulin classes and complement, is a feature of lupus nephritis but the distinctive clinical and serologic features usually make this diagnosis obvious).

Investigations

General Investigations

Assessment of renal function, urinary protein excretion and renal size should be undertaken in all patients under investigation for glomerulonephritis, as should an assessment of cardiovascular risk.

Raised serum IgA levels are found in 30–50 % of adult patients with IgAN. Serum IgA levels do not correlate with disease activity or severity.

Complement components C3, C4 and CH50 are usually normal.

Serum autoantibodies, IgA-rheumatoid factor and IgA-containing immune complexes may be found, but none appears to be disease specific. Likewise, measurement of undergalactosylated IgA1 *O*-glycoform levels are not sensitive or specific enough to be used as a diagnostic test in IgAN, although there is emerging evidence that high levels of undergalactosylated IgA1 *O*-glycoforms may correlate with a worse prognosis.

Laboratory tests for liver function and hepatitis B are sufficient to exclude the most common cause of secondary IgAN.

Renal Biopsy

IgAN can only be diagnosed with a renal biopsy; however, in some cases where IgAN is one of the most likely diagnoses, e.g. in isolated non-visible haematuria [5], many nephrologists would not now routinely perform a renal biopsy, although these patients will require careful follow-up (see below).

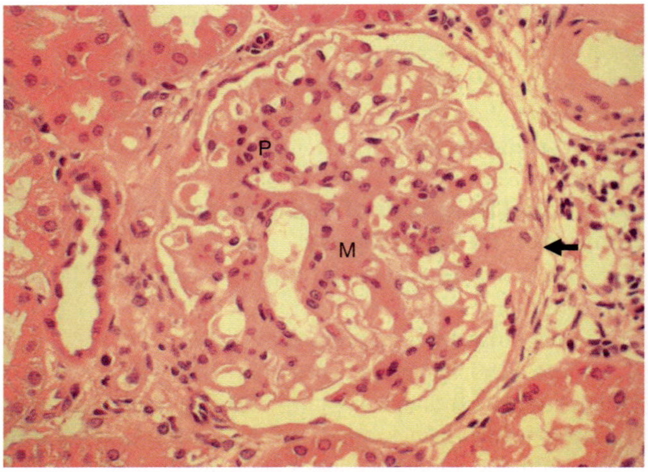

Fig. 19.2 A renal biopsy showing mesangial proliferation (*P*) and expansion of the mesangial extracellular matrix (*M*) in a patient with IgA nephropathy. *Arrow* indicates capsular adhesion

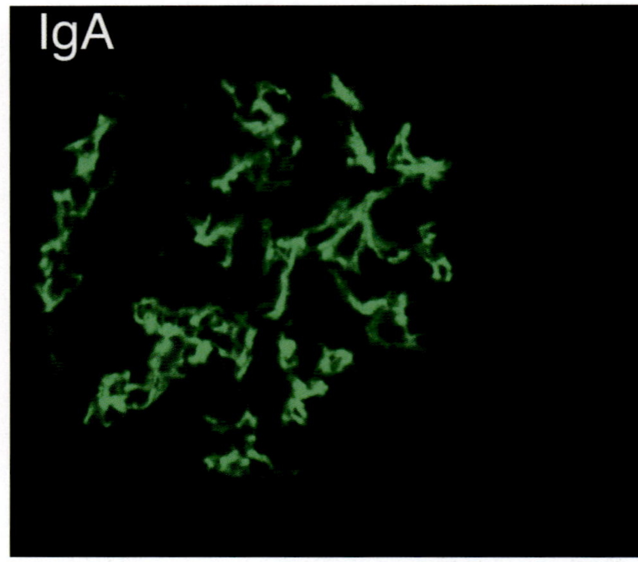

Fig. 19.3 A renal biopsy showing immunofluorescent staining for IgA in a patient with IgA nephropathy

When to Consider Doing a Renal Biopsy in Suspected IgAN

Most clinicians would consider performing a renal biopsy in the context of normal renal imaging and:

- Proteinuria >1 g/24 h ± haematuria without impaired renal function
- Impaired renal function with or without haematuria ± proteinuria (any level)
- Acute kidney injury

Occasionally, patients with IgAN develop acute or chronic renal failure, and a renal biopsy may be necessary to distinguish acute tubular necrosis (due to red cell cast tubular obstruction secondary to massive haematuria) from a crescentic transformation of IgAN.

Renal Biopsy Features

The hallmark of IgAN is mesangial IgA deposition, often accompanied by C3 and less frequently IgG and IgM. Deposition of IgA occurs in a diffuse and global pattern.

Light Microscopy

- May appear normal, even with heavy mesangial IgA deposition.
- Commonly shows mesangial hypercellularity in a focal or diffuse pattern and matrix expansion (Fig. 19.2).
- Crescentic change may be superimposed on mesangial hypercellularity.
- Crescents are more common in biopsies performed during episodes of visible haematuria.
- Tubulointerstitial changes are similar to other forms of progressive glomerulonephritis with tubular atrophy and interstitial fibrosis.

Immunohistology

- Mesangial staining for IgA is the defining feature of IgAN (Fig. 19.3).
- IgA deposits may extend beyond the mesangium to the glomerular capillaries. This finding is associated with a worse prognosis.
- IgA is the sole deposited immunoglobulin in 15 % of cases.
- Other immunoglobulins may also be deposited: IgG (50–70 % of cases) and IgM (31–66 % of cases), although staining is usually less intense than IgA. The presence of IgG and IgM has no prognostic significance.
- C3 deposition is usually also present.

Electron Microscopy

- Mesangial and para-mesangial electron-dense deposits are often seen and correspond to IgA immune complex deposition (Fig. 19.4).
- Capillary loop deposits may be seen and are usually subendothelial, but may be intramembranous or subepithelial. These are associated with a worse prognosis.
- The size, shape, quantity and density of the deposits vary between glomeruli.
- Glomerular basement membrane (GBM) abnormalities are seen in 15–40 % and are associated with heavy proteinuria, more severe glomerular changes and crescent formation.
- A group of patients have thinning of the GBM indistinguishable from thin membrane disease. It remains unclear whether the clinical course of these patients is altered.

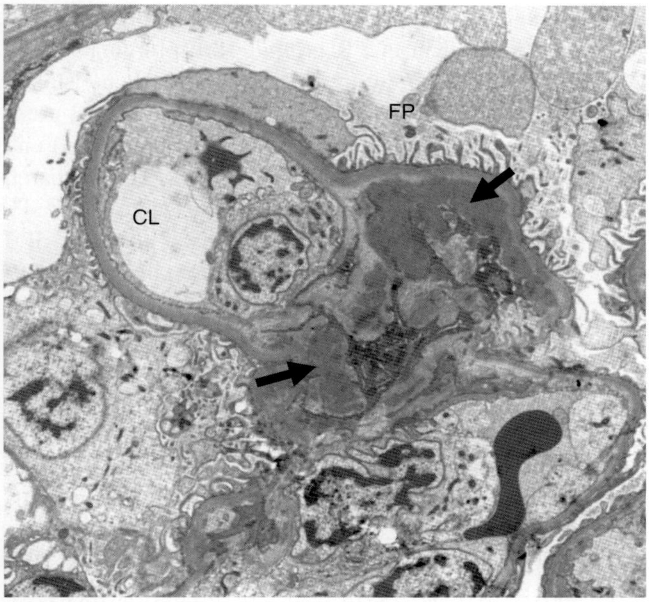

Fig. 19.4 An electron micrograph of a portion of a glomerulus (*CL* capillary lumen, *FP* foot processes) showing electron-dense immune complex deposits (*arrowed*) within the mesangium

The Oxford Classification of IgA Nephropathy

In 2009, a consensus on the pathologic classification of IgAN was published by the International IgA Nephropathy Network and the Renal Pathology Society. Clinical data and renal biopsies were obtained from 265 patients followed for a median of 5 years. The first part of this work identified histological variables which could be interpreted with a high degree of reproducibility between different pathologists [6]. The second part was a retrospective analysis identifying renal biopsy features that correlated most strongly with clinical outcome, independent of known clinical risk factors including the presence of hypertension, impaired renal function at diagnosis and degree of proteinuria (Table 19.1). The predictive value of these biopsy features was similar in both adults and children [7, 8]. Studies are ongoing to validate this classification in different patient populations and include the VALIGA study funded by the European Renal Association (ERA-EDTA).

Secondary IgAN

Mesangial IgA deposition may occur secondary to a number of other diseases and the renal biopsy appearances are often indistinguishable from primary IgAN [9]. The course of the renal disease is however typically very different with most patients rarely progressing to end-stage renal disease.

Diseases associated with mesangial IgA deposition include:

- Chronic liver disease, particularly alcoholic liver disease (possibly due to impaired clearance of IgA immune complexes by the liver)

Table 19.1 The Oxford classification of IgA nephropathy

Histological variable	Definition	Score
Mesangial hypercellularity	Mesangial hypercellularity score[a]	**M**0 ≤0.5 **M**1 >0.5
Endocapillary hypercellularity	Hypercellularity due to increased number of cells within glomerular capillary lumina causing narrowing of the lumina	**E**0 absent **E**1 present
Segmental glomerulosclerosis	Any amount of the tuft involved in sclerosis, but not involving the whole tuft or the presence of an adhesion	**S**0 absent **S**1 present
Tubular atrophy/ interstitial fibrosis	Percentage of cortical area involved by the tubular atrophy or interstitial fibrosis, whichever is greater	**T**0 0–25 % **T**1 26–50 % **T**2 >50 %

Scoring should be assessed on period acid-Schiff-stained sections
[a]For a precise definition of mesangial hypercellularity, see [7]

- HIV/AIDS (associated with a high serum IgA concentration)
- Coeliac disease (no clear explanation but a gluten-free diet may lead to a short-term reduction in proteinuria and improvement in renal function)
- Henoch-Schönlein purpura

Treatment of secondary forms of IgAN should be based on treating the primary disease.

Management

Despite advances in the understanding of the pathogenesis of IgAN, there is still no intervention available to prevent production of pathogenic IgA or its glomerular deposition. Treatment strategies therefore centre on modulating downstream immune and inflammatory events and can be thought of as generic strategies applicable to all chronic glomerulonephritides: reduction of proteinuria, use of renin-angiotensin blockade and control of hypertension. As with all other causes of CKD, cardiovascular risk factors should be addressed and advice should be given regarding smoking cessation, a healthy diet and exercise.

The Patient with Invisible Haematuria and <0.5 g/day Proteinuria

No specific therapy is advised, although long-term follow-up in primary care is recommended to identify development of increasing proteinuria, renal impairment and hypertension.

The Patient with Recurrent Visible Haematuria

No specific treatment is required for patients with recurrent visible haematuria, and there is no role for prophylactic antibiotics. Tonsillectomy reduces the frequency of acute episodes of visible haematuria where tonsillitis is the provoking factor and has its advocates, especially in Japan, as a treatment to reduce progression to ESRD. However, data from clinical trials is conflicting, and larger studies are needed before any conclusion can be drawn regarding the role of tonsillectomy in preserving long-term renal function in IgAN [10, 11].

The Patient with >0.5 g/day Proteinuria and Slowly Progressive IgAN

The risk of progressive IgAN correlates with the degree of proteinuria. Patients with less proteinuria have improved renal survival, and reducing proteinuria in patients with heavy proteinuria improves prognosis, according to registry data [12]. Several randomised controlled trials have shown that renin-angiotensin blockade, with an angiotensin-converting enzyme inhibitor (ACEi) or angiotensin II receptor blocker (ARB) to control hypertension and reduce proteinuria to less than 0.5 g/day, is beneficial in slowing progression of proteinuric IgAN [13, 14]. Therefore, an ACEi or ARB should be introduced and maximised to achieve this threshold. Although the combination of using both ACEi and ARB reduces proteinuria in IgAN, long-term beneficial effects on renal survival have not been demonstrated, and the safety of this approach has been questioned in the ONTARGET study [15].

There are a number of patients who will continue to have proteinuria in excess of 0.5 g/day and declining renal function despite maximal doses of ACEi and/or ARB. In these patients, current evidence regarding additional therapy is controversial.

Corticosteroids

A 6-month course of corticosteroids in patients with persistent proteinuria >1 g/day despite renin-angiotensin blockade and preserved renal function (eGFR >50 ml/min) may slow progression of renal decline.

Pozzi et al. showed that treatment of patients with IgAN with a course of corticosteroids reduced proteinuria and prevented progression to ESRD over a 10-year period [16]. However, the high-dose corticosteroid regimen used – 'pulsed' methylprednisolone (1 g daily for 3 days at induction and at the beginning of months 2 and 4) and alternate day prednisolone (0.5 mg/kg) for 6 months – is felt by many clinicians to carry unacceptable toxicity, although only minor side effects were reported in this study. Additionally, renin-angiotensin blockade was only used in a minority of patients in this study, although usage was evenly distributed between both treatment groups.

Studies by Manno et al. and Lv et al. evaluated the effect of corticosteroids plus renin-angiotensin blockade versus renin-angiotensin blockade alone in patients with preserved renal function (mean eGFR around 100 ml/min/1.73 m^2) and proteinuria (>1 g/day) [17, 18]. In the study by Manno et al., a combination of an ACEi and 6 months oral prednisolone led to fewer patients reaching the combined end point of doubling of serum creatinine or ESRD compared to those treated with ACEi alone. Lv et al. demonstrated a reduction of patients reaching the primary endpoint of a 50 % increase in serum creatinine in the combination ACEi and corticosteroid arm compared to ACEi alone (3 % versus 24 %).

These studies have, however, been criticised as they required ACEi and ARBs to be stopped prior to commencement in the trial and therefore there was a lack of a suitable run-in period to allow for optimisation of supportive treatment prior to administration of corticosteroids. Patients entering into the corticosteroid treatment arm may therefore have benefited from optimised supportive care alone. The STOP-IgAN trial has been designed to address this [19]. Patients with persistent proteinuria >0.75 g/day have initially been given optimised supportive therapy for 6 months, followed by randomisation to continue supportive therapy, or given additional immunosuppressive therapy (corticosteroids if eGFR ≥60 ml/min, corticosteroids plus cyclophosphamide/azathioprine if eGFR <60 ml/min). Results from this study are awaited.

Fish Oil

Conflicting data exists regarding the use of prescription strength fish oil. Fish oil is widely prescribed in IgAN in certain centres and appears to be safe, although tolerability is a major issue due to a fishy odour to the breath and perspiration and increased flatulence. In one RCT, patients randomised to receive fish oil (compared to placebo) had better preservation of renal function over a median of 6 years follow-up [20]. However, this finding has not been reproduced in other RCTs, and a meta-analysis concluded that the available evidence is inconclusive [21]. Further studies in this area are required before a definitive recommendation can be made.

Other Immunosuppressive Agents

There is currently insufficient evidence to support the routine use of cyclophosphamide and azathioprine in IgAN. Mycophenolate mofetil (MMF) has been studied in a number of small RCTs but results have been inconsistent, and a recent meta-analysis of these trials concluded that there is no significant benefit of MMF in reducing proteinuria in IgAN [22]. The most recent report providing longer follow-up data on 40 Chinese patients with mild histological lesions did show benefit in reducing the composite end points of doubling of serum creatinine or ESRD [23]. Further studies of MMF in IgAN are however ongoing.

The Patient with Acute Kidney Injury

In patients known to have IgAN who develop AKI and fail to respond to simple supportive measures, a renal biopsy is required to differentiate between the two most common causes of AKI in IgAN:

Acute Tubular Necrosis with Intratubular Erythrocyte Casts

This requires supportive care only. Recovery to baseline GFR is usual; however, some patients may be left with irreversible tubulointerstitial scarring.

Crescentic IgAN

Patients with rapidly progressive loss of renal function, active glomerular inflammation and crescents on renal biopsy and no significant chronic damage may be treated in a similar way to other forms of crescentic GN, i.e. high-dose corticosteroids, cyclophosphamide and plasma exchange. Evidence for treatment of crescentic IgAN is derived from small case-series and retrospective data [24]. Response to treatment is worse in crescentic IgAN than in other forms of crescentic glomerulonephritis, and renal survival is estimated to be only 50 % at 1 year and 20 % at 5 years. This may be the consequence of significant pre-existing chronic damage at the time of a crescentic transformation, thereby reducing the chances of a response to immunosuppression.

The Patient with Nephrotic Syndrome

Nephrotic syndrome in association with mesangial IgA deposition may be due to advanced glomerular scarring as a consequence of longstanding IgAN and therefore reflect established CKD or an acute podocyte injury indistinguishable from minimal change disease, occurring in a patient with coincidental IgAN. A renal biopsy is clearly the key to distinguishing between these two extremes and in particular electron microscopy should be performed. Patients with IgAN, nephrotic syndrome, minimal glomerular scarring and podocyte effacement typical of minimal change disease should be treated as minimal change disease [25].

Follow-up

Patients with IgAN and CKD1-3 may be followed up in primary care. On discharge from nephrology services, clear guidance should be provided to the primary care physician regarding frequency of renal function, urine dipstick and blood pressure monitoring. For the patient and primary care physician it may be worth pre-empting some of the common questions and concerns relating to IgA (see Box 19.1). This will be dictated by local guidelines; however, we would suggest that this should be performed at least annually.

Patients with CKD 4-5 require follow-up in a nephrology clinic.

Special Circumstances in IgAN

Transplantation

Recurrence of IgA deposition following renal transplantation is common, affecting up to 50 % of grafts within 5 years [26]. Graft failure due to recurrence of IgAN is however relatively rare and most often occurs in patients who have had a rapidly progressive course in their native kidneys, e.g. crescentic IgAN. There is little evidence that the choice of posttransplant immunosuppression protocol modifies the risk of recurrence, although a recently published analysis of the Australia and New Zealand Dialysis and Transplant Registry (ANZDATA) suggests recurrent disease is more common in patients who undergo steroid withdrawal [27]. There is also no evidence to support any specific therapy regimen once recurrent IgAN has been diagnosed following renal transplantation, although a single centre retrospective analysis has suggested that ACEi/ARB treatment may reduce the rate of decline of allograft function in recurrent IgAN [28] .

Pregnancy

As with other forms of glomerulonephritis, renal prognosis is worse in pregnancy (see Pregnancy and Renal Disease Chapter (G.Lipkin)) when there is:

- Renal impairment (serum creatinine >150 μmol/l)
- Proteinuria (>1 g/day)
- Hypertension (on treatment or BP >140/90)

Patients should receive appropriate preconception counselling. ACEi and ARBs along with teratogenic immunosuppressive agents (e.g. cyclophosphamide, MMF) should be stopped prior to planned conception or at the earliest indication of pregnancy. Once pregnant, patients should receive careful monitoring in a combined renal-obstetric clinic.

Box 19.1 IgA Nephropathy: Commonly Asked Questions

Can I diagnose IgA nephropathy without a renal biopsy?	You can only diagnose IgA nephropathy with a renal biopsy. Serum IgA level and measurement of IgA glycosylation are not sensitive or specific enough to be diagnostic
Does IgA nephropathy run-in families?	IgAN (& HSP) can be inherited but this is rare. Much more common causes of inherited haematuria (which can be episodically visible) are thin membrane nephropathy and Alport's disease
What should I do with young adults with recurrent visible haematuria?	Reassure them that the episodes will subside with time and that no specific treatment is required

Should my patient have a tonsillectomy?	There is no convincing evidence that tonsillectomy preserves renal function and should not therefore be recommended as a renoprotective strategy
Should my patient take fish oils?	The jury is out on any beneficial effect of fish oils and the most recent meta-analysis failed to confirm renoprotective efficacy. They are safe and many clinicians offer fish oils but patients need to expect to develop a 'fishy odour'
Should I give my patient steroids?	There is very much a split of opinion on this. I would only consider steroids in patients with proteinuria >1 g/24 h after maximal renin-angiotensin blockade and blood pressure <125/80 mmHg. The STOP-IgAN trial should definitively answer this question
What should I do if a patient with IgA nephropathy develops acute kidney injury?	The two things always to consider are tubular obstruction by red cell casts in heavy haematuria (resolves with supportive measures) and crescentic IgAN. Failure to improve with supportive measures should trigger an early renal biopsy and consideration of immunosuppression if crescentic IgAN identified
Should patients with IgA nephropathy be transplanted?	While there is a significant risk of recurrent IgA *deposition* in renal allografts, the actual risk of recurrent *disease* leading to graft loss is much smaller and therefore patients with IgA nephropathy should be offered a renal transplant
	It is reported that patients with IgAN who exhibited a rapid decline in renal function in their native kidneys are more likely to have similarly aggressive recurrent disease in their allograft. No specific immunosuppressive regimen has been shown to protect against recurrent IgAN

Henoch-Schönlein Purpura

HSP is the commonest form of systemic vasculitis in children and is characterised by IgA deposition in affected blood vessels. The renal lesion is a mesangioproliferative glomerulonephritis with mesangial IgA deposition, indistinguishable from IgAN.

Epidemiology

Although HSP may occur at any age, it is most common during childhood, between the ages of 3 and 15. There is a slight male predominance. Most cases occur in the winter, spring and autumn months, which may be due to its association with preceding upper respiratory tract infections.

Aetiology and Pathogenesis

The exact cause of HSP remains unknown. There are, however, many factors which suggest there are common pathogenic pathways operating in HSP and IgAN [29]:

- Identical twins have been reported, where one presents with IgAN and the other with HSP.
- HSP developing on a background of IgAN is described in both adults and children.
- Both diseases share similar findings on renal biopsy and also changes in the complement of serum IgA1 O-glycoforms.
- There is a similar association between mucosal infection and presentation of disease.

Natural History

The renal disease that accompanies HSP is often transient and self-limiting in nature, with haematuria or proteinuria typically resolving within weeks of presentation. AKI due to crescentic HSP nephritis is more common than crescentic IgAN (although still uncommon) and tends to occur early in the course of the disease. The long-term outlook of patients who have transient HSP is generally very good. However, up to 10 % of patients with HSP nephritis will develop ESRD [30].

Clinical Features

The classical tetrad of symptoms in HSP are:

1. Palpable purpuric rash
2. Arthritis/arthralgia
3. Abdominal pain
4. Renal disease

Symptoms appear in any order and can evolve over a few days to weeks [31].

The *rash* is classically distributed on extensor surfaces, with sparing of the trunk and face. It typically appears in crops and is symmetrically distributed (Fig. 19.5).

Polyarthralgia is common and is usually transient and migratory. There is often swelling and tenderness but without chronic destructive damage.

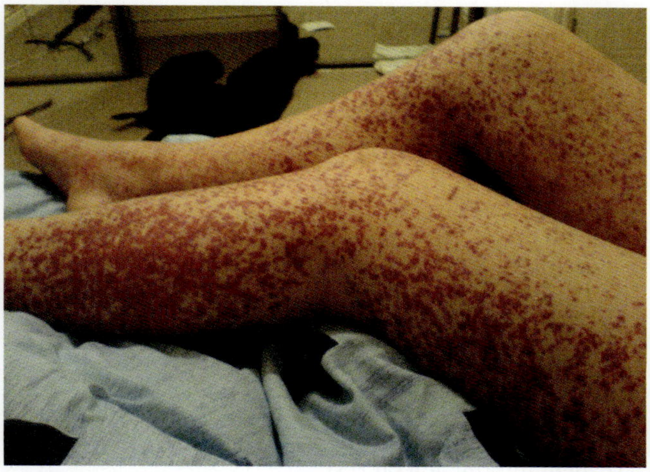

Fig. 19.5 Typical appearance of the leucocytoclastic vasculitis of Henoch-Schönlein purpura

Gastrointestinal symptoms often appear after the rash. Abdominal pain is usually mild and transient, but may be severe and lead to gastrointestinal haemorrhage, bowel ischaemia, intussusception and perforation (Fig. 19.6).

Renal involvement (HSP nephritis) typically manifests as transient asymptomatic invisible haematuria and/or proteinuria. More severe complications, such as nephrotic syndrome or rapidly progressive deterioration of renal function, occur less frequently and tend to occur in adults more often than in children.

Rarely, HSP can be associated with other features more commonly seen with the ANCA-associated small vessel vasculitides including pulmonary haemorrhage (Fig. 19.7).

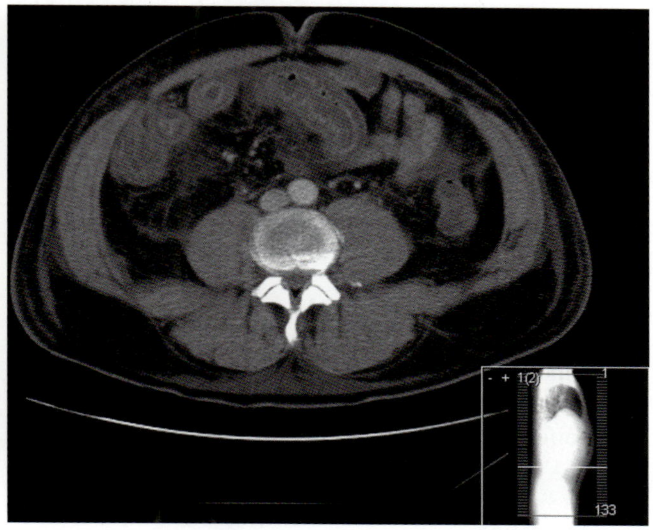

Fig. 19.6 CT scan showing marked oedema of the small bowel in a patient with Henoch-Schönlein purpura and abdominal pain

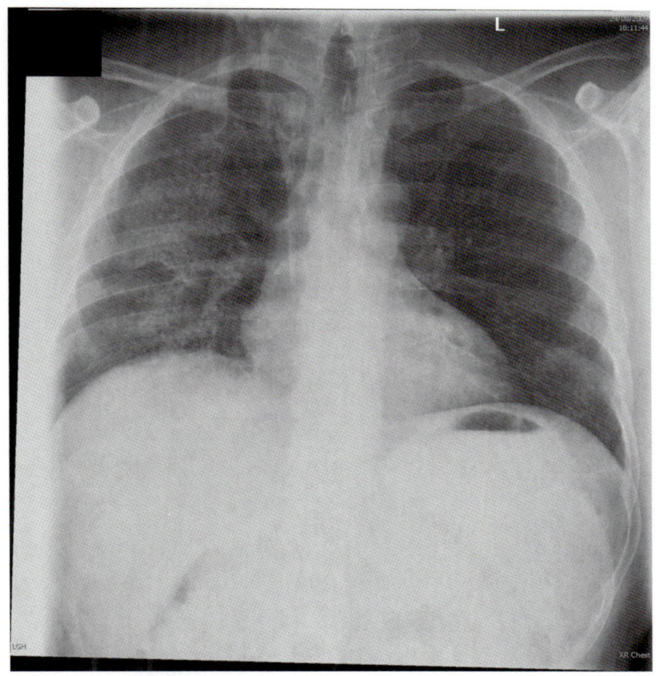

Fig. 19.7 Extensive right-sided alveolar shadowing due to pulmonary haemorrhage in a patient with HSP and crescentic glomerulonephritis (note the vascular catheter in place for dialysis and plasma exchange)

Differential Diagnosis

In children, a clinical diagnosis is often made without the need to proceed to a renal biopsy.

In adults, the differential diagnoses are wide and include other forms of small vessel vasculitides such as ANCA-associated vasculitis, cryoglobulinaemia and systemic lupus erythematosus. These should be distinguished on the basis of clinical, serological and histological findings.

Investigations

General Investigations

Assessment of renal function, urinary protein excretion and renal size should be undertaken in all patients under investigation for glomerulonephritis, as should an assessment of cardiovascular risk.

As in IgAN, raised serum IgA levels are found in 30–50 % of adult patients with HSP. Serum IgA levels do not correlate with disease activity or severity. Similarly, changes in the levels of undergalactosylated IgA1 *O*-glycoform levels are not sensitive or specific enough to be used as a diagnostic test in HSP.

Confirmation of the clinical diagnosis requires histological evidence of IgA deposition in affected tissue, often the skin or kidney.

Skin Biopsy

Biopsy of the skin rash typically shows a leucocytoclastic vasculitis. IgA immune complex deposition can be seen by immunofluorescent staining; however, detection of IgA is unreliable, and if a tissue diagnosis is required then a renal biopsy should be performed if there is clear evidence of nephritis.

Renal Biopsy

Renal biopsy is usually reserved for adult cases of diagnostic uncertainty or when a child presents with more severe renal involvement. Histological features are the same as those for IgAN; however, in HSP nephritis there will also be extrarenal manifestations of disease [32].

Management

There is little evidence to guide the treatment of HSP nephritis, and what there is derived from small retrospective case series [30].

Patients with haematuria, proteinuria and mild renal impairment do not require any specific treatment, and the nephritis usually resolves spontaneously.

In patients with crescentic HSP nephritis, typified by a rapidly progressive loss of renal function and systemic manifestations of small vessel vasculitis, there is limited evidence that high-dose corticosteroids may be beneficial. Regimes include pulsed methylprednisolone followed by a 3-month course of oral prednisolone. There is currently no conclusive evidence that other immunosuppressive agents, including cyclophosphamide or azathioprine or other interventions such as plasmapheresis, have any beneficial effect on outcome.

Follow-up

Patients should be monitored as for IgAN. As with other forms of glomerular disease, those patients with persistent proteinuria are at highest risk of developing progressive CKD [33].

Special Circumstances in HSP

Transplantation

Renal transplantation is the treatment of choice in patients with ESRD due to HSP nephritis. As with IgAN recurrence of mesangial IgA, deposition may occur [34] while loss of the graft due to recurrence is less common and tends to occur in patients who had an aggressive original disease [35]. Renal transplantation should be delayed for 12 months from date of presentation.

Pregnancy

Evidence from cohort studies of children with HSP suggests that all women with a history of HSP should be carefully monitored during pregnancy, even if they had no evidence of renal disease at the time of diagnosis as they are at increased risk of developing hypertension and proteinuria [36].

Internet Resources

The International IgA nephropathy network:
http://www.igan-world.org/main.htm.

Patient information on IgAN:
http://www.emrn.org.uk/documents/IgANephropathy.pdf.
http://www.gosh.nhs.uk/gosh_families/information_sheets/iga_nephropathy/iga_nephropathy_families.html.

Patient information on HSP:
http://www.gosh.nhs.uk/gosh_families/information_sheets/henoch_schonlein_purpura/henoch_schonlein_purpura_families.html.

References

1. D'Amico G. Natural history of idiopathic IgA nephropathy: role of clinical and histological prognostic factors. Am J Kidney Dis. 2000;36(2):227–37.
2. Suzuki K, Honda K, Tanabe K, Toma H, Nihei H, Yamaguchi Y. Incidence of latent mesangial IgA deposition in renal allograft donors in Japan. Kidney Int. 2003;63(6):2286–94.
3. Barratt J, Smith AC, Feehally J. The pathogenic role of IgA1 O-linked glycosylation in the pathogenesis of IgA nephropathy. Nephrology (Carlton). 2007;12(3):275–84.
4. Barratt J, Feehally J. Primary IgA nephropathy: new insights into pathogenesis. Semin Nephrol. 2011;31(4):349–60.
5. Topham PS, Harper SJ, Furness PN, Harris KP, Walls J, Feehally J. Glomerular disease as a cause of isolated microscopic haematuria. Q J Med. 1994;87(6):329–35.
6. Roberts IS, Cook HT, Troyanov S, Alpers CE, Amore A, Barratt J, et al. The Oxford classification of IgA nephropathy: pathology definitions, correlations, and reproducibility. Kidney Int. 2009;76(5):546–56.
7. Cattran DC, Coppo R, Cook HT, Feehally J, Roberts IS, Troyanov S, et al. The Oxford classification of IgA nephropathy: rationale, clinicopathological correlations, and classification. Kidney Int. 2009;76(5):534–45.
8. Coppo R, Troyanov S, Camilla R, Hogg RJ, Cattran DC, Cook HT, et al. The Oxford IgA nephropathy clinicopathological classification is valid for children as well as adults. Kidney Int. 2010;77(10):921–7.
9. Pouria S, Barratt J. Secondary IgA nephropathy. Semin Nephrol. 2008;28(1):27–37.
10. Piccoli A, Codognotto M, Tabbi MG, Favaro E, Rossi B. Influence of tonsillectomy on the progression of mesangioproliferative glomerulonephritis. Nephrol Dial Transplant. 2010;25(8):2583–9.
11. Wang Y, Chen J, Chen Y, Wang L, Lv Y. A meta-analysis of the clinical remission rate and long-term efficacy of tonsillectomy in patients with IgA nephropathy. Nephrol Dial Transplant. 2011;26(6):1923–31.
12. Reich HN, Troyanov S, Scholey JW, Cattran DC. Remission of proteinuria improves prognosis in IgA nephropathy. J Am Soc Nephrol. 2007;18(12):3177–83.

13. Coppo R, Peruzzi L, Amore A, Piccoli A, Cochat P, Stone R, et al. IgACE: a placebo-controlled, randomized trial of angiotensin-converting enzyme inhibitors in children and young people with IgA nephropathy and moderate proteinuria. J Am Soc Nephrol. 2007;18:1880–8.
14. Praga M, Gutierrez E, Gonzalez E, Morales E, Hernandez E. Treatment of IgA nephropathy with ACE inhibitors: a randomized and controlled trial. J Am Soc Nephrol. 2003;14(6):1578–83.
15. Mann JF, Schmieder RE, McQueen M, Dyal L, Schumacher H, Pogue J, et al. Renal outcomes with telmisartan, ramipril, or both, in people at high vascular risk (the ONTARGET study): a multicentre, randomised, double-blind, controlled trial. Lancet. 2008;372(9638):547–53.
16. Pozzi C, Andrulli S, Del Vecchio L, Melis P, Fogazzi GB, Altieri P, et al. Corticosteroid effectiveness in IgA nephropathy: long-term results of a randomized, controlled trial. J Am Soc Nephrol. 2004;15(1):157–63.
17. Lv J, Zhang H, Chen Y, Li G, Jiang L, Singh AK, et al. Combination therapy of prednisone and ACE inhibitor versus ACE-inhibitor therapy alone in patients with IgA nephropathy: a randomized controlled trial. Am J Kidney Dis. 2009;53(1):26–32.
18. Manno C, Torres DD, Rossini M, Pesce F, Schena FP. Randomized controlled clinical trial of corticosteroids plus ACE-inhibitors with long-term follow-up in proteinuric IgA nephropathy. Nephrol Dial Transplant. 2009;24(12):3694–701.
19. Eitner F, Ackermann D, Hilgers RD, Floege J. Supportive versus immunosuppressive therapy of progressive IgA nephropathy (STOP) IgAN trial: rationale and study protocol. J Nephrol. 2008;21(3):284–9.
20. Donadio Jr JV, Grande JP, Bergstralh EJ, Dart RA, Larson TS, Spencer DC. The long-term outcome of patients with IgA nephropathy treated with fish oil in a controlled trial. Mayo Nephrology Collaborative Group. J Am Soc Nephrol. 1999;10(8):1772–7.
21. Strippoli GF, Manno C, Schena FP. An "evidence-based" survey of therapeutic options for IgA nephropathy: assessment and criticism. Am J Kidney Dis. 2003;41(6):1129–39.
22. Xu G, Tu W, Jiang D, Xu C. Mycophenolate mofetil treatment for IgA nephropathy: a meta-analysis. Am J Nephrol. 2008; 29(5):362–7.
23. Tang SC, Tang AW, Wong SS, Leung JC, Ho YW, Lai KN. Long-term study of mycophenolate mofetil treatment in IgA nephropathy. Kidney Int. 2010;77(6):543–9.
24. Tumlin JA, Hennigar RA. Clinical presentation, natural history, and treatment of crescentic proliferative IgA nephropathy. Semin Nephrol. 2004;24(3):256–68.
25. Lai KN, Lai FM, Ho CP, Chan KW. Corticosteroid therapy in IgA nephropathy with nephrotic syndrome: a long-term controlled trial. Clin Nephrol. 1986;26(4):174–80.
26. Floege J. Recurrent IgA nephropathy after renal transplantation. Semin Nephrol. 2004;24(3):287–91.
27. Clayton P, McDonald S, Chadban S. Steroids and recurrent IgA nephropathy after kidney transplantation. Am J Transplant. 2011;11(8):1645–9.
28. Courtney AE, McNamee PT, Nelson WE, Maxwell AP. Does angiotensin blockade influence graft outcome in renal transplant recipients with IgA nephropathy? Nephrol Dial Transplant. 2006;21(12):3550–4.
29. Davin JC, Ten Berge IJ, Weening JJ. What is the difference between IgA nephropathy and Henoch-Schonlein purpura nephritis? Kidney Int. 2001;59(3):823–34.
30. Sanders JT, Wyatt RJ. IgA nephropathy and Henoch-Schonlein purpura nephritis. Curr Opin Pediatr. 2008;20(2):163–70.
31. Saulsbury FT. Henoch-Schonlein purpura in children. Report of 100 patients and review of the literature. Medicine. 1999;78(6):395–409.
32. Gedalia A. Henoch-Schonlein purpura. Curr Rheumatol Rep. 2004;6(3):195–202.
33. Sano H, Izumida M, Shimizu H, Ogawa Y. Risk factors of renal involvement and significant proteinuria in Henoch-Schonlein purpura. Eur J Pediatr. 2002;161(4):196–201.
34. Ponticelli C, Glassock RJ. Posttransplant recurrence of primary glomerulonephritis. Clin J Am Soc Nephrol. 2010;5(12):2363–72.
35. Meulders Q, Pirson Y, Cosyns JP, Squifflet JP, van Ypersele de Strihou C. Course of Henoch-Schonlein nephritis after renal transplantation. Report on ten patients and review of the literature. Transplantation. 1994;58(11):1179–86.
36. Ronkainen J, Nuutinen M, Koskimies O. The adult kidney 24 years after childhood Henoch-Schonlein purpura: a retrospective cohort study. Lancet. 2002;360(9334):666–70.

Table 20.2 Clinical manifestations of ANCA-associated systemic vasculitis

Organ system	Clinical manifestations
Kidney	Microscopic haematuria, proteinuria, progressive renal impairment, oligoanuric renal failure
Respiratory tract	Cough, haemoptysis, pulmonary infiltrates, cavitating lung granulomata, alveolar capillaritis with pulmonary haemorrhage
ENT	Nasal crusting, sinusitis, hearing loss (conductive and sensorineural), laryngotracheal granulomatous inflammation causing subglottic stenosis, chondritis of the auricle or nasal cartilage
Skin	Purpuric rash, painful erythematous nodules, focal skin necrosis/ulceration
Musculoskeletal	Myalgia and migratory arthritis
Ocular	Episcleritis, scleritis, orbital granuloma, proptosis
Gastrointestinal	Gastrointestinal bleeding, abdominal pain
Nervous system	Mononeuritis multiplex, peripheral neuropathy, stroke
Constitutional symptoms	Fever, general malaise, weight loss and anorexia

Classification of systemic vasculitis has traditionally been confusing with little consensus between centres. Criteria for diagnosis were developed by the ACR in 1990, but these do not recognise a small vessel subtype of polyarteritis nodosa [2]. The Chapel Hill Consensus Conference (CHCC) proposes definitions for AASV (GPA, MPA and CSS) that were primarily based on histology (not always practical to obtain), and not intended for use as diagnostic criteria in the clinical setting [1]. Although the ACR and CCHC criteria are widely used, there was no consensus on how they should be applied in diagnosing a patient with suspected AASV. A consensus methodology has since been published with a proposed diagnostic algorithm which incorporates the ACR and CHCC definitions and has been validated [3] (Fig. 20.1).

A nonspecific prodrome is common in AASV, which can precede other organ manifestations of the disease by several months, and delays in diagnosis are all too common. Constitutional symptoms include fever, anorexia, weight loss and general malaise, reflecting the underlying inflammatory nature of this disease. A purpuric vasculitic rash and arthralgia are also very common and often associated with symmetrical, migratory small joint polyarthritis.

The kidneys and lungs are the two organ systems most commonly and extensively injured in AASV. Hence, AASV is an important cause of the "pulmonary-renal syndrome". Vasculitis in the kidney may progress to a necrotising crescentic glomerulonephritis with haematuria (often with urinary red cell casts) and rapidly progressive renal failure. Lung involvement is varied depending on the particular clinico-pathological syndrome (see below) but, in its most severe form, leads to development of pulmonary capillaritis with consequent alveolar haemorrhage, an important cause of early mortality in this condition.

The different clinico-pathological syndromes of AASV may present with typical clinical features and different patterns of organ involvement at the time of diagnosis:

- *GPA* is classically associated with granulomatous inflammation of the upper respiratory tract, which produces a variety of ENT symptoms including nasal crusting, hearing loss (conductive and sensorineural), sinusitis and occasionally a saddle-shaped nasal deformity as a result of necrotising inflammation in the cartilaginous nasal septum. Seventy-seven per cent of patients with GPA have upper respiratory tract symptoms at the time of diagnosis compared to 29 % of patients with MPA [4]. Ultimately, 86 % of patients with GPA will develop renal disease at some point in their disease, although this is less common at presentation than in MPA (see below).
- If there is no clinical evidence of granulomatous inflammation or eosinophilic vasculitis, the AASV syndrome is termed *MPA*. It is important to note that granulomatous inflammation may emerge at a later time point, at which stage the diagnosis will change to GPA. Extrarenal organ involvement in MPA is generally less common than in GPA. Patients tend to present with renal disease, which is more common at the time of diagnosis in MPA than in GPA (92 % vs. 77 %), possibly as they present later in the disease because the renal disease is largely asymptomatic until advanced.
- Some patients may present with disease limited to the kidney (causing a pauci-immune crescentic glomerulonephritis). This renal limited disease is considered as MPA unless evidence of granulomatous inflammation develops subsequently.
- *EGPA* displays clinical features of (1) late onset asthma and wheeze (>95 %) with (2) variable peripheral blood eosinophilia accounting for >10 % of leucocytes (100 %, although disappears rapidly with treatment of asthma with glucocorticoids so may be missed) and evidence of (3) end-organ damage secondary to vasculitis. Rhinitis, with nasal polyposis and hearing loss, is often present. End-organ disease is manifested as skin granulomas or palpable purpura (60 %), mononeuritis multiplex (75 %), pauci-immune crescentic glomerulonephritis (25 %) and cardiac disease (pericarditis/myocarditis/valvular lesions, 40 %). It is not uncommon for patients to have chest symptoms with eosinophilia for months or years before developing overt vasculitis. Renal involvement is less common compared to GPA and MPA and the association with ANCA is much weaker, although those with renal disease tend to have a positive ANCA test.

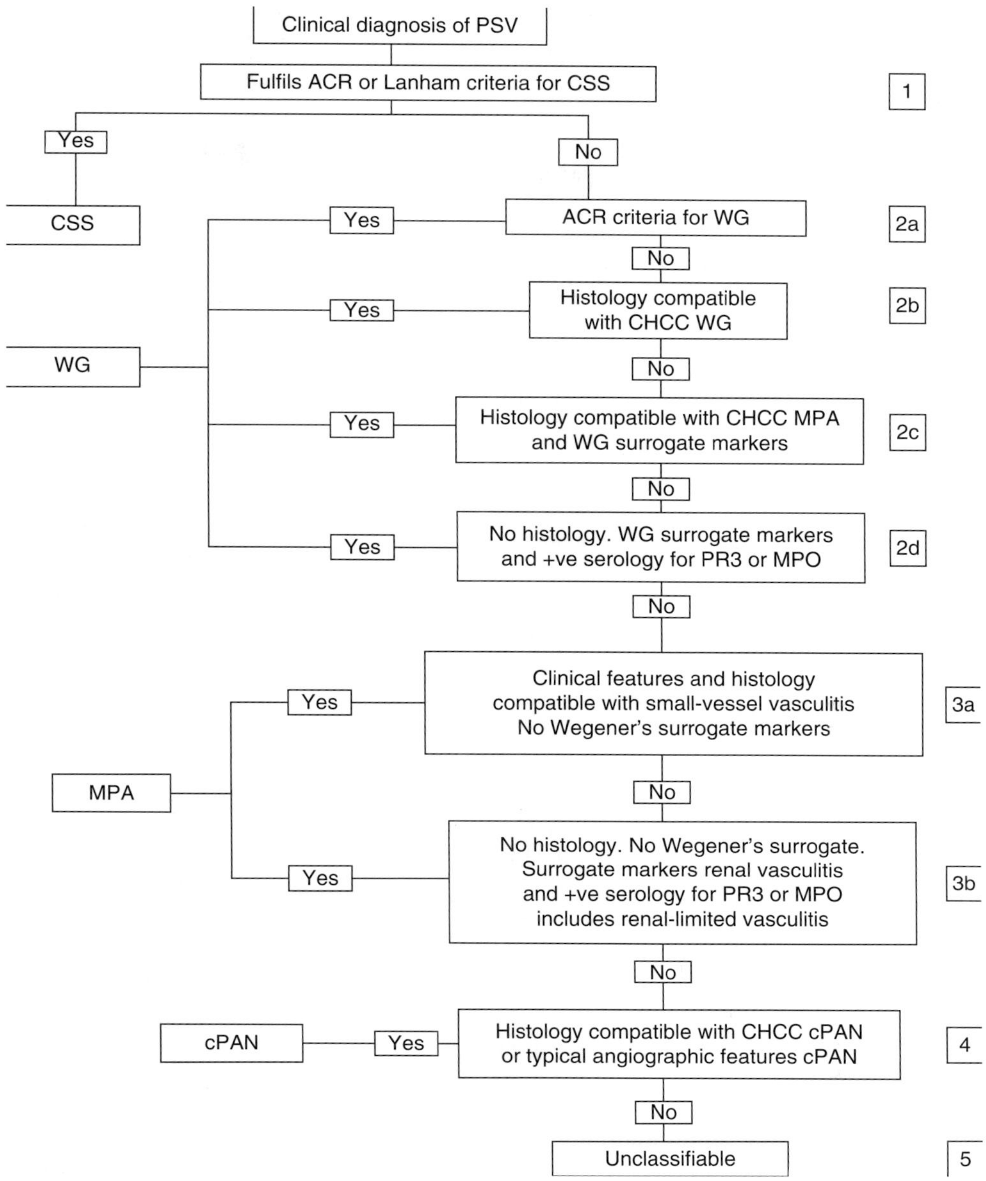

Fig. 20.1 A validated diagnostic algorithm for AASV developed by Watts et al. (Copyright © 2007 BMJ Publishing Group Ltd.)

Epidemiology

The estimated overall annual incidence of AASV is 10–20 cases/million, and most studies indicate a Caucasian preponderance. Incidence increases with age with a peak age of onset between 65 and 74 years [5]. Studies suggest that, in contrast to other autoimmune diseases, AASV does not display a female preponderance [5].

Some epidemiological studies indicate an increasing incidence of GPA and MPA. The reasons for this are not clear but are almost certainly partly due to increased awareness of the disease, better case definition and enhanced availability of ANCA testing. Clinician experience suggests that there appears to be a seasonal peak in incidence in Spring but this is not uniformly supported by formal epidemiological studies [6].

Although AASV is a rare disease, it is the most common cause of RPGN and causes 4 % of all cases of end-stage renal failure (ESRF). It carries a significantly greater mortality rate than other autoimmune diseases and many malignancies. It is generally fatal if left untreated with a 1-year mortality rate of 90 %. Even with modern treatment regimens, 15 % of patients die within 1 year and 36 % by 5 years. Treatment of the disease with immunosuppressive therapy is itself associated with a high rate of adverse events, a recent study finding that death within 1 year of presentation was three times more likely to be attributable to an adverse event related to treatment than to active vasculitis [7].

The costs of managing this group of patients are disproportionate to the frequency of the condition. The average first year costs to the NHS of treating AASV is £8,000 and £4,000/annum thereafter (Jayne D, 2009 unpublished data). Permanent renal replacement therapy is required by 14 % of patients in the first year and in 21 % by 10 years.

Diagnosis of ANCA-Associated Vasculitis

The diagnosis of AASV requires a combination of clinical, radiological, serological and pathological features. The histological hallmark is necrotising small vessel vasculitis and this is still considered necessary for definitive diagnosis.

Renal involvement with rapidly progressive glomerulonephritis (RPGN) carries a high risk of progression to irreversible end-stage renal failure and is associated with a high risk of patient death if not treated promptly. It is therefore essential to make an early and accurate diagnosis of AASV so that appropriate treatment can be administered without delay. Rapid loss of renal function in association with clinical features of glomerulonephritis should be considered a medical emergency.

All patients with suspected RPGN should therefore have appropriate urgent serological investigation and be considered for renal biopsy to obtain histological confirmation of the diagnosis, i.e. evidence of acute glomerular injury associated with a pauci-immune, necrotising small vessel vasculitis in AASV. If the kidneys are not involved, every effort should be made to obtain a sample of affected tissue for histological analysis, although this is seldom rewarding in cases of isolated sino-nasal disease, in which the often observed absence of a positive ANCA test may lead to significant diagnostic uncertainty.

Use of ANCA Testing in Diagnosis

Indirect Immunofluorescence

ANCA were originally described by the staining pattern produced by autoantibodies to neutrophil cytoplasmic proteins, as detected by indirect immunofluorescence (IIF) using ethanol-fixed neutrophils. Two distinct patterns of staining were identified: cytoplasmic staining (c-ANCA) and perinuclear (p-ANCA) staining. Additional ANCA-staining patterns are now recognised including "atypical c-ANCA" (with homogenous flat cytoplasmic fluorescence) and combination p- and c-ANCA staining.

c-ANCA positivity correlates with antibodies to proteinase 3 (PR3), a serine protease enzyme, and is associated with GPA. p-ANCA positivity correlates with antibodies to myeloperoxidase (MPO), a lysosomal peroxidase enzyme, and is associated with MPA and EGPA. Both the PR3 and MPO antigens are expressed in neutrophil cytoplasmic granules.

Table 20.3 Potential pitfalls with the ANCA test

Test finding	Potential pitfalls
Positive p-ANCA	In addition to anti-MPO antibodies, may be observed in the presence of antibodies to lactoferrin, elastase, cathepsin G, catalase, bactericidal permeability inhibitor, lysozyme and beta-glucuronidase
Positive p-ANCA	May be confused with a positive ANA
Positive p-ANCA	Associated with non-vasculitic conditions, e.g. inflammatory bowel disease, cystic fibrosis, autoimmune hepatitis
Negative ANCA with clinical vasculitis	Relatively common with ENT limited disease; 10 % of multisystem disease is also ANCA-negative
Positive c-ANCA	Usually indicative of systemic vasculitis but may be seen in chronic cocaine use with nasal septum destruction

Most of these can be overcome by combining the immunofluorescence test with an ELISA for anti-PR3 and anti-MPO antibodies, which greatly increases the sensitivity and specificity

Staining of the perinuclear region by p-ANCA in patients with AASV and anti-MPO antibodies is an artefact of ethanol fixation (Table 20.3). This makes the neutrophil granule membranes permeable and results in a redistribution of positively charged cytoplasmic granular proteins, i.e. MPO, onto the surface of the negatively charged nucleus, resulting in a perinuclear staining pattern which outlines the neutrophil multilobed nucleus. By comparison, patients with PR3 antibodies have a c-ANCA-staining pattern where the nucleus appears as a "ghost" and the cytoplasm between the lobes of the neutrophil nucleus is accentuated (Fig. 20.2).

This artefactual perinuclear staining caused by antibodies to MPO in ethanol-fixed neutrophils may closely resemble the staining pattern produced by anti-nuclear (ANA) antibodies, resulting in a "false-positive" p-ANCA result. Equally, p-ANCA-positive patients who are also strongly positive for ANA antibodies may have the subtle perinuclear staining masked by strong homogenous nuclear staining produced by the ANA antibody.

Enzyme-Linked Immunosorbent Assay (ELISA)

ELISA should *always* be used to confirm the identity of the target antigen in patients with a p- or c-ANCA positive staining pattern on IIF and to quantify the antibody level as serial antibody titres can be helpful in monitoring disease activity and response to treatment. The International Consensus Statement [8] on testing and reporting of ANCA proposes that ANCA is best demonstrated in AASV by using a combination of IIF *and* ELISA that detect ANCA specific for PR3 or MPO. All patients with a suspected new diagnosis of AASV should have IIF performed on serum (which is very sensitive) and any demonstrating ANCA, either cytoplasmic fluorescence or an ANA staining pattern should then be tested in ELISA for PR3 and

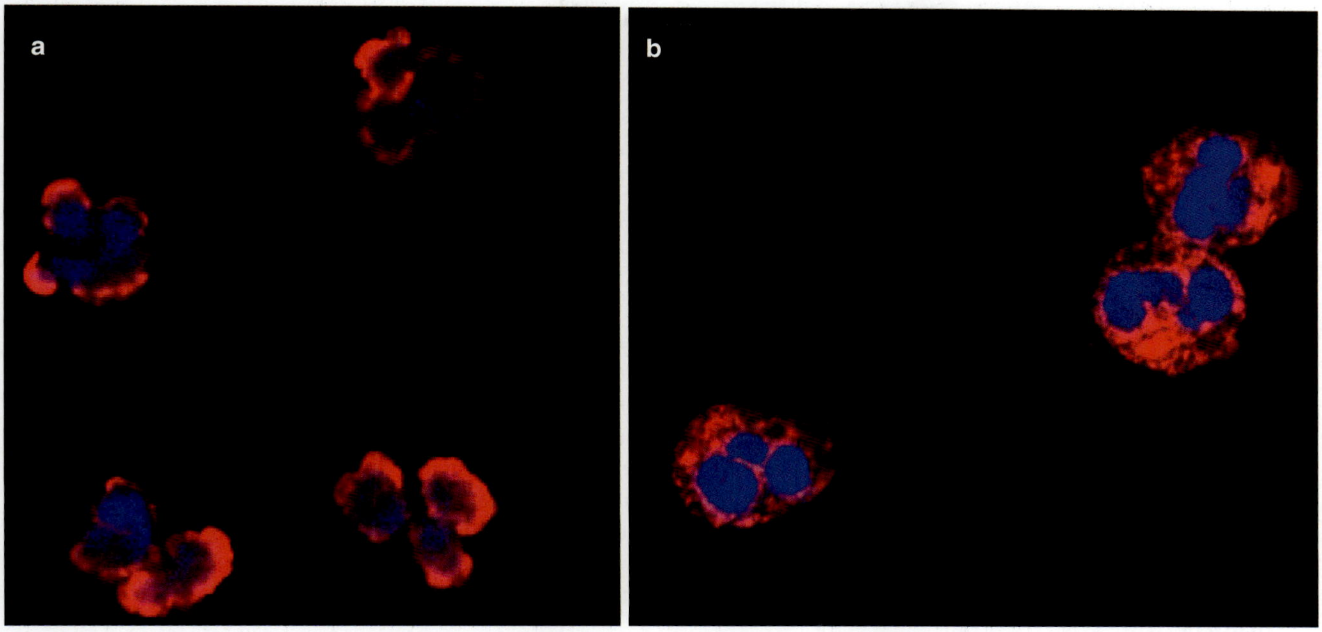

Fig. 20.2 Indirect immunofluorescence demonstrating c-ANCA and p-ANCA-staining patterns. (**a**) Perinuclear staining seen with p-ANCA. (**b**) Cytoplasmic staining seen with c-ANCA

MPO (which is very specific) to confirm the identity of the autoantigen.

Positive IIF alone is not specific for the diagnosis of GPA or MPA. However, when serological testing for ANCA combines IIF with ELISA specific for PR3 or MPO, the diagnostic specificity for ANCA-associated disease is close to 100 % in the appropriate clinical setting [9]. However, a significant number of patients with small vessel vasculitis, particularly those with disease limited to the nose and sinuses (and about 10 % of those with renal disease), are negative for ANCA (using combined testing with IIF and ELISA). Therefore, the overall sensitivity of combined serological testing for ANCA in patients with idiopathic, pauci-immune, small vessel vasculitis is 65–75 %.

False-positive ANCA results can occur in patients with (1) chronic infection (e.g. TB, HIV, infective endocarditis), (2) malignancies (e.g. lymphoma), (3) inflammatory bowel disease and, most notably, (4) chronic cocaine use. In fact, the main differential diagnosis of isolated destructive nasal lesions is chronic cocaine use. Therefore, decisions about treatment should not be based solely on the ANCA results: clinical, pathological and radiological features should all be considered, in addition to serological testing, to establish the correct diagnosis and guide appropriate treatment.

Renal Biopsy

A positive c-ANCA or p-ANCA result (using combined serological testing as above) in the context of clinical evidence of RPGN with active urinary sediment provides sufficient evidence to diagnose probable AASV and initiate treatment, and treatment must not be delayed in this context. However, renal biopsy is useful to:

1. Confirm the diagnosis of pauci-immune focal necrotising glomerulonephritis (i.e. associated with the paucity of immune deposits on immunofluorescence and/or electron microscopy)
2. Establish the activity and extent of glomerulonephritis
3. Assess the degree of chronic irreversible glomerular, interstitial and tubular damage, all of which will influence management with respect to the choice and intensity of induction immunosuppressive therapy

Classification of Disease Severity

At presentation, patients should have a clear assessment of disease severity in order to guide appropriate induction therapy. The EULAR recommendations on the management of AASV suggest that disease severity should be assessed according to the EUVAS categorisation system in order to guide treatment decisions (Table 20.4). Using this categorisation system, the EUVAS group have conducted a number of clinical trials to establish the most effective immunosuppression regimen for induction and maintenance of remission in patients with AASV (see section "Management").

During follow-up, it is important that patients' symptoms are attributed correctly to either current disease activity or organ damage in order to guide appropriate treatment. Given the rarity of AASV, patients should ideally receive expert assessment from specialists in dedicated vasculitis centres using standardised assessment tools to assess disease activity

Table 20.4 EUVAS disease categorisation of ANCA-associated vasculitis

Category	Defining features
Localised	Upper and/or lower respiratory tract disease without any other systemic involvement of constitutional symptoms
Early systemic	Any, without organ-threatening or life-threatening disease
Generalised	Renal or other organ-threatening disease, serum creatinine <500 μmol/L (5.6 mg/dL)
Severe	Renal or other vital organ failure, serum creatinine >500 μmol/L (5.6 mg/dL)
Refractory	Progressive disease unresponsive to glucocorticoids and cyclophosphamide

and damage, i.e. the Birmingham Vasculitis Activity Score (BVAS) and the Vasculitis Damage Index (VDI). (http://www.epsnetwork.co.uk/BVAS/bvas_flow.html)

Pathology

AASV is characterised histologically by necrotising small vessel vasculitis. Renal involvement by the vasculitic process results in fibrinoid necrosis of glomerular capillaries and arterioles supplying the glomerular tuft with consequent inflammatory glomerular necrosis and crescent formation (Fig. 20.3). Early lesions demonstrate segmental glomerular necrosis with or without adjacent small crescents. This may progress to global glomerular necrosis with large circumferential crescents in acute, severe disease. Glomerular capillaries rupture at sites of fibrinoid necrosis resulting in haemorrhage into Bowman's space, microscopic haematuria and the clinical appearance of urinary red cell casts. Patients with MPA tend to display more chronic, scarred lesions than those with GPA, perhaps reflecting the more frequent delay in diagnosis in the absence of granulomatous lesions.

Renal involvement in AASV is differentiated histologically from other causes of acute glomerulonephritis by the relative paucity or absence of glomerular deposits of immunoglobulin or complement demonstrated by immunofluorescent staining or electron microscopy (hence, the term "pauci-immune" vasculitis). It is also often possible to distinguish severe glomerulonephritis due to AASV from that due to anti-glomerular basement membrane disease by the focal nature of the glomerular lesion: it is not uncommon to find an entirely normal appearing glomerulus adjacent to one that has been completely destroyed, whereas other causes of RPGN tend to affect all glomeruli more or less equally. In addition, the glomerular lesions in AASV may vary significantly in age, with acute lesions interspersed with globally sclerosed glomeruli.

Fibrinoid necrosis of small vessels also occurs in other organs, resulting in tissue ischaemia which causes a range of other clinical manifestations. For example, alveolar capillaritis in the lung may result in pulmonary haemorrhage, inflammation of dermal venules in the skin results causes a palpable purpuric rash and involvement of epineural arteries causes a mononeuritis multiplex. The perivascular inflammatory infiltrate comprises neutrophils, macrophages and T cells; an infiltrate composed primarily of eosinophils ("eosinophilic vasculitis") is diagnostic of EGPA.

Patients with GPA and EGPA also display necrotising granulomatous inflammation. This is characterised by zones of tissue necrosis surrounded by a mixed inflammatory infiltrate consisting of neutrophils, lymphocytes, monocytes, macrophages and multinucleated giant cells. This inflammatory process causes tissue destruction in the upper respiratory tract in patients with GPA, resulting in sinusitis, conductive hearing loss and nasal deformity due to destruction of the cartilaginous nasal septum. Eosinophils may also be seen in the inflammatory infiltrate in these granulomatous lesions in both GPA and EGPA but are usually more prominent in the latter.

Pathogenesis

The aetiology of AASV is not fully understood. It is considered to be an autoimmune disease given the association with ANCA: autoantibodies directed against enzymes (PR3 and MPO) stored in the granules and lysosomes of neutrophils and monocytes.

Environmental Factors

Environmental factors are considered important in disease pathogenesis, as is infection and exposure to certain drugs.

Silica Exposure

Exposure to silica dust has been associated with a number of autoimmune disorders including AASV. Case–control studies suggest that 22–46 % of patients with AASV have previously been exposed to silica and there is an association between AASV and jobs such as farming, sandblasting, textile work and drilling, which are associated with high exposure to crystalline silica dust [10, 11]. Interestingly there was a significant rise in the incidence of AASV in the aftermath of the Kobe earthquake in 1996, and this has been attributed to the large quantities of silica and other industrial dusts released from the destroyed buildings.

The mechanism by which silica triggers AASV is not known but silica induces apoptosis of neutrophils in a dose-dependent manner [12] and silica may trigger an inflammatory reaction through accelerated apoptosis of neutrophils and alveolar macrophages. MPO released by neutrophils can

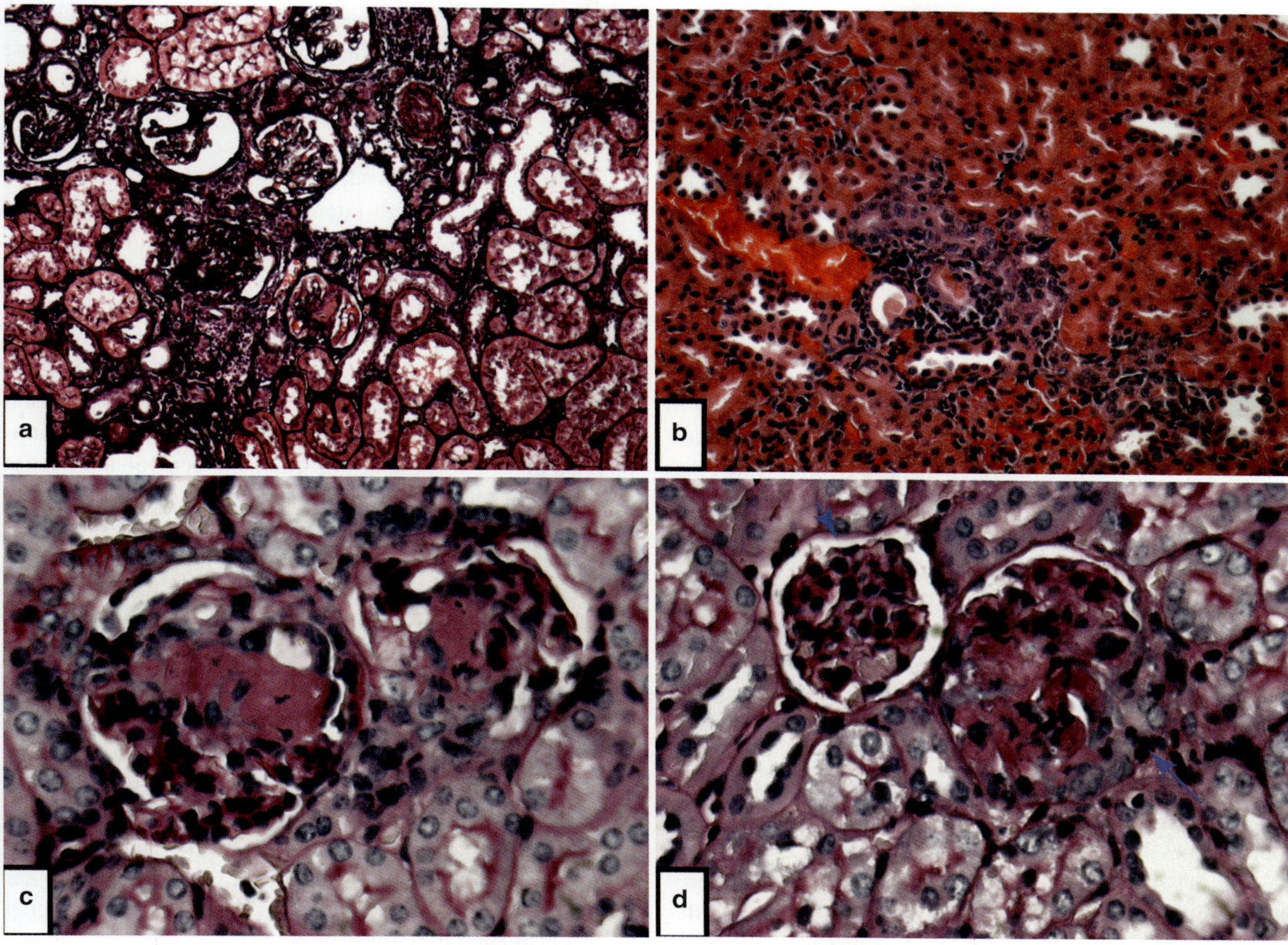

Fig. 20.3 Silver methenamine (**a**) and H&E (**b–d**) stains of renal biopsy specimens demonstrating histopathological features of AASV. (**a**) Glomerular sclerosis and collapse suggesting chronic, irreversible inflammation and scarring. (**b**) Interstitial inflammatory infiltrate with "tubulitis" and associated tubular epithelial damage. (**c**) Segmental necrotising glomerulonephritis with fibrinoid necrosis and periglomerular leucocyte infiltration. (**d**) Severe glomerular inflammation with segmental necrosis and "cellular crescent" (*arrow*) consisting of epithelial and inflammatory cells occupying Bowman's space. Note: comparatively normal neighbouring glomerulus (*arrow head*), emphasising focal nature of glomerular involvement in AASV

be taken up by activated alveolar macrophages and may be presented to T- and B-lymphocytes resulting in the development of anti-MPO antibodies and AASV [13].

Bacterial Infections

Bacterial infections, particularly with *Staphylococcus aureus*, have been associated with disease relapse in GPA. Patients with chronic nasal carriage of *S. aureus* are more likely to have disease relapses [14], and there is evidence that maintenance treatment with co-trimoxazole can reduce the frequency of disease relapse by 60 % in patients with GPA and granulomatous inflammation of the upper respiratory tract [15].

There is some evidence that patients with PR3-ANCA vasculitis have antibodies to complementary PR3 (cPR3, the peptide translated from the anti-sense DNA strand of the PR3 gene), as well as to the autoantigen PR3, found in the granules of neutrophils [16], although these findings have not been reproduced in other studies [17]. Peptides from cPR3 share strong homology with peptides from *S. aureus* and other infectious pathogens. It has therefore been proposed that infection with *S. aureus* may induce cPR3 antibodies and, subsequently, PR3-ANCAs by means of an antibody idiotypic network [13, 18].

Additional evidence for the role for infection and molecular mimicry with microbial peptides in the pathogenesis of AASV comes from the observation that 90 % of patients with active focal necrotising glomerulonephritis have intermittent autoantibodies to lysosomal membrane protein-2 (LAMP-2). These antibodies cross react with FimH, a bacterial adhesin which shares 100 % homology with an epitope of human LAMP-2. Infections with fimbriated pathogens (e.g. *E. coli* and *K. pneumoniae*) may therefore induce production of autoantibodies to LAMP-2 through molecular mimicry which may have a pathogenic role in the development of FNGN.

Drugs

A number of drugs have been associated with the development of ANCA and subsequent AASV, most notably propylthiouracil. Others include hydralazine, D-penicillamine and minocycline.

Role of ANCA in the Pathogenesis of AASV

There is increasing evidence from clinical, in vitro and in vivo studies that ANCA have a pathogenic role in the development of AASV. Numerous studies have demonstrated that ANCA activate neutrophils inappropriately and animal model work has proven that anti-MPO antibodies can cause systemic vasculitis in mice and rats.

Perhaps the most convincing evidence comes from a case report describing the development of pulmonary haemorrhage and glomerulonephritis associated with elevated MPO-ANCA titres in a neonate thought to be caused by transplacental transfer of IgG MPO-ANCA from a mother with active MPA [19].

Disease activity correlates well with ANCA titres in some patients with AASV [20] with some longitudinal observational studies suggesting that clinical remission is associated with falling ANCA titres, and increasing ANCA titres predict clinical relapse with a sensitivity of 79 % and a specificity of 68 % [13]. This is considered to provide supportive evidence of the pathogenic role of these antibodies, although much controversy exists in this area [13, 21–23] and there is no sufficient evidence to support the use of ANCA titre alone as a guide to therapy. Indeed, some patients can attain full clinical remission in the face of persistently elevated ANCA levels.

There is evidence from randomised trials that plasma exchange (which removes circulating IgG ANCA) and rituximab (monoclonal anti-CD20 antibody which depletes peripheral B cells) are effective in treating severe AASV. Treatment with rituximab is associated with a decline in ANCA titres and observational studies suggest that reconstitution of peripheral B cells may precede clinical relapse. The efficacy of these treatments, which are targeted at antibody removal, provides indirect evidence of the pathogenic role of ANCA in AASV.

Management

Morbidity and mortality is a result both of the destructive, inflammatory disease process itself and of the high-intensity immunosuppression required to induce and maintain remission of this disease. AASV, particularly GPA, is characteristically a relapsing disease with each relapse causing more destructive inflammation and organ damage. Hence, most patients with AASV require long-term immunosuppression to maintain remission, although the optimal duration of treatment is unknown.

Treatment of AASV is divided into two phases:

- *Induction* with high-intensity immunosuppression to induce remission as quickly as possible and avoid irreversible organ damage
- *Maintenance* of remission with lower intensity immunosuppression to prevent disease flares whilst minimising adverse effects of the treatment itself

Evidence-based management of AASV with significant renal involvement (generalised and severe disease) is summarised in an algorithm in Fig. 20.4, and general approaches are described in the following sections. Table 20.5 shows "Tips of the trade" in managing systemic vasculitis.

Induction Therapy

Conventional treatment of active AASV with renal involvement, aiming to induce disease remission, comprises high-dose corticosteroids and cyclophosphamide (CYP). This regimen induces remission in up to 80 % of patients but is associated with significant toxicity and infectious complications. Therefore, a number of clinical trials have been performed to establish effective treatment regimens using other immunosuppressive agents, with the aim of reducing treatment-related toxicity.

Generalised Disease

Patients with AASV presenting with generalised disease (see categorisation in Table 20.2) should receive induction therapy with oral prednisolone combined with CYP or rituximab [24]. The intensity and duration of induction therapy is an important factor in determining the risk of subsequent relapse. For example, pulsed cyclophosphamide regimens employ approximately half the dose of oral regimens [25]; this is associated with equivalent rates of remission but higher long-term relapse rates [26]. It is probable that most patients will do well with lower cumulative dose-pulsed CYP, although those at high risk of frequent relapses (anti-PR3 positive and/or large granulomatous disease burden) may benefit from a daily oral induction CYP regimen. The choice between rituximab and cyclophosphamide is guided by desire to protect fertility, perceived patient frailty or injured bone marrow (those at high risk of adverse events may do better not receiving cyclophosphamide, although clinical trials of rituximab have disappointingly failed to provide robust evidence in favour of this presumed safety benefit). Three months of intensive therapy with CYP following induction of remission is sufficient in the vast majority of cases.

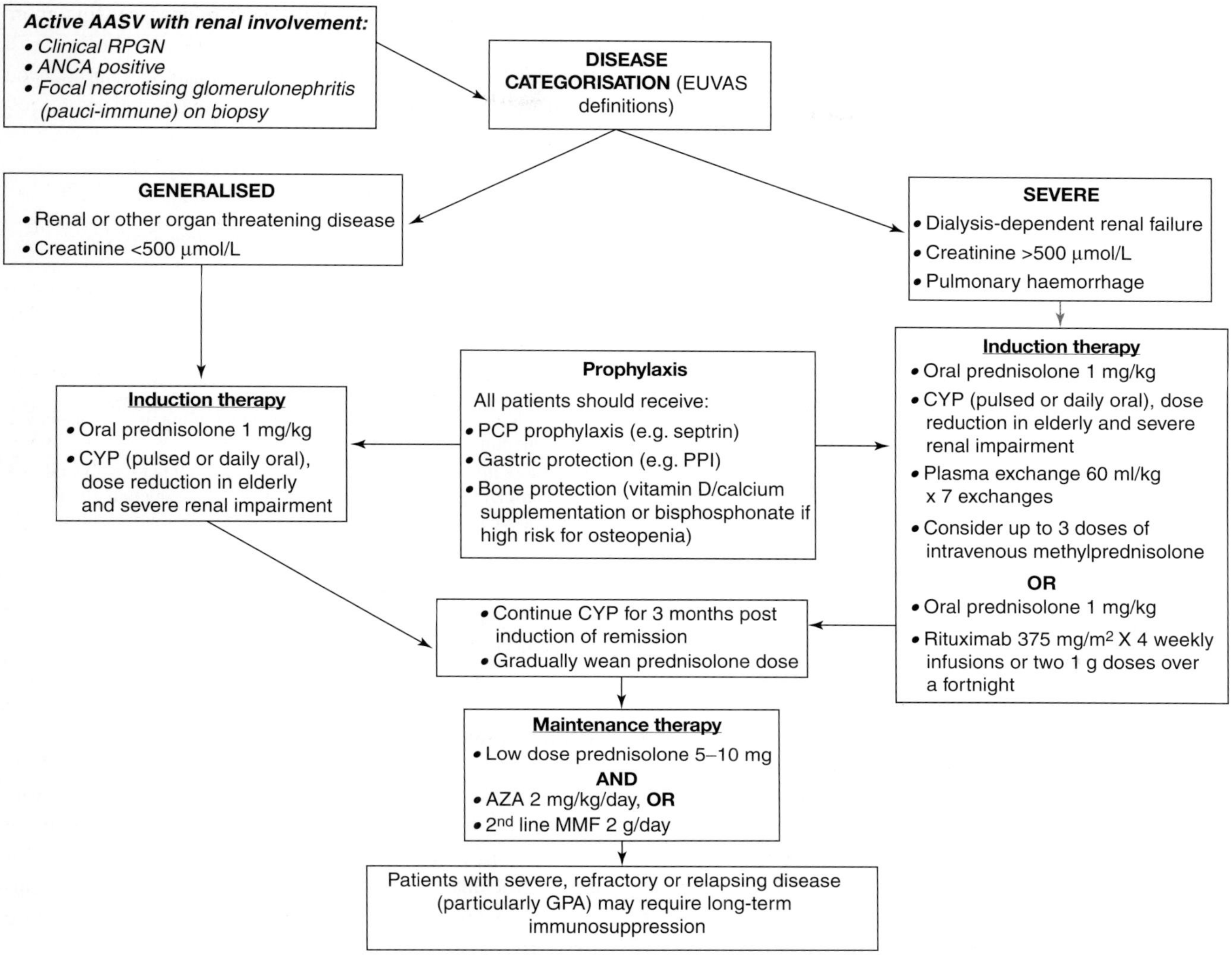

Fig. 20.4 Algorithm for management of generalised and severe AASV. *RPGN* rapidly progressive glomerulonephritis, *PPI* proton-pump inhibitor, *AZA* azathioprine, *CYP* cyclophosphamide, *MMF* mycophenolate mofetil, *PCP* pneumocystis (carinii) jiroveci pneumoniae, *GPA* granulomatosis with polyangiitis

Severe Disease

Patients presenting with dialysis-dependent renal failure, Cr>500 μmol/L or pulmonary haemorrhage may benefit from adjunctive therapy in addition to standard treatment with oral CYP and steroids, including:

- High-dose IV methylprednisolone (3 daily doses at 10–15 mg/kg)
- Plasma exchange (60 mL/kg × 7 exchanges)
- Rituximab (375 mg/m^2 per week for 4 weeks or two doses of 1 g over a fortnight)

The rationale for plasma exchange and rituximab is partially based on their antibody-depleting properties, which makes theoretical sense given the evidence for the pathogenic role of circulating ANCA. The full benefit, however, is clearly as a result of additional, more complex mechanisms. Their use is now supported by robust trial data. The MEPEX trial supported a benefit of plasma exchange over high-dose methylprednisolone [27], although this clear benefit has disappeared on long-term follow-up. Of note, no trial has examined the use of combined plasma exchange and high-dose methylprednisolone, a practice that is employed frequently in many centres in severely ill patients.

Unlike those with anti-GBM disease, patients presenting with dialysis-dependent renal failure often achieve renal recovery and independence from dialysis with appropriate high-intensity immunosuppression. However, there is a clear need to balance the risk of treatment-related toxicity with the potential benefit of organ recovery and histology on renal biopsy that is useful in assessing this risk/benefit ratio [28]. Severe tubular atrophy and a low percentage of normal glom-

Table 20.5 "Tips of the trade" in managing systemic vasculitis

Scenario	Salutary tips
A patient presenting with fever, systemic illness and positive anti-MPO serology	Look very carefully for endocarditis and tuberculosis: multiple blood cultures and echocardiography
Intensive induction therapy of a patient with dialysis requiring renal failure	Once the GFR drops below 15 mL/min, the risk of adverse event risk rises rapidly. If adverse events start accumulating, *pull back on therapy rapidly*
Young woman with dialysis requiring renal vasculitis who wants to maintain fertility	Consider using rituximab in place of CYP but do not compromise on therapy intensity; the priority is to recover renal function
Very scarred kidney in a patient requiring dialysis	Early withdrawal of immunosuppression but *beware of extrarenal disease*
Rapidly progressive renal vasculitis with lung disease	Measure anti-GBM antibodies as well as ANCA, up to 30 % of anti-MPO patients are also anti-GBM positive
ENT clinic	Introduce routine urine dipstick testing for patients with sino-nasal disease to pick up glomerulonephritis in a timely fashion
Multidisciplinary clinics	AASV affects many organs and patients probably have improved outcomes if cared for in a clinic setting that attempts to join up various services, such as rheumatology, nephrology, ENT, clinical psychology and immunology. This may involve running a joint clinic
Pulsed intravenous CYP	This is logistically more difficult to deliver than daily oral CYP but has several advantages: lower cumulative dose with equivalent remission induction efficacy and improved compliance (you know the patient has received it). It is worth setting up the infrastructure required
Want to use pulsed therapy but logistically difficult in a given unit	Oral pulses (given over 3 days) are probably as effective as intravenous
Rising ANCA in an asymptomatic patient	Increase vigilance to look for any evidence of new organ dysfunction; treat the clinical features, not the blood test

eruli on renal biopsy should prompt caution in administering high-intensity immunosuppression as the risk of treatment-related mortality likely exceeds the potential benefit in these patients.

Early Systemic Disease

Methotrexate (MTX) may be used with similar efficacy to CYP in the treatment of early systemic AASV without significant renal disease (serum creatinine <150 μmol/L). The NORAM trial [29] demonstrated reduced treatment-related toxicity with MTX but higher relapse rates compared to CYP. Patients should receive rescue therapy with folic acid to minimise MTX toxicity.

Standard Prophylaxis

All patients receiving induction immunosuppression for AASV should receive standard prophylaxis to minimise infection complications, gastric ulceration and bone resorption including:

- Trimethoprim/sulphamethoxazole (Septrin)
- Gastric protection agent, e.g. proton-pump inhibitor (PPI)
- Calcium/vitamin D supplementation

These medications should be administered as part of the induction therapy regimen in all patients. In women who wish to maximise subsequent fertility, ovarian protection with a GnRH agonist such as goserelin is employed by some centres, although without strong evidence to support the practice. Similarly, sperm banking can be used in younger men, if this can be arranged without delaying the induction therapy.

Maintenance Therapy

Up to 50 % of patients with AASV will relapse, despite appropriate high-intensity induction therapy. Maintenance therapy aims to reduce the risk of disease relapse whilst minimising the adverse events associated with long-term immunosuppression. Therapy generally consists of low-dose prednisolone with a second steroid-sparing agent:

- Azathioprine (2 mg/kg/day)
- Methotrexate (0.3 mg/kg/week increasing to 25 mg weekly) if tolerated.
- Mycophenolate mofetil (2 g/day)

The optimum duration of maintenance immunosuppression remains unclear. In general, given the relapsing nature of AASV, it should be continued for at least 2 years, although some centres stop after 6 months, and it may be required indefinitely in patients with frequent relapses.

Azathioprine is now widely used for maintenance therapy. It is as effective as CYP at maintaining remission and is a less toxic drug (CYCAZAREM trial [30]).

Methotrexate is as effective as azathioprine at maintaining disease remission and associated with a similar rate of adverse events [31]. It is contraindicated in patients with significant renal impairment and is therefore more frequently used as maintenance therapy in localised and early systemic disease.

Mycophenolate mofetil (MMF) has been used in AASV as maintenance therapy but data from the IMPROVE trial [32] suggest it is less effective (as well as being much more expensive) than azathioprine in maintaining disease remission, but associated with a similar rate of adverse events. It is recommended as second-line maintenance therapy in relapsing disease or patients intolerant of azathioprine.

In those patients that received rituximab induction therapy, a default scenario of remission maintenance using repeated dosing every 6–9 months is emerging. There are concerns regarding repeated use of rituximab, notably progressive hypogammaglobulinemia and a possible increased risk of progressive multifocal leukoencephalopathy. However, overall this appears to be a safe and effective strategy that is currently undergoing formal testing.

Patients with GPA with localised upper respiratory tract disease should receive trimethoprim/sulphamethoxazole (Septrin) in addition to other maintenance therapy as there is evidence that this decreases the frequency of disease relapse [15]. Treatment guidelines and links to current active trials are maintained on the EUVAS website (http://www.vasculitis.org).

Special Considerations

The Elderly or Frail Patient

Not surprisingly, the elderly have significantly higher early mortality rates in AASV compared to younger patients. In fact, age and serum creatinine at diagnosis are by far the strongest independent predictors of death and elderly patients are at particular risk of treatment-related toxicity. Therefore, the risk/benefit ratio of high-intensity treatment vs. the potential benefit of organ and patient survival should be considered prior to administration of induction therapy. Treatment regimens in most of the EUVAS trials used dose reduction of up to 50 % in those >70 years. It is worth noting that the risk/benefit equation almost always weighs on the side of administering some immunosuppression (rather than none) and that elderly patients also have a high risk of morbidity and death if they require long-term dialysis therapy.

The Young Woman Wishing to Have a Family

Women of child-bearing age may wish to avoid cyclophosphamide as prolonged exposure is associated with infertility. In these patients, rituximab may be used in preference to cyclophosphamide as part of induction therapy. However, the risk of infertility is smaller with modern low cumulative dose CYP regimens, compared to when the drug was administered for several years, and it is important to emphasise strongly the profound effect that severe chronic renal failure has on fertility. Most women who recover renal function after receiving CYP as treatment for vasculitis will subsequently be able to bear children. It is important not to compromise on treatment intensity when managing a young woman with severe systemic vasculitis.

The Septic Patient

The patient who presents with active AASV and coincident infection is extremely challenging to manage. Firstly, it is critical to ensure that the AASV is not occurring secondary to the infection. This is particularly true of patients with infectious endocarditis. In practice, this means treating both conditions and keeping an open mind as the condition evolves, with frequent reassessment of the vasculitis activity and spread of infection. If a suspicion lingers that the episode of vasculitis was secondary to infection, it may be possible to carefully withdraw immunosuppression early after the infection has been cured, with very close monitoring of vasculitis activity. In those who are overtly septic, intense immunosuppression is likely to lead to patient death from overwhelming sepsis. In these cases, intravenous immunoglobulin therapy (1–2 g/kg) may suppress vasculitis activity without compromising the immune response to the infection.

The Vasculitis Unit

AASV is a complex multisystem rare disease and consequently falls prey to many of the factors that hamper care in other rare diseases:

- Lack of awareness among clinicians leading to a delay in diagnosis
- Lack of access to the most recently developed therapies and diagnostic tools
- Poorly coordinated care with inadequate communication and integration between the specialties that a patient with vasculitis will encounter
- Requirement for the patient to travel to numerous clinics at different times
- Lack of ancillary support, such as clinical psychology and social work

Therefore, there is a strong rationale for the development of regional centres of excellence linked to local units ("hub and spoke" model) at which a patient can attend for a "one-stop shop" assessment with access to a multidisciplinary team. This includes:

- Ready access to ENT assessment with nasendoscopy
- An infusional therapy unit for administering CYP (with appropriate governance to ensure this is delivered safely)
- Respiratory team input with ability to provide rapid access to bronchoscopy
- Dermatology with facilities for diagnostic skin biopsy
- Ready access to neurology and facilities for sural nerve biopsy
- Excellent immunology services, with rapid turnaround of serological tests

The key person in coordinating such a clinical service efficiently and acting as a first port of call for patients is the clinical nurse specialist, who, with the assistance of carefully designed algorithmic protocols, would be able to manage the immunotherapy, provide initial clinical assessments and coordinate multi-specialist input. Procedures should be in place for recording the amount and type of immunosuppression delivered to an individual patient. This provides the capability to calculate cumulative CYP dose received and to audit the use of expensive biologic agents. The principal factor in determining treatment of relapsing vasculitis is the cumulative dose of CYP received previously.

References

1. Jennette JC, et al. Nomenclature of systemic vasculitides. Proposal of an international consensus conference. Arthritis Rheum. 1994;37(2):187–92.
2. Fries JF, et al. The American College of Rheumatology 1990 criteria for the classification of vasculitis. Summary. Arthritis Rheum. 1990;33(8):1135–6.
3. Watts R, et al. Development and validation of a consensus methodology for the classification of the ANCA-associated vasculitides and polyarteritis nodosa for epidemiological studies. Ann Rheum Dis. 2007;66(2):222–7.
4. Lane SE, et al. Primary systemic vasculitis: clinical features and mortality. QJM. 2005;98(2):97–111.
5. Watts RA, et al. Epidemiology of systemic vasculitis: a ten-year study in the United Kingdom. Arthritis Rheum. 2000;43(2):414–9.
6. Aries PM, et al. No seasonal variation in the onset of symptoms of 445 patients with Wegener's granulomatosis. Arthritis Rheum. 2008;59(6):904.
7. Little MA, et al. Early mortality in systemic vasculitis: relative contribution of adverse events and active vasculitis. Ann Rheum Dis. 2010;69(6):1036–43.
8. Savige J, et al. International consensus statement on testing and reporting of antineutrophil cytoplasmic antibodies (ANCA). Am J Clin Pathol. 1999;111(4):507–13.
9. Hagen EC, et al. Diagnostic value of standardized assays for anti-neutrophil cytoplasmic antibodies in idiopathic systemic vasculitis. EC/BCR Project for ANCA Assay Standardization. Kidney Int. 1998;53(3):743–53.
10. Beaudreuil S, et al. Occupational exposure in ANCA-positive patients: a case–control study. Kidney Int. 2005;67(5):1961–6.
11. Hogan SL, et al. Silica exposure in anti-neutrophil cytoplasmic autoantibody-associated glomerulonephritis and lupus nephritis. J Am Soc Nephrol. 2001;12(1):134–42.
12. Leigh J, et al. Silica-induced apoptosis in alveolar and granulomatous cells in vivo. Environ Health Perspect. 1997;105 Suppl 5:1241–5.
13. Chen M, Kallenberg CG. ANCA-associated vasculitides – advances in pathogenesis and treatment. Nat Rev Rheumatol. 2010;6(11):653–64.
14. Stegeman CA, et al. Association of chronic nasal carriage of Staphylococcus aureus and higher relapse rates in Wegener granulomatosis. Ann Intern Med. 1994;120(1):12–7.
15. Stegeman CA, et al. Trimethoprim-sulfamethoxazole (co-trimoxazole) for the prevention of relapses of Wegener's granulomatosis. Dutch Co-Trimoxazole Wegener Study Group. N Engl J Med. 1996;335(1):16–20.
16. Pendergraft 3rd WF, et al. Autoimmunity is triggered by cPR-3(105–201), a protein complementary to human autoantigen proteinase-3. Nat Med. 2004;10(1):72–9.
17. Tadema H, et al. Reactivity against complementary proteinase-3 is not increased in patients with PR3-ANCA-associated vasculitis. PLoS One. 2011;6(3):e17972.
18. Kallenberg CG, Tadema H. Vasculitis and infections: contribution to the issue of autoimmunity reviews devoted to "autoimmunity and infection". Autoimmun Rev. 2008;8(1):29–32.
19. Bansal PJ, Tobin MC. Neonatal microscopic polyangiitis secondary to transfer of maternal myeloperoxidase-antineutrophil cytoplasmic antibody resulting in neonatal pulmonary hemorrhage and renal involvement. Ann Allergy Asthma Immunol. 2004;93(4):398–401.
20. Boomsma MM, et al. Prediction of relapses in Wegener's granulomatosis by measurement of antineutrophil cytoplasmic antibody levels: a prospective study. Arthritis Rheum. 2000;43(9):2025–33.
21. Birck R, et al. Serial ANCA determinations for monitoring disease activity in patients with ANCA-associated vasculitis: systematic review. Am J Kidney Dis. 2006;47(1):15–23.
22. Kerr GS, et al. Limited prognostic value of changes in antineutrophil cytoplasmic antibody titer in patients with Wegener's granulomatosis. Arthritis Rheum. 1993;36(3):365–71.
23. Stegeman CA. Anti-neutrophil cytoplasmic antibody (ANCA) levels directed against proteinase-3 and myeloperoxidase are helpful in predicting disease relapse in ANCA-associated small-vessel vasculitis. Nephrol Dial Transplant. 2002;17(12):2077–80.
24. Stone JH, et al. Rituximab versus cyclophosphamide for ANCA-associated vasculitis. N Engl J Med. 2010;363(3):221–32.
25. de Groot K, et al. Pulse versus daily oral cyclophosphamide for induction of remission in antineutrophil cytoplasmic antibody-associated vasculitis: a randomized trial. Ann Intern Med. 2009;150(10):670–80.
26. Harper L, et al. Pulse versus daily oral cyclophosphamide for induction of remission in ANCA-associated vasculitis: long-term follow-up. Ann Rheum Dis. 2012;71:955–60.
27. Jayne DR, et al. Randomized trial of plasma exchange or high-dosage methylprednisolone as adjunctive therapy for severe renal vasculitis. J Am Soc Nephrol. 2007;18(7):2180–8.
28. de Lind van Wijngaarden RA, et al. Chances of renal recovery for dialysis-dependent ANCA-associated glomerulonephritis. J Am Soc Nephrol. 2007;18(7):2189–97.
29. De Groot K, et al. Randomized trial of cyclophosphamide versus methotrexate for induction of remission in early systemic antineutrophil cytoplasmic antibody-associated vasculitis. Arthritis Rheum. 2005;52(8):2461–9.
30. Jayne D, et al. A randomized trial of maintenance therapy for vasculitis associated with antineutrophil cytoplasmic autoantibodies. N Engl J Med. 2003;349(1):36–44.
31. Pagnoux C, et al. Azathioprine or methotrexate maintenance for ANCA-associated vasculitis. N Engl J Med. 2008;359(26):2790–803.
32. Hiemstra TF, et al. Mycophenolate mofetil vs azathioprine for remission maintenance in antineutrophil cytoplasmic antibody-associated vasculitis: a randomized controlled trial. JAMA. 2010;304(21):2381–8.

Goodpasture's or Anti-glomerular Basement Membrane (GBM) Disease

21

Alan D. Salama

Goodpasture's disease is the term for a pulmonary-renal syndrome associated with rapidly progressive glomerulonephritis* and anti-glomerular basement (GBM) membrane antibodies and is used alongside the term anti-GBM disease. The eponym was coined by Stanton and Tange in 1958 after their report of patients with the condition and their recognition that they were similar to the cases published 37 years earlier by Ernest Goodpasture, an American pathologist who described the clinical constellation of pulmonary haemorrhage and renal failure, during the 1918–1919 influenza pandemic. In the USA, Goodpasture's syndrome is often used to refer to any cause of pulmonary-renal syndrome while Goodpasture's disease is limited to those patients with anti-GBM antibodies.

Goodpasture's disease is a rare, rapidly progressive autoimmune condition leading to acute kidney injury and lung haemorrhage. It is vitally important to make a rapid diagnosis as early recognition and treatment can lead to significantly better clinical outcomes. Delayed therapy may make renal recovery unlikely and can be associated with significantly greater morbidity and higher mortality. There are many examples of delay in treatment resulting in irreversible renal failure, and it is thus critical to have robust processes for rapid diagnosis, transfer and treatment.

Clinical Features

Goodpasture's disease has a bimodal distribution with peaks of incidence in the third and sixth decades and has a slight male predominance [1]. It generally presents with a rapidly progressive decline in renal function in association with pulmonary haemorrhage in over half the patients, most frequently smokers (see Fig. 21.1) [2].

A.D. Salama, MA, PhD, FRCP
UCL Centre for Nephrology, Royal Free Hospital, Rowland Hill Street, London NW3 2PF, UK
e-mail: a.salama@ucl.ac.uk

> Rapidly progressive glomerulonephritis denotes a precipitous decline in renal function (doubling of creatinine) in less than 3 months due to crescentic glomerulonephritis.

While isolated glomerulonephritis is well recognised, it can also rarely present as isolated pulmonary haemorrhage, although urinary abnormalities may be detected if looked for carefully. Patients have limited systemic features, which mostly relate to anaemia and renal impairment and manifest as generalised fatigue or malaise but in some cases weight loss may also be found. This is in contrast to the main differential diagnosis of systemic anti-neutrophil cytoplasm antibody (ANCA)-associated vasculitis, in which systemic features are much more common (see Table 21.1).

Goodpasture's disease may present with complete anuria, in up to a fifth of cases [3] and this symptom should raise suspicion of the diagnosis (along with consideration of outflow obstruction and renal venous or arterial thrombosis). Rarely patients may present with macroscopic haematuria or loin pain related to renal oedema. Despite the target autoantigen being found in the lung, kidney, ear, eye and brain, symptoms are generally limited to the pulmonary-renal systems.

Goodpasture's disease rarely relapses, unlike ANCA-associated vasculitis, and in those few cases that do, there is more frequently a relapse of pulmonary haemorrhage in those with provoking factors such as infection or fluid overload or recurrent exposure to factors such as smoking or solvents/hydrocarbons [4, 5].

Epidemiology

Goodpasture's disease is 10–20 times less common than systemic ANCA-associated vasculitis, with an incidence of 0.5–1 cases/million population. However, it accounts for almost a fifth of the cases of rapidly progressive glomerulonephritis. It is common in white populations, but is clearly

M. Harber (ed.), *Practical Nephrology*,
DOI 10.1007/978-1-4471-5547-8_21, © Springer-Verlag London 2014

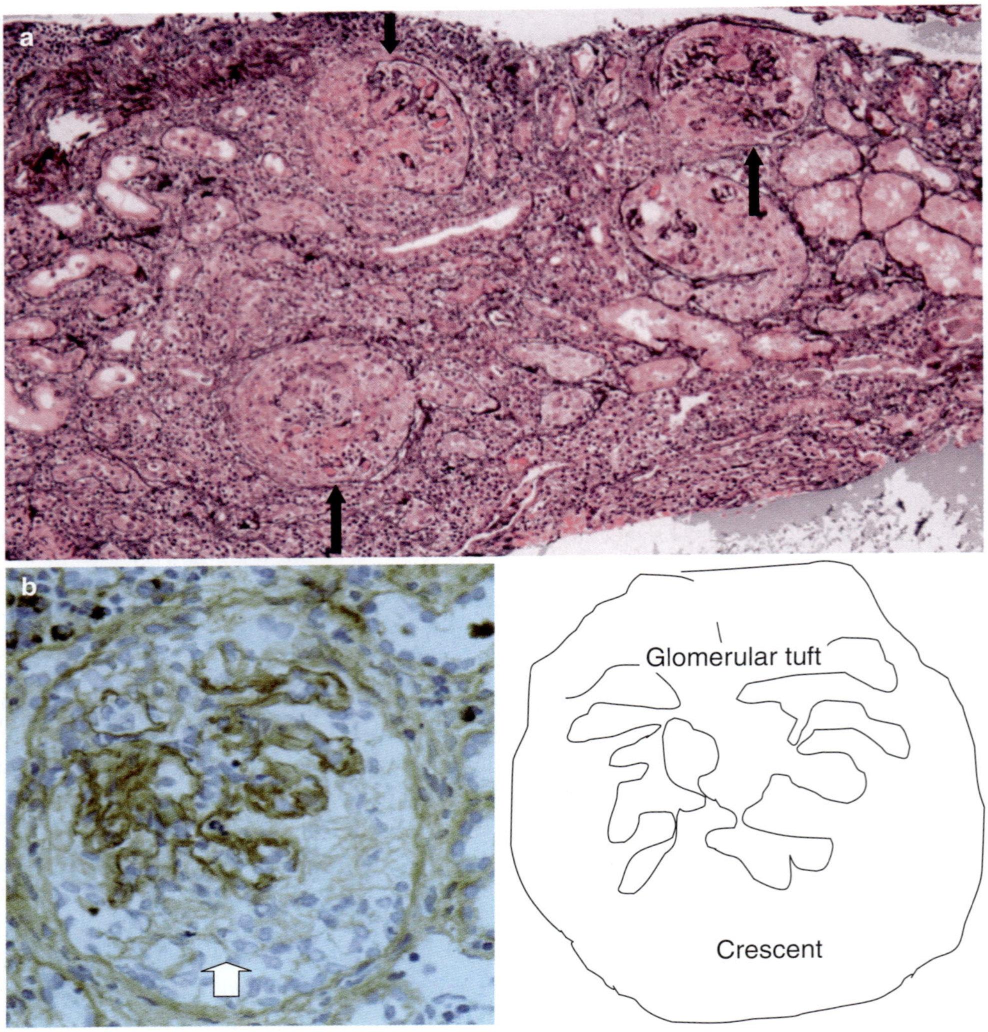

Fig. 21.1 (**a**) Low-power silver stain of a kidney biopsy from a patient with anti-GBM disease demonstrating widespread crescentic glomerulonephritis (*arrows*) with lesions all appearing of similar vintage (×100 magnification). (**b**) Immunoperoxidase staining for IgG on a renal biopsy from a patient with anti-GBM disease demonstrating fine smooth linear deposition along the basement membrane and a surrounding crescent (*arrowhead*) which is clearly compressing the glomerular tuft

Table 21.1 Renal outcome of Goodpasture's disease based on presenting creatinine

Goodpasture's disease	ANCA-associated vasculitis
May present with rapidly progressive renal failure and anuria	May present with rapidly progressive renal failure
Systemic prodromal symptoms uncommon	Systemic prodromal symptoms common, except in cases of renal limited vasculitis
Dialysis dependency at presentation rarely associated with renal recovery	Dialysis dependency at presentation associated with renal recovery in 40–60 % cases
Pulmonary haemorrhages in 50–70 % cases	Pulmonary haemorrhage in 25 %
Anti-GBM Ab positive Concurrent ANCA positivity in 30–47 % cases	Anti-GBM negative, ANCA positive in 95 % cases
Glomerular crescents of similar age	Glomerular lesions of various ages
Linear immunoglobulin deposition along GBM	Pauci-immune

found in other ethnic groups including Japanese and Chinese, in whom it appears to have similar genetic susceptibility traits. There are recognised genetic and environmental risk factors, with one of the strongest human leukocyte antigen (HLA) associations with disease, as over 90 % of patients carry the HLA DRB1*1501 or *0401 alleles [6]. There are also negative associations with HLA DRB1*01 and DRB1*07, with these alleles being underrepresented in the Goodpasture's patients. The reason for the relative susceptibility and protective effects of these alleles is not clear, as both DRB1*1501 and DRB1*0701 bind the Goodpasture antigen peptides. In addition, recent reports demonstrated polymorphisms in the inhibitory Fc (immunoglobulin) receptor FCγRIIB and copy number variation in activatory FcγRIIIA receptors in Chinese patients with anti-GBM disease, suggesting that these conferred increased risk of disease through augmented Fc receptor signalling. Despite these immunological susceptibility factors, Goodpasture's disease does not form part of a generalised autoimmune phenotype. However, in approximately 30 % of cases, there may be a concurrent ANCA detected, mostly a perinuclear (P)-ANCA with anti-myeloperoxidase reactivity [7]. Less often, Goodpasture's disease may follow on from membranous nephropathy [8] or systemic lupus erythematosus [9], while rare cases have also been reported following lithotripsy treatment for renal calculi [10]. It is assumed that in these cases, the primary damage to the glomerular basement membrane, which may have been mechanical or inflammatory, allows exposure of collagen chain neo-epitopes which then induces an immune response directed against the GBM.

Diagnosis

Diagnosis relies on renal biopsy demonstrating crescentic glomerulonephritis with linear immunoglobulin deposition along the basement membrane (see Fig. 21.2). This is predominantly IgG, but rare cases of other immunoglobulin classes predominating have been reported, some of which may bind alternative GBM antigens. Less intense linear basement membrane staining with IgG may occasionally be seen in patients with diabetes, systemic lupus erythematosus, myeloma or in transplanted kidneys, but these are not associated with crescent formation. Unlike ANCA-associated glomerulonephritis, crescents in anti-GBM disease appear of the same age without evidence of old and new lesions as it does not follow the same stuttering course as ANCA-associated disease.

Pulmonary haemorrhage in the absence of significant haemoptysis, maybe diagnosed on the basis of chest radiography with an elevated gas transfer coefficient (KCO) or by bronchoscopy. Suspicion should arise if there is an iron deficiency anaemia with no other obvious source of blood loss and a consistent chest radiograph. Serial KCO measurements may be useful in the monitoring of resolution of pulmonary haemorrhage. Serology to assay anti-GBM antibodies is helpful, as the assay is sensitive and specific. However, there are two common pitfalls. False positivity may occur in cases of polyclonal gammopathy such as in viral infections (often HCV or HIV) [11] and may require confirmation with Western blotting (not routinely performed in clinical laboratories); false negativity may rarely occur – for reasons that are not clear – but a small number of patients have been described in whom typical biopsy features are found, but circulating anti-GBM antibodies are not detected by standard methodology such as ELISA [12]. Finally, rare cases of IgA anti-GBM antibody-mediated disease have been reported and these would not be detected on standard anti-GBM ELISA. In all these cases, renal biopsy is critical to refute or confirm the diagnosis.

It is also critical to test all ANCA positive patients presenting with rapidly progressive glomerulonephritis for anti-GBM antibodies, as some will be double positive. This group of patients behaves like anti-GBM disease with regard to renal recovery (i.e. less likely to recover if presenting with dialysis dependency, unlike ANCA-associated vasculitis in which 50–60 % will recover independent renal function) but have extrarenal relapses like ANCA-associated vasculitis patients, which may necessitate maintenance immunosuppression. Curiously, there may be a dichotomy between the ANCA and anti-GBM autoantibodies, with the ANCA fluctuating during disease remission, but with the anti-GBM generally remaining negative.

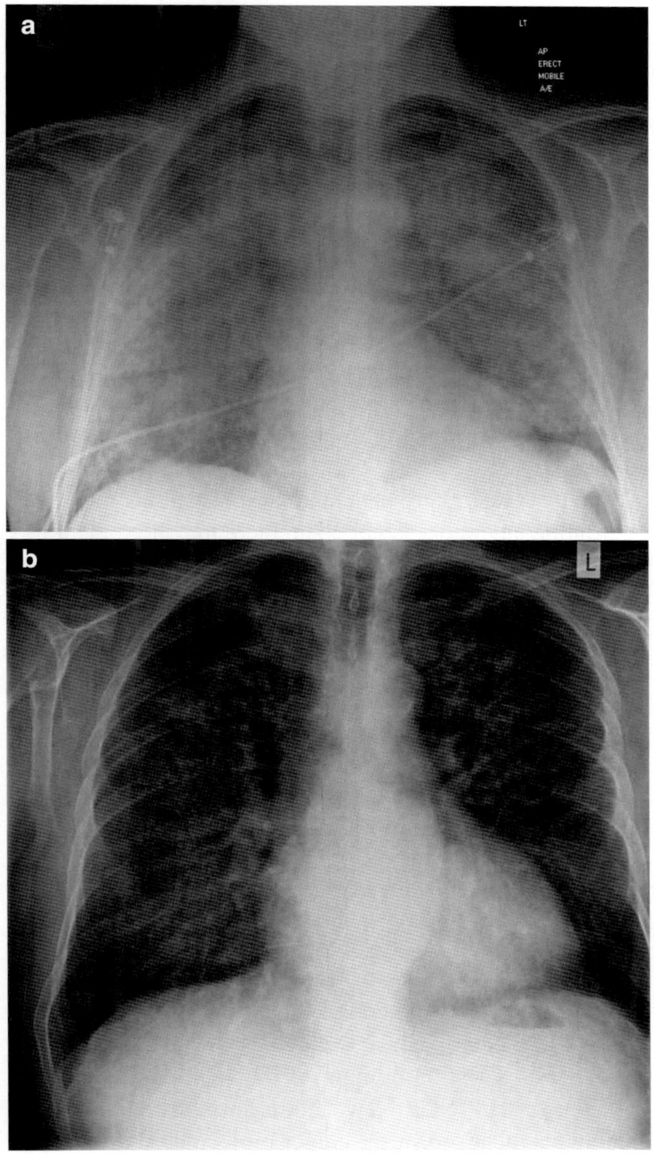

Fig. 21.2 (**a**) Chest radiograph of a patient with Goodpasture's disease demonstrating pulmonary haemorrhage with relative sparing of costophrenic angles and (**b**) 3 days later following immunosuppression with steroids and cyclophosphamide and plasmapheresis

Many laboratories batch sera for testing in immunological assays. This is clearly of no use if a timely diagnosis is to be made; therefore, it is important to discuss the urgency of the assay with the clinical immunology laboratory as many can perform rapid assays when requested if they appreciate the urgency of a particular clinical situation. All patients with a rapidly progressive AKI and an 'active urinary sediment' should have an urgent anti-GBM antibody assay (it is never a routine request in these circumstances) with a result within 24–48 h. Furthermore, it is worth establishing a standard operating procedure whereby the immunology laboratories within the Renal Unit's catchment urgently communicates any positive anti-GBM to the nephrologist on call, who can urgently discuss the case with the relevant clinical team.

Finally, since many patients may present at times when the routine laboratory is not open, there may be some utility in having rapid assay kits (such as the Quickcard which are also available for PR3- and MPO- ANCA) and resemble pregnancy test kits which require the addition of serum to a supplied buffer, which can be done on the wards, if there is an available centrifuge. These should not replace standard testing (formal confirmation with a standard laboratory assay is still required) as they are less reliable, but may represent a good interim measure to dictate whether emergency plasmapheresis should be instituted.

Immunology

The adult GBM is formed from a network of specialised type IV collagen molecules, consisting of α3, α4 and α5 chains. The Goodpasture antigen is present in the non-collagenous 1 (NC1) domain of the α3 chain of type IV collagen (α3(IV)NC1). Two main antibody epitopes are closely co-localised in the intact molecule, and these are sequestered under normal conditions, suggesting that tolerance is broken after exposure of the cryptic epitopes to the immune system. The anti-GBM antibodies are mostly IgG1, although some IgG4 antibodies are also found. Less commonly, other immunoglobulins may predominate such as IgA. The anti-GBM antibodies are almost never detected in normal individuals using conventional assays, making the test a highly sensitive and specific assay. Anti-GBM antibodies are closely associated with disease activity and were shown to transfer disease to experimental animals in classic experiments some 40 years ago. However, there is evidence for both humoral and cellular autoimmunity in patients, with both antibodies and T cells reactive to the α3(IV)NC1 [13]. In part the lack of disease relapse, unlike the high incidence in ANCA-associated vasculitis, is due to the early and persistent development of regulatory antigen-specific T-cell populations [14].

Treatment

Treatment consists of general measures such as avoiding fluid overload, stopping smoking and avoiding any potential occupational exposure to solvents – all of which may precipitate pulmonary haemorrhage. The rare cases of relapse, with pulmonary haemorrhage, were in patients who returned to smoking after their initial illness. The mainstay of treatment is with specific immunosuppression using oral corticosteroids and cyclophosphamide with additional plasmapheresis performed daily for 14 days or until antibody levels are undetectable, whichever comes first (Table 21.2). Steroids should be started at 1 mg/kg, maximum 60 mg, although there are no trial data to support this specific dosage regimen, and withdrawn by 6 months. Cyclophosphamide should be given for 2–3 months at a starting dose of 2–3 mg/kg/day, rounded down, and dose-adjusted in the elderly (over 60 years) to use 1–1.5 mg/kg. Prophylactic treatment to prevent infectious, metabolic and gastric complications is also required (see Table 21.2). Plasmapheresis was first introduced by the Hammersmith Hospital group in the 1970s, following their report of seven patients treated with steroids, cyclophosphamide and plasmapheresis [15], in which they demonstrated a rapid decline in anti-GBM antibodies and improvement in renal function in those patients who were not dialysis dependent at presentation. Surprisingly, there has only been one randomised trial investigating whether there is any additional benefit of plasmapheresis to conventional immunosuppressive therapy. This consisted of 17 patients, all treated with steroids and cyclophosphamide with eight receiving additional plasmapheresis, every 3 days. In these eight patients, antibody removal was more rapid, and renal function showed greater improvement. However, the two groups of patients were not well matched at onset, as serum creatinine and percentage crescent involvement on biopsy were lower in the plasmapheresis group [16]. The currently accepted protocol has evolved from these data based on the outcomes reported from institutions with significant experience in the management of such patients. Clearly, novel treatments may be of equal benefit but there have been no formal trials comparing intravenous pulsed cyclophosphamide, rituximab cyclosporine A or mycophenolate mofetil. However, there are anecdotal reports of all of these agents being used with variable outcomes [17–21], but these have tended to be used in patients in whom cyclophosphamide has failed or has led to complications and so they cannot be recommended as first-line therapies.

Outcomes

Retrospective cohort studies have confirmed that renal outcome is dependent on the severity of the renal damage at presentation, with those patients with greater severity

Table 21.2 Treatment of anti-GBM disease

Plasma exchange	Daily 50 ml/kg, maximum 4-l exchange, for 4.5 % human albumin solution. Replace 300–600 ml albumin with fresh plasma within 3 days after invasive procedure (e.g. biopsy) or in patients with pulmonary haemorrhage
	Continue for 14 days or until antibody levels are fully suppressed
	Withhold if platelet count is <70 × 10^9/ml, fibrinogen <1 g/l or haemoglobin is <9 g/dl. Watch for coagulopathy, hypocalcaemia and hypokalaemia
Cyclophosphamide	Daily oral dosing at 2–3 mg/kg/day (round down to nearest 50 mg; use 1–1.5 mg/kg/day in patients >60 years)
	Stop if white cell count is less than 4 × 10^9/ml and restart at lower dose when count increases to >4 × 10^9/ml
	Treat for 2–3 months; 2 months in elderly
	Pulsed IV cyclophosphamide has not been tested formally, but is equivalent in ANCA-associated vasculitis
Prednisolone	Daily oral dosing at 1 mg/kg/day (maximum, 60 mg)
	Reduce dose weekly to 20 mg by week 6, and then more slowly. Should be off steroids by 6 months
	There is no evidence of benefit of IV methylprednisolone, but consider if plasma exchange not immediately available
Prophylactic treatments	Use oral nystatin 1 ml qds or fluconazole 50 mg od to prevent oral thrush
	Use ranitidine or proton-pump inhibitor to prevent steroid-promoted gastric ulceration
	Use co-trimoxazole 480 mg daily or 960 mg three times a week to prevent *Pneumocystis jiroveci* pneumonia
	Use calcium-D3, two tablets a day as bone protection
Dialysis regimen	Avoid fluid overload by ensuring dry weight is carefully assessed and maintained. Albumin solutions contain significant sodium loads which should be factored in, when considering ultrafiltration volumes

Table 21.3

		Percentage with independent renal function at 1 year according to presenting serum creatinine (μmol/l)		
Study	Patients	<600	>600	Reference
Levy	71	95[a]	8[b]	[2]
Daly	40	20	0	[22]
Bouget	14	50	0	[23]
Walker	22	82	18	[3]
Johnson	17	69	0	[16]

[a]In this study <500 μmol/l and [b]dialysis dependent with creatinine >500 μmol/l

of glomerular disease (based on the crescent score) and worse renal function having the highest degree of end-stage renal failure at 1 year despite immunosuppressive therapy [2] (see Table 21.3). All series demonstrate that patients with serum creatinine levels greater than 600 mcmol/l had the worst outcome with regard to renal survival at 1 year. In the largest series reported by Levy et al. [2], those with presenting creatinine >500 mcmol/l and requiring dialysis at presentation fared the worst with few regaining independent renal function (See Table 21.3), despite treatment. Those with creatinine >500 mcmol/l but not requiring immediate (within 72 h of presentation) dialysis had better renal outcomes than those who required immediate dialysis upon presentation. Finally, those patients with less severe glomerular damage and better preserved renal function (creatinine <500 mcmol/l) have excellent short (1 year) and long-term (20 year) renal outcome following immunosuppressive therapy [2] and should be treated with standard therapy or modified regimens, if contraindications to standard therapy are found.

When Not to Treat?

Since data demonstrate that patients presenting with dialysis dependency and 100 % crescents, i.e. crescents in all glomeruli on the section, do not tend to recover independent renal function, if diagnosis is delayed and patients are already dialysis dependent with extensive crescentic change on biopsy, many practitioners would not treat with immunosuppression unless there was coexistent pulmonary haemorrhage. However, there are patients who do not present requiring dialysis but develop dialysis dependency in the early hospitalisation period. These may well benefit from immunosuppression and the decision should be made based on a balanced assessment of the individual risk of immunosuppression.

In some circumstances, such as those patients with a living kidney donor, even with dialysis dependency and 100 % crescents, treatment may be warranted to allow more rapid elimination of anti-GBM antibodies and early transplantation. In the absence of immunosuppressive therapy, anti-GBM antibodies may persist for up to 3 years [24].

Transplantation

Early experience of transplantation in the face of positive anti-GBM antibodies resulted in rapid disease recurrence [25]. It is therefore essential that transplantation is deferred until there has been a prolonged period of anti-GBM antibody negativity, and using this approach recurrence is rare [7]. Although there are no trial data to guide this period of time, we and others wait 6 months from the time of first antibody negativity, before proceeding. Persistent low-level anti-GBM antibody has been removed prior to transplantation by immunoadsorption, with those patients who could not have antibody successfully removed not undergoing transplantation [24]. Cases of late anti-GBM disease recurrence following cessation of transplant maintenance immunosuppressive therapy or following viral infection have been reported but are uncommon [26, 27]. If recurrence does occur, augmented immunosuppressive treatment may be used but is successful in only a minority of cases [27].

Anti-GBM Disease in Alport's Disease Following Transplantation

Alport's disease arises from mutations in the type IV collagen chains found in the glomerular basement membrane, which is the α5(IV) chain in the X-linked form of disease. Following transplantation of a kidney containing a normal α5(IV) chain, an alloimmune response to the collagen IV chain can arise and lead to development of anti-GBM antibodies. While this can be found in up to 20 % of patients, only 5–6 % go on to develop a crescentic glomerulonephritis which tends to be extremely difficult to treat, even with augmented immunosuppression [28]. Once this anti-collagen response has developed, subsequent transplantation is increasingly likely to result in disease recurrence.

Whilst monitoring Alport's patients who have undergone renal transplantation, it is important to realise that many anti-GBM assays are now using recombinant α3(IV) and not whole GBM as a substrate. They will therefore not detect anti-α5(IV) antibodies, to which the transplanted X-linked Alport's patient will react to [29].

References

1. Salama AD, Levy JB, Lightstone L, Pusey CD. Goodpasture's disease. Lancet. 2001;358(9285):917–20.
2. Levy JB, Turner AN, Rees AJ, Pusey CD. Long-term outcome of anti-glomerular basement membrane antibody disease treated with plasma exchange and immunosuppression. Ann Intern Med. 2001;134(11):1033–42.
3. Walker RG, Scheinkestel C, Becker GJ, Owen JE, Dowling JP, Kincaid-Smith P. Clinical and morphological aspects of the management of crescentic anti-glomerular basement membrane antibody (anti-GBM) nephritis/Goodpasture's syndrome. Q J Med. 1985;54(213):75–89.
4. Levy JB, Lachmann RH, Pusey CD. Recurrent Goodpasture's disease. Am J Kidney Dis. 1996;27(4):573–8.
5. Bowley NB, Steiner RE, Chin WS. The chest X-ray in antiglomerular basement membrane antibody disease (Goodpasture's syndrome). Clin Radiol. 1979;30(4):419–29.
6. Fisher M, Pusey CD, Vaughan RW, Rees AJ. Susceptibility to anti-glomerular basement membrane disease is strongly associated with HLA-DRB1 genes. Kidney Int. 1997;51(1):222–9.
7. Levy JB, Hammad T, Coulthart A, Dougan T, Pusey CD. Clinical features and outcome of patients with both ANCA and anti-GBM antibodies. Kidney Int. 2004;66(4):1535–40.
8. Sano T, Kamata K, Shigematsu H, Kobayashi Y. A case of anti-glomerular basement membrane glomerulonephritis superimposed on membranous nephropathy. Nephrol Dial Transplant. 2000;15(8):1238–41.
9. Savige JA, Dowling J, Kincaid-Smith P. Superimposed glomerular immune complexes in anti-glomerular basement membrane disease. Am J Kidney Dis. 1989;14(2):145–53.
10. Xenocostas A, Jothy S, Collins B, Loertscher R, Levy M. Anti-glomerular basement membrane glomerulonephritis after extracorporeal shock wave lithotripsy. Am J Kidney Dis. 1999; 33(1):128–32.
11. Szczech LA, Anderson A, Ramers C, Engeman J, Ellis M, Butterly D, et al. The uncertain significance of anti-glomerular basement membrane antibody among HIV-infected persons with kidney disease. Am J Kidney Dis. 2006;48(4):e55–9.
12. Salama AD, Dougan T, Levy JB, Cook HT, Morgan SH, Naudeer S, et al. Goodpasture's disease in the absence of circulating anti-glomerular basement membrane antibodies as detected by standard techniques. Am J Kidney Dis. 2002;39(6):1162–7.
13. Salama AD, Chaudhry AN, Ryan JJ, Eren E, Levy JB, Pusey CD, et al. In Goodpasture's disease, CD4(+) T cells escape thymic deletion and are reactive with the autoantigen alpha3(IV)NC1. J Am Soc Nephrol. 2001;12(9):1908–15.
14. Salama AD, Chaudhry AN, Holthaus KA, Mosley K, Kalluri R, Sayegh MH, et al. Regulation by CD25+ lymphocytes of autoantigen-specific T-cell responses in Goodpasture's (anti-GBM) disease. Kidney Int. 2003;64(5):1685–94.
15. Lockwood CM, Rees AJ, Pearson TA, Evans DJ, Peters DK, Wilson CB. Immunosuppression and plasma-exchange in the treatment of Goodpasture's syndrome. Lancet. 1976;1(7962):711–5.
16. Johnson JP, Moore Jr J, Austin 3rd HA, Balow JE, Antonovych TT, Wilson CB. Therapy of anti-glomerular basement membrane antibody disease: analysis of prognostic significance of clinical, pathologic and treatment factors. Medicine (Baltimore). 1985;64(4):219–27.
17. Uezu Y, Kiyatake I, Tokuyama K. A case of Goodpasture's syndrome with massive pulmonary hemorrhage ameliorated by cyclophosphamide pulse therapy. Nihon Jinzo Gakkai Shi. 1999;41(5):499–504.
18. Arzoo K, Sadeghi S, Liebman HA. Treatment of refractory antibody mediated autoimmune disorders with an anti-CD20 monoclonal antibody (rituximab). Ann Rheum Dis. 2002;61(10): 922–4.
19. Kiykim AA, Horoz M, Gok E. Successful treatment of resistant antiglomerular basement membrane antibody positivity with mycophenolic acid. Intern Med. 2010;49(6):577–80.
20. Merkel F, Weber M. Successful use of cyclosporin A in progressive anti-glomerular basement membrane nephritis. Nephrol Dial Transplant. 2000;15(10):1714–5.
21. Wechsler E, Yang T, Jordan SC, Vo A, Nast CC. Anti-glomerular basement membrane disease in an HIV-infected patient. Nat Clin Pract Nephrol. 2008;4(3):167–71.
22. Daly C, Conlon PJ, Medwar W, Walshe JJ. Characteristics and outcome of anti-glomerular basement membrane disease: a single-center experience. Ren Fail. 1996;18(1):105–12.
23. Bouget J, Le Pogamp P, Perrier G, Ramee MP, Rivalan J, Camus C, et al. Anti-basement-membrane antibody mediated, rapidly progressive, glomerulonephritis. Diagnostic and therapeutic strategy based on a retrospective study of 14 cases. Ann Med Interne (Paris). 1990;141(5):409–15.
24. Flores JC, Taube D, Savage CO, Cameron JS, Lockwood CM, Williams DG, et al. Clinical and immunological evolution of oligoanuric anti-GBM nephritis treated by haemodialysis. Lancet. 1986;1(8471):5–8.

25. Wilson CB, Dixon FJ. Anti-glomerular basement membrane antibody-induced glomerulonephritis. Kidney Int. 1973; 3(2):74–89.
26. Fonck C, Loute G, Cosyns JP, Pirson Y. Recurrent fulminant anti-glomerular basement membrane nephritis at a 7-year interval. Am J Kidney Dis. 1998;32(2):323–7.
27. Sauter M, Schmid H, Anders HJ, Heller F, Weiss M, Sitter T. Loss of a renal graft due to recurrence of anti-GBM disease despite rituximab therapy. Clin Transplant. 2009;23(1):132–6.
28. Browne G, Brown PA, Tomson CR, Fleming S, Allen A, Herriot R, et al. Retransplantation in Alport post-transplant anti-GBM disease. Kidney Int. 2004;65(2):675–81.
29. Dehan P, Van den Heuvel LP, Smeets HJ, Tryggvason K, Foidart JM. Identification of post-transplant anti-alpha 5 (IV) collagen alloantibodies in X-linked Alport syndrome. Nephrol Dial Transplant. 1996;11(10):1983–8.

Systemic Lupus Erythematosus, Antiphospholipid Syndrome and the Kidney

22

Neeraj Dhaun (Bean)†, Christopher O.C. Bellamy, and David C. Kluth

Systemic Lupus Erythematosus

Kidney involvement in systemic lupus erythematosus (SLE) is common and is a major contributor to disease morbidity and mortality. At presentation, up to 50 % of patients with SLE will have clinical evidence of renal involvement – abnormal renal function and haematuria with or without proteinuria. During follow-up renal involvement will be evident in >60 %, with an even greater representation among children and young adults.

Epidemiology

The majority of individuals affected by SLE are women of child-bearing age. The prevalence ranges from 20 to 150 cases per 100,000 population, with the highest prevalence reported in Brazil, and appears to be increasing as the disease is recognised more readily and survival increases. People of African, Hispanic or Asian ancestry, as compared with those of other ethnic groups, tend to have an increased prevalence of SLE and greater organ involvement. The 10-year survival is ~70 %, with the major causes of death being infections, atherosclerosis and cancer. Mostly, renal involvement occurs within the first 3 years following diagnosis. Treatment has improved 5-year renal survival to 50–95 %.

†Deceased

N. Dhaun (Bean)†, MD, PhD (✉) D.C. Kluth†, MD, PhD
Department of Renal Medicine,
Royal Infirmary of Edinburgh, The Queen's Medical Research Institute, 47 Little France Crescent, Edinburgh EH16 4TJ, UK
e-mail: bean.dhaun@ed.ac.uk; david.kluth@ed.ac.uk

C.O.C. Bellamy, MBBS, PhD, FRCPath
Department of Pathology,
Royal Infirmary of Edinburgh,
51 Little France Crescent, Edinburgh EH16 4SA, UK
e-mail: c.bellamy@ed.ac.uk

Pathophysiology

SLE is a multisystem autoimmune disease characterised by polyclonal B cell activation and the presence of autoantibodies, especially directed against nuclear components. The aetiology of SLE is unclear, but it is likely multifactorial incorporating several genetic, hormonal, environmental and immunoregulatory factors. Generation of autoantibodies and subsequent tissue deposition of immune complexes – some passively trapped in the glomeruli and others attached to glomerular structures – leads to glomerulonephritis, and complement fixation initiates an inflammatory and cytotoxic reaction. The autoantibodies may themselves be cytotoxic.

Histopathology of Lupus Nephritis

Renal lupus can manifest in several different ways, which may coexist. These include glomerulonephritis, vasculopathy and tubulointerstitial disease (see Table 22.1).

Glomerular Disease

The pattern of injury in lupus glomerulonephritis reflects the glomerular compartments in which immune deposits accumulate. This is in turn probably linked to physical–

Table 22.1 ISN/RPS histological classification of lupus nephritis

Class I	Normal glomeruli by light microscopy but mesangial immune deposits on immunofluorescence
Class II	Purely mesangial hypercellularity of any degree or mesangial expansion by light microscopy, with mesangial immune deposits
Class III	Focal proliferative lupus glomerulonephritis <50 % glomeruli affected
Class IV	Diffuse proliferative lupus glomerulonephritis >50 % glomeruli affected Disease may be segmental (IV-S or global IV-G)
Class V	Membranous lupus glomerulonephritis
Class VI	Advanced sclerotic lupus glomerulonephritis >90 % glomeruli globally sclerosed with no disease activity

M. Harber (ed.), *Practical Nephrology*,
DOI 10.1007/978-1-4471-5547-8_22, © Springer-Verlag London 2014

chemical properties of the immunoglobulins and their particular antigenic specificities. With immunofluorescence labelling of renal biopsies, it can usually be seen that the deposited immunoglobulins are of multiple classes and that they activate the classical pathway of complement activation with C1q deposition. The deposition of complexes in multiple glomerular compartments (mesangium, subendothelial, subepithelial) is very characteristic of lupus glomerulonephritis.

- *Mesangial* immune complex deposition alone is typical of milder disease and leads to a histological pattern similar to IgA nephropathy with mesangial hypercellularity and mesangial matrix accumulation. Clinically, this pattern of disease typically gives microscopic haematuria, subnephrotic range proteinuria and usually reasonably well-preserved renal function [1].
- *Subendothelial* immune deposits may excite leucocyte accumulation, endothelial cell injury and proliferation. Over time with repeated injury, remodelling of the glomerular capillary wall produces chronic changes of reduplication of the glomerular basement membrane and mesangial cell interposition into the capillary wall (mesangiocapillary pattern).
- *Subepithelial* immune deposits produce a membranous reaction in the capillary wall analogous to idiopathic membranous nephropathy. Clinically, this is associated with heavy proteinuria with initial preservation, but often a gradual decline, in glomerular filtration rate (GFR) [2].

Vasculopathy

Renal vascular complications are frequent in lupus nephritis, and their presence may profoundly alter the clinical course and treatment of the disease. They include:

- *Vascular immune complex deposits in the intima and media of small arteries and arterioles*: common and without prognostic significance [3].
- *Noninflammatory necrotising vasculopathy (lupus vasculopathy)*: intimal and luminal mixed immune deposits, fibrin and other plasma proteins; uncommon but associated with class IV nephritis and a poor prognosis [4].
- *Thrombotic microangiopathy*: may be seen independently of lupus glomerular disease, especially in those with the antiphospholipid syndrome. Variable prognosis [5].
- *Renal vasculitis*: inflammatory destructive vasculitis often with fibrin deposits. This is rare and not well characterised [6].
- *Renal vein thrombosis*: more common in the presence of the nephrotic and antiphospholipid syndromes.

Tubulointerstitial Disease

In ~50 % of individuals with lupus nephritis, immune complexes may be found in the tubular basement membrane [7]. The tubulitis – infiltration across the tubular basement membrane into the tubular epithelium by lymphocytes and monocytes, with a few B cells, plasma cells and natural killer cells – is common in active disease. In more chronic disease, the interstitium is expanded with collagen fibrosis. Rarely, acute tubulointerstitial nephritis may be the first presentation of lupus kidney disease presenting as acute renal failure.

Prognosis of Lupus Nephritis

Factors that predict poorer prognosis at disease presentation include:

Non-renal Factors

- Male sex
- Haematological features (thrombocytopenia and leucopenia)
- Younger age
- Persistent hypocomplementaemia
- Persistently raised dsDNA antibodies after treatment
- Antiphospholipid antibodies

Renal Factors

- Abnormal renal function at presentation
- Failure of renal response to treatment
- Renal flares of disease

Presentation of Lupus Nephritis

In general, the identification of lupus nephritis follows on from the diagnosis of SLE. Symptoms of SLE include arthralgia, mouth ulcers, alopecia, skin rash (discoid, malar or photosensitive rashes), haematological abnormalities (anaemia, thrombocytopenia), serositis, Raynaud's phenomenon or epilepsy. Hypertension is also often present.

The presence of autoantibodies supports the diagnosis. The majority of patients with SLE are positive for the antinuclear antibody (ANA), often with a titre of >1:160. However, ANA may also be positive in Sjögren's syndrome, scleroderma and rheumatoid arthritis, all of which may have renal involvement. Depending upon the titre of the ANA, the false-positive rate in healthy volunteers varies from ~30 % with ANA titres of 1:40 (high sensitivity, low specificity) to as little as 3 % with ANA titres of 1:320 (low sensitivity, high specificity). More specific serological tests are anti-double-stranded DNA antibody (anti-dsDNA) and anti-Smith antibody (anti-Sm). Compared to ANA, the sensitivity of these is much lower at about 75 and 25 %, respectively. The presence of a high titre of anti-dsDNA increases the risk of lupus nephritis. Hypocomplementaemia is often found at presentation with lupus nephritis (see

Cases 1–3), but is not a universal finding. It may also occur in other glomerulonephritides including postinfectious glomerulonephritis and cryoglobulinaemic vasculitis. It is not routine to follow complement levels to monitor disease progress.

The key test to identifying lupus nephritis is the urine dipstick with haematuria and proteinuria raising the possibility of lupus nephritis. Proteinuria can be quantified by a 24-h urine collection, protein-to-creatinine ratio or an albumin-to-creatinine ratio. Serum creatinine is frequently within the normal range at presentation even in the presence of significant inflammatory disease but may be elevated compared to baseline (see Cases 1–3). About 50 % of patients will present with a clinically overt reduction in GFR and occasionally with acute renal failure. Thus, lupus nephritis should be considered in multisystem disease (particularly in young females) with unexplained haematuria and proteinuria. Serology will help increase the likelihood of diagnosis but ultimately a renal biopsy with light, immunofluorescent and electron microscopy will be required to determine the class of disease and direct therapy.

Treatment of Lupus Glomerulonephritis

Although SLE may involve any compartment of the kidney, glomerular involvement is the best studied and correlates well with presentation, course and treatment of the disease [8]. In 2004 the International Society of Nephrology (ISN) and the Renal Pathology Society revised the World Health Organization (WHO) classification of lupus glomerulonephritis [9]. Current treatment for lupus glomerulonephritis – and studies of newer therapies – is guided by ISN/RPS histological disease class, with appropriate consideration given to clinical parameters and degree of renal impairment.

Conservative, Non-immunosuppressive Therapy Is Appropriate for ISN/RPS Class I and II Lupus Glomerulonephritis

Class I disease means that glomeruli look normal by light microscopy but have mesangial immune deposits on immunofluorescence and/or electron microscopy. Class II is similar but with mesangial proliferation now apparent on light microscopy [9]. In general, patients with class I and II disease do not require specific treatment directed against the kidney. Most will have an excellent prognosis. The only exception to this is the small group of lupus patients who develop minimal change disease or a lupus podocytopathy [10–12]. These patients respond well to a short course of high-dose corticosteroids (1 mg/kg/day to a maximum dose of 80 mg/day) similar to conventional minimal change disease.

Mycophenolate Mofetil for Proliferative Lupus Glomerulonephritis (ISN/RPS Classes III and IV)

Class III and IV diseases mean that glomerular capillaries show endocapillary or extracapillary proliferation or have sufficiently severe subendothelial immune deposits as to be appreciable by light microscopy alone. Mesangial disease is not a consideration. The differences between the classes are arbitrarily whether fewer (class III) or more than (class IV) half the glomeruli in an adequate biopsy sample show any of these changes. These abnormalities may affect some or most of each individual diseased glomerulus, but that does not affect the class. Instead each class is subclassified according to whether most of the diseased glomeruli have segmental (IV-S) or global (IV-G) disease. Cyclophosphamide (CYC) has been the cornerstone of immunosuppressive treatment for severe lupus nephritis for several decades. However, recent data support the use of mycophenolate mofetil (MMF) as first-line treatment for class III and IV lupus nephritis (see Case 1).

CYC is effective at treating lupus nephritis (see Case 2). It is unclear whether oral or intravenous CYC is more effective, but intravenous therapy is associated with a lower cumulative dose and less frequent cytopenias, enables enhanced bladder protection and avoids problems of non-adherence. Although earlier studies suggested that a greater cumulative CYC dose – usually alongside steroid treatment – may prevent more disease relapses and lead to a better long-term GFR [13], it was clear that this was associated with clinically unacceptable side effects such as infection, ischaemic and valvular heart disease, avascular necrosis, osteoporosis and premature menopause. Thus, more recent clinical studies have focused on achieving a high disease induction rate with fewer side effects.

The EuroLupus Group attempted to minimise CYC toxicity but maintain efficacy in their study of 90 patients with diffuse or focal proliferative lupus nephritis or membranous plus proliferative disease [14]. Patients were randomised to either 6 monthly pulses of intravenous CYC (0.5–1 g/m^2), followed by a pulse every third month or to a shorter treatment course of 500 mg of intravenous CYC every 2 weeks for six doses (cumulative dose 3 g), followed by azathioprine maintenance therapy thereafter. Both arms of the study were as effective in achieving the various renal and extrarenal endpoints, but the shorter treatment was associated with a lower rate of infections. It is noteworthy that this trial was mostly performed in white subjects and so the results can only be extrapolated to other populations with caution. However, the 10-year follow-up data continue to suggest no differences between the two groups [15].

MMF is the new standard of care for proliferative lupus nephritis [16–21]. The first good evidence of its efficacy was from a Chinese study in 42 patients randomised to receive either 12 months of MMF (2 g/day for 6 months followed by 1 g/day for 6 months) or 6 months of oral CYC

(2.5 mg/kg/day) followed by 6 months of azathioprine (1.5 mg/kg/day) [16]. Both groups received a tapering course of steroids. At 12 months there were no differences between the MMF and CYC groups in terms of complete remission (81 vs. 76 %), partial remission (14 vs. 14 %) and relapses (15 vs. 11 %). However, infections were less common with MMF, and mortality was associated with CYC alone (0 vs. 10 %). Longer-term follow-up has shown similar rates of CKD (defined as doubling of serum creatinine) as well as similar rates of relapse and relapse-free survival. Importantly, MMF is associated with lower infection rates than CYC (13 vs. 40 %), and mortality remained a feature of the CYC group [17].

A second study supporting the use of MMF was reported in 2005 [18]. The study was in 140 patients (of whom >50 % were African American) with proliferative (classes III and IV) and membranous (class V) lupus nephritis. There were two groups randomised to either monthly intravenous pulses of CYC or MMF up to 3 g/day, each with a tapering dose of corticosteroids over 6 months. Although this study was powered to be a non-inferiority study, complete and partial disease remissions were significantly more common with MMF at 6 months than with CYC (52 vs. 30 %). MMF had a better side effects profile, and there were no differences between the two treatments in terms of incidence of renal failure, ESRD or mortality at 3 years.

The most recent study supporting the use of MMF in lupus nephritis was published in 2009 [20]. This was a large, by lupus nephritis standards, international, multicentre study in 370 patients. It again compared monthly pulses of CYC against MMF up to 3 g/day. At 6 months, complete and partial remission rates were similar between the CYC and MMF arms (53 vs. 56 %), similar improvements in renal (GFR, serum creatinine, proteinuria and urine sediment) and non-renal parameters (reduction in dsDNA titres, normalisation of complement and increase in serum albumin). There was also no difference in mortality between the two groups.

Therefore, our current practice is to treat patients with class III or IV lupus nephritis with MMF and corticosteroids (see Case 1). However, intravenous cyclophosphamide may still have a role for those with more severe disease marked by crescentic changes on biopsy and more rapidly declining renal function (see Case 2).

Hydroxychloroquine for Lupus Nephritis

Hydroxychloroquine is often used to treat the skin and joint manifestations of SLE. There is also evidence that it protects against progression and relapse of all classes of lupus nephritis. It is our standard practice to put all patients with lupus nephritis on this adjunctive therapy (200–400 mg/day). Hydroxychloroquine is well tolerated but can cause retinopathy. Patients should have ophthalmology review before initiation of treatment and advised about changes in visual acuity. Ophthalmology follow-up should be every 3–5 years whilst on treatment.

Rituximab for Lupus Nephritis

Whilst azathioprine has been shown to not be as effective as intravenous CYC for induction therapy for lupus nephritis, with more disease relapses and less long-term benefit [22], the anti-CD20 monoclonal antibody, rituximab, that depletes B cells shows promise. It may be effective as rescue induction therapy for those patients who have failed with either CYC or MMF [23, 24]. Two recent randomised controlled trials investigated a role for rituximab as add-on therapy to standard of care with rather disappointing results. The first of these compared rituximab and placebo in 257 patients with moderate to severe active SLE but without clinically overt nephritis [25]. Patients studied were receiving equally distributed background treatment with azathioprine, MMF and methotrexate. No differences were seen between placebo and rituximab in any of the endpoints studied. The LUNAR study randomised 140 patients with severe lupus nephritis to either rituximab or placebo on a background of MMF and tapering corticosteroids. Although more patients achieved complete or partial remission in the rituximab arm than in the placebo, there were no differences in the primary clinical endpoint at 1 year [26]. Although the data currently available do not support the routine use of rituximab in lupus nephritis, this may be down to trial design – with rituximab added to standard therapy in reasonably small numbers of patients with a short follow-up period. Thus, rituximab may well have a role in treating resistant patients, in preventing flares or in reducing the number or doses of other immunosuppressive medication.

Maintenance Therapy for Proliferative Lupus Nephritis

Once remission has been achieved, the longer-term goals of maintenance therapy are:

- To prevent disease flares
- To avoid smouldering disease activity that may result in irreversible renal damage
- To prevent long-term side effects of treatment

Although the long-term use of immunosuppressive therapy is well established in lupus nephritis [21, 27, 28], the choice of agent, its dose, duration and potential for infertility and teratogenicity should be considered on an individual patient basis.

Corticosteroids remain the major component of maintenance therapy for lupus nephritis. However, given their potential side effects, the dose should be minimised and appropriate bone and gastric prevention given. Although there are no studies of maintenance therapy in lupus nephritis that do not include corticosteroids, there remain no data that tell us at which point these agents should be stopped. Provided the patient remains relapse-free and is receiving another steroid-sparing agent, stopping corticosteroids after 12–18 months is reasonable.

The long-term use of CYC is to be avoided given its risks of haemorrhagic cystitis, bladder cancer, infertility and early menopause. Both azathioprine and MMF are effective maintenance agents in lupus nephritis [29, 30]. Their equivalent efficacy has been shown in the results of the MAINTAIN trial, which looked at 105 patients with class III (31 %), class IV (58 %) and class V (10 %) lupus nephritis and followed them up for 3 years [31]. Here, induction was with intravenous CYC with patients randomised to azathioprine (mean maximum daily dose 124 mg) or MMF (mean maximum daily dose 2 g). The rates of all primary and secondary endpoints, including remission, steroid withdrawal and disease flares, were equal amongst the two groups. In contrast to this, the ALMS study published in 2011 showed MMF to be superior to azathioprine in terms of renal benefits [32]. This may be due to differences in racial contribution (MAINTAIN involved only Europeans, whereas ALMS a mixture of patients some of whom were non-Caucasians who may be more likely to respond to MMF) and the larger size of the ALMS study. Nevertheless, azathioprine in doses of 1–2.5 mg/kg/day is safe over a long period of time [33]. Macrocytosis, leucopenia and interactions with allopurinol are all potential side effects, alongside the obvious risk of infection with all immunosuppressive agents. Furthermore, azathioprine has only a small oncogenic potential, and pregnancy during maintenance azathioprine is relatively safe. Although MMF has a similar long-term toxicity profile, it should not be used during pregnancy. Given that many patients with lupus nephritis are women of child-bearing age, this difference between the two agents can help individualise therapy.

Treatment of Membranous (ISN/RPS Class V) Lupus Glomerulonephritis

Class V, or membranous, lupus nephritis is histologically characterised by widespread subepithelial immune deposits. A few such deposits are often present in class III or IV disease without particular clinical significance, but if they affect >50 % of the glomerular capillaries in >50 % of glomeruli, then class V disease is diagnosed alongside class III/IV. In that case they dictate treatment. The optimal management of pure class V membranous lupus nephritis remains unclear. Patients who have subnephrotic range proteinuria, or nephrotic range proteinuria but without the nephrotic syndrome, and pure class V disease do very well and often require no more than standard renin-angiotensin system blockade. For those with the nephrotic syndrome, treatment is often as for idiopathic membranous nephropathy.

In a study of 42 patients with membranous lupus nephritis, patients were randomised to cyclosporine and steroids for 11 months, monthly intravenous CYC for 6 months and steroids, or steroids alone [34]. At 1 year, the achieved remission rates were 27 % with steroids alone, 60 % with CYC and 83 % with cyclosporine. Remission occurred quicker with cyclosporine but there were fewer relapses with CYC [35]. Subgroups analyses of the MMF vs. CYC trials for induction therapy in lupus nephritis show that for those patients with pure membranous nephritis MMF is as effective as CYC in achieving disease control [18, 20]. Thus, although data are limited, there are several options for class V lupus nephritis associated clinically with the nephrotic syndrome. MMF is probably our best option overall but further trials are needed. Given the recent data supporting the use of rituximab in idiopathic membranous nephropathy [36], this may be another attractive option in class V lupus nephritis.

Clinical Follow-Up Following Initiation of Treatment

The frequency of clinical follow-up will vary depending on diagnosis and therapy. A response to treatment will be shown by a reduction in proteinuria; fall in, or stabilisation of, serum creatinine; and resolution of microscopic haematuria. Although it is encouraging to see a fall in anti-dsDNA antibodies, these have a relatively poor correlation with clinical response. As lupus nephritis has an indolent onset, it can take some months for maximum response to occur (unlike ANCA-associated systemic vasculitis). Whilst proliferative (classes III and IV) lupus nephritis may resolve completely, membranous nephropathy (class V) may show an even slower response to treatment, and residual proteinuria is common. Therefore, at least 1 year is required to determine the effectiveness of treatment and some patients may continue to improve after this. This is exemplified in Cases 1 to 3. If the response to therapy is considered inadequate, a repeat renal biopsy should be performed to establish the nature of any ongoing disease and to determine the extent of chronic renal damage. Clinic follow-up may well be in renal, rheumatology or dermatology clinics. In non-renal clinics, all patients should have their urinalysis and renal function checked. A change in either should trigger a referral to a specialist renal service.

Case 1: Mycophenolate Mofetil for the Treatment of Lupus Nephritis

A 19-year-old Caucasian female presented with swelling of her ankles and a purpuric rash over both legs. She had recently returned from a holiday in Spain and noticed feeling lethargic and having aching joints. She had recently been treated with an oral tetracycline for acne. Initial investigations showed:

Hb 10.9 g/dl WCC 5.6×10^9/l Platelets 109×10^9/l
Urea 6.2 mmol/l Creatinine 60 µmol/l ALT 225 U/l
Albumin 22 g/l
Isolated elevated APTT with subsequent isolation of the lupus anticoagulant
C-reactive protein 87 mg/l
Urinalysis blood +++ protein +++
Proteinuria 9 g/day
MSU negative
C3 0.81 g/l C4 0.21 g/l
ANA 1/640 speckled pattern dsDNA 22 U/ml ENA negative

A renal biopsy was performed (see slides) which showed a diffuse, segmental and global, necrotising and proliferative glomerulonephritis with one crescent. There was no evidence of chronic renal damage. These changes were consistent with WHO class IV lupus nephritis. The patient was treated with a tapering course of oral corticosteroids and MMF 2 g/day. She was also started on prophylactic low-dose aspirin. Clinical improvement was rapid alongside an improvement in renal function, liver enzymes and proteinuria (see Figure 22.1). MMF was tapered to 1 g/day after 2 years and all immunosuppression stopped after a total of 3 years treatment. The patient had a disease relapse 3 months following this and was recommenced on oral corticosteroids – which were gradually tapered to zero – and MMF on which she remains well at the last clinic review. Note that creatinine did not fall to baseline until 2 years after treatment was started.

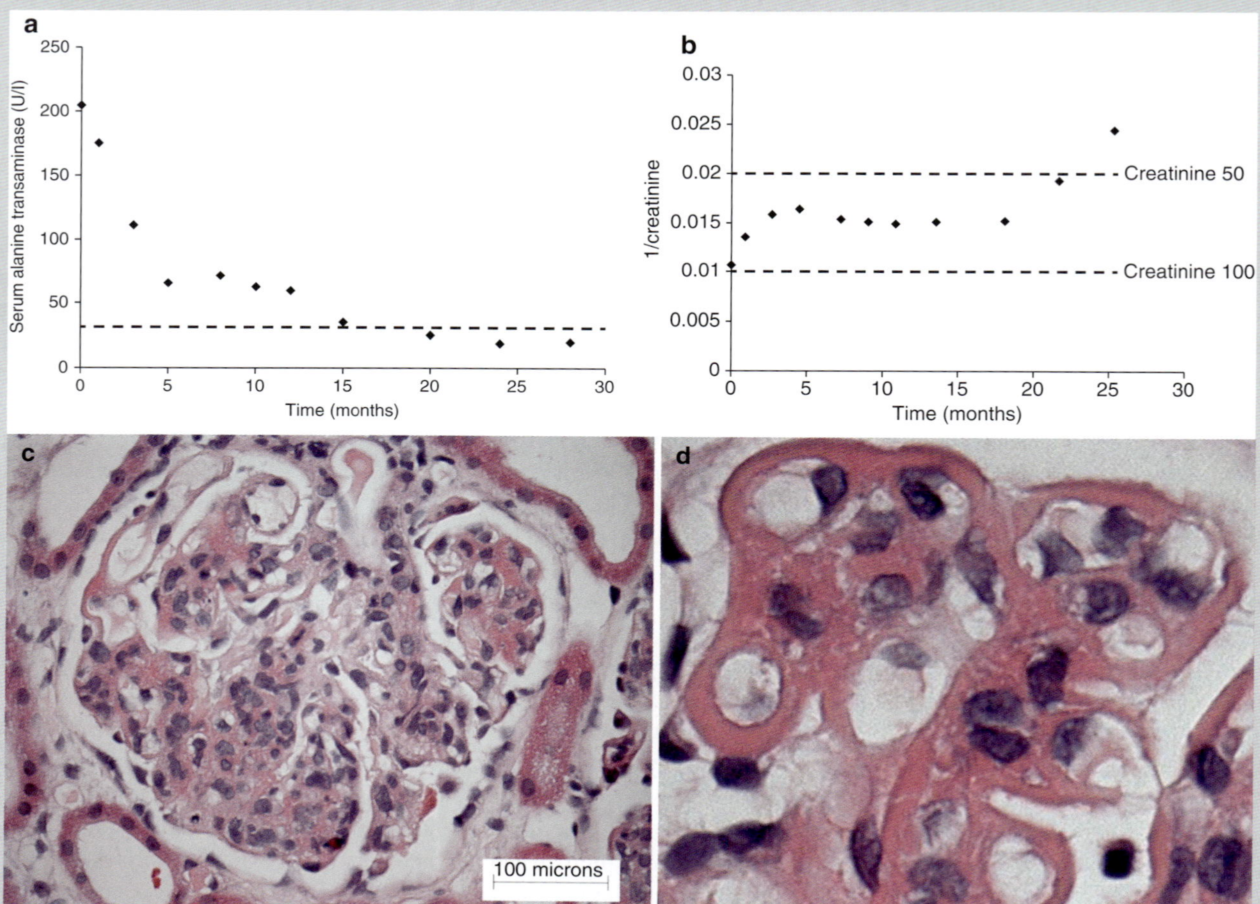

Fig. 22.1 (**a**) Improvement in hepatitis following treatment with steroids and MMF. (**b**) Change in serum creatinine following diagnosis. The serum creatinine falls even though originally in the normal range. (**c**) Glomerulus with global proliferation (>50 % of the tuft area) (H&E stain). (**d**) Glomerular tuft (H&E stain) showing "wire loop" capillary walls thickened due to immune deposits

Case Scenario 2: Cyclophosphamide for the Treatment of Lupus Nephritis

A 37-year-old female presented in 2007 with arthralgia, lethargy and alopecia. She was of Chinese extraction and had one child. She had been diagnosed 10 years earlier with idiopathic thrombocytopenic purpura, which had responded to treatment with oral corticosteroids alone. 5 years earlier she had presented with lethargy, night sweats, fevers, cough and mouth ulcers. She had a high titre of dsDNA antibodies and so was given a diagnosis of SLE and treated with oral corticosteroids and hydroxychloroquine. She had been well for the last 2 years. Initial investigations showed:

Hb 10.2 g/dl WCC 3.1×10^9/l Platelets 87×10^9/l
Urea 7.2 mmol/l Creatinine 90 μmol/l (previously 54)
C-reactive protein 34 mg/l
Urinalysis blood +++ protein +++
Proteinuria 6 g/day
MSU negative
C3 0.21 g/l C4 0.02 g/l
dsDNA >200 U/ml

A renal biopsy was performed (see slides) which showed a diffuse, segmental and global, necrotising and proliferative glomerulonephritis with crescents. There was no evidence of chronic damage. These changes were in keeping with WHO class IV lupus nephritis. The patient was treated with a tapering dose of oral corticosteroids alongside six monthly doses of intravenous CYC. The patient was then switched to MMF 2 g/day as maintenance therapy. There was a rapid and sustained improvement in the patient's symptoms and biochemical parameters (see Figure 22.2). After 12 months of MMF, the dose was reduced from 2 g to 1 g/day and the patient continued on this long term. She remains well at the last clinic review. Serum creatinine continues to improve and proteinuria falls further even after 12 months of treatment.

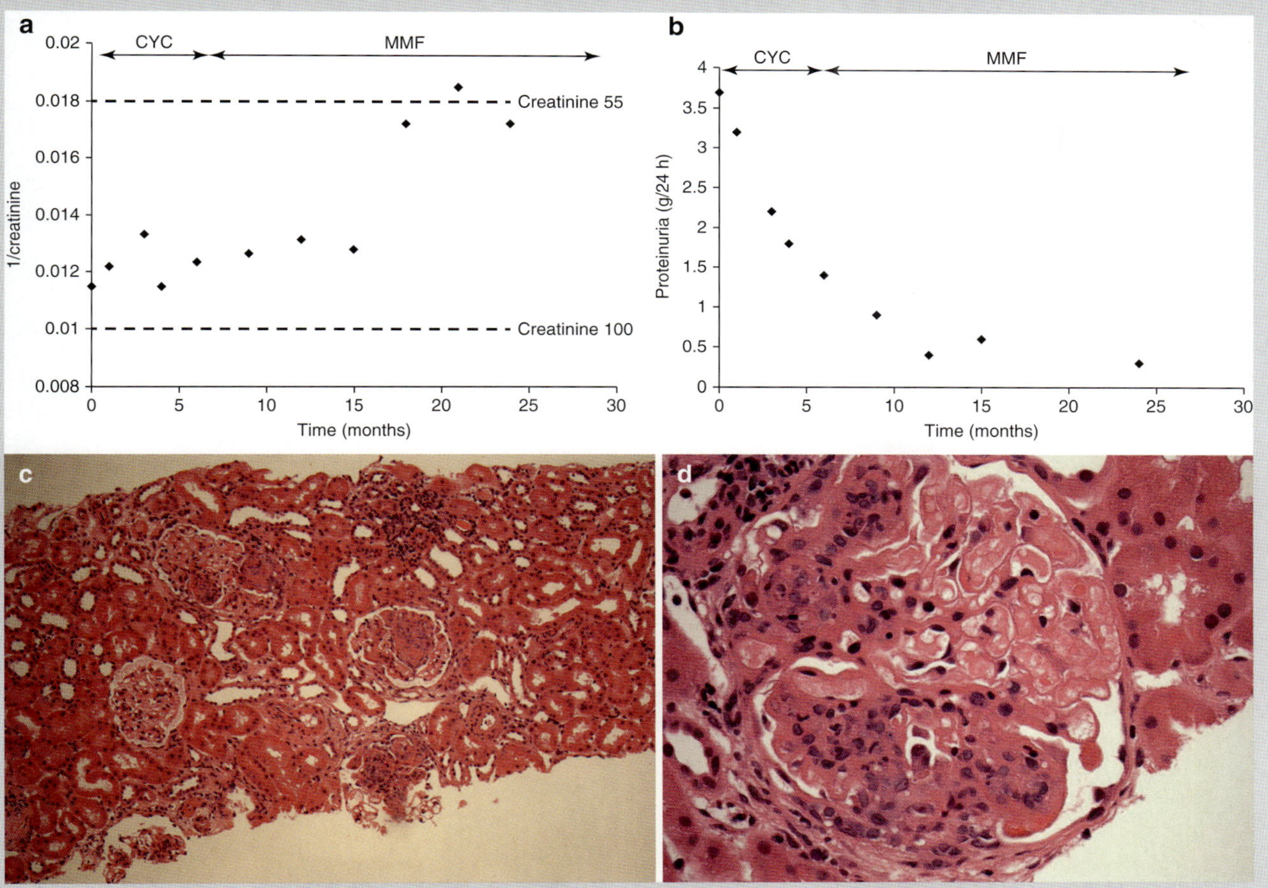

Fig. 22.2 (**a**) Improvement in serum creatinine following treatment with steroids and intravenous cyclophosphamide followed by MMF for maintenance treatment. (**b**) Reduction in proteinuria following treatment. (**c**) Kidney cortex (H&E stain) at low magnification, showing segmental abnormalities in 4 of 5 glomeruli but minimal chronic tubulointerstitial damage. (**d**) Glomerulus at high magnification (H&E stain), showing marked proliferation affecting just over 50 % of the tuft area (i.e. global)

Case 3: Rituximab for the Treatment of Lupus Nephritis

A 34-year-old female presented with fever, loin pain, worsening lethargy and arthralgia. She had a complicated past medical history. She had initially presented in 2003 with large and small joint arthralgia. She was noted to be ANA and dsDNA antibody positive and was given a diagnosis of SLE and successfully treated with hydroxychloroquine alone. She had a past history of intravenous drug use and in 2006 was diagnosed with hepatitis C. Investigations on admission showed:

Hb 9.7 g/l WCC 3.1×10^9/l Platelets 179×10^9/l
Urea 6.2 mmol/l Creatinine 86 μmol/l
C-reactive protein 82 mg/l
Urinalysis blood +++ protein +++
Proteinuria 2.5 g/24 h
C3 0.32 g/l C4 0.08 g/l
dsDNA 81 U/ml
Lupus anticoagulant positive and anticardiolipin IgG 82 U/ml
A renal vein thrombosis was excluded

A renal biopsy was performed which showed evidence of class IV lupus nephritis with interstitial inflammation as well as membranous nephropathy shown on silver staining (Figures 22.3c, d). As the patient was not keen on taking corticosteroids and there was also a concern about reactivation of hepatitis C, she was treated with a steroid-free regime incorporating intravenous rituximab and MMF 2 g/day. There were two doses of methylprednisolone given alongside the rituximab. The patient's symptoms gradually resolved alongside a fall in the dsDNA titre (81 to 37) and proteinuria. Proteinuria and serum creatinine fell progressively. The dose of MMF was halved at 2 years and stopped altogether after 4 years of treatment. The patient remains relapse-free at the last clinic visit.

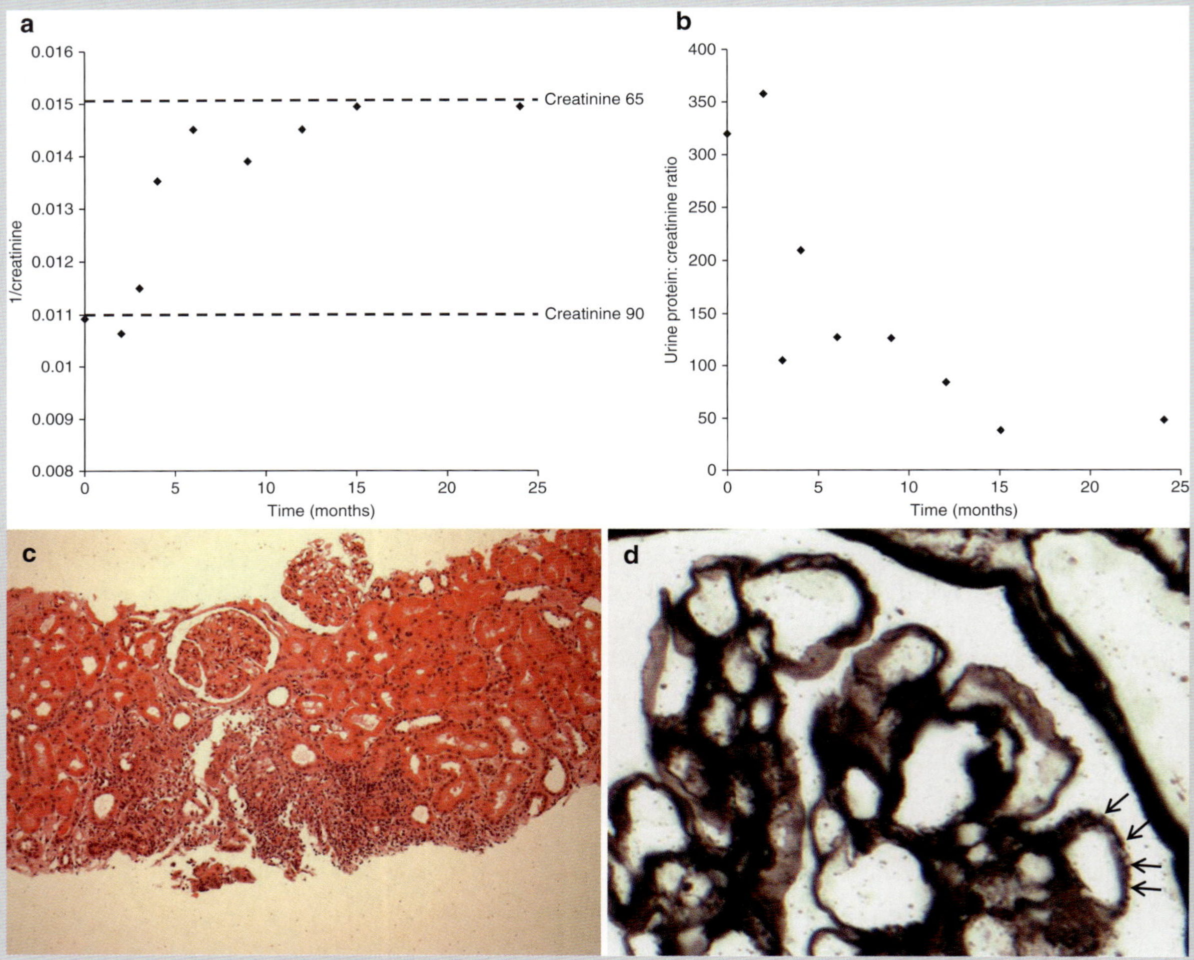

Fig. 22.3 (**a**) Improvement in serum creatinine following treatment with rituximab and MMF in a steroid-free regime. (**b**) Reduction in proteinuria following treatment. (**c**) Kidney cortex at low magnification (H&E stain), showing a discrete patch of interstitial inflammation. (**d**) Glomerulus at high magnification (silver stain) showing a capillary loop with glomerular basement membrane (GBM) lucencies and short spikes on the outer aspect (*arrows*), suggesting local membranous change (continuous stretches of subepithelial immune deposits). Some other capillary loops show reduplicated GBM and a couple look normal. Membranous change in lupus may be segmental or global. If global by light or fluorescence microscopy and associated with active class III/IV disease, then both diagnoses are reported together

Case Scenario 4: Antiphospholipid Syndrome

A 27-year-old girl presented with a lower abdominal pain, a skin rash and a temperature of 39 °C. Initial blood tests are shown below:

Hb 9.2 g/l WCC 3.4×10^9/l Platelets 87×10^9/l
Urea 10.2 mmol/l Creatinine 132 μmol/l
C-reactive protein 132 mg/l
Urinalysis blood +++ protein +++

She was admitted to the high dependency unit with a clinical diagnosis of sepsis and treated with broad-spectrum antibiotics. A CT scan revealed significant lymphadenopathy and a lymph node biopsy was performed. This showed a necrotising lymphadenitis without granulomas. She improved over the course of the next few weeks and was discharged home. Renal function on discharge showed a creatinine of 72 μmol/l.

She was readmitted 6 weeks later with worsening arthralgia, lethargy, some dysuria and shortness of breath. She had been taking ibuprofen for the joint discomfort. Investigations revealed:

Hb 7.3 g/dl WCC 4.2×10^9/l Platelets 87×10^9/l
Urea 9.2 mmol/l Creatinine 181 μmol/l
C-reactive protein 242 mg/l
Urinalysis blood +++ protein +++

A transthoracic echocardiogram revealed a global pericardial effusion 2 cm in depth.

Immunological tests performed on the previous admission showed:

C3 0.31 C4 0.02
ANA 1/160 homogenous staining pattern
dsDNA >200 Anti Ro >100 Anti La >100
ANCA negative
Anticardiolipin IgG >100
Lupus anticoagulant screen positive

The pericardial effusion was drained and the ibuprofen stopped. There was a rapid improvement in serum creatinine to 54 μmol/l. A renal biopsy was performed. This showed a mild increase in mesangial matrix. Immunofluorescence showed minimal C1q and C3 deposition (class II lupus nephritis).

The day following the biopsy, the patient complained of left arm discomfort. Neurological examination revealed some mild arm weakness. A Doppler ultrasound scan showed no evidence of thrombosis. However, an MRI of the brain showed evidence of both acute and subacute embolic foci of ischaemia/infarction.

The patient was started on prednisolone and MMF for her SLE (largely extrarenal involvement) and warfarinised lifelong for the antiphospholipid syndrome. There was a rapid improvement in clinical, biochemical and serological parameters.

There is no consensus on the length of immunosuppressive therapy. In part this will depend on the degree of response to treatment. Most patients will receive immunosuppression for 3–5 years, but with earlier discontinuation of steroids (after 1–2 years, if used). It is also sensible to perform a renal biopsy before stopping immunosuppression so that the extent of background injury and the presence of ongoing disease can be determined. This will help inform subsequent treatment decisions; 50 % of patients will experience disease relapses and so long-term follow-up is advised.

Newer Agents for the Treatment of Lupus Nephritis

A number of newer immunomodulatory agents are currently being studied for the treatment of lupus nephritis. These are largely for proliferative (classes III and IV) nephritis and as add-on therapy to current standard of care – either MMF or CYC.

Rituximab is a chimeric half murine-half human monoclonal antibody and so may be associated with the development, in around 10 % of cases, of human anti-chimeric antibodies. These are of uncertain significance but may limit the efficacy of rituximab. Ocrelizumab is a fully humanised anti-CD20 monoclonal antibody and was considered to have a potentially better outcome and safety profile than rituximab due to the absence of these antibodies. However, the trial investigating the potential benefits of ocrelizumab in lupus nephritis was stopped early due to an unexpected number of infections in the active treatment arm.

Abatacept is a selective T cell co-stimulation modulator, currently licensed for use in adult rheumatoid arthritis and juvenile idiopathic arthritis. It binds to a protein on antigen-presenting cells preventing them from stimulating and so activating T cells. T cell activation is a crucial step in the development of glomerulonephritis. There are currently two studies looking at the potential benefits of abatacept in lupus nephritis as add-on therapy to either the MMF or the EuroLupus CYC regime.

Belimumab is a fully humanised monoclonal antibody that binds to soluble B lymphocyte stimulator. This contributes to

B cell proliferation and differentiation, and thus belimumab, similar to rituximab, is another anti-B cell therapy. Recently published data show belimumab efficacy in both serological markers of disease activity and SLE disease activity scores [37]. This study did not include patients with overt lupus nephritis, so the potential for belimumab efficacy in this setting remains unclear and should be the focus of future clinical trials [38].

Finally, laquinimod is an oral agent that in animal models reduces leucocyte infiltration into target tissues (glomeruli in SLE, optic nerves in multiple sclerosis), downregulates MHC class II gene expression (and hence antigen presentation) and modulates circulating cytokines. It is currently being studied for the treatment of lupus nephritis.

Cardiovascular Risk in SLE and Lupus Nephritis

Cardiovascular disease (CVD) burden is significantly increased in patients with chronic inflammatory conditions. The risk of a woman under the age of 45 with SLE (in the absence of renal involvement) developing atherosclerosis is 50-fold greater than that of an age-matched control. It is also now well established that the development and progression of chronic kidney disease (CKD) is associated with an increased cardiovascular risk. Whilst many patients with CKD have other traditional risk factors for CVD such as diabetes mellitus, smoking and hypertension, a significant part of the increased risk appears to be attributable to CKD itself. Such findings have led the US National Kidney Foundation Task Force on CVD in Chronic Renal Disease to recognise that patients with CKD should be considered in the very-high-risk group for subsequent cardiovascular events. Thus, alongside immunosuppressive treatment of the nephritis, all patients with SLE, with or without nephritis, CVD risk should be assessed and treated aggressively.

We recommend all patients with SLE (both with and without nephritis) be treated with an angiotensin-converting enzyme (ACE) inhibitor or an angiotensin receptor blocker. These agents are first line for achieving optimum blood pressure (BP) control in proteinuric CKD. These drugs reduce intraglomerular pressure, lower systemic BP, reduce proteinuria and delay CKD progression. Emerging data suggest that ACE inhibitors may also delay the development of renal involvement in SLE. In this study, use of ACE inhibitors was also associated with a decreased risk of disease activity.

Pregnancy in SLE and Lupus Nephritis

There are a number of factors to consider when a patient with SLE wants to have a baby. The prognosis for both mother and child is best when the disease, including renal disease, has been quiescent for at least 6 months prior to the pregnancy. We would recommend a pre-pregnancy renal biopsy to confirm the state of the histological disease. If the patient is prescribed maintenance therapy, this should be converted to azathioprine with or without corticosteroids. Pregnancy in women with lupus nephritis is associated with an increased risk of foetal loss and with worsening of the renal and extrarenal manifestations of SLE. Preeclampsia is also a frequent complication of pregnancy in SLE. Maternal SLE is also associated with an increased risk of premature delivery and intrauterine growth restriction. There may be an increased risk of learning disabilities in the offspring, especially in males. Breast-feeding is feasible for most women with SLE. However, some medications may enter the breast milk.

Antiphospholipid Syndrome (APLS)

This is a unique form of autoantibody-induced thrombophilia, characterised by recurrent (arterial and venous) thrombosis and pregnancy complications. The syndrome arises due to endothelial cell, monocyte and platelet activation by antiphospholipid antibodies with anti-β2-glycoprotein-1 activity. Endothelial cells then express a number of adhesion molecules and together with monocytes upregulate the production of tissue factor. Activation of platelets results in an increase in their expression of glycoprotein 2b-3a and synthesis of thromboxane A2. Endothelial cell, monocyte and platelet activation results in a prothrombotic state and, alongside complement activation, provokes thrombosis, often in the presence of a second hit. Traditional cardiovascular risk factors such as smoking, inflammation or oestrogen therapy may play an important role at this point – such factors are present in >50 % of patients with the APLS.

Epidemiology

About 40 % of patients with SLE have antiphospholipid antibodies, but <40 % of them will eventually have thrombosis. However, thrombotic APLS is regarded as a major adverse prognostic factor in SLE. Recurrent miscarriage occurs in ~1 % of the general population. About 10–15 % of these women are diagnosed with the APLS. Foetal death occurs in up to 5 % of unselected pregnancies. Although this may be linked to the APLS, the overall contribution of this syndrome is uncertain, partly because of the effect of other contributing factors such as hypertension, SLE or CKD.

Clinical Manifestations

Thromboses, in particular venous thromboembolism, are the most frequent manifestation of the APLS. Importantly, by comparison to other thrombophilias, thrombosis associated with the APLS may occur in any vascular bed. Arterial thrombosis occurs most frequently in the central nervous system, usually in the form of a stroke or transient ischaemic attack, as shown in Case 4. Less common presentations include venous sinus thrombosis, myelopathy, chorea, migraine and epilepsy. Anticardiolipin antibodies are associated with cognitive impairment in SLE. Considerable interest, and controversy, has focused on the relationship between APLS and cognitive impairment. Cognitive deficits range from subtle findings to transient global amnesia to permanent and profound cognitive functioning. The cognitive deficits reported in APLS are sometimes but not always associated with white matter lesions.

Other clinical manifestations of the APLS include the cardiac valvular disease – mitral valve more commonly affected than the aortic, regurgitation more common than stenosis. Renal involvement in the APLS has only been described relatively recently [39]. Thrombotic microangiopathy is the commonest feature of APLS nephropathy, but other histological findings include fibrous intimal hyperplasia and focal cortical atrophy. A typical presentation of APLS nephropathy is hypertension with (often subnephrotic range) proteinuria and renal insufficiency. Other clinical features of the APLS include haemolytic anaemia, thrombocytopenia, skin involvement with livedo reticularis – present in ~25 % of patients with APLS and a marker of patients at risk of arterial thrombosis – avascular bone necrosis and adrenal insufficiency. Obstetric complications of the APLS include recurrent miscarriage, foetal death, severe preeclampsia and placental insufficiency.

Clinically the most severe, but fortunately the most infrequent, form of the syndrome is catastrophic APLS characterised by widespread small vessel thrombosis with multi-organ failure. Catastrophic APLS is associated with a >50 % mortality.

Investigations and Diagnosis

Diagnosis of APLS relies on a clinical manifestation alongside laboratory evidence of a circulating antiphospholipid antibody [40].

Clinical Criteria

- Vascular thrombosis – arterial, venous or small vessel
- Pregnancy morbidity – one or more of:
  - One or more deaths of a healthy foetus at 10 or more weeks' gestation
  - One or more premature births of a healthy baby before 34 weeks' gestation because of eclampsia or preeclampsia
  - Three or more unexplained consecutive spontaneous abortions before 10 weeks' gestation

Laboratory Criteria

Demonstration on two more occasions at least 12 weeks apart of:

- Lupus anticoagulant
- Anticardiolipin antibody (IgM or IgG)
- Anti-β2-glycoprotein 1 antibody (IgM or IgG)

Note, antibodies directed against phosphatidylserine-prothrombin complex, those of IgA subtype, and antiprothrombin antibodies currently remain excluded from these criteria. Also, the IgG subclass of antibody confers a greater risk of thrombosis than do those of IgM or IgA subtype.

Management

The goal of therapy is to prevent thrombosis either in those individuals with antiphospholipid antibodies who have already had a thrombotic event (secondary prevention) or in those without previous thrombosis (primary prevention).

Current treatment for secondary prevention in those individuals presenting with a first venous thrombosis is with lifelong anticoagulation, usually with warfarin, with a target INR of 2.0–3.0. For those who have had recurrent venous thrombosis or arterial thrombosis, a higher INR may be desirable.

Current recommendations for primary prevention of APLS are not clear. However, the annual thrombotic risk of patients with SLE and antiphospholipid antibodies is about 3–4 %, and so we would recommend the use of low-dose daily aspirin in these patients. Importantly, other vascular risk factors should be treated aggressively in all patients with antiphospholipid antibodies.

Potential Future Therapies

1. *Combination antiplatelet therapy*: low-dose aspirin with clopidogrel or dipyridamole. This may be of benefit in patients intolerant of warfarin or in whom this is not safe.
2. *Oral antifactor Xa agents (rivaroxaban, apixaban)* and *direct thrombin inhibitors (dabigatran)*: as yet not studied in APLS.
3. *B cell depletion (rituximab)*: case reports suggest this may be effective but no trials of its use in APLS yet.
4. *Statins and hydroxychloroquine*: these may have off-target effects in reducing thrombotic risk.

Useful Websites

For Professionals

http://www.rheumatology.org/practice/clinical/classification/
http://www.eular.org/index.cfm?framePage=/recommendations_management.cfm

For Patients

http://www.lupusuk.org.uk
http://www.arthritiscare.org.uk

References

1. Berden JH. Lupus nephritis. Kidney Int. 1997;52:538–58.
2. Austin HA, Illei GG. Membranous lupus nephritis. Lupus. 2005;14:65–71.
3. Pirani CL, Olesnicky L. Role of electronmicroscopy in the classification of lupus nephritis. Am J Kidney Dis. 1982;2:150–63.
4. Tsumagari T, Fukumoto S, Kinjo M, Tanaka K. Incidence and significance of intrarenal vasculopathies in patients with systemic lupus erythematosus. Hum Pathol. 1985;16:43–9.
5. Banfi G, Bertani T, Boeri V, et al. Renal vascular lesions as a marker of poor prognosis in patients with lupus nephritis. Gruppo Italiano per lo Studio Della Nefrite Lupica (GISNEL). Am J Kidney Dis. 1991;18:240–8.
6. Grishman E, Venkataseshan VS. Vascular lesions in lupus nephritis. Mod Pathol. 1988;1:235–41.
7. Cameron JS. Lupus nephritis. J Am Soc Nephrol. 1999;10:413–24.
8. Markowitz GS, D'Agati VD. Classification of lupus nephritis. Curr Opin Nephrol Hypertens. 2009;18:220–5.
9. Weening JJ, D'Agati VD, Schwartz MM, et al. The classification of glomerulonephritis in systemic lupus erythematosus revisited. J Am Soc Nephrol. 2004;15:241–50.
10. Dube GK, Markowitz GS, Radhakrishnan J, Appel GB, D'Agati VD. Minimal change disease in systemic lupus erythematosus. Clin Nephrol. 2002;57:120–6.
11. Kraft SW, Schwartz MM, Korbet SM, Lewis EJ. Glomerular podocytopathy in patients with systemic lupus erythematosus. J Am Soc Nephrol. 2005;16:175–9.
12. Han TS, Schwartz MM, Lewis EJ. Association of glomerular podocytopathy and nephrotic proteinuria in mesangial lupus nephritis. Lupus. 2006;15:71–5.
13. Illei GG, Austin HA, Crane M, et al. Combination therapy with pulse cyclophosphamide plus pulse methylprednisolone improves long-term renal outcome without adding toxicity in patients with lupus nephritis. Ann Intern Med. 2001;135:248–57.
14. Houssiau FA, Vasconcelos C, D'Cruz D, et al. Immunosuppressive therapy in lupus nephritis: the Euro-Lupus Nephritis Trial, a randomized trial of low-dose versus high-dose intravenous cyclophosphamide. Arthritis Rheum. 2002;46:2121–31.
15. Houssiau FA, Vasconcelos C, D'Cruz D, et al. The 10-year follow-up data of the Euro-Lupus Nephritis Trial comparing low-dose and high-dose intravenous cyclophosphamide. Ann Rheum Dis. 2010;69:61–4.
16. Chan TM, Li FK, Tang CS, et al. Efficacy of mycophenolate mofetil in patients with diffuse proliferative lupus nephritis. Hong Kong-Guangzhou Nephrology Study Group. N Engl J Med. 2000;343:1156–62.
17. Chan TM, Tse KC, Tang CS, Mok MY, Li FK. Long-term study of mycophenolate mofetil as continuous induction and maintenance treatment for diffuse proliferative lupus nephritis. J Am Soc Nephrol. 2005;16:1076–84.
18. Ginzler EM, Dooley MA, Aranow C, et al. Mycophenolate mofetil or intravenous cyclophosphamide for lupus nephritis. N Engl J Med. 2005;353:2219–28.
19. Walsh M, James M, Jayne D, Tonelli M, Manns BJ, Hemmelgarn BR. Mycophenolate mofetil for induction therapy of lupus nephritis: a systematic review and meta-analysis. Clin J Am Soc Nephrol. 2007;2:968–75.
20. Appel GB, Contreras G, Dooley MA, et al. Mycophenolate mofetil versus cyclophosphamide for induction treatment of lupus nephritis. J Am Soc Nephrol. 2009;20:1103–12.
21. Lee YH, Woo JH, Choi SJ, Ji JD, Song GG. Induction and maintenance therapy for lupus nephritis: a systematic review and meta-analysis. Lupus. 2010;19:703–10.
22. Grootscholten C, Ligtenberg G, Hagen EC, et al. Azathioprine/methylprednisolone versus cyclophosphamide in proliferative lupus nephritis. A randomized controlled trial. Kidney Int. 2006;70:732–42.
23. Lu TY, Ng KP, Cambridge G, et al. A retrospective seven-year analysis of the use of B cell depletion therapy in systemic lupus erythematosus at University College London Hospital: the first fifty patients. Arthritis Rheum. 2009;61:482–7.
24. Melander C, Sallee M, Trolliet P, et al. Rituximab in severe lupus nephritis: early B-cell depletion affects long-term renal outcome. Clin J Am Soc Nephrol. 2009;4:579–87.
25. Merrill JT, Neuwelt CM, Wallace DJ, et al. Efficacy and safety of rituximab in moderately-to-severely active systemic lupus erythematosus: the randomized, double-blind, phase II/III systemic lupus erythematosus evaluation of rituximab trial. Arthritis Rheum. 2010;62:222–33.
26. Rovin BH, Furie R, Latinis K, et al. Efficacy and safety of rituximab in patients with active proliferative lupus nephritis: the Lupus Nephritis Assessment with Rituximab study. Arthritis Rheum. 2012;64:1215–26.
27. Flanc RS, Roberts MA, Strippoli GF, Chadban SJ, Kerr PG, Atkins RC. Treatment of diffuse proliferative lupus nephritis: a meta-analysis of randomized controlled trials. Am J Kidney Dis. 2004;43:197–208.
28. Zhu B, Chen N, Lin Y, et al. Mycophenolate mofetil in induction and maintenance therapy of severe lupus nephritis: a meta-analysis of randomized controlled trials. Nephrol Dial Transplant. 2007;22:1933–42.
29. Contreras G, Pardo V, Leclercq B, et al. Sequential therapies for proliferative lupus nephritis. N Engl J Med. 2004;350:971–80.
30. Contreras G, Tozman E, Nahar N, Metz D. Maintenance therapies for proliferative lupus nephritis: mycophenolate mofetil, azathioprine and intravenous cyclophosphamide. Lupus. 2005;14 Suppl 1:s33–8.
31. Houssiau FA, D'Cruz D, Sangle S, et al. Azathioprine versus mycophenolate mofetil for long-term immunosuppression in lupus nephritis: results from the MAINTAIN Nephritis Trial. Ann Rheum Dis. 2010;69:2083–9.
32. Dooley MA, Jayne D, Ginzler EM, et al. Mycophenolate versus azathioprine as maintenance therapy for lupus nephritis. N Engl J Med. 2011;365:1886–95.
33. Ginzler E, Sharon E, Diamond H, Kaplan D. Long-term maintenance therapy with azathioprine in systemic lupus erythematosus. Arthritis Rheum. 1975;18:27–34.
34. Austin 3rd HA, Illei GG, Braun MJ, Balow JE. Randomized, controlled trial of prednisone, cyclophosphamide, and cyclosporine in lupus membranous nephropathy. J Am Soc Nephrol. 2009;20:901–11.
35. Cattran DC, Alexopoulos E, Heering P, et al. Cyclosporin in idiopathic glomerular disease associated with the nephrotic syndrome: workshop recommendations. Kidney Int. 2007;72:1429–47.
36. Waldman M, Austin 3rd HA. Treatment of idiopathic membranous nephropathy. J Am Soc Nephrol. 2012;23:1617–30.

37. Navarra SV, Guzman RM, Gallacher AE, et al. Efficacy and safety of belimumab in patients with active systemic lupus erythematosus: a randomised, placebo-controlled, phase 3 trial. Lancet. 2011; 377:721–31.
38. Dhaun N, Kluth DC. Belimumab for systemic lupus erythematosus. Lancet. 2011;377:2079–80; author reply 80–1.
39. Amigo MC, Garcia-Torres R, Robles M, Bochicchio T, Reyes PA. Renal involvement in primary antiphospholipid syndrome. J Rheumatol. 1992;19:1181–5.
40. Miyakis S, Lockshin MD, Atsumi T, et al. International consensus statement on an update of the classification criteria for definite antiphospholipid syndrome (APS). J Thromb Haemost. 2006;4:295–306.

Practical Immunosuppression Guidelines for Patients with Glomerulonephritis

23

Ruth J. Pepper and Alan D. Salama

Many forms of glomerular disease are immune mediated and are therefore treated with immunosuppression. The particular regimen that is used may vary depending on the underlying condition, but many protocols are based on combination therapy using glucocorticoids and a second agent, which has historically often been cyclophosphamide. With the introduction of newer immunosuppressive agents, including biologics, these protocols have been modified for different conditions and, in only some cases, tested in randomised controlled trials. Certain protocols are based on oral therapies and can easily be delivered safely as outpatients; others require infusions which necessitate careful co-ordination of day case admissions and outpatient monitoring to allow early recognition of potential adverse events. Regardless of the actual regimen used, there are some general principles that apply to delivering a safe immunosuppressive service. In this chapter, we discuss practical issues surrounding immunosuppression in glomerular disease.

Protocol Constituents

Cyclophosphamide

The risks of cyclophosphamide are believed to be outweighed in severe life- or organ-threatening conditions; however, it is important to make patients aware of potential toxicities (see Appendix 1, e.g. of a cyclophosphamide consent sheet). Limiting the patient's total exposure is desirable, as adverse events are related to cumulative dose and there are significant increases in haematological and bladder malignancies once total exposure exceeds 36 g [1].

Cyclophosphamide may be used orally (at doses of 2–3 mg/kg), for example, in anti-GBM disease or intravenously as pulses every 2–3 weeks depending on the protocol, for example, in the Eurolupus regimen or the CYCLOPS vasculitis regimen.

There is ample evidence that pulsed intravenous treatment induces remission as rapidly in as many patients as daily oral therapy but exposes the patients to lower drug levels and thus is associated with fewer leucopenic episodes [2]. Long-term lower doses of cyclophosphamide are associated with higher relapse rates, in certain conditions [3, 4]. While the data are available to confirm benefit in SLE and ANCA-associated vasculitis (AAV), no direct comparisons have, or will likely to be, performed in anti-GBM disease. Therefore, many practitioners still utilise oral cyclophosphamide in anti-GBM disease based on established protocols.

With modern dosage regimens of cyclophosphamide, the incidence of haemorrhagic cystitis is low and the use of MESNA as a bladder protectant may be unnecessary [5]. In addition there may be reactions to the MESNA itself and thus some units have abandoned the routine use of MESNA. Encouraging oral input (assuming the patient is not oligo-anuric) to maintain a good urine output and reduce the concentration of bladder accumulating metabolites is useful.

Dose adjustments should be made based on age and renal function. A schema for dose reduction of pulsed intravenous cyclophosphamide as used in ANCA-associated vasculitis is shown in Table 23.1, while if daily oral treatment is used, the dose should be reduced by 25 % if >60 years and 50 % if >70 years.

Cyclophosphamide should be withheld if the total WCC is less than 4×10^9, and oral doses should be reduced by 50 mg if the white count is trending downwards, to avoid development of episodes of leucopenia. Weekly WCC checks are mandatory whilst on oral cyclophosphamide for the first month, twice weekly for the second month and monthly thereafter for the first year.

R.J. Pepper, MRCP, PhD (✉)
Department of Nephrology, Royal Free Hospital, Pond Street, London NW3 2PF, UK
e-mail: r.pepper@ucl.ac.uk

A.D. Salama, MA, PhD, FRCP
UCL Centre for Nephrology, Royal Free Hospital, Rowland Hill Street, London NW3 2PF, UK
e-mail: a.salama@ucl.ac.uk

M. Harber (ed.), *Practical Nephrology*,
DOI 10.1007/978-1-4471-5547-8_23, © Springer-Verlag London 2014

Table 23.1 Intravenous cyclophosphamide regime used in systemic vasculitis demonstrating dose adjustment for both age and renal function

	Creatinine μmol/l	
Age (years)	<300	300–500
<60	15 mg/kg/pulse	12.5 mg/kg/pulse
60–70	12.5 mg/kg/pulse	10 mg/kg/pulse
>70	10 mg/kg/pulse	7.5 mg/kg/pulse

Taken from [2]
Patients with a nadir leucocyte count of $2–3 \times 10^9$/l had a dose reduction of 20 %. Dose reduced by 40 % in those who had a nadir leucocyte count of $1–2 \times 10^9$/l. Omit pulse if WBC nadir $<1 \times 10^9$/l and consider g-CSF administration and antibiotic prophylaxis

Table 23.2 Steroid reducing protocol. If pulsed methylprednisolone is given, starting dose of steroid could be reduced

Prednisolone (non-enteric-coated) protocol	Starting dose: 1 mg/kg daily orally (maximum 60 mg/day)
Week 1	60 mg/day
Week 2	45 mg/day
Week 3	30 mg/day
Week 4	25 mg/day
Week 5	20 mg/day
Thereafter steroid reductions depending on patient's response	2.5 mg dose reduction every 2 weeks
Month 3–4	10 mg/day

Pulsed therapy dosage should be adjusted depending on nadir WCC, checked 7–10 days after treatment. We ensure that a recent (within 1 week) blood test is available prior to delivering the next dose.

Prophylaxis for pneumocystis jiroveci with low-dose co-trimoxazole is required in CYP-treated patients. This can be delivered as 480 mg daily or 960 mg three times a week. In cases of co-trimoxazole allergy monthly nebulised pentamidine may be used instead. Anti-emetics, such as ondansetron 8 mg or granisetron 1–2 mg, should be given 30 min pre- and 12 h post-infusion.

Glucocorticoids

Steroids (glucocorticoids) have been the mainstay of treatment for nearly all immune-based diseases, and this is true of most glomerular diseases. The dose regimens used in glomerular diseases have been highly variable and mostly decided on empirically without any comparative trial data. There are two main ways of delivering steroids by intravenous bolus (using methylprednisolone or dexamethasone) or by daily or alternate-day oral medication (using prednisolone or methylprednisolone). These are clearly not mutually exclusive. Conventionally, in adult practice, steroids are taken daily and doses of 1 mg/kg, with a maximum starting dose of 60 mg, of prednisolone are commonly used to induce remission. The speed of taper and decision to wean completely or not are highly variable in clinical practice. One current strategy commonly used for weaning is shown in Table 23.2. If pulses of methylprednisolone are used, then it seems sensible to reduce the initial dose of oral prednisolone, to start at 30 mg/day although there are no available trial data to support this approach at present. Pulsed methylprednisolone has been delivered at doses of 250–1,000 mg/day over three consecutive days, again without ever comparing efficacy of differing doses. It is probably reasonable to limit pulses to a total of 1.5 g of methylprednisolone, as it is generally believed that much of the early morbidity following immunosuppression induction may relate to steroid usage. Pulsed steroid use may be a reasonable temporising measure if plasmapheresis is not immediately available, although the latter is preferable based on randomised trials, at least in management of systemic vasculitis and anti-GBM disease [6, 7].

Infection, Bone and Gastric Prophylaxis

Prevention of steroid side effects warrants prophylactic treatment with regard to gastric, bone and fungal complications. All patients on high-dose steroids should receive gastric protection with proton pump inhibitors or H2 antagonists. Bone protection with calcium D3 combination (1 g of calcium/day) and consideration for bisphosphonate use if renal function allows and if there is any pre-existing bone mineral density loss. Fungal prophylaxis may be in the form of nystatin suspension or low-dose fluconazole (but confirm no possible drug interaction with other immunosuppressants such as calcineurin inhibitors).

Plasmapheresis

Plasmapheresis removes a number of plasma proteins that may contribute to disease pathogenesis, including autoantibodies, immune complexes, complement components, clotting factors and microparticles derived from inflammatory or endothelial cells. There are two main ways of performing plasmapheresis, using a plasma filter or a centrifugal bowl. The advantage of the former is that it is easily performed by most dialysis nurses, but the filter may limit removal of larger molecules such as IgM; by contrast bowl centrifugation has the advantage of removing all plasma components but may be limited in availability in certain units. Further modifications of these techniques exist including the double-filtration plasmapheresis method (DFPP), which returns some of the smaller plasma molecules (such as albumin) to the patient, necessitating less replacement fluid; cryofiltration which is when the plasmapheresis is performed at lower temperatures in an attempt to increase removal of immune complexes; and plasma absorption when specific affinity columns are used to allow greater removal of certain molecules such as immunoglobulin (using protein A columns).

Replacement fluid should be in the form of 4.5 % albumin, unless there is a bleeding tendency; a recent invasive procedure or the procedure is aimed at replacing a missing factor, such as in atypical HUS where an abnormal complement factor may be contributing to disease. In those oligoanuric or anuric patients, the salt load from the 4.5 % albumin solution can be considerable, and increased fluid removal with subsequent dialysis may be necessary to prevent fluid overload.

The dose of plasmapheresis should be calculated based on plasma volume or body weight, and typically 1–1.5 plasma volumes are exchanged per session (generally 50–60 ml/kg). It is important to review the delivered dose that is achieved, as failure to respond may be due to inadequate plasma exchange.

Plasmapheresis has been shown to be of benefit in anti-GBM disease, when it is delivered for 14 exchanges or until the anti-GBM antibody is negative, and in patients with ANCA-associated vasculitis (AAV) and severe renal involvement (creatinine > 500 μmol/l) [6, 7]. It may be of benefit in less severe forms of AAV, and this is currently being tested in a randomised clinical trial (see www.vasculitis.org). There is no evidence for a benefit in SLE [8] or in other forms of rapidly progressive glomerulonephritis, but it is often used in such patients with renal deterioration in the hope that there may be some benefit (see RPGN below).

Fertility Sparing Measures and Pregnancies

Fertility impairment is related to use of cyclophosphamide and is in part related to the age of the patient and the pre-treatment sperm viability or ovarian function. It is therefore always best to sperm bank men of child-bearing age, prior to cyclophosphamide treatment, and discuss ovarian protection or egg harvesting in women. Practically, the induction therapy for egg harvesting is not suited to acutely ill patients who may need to start cyclophosphamide therapy urgently, and so a more favoured approach is the use of gonadotropin-releasing hormone (GnRH) analogues prior to the use of cyclophosphamide treatment, which may be appropriate in female patients up to the age of 40 years [9]. Use of Goserelin monthly (3.6 mg) or three monthly is generally adequate for induction of chemical menopause. There are no data however confirming that this approach results in a better proportion of patients with preserved fertility, but many practitioners use such an approach nonetheless.

In those planning a pregnancy, this should be ideally delayed for a period such as 6 months following the last dose of cyclophosphamide. The patient should also have had a period of disease remission for several months before planning a pregnancy. Certain maintenance immunosuppressives can be continued, while others need to be stopped or switched to more appropriate equivalents. Examples of drugs that can be or cannot be continued in pregnancy are shown in Table 23.3.

Table 23.3 Drug modifications in those planning pregnancy

Can be continued in pregnancy	Needs to be discontinued	Uncertain
Azathioprine	Mycophenolate mofetil/MPA	Rituximab
Steroids	Cyclophosphamide	
Tacrolimus or cyclosporin A	ACE inhibitors/ARB	
Hydroxychloroquine	Proton pump inhibitors	

Rituximab

This anti-CD20 monoclonal antibody, first introduced for treatment of lymphoma, is now extensively used in autoimmunity and in many forms of glomerular disease. It is administered as a slow intravenous infusion with steroid and antihistamine premedication (methylprednisolone 125 mg and chlorpheniramine). Infusion reactions are the most common adverse event. B-cell depletion is generally achieved after one dose but may be less efficacious if significant monoclonal is lost in the urine, in nephrotic states. B-cell numbers should be checked following administration. It may be administered as two infusions 2 weeks apart (each of 1g) or as a four-dose weekly regimen of 375 mg/m^2. Both appear to be equally efficacious in glomerular disease.

Secondary hypogammaglobulinaemia may result and the more severe this is, the more likely the patient will develop an infectious complication. IgG levels should be monitored in case levels are low and replacement immunoglobulin may be required. Rituximab is also currently being trialled as a maintenance therapy in two randomised vasculitis trials.

MMF and Azathioprine

MMF is extensively used as induction therapy in SLE and has been shown to be of equal efficacy in inducing remission in lupus nephritis as cyclophosphamide – with better tolerability in certain ethnic groups (such as African-Americans and Hispanics). Some centres advocate therapeutic drug monitoring, although many trials treated to a particular dose. Starting at a lower dose and increasing rapidly may allow for fewer gastrointestinal side effects.

Azathioprine requires no such dose adjustments, but TPMT levels should be checked prior to commencing therapy as this may allow dose adjustment in patients likely to suffer bone marrow toxicity, with low TPMT activity. Care should be taken if patients are on allopurinol as this increases azathioprine toxicity. Monitoring of liver function tests and a full blood count regularly will help prevent hepatitis and leucopenia. Azathioprine is infrequently used for induction therapy, but rather as a common maintenance agent. It is more effective than MMF in vasculitis maintenance, with significantly less time to relapse.

Table 23.4 Treatment regime for anti-GBM disease [14]

Drug/treatment	Dose	Duration
Corticosteroids	1 mg/kg/day (max 60 mg/day)	6–9 months
Cyclophosphamide	Oral: 2–3 mg/kg Dose reduction in >55 years	2–3 months
Plasma exchange	Human albumin solution; 50 ml/kg max 4 l	At least 14 days or till anti-GBM antibody normalised
Prophylaxis	Nystatin or fluconazole Calcium D3 PPI or H2 antagonist	For duration of high-dose steroids
	Septrin 480 mg daily or 960 mg three times a week	For duration of cyclophosphamide

Protocols for Particular Glomerular Diseases

Rapidly Progressive Glomerulonephritis

Rapidly progressive glomerulonephritis (RPGN) is defined as sudden loss of renal function, with halving of GFR within 3 months. Prompt diagnosis and treatment is crucial to prevent irreversible loss of renal function. Histologically, RPGN is caused by a crescentic glomerulonephritis, which is due to severe glomerular injury, as a result of rupture of the glomerular capillary loop basement membrane. Crescentic glomerulonephritis is generally defined as having more than 50 % of glomeruli involved with crescents, which are identified by the presence of at least two layers of cells in Bowman's space.

RPGN can be commonly categorised into being caused by:

- Anti-glomerular basement membrane (GBM) disease
- Immune-complex glomerulonephritis
- Pauci-immune glomerulonephritis, associated with ANCA in most cases

The standard of care has long been steroids and cyclophosphamide, with trials in pauci-immune GN demonstrating that newer regimens using lower doses of cyclophosphamide delivered as intravenous pulses provide equal efficacy and fewer adverse events such as leucopenia. New trials in ANCA-associated vasculitis have demonstrated that induction therapy with rituximab is as effective as cyclophosphamide [10, 11], while studies in SLE have failed to demonstrate benefit of additional RTX therapy above standard treatment [12, 13]. Since there have been few randomised studies of treatment of other causes of RPGN, we are left to extrapolate protocols from these studies.

Anti-GBM Disease

Treatment should be initiated immediately in those in whom it is appropriate. Recommendations are to initiate daily plasma exchange for a total of 14 sessions or until the anti-GBM antibody has disappeared. Plasma exchange should be against human albumin solution, unless there has been a recent renal biopsy or active bleeding, and then it should be replaced in part (300–600 ml) with fresh frozen plasma (FFP) [14]. Long-term immunosuppression is not required due to the monophasic nature of the disease, with cyclophosphamide treatment recommended for 2–3 months and steroid for no more than 6–9 months (see Table 23.4).

Immune-Complex Glomerulonephritis

This describes the formation of immune deposits, which contain immunoglobulins, complement and other proteins within the glomerulus resulting in glomerular injury. There are several underlying causes of a RPGN with immune-complex deposition histologically.

IgA Nephropathy (IgAN)

While there are data demonstrating efficacy of immunosuppression with steroids in patients with IgAN with moderate proteinuria (1–3.5 g/day) and mild renal impairment (serum creatinine ≤1.5 mg/dl) [15], evidence is lacking for treatment of a crescentic IgAN. A rapidly progressive course with crescents has been treated with a regimen based on that for systemic vasculitis using combination steroids and cyclophosphamide. A small study of 12 patients with a crescentic, progressive disease treated with pulsed steroids and monthly cyclophosphamide resulted in a reduction in proliferative lesions and proteinuria and stabilisation in renal function [16]. In some young patients with crescentic IgA and a rapid renal decline, plasmapheresis has also been used with variable results.

Lupus Nephritis

Renal involvement frequently occurs in SLE, with proliferative lesions (class III and IV) having a poorer outcome, than mesangial lesions (class II). The treatment regimen can be considered in two parts: induction therapy and maintenance. However, there are limited published data on treating crescentic lupus nephritis or SLE causing a RPGN.

The old NIH high-dose pulsed cyclophosphamide (CYP) regimen [17] has for the most part been abandoned, and there are now two significant protocols to consider. The first

Table 23.5 Treatment in lupus nephritis (class III, IV)

Drug	Dose	Investigations	Caution
MMF	Titrate aiming to 3 g/day (induction) 2 g/day (maintenance)	WCC: stop if neutropenic	Teratogenic
Cyclophosphamide Eurolupus: outpatient infusions	500 mg IV every 2 weeks for 3 months	WCC: 10–14 days after last dose. Hold dose if WCC<4	Mesna optional, dose 20 % of CYP dose Ovarian protection with GnRHa may be beneficial
Corticosteroids	60 mg/day: taper decreasing to ≤10 mg by 24 weeks		Gastric protection Bone protection
Azathioprine	2 mg/kg	TPMT (thiopurine methyltransferase) activity: low levels will require decreasing the dose FBC, LFTs: monitor after initiation of therapy	Can replace MMF as maintenance therapy if pregnancy being considered
Consider:			
Rituximab	1 g day 1 and 15	Peripheral B count (CD19) to assess depletion	Prevention of transfusion reaction give methylprednisolone 100 mg
Belimumab	Day 0, 14 and 28 then every 28 days		

is the Eurolupus protocol [18]. The Eurolupus trial consisted of predominantly Caucasian patients with proliferative lupus nephritis, including those patients with glomerular crescents, and compared low-dose CYP with standard high dose (NIH) CYP. This trial provided evidence for a short, low-dose course of intravenous cyclophosphamide (500 mg every 2 weeks for 3 months) followed by azathioprine (2–2.5 mg/kg/day) which was initiated 2 weeks after the last dose of CYP, as well as corticosteroids [18]. The dose of steroids was initially started at 1 mg/kg/day, with a gradual taper down to 5–7.5 mg after approximately 6 months of therapy.

The second is based on the use of mycophenolate mofetil (MMF) at a target dose of 3 g/day [19], in conjunction with prednisolone starting at 60 mg/day. Although a recent multicentre trial failed to demonstrate MMF *superiority* over intravenous cyclophosphamide (0.5–1 g/m^2 6 monthly pulses), the two drugs induced similar rates of remission and MMF treatment was associated with significantly fewer serious adverse events. In addition, differences in response to these immunosuppressants were found in different ethnic groups, with MMF proving more effective than cyclophosphamide in black and Hispanic patients [19].

After the completion of induction therapy, patients are prescribed maintenance treatment to reduce the risk of flares. This treatment should be continued for some time although exactly how long is debated. Similar to the induction treatment trials, there seems to be an ethnic variation in the response to treatment. In a predominantly Caucasian cohort, MMF (2 g/day) was not superior to azathioprine (2 mg/kg per day) with respect to renal flares, doubling of creatinine or infectious complications [20]. However, in the ALMS study, which included more of the high-risk black patients, MMF was superior to azathioprine at maintaining disease remission [21].

Various uncontrolled studies have demonstrated promising results with rituximab for patients with lupus nephritis [22] including those with refractory/relapsing disease [23]. However, a large multicentre, randomised trial (LUNAR), investigating the use of rituximab alongside steroids and MMF in proliferative lupus nephritis, failed to demonstrate additional impact of rituximab [13]. Currently, rituximab may be considered an option for those with refractory, relapsing disease or intolerant of first-line therapies. However, an anti-Blys (B-lymphocyte stimulator)monoclonal antibody, belimumab, has been shown to be effective in a recent SLE trial demonstrating improvements in a number of disease domains and has recently been licensed for treatment of SLE [24]. The treatment options are summarised in Table 23.5.

Postinfectious Glomerulonephritis (PIGN)

Infections can result in glomerulonephritis, with a variety of different histological manifestations. Bacteria such as *Staphylococcus aureus* and Streptococci as well as infective endocarditis are well recognised as underlying causes of an infection-related glomerulonephritis, which may manifest as a RPGN with crescentic or vasculitic lesions seen on renal biopsy. The association between staphylococcal infections and IgA rich PIGN is now well established. Antibiotic therapy is clearly crucial in these infectious diseases, while there may be a role for corticosteroids under certain circumstances. However, overall no correlation between steroid use and renal outcome has been demonstrated [25], so this issue remains controversial.

Pauci-Immune Glomerulonephritis

This describes the appearance on renal biopsy in which there is little or no glomerular staining of immunoglobulins, which most commonly is associated with anti-neutrophil cytoplasm antibody (ANCA), and represents the most likely cause of a RPGN in adults [26]. Like treatment of SLE, treatment of AAV consists of induction and maintenance. Renal function and age are important predictors of outcome. Cyclophosphamide has been part of the gold standard induction agent for many years, although its use at high doses for prolonged periods resulted in significant adverse effects. Treatment regimens have been refined over the years to reduce the total cumulative dose of cyclophosphamide. Numerous EUVAS (European Vasculitis Study Group) trials have investigated optimal regimens for different disease states. The CYCLOPS trial included patients with a serum creatinine <500 μmol/l and demonstrated that the combination of pulsed intravenous cyclophosphamide and oral steroids was as effective at inducing disease remission as an oral cyclophosphamide regimen but induced fewer episodes of leucopenia [2], although long-term follow-up has shown that this intravenous regime is associated with increased relapses [3]. Table 23.1 demonstrates the intravenous dosing regimen used in this study.

The MEPEX study investigated patients with more advanced renal failure (serum creatinine >500 μmol/l) and demonstrated the benefits of plasma exchange, alongside oral cyclophosphamide and corticosteroids in renal recovery at 3 months and 1 year [6]. There is now increasing use of intravenous cyclophosphamide in this group of patients with severe renal failure to reduce the incidence of leucopenia, with patients receiving 6–10 pulses of cyclophosphamide. The dose of steroids is usually started at 1 mg/kg, with tapering to a dose of 10–15 mg/day by 3 months and 5 mg by 1 year. Maintenance therapy consists of long-term immunosuppression following the period of induction therapy. The CYCAZAREM trial demonstrated that cyclophosphamide at 3–6 months could be safely substituted for azathioprine (2 mg/kg/day) [27], while a recent study demonstrated that MMF is not as effective as azathioprine in maintenance therapy [28], so should be reserved for patients who cannot tolerate azathioprine.

There is increasing use of rituximab in patients with AAV, with 2 randomised trials providing evidence that its use as induction therapy is equivalent to that of cyclophosphamide [10, 11]. The RAVE trial compared oral cyclophosphamide with rituximab, excluding those with severe renal failure (creatinine>4 mg/dl), although patients with less severe renal disease were included [10] and demonstrated equivalence of RTX and CYP but superiority of RTX for those with relapsing disease. RITUXVAS included those with severe (dialysis dependent) renal involvement and demonstrated the rituximab regime not to be inferior [11]. Both the 375 mg/m^2 × 1/week for 4 weeks (regime in RAVE and RITUXIVAS) and 1 g repeated after 2 weeks appeared equally effective. Table 23.6 shows the treatment options in AAV.

Table 23.6 Induction and maintenance doses of immunosuppressive agents in ANCA-associated vasculitis

Therapy	Dose	Specific investigations that modify dose/therapy
Cyclophosphamide	MEPEX oral: 2–3 mg/kg	WCC: <4 withhold drug
	Age>60 years 2 mg/kg	WCC: 4–5 reduce dose
		Prophylaxis as for anti-GBM disease
Rituximab	Either 375 mg/m^2 × 1/week for 4 weeks	Monitor CD19 count: adequate peripheral blood depletion <0.005 × 10^9
	Or 1 g at day 1 and day 15	WCC: neutropenia reported following chronic use
		Monitor immunoglobulins
Azathioprine	1–2 mg/kg	TPMT (thiopurine methyltransferase) activity: low levels require decreasing the dose to 1 mg/kg
		FBC, LFTs: monitor after initiation of therapy
Mycophenolate mofetil	2 g/day	WCC: stop if neutropenic
		Reduce dose WCC<4
Methotrexate	0.03 mg/kg/week	Check LFT, WCC alt weeks to begin with
		Annual CXR
	Starting at 10–15 mg/week	Procollagen III may be helpful in monitoring for liver damage
		Add folic acid 5 mg weekly taken 2 days after MTX

Appendix 1: Information for Renal Patients Receiving Cyclophosphamide Therapy

This information sheet describes cyclophosphamide, how it is administered and some of the side effects it may cause. Please ask a member of staff if you want information about other alternatives to treatment with cyclophosphamide or if you have any other questions.

How Is It Given?

Cyclophosphamide can be given by injection into a vein (intravenously) or as a tablet. Your doctor will agree with you as to which the best route is for you to receive the drug.

Tablets may have to be taken for a number of months; the intravenous infusion is generally given every 2–4 weeks. The length of the treatment will depend on your condition and response to treatment, but it generally lasts 3–4 months.

If you are receiving the intravenous infusion, you will attend the renal day ward (3 East). You will need to stay for up to 2 h, although generally it takes less time.

How Does Cyclophosphamide Work?

Cyclophosphamide works by depressing ('damping down') your immune system. The aim of the treatment is to reduce the inflammation that is causing the problem with your affected organs such as kidneys, lungs or nose.

What Are the Possible Side Effects?

Nausea and vomiting may occur if you take cyclophosphamide. This can be controlled by giving you anti-sickness (anti-emetic) tablets as needed.

Increased risk of infection is a result of the suppression of white blood cell production in your bone marrow. White blood cells help to fight infection. Your levels of white blood cells will be monitored. If you develop a temperature, fever or any signs of infection, please contact either the ward or your GP. You should also report any bruising/bleeding or excessive tiredness. You will be given an antibiotic tablet (or nebuliser if you cannot tolerate the tablets) to stop certain infections, but this will not prevent all infections.

Bladder irritation is a possible side effect if you are receiving intravenous cyclophosphamide. Symptoms include blood in the urine and symptoms of cystitis. You may be given a drug called mesna during the intravenous infusion that will help to prevent this occurring. If you notice any blood in your urine after discharge home, please contact the ward.

Hair thinning may occur. This is not permanent and will grow back after treatment.

Mouth sores may develop if you are taking the tablets, and you will be given a supply of mouth lozenges to help prevent this. Good oral and dental hygiene is important.

Contraception and fertility should be discussed with your doctor or nurse as cyclophosphamide may affect your ability to conceive or father a child. With a standard treatment course, the risk of this happening is relatively small. Women may find their periods altered and men may wish to discuss sperm banking.

Cyclophosphamide and Pregnancy

Cyclophosphamide may cause several different birth defects if it is either taken at the time of conception or during pregnancy. Be sure that you practice effective birth control with a barrier method of contraception while you are being treated with cyclophosphamide. Tell your doctor right away if you think you have become pregnant while taking cyclophosphamide.

If You Become Unwell While Being Treated with Cyclophosphamide

If you become unwell or develop a temperature above 37.5 °C, you must let your doctors know. Please contact your clinic consultant (through switchboard) or the renal day ward during working hours or the on-call renal registrar out of hours, who can be reached through switchboard.

If you require any further information or advice, please ask either your doctor or nurse.

References

1. Faurschou M, Sorensen IJ, Mellemkjaer L, Loft AG, Thomsen BS, Tvede N, et al. Malignancies in Wegener's granulomatosis: incidence and relation to cyclophosphamide therapy in a cohort of 293 patients. J Rheumatol. 2008;35(1):100–5.
2. de Groot K, Harper L, Jayne DR, Flores Suarez LF, Gregorini G, Gross WL, et al. Pulse versus daily oral cyclophosphamide for induction of remission in antineutrophil cytoplasmic antibody-associated vasculitis: a randomized trial. Ann Intern Med. 2009;150(10):670–80.
3. Harper L, Morgan MD, Walsh M, Hoglund P, Westman K, Flossmann O, et al. Pulse versus daily oral cyclophosphamide for induction of remission in ANCA-associated vasculitis: long-term follow-up. Ann Rheum Dis. 2012;71(6):955–60.
4. Pepper R, Chanouzas D, Tarzi R, Little MA, Caisian A, Walsh M, et al. Intravenous cyclophosphamide and plasmapheresis in dialysis dependent ANCA associated vasculitis. Clin J Am Soc Nephrol. 2011;22:560A.
5. Monach PA, Arnold LM, Merkel PA. Incidence and prevention of bladder toxicity from cyclophosphamide in the treatment of rheumatic diseases: a data-driven review. Arthritis Rheum. 2010;62(1):9–21.
6. Jayne DR, Gaskin G, Rasmussen N, Abramowicz D, Ferrario F, Guillevin L, et al. Randomized trial of plasma exchange or high-dosage methylprednisolone as adjunctive therapy for severe renal vasculitis. J Am Soc Nephrol. 2007;18(7):2180–8.
7. Johnson JP, Moore Jr J, Austin 3rd HA, Balow JE, Antonovych TT, Wilson CB. Therapy of anti-glomerular basement membrane antibody disease: analysis of prognostic significance of clinical, pathologic and treatment factors. Medicine (Baltimore). 1985;64(4):219–27.
8. Lewis EJ, Hunsicker LG, Lan SP, Rohde RD, Lachin JM. A controlled trial of plasmapheresis therapy in severe lupus nephritis. The Lupus Nephritis Collaborative Study Group. N Engl J Med. 1992;326(21):1373–9.
9. Henes M, Henes JC, Neunhoeffer E, Schmalzing M, von Wolff M, Kotter I, et al. Fertility preservation methods in young women with systemic lupus erythematosus prior to cytotoxic therapy – Experiences from the FertiProtekt network. Lupus. 2012;21(9):953–8.
10. Stone JH, Merkel PA, Spiera R, Seo P, Langford CA, Hoffman GS, et al. Rituximab versus cyclophosphamide for ANCA-associated vasculitis. N Engl J Med. 2010;363(3):221–32.
11. Jones RB, Tervaert JW, Hauser T, Luqmani R, Morgan MD, Peh CA, et al. Rituximab versus cyclophosphamide in ANCA-associated renal vasculitis. N Engl J Med. 2010;363(3):211–20.
12. Merrill JT, Neuwelt CM, Wallace DJ, Shanahan JC, Latinis KM, Oates JC, et al. Efficacy and safety of rituximab in moderately-to-severely active systemic lupus erythematosus: the randomized, double-blind, phase II/III systemic lupus erythematosus evaluation of rituximab trial. Arthritis Rheum. 2010;62(1):222–33.
13. Rovin BH, Furie R, Latinis K, Looney RJ, Fervenza FC, Sanchez-Guerrero J, et al. Efficacy and safety of rituximab in patients with active proliferative lupus nephritis: the Lupus Nephritis Assessment with Rituximab study. Arthritis Rheum. 2012;64(4):1215–26.
14. Levy JB, Turner AN, Rees AJ, Pusey CD. Long-term outcome of anti-glomerular basement membrane antibody disease treated with plasma exchange and immunosuppression. Ann Intern Med. 2001;134(11):1033–42.
15. Pozzi C, Andrulli S, Del Vecchio L, Melis P, Fogazzi GB, Altieri P, et al. Corticosteroid effectiveness in IgA nephropathy: long-term results of a randomized, controlled trial. J Am Soc Nephrol. 2004;15(1):157–63.
16. Tumlin JA, Lohavichan V, Hennigar R. Crescentic, proliferative IgA nephropathy: clinical and histological response to methylprednisolone and intravenous cyclophosphamide. Nephrol Dial Transplant. 2003;18(7):1321–9.
17. Austin 3rd HA, Klippel JH, Balow JE, le Riche NG, Steinberg AD, Plotz PH, et al. Therapy of lupus nephritis. Controlled trial of prednisone and cytotoxic drugs. N Engl J Med. 1986;314(10):614–9.
18. Houssiau FA, Vasconcelos C, D'Cruz D, Sebastiani GD, Garrido Ed Ede R, Danieli MG, et al. Immunosuppressive therapy in lupus nephritis: the Euro-Lupus Nephritis Trial, a randomized trial of low-dose versus high-dose intravenous cyclophosphamide. Arthritis Rheum. 2002;46(8):2121–31.
19. Appel GB, Contreras G, Dooley MA, Ginzler EM, Isenberg D, Jayne D, et al. Mycophenolate mofetil versus cyclophosphamide for induction treatment of lupus nephritis. J Am Soc Nephrol. 2009;20(5):1103–12.
20. Houssiau FA, D'Cruz D, Sangle S, Remy P, Vasconcelos C, Petrovic R, et al. Azathioprine versus mycophenolate mofetil for long-term immunosuppression in lupus nephritis: results from the MAINTAIN Nephritis Trial. Ann Rheum Dis. 2010;69(12):2083–9.
21. Dooley MA, Jayne D, Ginzler EM, Isenberg D, Olsen NJ, Wofsy D, et al. Mycophenolate versus azathioprine as maintenance therapy for lupus nephritis. N Engl J Med. 2011;365(20):1886–95.
22. Pepper R, Griffith M, Kirwan C, Levy J, Taube D, Pusey C, et al. Rituximab is an effective treatment for lupus nephritis and allows a reduction in maintenance steroids. Nephrol Dial Transplant. 2009;24(12):3717–23.
23. Melander C, Sallee M, Trolliet P, Candon S, Belenfant X, Daugas E, et al. Rituximab in severe lupus nephritis: early B-cell depletion affects long-term renal outcome. Clin J Am Soc Nephrol. 2009;4(3):579–87.
24. Manzi S, Sanchez-Guerrero J, Merrill JT, Furie R, Gladman D, Navarra SV, et al. Effects of belimumab, a B lymphocyte stimulator-specific inhibitor, on disease activity across multiple organ domains in patients with systemic lupus erythematosus: combined results from two phase III trials. Ann Rheum Dis. 2012;71:1833–8.
25. Nasr SH, Markowitz GS, Stokes MB, Said SM, Valeri AM, D'Agati VD. Acute postinfectious glomerulonephritis in the modern era: experience with 86 adults and review of the literature. Medicine (Baltimore). 2008;87(1):21–32.
26. Jennette JC. Rapidly progressive crescentic glomerulonephritis. Kidney Int. 2003;63(3):1164–77.
27. Jayne D, Rasmussen N, Andrassy K, Bacon P, Tervaert JW, Dadoniene J, et al. A randomized trial of maintenance therapy for vasculitis associated with antineutrophil cytoplasmic autoantibodies. N Engl J Med. 2003;349(1):36–44.
28. Hiemstra TF, Walsh M, Mahr A, Savage CO, de Groot K, Harper L, et al. Mycophenolate mofetil vs azathioprine for remission maintenance in antineutrophil cytoplasmic antibody-associated vasculitis: a randomized controlled trial. JAMA. 2010;304(21):2381–8.

Infectious Diseases and the Kidney

24

Elizabeth Williams, Sanjay Bhagani, and Mark Harber

Infections are an important cause of renal dysfunction and can provoke this in a variety of ways (see Table 24.1). Most commonly this is in the form of acute kidney injury (AKI) as collateral damage in (1) acute severe sepsis but also may occur due to (2a) direct infection of the urinary tract, e.g. bacterial UTI or tuberculosis of the renal parenchyma (see Chap. 35), or (2b) obstruction secondary to involvement of lower urinary tract (typically schistosomiasis and TB). Alternatively renal impairment may result as a secondary phenomenon which can either be (3a) postinfectious (classically poststreptococcal GN) or as a result of (3b) persistent infection such as endocarditis, shunt nephritis and chronic viral infections (hepatitis B and C and HIV have such a profound and complex global impact that they are discussed separately in the following chapter). There is often a significant degree of overlap in these processes, but distinguishing the underlying infective agent and whether it is still present is very important for treatment and prognosis. Secondary effects of infection can result in glomerulonephritis, interstitial nephritis or obstruction and, worldwide, are responsible for a huge burden of renal disease offering enormous potential for prevention. While the role of many infections and secondary renal disease is well established, reports of other infectious associations are based on little more than case reports and circumstantial evidence often published before or without the full range of modern diagnostics so remain fairly speculative.

E. Williams, MBBS, MRCP
Genito-Urinary Medicine, Royal London Hospital,
Whitechapel Road, London E1 1BB, UK
e-mail: eawilliams@doctors.org.uk

S. Bhagani, BSc (Hons), MBChB, FRCP (UK)
Department of Infectious Diseases/HIV Medicine,
Royal Free Hospital, Pond Street, London NW3 2QG, UK
e-mail: s.bhagani@nhs.net

M. Harber, MBBS, PhD, FRCP (✉)
UCL Department of Nephrology,
Royal Free London NHS Foundation Trust,
Pond Street, Hampstead, London NW3 2QG, UK
e-mail: mark.harber@nhs.net

Table 24.1 Mechanisms of renal impairment secondary to infection

1.AKI secondary to indirect consequence of acute sepsis	Usually bacterial but can occur as a consequence of severe viral infection, e.g. viral haemorrhagic fevers, fungaemia or protozoal infection, e.g. falciparum malaria. Associated with exotoxins and endotoxins (such as myoglobin or haemoglobinuria)
2a. Direct infection of the kidney	Usually acute or chronic bacterial pyelonephritis but particularly in the immunocompromised can be viral, fungal or mycobacterial, typically causing interstitial nephritis
2b. Direct infection of the urinary tract	Obstruction secondary to schistosomiasis or tuberculosis
3a. Indirect effects of infection – postinfectious	Usually immune complex mediated following successful immune response, classically poststreptococcal glomerulonephritis but may also cause interstitial nephritis, HUS (*E. coli* O157-H7) typically spontaneous resolution. Possibly vasculitis secondary to molecular mimicry
3b. Indirect effects of infection – ongoing	Usually immune complex mediated from persistent chronic antigen exposure and resulting in glomerulonephritis classically secondary to subacute bacterial (or fungal) infection such as endocarditis, shunt nephritis and osteomyelitis but also secondary to chronic viral infections such as hepatitis B and C and HIV. Spontaneous resolution does not occur until underlying pathogen is eradicated. Long-term infection may also result in AA amyloid, immunotactoid, cryoglobulinaemia and fibrillary involvement

Many of the infections causing renal disease are not commonly seen in industrialised nations, but expanding global population and travel is likely to increase the incidence of infection-related renal diseases. In this chapter we list the documented infections associated with renal disease and focus on a few diseases with significance either because of their severity or global incidence.

M. Harber (ed.), *Practical Nephrology*,
DOI 10.1007/978-1-4471-5547-8_24, © Springer-Verlag London 2014

A detailed assessment is very important in cases of AKI related to infection (see Table 24.2). Important points in the history include: recent unwell contacts foreign travel; specific activities, e.g. water sports, hiking/camping, caving; sexual history; and if any prophylactic medication has been taken, e.g. antimalarials or antibiotics. Significant examination findings include bite marks, rashes, hepatosplenomegaly and lymphadenopathy. As discussed below it is important to have a high index of suspicion and where possible distinguish between postinfectious and ongoing infection as the management is very different.

Table 24.2 Key features in history and examination in a patient suspected of infection-related renal disease

History
Details of travel, particularly in the previous 12 months, but also country of origin/birth (e.g. schistosomiasis may be asymptomatic for decades). Particular attention should be paid to the following:
Pretravel vaccinations and malaria prophylaxis
Rural versus urban
Unwell contacts
Time period between return and onset of symptoms
Accommodation and food/drink exposures
Freshwater swimming
Animal contacts or tick bites
Unwell contacts
Occupation and hobbies – e.g. water sports or agricultural employment
Recent dental work, surgical procedures
Tick, animal, bird or bat bites and scratches
Sexual history
Symptoms
Fevers and rigours (pattern of fever not particularly helpful)
Night sweats
Skin rashes
Arthralgia, myalgia or arthritis
Mouth ulcers, pharyngitis, cough
Headaches, especially if associated with fevers and/or accompanied by focal neurological symptoms, meningeal irritation symptoms
Diarrhoea
Urinary symptoms suggestive of infection – dysuria, frequency, haematuria, abdominal or flank pain
Urethral discharge and/or perineal ulcers
Signs and examination findings
SIRS response
Peripheral stigmata of infective endocarditis
Skin rash or changes (e.g. purpuric rash or mottled skin changes of severe sepsis)
Choroidoretinitis
Oropharyngeal ulcers or candidiasis
Palpable lymphadenopathy
New cardiac murmurs
Hepatosplenomegaly
Acute arthritis, especially mono-arthritis involving large joints
Meningism, focal neurological deficits, abrupt change in mental status

Non-specific Acute Kidney Injury

AKI secondary to the effects of sepsis is common and broadly correlates with the severity of the insult and or volume loss if associated with diarrhoea. For example, fulminant streptococcus A infection in previously healthy young adults may result in marked AKI accompanied by thrombocytopenia and shock. Similarly profound shock secondary to *Neisseria meningitidis* (C>B) can result in severe AKI or cortical necrosis. With the exception of hantavirus, AKI is not the predominant feature of viral haemorrhagic fevers, but AKI is common in severe cases and associated with marked acute tubular injury (and mild self-limiting mesangial proliferation). Falciparum malaria (almost exclusively although very rarely reported with plasmodium vivax) is an important, potentially avoidable cause of AKI [1]. Nonimmune adults are particularly at risk, with AKI rates of 30–40 % in Europeans with a parasitaemia of >5 %, the level of parasitaemia being an important risk factor. The rates of AKI secondary to falciparum malaria in endemic areas are less well defined but appear to be much lower at around 3–5 % in adults; however, because of the prevalence of malaria, this still represents a significant cause of AKI and if present augurs a poor prognosis. Hypotension, hyperbilirubinaemia, intravascular haemolysis and hypoxia (although, unlike in the cerebral vessels, schizonts do not adhere to and block renal vasculature) all contribute to the acute tubular injury which is the predominant finding; however, mild mesangial proliferation with transitory glomerular proteinuria and tubulointerstitial nephritis do occur. Finally, blackwater fever, massive intravascular haemolysis secondary to the use of quinine for the treatment of malaria, is still reported, often associated with AKI. Early diagnosis, rapid transfer for supportive care and prompt institution of alternative antimalarials are critical.

Direct Involvement

The most common infective invasion of the kidneys is by uropathogenic bacteria in the form of pyelonephritis and covered along with tuberculosis and fungal infections in Chap. 35. Less commonly the kidney can be directly infected by other organisms usually resulting in an acute or subacute interstitial nephritis. The infective causes of interstitial nephritis are listed in Table 24.3 and include examples where the pathological process is driven by direct infiltration but also others where the interstitial nephritis may be a postinfectious phenomenon without direct involvement.

It is often difficult to differentiate an interstitial nephritis secondary to a primary infection from an antibiotic-induced interstitial nephritis. Identification of granulomata may help guide the diagnosis but is often not a great discriminator as

Table 24.3 Infectious causes of interstitial nephritis

	Investigations and associations
Viruses:	
1. HIV	HIV RNA
2. Hepatitis A, B and C	Hepatitis A serology, BsAg or hepatitis B DNA, hepatitis C RNA
3. Cytomegalovirus[a]	CMV PCR
4. Hantavirus	Serology in reference lab, interstitial haemorrhage
5. Epstein-Barr virus[a]	EBV PCR, may involve granulomata
6. Adenovirus[a]	Adenovirus DNA
7. Herpes simplex[a]	HSV DNA
8. Measles[a]	Clinical features usually clear
9. Polyoma virus[a]	Typically in significantly immunocompromised, may involve granulomata, BKV PCR and SV40 large T cell stain
Bacteria:	
1. *Mycobacterium tuberculosis*	Classically associated with caeseating granulomata (AFB rarely seen but diagnostic)
2. Brucellosis	Serology, may involve granulomata
3. Leptospirosis	Usually apparent from clinical picture, may be associated with tubular defect polyuria
4. *Campylobacter jejuni*	Usually history of significant diarrhoea, stool culture positive
5. *Legionella*	Usually associated with pneumonia
6. Salmonellosis	May involve granulomata
7. *Yersinia pseudotuberculosis*	Stool culture
8. *Escherichia coli*	Blood, urine or stool culture depending on source
9. *Streptococci* species	Blood cultures
10. *Staphylococci* species	Blood cultures
11. *Chlamydia* species	
12. *Mycoplasma* species	Paired serology may be helpful
Parasites:	
1. *Toxoplasma*	May involve granulomata
2. *Leishmania donovani*	Associated with concentrating defect and polyuria

[a]Typically clinically significant disease only in immunocompromised patients

can occur with some antibiotic reactions and usually not present with most infective causes. Ultimately, thorough dissection of drug history and sequential blood results may be the only way to prevent repeating renal injury or avoiding antibiotics inappropriately.

Viral infection of the kidney in the immunocompromised is covered in the Chapter 71 on post-transplant infection, and with the exception of hantavirus and hepatitis viruses, it is very unusual in immunocompetent individuals for viral infections to cause a clinically significant interstitial nephritis. The finding of normally opportunistic organisms causing renal infection in non-transplant patients warrants exclusion of HIV, lymphopenia and hypogammaglobulinaemia of other causes and congenital immunodeficiency syndromes. Very rarely primary EBV and CMV infections can lead to AKI as part of the acute sepsis syndrome seen in a minority of immunocompetent patients.

Hantavirus

As mentioned AKI is common in patients with viral haemorrhagic fevers although usually as collateral damage of severe sepsis in dengue, Lassa fever and Crimean-Congo haemorrhagic fever, whereas *Hantavirus* spp. (zoonotic RNA viruses of the Bunyaviridae family) cause a clinical syndrome in which renal failure predominates.

There are various subtypes of hantavirus, with prevalence differing depending on geographical area with specific rodent reservoirs and disease spectrums and severity. Two main severe syndromes predominate: haemorrhagic fever with renal syndrome (HFRS also nephropathia epidemica, NE) (Asia and Europe) which will be discussed here and hantavirus cardiopulmonary syndrome (HCPS or HPS) (Americas) which is much less common than HFRS but has a higher mortality [2].

Hantavirus is spread by rodents, and the virus is transmitted from rodent to human by contact with an infected rodent's urine or faeces, whereas human-to-human transmission is extremely rare. Commonly subtypes Puumala (Scandinavia and Western Europe) and Dobrava (Balkans) are carried by the bank mole and yellow-necked field mouse, respectively, whereas Hantaan and Seoul are found in China and South Korea (striped field mouse and rats, respectively). The WHO estimates that 150,000–200,000 people worldwide are hospitalised due to HFRS each year (men more commonly than women), and surveillance suggests that HFRS incidence is increasing [2–4]. Occupational history may be important as sewage workers, forest workers and farmers have a high rate of seropositivity as do water sports enthusiasts suggesting that subclinical infections are much more common than overt HFRS.

Clinically, there are various clinical presentations varying from a mild form with flu-like symptoms to life-threatening illness, with an incubation period usually 2–4 weeks but ranging from 4 to 42 days. As the name suggests there may be signs of bleeding, mainly petechiae or bleeding from the GI tract, and patients can have disseminated intravascular coagulopathy and thrombocytopaenia [2]. HFRS typically has five phases:

1. Febrile phase: non-specific flu-like symptoms such as headache, myalgia, back pain, abdominal pain, fevers, nausea and vomiting, lethargy and blurred vision. Usually lasting 3–7 days.
2. Hypotensive/septic phase: patients often will have degree of renal impairment at this stage. Usually lasts a few hours up to 2 days.

3. Oliguric phase: oliguric acute renal failure, there may also be evidence of haemorrhage (e.g. conjunctival haemorrhage), usually lasts 3–7 days.
4. Diuretic phase: the patient becomes polyuric. Can last from a few days to several weeks.
5. Convalescent phase: blood results and urine output normalise. This last phase can last a few months.

Whilst a useful description, not all patients neatly fit this pattern; cases vary in severity and patients presenting late may offer few clues but except a history of viral illness. Beyond abnormal renal tests a raised WBC, moderate elevation in transaminases, microscopic haematuria and proteinuria are common, and complement may be low. The biggest clue is the presence of marked thrombocytopenia in the presence of normal clotting with no evidence of thrombotic microangiopathy (although leptospirosis can present in a similar way). However, if the patient presents later, the platelet count may have recovered, and some degree of abnormal clotting is not uncommon. There is a marked increase in vascular permeability, endothelial dysfunction, acute tubular injury, interstitial oedema and classically with interstitial haemorrhage in the outer medulla, which is highly suggestive of the diagnosis [5] (see Fig. 24.1). Serological tests for IgM and IgG against hantavirus are confirmatory, and in the early phase peripheral blood RT-PCR may detect virus. Microscopic haematuria (a) raised AST level (b) and raised leucocyte count at time of admission (c) are useful predictors of patients who are at risk of developing oliguric renal failure [6].

Management consists of excluding other causes of viral haemorrhagic fevers, bacterial sepsis and MAHA, and treatment is supportive with renal replacement therapy in ~10 % there is some suggestion that ribavirin may be helpfu [2]. Most patients' renal function and blood pressure return to baseline, but some remain with a degree of renal impairment and hypertension. Mortality from HFRS is between 1 and 15 %, dobravirus having a worse prognosis than puumala virus infections.

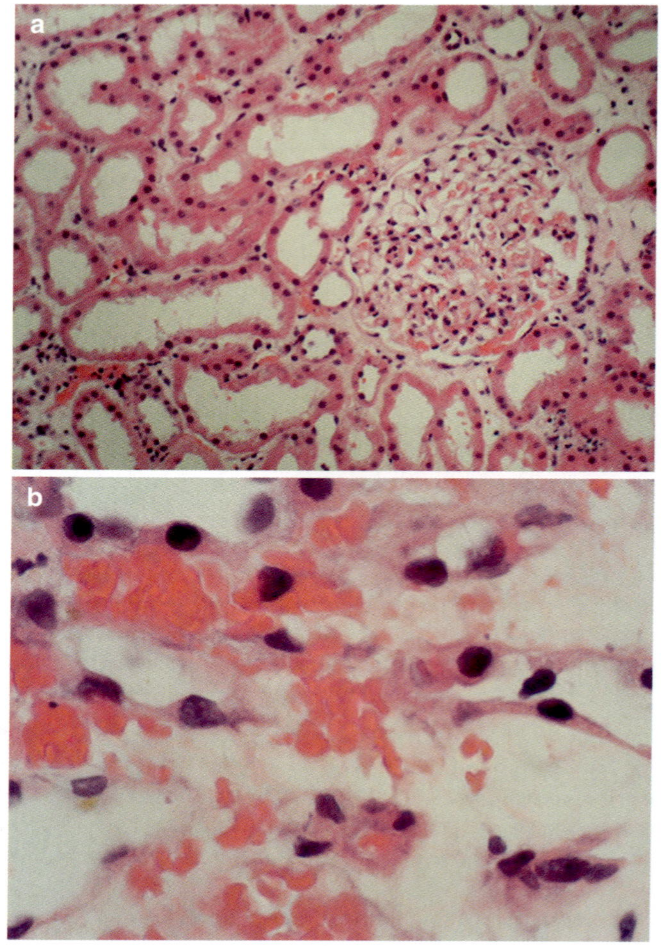

Fig. 24.1 Renal biopsy of a patient with hantavirus infection: (**a**) low power showing marked acute tubular injury and some erythrocytes in the interstitium and (**b**) high power of interstitial haemorrhage

Leptospirosis

Leptospirosis is a zoonosis caused by the spirochete (gram-negative bacteria) *Leptospira interrogans*. Leptospirosis should be suspected in a patient with non-specific prodrome who then develops AKI and disproportionate hyperbilirubinaemia, particularly if 'at-risk' history. A variety of mammals can host the infection, but usually infections in humans are transmitted from rats and domesticated livestock. Humans acquire infection through contact with animal urine usually in contaminated water through breaches in the skin or mucous membranes. *Leptospira interrogans* is almost ubiquitous, but leptospirosis is more common in the tropics due to farming practices, flooding and infection and is more common during rainy seasons where it can be a common cause of AKI. There is a significant male preponderance (4:1). The incidence in Western countries is falling but does still occur. In England and Wales there are approximately 50–60 cases (50 % acquired abroad) each year and 2–3 deaths. In Western countries the proportion of cases that are travel acquired is increasing significantly, with a shift from work-related to leisure-acquired infection particularly in those partaking in adventure sports, e.g. outbreaks have been reported after triathlons.

Incubation period can range from 2 to 26 days (average 10 days) with the length of illness averaging 14 days. Symptoms are often non-specific in the first week with fevers, malaise, headache, meningism, anorexia, nausea, vomiting, diarrhoea and abdominal, chest and back pain. Physical signs such as hepatomegaly, splenomegaly, rash, jaundice and conjunctival suffusion typically occur in the second week [7]. Weil's disease is the presence of jaundice and AKI in a patient with serologically confirmed leptospirosis infection and occurs in around 5–10 % of those infected, less commonly in children. The second phase of the disease is immunologically mediated and may be associated with a myositis, AKI, myocarditis and pulmonary and gastrointestinal haemorrhage. Thrombocytopenia occurs in 50 % often associated with a neutrophilia, but leucocytopenia can also occur. Liver transaminases are often minimally to moderately raised (<200 U/l), but hyperbilirubinaemia is disproportionate and an important clue. Low-level proteinuria and haematuria are common, and AKI is non-oliguric in about 50 %, often with hypokalaemia (45 %) [8]. Creatinine kinase is elevated in roughly 50 % sometimes substantially so. Diagnosis is made on culture from the blood early in the disease or by serology. Urine cultures may become positive from the second week of illness and may remain so for up to 30 days after resolution of symptoms. Newer PCR-based assays are increasingly being used to diagnose infection.

Secondary factors for the development of AKI in leptospirosis include hypotension, hypovolaemia, jaundice and rhabdomyolysis. The main finding on biopsy is interstitial nephritis, oedema and acute tubular injury; mild mesangial proliferation in common with many infectious diseases may be present early on [8]. The predominant site of direct injury by leptospira in the kidney is the proximal convoluted tubule with decreased activity of the sodium-hydrogen co-transporter proximally and NKCC co-transporter in the thick ascending limb. Therefore sodium and water transport across the tubule wall is impaired causing polyuria and hypokalaemia secondary to more potassium (and magnesium) being excreted distally.

Treatment is largely supportive as the condition is usually self-limiting. The role of antibiotics is controversial, and the recent Cochrane database review [9] of 7 RCTs concluded that there was insufficient evidence to indicate the benefit of antibiotics in established disease. In practical terms if antibiotics are prescribed then it should be in the early phase of the disease. If the patient is able to take oral medications, then doxycycline 100 mg bid is a good choice as it also covers rickettsial diseases which are an important differential diagnosis. Cefotaxime or ceftriaxone are good intravenous alternatives, whereas benzylpenicillin is no longer recommended as first-line therapy since it will not cover rickettsiosis. Antibiotic therapy is usually given for 5–7 days.

Mortality figures for Weil's disease vary significantly depending on the series and case mix but amounts to roughly 20 % and thus is a serious condition. Advanced age, alcohol abuse, oliguria, presence of arrhythmias and jaundice have been shown to be predictors of severe leptospirosis infection [10], but even the young and fit can succumb. For those who survive, good renal recovery is the norm.

Brucellosis

Brucellosis is a zoonosis caused by *Brucella* spp. most commonly *Brucella melitensis*. Human infection is normally acquired after contact with fluids from infected domestic animals and livestock or derived food products such as unpasteurised milk and cheese. Renal involvement in brucelosis is relatively uncommon but because the multitude. Because the multitude of symptoms associated with brucellosis such as fevers, malaise, sweating, headaches and bone and joint pain may mimic other autoimmune or malignant causes, the diagnosis may be missed. There is little literature on brucellosis with renal involvement, with what there is coming from small case series, and on the basis of this literature, there seem to be no risk factors beyond the ingestion of unpasteurised products or stock keeping in the Mediterranean area. Renal involvement is predominantly a granulomatous tubulointerstitial nephritis but can also be associated with cystitis, renal abscess indirect involvement secondary to persistent infection in the form of a glomerulopathy associated with *Brucella endocarditis* or MPGN sometimes appearing many months after initial symptoms [11].

Diagnosis can normally be confirmed by culture or serology. Brucella can be cultured from blood, bone marrow or other appropriate fluids with bone marrow aspirate having the highest yield for positive cultures. There is a significant risk of laboratory infections, and so laboratory staff must be informed of the possibility of brucellosis so that the cultures can be incubated in appropriate isolation facilities and appropriately prolonged. A diagnosis can also be made on the basis of an appropriate clinical syndrome together with rising antibody titres on serological tests. Brucella antibodies may persist long after recovery of infection so caution is needed in interpreting serological tests in the context of chronic infection and relapsing infection and in patients from endemic areas.

Treatment is generally with a combination of antibiotics that include doxycycline, rifampicin and aminoglycoside.

Syphilis

The incidence of syphilis caused by *Treponema pallidum* is on the increase in Western Europe and the USA particularly in men who have sex with men. There are well-documented cases of renal involvement associated with secondary syphilis although this does not result in a high incidence of renal disease. Patients, who may have the classical maculopapular rash involving palms and soles, present with proteinuria which may be nephrotic range. The most common histological pattern is membranous GN, but MPGN, PRGN and interstitial nephritis have been described as having solid renal lesions due to syphilitic gumma. Although rare it is important to exclude treponemal infection as part of the screening for unexplained renal involvement as the treatment is simple/effective and the diagnosis important not to miss. Diagnosis is established by the presence of IgM/IgG by ELISA tests. IgG antibodies persist for life. Positive ELISA IgM needs to be interpreted with care; although a positive IgM reflects active infection, IgM antibodies can persist for 12–18 months post-

Postinfectious

Renal dysfunction as an indirect effect of the immune response to infection is classically exemplified by acute poststreptococcal glomerulonephritis but also occurs as the phenomenon of haematuria following upper respiratory tract infections (as with IgA nephropathy) and more rarely following pneumonia or gastroenteritis secondary to other infectious agents such as *Streptococcus pneumoniae*, salmonellosis and *Mycoplasma pneumoniae*. It is worth reiterating that haematuria (and proteinuria) occurs rapidly (within 1–3 days) of upper respiratory tract infections with IgA, whereas postinfectious glomerulonephritis from other causes typically occurs 1–2 weeks after the primary infection, and postinfectious glomerulonephritis is likely to be accompanied by hypocomplementaemia and a raised antistreptolysin O (ASO titre) if due to a streptococcal infection.

Acute Poststreptococcal Glomerulonephritis (APSGN)

It is 200 years since the association between scarlet fever and subsequent 'dropsy' was first described, and APSGN remains the most common cause of nephritis worldwide, but the epidemiology has changed significantly over the past four decades, and it is now relatively rare as a childhood infection in industrialised countries. It is estimated that there are nearly half a million cases of APSGN globally with an incidence of 10–30 per 100,000/year although severe cases of rapidly progressive glomerulonephritis represent <1 %. The vast majority of these cases occurring in children at a mean age of 7 and in the developing world, although interestingly it is rare in children below the age of 2. There is a second peak in those over 60 particularly in industrialised countries with a predisposition to those with comorbidity and alcohol or parenteral drug abuse. APSGN is strongly associated with social deprivation. Rates are falling significantly in China and South America with persistently high rates in Sub-Saharan Africa and the Indian subcontinent [16, 17].

APSGN occurs secondary to nephritogenic strains of group A streptococcal infection such as pharyngitis/tonsillitis and upper respiratory tract or skin infection, but there have been reported outbreaks due to group C streptococcal infection (*S. zooepidemicus*) from unpasteurised milk. Typically APSGN is a disease of the socioeconomically disadvantaged and frequently occurs in clusters and epidemics especially following skin infection and commonly associated with scabies and skin sores.

Aetiopathogenesis

Only some strains of *S. pyogenes* have nephritogenic potential, and this is attributable to two nephritogenic antigens: nephritis-associated plasmin receptor (NAPlr) and streptococcal pyogenic exotoxin B (SPEB). Both of these are capable of activating complement via the alternative pathway, inducing production of IL-6 and MCP-1 by mesangial cells (promoting immune recruitment) and both capable of inducing an antibody response in the host. It has been assumed that the pathogenesis of APSGN is akin to serum sickness with circulating immune complexes to the nephritogenic antigens depositing in the kidney; however, there is still debate about the precise mechanism of the damage to the kidney as C3 (alternative pathway activation) is deposited before IgG complexes. Other possibilities include IgG binding to the GBM secondary to molecular mimicry or in situ deposition of IgG to streptococcal antigens trapped in the kidney [18].

Clinical Features

Typically there is a latency of 1–2 weeks after pharyngitis before features of APSGN develop but it is usually later after skin infections at around 3–6 weeks. However, approximately 20 % of serologically positive household contacts in APSGN epidemics do not show signs of the original streptococcal infection. Patients usually present with oedema, haematuria which may be macroscopic (classically cola coloured) and the features of hypertension (80–90 %). Hypertensive crises including encephalopathy are relatively common in childhood presentations. Autoimmune haemolytic anaemia is also reported but a relatively rare complication of APSGN. Proteinuria is usually subnephrotic with nephrotic syndrome in <4 % although said to be more common in adults. Less than 1 % develop rapidly progressive glomerulonephritis with crescent formation; however, renal impairment is common especially in the elderly, and patients may present with congestive cardiac failure. For most patients symptoms resolve spontaneously within 2 weeks although the microscopic haematuria persists a little longer.

Blood cultures and swabs may be positive for *S. pyogenes*, but ASOT, anti-hyaluronidase and anti-DNAse antibodies are more sensitive. Glomerular haematuria is universal and red blood cells casts common. One of the most useful pointers is a depressed C3 level (typically C4 are normal) which frequently falls before the onset of any clinical features of APSGN and is one of the last tests to return to normal so may suggest the diagnosis in a late presentation and help differentiate from IgA or pauci-immune vasculitis.

A renal biopsy is rarely necessary, but if performed typically demonstrates a diffuse hypercellularity (proliferative) of the endothelium (resulting in reduced perfusion) and mesangium with infiltration of the tuft with neutrophils (see Fig. 24.2). Immunohistochemistry reveals deposits of IgG, C3 (but not C4 or C1q) in the mesangium and glomerular capillary wall with pathognomonic subepithelial humps on

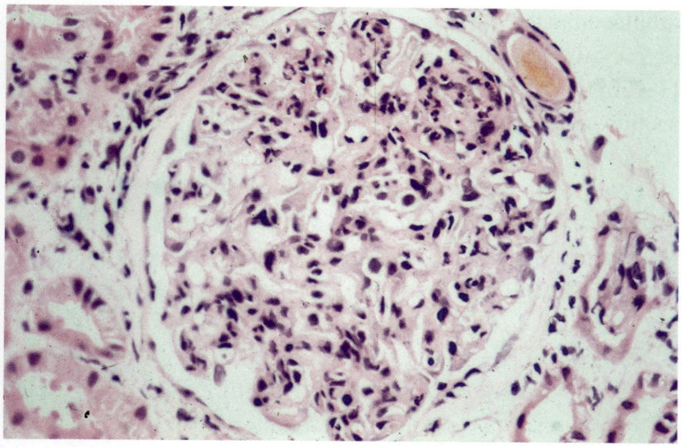

Fig. 24.2 Light microscopy of poststreptococcal glomerulonephritis with proliferative, hypercellular glomerulus rich in neutrophils

electron microscopy, although subendothelial deposits can occur in the disease. A small proportion of patients can have a more fulminant course with >50 % crescents and a RPGN.

Management is largely supportive with sodium and water restriction and diuretics. Haemodialysis is rarely required but may be needed in severe acute renal failure. Appropriate antibiotic therapy such as penicillin is sometimes given to those with APSGN as often it is difficult to know if the streptococcal infection is ongoing although there is currently no convincing evidence of benefit. Prophylactic antibiotics, however, are indicated in epidemic areas and in close contacts of those affected as early antibiotic therapy in group A streptococcal infections appears to reduce risk of developing PSGN.

Overall mortality is less than 1 % globally representing about 5,000 (potentially preventable) deaths per year, 97 % of which are in the developing world. Thus the prognosis for the majority is usually very good in children but worse in the elderly especially when they have other health problems. In these patients mortality can be up to 25 %. Of the elderly patients that do survive but have persistent nephrotic range proteinuria, around 75 % will go on to have chronic renal failure. Progression to end-stage renal failure occurs in less than 2 % of all patients with PSGN, with less than 1 % of children progressing to ESRF after PSGN. Although largely considered benign, it has been speculated that APSGN might contribute to the huge burden of CKD in communities such as indigenous Australians that also have a high burden of diabetes and hypertensive renal disease. Recurrence of PSGN is uncommon but has been reported.

Parvovirus

Although the incidence of parvovirus B19 infection in industrialised countries is falling, it is increasingly recognised as a cause (albeit rare) of postinfection (and possibly persistent infection)-related glomerulonephritis, perhaps related to the viruses' predilection for vascular endothelium. Nephrotic and nephritic presentations have been described a week or so after initial flu-like symptoms, often associated with arthralgia, but in adults less commonly associated with the classical rash. A wide range of histological patterns that have been described include collapsing FSGS, MPGN, endocapillary proliferative glomerular lesions, HSP, thrombotic microangiopathy vasculitis and mixed essential cryoglobulinaemia. Deposition of IgM, IgG, C3 and C1q has all been reported. Part of the evidence relating parvovirus B19 to the collapsing variant of FSGS was the association of viral DNA in a retrospective biopsy study [19] but (in common with case reports of other glomerulonephritides) does not prove causality. Nonetheless the spectrum of histological patterns associated with parvovirus B19 infection makes it worth considering screening for this infection. The outcome of postinfectious GN secondary to parvovirus seems to be excellent and largely self-limiting although mixed essential cryoglobulinaemia may require further treatment.

Persistent Infection

In contradiction to self-limiting postinfectious renal disease, which is a consequence of the successful immunological response to a pathogen, renal disease secondary to persistent infection is a result of ongoing immunological defence and unlikely to resolve until the infection is treated. Common causes include hepatitis B and C and HIV and are shown in Table 24.5; worldwide some tropical diseases such as filariasis are also implicated.

Malaria

In the 1970s, it was felt that a significant proportion of childhood nephrotic syndrome in Sub-Saharan Africa was related to chronic malarial infection principally with *Plasmodium malariae* (quartan malarial nephropathy (QMN)). The evidence for this was largely circumstantial, and even if QMN was a significant clinical entity, it seems a rare beast these days. In practical terms any patient with nephrotic syndrome in the tropics ought to have a malaria screen and positive results treated, but it should no longer be assumed that malaria is the principle cause of the nephrotic syndrome [20].

Filariasis

A variety of filarial infections can result in a variety of renal diseases mostly via indirect effects, although as mentioned above, *Wuchereria bancrofti* can result in renal lymphatic obstruction with chyluria and significant proteinuria. *Onchocerca volvulus*, *Loa loa*, *Wuchereria bancrofti* and *Brugia malayi* have all been associated with glomerular

Table 24.5 Renal disease as indirect consequence of persistent infection

Viruses:	
1. HIV	HIVAN collapsing FSGS, immune complex GN (MPGN, lupus-like) FSGS, thrombotic microangiopathy, IgA
2. Hepatitis B	Membranous GN, MPGN (with or without cryoglobulinaemia), polyarteritis nodosa
3. Hepatitis C	MPGN (with or without cryoglobulin), membranous GN, cryoglobulinaemic vasculitis, fibrillary GN
4. *Cytomegalovirus*	Rarely associated with cryoglobulinaemia
Bacterial:	
1. *Staphylococcus* species	Especially *S. aureus*: cellulitis; endocarditis; osteomyelitis; line, wire and shunt infections; pneumonia
2. *Streptococcus*	Cellulitis, endocarditis, pneumonia
3. Other bacteria	Visceral abscess; endocarditis; osteomyelitis; line, wire and shunt infections
4. *Mycobacterium tubercle, leprae*	Amyloid
Fungal	
Spirochetes	
Parasites	Filarial infection

lesions although the incidence of significant renal involvement is probably very low. MPGN, diffuse proliferative, minimal change and membranous and collapsing FSGS have all been documented, with occasional microfilariae seen in the all parts of the kidney.

Chronic bacterial infection

The other common scenario in which glomerulonephritis results from ongoing infection relates to chronic bacterial infection such as endocarditis, osteomyelitis, visceral abscess as well as infections of foreign bodies previously personified by 'shunt nephritis' but increasingly likely to result from infected pacing wires, defibrillators, tunnelled central venous catheters or other foreign bodies. Glomerulonephritis secondary to chronic bacterial infection has a changing demographic and is increasingly likely to occur in older patients with comorbidity including diabetes, those hospitalised for prolonged periods and those with medium-term medical implants such as central venous lines. It is also increasingly common secondary to intravenous and subcutaneous drug abuse.

Renal involvement may take weeks to develop and may be underdiagnosed as these patients, particularly hospitalised ones, often have multiple renal insults including potentially nephrotoxic medication and sepsis. Declining renal function especially associated with de novo haematuria and proteinuria should raise suspicion even in patients with low-grade infections such as diabetic osteomyelitis. The differential diagnosis of AKI in patients with chronic bacterial infection is complicated by raised inflammatory markers, anaemia, false-positive and secondary ANCA and general noise but includes (1) acute tubular injury from whatever cause (most common), (2) TIN (especially drug induced), (3) vasculitis (GPA/MPA), (4) IgA/HSP, (5) cryoglobulinaemia, (6) postinfectious GN and (7) GN secondary to persistent infection (including *Staphylococcus aureus*-associated glomerulonephritis (SAAGN).

Features in favour of GN secondary to persistent bacterial infection such as endocarditis include polyclonal increase in Igs especially IgG, hypocomplementaemia, splenomegaly and circulating immune complexes, and if an ANCA is positive then anti-PR3 is relatively low titre (see Table 24.6).

A renal biopsy is often a challenge in septic patients, and urine microscopy may be helpful in differentiating ATI or TIN from an active proliferative glomerular lesion.

Infective endocarditis is an important cause of secondary glomerulonephritis with approximately a quarter of patients developing an acute glomerulonephritis although a much higher incidence has been reported particularly in the setting of *Staphylococcus aureus* infections. The demographic of IE is changing in industrialised countries, and *S. aureus* infection is now more common than *viridans* group streptococcal infections in part due to intravenous drug use and medical use, or misuse, of central venous access. Haemodialysis patients, in particular, have very high risk of IE. A multitude of other organisms causing IE with glomerulonephritis have been documented including *Coxiella burnetii* (Q fever), *Streptococcus bovis* (associated with bowel pathology), *S. pyogenes*, *S. mitis*, *S. mutans*, *S. epidermidis*, *Pseudomonas* spp., *Chlamydia psittaci*, *brucellosis*, *bartonellosis*, *Enterococcus faecalis* and *Candida* species. Renal involvement is manifest with microscopic haematuria, subnephrotic range proteinuria and usually renal impairment although this may be subtle if previously normal function. Patients may have episodes of macroscopic haematuria and flank pain suggesting emboli which are common. A third of necropsy specimens demonstrate embolic damage which may result in cortical necrosis and scarring or renal abscesses. Microscopically lesions range from focal segmental proliferative glomerulonephritis to a diffuse exudative proliferative GN with crescents although MPGN and membranous GN have been described. IgM, IgG and C3 are ubiquitous with subendothelial and subepithelial deposits.

The prognosis is very variable and largely dependent on early identification and effective treatment of the IE. There is no specific treatment of the secondary glomerulonephritis apart from avoiding nephrotoxins and maintaining vigilance for drug-induced interstitial nephritis. There are case reports and small series advocating the use of steroids or plasma exchange in diffuse proliferative GN, but there is no substantial evidence to support either. In practical terms some nephrologists do treat aggressive endocarditis with either or both, and it boils down to individual risk versus potential benefit.

As alluded to above, acute glomerulonephritis with IgA deposition is increasingly recognised as a unique complication of staphylococcal infections [21–23]. Known

Table 24.6 Discriminating findings in setting of AKI

	Splenomegaly	Polyclonal IgG	C3	C4	Circulating immune complexes	Serology
Endocarditis	Yes	Yes	Low	Low	Yes	Secondary ANCA (low titre), RhF and cryoglobulins very common
SAAGN	No	Yes	Normal in 70 %	Normal	Yes	Polyclonal Ig increase
GPA/MPA	No	No	Normal	Normal	No	Primary ANCA
IgA/HSP	No	No	Normal	Normal	No	Negative, IgA may be raised
Postinfectious	Occasionally	No	Low	Low/N	Yes	ASO if *streptococcus* IgM response to other infections
Cryoglobulinaemia	Occasionally	Yes	Normal	Low	Yes	RhF
SLE	Yes	Yes	Low	Low	Yes	ANA, dsDNA, ENA, polyclonal
Drug-induced TIN	No	No	Normal	Normal	No	Nil
Acute tubular injury	No	No	Normal	Normal	No	Nil

as *Staphylococcus aureus*-associated glomerulonephritis (SAAGN), this recently identified clinical entity is almost certainly increasing and significantly underdiagnosed. The emerging prevalence is associated with an aging population with comorbidity and in the setting of chronic or subacute infections such as cellulitis, line infection, osteomyelitis or visceral abscesses. Renal involvement may occur weeks after the start of the infection and is usually manifest as haematuria, proteinuria (sometimes nephrotic range) and renal dysfunction, often acute renal failure. It may also be associated with palpable purpura which can be confused with vasculitis, HSP or drug-induced cause of renal injury. Although SAAGN is associated with a polyclonal increase in IgM, IgG and IgA (possibly related to the superantigen stimulation of *S. aureus* on T cells), complement levels are normal in 70 % of cases, and this may be an important discriminator. While IgG, C3 and IgM may also be present, IgA is predominant, and the histological appearances can be almost indistinguishable from IgA nephropathy with mesangial hypercellularity with or without crescents. Subendothelial humps indicate SAAGN rather than IgA; thus electron microscopy may be helpful in differentiating the two conditions. The management consists of considering and making the diagnosis in the first place and excluding other potential causes of AKI. This is important for a variety of reasons not least as it may alert the clinician to the possibility of subclinical low-grade infection such as osteomyelitis and the importance of eradicating an ongoing infection, which is the treatment of this condition.

Shunt nephritis is immune complex-mediated GN secondary to chronic infection of ventriculoatrial or ventriculojugular shunts. It occurs in about 1 % of those with ventriculovascular shunts (much less so with ventriculoperitoneal shunts) and thus is rare but important to consider in any patient with ventriculovascular access. *S. aureus* or *S. epidermidis* and also other less virulent skin commensals are the main culprits.

Clinically, renal involvement is with microscopic haematuria, proteinuria, hypertension and AKI usually in the setting of low-grade fevers and hypocomplementaemia (cryoglobulins and rheumatoid factor may also be present). Glomerulonephritis may occur weeks or years after the insertion of the shunt, and as fairly indolent organisms may be involved, the diagnosis may be delayed and significant damage accrued.

Typically the renal pattern is that of MPGN with IgM, IgG and C3; mesangial proliferation; and subendothelial deposits. Management relies on making the diagnosis and treating the primary infection, often entailing removal and replacement of the shunt. There is no specific treatment for the renal lesion, and thus it makes sense for patients with VA/VJ shunts to have their urine dipped, especially if they become unwell.

Glomerulonephritis associated with persistent infection also occurs secondary to bacteria other than *S. aureus* in the setting of visceral abscesses, osteomyelitis and line infections. The clinical history is similar to that of SAAGN, and renal involvement is usually weeks after the onset of the infection and may be mild or severe. Almost all histological patterns have been associated with this, but diffuse or focal proliferative lesion and MPGN seem the most common.

While antibiotics have no role in the treatment of postinfectious renal disease, they are critical in the resolution of renal disease secondary to persistent infection – thus identification of an ongoing infective cause is essential, and aggressive pursuit of culture-negative endocarditis or other deep-seated infection with repeated sampling, biopsies for culture and 16 s ribosomal RNA analyses are all important.

Summary

The causes of acute kidney injury described in this chapter are relatively uncommon in industrialised nations, but the epidemiology of some of these conditions is changing with global demographics and travel, and a high index of suspicion is required in unexplained renal disease. A thorough history when the patient is first seen, particularly noting any travel history and activities that may have exposed the patient to these infections, will help list the differential diagnosis and therefore aid appropriate investigations. On a world scale renal disease secondary to infection is responsible for a huge burden of potentially avoidable or recoverable kidney disease and represents an important challenge for the renal community.

References

1. Ehrich JH, Eke FU. Malaria-induced renal damage: facts and myths. Pediatr Nephrol. 2007;22(5):626–37.
2. Jonsson CB, Figueiredo LT, Vapalahti O. A global perspective on hantavirus ecology, epidemiology, and disease. Clin Microbiol Rev. 2010;23(2):412–41. doi:10.1128/CMR.00062-09.
3. Heyman P, Ceianu CS, Christova I, Tordo N, Beersma M, Joao Alves M, Lundkvist A, Hukic M, Papa A, Tenorio A, Zelena H, Essbauer S, Visontai I, Golovljova I, Connell J, Nicoletti L, Van Esbroeck M, Gjeruldsen Dudman S, Aberle SW, Avsic-Zupanc T, Korukluoglu G, Nowakowska A, Klempa B, Ulrich RG, Bino S, Engler O, Opp M, Vaheri A. A five-year perspective on the situation of haemorrhagic fever with renal syndrome and status of the hantavirus reservoirs in Europe, 2005–2010. Euro Surveill. 2011;16(36).
4. Vapalahti O, Mustonen J, Lundkvist A, Henttonen H, Plyusnin A, Vaheri A. Hantavirus infections in Europe. Lancet Infect Dis. 2003;3(10):653–61.
5. Ferluga D, Vizjak A. Hantavirus nephropathy. J Am Soc Nephrol. 2008;19(9):1653–8.
6. Kim YK, Lee SC, Kim C, Heo ST, Choi C, Kim JM. Clinical and laboratory predictors of oliguric renal failure in haemorrhagic fever with renal syndrome caused by Hantaan virus. J Infect. 2007;54(4):381–6.
7. Regina C. R. M. Abdulkader, Marcos Vinicius Silva. The kidney in leptospirosis. Pediatr Nephrol. 2008;23:2111–20.
8. Katz AR, Ansdell VE, Effler PV, Middleton CR, Sasaki DM. Assessment of the clinical presentation and treatment of 353 cases of laboratory-confirmed leptospirosis in Hawaii, 1974–1998. Clin Infect Dis. 2001;33(11):1834–41.
9. Brett-Major DM, Coldren R. Antibiotics for leptospirosis. Cochrane Database Syst Rev. 2012;2, CD008264.
10. Dassanayake DL, Wimalaratna H, Nandadewa D, Nugaliyadda A, Ratnatunga CN, Agampodi SB. Predictors of the development of myocarditis or acute renal failure in patients with leptospirosis: an observational study. BMC Infect Dis. 2012;12:4.
11. Turunc T, Demiroglu YZ, Aliskan H, Colakoglu S, Timurkaynak F, Ozdemir N, Arslan H. Brucellosis in cases of end-stage renal disease. Nephrol Dial Transplant. 2008;23:2344–9.
12. Dutra M, Martinelli R, Carvalho EM, Rodrigues LE, Brito E, Rocha H. Renal involvement in visceral leishmaniasis. Am J Kidney Dis. 1985;6(1):22–7.
13. Barsoum RS. Schistosomiasis and the kidney. Semin Nephrol. 2003;23(1):34–41.
14. KDIGO. Chapter 9: Infection-related glomerulonephritis. Kidney Int Suppl. 2012;2: 200–8; doi:10.1038/kisup.2012.22.
15. Mahmoud KM, Sobh MA, El-Agroudy AE, Mostafa FE, Baz ME, Shokeir AA, Ghoneim MA. Impact of schistosomiasis on patient and graft outcome after renal transplantation: 10 years' follow-up. Nephrol Dial Transplant. 2001;16(11):2214–21.
16. Carapetis JR, Steer AC, Mulholland EK, Weber M. The global burden of group A streptococcal diseases. Lancet Infect Dis. 2005;5(11):685–94.
17. Rodigueiz-Iturbe B, Musser JM. The current state of poststreptococcal glomerulonephritis. J Am Soc Nephrol. 2008;19:1855–64.
18. Eison TM, Ault BH, Jones DP, Chesney RW, Wyatt RJ. Post-streptococcal acute glomerulonephritis in children: clinical features and pathogenesis. Pediatr Nephrol. 2011;26:165–80.
19. Moudgil A, Nast CC, Bagga A, Wei L, Nurmamet A, Cohen AH, Jordan SC, Toyoda M. Association of parvovirus B19 infection with idiopathic collapsing glomerulopathy. Kidney Int. 2001;59(6):2126–33.
20. Doe JY, Funk M, Mengel M, Doehring E, Ehrich JH. Nephrotic syndrome in African children: lack of evidence for 'tropical nephrotic syndrome'? Nephrol Dial Transplant. 2006;21(3):672–6.
21. Koyama A, Kobayashi M, Yamaguchi N, Yamagata K, Takano K, Nakajima M, Irie F, Goto M, Igarashi M, Iitsuka T, et al. Glomerulonephritis associated with MRSA infection: a possible role of bacterial superantigen. Kidney Int. 1995;47(1):207–16.
22. Satoskar AA, Nadasdy G, Plaza JA, Sedmak D, Shidham G, Hebert L, Nadasdy T. Staphylococcus infection-associated glomerulonephritis mimicking IgA nephropathy. Clin J Am Soc Nephrol. 2006;1(6):1179–86.
23. Nadasdy T. Infection-related glomerulonephritis: understanding mechanisms. Semin Nephrol. 2011;31(4):369–75.

Blood-Borne Viruses and the Kidney

25

John W.R. Booth, Sanjay Bhagani, and Mark Harber

The main blood-borne viruses, HIV and hepatitis B and C, are responsible for a huge burden of renal disease worldwide. These chronic infections produce a complex and fascinating spectrum of kidney diseases which have the potential to cause end-stage renal disease. Advances in the development of antivirals are altering the epidemiology of these diseases and permitting near-normal life expectancy. With this has come some renal disease secondary to antivirals and an increasing population of well patients with ESRD and chronically suppressed viruses raising new challenges for transplantation.

Human Immunodeficiency Virus

Widespread use of combination antiretroviral therapy (cART) in HIV has dramatically enhanced patient survival and reduced the incidence of AIDS but also altered the spectrum of renal disease encountered in Western populations (Table 25.1) [1]. Rates of HIV-associated acute kidney injury (AKI) have more than halved in the post-cART era, parallel to a decline in severe infection episodes [2, 3]. The incidence of HIV's archetypal renal lesion, HIVAN, has also diminished. In turn, rates of multifactorial CKD have risen, driven by increasing patient age and higher prevalence of common comorbidities such as hypertension and diabetes. Specific nephrotoxicities of cART have also emerged.

HIV-positive patients should be screened for renal disease by means of eGFR measurement, urinalysis and protein/creatinine ratio at diagnosis, prior to starting cART and at periodic intervals no greater than 1 year [4]. Patients with risk

Table 25.1 The spectrum of renal disease encountered in patients infected with HIV

HIV associated	**Examples**
HIVAN	
Immune complex kidney disease	See Table 25.3
Thrombotic microangiopathy	
Diffuse infiltrative lymphocytic syndrome	
HIV treatment associated	
ART nephropathy	Proximal tubulopathy with tenofovir
	Crystallopathy with indinavir
Immune reconstitution inflammatory syndrome	
Immunodeficiency associated	See Table 25.4
Antimicrobial toxicity	Tubulointerstitial nephritis or ATI with antibiotics
Renal parenchymal infection	Tuberculous granulomatous interstitial nephritis
	Viral nephropathies, e.g. CMV
Neoplasia	Infiltration, e.g. by lymphoma
Other commonly encountered conditions	
Immune complex kidney disease	HBV-associated membranous nephropathy
	HCV-associated mesangiocapillary GN
Non-collapsing FSGS (NOS or hilar variants)	
Acute tubular injury	Hypovolaemia, sepsis, nephrotoxic drugs
Diabetic or hypertensive kidney disease	
AA amyloid	Associated with injection drug use

J.W.R. Booth, MA, MRCP (✉)
UCL Centre for Nephrology, Royal Free Campus, Pond Street, London NW3 2PF, UK
e-mail: johnwrbooth@doctors.org.uk

S. Bhagani, BSc (Hons), MBChB, FRCP (UK)
Department of Infectious Diseases/HIV Medicine, Royal Free Hospital, Pond Street, London NW3 2QG, UK
e-mail: s.bhagani@nhs.net

M. Harber, MBBS, PhD, FRCP
UCL Department of Nephrology, Royal Free London NHS Foundation Trust, Pond Street, Hampstead, London NW3 2QG, UK
e-mail: mark.harber@nhs.net

M. Harber (ed.), *Practical Nephrology*,
DOI 10.1007/978-1-4471-5547-8_25, © Springer-Verlag London 2014

Table 25.2 Common nephrotoxic medications encountered in management of HIV

Drug	Renal adverse effect
Antibiotics	
Co-trimoxazole (Septrin)	Acute TIN, ATI, hyperkalaemia
Aminoglycosides, e.g. gentamicin	ATI
Sulphadiazine	Crystalluria, nephrolithiasis
Rifampicin	Acute TIN
Antivirals	
Acyclovir	Crystallisation with tubular obstruction
Foscarnet	ATI, crystalline glomerulonephritis, RTA
Antifungals	
Amphotericin	ATI, proximal tubular dysfunction
Antiretrovirals	
Indinavir	Nephrolithiasis, chronic TIN
Atazanavir	Nephrolithiasis
Tenofovir (NtRTI)	Proximal tubular dysfunction, ATI
NRTIs, e.g. didanosine	Lactic acidosis

TIN tubulointerstitial nephritis, *ATI* acute tubular injury, *RTA* renal tubular acidosis

factors for CKD (black race, hypertension or cardiovascular disease, diabetes, viral hepatitis, family history or potentially nephrotoxic mediations) need enhanced surveillance.

Acute Kidney Injury (AKI)

Common precipitants for AKI in HIV include sepsis, hypovolaemia or exposure to potentially nephrotoxic medication, often during treatment for opportunistic infection (Table 25.2); risk factors include prior chronic kidney disease and greater degree of immunodeficiency [5]. Less common causes include acute presentations of HIVAN or HIV immune complex glomerulonephritis, HIV-associated thrombotic microangiopathy and non-drug-induced tubulointerstitial nephritis or parenchymal infection (see below). Diagnostic kidney biopsy may be required when injury is severe or sustained and a clear cause is not identifiable. Indications for renal replacement therapy in AKI are the same as those for non-infected individuals.

HIV-Associated Thrombotic Microangiopathy

Thrombotic microangiopathy (TMA) is an uncommon but well-recognised complication of HIV, typified by the presence of microangiopathic haemolytic anaemia, thrombocytopaenia, elevated lactate dehydrogenase and renal impairment and/or neurological symptoms. TMA may present at any stage of HIV infection but is more common in advanced disease. HIV p24 antigen has been detected within endothelial cells during TMA, suggesting that HIV may directly incite endothelial injury [6]. ADAMTS13 activity may be depressed, typically in conjunction with detectable anti-ADAMTS13 antibodies. Other potential secondary causes of TMA may coexist, including CMV viraemia or drug exposures (e.g. rifampicin).

Where possible, a kidney biopsy should be performed to confirm thrombotic microangiopathy as the cause of renal failure. Management is based on treatment strategies for TMA in non-infected individuals as no prospective trials have been performed in HIV. Plasma exchange (with plasma replacement) is widely used as first-line therapy albeit with inconsistent outcomes among published studies. Antiretroviral therapy should be initiated early to counteract any ongoing endothelial injury attributable to the virus and should be administered post-plasma exchange. Excellent outcomes have been reported for a regimen of plasma exchange, corticosteroids and early antiretroviral therapy in a cohort of patients with TMA and low ADAMTS13 activity [7].

HIV-Associated Nephropathy (HIVAN)

First described among the AIDS populations of New York and Miami in 1984, the 'collapsing glomerulopathy' of HIVAN is almost exclusively seen in HIV-infected patients of black African or Caribbean ancestry. Although HIVAN has declined in the era of widespread cART use, the prevalence among black HIV-infected patients in the UK remains 1 %, with estimates among Sub-Saharan African populations significantly higher [8, 9].

Aetiology and Pathogenesis

Viral nucleic acids can be identified in human renal epithelial cells in biopsies from patients with HIVAN, and these cells appear to be able to support local replication, although virus can also be detected in the absence of clinical disease.

Virtual confinement of disease to those of African ancestry suggests a marked genetic predisposition, and a strong association has been found with polymorphisms in *APOL1*, the gene encoding apolipoprotein L1 (Apol1), with disease risk following a recessive pattern of inheritance. Only kidney disease-associated Apol1 variants lyse the parasite *Trypanosoma brucei rhodesiense* in vitro, suggesting that these variants may have proliferated under pressure of positive selection [10].

Clinicopathologic Characteristics

Classical disease comprises heavy proteinuria (often nephrotic range) with renal impairment, minimal oedema and relative normotension. CD4 count is typically <200 at presentation although cases have been described early in disease,

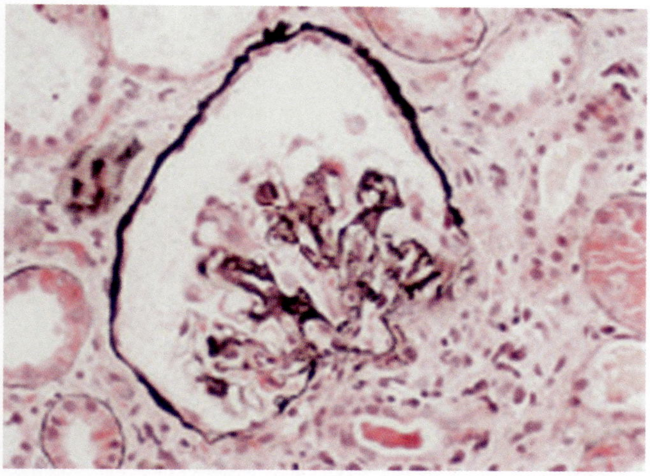

Fig. 25.1 Collapsing glomerulopathy of HIVAN

Table 25.3 Immune complex kidney disease in HIV

Histological pattern	Important secondary causes/ associations in HIV
HIV immune complex kidney disease (HIVICK)	
Membranous GN	Syphilis, HBV, neoplasia
IgA nephropathy	Chronic liver disease
Post-infectious GN	Streptococcal infection, staphylococcal infection (IgA predominant?), other bacterial, fungal, viral or parasitic disease
Mesangiocapillary GN	HCV, HBV, chronic infection (e.g. SBE), SLE, drugs (e.g. interferon-alpha)
Immunotactoid or fibrillary GN	HCV, neoplasia
Lupus-like nephritis	SLE

HBV hepatitis B virus, *HCV* hepatitis C virus, *SBE* subacute bacterial endocarditis, *SLE* systemic lupus erythematosus

including at seroconversion. Recent studies have shown that typical histological lesions of HIVAN may be found on biopsy in patients exhibiting only microalbuminuria, although the natural history of disease in such cases is unknown. Ultrasound classically shows bilaterally enlarged echogenic kidneys. No non-invasive test has sufficient specificity for HIVAN and definitive diagnosis requires renal biopsy.

The hallmark histologic lesion of HIVAN is 'collapse' of the glomerular tuft, defined by severe retraction of glomerular capillary walls resulting in loss of patency of capillary lumens and often best appreciated on silver stain (Fig. 25.1). This is accompanied by podocyte swelling and hyperplasia, often sufficiently florid to obliterate Bowman's space as 'pseudocrescents'. Lesions may evolve into a more typical pattern of FSGS (NOS) over time. Tubulointerstitial disease is a prominent feature, with 'microcyst' formation – cylindrically dilated tubules containing large proteinaceous casts – and a lymphocyte-rich interstitial infiltrate. Positive immunostaining is confined to variable IgM and complement deposition in collapsed segments and, to a lesser extent, the mesangium, without significant electron-dense deposits on electron microscopy. Endothelial tubuloreticular inclusion bodies are frequently seen.

Treatment and Prognosis

No randomised controlled treatment trials have been conducted in HIVAN. General measures include careful control of blood pressure, aiming for levels <130/80 ideally with ACEi or ARB. Despite current best therapy, rates of progression to ESRF remain high.

Antiretroviral Therapy

HIVAN incidence has fallen markedly since widespread introduction of cART, and new cases among patients in stable care in the UK are rare [8]. Numerous published cases have reported stabilisation or improvement of disease, including histological changes, with the commencement of cART. Cohort studies examining the effect of cART on renal outcomes in HIVAN have yielded conflicting results, however. The benefits of treatment are likely to be greatest in those with less established interstitial fibrosis and atrophy, and failure to stratify for this may explain some of the heterogeneity in study outcomes. Current guidance is for initiation of cART in all patients where HIVAN is confirmed, regardless of CD4 count [4].

Corticosteroids

The majority of published studies examining the effect of steroids on disease progression in HIVAN have reported benefit, but most were conducted before the routine administration of cART or consider small patient numbers in retrospective analyses. Cases where serial biopsy has been performed before and after steroid therapy suggest a particular amelioration of tubulointerstitial inflammation. Concerns regarding an increased infection risk with steroid use in HIV have not been borne out in studies where steroids have been used as part of initial HIV therapy. Current guidelines suggest reserving therapy for those in whom concomitant opportunistic infection has been excluded and with progressive decline in renal function despite cART [11].

Immune Complex Kidney Disease

Immune complex kidney disease (ICKD) is characterised by the presence of immune deposits on immunostaining, typically accompanied by electron-dense deposits on electron microscopy. A variety of glomerular histological patterns have been described in association with HIV infection (Table 25.3). Patients are more likely to be non-black or coinfected with viral hepatitis although ICKD does occur in black populations and can coexist with HIVAN. Clinical presentations mirror the spectrum seen in glomerulonephritis in the non-HIV population: from asymptomatic dipstick haemo-proteinuria in early IgA or mesangial proliferative lesions, to nephrotic syndrome in membranous nephropathy, to hypertension and rapidly progressive renal failure in crescentic proliferative disease.

Patients with HIV are frequently hypergammaglobulinaemic, and circulating immune complexes can be detected in the majority of patients. Immune complexes eluted from biopsy material of patients with ICKD have confirmed the presence of HIV antigens such as P24 within the kidney, and it is likely that HIV represents the primary pathogenic factor in some cases [12]. However, ICKD may precede acquisition of HIV (e.g. IgA disease, lupus nephritis) or may be precipitated by factors other than the HIV virus (e.g. hepatitis B and C, other opportunistic infections or drugs), meaning a careful evaluation is required to formulate the most appropriate management plan.

HIVICK (HIV Immune Complex Kidney Disease)

The term HIVICK has been used to describe a unique histological pattern observed in HIV, characterised predominantly by mesangial hyperplasia with mesangial and subepithelial immune deposits, with features intermediate between post-infectious and incompletely expressed membranous glomerulopathies [13]. Subepithelial deposits may be large and produce a characteristic 'ball in cup' appearance on light and electron microscopy, while immunohistochemistry shows variable staining of deposits for IgA, IgM, IgG and C3. Lack of consensus when classifying HIV ICKD in studies has limited understanding of the clinical characteristics and natural history of this lesion and, indeed, of whether it represents a discrete disease entity.

Lupus-Like Nephritis

Several small studies have described cases of ICKD in HIV resembling lupus nephritis with 'full-house' immunoglobulin and complement deposits (including C1q), but in the absence of serological evidence of SLE. Histological features overlap those of HIVICK but frequently include prominent subendothelial deposits (sometimes forming 'wire loops') and diffuse or focal endocapillary proliferation (Fig. 25.2a, b). Patients are typically nephritic with microscopic haematuria and marked renal impairment at presentation. Lupus-like nephritis is associated with a high incidence of ESRD by 1 year of diagnosis.

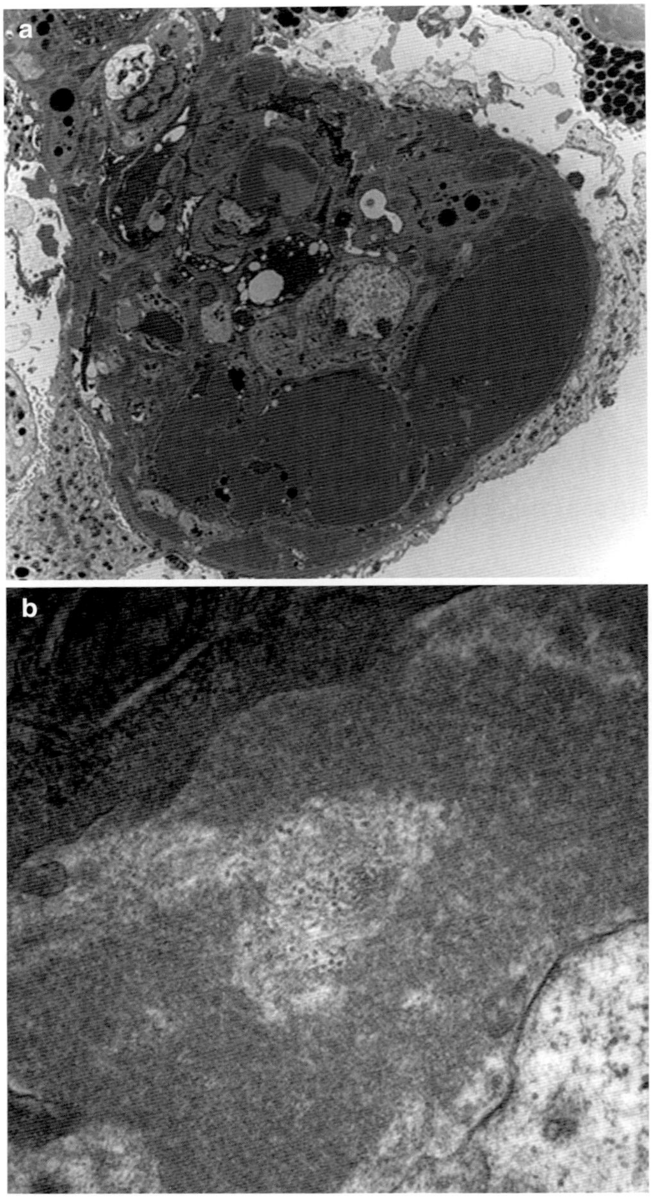

Fig. 25.2 (**a**) The electron microscopy images ×3,000 show massive electron-dense deposits in the subendothelial space and associated with endocapillary-type closure of the capillary lumina. The impression of a substructure to the deposits is apparent from low power (Courtesy of Dr Catherine Horsfield). (**b**) Electron microscopy image ×80,000 shows the detail of the substructure to the deposits, which in cryoglobulins can vary but can include fibrils including those with a curvilinear appearance (Courtesy of Dr Catherine Horsfield)

Treatment

Management should begin with careful consideration of alternative causes for an immune complex lesion beyond HIV per se which may direct specific treatment (Table 25.2).

No controlled trials have examined specific treatment strategies in HIV ICKD. While initiation of cART has been reported to retard or reverse ICKD in published case reports, cohort studies do not robustly demonstrate a benefit. Such studies have featured small numbers or considered ICKD grouped with other miscellaneous non-HIVAN disease, preventing identification of ICKD subgroups which may potentially benefit from control of replication. In light of data supporting a pathogenic role for HIV in some cases of ICKD, and the prevailing immune dysregulation attributable to disease, most physicians would currently start cART on diagnosis regardless of CD4 count or VL. Other immunomodulatory drugs, including corticosteroids, have not been systematically tested in this area.

Tubulointerstitial Pathology

Tubulointerstitial disease encountered in HIV includes acute tubular injury, frequently attributable to drugs or ischaemic injury consequent on infection, tubulointerstitial nephritis (TIN), drug crystallopathy or functional tubular abnormalities such as that seen with tenofovir (see below).

A broad range of conditions may incite acute or chronic tubulointerstitial inflammation in HIV including drug exposures, opportunistic infection, neoplasia and certain specific immune dyscrasias (Table 25.4). Clinical assignment of disease to the tubulointerstitial compartment is often difficult as patients frequently exhibit heavy proteinuria (>1 g/day) and microscopic haematuria, even in the absence of a discernible glomerular lesion [14]. The classic triad of fever, rash and pyuria seen with drug-induced acute TIN is rare in the context of HIV, although peripheral eosinophilia is frequent [14]. Diagnosis of TIN in HIV requires careful consideration of the prevailing degree of immunodeficiency, temporal relationship to drug exposures and workup for systemic disease present in other organ systems to ensure the correct treatment is instigated.

Diffuse Infiltrative Lymphocytosis Syndrome (DILS)

DILS is a Sjögren-like multisystem disorder of HIV characterised by oligoclonal CD8+ T cell expansion and consequent organ infiltration [15]. Affected individuals may be of any ethnicity or gender, often present some years after HIV diagnosis and typically have preserved CD4 cell counts and a low incidence of opportunistic infection. DILS incidence has fallen markedly in the post-cART era suggesting a protective effect of viral suppression. Parotid enlargement, often accompanied by sicca symptoms, is almost universal, while extra-glandular disease may include lymphadenopathy, lymphocytic interstitial pneumonitis, cranial or peripheral neuropathies, hepatitis and renal involvement. Renal disease manifests as florid tubulointerstitial infiltration of CD8+ T cells with progressive renal impairment and subsequent fibrosis if untreated. Treatment should include instigation or optimisation of cART to attain viral suppression, theoretically diminishing the stimulus for CD8+ T cell proliferation. Most clinicians will also use adjunctive corticosteroids in the presence of significant renal disease.

Immune Reconstitution Inflammatory Syndrome (IRIS)

IRIS describes a syndrome of 'paradoxical' organ inflammation seen while adaptive immunity recovers during antiretroviral treatment, targeted most frequently against residual or occult infectious antigens [16]. Clinical presentation largely corresponds to target organs involved by the inciting infection (e.g. ocular disease with CMV, pneumonitis with pneumocystis) where disease appears to worsen after initial improvement with antimicrobials. Affected patients typically have low (<50) CD4 counts when cART is initiated with rapid viral suppression and immune reconstitution; median time of presentation in the largest retrospective cohort was 46 days [17]. While as many as 30 % of patients experience some form of IRIS, renal involvement is rare and largely

Table 25.4 Differential diagnosis of tubulointerstitial inflammation in HIV

Cause	Clinical or histological pointers to diagnosis
Drugs	
Antimicrobials (e.g. Septrin, rifampicin, β-lactams)	Temporal relationship to drug introduction
Antiretrovirals (abacavir, indinavir)	Clinical response to drug withdrawal
General, e.g. NSAIDs, PPIs	Fever and rash unusual, eosinophilia common
	Often eosinophil infiltrate on biopsy
	Chronic scarring inflammation and leucocyturia with indinavir
Bacterial infection	
Mycobacterial disease	May be signs of extrarenal disease (e.g. pulmonary infiltrates, lymphadenopathy). Granulomatous inflammation on biopsy. Specific mycobacterial stains and PCR may be negative despite active disease
Ascending urinary tract infection	Positive urine cultures. Neutrophil-rich infiltrate in acute infection with tubular casts
Viral infection	
CMV Adenovirus EBV BK virus (rare in HIV)	CD4 often <100. Extrarenal disease may be evident (e.g. retinitis, pneumonitis with CMV). Viral inclusion bodies often seen on biopsy and specific immunohistochemistry or in situ hybridisation for viral nucleic acids are diagnostic
Fungal and parasitic infections	
Cryptococcus Candida Microsporidia	Occur in conjunction with disseminated disease in context of severe immunodeficiency (CD4 < 100)
Lymphoma	Often extrarenal disease (e.g. lymphadenopathy). Infiltrating lymphocytes atypical in morphology
HIVAN	Associated microcystic tubular dilatation, typical collapsing glomerular lesion usually evident
Immune disorders of HIV	
DILS	Parotid enlargement. CD4 often >200. CD8-dominant lymphocytic infiltrate
IRIS	Recent introduction of cART. Usually underlying mycobacterial infection. Often granulomatous inflammation with CD4+ lymphocytic infiltrate

reported in the context of mycobacterial infection. Histology shows a tubulointerstitial mononuclear cells infiltrate, which may be granulomatous, with CD4+ T cells predominating. cART can usually be continued in such circumstances with addition of oral corticosteroids, which may be tapered after robust clinical improvement. Antimicrobial therapy should be continued if active infection persists.

Renal Complications of Antiretroviral Therapy

Widespread use of cART has revolutionised outcomes in HIV, but with it has come a broad range of adverse effects including renal toxicities. Three drugs have received most attention: tenofovir, indinavir and atazanavir. All three have been associated with an increased risk of developing CKD in a recent large European cohort study, and periodic monitoring for emergence of kidney disease should be performed in all patients on cART [18].

Indinavir

Nephrolithiasis is a common and well-recognised side effect of the protease inhibitor indinavir, with crystalluria present in up to 65 % of patients. Manifestations include classical renal colic with radiolucent stones, a syndrome of flank pain and dysuria in the absence of discrete calculi and a more sinister insidious scarring tubulointerstitial nephritis associated with persistent pyuria and driven by intraparenchymal crystallisation. Nephrolithiasis can in part be combated by maintenance of good oral water intake (>1.5 l/day), while persistent leucocyturia or new renal impairment should prompt discontinuation.

Atazanavir

Atazanavir is a well-tolerated and commonly used once-daily protease inhibitor. Like indinavir, it has the potential to crystallise and form calculi albeit much less frequently (around 1 %). Tubulointerstitial nephritis with atazanavir is correspondingly rare.

Tenofovir

Tenofovir is an acyclic nucleotide reverse transcriptase inhibitor (NtRTI) with activity against both HIV and hepatitis B virus, frequently used in first-line cART regimens. Biochemical features of toxicity are those of a partial or complete Fanconi syndrome, variably comprising glycosuria, phosphaturia, hypouricaemia, aminoaciduria, renal tubular acidosis and low-molecular-weight proteinuria. Reduced eGFR is a variable finding and may reflect reversible impairment of tubular creatinine secretion, AKI, or established CKD with persistent severe toxicity. Risk factors for tenofovir toxicity include older age, lower BMI, prior CKD and use of other nephrotoxic medication. Concomitant use of the NRTI didanosine may enhance tenofovir toxicity and is not recommended, while ritonavir-boosted protease inhibitor regimens have also been associated with increased tenofovir plasma levels and toxicity, requiring vigilance when used [19].

Table 25.5 Schema for monitoring of proximal tubular function during tenofovir therapy

Screening tests	Frequency
1. eGFR	Baseline
2. Urine protein/creatinine ratio	3 monthly for 1 year
3. Urine glucose	Twice yearly thereafter
4. Urinary fractional excretion of phosphate[a]	
5. Tubular proteinuria (e.g. retinol-binding protein)[b]	
Additional survey for proximal renal tubulopathy if any of 1–5 abnormal:	
Serum bicarbonate and urinary pH (bicarbonate <21 and urinary pH >5.5 suggest RTA[c])	
Urinary fractional excretion of uric acid (abnormal >0.1 on a fasted morning spot urine sample)	
Serum potassium and urinary potassium excretion	
Consider DEXA scan if evidence of renal phosphate wasting	
Consider stopping if:	
Significant and sustained changes in 1–4	
Syndrome of proximal renal tubulopathy with no other cause	
Progressive deterioration in tubular proteinuria	

Adapted from Hall et al. and European Aids Clinical Society Guidelines

[a]Abnormal >0.2 (>0.1 if serum phosphate <0.8 mmol/l). Monitoring fractional excretion of phosphate is preferable to serum phosphate, as hypophosphataemia may be a late event and accompanied by established bone demineralisation. It is important to exclude vitamin D deficiency which may provoke phosphaturia through secondary hyperparathyroidism

[b]Retinol-binding protein (RBP) is a low-molecular-weight protein, freely filtered by the glomerulus and reabsorbed in the proximal tubule. Elevated levels reflect proximal tubular dysfunction and may be grossly deranged in tenofovir toxicity

[c]Urinary pH may still fall below 5.5 in proximal RTA as distal urinary acidification mechanisms remain intact. An elevated urinary pH in the context of systemic acidaemia would however suggest a renal acidosis

Mild toxicity is frequently asymptomatic but manifestations of severe injury include osteomalacia with bone pain (consequent on phosphate wasting) or AKI. Renal biopsy in AKI reveals acute proximal tubular damage with giant and misshapen mitochondria on electron microscopy, suggesting this organelle as the primary target for toxicity.

Tenofovir-induced proximal tubular dysfunction is typically reversible if detected promptly and the drug withdrawn. Monitoring eGFR and urinalysis alone are insufficient and must be combined with more specific tests of proximal tubular function (see Table 25.5).

Hepatitis C

The global prevalence of hepatitis C is vast with an estimated 170 million (2–3 % of the world's population) infected; estimated prevalence is 1.6 % in the USA of which 1.3 % are viraemic. There is a particularly high prevalence in the Far East, Mediterranean countries, the Middle East and North Africa. It is estimated that in some regions of Egypt, 20 % of the adult population is chronically infected. Since the discovery of the virus in 1988, reports rapidly emerged of associated renal disease as well as cryoglobulinaemia, Sjögren's syndrome and lymphoproliferative disorders. The association with cryoglobulinaemia is particularly striking with evidence of type II monoclonal IgM to polyclonal IgG (or type III polyclonal IgM to polyclonal IgG) cryoglobulinaemia in 20–56 % of those with hepatitis C and 90 % of all type II cryoglobulinaemia being attributable to hepatitis C. However, cryoglobulinaemia tends to be a late presentation of hepatitis C, and curiously only a minority (≤25 %) of those patients who develop cryoglobulinaemia develop overt renal disease. This may not tell the whole story as hepatitis C can affect the kidney in the absence of cryoglobulinaemia, and in one study 25 out of 30 patients undergoing a protocol renal biopsy at the time of liver transplant for hepatitis C had evidence of immune complex glomerular disease (mostly MPGN), but frequently this was not clinically apparent.

The natural history of HCV is variable. It is estimated that 5–40 % of adults infected with HCV clear virus spontaneously. Spontaneous clearance is almost always within the first 6 months after infection and rarely occurs after the first year of infection. Of those with chronic infection, 20–30 % will progress to end-stage liver disease in 20–30 years time.

Clinical Presentation

Hepatitis C-related renal disease tends to present in the fifth and sixth decade and in the setting of chronic infection. There are a variety of renal pathologies associated with hepatitis C (see Table 25.6), and the clinical manifestations of HCV-associated renal disease depend on the renal lesion. Typically presentations are associated with microscopic haematuria, proteinuria and renal impairment, but RPGN, AKI and nephrotic syndrome can also occur. Patients with cryoglobulinaemia-related renal disease may present with vasculitis-associated signs and symptoms such as arthralgia, abdominal pain (mesenteric vasculitis), purpura and neuropathy.

Polyclonal gammopathy is common, with low C4, C1q and CH50 with variably depressed C3 and cryoglobulinaemia present in 60–70 %, the presence of rheumatoid factor and low complement being a strong pointer. It is also important to note that hepatitis C Ab assay can have false negatives particularly in patients with renal failure, cryoglobulinaemia or immunosuppressed [20]. Where there is an index of suspicion about HCV infection and the HCV-Ab test is negative, an HCV RNA test should be carried out.

Table 25.6 Renal involvement in hepatitis C

Renal involvement
Glomerular
Cryoglobulin positive
MPGN
Fibrillary
Immunotactoid
Amyloid
Cryoglobulin negative
MPGN
Membranous GN (exclude hepatocellular carcinoma)
FSGS
Mesangial deposits
Amyloid (if associated with IV or SC drug abuse)
Vasculitic
Thrombotic microangiopathy (post-transplant)
Tubulointerstitial nephritis
Interstitial nephritis secondary to virus
Interstitial nephritis secondary to Interferon

Pathology

The predominant renal lesion is MPGN which can be associated with cryoglobulinaemia or be independent and in Japan 60 % of MPGN is associated with chronic hepatitis C infection, but other glomerular lesions, interstitial nephritis and small vessel vasculitis (especially in association with cryoglobulinaemia) have all been reported [21, 22] (see Table 25.6). If membranous GN is apparent, then it is worth checking α-fetoprotein level to exclude hepatocellular carcinoma, and lymphoma is said to develop in 10 % of patients with essential cryoglobulinaemia, which may present as minimal change disease. MPGN is usually associated with deposition of IgM, IgG and C3 in the mesangium and capillary walls, and electron microscopy is important in establishing the diagnosis demonstrating subendothelial deposits and may also reveal cryoglobulin deposition. Fibrillary and immunotactoid glomerulonephritis, although rare, have both been documented with hepatitis C (hepatitis C is an important cause of fibrillary GN) and again emphasise the importance of electron microscopy in the assessment. RPGN can occur in the setting of underlying MPGN or in the context of a vasculitis (usually cryoglobulin associated) or fibrillary GN. Thrombotic microangiopathy has been reported (predominantly post-transplant), and hepatitis C is a cause of isolated interstitial nephritis. It has been difficult to demonstrate hepatitis C antigens histologically although this has been done; although the presence of antigens in the kidney clearly does not prove causality, they have been detected in patients with MPGN. The majority of renal pathology relates to immune complex disease either in the form of cryoglobulins or presumably hepatitis C Ab/Ag complexes, but there is also evidence of direct cytotoxicity of the podocytes (FSGS), the endothelium (thrombotic microangiopathy) and interstitium (with cell-mediated response).

Treatment and Outcome

MPGN secondary to hepatitis C is said to resolve spontaneously in a third of patients, stabilise in a third and progress to overt nephritic/nephrotic syndrome in the remaining third. Patients with HIV have a worse renal outcome if coinfected with hepatitis C in terms of ESRD (RR 1.8) and have a greater likelihood of immune complex glomerular disease [23, 24]. There appears to be no correlation between absolute viral load and risk of nephropathy, but clearing of the virus is usually associated with renal remission and recurrence of viraemia universally results in relapse.

The state of the literature is nicely reviewed by Fabrizi and colleagues [22], and the current advice for the treatment of hepatitis C-associated glomerulonephritis is summarised in the recent KDIGO guidelines [25], the authors quite rightly emphasising how dreadfully poor the evidence base is for any treatment. However, drawing from the experience of HIV and the fact that chronic antigenaemia is clearly the driving force and that the best long-term predictor of outcome is sustained virological remission, eradication of the virus should be the treatment of choice in any patient with hepatitis C-driven renal disease or cryoglobulinaemia. Currently this is with pegylated interferon and ribavirin (with appropriate dose reduction) and under the supervision of a hepatologist. In patients with a normal GFR, this combination can expect a 75 % sustained virological response (SVR, cure) rate in genotypes 2 and 3 with an SVR rate of 45–50 % for genotypes 1 and 4 (those RNA negative at 4 and 12 weeks have an 80 % chance of an SVR) [26]. A meta-analysis comparing antiviral therapy with immunosuppression (steroids plus or minus cyclophosphamide) was strongly in favour of antivirals in terms of reduced proteinuria (but with no difference in renal function). However, interferon-α itself can cause minimal change glomerulonephritis (and TIN), and interferon and ribavirin are poorly tolerated in CKD, requiring significant dose reduction. There is little published evidence on the cure rates in ESRD.

While the anti-HCV activity of IFN and ribavirin is mostly immunomodulatory, over the recent years there has been a huge interest in antivirals that target virally encoded enzymes or processes involved in HCV replication. There are numerous directly acting antivirals (DAAs) against HCV undergoing clinical evaluation. The first two NS3/4 protease inhibitors, telaprevir and boceprevir, have recently been licenced in combination with IFN and ribavirin, for the treatment of genotype 1 HCV. These triple combinations have increased SVR rates up to 70–80 % for these difficult-to-treat patients. The new DAAs are not licenced for use in renal failure but offer huge potential if truly effective in suppressing viral replication and trials in this setting are urgently needed.

Given that a proportion of patients go into spontaneous remission and proteinuric renal disease should be treated as such, it seems sensible to aim for good blood pressure control and inhibition of the renin-angiotensin system with ACEI/ARB.

In the absence of viral remission and progressive nephropathy, the usual suspects have been tried including most commonly pulsed and oral steroids, cyclophosphamide, MMF, plasma exchange and more recently anti-CD20mAb. The evidence base for any of the above is almost non-existent, but given that much of the renal pathology relates to pathological deposition of antibodies, there is a logic at least in targeting B cells in patients with severe aggressive disease such as RPGN or cryoglobulinaemic vasculitis. Rituximab is effective at treating non-virally associated mixed essential cryoglobulinaemia, and there is accumulating evidence of short-term benefit in patients with hepatitis C-associated MPGN. Remission rates of 80 % have been reported, but relapse at a mean of 6 months is very common following treatment. Care needs to be exercised with respect to immunosuppression withdrawal hepatic flares that may occur [27]. As with all immunosuppression in this setting, there is no data on long-term outcomes for liver disease. There are a few case reports claiming marked reduction in cryoglobulins and clinical improvement with plasma exchange; again the evidence base is very limited and plasma exchange not without its risks, but it may be worth considering in patients with very aggressive disease while awaiting a response from antivirals or anti-B cell agents.

Hepatitis B

Approximately 400 million people are chronically infected with hepatitis B worldwide exceeding the prevalence even of hepatitis C (see Fig. 25.3). In Africa exposure to hepatitis B is approaching 100 % and (depending on age of exposure) roughly 10 % go on to develop chronic disease and of these 3 % develop nephropathy.

Table 25.7 shows the relationship between the different phases of disease and the serological tests, HBV DNA levels and serum ALT.

As with hepatitis C there are major infection control issues for patients and staff as hepatitis B is highly transmissible. Similarly, active hepatitis B infection has implications for donor and transplant recipients and clear guidelines for both.

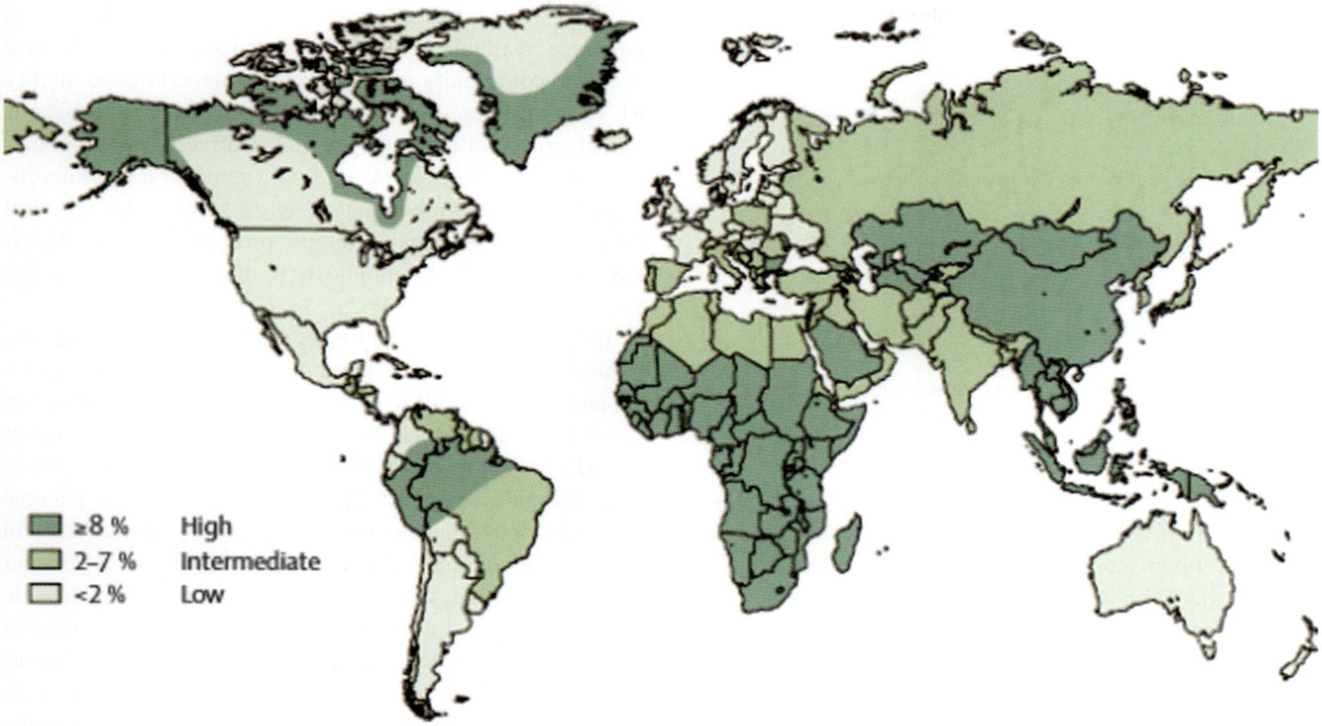

Fig. 25.3 Global distribution of HBV. The *shades of green* represent HBsAg prevalence (Reproduced with permission from Hoffmann and Thio [28])

Table 25.7 Natural histories of hepatitis B infection as measured by antigenaemia, antibodies, viral DNA and ALT

Stage of infection	Surface antigen (HBsAg)	'e' antigen (HBeAg)	IgM anti-core antibody	IgG anti-core antibody	Hepatitis B virus DNA	Anti-HBe	Anti-HBs	ALT
Acute (early)	+	+	+[a]	+	+	–	–	↑↑↑
Acute (resolving)	+	–	+	+	–	+/–	–	↑↑
Chronic (immune tolerant)	+	+	–	+	++	–	–	N[b]
Chronic (immune active)	+	+	–	+	+	–	–	↑
Chronic (e-Ag negative)	+	+	–	+	+	–	–	↑
Chronic (inactive carrier)	+	–	–	+	–	+	–	N
Resolved (immune)	–	–	–	+	–	+/–	+/–	N
Successful vaccination	–	–	–	–	–	–	+	N

[a] In very early infection the IgM anti-core can be negative and by definition so can the IgG
[b] *N* normal

Clinical Manifestations

Renal involvement secondary to hepatitis B can manifest in a variety of ways (see Table 25.8), classically with blood and proteinuria secondary to membranous glomerulonephritis and less frequently MPGN [29]. Membranous GN is much more common in children and has a marked, and unexplained, male predominance. Presentation may be with nephrotic range proteinuria, oedema, less commonly hypertension and renal impairment whereas a history of clinically overt hepatitis is rare. In children the prognosis is good with most cases resolving spontaneously, but this appears less likely to happen in adults unless resolution of the viraemia occurs; remission of membranous tends to correlate well with the disappearance of e antigenaemia.

Complement levels may be low in both MPGN and membranous GN. Cryoglobulinaemia is much less common than with hepatitis C but does occur and can be associated with MPGN.

In addition to these presentations of chronic hepatitis B infection, serum sickness (comprising arthralgia, fever, maculopapular rash, acute hepatitis and microscopic haematuria

Table 25.8 Renal involvement in hepatitis B

Glomerular
Cryoglobulin negative
Membranous GN
MPGN
Mesangial proliferation (with serum sickness)
IgA
Cryoglobulin positive
MPGN
Vasculitic
Polyarteritis nodosa
Treatment related
Proximal tubular dysfunction/Fanconi syndrome secondary to tenofovir

and proteinuria–the latter which may come to the attention of the nephrologist) can develop at the time of seroconversion, usually resolving spontaneously within 2 weeks.

The other fairly unique presentation of hepatitis B infection is polyarteritis nodosa (PAN) which occurs in a tiny proportion of patients recently infected, possibly as a result of molecular mimicry (there have been case reports of PAN following hepatitis B vaccination). The French vasculitis study group reviewed the clinical findings of 384 patients with PAN presenting over a 30-year period of which 123 patients had hepatitis B-associated PAN. They noted 66 % of patients had renal involvement which was universally an ANCA-negative large vessel vasculitis and no patients in this cohort had glomerulonephritis. Hepatitis B-associated PAN had a stronger association with neuropathy, orchitis and hypertension. It is worth noting that even with the use of antivirals, this group had a mortality of 34 % (which was worse than non-hepatitis B-associated PAN), with age >65, hypertension and abdominal pain being adverse prognostic indications [30].

Pathology

There seems to be a strong association with hepatitis B e antigenaemia and MGN, whereas both hepatitis e and s antigens are thought to contribute to the aetiopathology of MPGN. The appearance of hepatitis B-associated membranous GN is similar to IMN, but there may be more mesangial expansion. With hepatitis B-associated MN, MPGN or IgA, it may be possible to detect hepatitis B antigens by PCR and may help to distinguish between primary and secondary GN.

Treatment and Outcome

The KDIGO guidelines [17] point out that there are no randomised controlled trials on the treatment of hepatitis B-associated glomerulonephritis, and therefore there is no guidance available. This depressing fact should galvanise the renal community to design and implement good quality RCTs in this area. In the meantime a pragmatic approach is that clearance of hepatitis B e and s antigenaemia, together with HBV DNA, is associated with remission of glomerulonephritis, and thus it makes sense to consider antiviral treatment (in addition to blood pressure control, ACEI/ARB) as soon as the diagnosis is made and other causes excluded.

IFN and nucleoside analogues (lamivudine, emtricitabine, telbivudine and entecavir) and nucleotide analogues (adefovir and tenofovir) all have activity against HBV. Finite (48 weeks) of IFN-alpha is associated with consistently higher anti-HBe seroconversion than with the nucleoside/nucleotide analogues. However, IFN is contraindicated in patients with decompensated cirrhosis and may only have efficacy in patients with certain HBV genotypes (A/B) and in younger patients with high liver necro-inflammation. The nucleoside analogues lamivudine, emtricitabine and telbivudine all have a low genetic barrier and therefore should be avoided as monotherapy. Adefovir and tenofovir have both been associated with Fanconi syndrome and cumulative renal toxicity. For oral therapy, entecavir or tenofovir (with careful renal monitoring) are the agents of choice. Therapy may need to be lifelong for many patients, although finite therapy may be possible for patients who achieve HBsAg loss or HBeAg loss and anti-HBe seroconversion in HBeAg+ [31].

On the positive side there is hugely encouraging data showing almost complete eradication of childhood MN secondary to hepatitis B following universal vaccination programmes [32], and a similar approach to control other infective agents may well have comparable benefits.

HTLV1 and 2

There are a smattering of case reports of glomerular lesions in patients with HTLV1 and 2 infection including lupus-like nephropathy, TINU and MPGN. It is difficult to be clear if these are genuine associations, and although one might expect glomerular disorders in patients with chronic viraemia, the rarity of these reports given the global prevalence of HTLV infection (3.8 % of Japanese dialysis patients) suggests HTLV-associated renal disease is rare.

Summary

In summary hepatitis B and C and HIV contribute significantly to global renal disease, and glomerulonephritis secondary to these blood-borne viruses should be considered in the diagnostic work of all patients with glomerulonephritis or unexplained AKI. The treatment of these secondary glomerulonephritides is primarily control or eradication of virus and should be undertaken in collaboration with specialists.

References

1. Palella Jr FJ, Delaney KM, Moorman AC, Loveless MO, Fuhrer J, Satten GA, Aschman DJ, Holmberg SD. Declining morbidity and mortality among patients with advanced human immunodeficiency virus infection. HIV Outpatient Study Investigators. N Engl J Med. 1998;338:853–60.
2. Li Y, Shlipak MG, Grunfeld C, Choi AI. Incidence and risk factors for acute kidney injury in HIV Infection. Am J Nephrol. 2012;35:327–34.
3. Buchacz K, Baker RK, Palella Jr FJ, Chmiel JS, Lichtenstein KA, Novak RM, Wood KC, Brooks JT. AIDS-defining opportunistic illnesses in US patients, 1994-2007: a cohort study. AIDS. 2010;24: 1549–59.
4. EACS (European AIDS Clinical Society) Guidelines for treatment of HIV infected adults in Europe. 2011. http://www.europeanaidsclinicalsociety.org/images/stories/EACS-Pdf/EACSguidelines-v6.0-English.pdf.
5. Ibrahim F, Naftalin C, Cheserem E, Roe J, Campbell LJ, Bansi L, Hendry BM, Sabin C, Post FA. Immunodeficiency and renal impairment are risk factors for HIV-associated acute renal failure. AIDS. 2010;24:2239–44.
6. del Arco A, Martinez MA, Pena JM, Gamallo C, Gonzalez JJ, Barbado FJ, Vazquez JJ. Thrombotic thrombocytopenic purpura associated with human immunodeficiency virus infection: demonstration of p24 antigen in endothelial cells. Clin Infect Dis. 1993;17:360–3.
7. Hart D, Sayer R, Miller R, Edwards S, Kelly A, Baglin T, Hunt B, Benjamin S, Patel R, Machin S, Scully M. Human immunodeficiency virus associated thrombotic thrombocytopenic purpura – favourable outcome with plasma exchange and prompt initiation of highly active antiretroviral therapy. Br J Haematol. 2011;153:515–9.
8. Post FA, Campbell LJ, Hamzah L, Collins L, Jones R, Siwani R, Johnson L, Fisher M, Holt SG, Bhagani S, Frankel AH, Wilkins E, Ainsworth JG, Larbalestier N, Macallan DC, Banerjee D, Baily G, Thuraisingham RC, Donohoe P, Hendry BM, Hilton RM, Edwards SG, Hangartner R, Howie AJ, Connolly JO, Easterbrook PJ. Predictors of renal outcome in HIV-associated nephropathy. Clin Infect Dis. 2008;46:1282–9.
9. Wyatt CM, Meliambro K, Klotman PE. Recent progress in HIV-associated nephropathy. Annu Rev Med. 2012;63:147–59.
10. Genovese G, Friedman DJ, Ross MD, Lecordier L, Uzureau P, Freedman BI, Bowden DW, Langefeld CD, Oleksyk TK, Uscinski Knob AL, Bernhardy AJ, Hicks PJ, Nelson GW, Vanhollebeke B, Winkler CA, Kopp JB, Pays E, Pollak MR. Association of trypanolytic ApoL1 variants with kidney disease in African Americans. Science. 2010;329:841–5.
11. Gupta SK, Eustace JA, Winston JA, Boydstun II, Ahuja TS, Rodriguez RA, Tashima KT, Roland M, Franceschini N, Palella FJ, Lennox JL, Klotman PE, Nachman SA, Hall SD, Szczech LA. Guidelines for the management of chronic kidney disease in HIV-infected patients: recommendations of the HIV Medicine Association of the Infectious Diseases Society of America. Clin Infect Dis. 2005;40:1559–85.
12. Kimmel PL, Phillips TM, Ferreira-Centeno A, Farkas-Szallasi T, Abraham AA, Garrett CT. Brief report: idiotypic IgA nephropathy in patients with human immunodeficiency virus infection. N Engl J Med. 1992;327:702–6.
13. Gerntholtz TE, Goetsch SJ, Katz I. HIV-related nephropathy: a South African perspective. Kidney Int. 2006;69:1885–91.
14. Parkhie SM, Fine DM, Lucas GM, Atta MG. Characteristics of patients with HIV and biopsy-proven acute interstitial nephritis. Clin J Am Soc Nephrol. 2010;5:798–804.
15. Kazi S, Cohen PR, Williams F, Schempp R, Reveille JD. The diffuse infiltrative lymphocytosis syndrome. Clinical and immunogenetic features in 35 patients. AIDS. 1996;10:385–91.
16. Hirsch HH, Kaufmann G, Sendi P, Battegay M. Immune reconstitution in HIV-infected patients. Clin Infect Dis. 2004;38:1159–66.
17. Shelburne SA, Visnegarwala F, Darcourt J, Graviss EA, Giordano TP, White Jr AC, Hamill RJ. Incidence and risk factors for immune reconstitution inflammatory syndrome during highly active antiretroviral therapy. AIDS. 2005;19:399–406.
18. Mocroft A, Kirk O, Reiss P, De Wit S, Sedlacek D, Beniowski M, Gatell J, Phillips AN, Ledergerber B, Lundgren JD. Estimated glomerular filtration rate, chronic kidney disease and antiretroviral drug use in HIV-positive patients. AIDS. 2010;24:1667–78.
19. Hall AM, Hendry BM, Nitsch D, Connolly JO. Tenofovir-associated kidney toxicity in HIV-infected patients: a review of the evidence. Am J Kidney Dis. 2011;57:773–80.
20. Barsoum R. Hepatitis C virus: from entry to renal injury - facts and potentials. Nephrol Dial Transplant. 2007;22:1840–8.
21. Kamar N, Izopet J, Alric L, Guilbeaud-Frugier C, Rostaing L. Hepatitis C virus-related kidney disease: an overview. Clin Nephrol. 2008;69:149–60.
22. Fabrizi F, Plaisier E, Saadoun D, Martin P, Messa P, Cacoub P. Hepatitis C virus infection, mixed cryoglobulinemia, and kidney disease. Am J Kidney Dis. 2013;61:623–37.
23. George E, Nadkarni GN, Estrella MM, Lucas GM, Sperati CJ, Atta MG, Fine DM. The impact of hepatitis C coinfection on kidney disease related to human immunodeficiency virus (HIV): a biopsy study. Medicine (Baltimore). 2011;90:289–95.
24. Tsui J, Vittinghoff E, Anastos K, Augenbraun M, Young M, Nowicki M, Cohen MH, Peters MG, Golub ET, Szczech L. Hepatitis C seropositivity and kidney function decline among women with HIV: data from the Women's Interagency HIV Study. Am J Kidney Dis. 2009;54:43–50.
25. Kidney International Supplements. KDIGO clinical practice guidelines for glomerulonephritis, 2012;2:200–208.
26. McHutchison JG, Lawitz EJ, Shiffman ML, Muir AJ, Galler GW, McCone J, Nyberg LM, Lee WM, Ghalib RH, Schiff ER, Galati JS, Bacon BR, Davis MN, Mukhopadhyay P, Koury K, Noviello S, Pedicone LD, Brass CA, Albrecht JK, Sulkowski MS; IDEAL Study Team. Peginterferon alfa-2b or alfa-2a with ribavirin for treatment of hepatitis C infection. N Engl J Med. 2009;361:580–93.
27. Sagnelli E, Pisaturo M, Sagnelli C, Coppola N. Rituximab-based treatment, HCV replication, and hepatic flares. Clin Dev Immunol. 2012. doi: 10.1155/2012/945950.
28. Hoffmann CJ, Thio CL. Clinical implications of HIV and hepatitis B co-infection in Asia and Africa. Lancet Infect Dis. 2007;7:402–9.
29. Bhimma R, Coovadia HM. Hepatitis B virus-associated nephropathy. Am J Nephrol. 2004;24:198–211.
30. Pagnoux C, Seror R, Henegar C, Mahr A, Cohen P, Le Guern V, Bienvenu B, Mouthon L, Guillevin L; French Vasculitis Study Group. Clinical features and outcomes in 348 patients with polyarteritis nodosa: a systematic retrospective study of patients diagnosed between 1963 and 2005 and entered into the French Vasculitis Study Group Database. Arthritis Rheum. 2010;62:616–26.
31. European Association For The Study Of The Liver. EASL clinical practice guidelines: Management of chronic hepatitis B virus infection. J Hepatol. 2012;57:167–85.
32. Liao MT, Chang MH, Lin FG, Tsai IJ, Chang YW, Tsau YK. Universal hepatitis B vaccination reduces childhood hepatitis B virus-associated membranous nephropathy. Paediatrics. 2011;128(3): e600–4.

Table 26.1 Common causes of biopsy proven AIN

Aetiological agent	Frequency in renal biopsy series (%)
Medications	50–75
Multisystem inflammatory disease	5–15
Infection	1–10
Unknown	10–30

Table 26.2 Clinical and laboratory features in drug-induced AIN [20]

Aetiological agent	Frequency in renal biopsy series (%)
Acute KI	100
Acute KI requiring dialysis	40
Arthralgia	45
Skin rash	22
Pyrexia	36
Non-visible haematuria	67
Visible haematuria	5
Proteinuria	93
Nephrotic range proteinuria	2.5
Nephrotic syndrome	0.8
Eosinophilia	35
Eosinophiluria	66

(AKI). A multicentre study from Spain published in 2012 reports that in recent years this is particularly so in those aged over 65 years (12.3 %) [1]. Although this could be accounted for by increasing use of renal biopsy in modern practice, it may be that there is a real increase in AIN, possibly consequent upon increasingly widespread use of medications such as proton pump inhibitors (PPIs) and non-steroidal anti-inflammatory drugs (NSAIDs). Although AIN is a rare complication of these medications, they are used by millions and are therefore amongst the most common agents implicated in the causation of AIN. PPI use is approximately three times more common and NSAID use twice as common in patients with AIN than in controls [2]. These findings together with reports identifying plausible temporal relationships between drug exposure and presentation, deffervescence post cessation and recurrence on occasional rechallenge support their aetiological importance.

The likelihood of AIN underlying an episode of AKI is of course significantly increased by prior exposure to relevant drugs or evidence of multisystem inflammatory diseases. Specific causes of AIN also exhibit ethnic variability: mycobacterial AIN is most commonly seen in the South Asian community in the United Kingdom as is interstitial nephritis with no determined cause. AIN in sarcoidosis is also reportedly associated with black ethnicity however this may not be any greater than the underlying disease itself. There are few data to suggest ethnic disparities in the occurrence of drug-induced interstitial nephritis, but it seems increasingly likely that there are HLA associations.

Clinical Manifestations

The precise mode of presentation differs between AIN of different causes. In multisystem disease and acute infectious illnesses, biochemical derangement is often detected during routine monitoring. In other situations such as idiosyncratic responses to commonly used medications, there may be a presentation with uraemia, fluid overload and hypertension. There *may* be extrarenal manifestations such as a (1) pyrexia, (2) rash, (3) arthralgia and (4) eosinophilia accompanying these idiosyncratic responses, reflecting a hypersensitivity reaction. The mode of presentation in two large series from Ireland and Spain in which drugs were the causative agent in 116/121 is shown in Table 26.1. In the United Kingdom, at least in the 1980s [3] and 1990s [4, 5], reports from centres serving populations of diverse ethnicity suggest only a third of cases of AIN were associated with idiosyncratic drug reactions and in these series extrarenal manifestations were significantly less common.

In the case of drug-induced AIN, clinical presentation generally occurs within 4 months of drug exposure [6]. An early presentation within days of drug initiation seems likely to represent a secondary response. There are no hard and fast rules, but since many cases arise in the setting of polypharmacy, deduction of plausible temporal relationships provides some evidence of likely causation. It is therefore important to get a clear drug history, if necessary from the primary practitioner or other third parties, ideally with previous exposure and preceding renal tests.

Investigation

Urinary Analysis

Low molecular weight proteinuria is common and the uPCR can be disproportionally higher than the uACR. If available, analysis of low molecular weight proteins (such as urinary retinal binding protein (uRBP), beta-2 microglobulin (β_2M) or α_1-microglobulin) may indicate a tubular origin and be strongly suggestive. The nephrotic syndrome is rare (<1 %) but can occur in particular with NSAIDs, in which case the glomerular lesion is generally minimal change [7]. Similarly haematuria is usually non-visible and low level on conventional stick urinalysis. Visible haematuria was reported in early reports of methicillin-induced AIN but is now rare. Critically this means that patients sometimes present with a raised creatinine but 'quiet urine' the assumption being that there is not an acute inflammatory process; identification of sterile pyuria may be the only clue to an acute pathology (eosinophiluria has a poor predictive value).

There may be defects in tubular handling of water, sodium and hydrogen ions resulting in nephrogenic diabetes insipidus, salt-losing nephropathy and renal tubular acidosis

(RTA), which can all lead to the initial presentation. In particular type 1 RTA is a relatively common (~10 %) manifestation of Sjögren's syndrome (a lower than expected venous bicarbonate and relatively alkaline urine may hint at this), whilst impaired renal function is less common [8].

Renal Imaging

The renal ultrasound in cases of AIN may show increased cortical echogenicity but is otherwise non-contributory. ^{67}Ga scanning has been reported to distinguish between AIN and acute tubular injury (ATI), which may be of some use in special cases in which renal biopsy is contraindicated and the likely differential diagnosis is ATI.

Histology

None of the clinical manifestations or investigations are diagnostic of AIN. In patients presenting de novo with renal impairment, this is not a significant challenge because in practice, presentation with unexplained renal failure and normal-sized kidneys would indicate a renal biopsy, providing the diagnosis.

On biopsy inflammatory cells can be seen invading the interstitium, breaching the tubular basement membrane, manifestations of a tubulitis (Fig. 26.1). The process is often patchy except in severe cases. It does not involve the glomeruli or vessels, an important discriminatory feature in most cases of SLE or vasculitis-induced AIN. Cells are predominantly T cells and macrophages, but classically eosinophils may be present (although are not specific); B cells and neutrophils are also often present. Granulomas and giant cells may occur and suggest particular underlying aetiologies (see Tables 26.3 and 26.4) (Figs. 26.1 and 26.2).

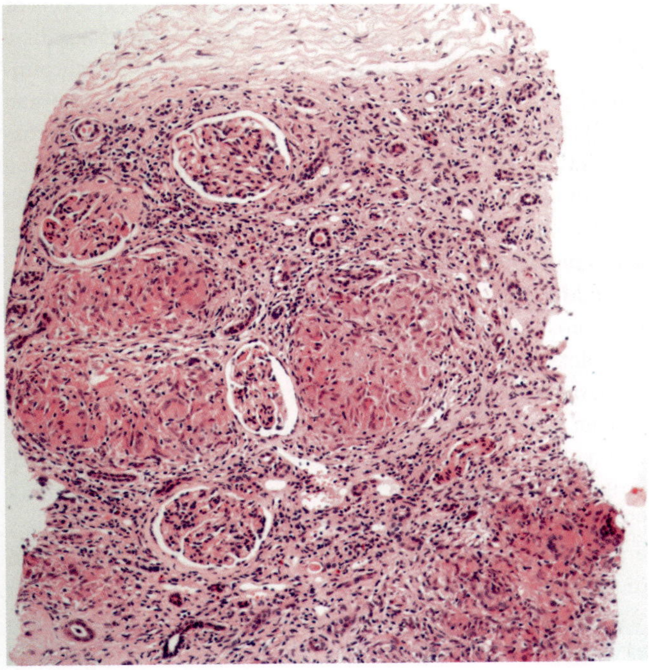

Fig. 26.1 Medium power renal biopsy showing intense acute TIN with diffuse inflammatory cells and gross granulomata in patients with AKI and a calcium of 3.9 mmol/L detected after starting vitamin D supplements

Blood Analysis

In most cases renal histology does not identify an underlying aetiology. Even Mycobacterium tuberculosis-associated AIN rarely demonstrates caseating granulomata with positive Ziehl-Neelsen staining. Consideration of the clinical context, the precise histology and corroborating information including screening for autoimmune and infectious aetiologies is required. This will generally include a screen for ANCA, ANA, ENA (including SS-A and SS-B (anti-Ro and anti-La), Igs, protein electrophoresis (polyclonal gammopathy being an important clue to autoimmune or infectious causes) and serum ACE, a chest x-ray, additional imaging according to symptoms and screening for mycobacterial (EMU and ELISPOT) and other causative organisms outlined in Table 26.4.

The finding of eosinophilia in patients with AIN, even drug induced, has insufficient predictive value to contribute significantly to the initial diagnostic algorithm. If present it can though help define a likely aetiology when there are multiple candidate drugs, particularly in patients who have spent significant time in secondary care. Retrospective analysis of the eosinophil count can be used to define a likely timeframe for the immune response often more precisely than renal function in patients who have been critically ill. For example, in patients found to have AIN following prolonged illness and AKI initially attributed to acute tubular injury, a retrospective finding of progressive eosinophilia can help identify candidate drugs and perhaps more importantly help exclude others. This has real value since these patients have often been exposed to multiple agents.

Multisystem diseases associated with AIN

AIN is often part of a multisystem disease, and renal manifestations may be the quickest route to the diagnosis. Many of these conditions are covered elsewhere in more detail but it is worth noting that renal limited AIN can occur as an early manifestation of what might subsequently be classified a multisystem disease.

Sarcoidosis is associated with renal granulomata very commonly; however, clinical manifestation of AIN is relatively uncommon [9]. A more common cause of renal impairment is hypercalcaemia. There are reports that some forms of glomerular disease are more common in those with sarcoidosis; however, this remains to be proved. In recent years a sarcoid-like illness has been associated with the use of anti-TNF therapy, and this has been documented to cause a granulomatous interstitial nephritis. Although evidently rare, given increasingly widespread use of this class of agents then

Table 26.3 Medications and AIN

NSAIDs	Antimicrobials	Anticonvulsants	Others
Ibuprofen	Penicillins	Phenytoin	Allopurinol[a]
Indomethacin	Sulphonamides	Valproate	H_2 receptor antagonists, e.g. cimetidine[a]
Diclofenac	Rifampicin	Lamotrigine	Phenindione[a]
Piroxicam	Quinolones	Carbamazepine	Furosemide and other loop diuretics
COX-2 inhibitors	Vancomycin	Phenobarbitone	Proton pump inhibitors
Salicylates (aspirin)	Teicoplanin		TNF inhibitors
Mefenamic acid	Tetracyclines		Azathioprine
Naproxen	Cephalosporins		Quinine
Celecoxib and rofecoxib	Isoniazid		Thiazides
Mesalazine	Ethambutol Nitrofurantoin[a] Tetracyclines		Phenindione and warfarin Calcium channel blockers

A wide range of medications have been implicated in AIN; therefore any medication should be considered as a potential cause. Those shown have consistently been reported in case series and or case control studies
[a]Reported association with granulomatous AIN

Table 26.4 Infections causing tubulointerstitial nephritis

Virus	Bacteria	Others
Hantaviridae	Legionella	Leishmania
Epstein-Barr virus	Leptospira	Toxoplasma
HIV	Mycobacteria tuberculosis	
Measles	Streptococci	
Polyomavirus	Brucella	
Cytomegalovirus	Mycoplasma	
Adenovirus	Chlamydia	
Herpes simplex virus	Salmonella	
Hepatitis A	Yersinia	
Hepatitis B	Campylobacter	
Hepatitis C	Rickettsia Strep species Staph species	

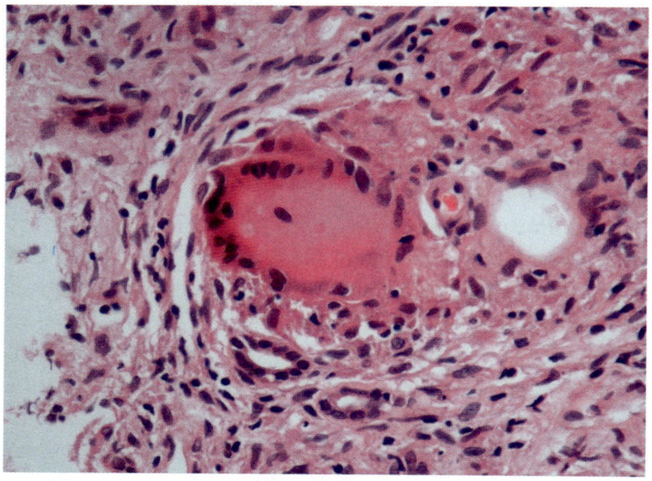

Fig. 26.2 High-power image of a giant cell in a patient with acute TIN

this may be increasingly recognised in patients with rheumatoid and inflammatory bowel disease, in both of which there are a number of other potential causes of renal impairment.

Sjögren's syndrome is commonly associated with renal tubular acidosis but approximately 4 % of patients with primary Sjögren's syndrome develop overt renal disease, half of whom have AIN and the other glomerular diseases [10]. Thus it is important to enquire about dry eyes or mouth, the predominant presenting system and an important clue.

IgG4-related disease is characterised by elevated levels of serum IgG4 and IgG4 plasma cell positive infiltrates in a range of organs. It is most often associated with 'autoimmune' pancreatitis; however, there can be widespread organ involvement with inflammatory masses, sialadenitis, sclerosing cholangitis, aortitis and retroperitoneal fibrosis [11]. One third of cases are associated with an AIN that manifests most often with AKI, however can present as a renal mass. There is a typical pattern of progressive expansile interstitial fibrosis in affected tissues and a plasma cell-rich TIN frequently with eosinophils. Tubular basement membrane immune complexes are also common.

Systemic lupus erythematosus Tubulointerstitial inflammation is a common and prognostically significant manifestation of the SLE which correlates highly with renal progression but not with other features of disease activity [12]. In a small number of patients, interstitial nephritis is a predominant feature, and this is commonly associated with a renal tubular acidosis.

Granulomatosis with polyangiitis (*GPA*) (*formally known as Wegener's granulomatosis*) may also manifest as an AIN usually in association with, but sometimes without, glomerular inflammation [13].

TIN with uveitis (*TINU*) syndrome is rare, has a female bias (3:1) and a median age of onset of 15, although cases presenting in middle age are well documented. Presentation is initially with TIN in 2/3rds of patients, 20 % TIN with uveitis and only 15 % initially as uveitis. In some cases onset seems to be drug induced. Clinically, fever and weight loss are present in 50 % rash arthralgia, myalgia, anorexia, and malaise are common. Renal involvement may manifest as renal impairment, concentrating defects or features of the Fanconi syndrome. The presumed aetiology is immune dysregulation with T-cell infiltration, but recently IgG antibodies have been demonstrated against tubular epithelial cells and HLA associations are emerging. The TIN of TINU is usually treated with steroids but may resolve spontaneously and generally has a good prognosis although in one report 15 % of patients developed CKD. The prognosis of the uveitis (which is usually anterior) is less good in that it is much more likely to relapse chronically.

Infectious Diseases Associated with AIN

A myriad of infectious diseases have been reported causing renal disease and specifically AIN (see Chap. 24). While with some diseases such as tuberculosis, hantavirus and leptospirosis the aetiology is clear, causality with some other infectious agents is not yet proven.

Acute pyelonephritis is characterised by neutrophil inflammation centred on tubules generally considered to be consequent upon an ascending bacterial infection, although this may not always be proven. Although this could reasonably be considered a form of interstitial nephritis, it is by convention considered separately.

Tubulointerstitial nephritis can complicate various systemic infections (see Table 26.4). In a large ethnically diverse urban UK practice, over the course of the last 10 years, we have observed relatively few cases definitely attributable to infection; these have been due to *Mycobacterium tuberculosis* and leptospirosis. The causation of AIN will however inevitably be significantly affected by the location and population served by any centre.

Mycobacterium tuberculosis can affect the urinary tract in various ways; however, one important manifestation is as a granulomatous interstitial nephritis. This may present with unexplained renal impairment usually with a fever, but sometimes remarkably few other symptoms. The microbiological diagnosis may not be immediately established, the granulomas are not necessarily caseating and the Ziehl-Neelsen stain is usually negative. The diagnosis may only become apparent at a later date or be inferred from a beneficial response to antituberculous chemotherapy.

Leptospirosis can result in AIN. The incidence of renal failure varies widely in different series but is common. Other features include presentation with a 'flu-like illness', particularly with disproportionate jaundice, thrombocytopenia in some with a bleeding diathesis and multisystem involvement including pulmonary and central nervous system involvement.

Hantavirus in Europe typically causes nephropathia epidemica, in which a 'flu-like illness' is accompanied by AKI and thrombocytopenia. Travel to endemic areas may identify the risk [14], perhaps most likely from central and eastern Europe. AIN can be striking and is often associated with interstitial haemorrhage.

In *HIV infection*, a post-mortem series of HAART-experienced patients found interstitial nephritis in 5/89; however, only one of these has the evidence of having chronic kidney disease. The most common cause of IN appears to be drug associated but only rarely is this attributable to components of HAART, more commonly to NSAIDs and to cotrimoxazole.

Epstein-Barr virus is occasionally associated with an AIN, usually as part of a systemic disease [15]. Reports that AIN of undetermined cause may be significantly contributed to by EBV infection [16] seem not to have been supported by subsequent studies [17].

BK virus is a polyomavirus that causes interstitial nephritis sometimes granulomatous in renal transplant patients and occasionally in other immunosuppressed patients (in whom it may also cause a haemorrhagic cystitis). The diagnosis is made by renal biopsy; however, quantification of viral DNA in the plasma by polymerase chain reaction (PCR) or examination of the urine for decoy cells provides noninvasive means of predicting those at risk. It presents with deteriorating renal function and the diagnosis is made by renal biopsy. The backbone of treatment is reduction of immunosuppression. Various other treatments have been tried although none have yet been proven to be effective.

Treatment of AIN

The treatment of AIN depends upon a thorough clinical investigation of potential underlying causes some of which have been discussed above. AIN associated with the aforementioned multisystem inflammatory diseases is invariably treated with corticosteroids, in some instances with additional immunosuppression.

Drug-induced AIN requires immediate withdrawal of the likely offending agent. The use of corticosteroids to shorten and enhance recovery has been reported in a number of uncontrolled, retrospective studies that were generally small in size. More recently a study of 61 patients with drug-induced AIN undertaken in Spain has suggested that better outcome was associated with earlier corticosteroid treatment [18]; however, the retrospective nature of this analysis means that no recommendation can be conclusive, and indeed a similar-sized study from Ireland suggests no benefit [19]. It seems reasonable to recommend that if used, corticosteroids should be introduced early. Gonzalez and colleagues have recommended an early pulse of corticosteroids for 3 days followed by a reducing course of oral prednisone (0.5–1 mg/kg/day) over ~6 weeks [20]. If a drug is suspected of causing AIN, then it is imperative that the patient is aware they are allergic to this drug, and if there is doubt about an important agent, such as penicillin, then it is critical that the practitioner is aware and monitors renal function within a few days of any rechallenge. Nephrologists have the responsibility of ensuring that this information is clearly imparted.

Chronic Interstitial Nephritis

CIN is also extremely heterogeneous in its aetiology and pathology. In broad terms it can be considered as a feature of localised tissue damage consequent direct toxicity or other causes of cell necrosis and inherited disorders of tubular proteins (nephronophthisis), which are associated with an inflammatory response of varying degrees. This can be explained by the activation of innate immune mechanisms in the context of tissue damage. As discussed above, the distinction between the features of inflammation in disorders of the renal vasculature, glomeruli or urinary drainage and CIN is one of degree, contextualised by the presence of a plausible underlying aetiology. A separate mechanistic group is represented by inflammation consequent upon a dysregulated immune response that targets the kidney. This can for most purposes be considered as the late stage of the mechanisms described for AIN. Important causes of CIN are discussed below.

Aristolochic Acid Nephropathy

The role of aristolochic acid in chronic interstitial nephritis came to light as Chinese herbs nephropathy in 1992 in a group of Belgian women taking slimming pills contaminated with *Aristolochia fangchi*. The similarities to Balkan nephropathy have suggested that this is also highly likely to be a form of aristolochic acid nephropathy, associated with wheat contaminated with seeds of *Aristolochia clematitis*. Furthermore aristolochic acid DNA adducts are found in the kidneys of those with Balkan nephropathy and in transitional cell cancers, which are a frequent complication of these diseases [21]. These mechanisms may well be relevant to endemic nephropathy in other geographical locations. Identifying exposure to aristolochic acid is very important, in part to prevent further exposure but also because of the risk of subsequent uroepithelial cancer. These patients should be referred onto a uroepithelial cell cancer screening programme.

Lithium

Lithium treatment for affective disorders can be complicated by a variety of renal disorders including nephrogenic diabetes insipidus (40 %) (which can be acute (occurring within 8 weeks) and reversible or chronic and irreversible) and other tubular dysfunctions (metabolic hyperchloraemic acidosis, renal tubular acidosis and acute tubular injury, as well as hypercalcemia associated with hyperparathyroidism). Following long-term use, CIN and CKD can result, but absolute risk of end-stage renal failure appears to be low (perhaps 0.5 % [22]) and is unusual before 10–20 years of treatment. However, one study screening lab requests for lithium levels identified nearly 40 % of 20–39-year-olds and 85 % of patients over 70 with eGFR <60 [23]. Another study revealed a raised creatinine in only 4 % 6.5 years after initiation of treatment compared with 12–21 % at around 18 years and suggested that chronic lithium use is associated with a sixfold relative risk of ESRD [24]. The mechanism of injury is not clear but lithium is freely filtered and mostly reabsorbed by the PCT with small quantities being taken up via the epithelial cation channel ENaC on the principal cell. The accumulation of cytosolic lithium dysregulates aquaporin 2 which results in NDI [25].

Histologically the predominant finding is non-specific interstitial fibrosis which may be detectable within a few years and significantly before a rising creatinine. Cysts originating from the collecting duct and distal tubule are commonly seen, suggestive but not diagnostic.

As with most CIN, that due to lithium is usually asymptomatic although polyuria and polydipsia may be prominent. Haematuria is absent, proteinuria usually trivial and hypertension not a significant feature. MRI scanning may demonstrate medullary cysts which is consistent with the diagnosis.

There is no specific treatment for lithium-induced CIN but early identification is important and there is evidence that annual screening of patients on lithium could be considerably better than it is. Avoiding other nephrotoxic agents, surveillance and early treatment of hypercalcaemia would seem prudent. There is some evidence that amiloride which inhibits ENaC can help treat lithium-induced NDI, but there is as yet no data that it reduces the risk of CIN [25]. Fortunately the rate of renal decline tends to be slow in part because of the absence of proteinuria and significant hypertension. The decision to withdraw lithium from a patient whose disease is well controlled should not be taken lightly or in isolation; the balance of risks should be weighed in collaboration with the patient's psychiatrist.

Heavy-Metal Intoxification

CIN from heavy-metal intoxification may arise following industrial exposure (those in the smelting industries) or environmental sometimes on an epidemic level as in groundwater contamination by arsenic in Bangladesh or cadmium in Japan. Heavy-metal intoxication particularly with arsenic, mercury and lead has also been documented in traditional Chinese and Indian Ayurvedic remedies. Many heavy metals can cause renal damage mostly by causing tubular injury, and secondary inflammatory changes may arise as a consequence of heavy-metal exposure. The precise mechanisms of toxicity of heavy metal are undetermined but involve direct toxicity, for example, by interfering with mitochondrial function and inducing oxidative stress. This is followed by activation of innate immune mechanisms and a resulting low grade inflammatory infiltrate.

The proximal tubular injury secondary to lead, cadmium, mercury and arsenic typically result in a renal tubular acidosis and Fanconi syndrome (with low level tubular proteinuria). Clinically chronic exposure is often associated with very non-specific symptoms of malaise, disproportionate anaemia, abdominal pain, weight loss and rashes.

Heavy-metal poisoning is thus worth considering in anyone with unexplained proximal RTA or Fanconi syndrome and CKD if from an endemic area, working in high-risk occupation or with a history of herbal remedies, particularly if associated with non-specific symptoms above. The diagnosis may be made on blood or urine levels, but if exposure has stopped a clever diagnosis can be made by hair analysis.

The compound effect is usually chronic irreversible interstitial damage but not before patients have sought medical advice for chronic non-specific symptoms.

Eating Disorders

Chronic renal impairment may arise in patients with eating disorders [26]. A CIN may be identified if the kidneys are biopsied. Long-standing or recurrent hypovolaemia and hypokalaemia may contribute to tubular injury and secondary inflammation. This tubular injury can itself contribute to the complex electrolyte disturbances, which may, for example, fluctuate between alkalosis during periods of vomiting and renal tubular acidosis at other times.

Radiation Nephritis

Renal disease may be caused by radiotherapy. This applies both to external beam irradiation and targeted radionuclide therapy. The effects of external beam irradiation may be ameliorated by shielding and dose fractionation. Targeted radiopharmaceuticals may be in fact concentrated in the collecting system and the kidney may therefore be particularly sensitive to the effects of this therapy. An understanding of the handling of these agents may identify means by which to minimise this accumulation and its consequences. It is likely that this particular complication will become more frequent as new agents are developed.

The pathology of radiation nephropathies varies from a thrombotic microangiopathy of varying degree, a glomerulopathy with proteinuria and CIN. In fact more often than not, CIN is dominated by interstitial fibrosis and tubular atrophy with relatively little inflammation.

Analgesic Nephropathy (AN)

Beyond the role of NSAIDs in causing AIN, minimal change nephrotic syndrome and AKI, the phenomenon of AN can result from the ingestion of large quantities of compound analgesics containing phenacetin (5,000 doses confer a RR of 8.8 for ESRD). The role of non-phenacetin-containing analgesics is plausible but unproven. It presented as an epidemic in the 1970s in Australia with roughly a fifth of all patients starting dialysis being diagnosed with analgesic nephropathy and were associated with high national rates of phenacetin sales. Restriction on phenacetin sales resulted in a drop of AN-induced ESRD from 20 to 9 % in the 1990s with rates in Europe and America approximately 1–3 %; however, rates in Eastern Europe seem to be rising. Presentation is typically in the 6th and 7th decade after a minimum of 5 years (or roughly 3,000 doses). AN is usually clinically silent and picked up on routine blood tests of investigation of ESRD symptoms but may manifest with concentrating defects or rarely with passage of a necrosed papilla. Non-contrast CT scanning has a good sensitivity and high specificity for AN if the kidneys are small and have papillary calcification and a lumpy renal contour [3, 27]. The typical pathology is centred on the medulla with overlying scarring, calcification and papillary necrosis. (Papillary necrosis may also complicate sickle cell nephropathy, which resembles CIN.) There is prominent tubular dysfunction arising from medullary ischaemia.

There is no known effective treatment, but AN is an important diagnosis to make in part because of the associated risk of uroepithelial cancer. Non-contrast CT is worth thinking about in a patient with unexplained ESRD; a diagnosis of AN should prompt referral for uroepithelial cell cancer screening programme.

Idiopathic CIN

A significant number of cases of both AIN and CIN have no immediately attributable cause. These appearances have been particularly observed in the south Asian population in the United Kingdom, and it has been suggested that this may account for the high proportion of patients from this ethnic group presenting with relatively advanced but unsuspected renal failure, with unscarred, small kidneys and little albuminuria [28]. The underlying aetiology in these cases remains to be determined, although in these cases it a complete history should be taken that includes direct questioning on the subject of non-prescription medication.

Diagnostic Challenges

The most frequent diagnostic challenge is to consider AIN in patients who have other causes of CKD or AKI and to thereby expedite investigation by renal biopsy.

In the case of CKD, the presence of proteinuria gives useful information. The presence of proteinuria with renal dysfunction would usually indicate renal biopsy; conversely, in diabetes mellitus it may be the absence of proteinuria that suggests an alternative diagnosis such as AIN. There may be little proteinuria in hypertensive ischaemic nephropathy, and the indications for renal biopsy will be informed by the history, rate of change of renal function, renal size and the presence of a candidate cause of AIN.

In the case of AKI with a putative diagnosis of ATN, alternative diagnoses should be considered if renal failure is out of keeping with degree of physiological disturbance or unexpectedly prolonged. This would indicate further investigation by renal biopsy. An unexpected rash or eosinophilia might also lower the threshold for early biopsy in patients otherwise thought to have ATN.

As mentioned previously, on rare occasions where renal biopsy is precluded (generally by an absolute need for anticoagulation), then a gallium scan may give some valuable information; however, this is rare.

Summary

AIN and CIN represent diverse pathologies with a range of aetiologies. The main diagnostic challenge lies in considering these potential pathologies, particularly in an older population with underlying CKD associated with hypertension and renal ischaemia. Supportive therapy, rapid identification and removal of potential drug causes while excluding autoimmune or infectious causes are the mainstay of management. Proper randomised controlled trials of treatments for AIN are sorely needed.

References

1. Goicoechea M, Rivera F, Lopez-Gomez JM. Increased prevalence of acute tubulointerstitial nephritis. Nephrol Dial Transplant. 2013;28:112–5.
2. Leonard CE, Freeman CP, Newcomb CW, Reese PP, Herlim M, Bilker WB, et al. Proton pump inhibitors and traditional nonsteroidal anti-inflammatory drugs and the risk of acute interstitial nephritis and acute kidney injury. Pharmacoepidemiol Drug Saf. 2012;21:1155–72.
3. Farrington K, Levison DA, Greenwood RN, Cattell WR, Baker LR. Renal biopsy in patients with unexplained renal impairment and normal kidney size. Q J Med. 1989;70(263):221–33. Epub 1989/03/01.
4. Ball S, Cook T, Hulme B, Palmer A, Taube D. The diagnosis and racial origin of 394 patients undergoing renal biopsy: an association between Indian race and interstitial nephritis. Nephrol Dial Transplant. 1997;12(1):71–7. Epub 1997/01/01.
5. Ball S, Lloyd J, Cairns T, Cook T, Palmer A, Cattell V, et al. Why is there so much end-stage renal failure of undetermined cause in UK Indo-Asians? QJM. 2001;94(4):187–93. Epub 2001/04/11.
6. Harmark L, van der Wiel HE, de Groot MC, van Grootheest AC. Proton pump inhibitor-induced acute interstitial nephritis. Br J Clin Pharmacol. 2007;64(6):819–23. Epub 2007/07/20.
7. Ravnskov U. Glomerular, tubular and interstitial nephritis associated with non-steroidal antiinflammatory drugs. Evidence of a common mechanism. Br J Clin Pharmacol. 1999;47(2):203–10. Epub 1999/04/06.
8. Maripuri S, Grande JP, Osborn TG, Fervenza FC, Matteson EL, Donadio JV, et al. Renal involvement in primary Sjogren's syndrome: a clinicopathologic study. Clin J Am Soc Nephrol. 2009;4(9):1423–31. Epub 2009/08/15.
9. Gobel U, Kettritz R, Schneider W, Luft F. The protean face of renal sarcoidosis. J Am Soc Nephrol. 2001;12(3):616–23.
10. Goules A, Masouridi S, Tzioufas AG, Ioannidis JP, Skopouli FN, Moutsopoulos HM. Clinically significant and biopsy-documented renal involvement in primary Sjogren syndrome. Medicine (Baltimore). 2000;79(4):241–9. Epub 2000/08/15.
11. Raissian Y, Nasr SH, Larsen CP, Colvin RB, Smyrk TC, Takahashi N, et al. Diagnosis of IgG4-related tubulointerstitial nephritis. J Am Soc Nephrol. 2011;22(7):1343–52. Epub 2011/07/02.
12. Hsieh C, Chang A, Brandt D, Guttikonda R, Utset TO, Clark MR. Predicting outcomes of lupus nephritis with tubulointerstitial inflammation and scarring. Arthritis Care Res. 2011;63(6):865–74. Epub 2011/02/11.
13. Banerjee A, McKane W, Thiru S, Farrington K. Wegener's granulomatosis presenting as acute suppurative interstitial nephritis. J Clin Pathol. 2001;54(10):787–9.
14. Fhogartaigh CN, Newsholme W, Kinirons M, Tong W. An emerging infectious cause of renal impairment in the UK. BMJ case reports. 2011. Epub 2011/01/01.
15. Cataudella JA, Young ID, Iliescu EA. Epstein-Barr virus-associated acute interstitial nephritis: infection or immunologic phenomenon? Nephron. 2002;92(2):437–9. Epub 2002/09/10.
16. Becker JL, Miller F, Nuovo GJ, Josepovitz C, Schubach WH, Nord EP. Epstein-Barr virus infection of renal proximal tubule cells: possible role in chronic interstitial nephritis. J Clin Invest. 1999;104(12):1673–81.
17. Mansur A, Little MA, Oh WC, Jacques S, Nightingale P, Howie AJ, et al. Immune profile and Epstein-Barr virus infection in acute interstitial nephritis: an immunohistochemical study in 78 patients. Nephron Clin Pract. 2011;119(4):c293–300. Epub 2011/09/29.
18. Gonzalez E, Gutierrez E, Galeano C, Chevia C, de Sequera P, Bernis C, et al. Early steroid treatment improves the recovery of renal function in patients with drug-induced acute interstitial nephritis. Kidney Int. 2008;73(8):940–6. Epub 2008/01/11.
19. Clarkson MR, Giblin L, O'Connell FP, O'Kelly P, Walshe JJ, Conlon P, et al. Acute interstitial nephritis: clinical features and response to corticosteroid therapy. Nephrol Dial Transplant. 2004;19(11):2778–83. Epub 2004/09/02.

20. Praga M, Gonzalez E. Acute interstitial nephritis. Kidney Int. 2010;77(11):956–61. Epub 2010/03/26.
21. Jelakovic B, Karanovic S, Vukovic-Lela I, Miller F, Edwards KL, Nikolic J, et al. Aristolactam-DNA adducts are a biomarker of environmental exposure to aristolochic acid. Kidney Int. 2012;81(6):559–67. Epub 2011/11/11.
22. McKnight RF, Adida M, Budge K, Stockton S, Goodwin GM, Geddes JR. Lithium toxicity profile: a systematic review and meta-analysis. Lancet. 2012;379(9817):721–8. Epub 2012/01/24.
23. Bassilios N, Martel P, Godard V, Froissart M, Grunfeld JP, Stengel B, et al. Monitoring of glomerular filtration rate in lithium-treated outpatients–an ambulatory laboratory database surveillance. Nephrol Dial Transplant. 2008;23(2):562–5.
24. Bendz H, Schon S, Attman PO, Aurell M. Renal failure occurs in chronic lithium treatment but is uncommon. Kidney Int. 2010;77(3):219–24.
25. Grunfeld JP, Rossier BC. Lithium nephrotoxicity revisited. [Review]. Nat Rev Nephrol. 2009;5(5):270–6.
26. Bouquegneau A, Dubois BE, Krzesinski JM, Delanaye P. Anorexia nervosa and the kidney. Am J Kidney Dis. 2012;60(2):299–307. Epub 2012/05/23.
27. De Broe ME, Elseviers MM. Analgesic nephropathy. [Review]. N Engl J Med. 1998;338(7):446–52.
28. Ball ST, Lapsley M, Norden AG, Cairns TD, Palmer AB, Taube DH. Urinary retinol binding protein in Indo-Asian patients with idiopathic interstitial nephritis. QJM. 2003;96(5):363–7.

27 Rheumatological Conditions and the Kidney

Bernadette Lynch and Aine Burns

Systemic sclerosis (SSc) is a debilitating, chronic, systemic, autoimmune disease of unknown cause. It is classified as limited or diffuse dependent on skin involvement. The incidence and prevalence of SSc vary in different populations where it seems to be more prevalent in the United States (286 cases per million adults) than in Europe (31 cases per million adults) with an annual incidence of 1–20 cases per million. SSc is three times more common in females than males and typically presents between the ages of 30 and 60 years. Typical skin features of SSc are well described and include skin thickening, sclerodactyly, finger pulp pitting, fingertip ulceration, digital gangrene and telangiectasia; some of which are illustrated in Figs. 27.1 and 27.2. SSc causes vascular damage, immune activation and inflammation, culminating in fibrosis which is responsible for the clinical manifestations of the disease. Table 27.1 summarizes the prevalence of extrarenal clinical manifestations seen in SSc.

Definition of SRC

Scleroderma renal crisis (SRC) is characterized by the development of accelerated hypertension and acute kidney injury (AKI) and is a highly dangerous development in a scleroderma patient. The definition of SRC is summarized in Table 27.2 [3]. SRC usually occurs relatively early (within the first 4 years) in the course of aggressive skin disease but has also, rarely, been reported to occur in those without obvious or occasionally preceding skin change and is the presenting feature of this disease in 22 % of SSc patients. Although modulators of the renin-angiotensin system have improved the outcome in SRC, this complication still carries very significant morbidity with many patients rendered permanently dependent on dialysis, and mortality still approaches 25 % even in specialist centres.

Epidemiology of Scleroderma Renal Crisis

The reported incidence of scleroderma renal crisis (SRC) in SSc patients varies depending on whether limited disease is included in the denominator but is likely to occur in approximately 10 % of patients with diffuse systemic disease. The presence of RNA-polymerase antibodies and recent initiation or intensification of steroid therapy (>15 mg/day) together with rapidly progressing skin scores are all recognized as risk factors. The prevalence of RNA-polymerase antibodies in patients whose disease is progressing to renal crisis is at least five times as high as the prevalence in patients without disease progression. Conversely, the presence of anti-Scl-70 antibodies though typically present in 70 % of SSc patients is under represented in this group occurring in only approximately 30 %.

Clinical Presentation of SRC

A typical patient undergoing an SRC presents with new or worsening hypertension or its consequences such as headache, blurred vision (with grade 3–4 retinopathy) and hypertensive encephalopathy including cortical blindness, altered consciousness and seizures. Hypertensive encephalopathy is due to the failure of the upper limit of cerebral autoregulation and can occur with or without hypertensive retinopathy. If not adequately treated, hypertensive encephalopathy can

B. Lynch, MD, MRCPI, BA Physiology (✉)
Rheumatology Department, Royal Free Hospital, Pond Street, London NW3 2QG, UK
e-mail: bernadettemlynch@gmail.com

A. Burns, MD, FRCP, MSc Med Ed
UCL Department of Nephrology, Royal Free London NHS Foundation Trust, Pond Street, Hampstead, London NW3 2QG, UK
e-mail: aine.burns@nhs.net

M. Harber (ed.), *Practical Nephrology*,
DOI 10.1007/978-1-4471-5547-8_27,

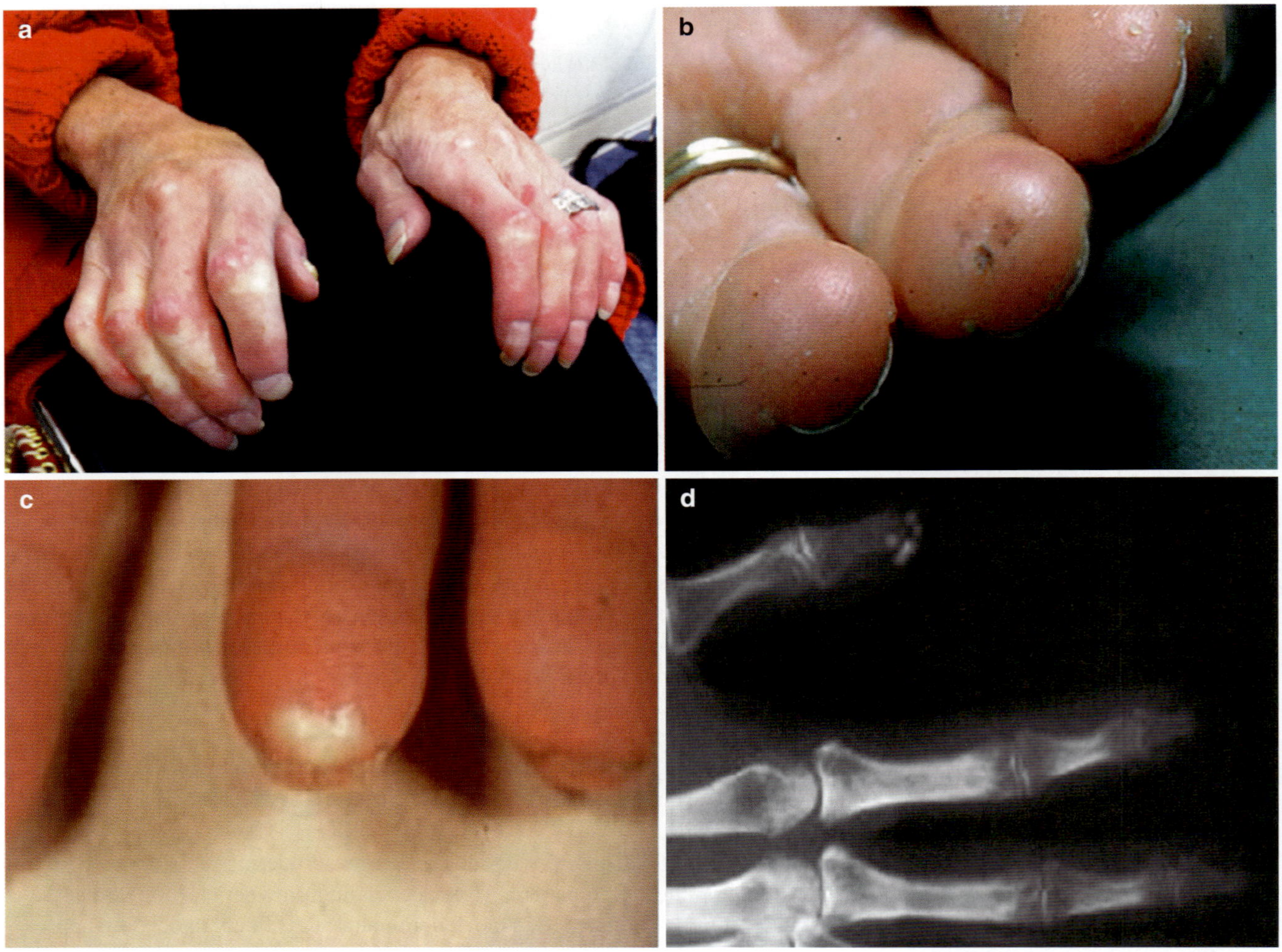

Fig. 27.1 Clinical features of scleroderma showing typical shiny, atrophic skin and Raynauds of hands (**a**) with dry ulcers at the tip of middle finger (**b**) and calcinosis (**c**) which is illustrated on plain radiograph of the hand at the thumb (**d**)

progress to cerebral haemorrhage, coma and death. However, with timely and appropriate management, hypertensive encephalopathy and its clinical and neuroimaging consequences are potentially fully reversible. During an SRC a patient can also present with progressive breathlessness (pulmonary oedema or congestive heart failure) and/or palpitations with evidence of biochemical renal impairment. Oligo-anuria, low urinary sodium and high urine specific gravity may be present in early, untreated stages. The hypertensive crisis usually, but not exclusively, occurs in a patient with known SSc during a phase of rapidly worsening skin disease. Extreme shut down of the peripheral circulation with severe (marble like) coldness of the extremities is a strong indicator. Table 27.3 outlines the presenting features of 110 patients undergoing SRC in a large cohort of British SRC patients. Systemic vascular resistance is up to five times normal, and stroke volume may be reduced by as much as 50 %. Consequently (although restrictive cardiomyopathy and myocardial ischaemia may also be important), in an effort to maintain cardiac output, the patient often develops extreme tachycardia. Pulmonary arterial wedge pressures are high and pulmonary oedema may ensue. Proteinuria may be present on urine analysis. Some patients undergoing a renal crisis have evidence of the underlying profound vasculopathy with digital gangrene developing in tandem with the SRC.

Aetiology and Pathogenesis of SRC

The sequence of events leading to an SRC is not fully understood. A number of risk factors for the development of SRC have been identified (Table 27.4). Patients with specific autoantibody profiles are over represented. Steroids and cyclosporin are well recognized to precipitate crises. This may reflect increased vascular sheer stresses consequent on salt and water retention and vascular endothelial injury, respectively. Analgesics (NSAIDS) arguably via their anti-prostaglandin effects together with pain secondary to digital ischaemia (perhaps mediated by

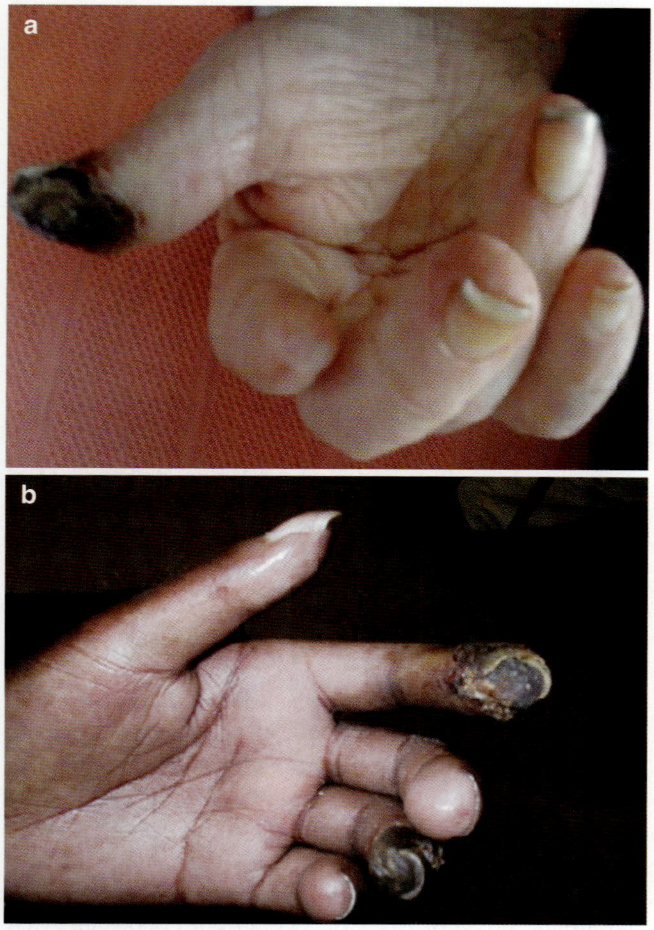

Fig. 27.2 Gangrenous thumb (**a**) and index and ring finger with telangiectasia of the palm and thumb (**b**)

Table 27.1 Prevalence of extrarenal manifestations of SSc

Clinical manifestation	Prevalence (%)
Interstitial lung disease	40
Pulmonary arterial hypertension	7–12
Cardiac	20–25
Oesophageal dysmotility	75–90
Stomach involvement	≥50
Small bowel	40–70
Colon	20–50
Anorectal	50–70

adrenaline or other vasoactive substances) as well as increased sensitivity to cold stimuli or temperature changes are all reported as relevant.

Diagnosis

The cardinal feature of SRC is sustained (usually severe) hypertension, and evidence of AKI may be present. Intravascular haemolysis has been found in 50 % of SRC patients and is confirmed by the presence of reduced platelet counts, anaemia, reduced haptoglobin levels, red cell fragments and schistocytes on blood film together with very elevated lactate dehydrogenase (LDH) levels (often >2,000) and normal clotting.

CXR may reveal evidence of pulmonary oedema or background pulmonary fibrosis. An enlarged cardiac silhouette might result from a pericardial effusion. Echocardiography is useful to exclude clinically significant effusions, assess pulmonary pressures, measure ejection fractions and identify any coexisting valvular abnormalities. Most patients presenting with SRC have nonsignificant pericardial effusions.

Table 27.2 Renal crisis classification

Definition of SRC
New onset of blood pressure >150/85 mmHg obtained at least twice over a 24-h period
Documented decrease in the renal function as defined by a decrement of >30 % in the calculated glomerular filtration rate (eGFR)
Corroborative features
Microangiopathic haemolytic anaemia
Hypertensive retinopathy
New onset of urinary RBCs (other causes having been excluded)
Flash pulmonary oedema
Oliguria or anuria
Typical renal biopsy features (Fig. 27.4)

Reproduced with permission from Penn et al. [3]

Table 27.3 Presenting features of 110 patients undergoing SRC in a British cohort [3]

General observations
Frequency of SRC – 12 % dcSS and 2 % lcSS
Median duration of SSc at time of SRC was 7.5 months (0–200)
66 % had SRC within 1 year of diagnosis of SSc
SRC was the presenting feature in 22 %
59 % treated with steroids within 1 month prior to diagnosis
Presenting statistics
Mean BP 193/114
Median creatinine 200 mmol/L
50 % thrombocytopenia
31 % ECHO EF<55 %

Table 27.4 Published risk factors for developing SRC [3]

Anaemia
New cardiac events
Steroid usage >15 mg
Cyclosporin A treatment
Diffuse skin disease, high skin score or large joint contractures
Rapidly progressive skin disease
RNA polymerase antibodies
<4 years since scleroderma onset (rare in patients >4 years)
ACE gene polymorphism
? cocaine

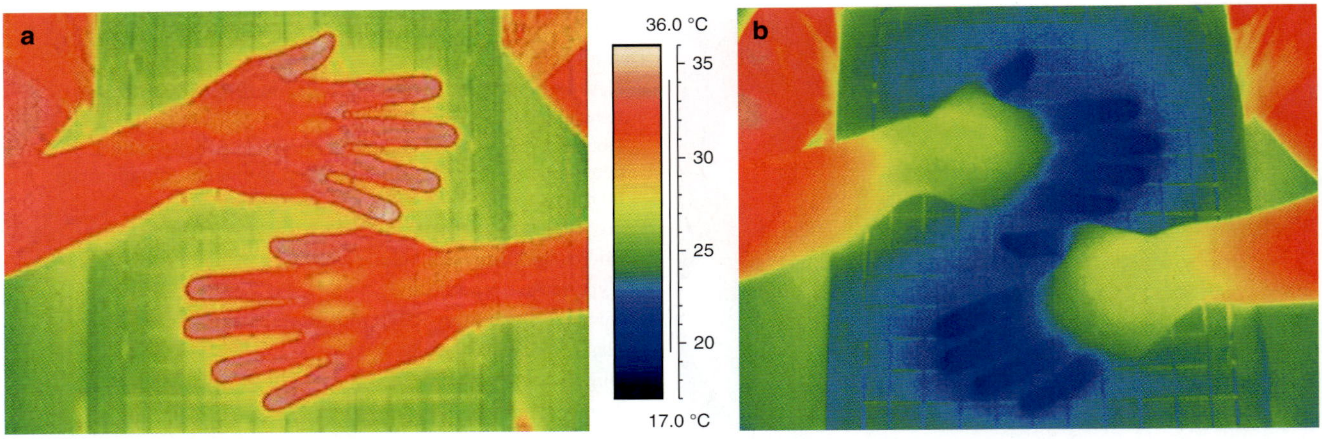

Fig. 27.3 Cold pressor testing, performed by asking a patient to immerse their hands in cold water for 1 min, and a thermography study is performed after 10 min to assess rewarming. Normal (**a**) and abnormal response (**b**) suggestive of Raynauds (Courtesy of Kevin Howell, Department of Rheumatology, Royal Free Hampstead)

Troponin and BNP may be useful indicators of myocardial ischaemia and failure, respectively.

Nailfold capillaroscopy and cold pressor testing (Fig. 27.3) can be very helpful in those patients who do not have a known or obvious diagnosis of SSc at presentation or in whom the skin changes are minimal or absent.

Pathology

The renal pathological findings in SRC are indistinguishable from any other cause of accelerated hypertension [1]. Vessels show profound intimal proliferation that may occlude the vessel lumen completely and fibrinoid necrosis may be present in vessel walls. Glomeruli become collapsed with wrinkling of basement membrane (Fig. 27.4). The prognostic value of measurements of renal scarring does not seem to follow the patterns seen in other renal diseases [3].

Pathogenesis

The aetiology of SSc is unknown but much evidence supports an autoimmune basis for its development. Vascular dysfunction is thought to be one of the initiating steps in SSc and is mediated by cytokines produced by activated lymphocytes and by antibodies against endothelial cells. It is believed that this immunological activity leads to an exaggerated production of fibroblasts and abnormal collagen build-up. Genetic and environmental factors are likely to be relevant but their exact role has yet to be determined.

The autoantibodies identified in scleroderma patients correlate with distinct subsets of the disease. These autoantibodies often have a relative high specificity, but their sensitivity is moderate. Table 27.5 summarizes these autoantibodies and their correlation with disease subsets. Anti-RNA polymerase III autoantibodies (ARA) are strongly associated with SRC (odds ratio 11), 30 % of ARA positive cases develop SRC and around 60 % of cases of SRC in our cohort are ARA positive.

Management

The outcome of SRC has greatly improved in the last half century. Increased awareness of this complication with regular BP measurements (especially in susceptible groups) allows earlier diagnosis with improved outcomes. Renal biopsies are considered to be helpful (to exclude other pathologies and assess prognosis) but clearly needs to be delayed until the patient's BP is well controlled and platelet counts have recovered.

In the era before treatment with inhibitors of the renin-angiotensin-aldosterone system, 1-year mortality approached 100 % although. More recent series report survival rates of 70–80 % although significant numbers still become dialysis dependent following SRC. Interestingly, many authors have reported spontaneous improvement in skin scores following a SRC. In one series 36 % did not require dialysis during SRC (3 subsequently needed dialysis, 7, 8 and 10 years later), 23 % recovered

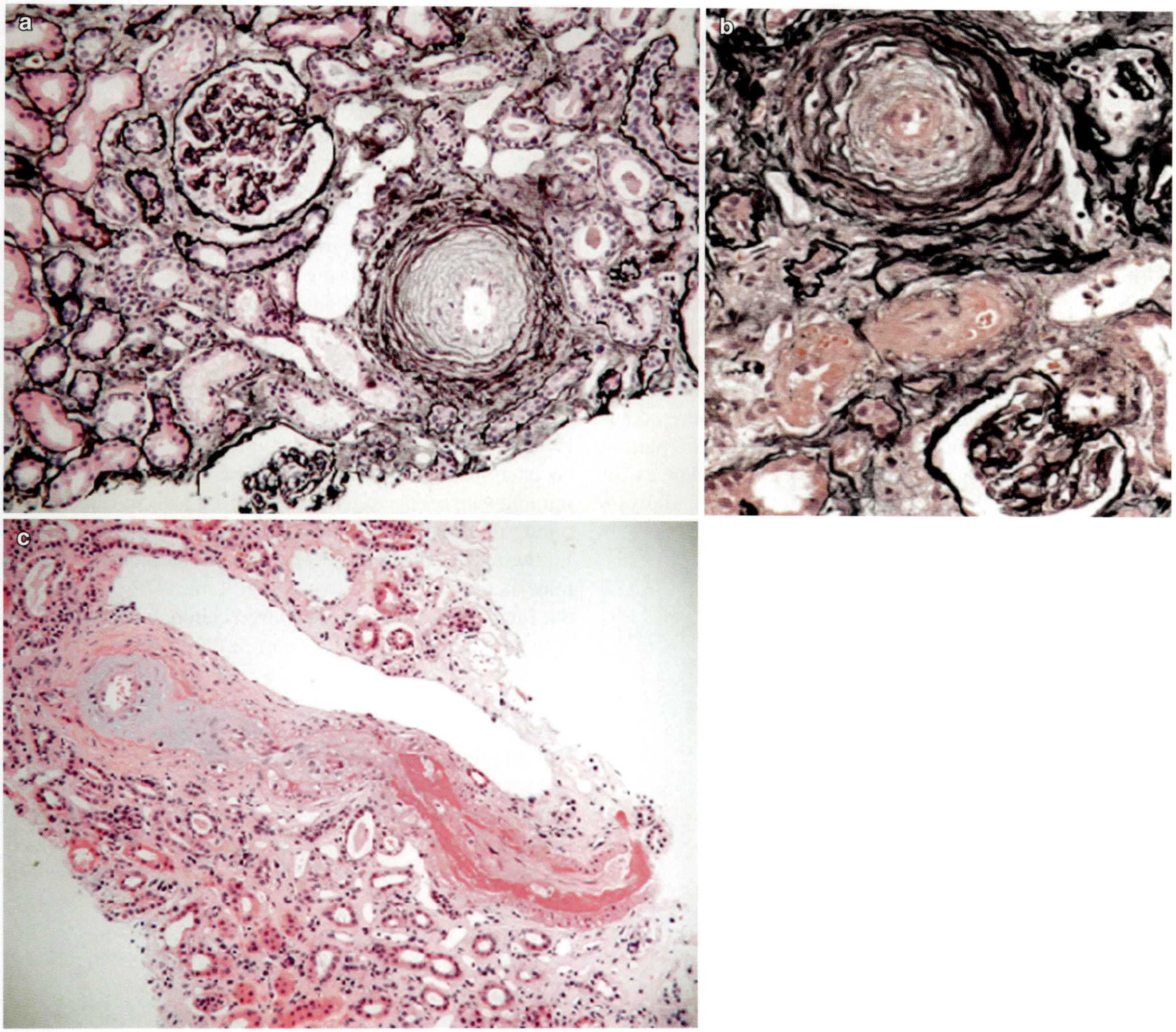

Fig. 27.4 Histological appearances of a typical renal biopsy taken following a SRC. Severe acute small vessel vasculopathy: Panels (**a**) and (**b**) (silver stain) show shrunken collapsed glomeruli with wrinkling of basement membranes particularly Panel (**b**). Interlobular arteries show virtual occlusion by loose concentric intimal thickening (onion skinning). Panel (**c**) (haematoxylin & eosin stain) is a longitudinal section through a very abnormal, almost completely occluded vessel (Images courtesy of Professor AJ Howie, Department of Histopathology, Royal Free Hampstead)

Table 27.5 Frequency and clinical associations of hallmark systemic sclerosis (SSc) associated autoantibodies

Autoantibodies	Frequency (%)	Subset associations	Organ complication associations
Anti-centromere	16–40	lcSSc	Protective for PF and SRC
Anti-topoisomerase I	9–39	dcSS > lcSS	PF; SDV
Anti-RNA polymerase	4–25	dcSSc	SRC
Anti-Th/To	0.2–7	lcSSc	PF; PH
Anti-U3RNP	1–6	dcSSc > lcSSc; SSc overlap with PM/DM	PH
Anti-U11/U12 RNP	1.6–5	dcSSc = lcSSc	PF, GI involvement
Anti-PM-Scl	0–7	SSc overlap with PM/DM or RA	PF

Reproduced with permission from Moinzadeh et al. [2]

dcSSc diffuse cutaneous systemic sclerosis, *lcSSc* limited cutaneous systemic sclerosis, *PH* pulmonary hypertension, *PF* pulmonary fibrosis, *PM/DM* polymyositis/dermatomyositis, *SDV* severe digital vasculopathy, *SRC* scleroderma renal crisis, *RA* rheumatoid arthritis, *GI* gastrointestinal sufficient function to discontinue dialysis (2 required dialysis again) and 42 % continued dialysis without recovery. Renal recovery typically occurs very slowly with median time to dialysis independence of 9 months (1–34 months). Following discontinuation of dialysis, Penn et al. have documented further improvement in renal function (3 ml/min/pa) occurring in their long-term follow-up study of a UK cohort.

Acute management involves general supportive care with thoughtful BP control. Prompt BP control is essential if hypertensive encephalopathy or cardiac decompensation dictate it. Otherwise, moderate steady reduction in BP (10 % reduction in systolic BP per day) is likely to optimize chances of renal recovery. The use of an ACEI or ARB in the early stages is now standard, and there is evidence that continuation of these agents even if the patient becomes dialysis dependent improves the chances of recovering sufficient renal function to become dialysis independent. Intravenous vasodilators especially prostaglandin inhibitors are effective in the short term, and the latter may have the added advantage of discouraging platelet/vascular endothelial activation. Such agents can be titrated effectively in very sick patients to reduce systemic vascular resistance (SVR), increase stroke volume (SV) with consequent slowing of heart rate and improvement of cardiac index and cardiac failure. Such careful management can be facilitated using oesophageal Doppler or Swann Ganz monitoring in an ITU setting. In severely tachycardiac patients beta blockers may be contraindicated as the increased heart rate maintains cardiac output in the setting of such high SVR and reduced SV.

Long term, in dialysis-dependent patients, renal transplantation is an option, but careful consideration needs to be given to the timing of transplantation as renal recovery can occur up to 2 years following a SRC. Similarly, a suitable immunosuppressive agent needs to be selected bearing in mind that cyclosporine (CYA) can precipitate SRC. Furthermore, coexisting cardiac and pulmonary disease may dictate suitability for listing. Table 27.6 summarizes the long-term outcomes of a large cohort from one centre with a SRC.

Table 27.6 Long-term outcome of SRC [3]

Long-term survival following SRC
82 % – 1 year
74 % – 2 years
71 % – 3 years
59 % – 5 years
47 % – 10 years
Commonest in the dialysis recovery group
The dialysis and recovery group had the best prognosis
No correlation between age at time of SRC and death
Prognosis was worse in males (17 % 10-year survival)

Renal Disease in SSc Other than SRC

Clinically, SRC should be suspected when AKI develops in SSc patients. Nevertheless, AKI occurring in SSc patients is not always due to SRC. Table 27.7 summarizes other causes of renal disease in SSc.

Table 27.7 Renal disease in SSc other than SRC

Renal disease	Clinical findings	Renal biopsy
ANCA-associated GN	Progressive renal failure Mild hypertension Proteinuria MPO antigen	Crescentic GN
Penicillamine-associated renal Dx	Rare Progressive renal failure 40 % mortality	Membranous GN
Asymptomatic renal injury	10–55 % of SSc patients Proteinuria seen in 25 % Co-morbidities contributing to renal failure include CCF, GI involvement, medication exposure, dehydration	

ANCA antineutrophil cytoplasmic antibodies, *GN* glomerulonephritis, *MPO* myeloperoxidase, *CCF* congestive cardiac failure, *GI* gastrointestinal

Tips and Tricks in Managing Scleroderma Renal Crisis SRC

Scenario	Salutary tip
Any patient with accelerated or malignant hypertension	Consider scleroderma renal crisis. This can happen with little or no skin disease which may develop later. You may see a few telltale telangiectasia. 22 % of patients are diagnosed with scleroderma at the same time as they present with SRC
Who might develop SRC	About 10 % of SSC patients develop SRC (2 % with lcSSc and 12 % with dcSSc). Rapidly progressive skin disease and autoantibody profiles (RNA polymerase III) may help predict which patients are more likely to develop SRC
A scleroderma patient who has recently been prescribed steroids for rheumatological overlap symptoms	Steroids are known to trigger SRC. Any scleroderma patient starting steroids or taking an increased dose should have their BP carefully monitored and controlled, preferably with ACEI or ARB
During a scleroderma crisis the patient's vasculature is very stiff and cannot tolerate large shifts in intravascular fluid. A patient's systemic vascular resistance may increase very radially and dramatically reducing cardiac output	Be very careful when administering fluids as pulmonary oedema can be precipitated very easily. Give very slowly preferably while paying attention to physiology: CVP, pulse rate, stroke volume, cardiac output
New patients with SRC	Aim to reduce BP relatively slowly (10 % per day) unless the patient is fitting or in pulmonary oedema when BP needs to be reduced rapidly (lower MAP by 20 % or to a diastolic pressure of 100–110 mmHg during the first hour). This will improve the chances of inducing recovery of renal function
A new SRC patient. What agents should I use to bring down BP during the immediate crisis	Systemic vascular resistance is very high. This is usually renin and angiotensin mediated; hence, ACEI and ARBs are the most appropriate treatment although iloprost works well to reduce BP and inhibit platelet aggregation as well as smooth vascular endothelium. The dose of iloprost can easily be titrated to target BP. Short-acting ACEs, e.g. captopril, can also be useful as doses can be titrated more rigidly but don't worry any ACEI is better than none. GTN and labetalol can be used but avoid cardioselective beta blockers for reasons outlined below
Tachycardia during an SCC	Many patients undergoing SRC develop marked sinus tachycardia. This is a physiological response to the very reduced stroke volumes as the ventricle aims to pump against massive SVR. Aim to reduce the SVR and the tachycardia will settle. Don't use beta blockers as CO will be reduced and your patient may collapse!
Low platelet counts with evidence of microangiopathic haemolytic anaemia (MAHA)	Don't be tempted to transfuse with platelets. This will resolve when BP settles and transfused platelets can aggravate the MAHA
Nutrition	Gut involvement in scleroderma is very common as is bacterial overgrowth. During an SRC pay attention to nutrition from an early stage. A PEG may be beneficial. Consider early and sometimes repeated eradication of bacterial overgrowth
In the months after an SRC BP seems to be settling	You may need to reduce the amount of antihypertensive medication a patient is taking (as renal blood vessels remodel). Get the patient to monitor their own BP and aim to titrate the BP meds to achieve target BP. Stop Ca channel blockers and alpha blockers retaining the ACEI or ARB if possible as the latter drugs encourage vascular remodelling and the evidence suggests that renal recovery is more likely to occur if these agents are continued
A patient who remains dialysis dependent following a renal crisis	Recovery of renal function occurs in approx 40 % of dialysis dependent post SRC patients, but recovery is very slow and can occur up to 18–24 months after starting dialysis. You may want to delay listing on renal transplant waiting list
Which modality of dialysis to use in the event of AKI	Continuous therapies (CVVHD/CVVHF) are very useful during an acute crisis. Peritoneal dialysis provides a gentle therapy which has the advantage of avoiding intravascular volume fluid shifts but individual patient's hands (contractures) or occasionally the severely thickened abdominal skin may preclude this choice

Table 27.8 Types of renal disease in MCTD

Membranous glomerulonephritis (commonest)
Mesangial proliferative glomerulonephritis (common)
Membranoproliferative glomerulonephritis
Focal and segmental glomerulosclerosis
Scleroderma renal crisis
Renal infarcts (associated with anti-cardiolipin antibody syndrome) (rare)
Renal amyloidosis (rare)
Minimal change disease (rare)
Collapsing glomerulopathy (very rare)

Renal Disease in Mixed Connective Tissue Disease

Criteria for the diagnosis of mixed connective tissue disease (MCTD) include the presence of a positive anti-U1-RNP autoantibody, the presence of either swollen fingers or Raynaud syndrome and features of at least two of the following connective tissue diseases: systemic lupus erythematosus (SLE), systemic sclerosis (SSc) and polymyositis (PM).

Renal manifestations of MCTD have been reported in 11–40 % of patients (most commonly membranous glomerulonephritis), but severe renal disease is rare. Anti-U1-RNP antibodies, which are present in all patients with MCTD by definition, may be protective against the development of diffuse proliferative glomerulonephritis. Patients who have renal disease in MCTD have more systemic manifestations than those without. Table 27.8 outlines the types of renal disease seen in patients with MCTD. Overlap in scleroderma patients and a few cases of renal crisis, with abrupt onset of severe hypertension and renal dysfunction, have been reported. The histological findings on renal biopsy of these patients are identical to that seen in scleroderma renal crisis, similarly patients with scleroderma and MCTD may develop membranous nephropathy. There are a few case reports of patients who developed acute renal failure contemporaneously with an exacerbation of MCTD.

Renal Disease in Polymyositis and Dermatomyositis

The inflammatory myopathies, polymyositis (PM), dermatomyositis (DM) and inclusion body myositis (IBM), are rare diseases with an annual incidence of 2–7 per 1 million people with a female preponderance (3:1) and a peak incidence at 50–60 years.

Renal involvement is rare in patients with PM/DM and predominantly secondary to rhabdomyolysis causing acute tubular injury. The glomerular lesion most commonly associated with PM is mesangial proliferative glomerulonephritis. However, there are reports of patients with PM who developed rapidly progressive GN. Membranous GN is more commonly associated with DM and highly unlikely in PM. Proteinuria and microscopic haematuria are observed in renal disease associated with PM. Table 27.9 summarizes the common findings observed in renal disease in myositis.

Table 27.9 Findings observed in renal disease in PM and DM

	Polymyositis	Dermatomyositis
Acute tubular injury Rhabdomyolysis	Yes	Yes
Type of GN	Mesangioproliferative GN	Membranous GN
Immune deposits in kidney	Yes	Yes
Onset of myositis and GN concurrent	Yes	Yes

Renal Disease in Sjogren's Syndrome

Sjogren's syndrome (SS) is characterized by lymphocytic infiltrates of salivary and tear glands leading to ocular and mouth dryness. It is reported to affect 0.1–0.6 % of the general adult population with a female preponderance (female-to-male ratio at least 9:1). The peak incidence of the disease occurs after the menopause in the mid-50s.

Renal involvement in SS is frequent and 16–67 % of patients have manifestations such as interstitial nephritis or glomerulonephritis. Interstitial nephritis is the commonest renal lesion in primary SS and occurs early in the disease process with lymphocytic infiltration into and subsequent tubular atrophy and fibrosis. Glomerulonephritis (GN) is rare in primary SS and usually occurs late in the disease. It is thought to be due to immune complex deposition in the glomeruli. Three histological types of GN have been reported in SS: membranoproliferative (MP) GN, mesangioproliferative GN and membranous GN. The histology of each of these is summarized in Table 27.10.

Table 27.11 summarizes the types of renal disease in SS, their clinical presentation and outcome. Interstitial disease typically manifests as hyposthenuria (excretion of urine of low specific gravity due to an inability of the tubules of the kidneys to produce concentrated urine) and type I or type II renal tubular acidosis. Type I renal tubular acidosis is commoner. There is no consensus on the treatment of tubulointerstitial nephritis (TIN) in SS, but our local practice is to use medium dose steroids and a steroid-sparing agent such as azathioprine, using the acute phase response, IgG level and pyuria as markers of disease activity.

GN is rare in SS. The outcomes in these patients are diverse, but patients tend to have a less favourable outcome. Renal failure is common and it is often associated with cryoglobulinaemia

Table 27.10 Renal histological subtypes in SS

Type	Histology
Interstitial nephritis	Interstitial infiltrate which can develop into interstitial atrophy and fibrosis
Type I MPGN	Predominance of subendothelial deposits
Type II MPGN	Predominance of intramembranous deposits
Type III MPGN Burkholder type	Subepithelial and subendothelial deposits and mesangial dense deposits
Type III MPGN Strife type	Intramembranous and subendothelial deposits with marked basement membrane irregularities
Mesangioproliferative GN	
Membranous GN	

Table 27.11 Types of renal disease in SS, associations and outcome

Type	Interstitial nephritis	Glomerulonephritis
Incidence	Most frequent	Very rare
Associations	Renal tubular acidosis	Cryoglobulinaemia and vasculitis
Renal failure	Infrequent	Common
Outcome	Good	Associated with increased morbidity and mortality

and vasculitis. There are no controlled studies about treatment of secondary glomerulonephritis in SS.

Renal Disease in Sarcoidosis

Sarcoidosis is a multisystemic inflammatory disorder of unknown aetiology characterized by the presence of epithelioid non-caseating granulomas in involved organs. It has a worldwide distribution, with the highest geographic prevalence in Northern Europe. Sarcoidosis is slightly more prevalent in women with a peak incidence between 20 and 40 years of age, with a second peak in women over the age of 50.

Kidney involvement in sarcoidosis is rare (0.7–1 %) and is usually diagnosed after lung disease is already evident. It occurs in chronic sarcoidosis and is very rare in acute sarcoidosis. Renal sarcoidosis can result in nephrotic syndrome, tubulointerstitial disease or glomerulonephritis (Table 27.12).

Hypercalcaemia and Hypercalciuria (See Stone Chapter)

Hypercalcaemia and hypercalciuria are the commonest renal abnormalities seen in sarcoidosis. Hypercalcaemia affects 10–20 % of patients and can cause AKI or CKD secondary to nephrocalcinosis. Dysregulated calcium and vitamin D metabolism can occur in sarcoidosis as pulmonary macrophages often express 1-α hydroxylase not subject to the normal feedback mechanisms observed in calcium metabolism. Hypercalcaemic episodes can be precipitated by sun exposure because of vitamin D synthesis in skin. Hypercalcaemia causes afferent arteriolar vasoconstriction, decreasing renal blood flow and GFR. It can cause tubular necrosis leading to urinary sodium wasting and symptomatic polyuria and dehydration. Untreated, hypercalcaemia can lead to nephrocalcinosis and CKD.

Table 27.12 Types of renal dysfunction in sarcoidosis

Renal involvement	Prevalence (%)
Hypercalcaemia	Common
Hypercalciuria (± stones)	Very common
Renal tubular dysfunction	Common
Granulomatous interstitial nephritis	Very small percentage of clinically relevant cases
Glomerular disease	Rare
Renovascular disease	Rare
Obstructive uropathy	Rare

Hypercalciuria is the commonest renal abnormality in sarcoidosis. It is due to an increased calcium load at the glomerulus, along with suppression of PTH secretion by calcitriol, thus diminishing tubular reabsorption of calcium. Hypercalciuria predisposes to calcium oxalate nephrolithiasis.

Renal Tubular Dysfunction

Tubular function may be affected with impaired concentrating ability and water reabsorption with abnormal renal acidification. This may cause polyuria or frank nephrogenic diabetes insipidus. Tubular abnormalities and polyuria usually improve with corticosteroid treatment.

Granulomatous Interstitial Nephritis

Granulomatous interstitial nephritis (GIN) represents the classic renal lesion of sarcoid with non-caseating granulomatous inflammation. Although it is found in a large number of kidneys at autopsy in patients with sarcoidosis, it only represents a very small percentage of clinically relevant cases of renal failure. GIN can present as either AKI or CKI. The granulomatous inflammatory infiltrate is confined primarily to the renal cortex. GIN responds well to corticosteroids. There is no standard dosing protocol, but 1 mg/kg/day of oral prednisolone is the most frequent starting regimen. In one case series of 94 patients, only seven patients required dialysis therapy either initially or shortly after presentation, despite treatment with corticosteroids.

Glomerular Disease

Glomerular disease in sarcoidosis is very rare and can present with different associated lesions; the commonest is membranous nephropathy. Sarcoidosis has been reported with many glomerulonephritides, including immunoglobulin A nephropathy, crescentic glomerulonephritis, minimal change disease and focal segmental glomerulosclerosis. Renal amyloid can also occur. There are no particular guidelines for treatment but corticosteroids are often used.

Renovascular and Obstructive Uropathy

Renovascular disease is rare in sarcoidosis and can be associated with severe hypertension caused by renal artery stenosis from granulomatous angiitis or renal artery encasement by an external inflammatory mass. Urethral, ureteral or bladder obstruction caused by direct sarcoid involvement of these structures is rare.

Renal Disease in Rheumatoid Arthritis

Rheumatoid arthritis (RA) has a prevalence of approximately 1–2 % and is two to three times more prevalent in females than males. The kidney is rarely directly involved in RA but may be compromised by therapies such as non-steroidal anti-inflammatory drugs (NSAIDs) and disease modifying anti-rheumatic drugs (DMARDs) such as gold and penicillamine. Renal involvement in RA is characterized principally by secondary amyloidosis and side effects of medication. Renal lesions directly due to the disease itself are infrequent.

Glomerulonephritis and interstitial renal disease are uncommon in the absence of vasculitis (Table 27.13).

Table 27.13 Types of renal disease in rheumatoid arthritis

Renal disease	
AA amyloidosis	
Type 1	Rapid decline in function
Type 2	Insidious decline in function
IgA mesangial GN	Commonest histopathological type
Membranous GN	Secondary to gold or penicillamine
Interstitial renal disease	Associated with drugs
Type 2 mixed cryoglobulinaemia	Rare
Rheumatoid vasculitis	Very rare. Diffuse necrotizing GN

GN glomerulonephritis

The frequency of amyloidosis in RA has been reported to range from 5 to 13.3 % in cases confirmed by biopsy and from 14 to 26 % in cases confirmed by autopsy. A clinical diagnosis of amyloidosis is usually suspected with the onset of proteinuria, renal insufficiency and diarrhoea. Renal impairment may progress to end-stage renal disease which is a major contributor to death in this disease.

In patients with RA and AA amyloidosis, two distinct clinical courses in terms of renal function have been identified. In type 1 disease, renal function deteriorates rapidly reaching ESRF within 5 years. Type 2 disease is more insidious and renal function does not worsen significantly in 5 years. In type 2 disease, amyloid deposits were found around blood vessels and were absent in the glomerulus [4].

The relationship between IgA, IgA-RF and renal disease in patients with RA is not clear, but the affinity of IgA for mesangium, skin and synovium might explain the clinical presentation of RA with mesangial IgA glomerulonephritis. A striking association of IgM-RF with mesangial glomerulonephritis has been described. It is suggested that a functional deficiency or defect in the renal mesangium to remove IgM-RF-IgG complexes could lead to these mesangial lesions.

Renal involvement due to cryoglobulins is very rare in patients with RA. Type II mixed cryoglobulinemia is the commonest type. It occurs when cryoglobulins form circulating immune complexes. Rheumatoid vasculitis, a severe necrotizing polyangiitis, may sometimes complicate the course of longstanding RA, but renal involvement (diffuse necrotizing GN) is less common in this form of vasculitis.

Treatment of Renal Disease in RA

It is important to distinguish between renal dysfunction secondary to active rheumatoid arthritis, a drug reaction or other unrelated causes of AKI or CKD, and often this can only be achieved by renal biopsy. In essence, treatment of the former is by control of disease activity. There are a number of case reports and series that have successfully used etanercept in the treatment of AA amyloidosis with renal involvement [5]. There are no guidelines for the treatment of IgA nephritis, but cyclophosphamide has been used successfully in cases of deteriorating renal function and IgA nephritis.

Renal Disease in Ankylosing Spondylitis (AS)

Renal disease in AS is relatively common with a reported prevalence of 10–35 %. Table 27.14 outlines the different types of glomerular involvement seen in AS. Renal disease can also be caused by treatments such as NSAIDs, sulphasalazine and azathioprine, which can cause tubulointerstitial nephritis.

Amyloidosis is more prevalent in aggressive and active AS and in older patients with long-standing disease. Clinically, amyloid nephropathy causes proteinuria, which can progress to nephrotic syndrome and renal insufficiency. There is very little data available on the treatment of renal amyloidosis; some case reports suggest a potential role of

Table 27.14 Types of renal disease seen in AS

Type of renal disease	Prevalence
Secondary amyloidosis (AA)	Commonest
IgA nephropathy	Second commonest
Mesangioproliferative GN	Rare
Focal segmental GS	Very rare
Focal proliferative GN	Very rare

GN glomerulonephritis, *GS* glomerulosclerosis

TNF inhibitors in improving AA amyloidosis, but probably the most effective intervention is early detection by ensuring screening for proteinuria in rheumatology clinics and getting control of inflammatory process.

References

1. Batal I, Domsic RT, Shafer A, Medsger Jr TA, Kiss LP, Randhawa P, Bastacky S. Renal biopsy findings predicting outcome in scleroderma renal crisis. Hum Pathol. 2009;40(3):332–40.
2. Moinzadeh P, Nihtyanova SI, Howell K, Ong VH, Denton CP. Impact of hallmark autoantibody reactivity on early diagnosis in scleroderma. Clin Rev Allergy Immunol. 2012;43(3):249–55.
3. Penn H, Howie AJ, Kingdon EJ, Bunn CC, Stratton RJ, Black CM, et al. Scleroderma renal crisis: patient characteristics and long-term outcomes. QJM. 2007;100(8):485–94.
4. Uda H, Yokota A, Kobayashi K, et al. Two distinct courses of renal involvement in rheumatoid patients with AA amyloidosis. J Rheumatol. 2006;33:1482–7.
5. Nakamura T, Higashi S, Tomoda K, Tsukano M, Baba S. Efficacy of etanercept in patients with AA amyloidosis secondary to rheumatoid arthritis. Clin Exp Rheumatol. 2007;25(4):518–22.

Table 28.2 The published evidence for the use of plasma exchange for light chain removal

Study	Inclusion criteria	Patient numbers	Outcome measures	Results
Clark et al. [24]	Newly diagnosed MM (>10 % plasma cells in bone marrow aspirate), serum creatinine >200 mmol/L	104	Composite of death, dialysis dependence and eGFR <30 mL/min	The composite end point was met in 57.9 % of the plasma exchange group and 69.2 % of the control group with wide confidence intervals
Zucchelli et al. [25]	Acute renal failure, new or previously diagnosed MM	29	Independence from dialysis, serum creatinine	More patients in the plasma exchange group recovered renal function (13/15 versus 2/14), the 1-year survival was higher in the plasma exchange group (66 % versus 28 %)
Johnson et al. [26]	Active myeloma, progressive renal failure	21		Plasmapheresis and chemotherapy lowered the serum protein more rapidly than chemotherapy alone; of the 5 patients who were dialysis dependent, only 3 who received plasmapheresis recovered

High Cut-Off Dialysis

To overcome the limitations of plasma exchange, interest has grown in a novel technique for the removal of light chains, using a large-pore (high cut-off (HCO)) dialysis membrane originally developed for cytokine removal in critically ill patients on continuous dialysis in the intensive care setting. Subsequently, both in vivo and in vitro studies have shown that both FLC isotypes are cleared through this membrane, with major reductions in sFLC levels in patients with MM [27, 28].

A pilot study in patients with biopsy-proven cast nephropathy received HCO dialysis and chemotherapy and reported dramatic early reductions in circulating light chains, and 74 % of patients recovered independent renal function [3]. To further investigate the potential benefit of HCO dialysis, two randomised controlled trials, acronymed EuLITE [29] and MYRE (ClinicalTrials.gov Identifier: NCT01208818), are in recruitment, patients are randomised to either extended HCO dialysis or conventional haemodialysis and all participants will receive the same chemotherapy regimen.

Supportive Care

Careful attention to fluid balance and electrolytes, infection, drug use and bone management is mandatory. An individualised approach is required for provision of supportive care. For example, whilst a high oral fluid intake is important for the dilution of light chains to decrease the likelihood of cast formation and direct tubular toxicity, in patients with advanced renal impairment and or pre-existing cardiac disease, this may require meticulous attention and fluid requirements may change from day to day.

Fluid Balance and Acid-Base Status

As long as there are no major contraindications, patients should be encouraged to drink at least 3 L of fluid a day. Salt loading (with iv NaCL) should be avoided, as increased tubular NaCl concentrations can precipitate cast formation. Loop diuretics are contraindicated as they both increase intratubular sodium and lower intratubular pH.

Animal and in vitro studies indicated that casts are more likely to precipitate with more acidic milieu. Therefore maintenance of adequate hydration, tissue oxygenation, avoidance of infection and timely commencement of dialysis treatment should prevent the development of systemic acidosis.

Drugs

Whilst all nephrologists recognise the importance of thoughtful and accurate use of drugs in patients with AKI, this is crucial in the setting of MM. Drugs that can decrease renal perfusion are contraindicated and all medications should be justified as clinically appropriate for the patient.

Data sheets should be consulted and adjusted for renal impairment; clinicians often overlook that most drug dose adjustments based on kidney function utilise the Cockroft-Gault calculation, not MDRD. In patients with rapidly progressive AKI, there should be an assumption that the GFR is <15 mL/min.

Bone Disease, Hypercalcaemia and Bisphosphonates

Bone destruction and hypercalcaemia are very common and arer consequences of osteoclast-mediated osteolysis and inhibition of osteoblast function [30]. In addition myeloma cells produce substances that make the bone marrow itself even more conducive to myeloma growth and accelerating disease progression [31].

In addition to treatment of hypercalcaemia, bisphosphonates have a role in the stabilisation of bone, and there is also great interest in a potential synergistic action with bortezomib, which could contribute directly to improved outcomes from disease activity itself [32]. Whilst the Myeloma IX study showed that zoledronic acid was associated with better outcomes than clodronate, this bisphosphonate should be avoided in advanced renal impairment because it has high renal toxicity. At present intravenous pamidronate at an adjusted dose should be used for the management of hypercalcaemia and to facilitate immediate bone stabilisation. If the kidney function does not improve to an eGFR of ≥30 mL/min, we would recommend dialogue with haematology colleagues to produce an individualised risk assessment that can then be discussed with the patient.

Infections

Guidelines for the management of infections are available [33]. Patients with MM are at high risk because of global suppression of immunity. Humoral immunity can be overestimated by not accounting for the M-protein when interpreting the levels of intact Ig isotype. For example, patients with an intact IgG clone may have 'normal IgG' levels, but the major component of IgG may be clonal, and there may be profound depression of humoral immunity. The role of intravenous immunoglobulin infusions is unclear; some centres use these for patients with hypogammaglobulinemia and recurrent serious infections; however, there is no prospective evidence base to support this.

Both bacterial infections including *Streptococcus pneumonia* and *Haemophilus influenza* and viral infections such as herpes zoster are common. A role for primary antibiotic prophylaxis is uncertain; however, most clinicians would use antibiotic prophylaxis if there are one or more serious bacterial infections. A randomised controlled trial of antibiotic prophylaxis for patients with MM is required. Antiviral prophylaxis with aciclovir is recommended during treatment.

Patients with MM develop suboptimal antibody responses; however, immunisation with pneumococcal and influenza vaccine should still be given.

Multidisciplinary Working in MM

Although MM is a haematological malignancy, it may present to a variety of specialties and when diagnosed will often require the input of a multiprofessional and multidisciplinary team. Only when all members of this team are aware of MM as a potential diagnosis and the treatment options for patients with MM will optimal care be delivered, there is evidence that the diagnosis of MM may be delayed when patients' initial presentation is to a nephrologist [34]. The multiprofessional/multidisciplinary team who may be involved in the diagnosis and management of MM are shown in Fig. 28.5.

Multi - disciplinary specialists

- Haematology clinical nurse specialists
- Dialysis nurses
- Research nurses
- Pharmacists
- Physiotherapists
- Occupational therapists

Medical Specialties

- General Practitioners
- Haematologists
- Nephrologists
- Neurosurgeons (to manage spinal cord compression....)
- Clinical oncologists (radiotherapy to bone lesions...)
- Palliative care specialists
- Pain control specialist

Fig. 28.5 Multidisciplinary and medical specialty involvement in the diagnosis and management of MM

Patient Information in MM

A diagnosis of MM may be a shattering event for a patient, and there are a number of different areas where detailed and carefully targeted patient information will be required; these include:

- Information about the causes of the disease
- Information about the consequences of the disease (e.g. renal failure, bone disease, anaemia)
- Information about the supportive treatment of the consequences of MM (e.g. pain control)
- Information about chemotherapy, the various options available and the side effects they may experience
- Information about renal impairment, including information about aspects of dialysis if required
- Information about clinical trials if relevant
- General supportive information that any patient with a potentially life-limiting condition might require (relating to social, psychological or other palliative care issues)

There are a number of sources of such information and support for patients diagnosed with MM. Myeloma UK has a series of info guides which are available on line and are a useful resource for patients and health-care professionals (www.myeloma.org.uk).

References

1. Kumar SK, Rajkumar SV, Dispenzieri A, Lacy MQ, Hayman SR, Buadi FK, et al. Improved survival in multiple myeloma and the impact of novel therapies. Blood. 2008;111(5):2516–20.
2. Haynes RJ, Read S, Collins GP, Darby SC, Winearls CG. Presentation and survival of patients with severe acute kidney injury and multiple myeloma: a 20-year experience from a single centre. Nephrol Dial Transplant. 2010;25(2):419–26.
3. Hutchison CA, Bradwell AR, Cook M, Basnayake K, Basu S, Harding S, et al. Treatment of acute renal failure secondary to multiple myeloma with chemotherapy and extended high cut-off hemodialysis. Clin J Am Soc Nephrol. 2009;4(4):745–54.
4. Hutchison CA, Heyne N, Airia P, Schindler R, Zickler D, Cook M, et al. Immunoglobulin free light chain levels and recovery from myeloma kidney on treatment with chemotherapy and high cut-off haemodialysis. Nephrol Dial Transplant. 2012;27(10):3823–8.
5. Basnayake K, Stringer SJ, Hutchison CA, Cockwell P. The biology of immunoglobulin free light chains and kidney injury. Kidney Int. 2011;79(12):1289–301.
6. Kyle RA, Therneau TM, Rajkumar SV, Larson DR, Plevak MF, Offord JR, et al. Prevalence of monoclonal gammopathy of undetermined significance. N Engl J Med. 2006;354(13):1362–9.
7. Kyle RA, Therneau TM, Rajkumar SV, Offord JR, Larson DR, Plevak MF, et al. A long-term study of prognosis in monoclonal gammopathy of undetermined significance. N Engl J Med. 2002;346(8):564–9.
8. Dispenzieri A, Katzmann JA, Kyle RA, Larson DR, Melton 3rd LJ, Colby CL, et al. Prevalence and risk of progression of light-chain monoclonal gammopathy of undetermined significance: a retrospective population-based cohort study. Lancet. 2010;375(9727):1721–8.
9. International Myeloma Working Group. Criteria for the classification of monoclonal gammopathies, multiple myeloma and related disorders: a report of the International Myeloma Working Group. Br J Haematol. 2003;121(5):749–57.
10. Tsakiris DJ, Stel VS, Finne P, Fraser E, Heaf J, de Meester J, et al. Incidence and outcome of patients starting renal replacement therapy for end-stage renal disease due to multiple myeloma or light-chain deposit disease: an ERA-EDTA Registry study. Nephrol Dial Transplant. 2010;25(4):1200–6.
11. Haynes R, Hutchison CA, Emberson J, Dasgupta T, Wheeler DC, Townend JN, et al. Serum free light chains and the risk of ESRD and death in CKD. Clin J Am Soc Nephrol. 2011;6(12):2829–37.
12. Eleutherakis-Papaiakovou V, Bamias A, Gika D, Simeonidis A, Pouli A, Anagnostopoulos A, et al. Renal failure in multiple myeloma: incidence, correlations, and prognostic significance. Leuk Lymphoma. 2007;48(2):337–41.
13. Hutchison CA, Plant T, Drayson M, Cockwell P, Kountouri M, Basnayake K, et al. Serum free light chain measurement aids the diagnosis of myeloma in patients with severe renal failure. BMC Nephrol. 2008;9:11.
14. Pratt G. The evolving use of serum free light chain assays in haematology. Br J Haematol. 2008;141(4):413–22.
15. Hutchison CA, Cockwell P, Harding S, Mead GP, Bradwell AR, Barnett AH. Quantitative assessment of serum and urinary polyclonal free light chains in patients with type II diabetes: an early marker of diabetic kidney disease? Expert Opin Ther Targets. 2008;12(6):667–76.
16. Herrera GA, Joseph L, Gu X, Hough A, Barlogie B. Renal pathologic spectrum in an autopsy series of patients with plasma cell dyscrasia. Arch Pathol Lab Med. 2004;128(8):875–9.
17. Pirani CL, Silva F, D'Agati V, Chander P, Striker LM. Renal lesions in plasma cell dyscrasias: ultrastructural observations. Am J Kidney Dis. 1987;10(3):208–21.
18. Basnayake K, Cheung CK, Sheaff M, Fuggle W, Kamel D, Nakoinz S, et al. Differential progression of renal scarring and determinants of late renal recovery in sustained dialysis dependent acute kidney injury secondary to myeloma kidney. J Clin Pathol. 2010;63(10):884–7.
19. Sanders PW, Herrera GA, Lott RL, Galla JH. Morphologic alterations of the proximal tubules in light chain-related renal disease. Kidney Int. 1988;33(4):881–9.
20. Alexanian R, Dimopoulos MA, Delasalle K, Barlogie B. Primary dexamethasone treatment of multiple myeloma. Blood. 1992;80(4):887–90.
21. Dimopoulos MA, Terpos E, Chanan-Khan A, Leung N, Ludwig H, Jagannath S, et al. Renal impairment in patients with multiple myeloma: a consensus statement on behalf of the International Myeloma Working Group. J Clin Oncol. 2010;28(33):4976–84.
22. Popat R, Joel S, Oakervee H, Cavenagh J. Bortezomib for multiple myeloma. Expert Opin Pharmacother. 2006;7(10):1337–46.
23. Stringer S, Basnayake K, Hutchison C, Cockwell P. Recent advances in the pathogenesis and management of cast nephropathy (myeloma kidney). Bone Marrow Res. 2011;2011:493697.
24. Clark WF, Stewart AK, Rock GA, Sternbach M, Sutton DM, Barrett BJ, et al. Plasma exchange when myeloma presents as acute renal failure: a randomized, controlled trial. Ann Intern Med. 2005;143(11):777–84.
25. Zucchelli P, Pasquali S, Cagnoli L, Ferrari G. Controlled plasma exchange trial in acute renal failure due to multiple myeloma. Kidney Int. 1988;33(6):1175–80.
26. Johnson WJ, Kyle RA, Pineda AA, O'Brien PC, Holley KE. Treatment of renal failure associated with multiple myeloma. Plasmapheresis, hemodialysis, and chemotherapy. Arch Intern Med. 1990;150(4):863–9.
27. Hutchison CA, Cockwell P, Reid S, Chandler K, Mead GP, Harrison J, et al. Efficient removal of immunoglobulin free light chains by hemodialysis for multiple myeloma: in vitro and in vivo studies. J Am Soc Nephrol. 2007;18(3):886–95.
28. Hutchison CA, Harding S, Mead G, Goehl H, Storr M, Bradwell A, et al. Serum free-light chain removal by high cutoff hemodialysis: optimizing removal and supportive care. Artif Organs. 2008;32(12):910–7.
29. Hutchison CA, Cook M, Heyne N, Weisel K, Billingham L, Bradwell A, et al. European trial of free light chain removal by extended haemodialysis in cast nephropathy (EuLITE): a randomised control trial. Trials. 2008;9:55.
30. Oyajobi BO. Multiple myeloma/hypercalcemia. Arthritis Res Ther. 2007;9 Suppl 1:S4.
31. Terpos E, Dimopoulos MA. Myeloma bone disease: pathophysiology and management. Ann Oncol. 2005;16(8):1223–31.
32. Terpos E, Sezer O, Croucher PI, Garcia-Sanz R, Boccadoro M, San Miguel J, et al. The use of bisphosphonates in multiple myeloma: recommendations of an expert panel on behalf of the European Myeloma Network. Ann Oncol. 2009;20(8):1303–17.
33. Kyle RA, Rajkumar SV. Treatment of multiple myeloma: a comprehensive review. Clin Lymphoma Myeloma. 2009;9(4):278–88.
34. Kariyawasan CC, Hughes DA, Jayatillake MM, Mehta AB. Multiple myeloma: causes and consequences of delay in diagnosis. QJM. 2007;100(10):635–40.

29 Amyloidosis

Julian David Gillmore and Helen J. Lachmann

Amyloidosis is a generic term for a group of diseases caused by misfolding and extracellular accumulation of certain proteins as fibrillar deposits that stain with Congo red and produce pathognomonic green birefringence when viewed by microscopy under crossed polarised light. The process of amyloid formation and deposition causes progressive organ dysfunction. Amyloidosis is remarkably diverse and can be hereditary or acquired, localised or systemic and lethal or merely an incidental finding. So far, 27 different human proteins with in vivo amyloidogenic potential have been identified of which 15 cause systemic amyloidosis. The classification of amyloid is based on the fibril protein, and different amyloidogenic proteins give rise to distinct but frequently overlapping clinical syndromes. The kidneys are frequently involved in systemic amyloidosis (Table 29.1) which, without treatment, is usually fatal. Current management of amyloidosis is dependent upon determining the fibril protein and reducing its abundance. This can result in regression of amyloid deposits, prevention or recovery of organ failure and improved survival.

Aetiology and Pathogenesis

Amyloid formation occurs when a protein or peptide loses, or fails to acquire, its physiologic, functional folding and, in its misfolded state, undergoes fibril formation and extracellular deposition. Amyloid deposits display distinctive ultrastructural (beta-sheet conformation) and tinctorial properties. The process of amyloid formation and deposition ultimately results in tissue damage and organ dysfunction (Fig. 29.1). The propensity of proteins to form amyloid fibrils in vivo is enhanced by the following:

- A pathologic and sustained increase in concentration of the protein. This is the case of the acute-phase reactant serum amyloid A protein (SAA) in chronic inflammation and of β2-microglobulin in patients with end-stage renal disease (ESRD).
- Presence of an unstable mutant protein, favouring its misfolding and aggregation, as occurs in hereditary amyloidoses.
- Proteolytic remodelling of a protein as in the case of the protease furin cleaving ABri and gelsolin and the β- and γ-secretases releasing amyloid-β (Aβ) peptides.
- Advancing age as in the case of wild-type transthyretin and apolipoprotein A-I both of which have intrinsic amyloidogenic properties and are associated with age-related amyloid deposition.

Frequently, a combination of these factors determines the amyloidogenicity of an individual protein. However,

Table 29.1 Systemic amyloidoses commonly associated with kidney involvement

Amyloid type	Fibril precursor	Note
AL	Light chain V region fragments	Primary, myeloma associated
AA	Serum amyloid A protein (SAA)	Secondary, reactive to chronic inflammation
ALect2	Leukocyte chemotactic factor 2	Sporadic, more common in Mexican Americans and South Asians
AApoAI	Apolipoprotein A-I	Familial
AApoAII	Apolipoprotein A-II	Familial
ALys	Lysozyme	Familial
AFib	Fibrinogen Aα-chain	Familial
AGel	Gelsolin	Familial
ATTR	Transthyretin	Familial, kidney involvement/dysfunction unusual until late stage of disease

J.D. Gillmore, MBBS, MD, PhD, FRCP (✉)
Division of Medicine, National Amyloidosis Centre, UCL Medical School, Rowland Hill Street, London NW3 2PF, UK
e-mail: j.gillmore@ucl.ac.uk

H.J. Lachmann, MA, MBBChir, MD, FRCP
Division of Medicine, National Amyloidosis Centre, UCL Medical School and Royal Free London NHS Foundation Trust, Royal Free Campus, Rowland Hill Street, London NW3 2PF, UK
e-mail: h.lachmann@ucl.ac.uk

M. Harber (ed.), *Practical Nephrology*,
DOI 10.1007/978-1-4471-5547-8_29,

effective. Eculizumab is a monoclonal antibody that inhibits activation of C5 and has recently been licenced for the treatment of aHUS. The first beneficial effects of eculizumab in aHUS were reported in 2009 [13, 14], and subsequently two phase II trials have been completed although only published in abstract form [15]. Thirty-seven adolescent or adults patients with aHUS were enrolled in the trials with either plasma-resistant or plasma-sensitive aHUS. All treated patients responded to eculizumab assessed by stopping ongoing or preventing further episodes of TMA. Kidney function also improved after eculizumab treatment. In these trials approximately 30 % of patients did not have an identifiable defect in complement control but responded to treatment with eculizumab. A high relapse rate has been reported in patients who discontinued eculizumab. Inhibition of C5 activity with eculizumab increases susceptibility to meningococcal infection. Vaccination is mandatory prior to eculizumab use, but current meningococcal vaccinations do not prevent infection with serotype b, the commonest cause of meningococcal meningitis in the UK. Long-term prophylactic antibiotics should also be considered.

Prognosis

The prognosis of aHUS is worse than in STEC-HUS with over 50 % of patients either dying or developing end-stage renal disease 3 years after diagnosis [11]. The likelihood of patient and renal survival after the first episode of aHUS depends upon the mutation that is present (see Table 30.3). Patients with mutations in factor H or factor I develop severe disease with high rates of death or renal failure after the first presentation. In contrast patients with mutations in CD46 have a more benign disease and can run a remitting, relapsing course without loss of renal function. Once patients have established renal failure, the TMA tends to remit although ongoing haematological evidence for TMA can be found. Although accelerated vascular disease is reported in this patient group, this is difficult to distinguish from the effects of chronic kidney disease.

Kidney transplantation is associated with a high risk of recurrence of aHUS (Table 30.4) and transplantation is generally contraindicated in these patients. Patients with mutations in CD46 have a lower rate of recurrence as CD46 is expressed on the endothelial cell surface and therefore converts to donor type after transplantation [16]. Combined liver and kidney transplantation has been used successfully in this patient group. Factors H and I are synthesised in the liver; therefore, liver transplantation results in production of normal protein, protecting the recipient from recurrent aHUS. There is a high morbidity and mortality associated with this procedure. Although early outcomes were poor, the results of recent combined transplants with aggressive pre-transplant plasma exchange have been encouraging. In the future therapeutic complement inhibition will allow these patients to receive kidney transplants by controlling complement activation and preventing TMA.

Table 30.4 Recurrence of aHUS after isolated kidney transplantation

	Transplants	% Recurrence	% Graft loss after recurrence
Factor H mutations	42	76	86
Factor H antibodies	5	20	2/2
Factor I mutations	12	92	85
CD46 mutations	10	20	1/2
C3 mutations	7	57	80
CFB mutations	3	3/3	2/3
Thrombomodulin mutations	1	1/1	1/1

Ref. Noris and Remuzzi [16]

Thrombotic Thrombocytopenic Purpura

TTP is closely associated with a severe deficiency in the protease enzyme, known as ADAMTS13, responsible for cleaving von Willebrand factor (vWF). vWF is produced by endothelial cells and is involved in haemostasis, inducing platelet aggregation and thrombus formation. vWF is initially secreted as large multimers which are gradually degraded by ADAMTS13. Large multimers of vWF are prothrombogenic and accumulate in TTP, implying a defect in ADAMTS13 function [17].

Congenital TTP is rare accounting for 5 % of all cases of TTP. It is due to a homozygous (or compound heterozygous) mutation in the *ADAMTS13* gene, and there is a high degree of penetrance. More commonly (>90 % of cases) TTP is due to an autoantibody that inhibits the function of ADAMTS13.

TTP has also been linked to the platelet inhibitors ticlopidine and clopidogrel. This is a rare side effect which usually develops in the first few weeks after starting treatment. Autoantibodies to ADAMTS13 have been reported in some cases and plasma exchange improves the outcome.

Clinical Features

With the exception of the congenital form which usually occurs early in childhood, TTP occurs predominantly in adults. The features of TMA are present, and the thrombocytopenia is often profound, with platelet counts lower than are typically seen in HUS. Neurological symptoms and signs are usually present and often severe and can include focal neurological deficit, seizures and reduced level of consciousness. Fever is frequently present and renal impairment, including an abnormal urinary sediment, can be present.

Diagnosis

Initial diagnosis is based on the typical clinical features in the presence of a TMA. The diagnosis is confirmed by testing ADAMTS13 activity, with severe deficiency (<5 % activity) being associated with disease. ADAMTS13 activity can also be low in TMA associated with autoimmune disease and pregnancy and can be low in patients with malignancy or chronic infection without features of TMA. If low ADAMTS13 activity is found, the patient should be screened for autoantibodies to ADAMTS13 or mutations in the *ADAMTS13* gene.

Treatment

Without treatment mortality in patients with TTP is high (over 90 %). Plasma-based therapy, either exchange or infusion, is the mainstay of treatment, with plasma exchange generally being preferred because of better outcomes [18]. Despite treatment, mortality rate remains high (20–40 %). Early treatment is important, and treatment should begin before ADAMTS13 activity is known or STEC-HUS excluded. Plasma infusion can be started if plasma exchange is not immediately available. It is less important to exclude aHUS as plasma therapy is an appropriate treatment for this condition. Plasma exchange should be with fresh frozen plasma (or equivalent product) and should be at least 1 plasma volume on a daily basis until a response is seen. Increasing the volume of exchange or twice daily exchanges should be considered if no response is seen. Relapse after remission occurs in up to 30 % of patients.

Immunosuppression is frequently used in patients with TTP. In a trial comparing high-dose intravenous followed by oral steroids with lower-dose oral steroid a beneficial effect of high-dose steroids was seen [19]. A beneficial effect of rituximab (anti-CD20) has been reported in a number of case series and one non-randomised phase II study in patients with resistant or refactory TTP. Other drugs, including vincristine, cyclophosphamide and cyclosporine A, have been used to treat TTP, but there is little evidence of benefit.

Defective Cobalamin metabolism

An autosomal recessive abnormality in cobalamin C (B12) metabolism leads to hyperhomocysteinaemia and methylmalonic aciduria. This usually presents in the first few months of life with TMA, respiratory, hepatic and renal failure. The vascular injury inducing the TMA may be due to hyperhomocysteinaemia. Although usually a fulminant disease, a more chronic TMA can be seen in older children. The metabolic abnormalities correct with daily hydroxycobalamin treatment.

Quinine

In a series of patients with TMA, 11 % reported taking quinine [20]. Typically quinine-induced TMA starts abruptly after taking the drug with systemic symptoms, evidence of a TMA and acute renal failure. Patients have circulating antibodies that recognise a glycoprotein on platelets, erythrocytes and leucocytes only in the presence of quinine. Binding of quinine to this glycoprotein creates a neoepitope, inducing antibody binding and cell activation. Treatment of the acute episode is with plasma exchange followed by avoidance of quinine.

Associations with HUS/TTP

HIV Infection

HUS is more common in patients with HIV infection. Although other forms of HUS (e.g. STEC related) can occur in patients infected with HIV, there appears to be a specific HIV-related form of HUS. The mechanism by which HIV induces a TMA is not known but is hypothesised that virus infection causes endothelial activation inducing a pro-thrombotic state.

Malignancy and Its Treatment

HUS and TTP-like syndromes are associated with disseminated adenocarcinoma (gastric, colonic and prostatic). Although this HUS/TTP can predate the diagnosis of cancer, many of these patients will have received mitomycin, gemcitabine or irradiation. These treatments have been reported to cause HUS/TTP and it can be difficult to determine whether the TMA is due to malignancy or its treatment. There is some evidence of a response to steroids and plasma exchange.

Transplantation

TMA has been reported after kidney, liver, heart and bone marrow transplantation but is probably most common after kidney transplantation. Both cyclosporine A and tacrolimus have been implicated as causal drugs with one report suggesting TMA occurs in 14 % of patients on cyclosporine A and 1–5 % of patients on tacrolimus [21]. This is probably an overestimate of incidence. These drugs are vasoconstrictive and may directly damage the renal endothelium inducing a pro-thrombotic state. This effect is idiosyncratic and does not necessarily relate to drug levels. Patients may improve with dose reduction or a switch from cyclosporine A to tacrolimus (or vice versa), although avoidance of calcineurin inhibitors is preferable switching to sirolimus is of unproven benefit. Plasma exchange is frequently used in this situation and positive results have been reported.

Post-transplant HUS may represent recurrence of aHUS in the transplanted kidney. HUS may have been the initial cause of renal failure which may have not been diagnosed or the risk of recurrence not recognised. In one series 30 % or patients with post-transplant HUS had mutations in factor H or factor I [22]. Eculizumab can be useful in post-transplant HUS even in the absence of a complement gene mutation [23].

Pregnancy

HUS and TTP are more common in women, particularly in pregnancy. Presentation can occur anytime in pregnancy but is most common in the third trimester, and it can be difficult to distinguish from pre-eclampsia. It is clear that pregnancy is one factor that can trigger aHUS, and this will explain some cases [24]. Low levels of ADAMTS13 protease activity have also been reported in pregnancy-related TMA. In the majority the cause of TMA is not known.

Other Autoimmune Disease

TMA has been reported to effect up to 8 % of patients with systemic lupus erythematosus (SLE), but experience would suggest a much lower incidence. Autoantibodies to ADAMTS13 and platelets have been reported in patients with SLE, and this may explain the prothrombotic phenotype that leads to TMA. Treatment is usually with plasma exchange and immunosuppressive regimes with reported efficacy in SLE. TMA can develop in patients with anti-phospholipid syndrome probably due to antibody binding to and activation of platelets and endothelial cells.

References

1. Besbas N, et al. A classification of hemolytic uremic syndrome and thrombotic thrombocytopenic purpura and related disorders. Kidney Int. 2006;70(3):423–31.
2. Frank C, et al. Epidemic profile of Shiga-toxin-producing Escherichia coli O104:H4 outbreak in Germany. N Engl J Med. 2011;365(19):1771–80.
3. Menne J, et al. Validation of treatment strategies for enterohaemorrhagic Escherichia coli O104:H4 induced haemolytic uraemic syndrome: case-control study. BMJ. 2012;345:e4565.
4. Michael M, et al. Interventions for haemolytic uraemic syndrome and thrombotic thrombocytopenic purpura. Cochrane Database Syst Rev. 2009;(1):CD003595.
5. Lapeyraque AL, et al. Eculizumab in severe Shiga-toxin-associated HUS. N Engl J Med. 2011;364(26):2561–3.
6. Garg AX, et al. Long-term renal prognosis of diarrhea-associated hemolytic uremic syndrome: a systematic review, meta-analysis, and meta-regression. JAMA. 2003;290(10):1360–70.
7. Copelovitch L, Kaplan BS. Streptococcus pneumoniae-associated hemolytic uremic syndrome. Pediatr Nephrol. 2008;23(11): 1951–6.
8. Warwicker P, et al. Genetic studies into inherited and sporadic hemolytic uremic syndrome. Kidney Int. 1998;53(4):836–44.
9. Sanchez-Corral P, Melgosa M. Advances in understanding the aetiology of atypical haemolytic uraemic syndrome. Br J Haematol. 2010;150(5):529–42.
10. Esparza-Gordillo J, et al. Predisposition to atypical hemolytic uremic syndrome involves the concurrence of different susceptibility alleles in the regulators of complement activation gene cluster in 1q32. Hum Mol Genet. 2005;14(5):703–12.
11. Noris M, et al. Relative role of genetic complement abnormalities in sporadic and familial aHUS and their impact on clinical phenotype. Clin J Am Soc Nephrol. 2010;5(10):1844–59.
12. Delvaeye M, et al. Thrombomodulin mutations in atypical hemolytic-uremic syndrome. N Engl J Med. 2009;361(4):345–57.
13. Gruppo RA, Rother RP. Eculizumab for congenital atypical hemolytic-uremic syndrome. N Engl J Med. 2009;360(5):544–6.
14. Nurnberger J, et al. Eculizumab for atypical hemolytic-uremic syndrome. N Engl J Med. 2009;360(5):542–4.
15. Cohen DJ, et al. The terminal complement inhibitor eculizumab for treatment of atypical haemolytic uraemic syndrome. N Engl J Med. 2013;368(23):2169–81.
16. Noris M, Remuzzi G. Thrombotic microangiopathy after kidney transplantation. Am J Transplant. 2010;10(7):1517–23.
17. Furlan M, et al. Deficient activity of von Willebrand factor-cleaving protease in chronic relapsing thrombotic thrombocytopenic purpura. Blood. 1997;89(9):3097–103.
18. Michael M, et al. Interventions for hemolytic uremic syndrome and thrombotic thrombocytopenic purpura: a systematic review of randomized controlled trials. Am J Kidney Dis. 2009;53(2): 259–72.
19. Balduini CL, et al. High versus standard dose methylprednisolone in the acute phase of idiopathic thrombotic thrombocytopenic purpura: a randomized study. Ann Hematol. 2010;89(6):591–6.
20. Kojouri K, Vesely SK, George JN. Quinine-associated thrombotic thrombocytopenic purpura-hemolytic uremic syndrome: frequency, clinical features, and long-term outcomes. Ann Intern Med. 2001;135(12):1047–51.
21. Zarifian A, et al. Cyclosporine-associated thrombotic microangiopathy in renal allografts. Kidney Int. 1999;55(6):2457–66.
22. Le Quintrec M, et al. Complement mutation-associated de novo thrombotic microangiopathy following kidney transplantation. Am J Transplant. 2008;8(8):1694–701.
23. Wilson CH, et al. Successful treatment of de novo posttransplant thrombotic microangiopathy with eculizumab. Transplantation. 2011;92(8):e42–3.
24. Salmon JE, et al. Mutations in complement regulatory proteins predispose to preeclampsia: a genetic analysis of the PROMISSE cohort. PLoS Med. 2011;8(3):e1001013.

31 Sickle Cell Disease and Other Haematological Disorders Involving the Kidney

Claire Sharpe, Catherine J. Horsfield, and Mark Harber

Several haematological conditions have significant renal sequelae perhaps most notably multiple myeloma and the haemolytic uraemic syndrome spectrum of conditions, which are covered elsewhere. Renal disease is also associated with several red cell disorders including the haemoglobinopathies and other disorders that result in acute or chronic intravascular haemolysis. Aside from myeloma, most renal diseases related to white cell disorders are secondary to the systemic effects, direct infiltration or treatment of lymphoma or leukaemia.

Haemoglobinopathies

Sickle Cell Disease

Worldwide, sickle cell disease (SCD) is the most common congenital haematological condition and is a major cause of renal impairment, probably second only to myeloma overall.

Epidemiology

Sickle cell disease is endemic in malaria-prevalent (or previously prevalent) regions due to the protective nature of the carrier state. Across equatorial Africa, the prevalence of the sickle cell trait (SCT, heterozygous carriers) ranges between 10 and 40 % and decreases to between 1 and 2 % on the north African coast and <1 % in South Africa. However, migration has led to SCD becoming increasingly common in non-endemic regions, for example, there are currently over 12,000 sufferers of sickle cell disease living in the UK and approximately 72,000 in the USA. Renal involvement in SCD is well recognised, and chronic kidney disease (CKD) secondary to sickle cell nephropathy (SCN) is becoming more prevalent as the life expectancy of patients with SCD improves.

SCN increases with age and it is, in general, more common and severe in those with HbSS and HBSβ^0-thalassaemia than in those with the more mild forms of SCD such as HbSC [1]. The onset is insidious, and microalbuminuria, an early manifestation of SCN, reaches a prevalence of approximately 60 % in those over 45 although only 4–12 % of patients with SCD will develop end-stage renal disease.

Pathogenesis

The pathogenesis of SCN is intimately related to the circulation of the kidney. Although in health the kidneys receive approximately 25 % of the cardiac output, the vessels (vasa recta) that supply the medulla of the kidney branch off early from the efferent arteriole taking only a fraction of the total renal blood flow with them. The relatively sluggish but intricate circulation of the inner medulla is critical to maintaining the countercurrent multiplier system of the loop of Henle which drives water and solute reabsorption and allows for effective urinary concentration. The resulting hypoxia (partial pressure of oxygen 10–35 mmHg), acidosis and hyperosmolarity of the inner medulla make it an ideal environment for the polymerisation of deoxygenated haemoglobin S and subsequent sickling of red blood cells. Over time, repeated cycles of sickling and sludging cause micro-infarcts and ischaemic injury leading to the chronic microvascular disease that is apparent in established SCN. In parallel with this, cortical renal blood flow and glomerular filtration rate (GFR) are increased in response to anaemia and vasodilation.

C. Sharpe, MBBS, PhD, FRCP (✉)
Department of Renal Medicine, King's College London and King's College Hospital NHS Foundation Trust, 10 Cutcombe Road, London SE5 9RJ, UK
e-mail: claire.sharpe@kcl.ac.uk

C.J. Horsfield, FRCPath
Department of Histopathology, Guy's & St Thomas' NHS, St Thomas' Hospital, Lambeth Palace Road, London SE1 7EH, UK
e-mail: catherine.horsfield@gstt.nhs.uk

M. Harber, MBBS, PhD, FRCP
UCL Department of Nephrology, Royal Free London NHS Foundation Trust, Pond Street, Hampstead, London NW3 2QG, UK
e-mail: mark.harber@nhs.net

M. Harber (ed.), *Practical Nephrology*,
DOI 10.1007/978-1-4471-5547-8_31, © Springer-Verlag London 2014

The subsequent hyperfiltration eventually results in proteinuria and glomerulosclerosis, which together with tubulointerstitial fibrosis herald the onset of progressive CKD [2]. In addition, when red blood cells haemolyse, free haemoglobin, a highly potent nitric oxide scavenger, is released into the circulation. The reduction in free nitric oxide leads to localised vasoconstriction, which is thought to underlie the pathogenesis of pulmonary hypertension, priapism, leg ulceration and stroke and is also likely to be involved in the progression of CKD.

Clinical Features

Hyperfiltration

Histological analysis of the kidneys postmortem has revealed the presence of abnormally large and distended glomeruli in people with sickle cell disease as young as 2 years old, which is associated with increased total renal blood flow and GFR [3]. The recently reported BABY HUG trial showed a significantly elevated GFR in infants with a mean age of 13.6 months [4]. Glomerular filtration rate continues to rise throughout childhood and early adulthood, often reaching 200 mL/min/1.73 m^2. This may be partially accounted for by an increased cardiac output driven by anaemia, although the elevated GFR is not reversed by repeated red cell transfusion [7]. Localised prostaglandin release and an increase in nitric oxide synthase in response to hypoxia both result in an increase in total renal blood flow, and inhibition of prostaglandin synthesis with indomethacin has a significant negative impact on GFR. In contrast to the hyperfiltration associated with diabetic nephropathy, however, patients with sickle cell disease tend to have a lower mean arterial pressure when compared with age and ethnicity-matched controls. Heme oxygenase-1 (HO-1) has also been demonstrated to be up-regulated in injured kidneys in response to ongoing haemolysis in SCD. HO-1 is responsible for the conversion of heme to biliverdin with the subsequent release of carbon monoxide (CO). Both biliverdin and CO at these levels are potent antioxidants, and the carbon monoxide acts locally as a vasorelaxant thus increasing both total renal blood flow and GFR.

Although it is not clear whether early or prolonged hyperfiltration is pathogenic in the aetiology of CKD, it is very common. Seventy-one per cent of adults were found to have an estimated GFR (eGFR) ≥140 mL/min/1.73 m^2 in a cross-sectional study of our own patient group, a finding in keeping with that of others [6]. Although only a small proportion of these patients would be expected to develop progressive CKD, GFR does begin to decline in most people with SCD over the age of 30, and in a recent study of an elderly cohort of patients in Jamaica, those who had died over the age of 60, chronic renal failure was cited as the major cause of death in 43 % making CKD the most frequent fatal complication in this age group [7]. Although this is a circumstantial evidence, in CKD due to SCN, it is probable that hyperfiltration plays a role in the pathogenesis of progressive renal dysfunction, as it does in other renal diseases such as diabetic nephropathy.

Microalbuminuria and Proteinuria

The appearance of albumin in the urine at levels above those detected in normal individuals is another early manifestation of SCN and can be detected in some patients from late childhood. In our own cohort, microalbuminuria (as defined as a urinary albumin/creatinine ratio of ≥4.5 mg/mmol) is detectable in approximately 28 % of patients in the 15–26 age group, 38 % in the 26–35 s, 50 % in the 36–45 s and >60 % in the over 46 s [6]. In some patients, microalbuminuria can develop into frank proteinuria (protein/creatinine ratio (PCR) >50 mg/μmol) occasionally reaching the nephrotic range (>3 g total protein/24 h). Although full-blown nephrotic syndrome is uncommon (at about 4 %), when it does occur, it is associated with a very poor renal prognosis. One rare but recognised cause of sudden-onset nephrotic syndrome that has been described in patients with SCD is recent infection with human parvovirus B19 (HPV B19). In cases that have been biopsied early, the collapsing variant of focal segmental glomerulosclerosis (FSGS) has been found (with or without evidence of direct HPV B19 infection) which is the classical lesion associated with virus-induced glomerulopathy. Although the nephrotic syndrome spontaneously resolves, it often results in progressive renal dysfunction.

Tubular Abnormalities

Hyposthenuria (inability to concentrate urine under conditions of water deprivation) is a phenomenon that is almost universal in people with SCD and also occurs in older people with SCT. It often leads to enuresis in children and can cause marked dehydration. It is primarily caused by sickling in the vasa recta leading to microthrombi, infarction and collateral formation of blood vessels. As a consequence, there is a defect in zonation and countercurrent exchange. Increased endothelin-1 (ET-1) release, results in vasoconstriction but also promotes natriuresis via stimulation of ET type b receptors in the renal-collecting ducts [8]. Although hyposthenuria is reversible by blood transfusion until the age of 10, after this age it becomes irreversible and is associated with a permanently damaged microvasculature [5].

SCD is also associated with both proximal and distal tubular abnormalities. The increase in sodium and water loss from the collecting ducts leads to a reactive increase in sodium and water reabsorption by the proximal tubule. This reabsorption of sodium is the driving force for the reabsorption of other solutes such as phosphate and β2-microglobulin and hence many patients have hyperphosphataemia. Other solutes have a marked increase in proximal tubular secretion, such as creatinine and uric acid. Up to 30 % of the total creatinine excretion can arise from tubular secretion and so creatinine-based formulas for GFR can significantly overestimate renal function in SCD. Cystatin C has been demonstrated to be a more accurate surrogate marker of renal function in both adults and children with SCD, and hence its use is more likely to detect early decline in renal function [9].

Distal tubule function is often impaired leading to reduced potassium and hydrogen ion excretion and an incomplete type IV renal tubular acidosis. Although in steady state this is not normally clinically apparent, unwell patients are often disproportionately acidotic and hyperkalaemic. In most patients, the potassium abnormality is associated with a normally functioning renin/angiotensin/aldosterone pathway, but a few patients have been shown to have hyporeninaemic hypoaldosteronism.

Haematuria

Haematuria is common in both SCD and SCT. It can range from microscopic and painless through visible and painless to visible and painful. It is usually self-limiting but can occasionally be severe enough to require transfusion. Small microinfarcts are often the cause of minor bleeding, but full renal papillary necrosis (RPN) with sloughing of the ischaemic papilla can lead to severe haemorrhage and obstruction and may be complicated by superadded infection. The renal papillae are dependent upon the vasa recta for their blood supply and are therefore particularly susceptible to ischaemic insults due to localised sickling. RPN can sometimes be diagnosed by ultrasonography but CT urography (or intravenous urography if CT is unavailable) and direct ureterorenoscopy have a much higher diagnostic rate. Due to its self-limiting nature, the management of haematuria is usually conservative and limited to good hydration, pain relief and antibiotics if necessary.

Renal medullary carcinoma is a rare but devastating complication specific to patients with sickle haemoglobinopathies. It is a highly aggressive cancer that can occur in children as young as 2. It is most often metastatic at presentation, and although it may initially respond to chemotherapy, it has so far proven to be universally fatal within 2 years of presentation [10].

Investigations

Renal Histology

There is no pathognomonic lesion that defines SCN. Glomerular hypertrophy with distended capillaries is universally found, but is not confined to those who have developed microalbuminuria or proteinuria. Focal and segmental glomerular sclerosis (FSGS) is the most common lesion associated with proteinuria, but is not specific to SCN. Other lesions that have been noted on biopsy include thrombotic microangiopathy (TMA) and membranoproliferative glomerulonephritis (MPGN), lesions also not exclusive to SCN. The only frequently demonstrated interstitial lesion is the presence of abundant haemosiderin granules in proximal tubular epithelial cells. Renal iron deposition has also been noted on magnetic resonance scans in patients with SCD but appears not to be related to total body iron load. Renal iron, however, does appear to be correlated with markers of haemolysis but so far has not been shown to be associated with renal dysfunction or degree of albuminuria.

Management of Sickle Cell Nephropathy

The management of sickle cell nephropathy can be divided into specific therapies targeting sickle cell disease and the general management of chronic kidney disease.

Therapies for Treating Sickle Cell Disease

Sickle cell nephropathy is a chronic complication of SCD; therefore, strategies designed to alleviate the severity of SCD are likely to impact upon the development of SCN.

Blood transfusions, either intermittent or regular, are an established treatment for the management of both acute and chronic complications of sickle cell disease and are regularly used for stroke prevention and in the treatment of acute chest crisis and pulmonary hypertension. However, there is little evidence for the benefits of long-term blood transfusions for the prevention of renal complications. In a retrospective analysis of 120 children with sickle haemoglobinopathies, Alvarez et al. concluded that chronic transfusion protected against the onset of microalbuminuria when commenced before the age of 9 [11]. Becton and colleagues, however, found no difference in the number of children receiving chronic transfusion when comparing those with microalbuminuria to those without [12].

Hydroxycarbamide (HC, also known as hydroxyurea) is a cytotoxic, antimetabolite and the only agent approved for use in SCD although the mode of action is not clear. Clinical benefits include lower rates of pain, acute chest syndrome and need for blood transfusion. Long-term usage has been associated with improved growth and development in children and reduced overall mortality and morbidity in adults. Although some small studies have suggested that it may also be efficacious both in the treatment of children with established SCN and also in preventing its onset, the BABY HUG study (a phase III randomised, placebo-controlled, double-blind study of 193 patients starting HC in infancy between 9 and 17 months) was unable to prove this. It did demonstrate a marked reduction in vasoocclusive crises and hospitalisation episodes in the HC group, but no prevention of hyperfiltration. HC was associated with better urine concentrating ability and less renal enlargement suggesting some benefits to renal function [13].

The only curative treatment currently available for sickle cell disease is allogeneic haematopoietic cell transplantation (HCT). It is usually reserved for children with major complications such as stroke and is not widely available. Although it is probable that HCT recipients who have a good outcome are likely to be protected from developing SCN, most published studies exclude those with established renal disease from receiving this treatment. One small study evaluating the use of HCT in 10 adults with SCD showed no change in renal progression of renal disease at 30 months [14]. From a different perspective, there have been case reports describing HCT as safe in adults with end-stage renal failure suggesting that the presence of advanced SCN should not exclude patients from receiving this treatment if indicated.

Whilst not a treatment for SCD per se, the management of acute painful crises and chronic pain due to disease complications is of paramount importance to patients and clinicians alike. Conflicts over choice and frequency of medications frequently lead to a loss of trust and breakdown of relations, and so it is vitally important to plan ahead and have mutual agreement of pain management strategies in advance. The added burden of CKD has implications for the use of numerous analgesics including nonsteroidal anti-inflammatory drugs (NSAIDs) (which may exacerbate medullary ischaemia accelerating renal decline) and opiate-based medications. Opiates, valuable in the management of SCD, can accumulate in CKD, so careful choice of opiates and monitoring of dose and side effects is required. Advance pain-management planning involving both haematologists and nephrologists is the ideal situation.

Therapies for Treating Chronic Kidney Disease

In common with all causes of CKD, it seems logical to attempt aggressive treatment of hypertension and reduction of proteinuria with blockade of the renin-angiotensin system. Although studies designed to demonstrate the benefit of ACE inhibition in SCN have been small and short-term, the results of these have been positive in reducing proteinuria and hyperfiltration. Although there are no published guidelines, in our own practice we generally recommend the introduction of an ACEi or angiotensin receptor blockers (ARBs) when a patient has a urinary protein/creatinine ratio persistently above 100 mg/μmol. Some patients report a reduction in their frequency of nocturia, presumably as a result of the reduction in GFR that these drugs impart.

Management of Advanced Chronic Kidney Disease

Despite optimal treatment as outlined above, a proportion of patients with SCN will develop progressive CKD. Chronic anaemia and tissue hypoxia are strong drivers for epo synthesis, and SCD patients with normal kidney function often have epo levels well-above the normal range. However when the GFR falls below approximately 60 mL/min, their ability to produce sufficient levels of endogenous epo also begins to decline. Erythropoiesis-stimulating agents (ESAs) can be useful, particularly in combination with HC in patients who are intolerant of HC alone due to reticulocytopenia. Patients with CKD stages 3–4 often require very high doses of ESAs to have an impact on haemoglobin (Hb) levels. Although Hb targets should be lower than in the general CKD population (<10 mg/dL) due to the increased risk of triggering vasoocclusive crises, they are still rarely achieved and most patients become transfusion dependent by the time they reach end-stage renal disease (ESRD). It is often beneficial to continue ESA therapy after the commencement of RRT, however, as this can prolong the interval between red cell transfusions and minimise the risks of iron overload.

In patients who develop progressive renal dysfunction secondary to SCN, the rate of decline can be quite rapid once the GFR falls below 40 mL/min/1.73 m^2 and so timely preparation for renal replacement therapy (RRT) is very important. Multiple admissions to hospital often result in very poor peripheral veins, so access planning needs to be expert. Outcome data for patients with SCN on dialysis are few, but Powars reported that ESRD is associated with a very poor prognosis as not only was the average age of those reaching ESRD is very young (23.1 in those with HbSS disease), but the mean time to death after reaching ESRD was only 4 years despite being on haemodialysis [15]. Saxena et al. who retrospectively compared a group of 11 patients with SCD in Saudi Arabia to 192 patients with renal failure due to other causes, reported a similar finding. Those with SCD suffered more infectious complications, lived on average for only 27 months after commencing RRT and were significantly younger when they died (31 versus 47.8) [16]. A larger scale comparison was done by Abbott et al. using the US Renal Data System looking at all patients who commenced RRT between 1992 and 1997. They found that not only was SCN an independent risk factor for death, worse even than diabetes, but patients with SCD were much less likely to receive a kidney transplant [17].

Although there may be many obstacles in the path to kidney transplantation, it is probably the modality that offers the best outcome for patients with SCD requiring RRT. In Abbott's study, SCN ceased to be an independent risk factor for death after transplantation. Scheinman and colleagues also report an analysis of the US data system and conclude that although long-term graft and patient survival were not quite as good as for patients with other causes of renal failure, the prognosis for individuals with SCN is far better after transplantation with a projected 7-year survival of 67 % (versus 83 % for other African American) when compared with a 10-year survival of only 14 % for those who remain on dialysis [2].

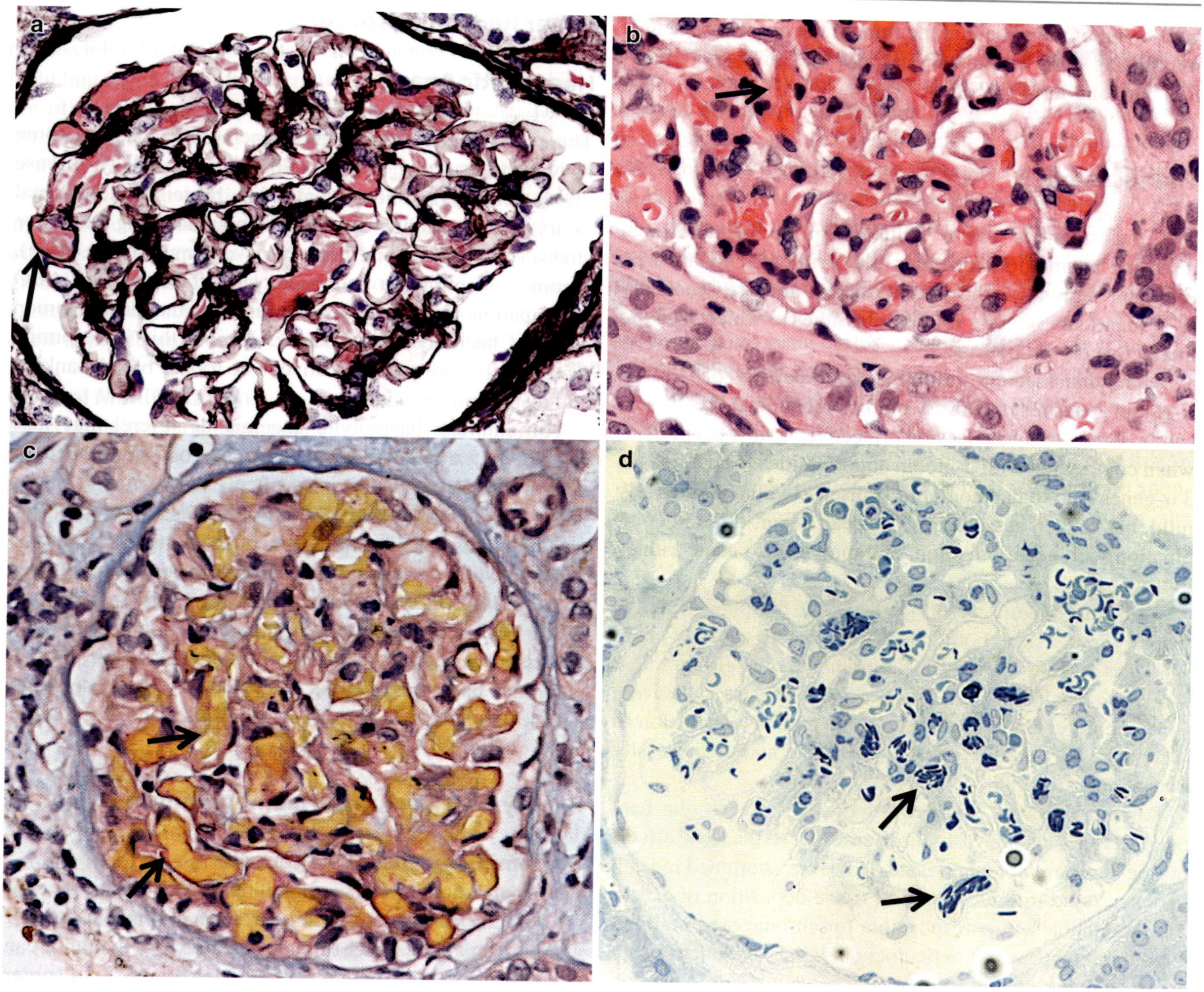

Fig. 31.1 Acute sickle glomerulopathy: a biopsy of a kidney transplant demonstrating glomerular capillary tufts congested with sickle-shaped red blood cells (*arrow heads*). (**a**) Silver stain; (**b**) haemotoxylin and eosin; (**c**) picro-Mallory trichrome; and (**d**) toluidine blue

Management of the Transplanted Patient

In our experience, the major complications following transplantation in patients with SCD are sepsis, an increase in painful crises and acute renal sickling, and their increased susceptibility to infection should be borne in mind when considering the management of acute rejection. Patients with ESRD receiving RRT experience very few painful crises, probably as a result of severe anaemia and relatively frequent blood transfusions. Following transplantation, there is a significant rise in the haemoglobin, and this has been accompanied by an increase in the number of painful crises experienced by the patients. Acute intrarenal sickling has been demonstrated as a cause for a sudden deterioration in renal function posttransplantation in homozygote SCD and interestingly also in heterozygotes (Fig. 31.1). To minimise the risk, we recommend that patients with SCD receive a top-up transfusion preoperatively if very anaemic or red cell exchange with a view to reducing the HbS to <30 % prior to transplantation. Although no evidence base exists, we feel it is reasonable to offer regular, preferably exchange transfusion postoperatively to patients with either evidence of acute sickle nephropathy in their transplanted kidney or to those who have lost a graft previously to recurrent SCN. Some physicians would offer long-term regular exchange transfusion postoperatively to all patients, regardless of previous history, with a view to preserving allograft function. For this reason, it is important that there is good communication between the haematologists and nephrologists caring for patients who are being prepared for renal transplantation. Advanced, individualised planning can both increase the remaining patients is haematopoietic cell transplantation. However, the treatment of PNH has recently been transformed by the development of eculizumab, a humanised monoclonal antibody that binds to the C5 component of complement and inhibits terminal complement activation. This drug not only improves the signs and symptoms associated with the disease, it also improves life expectancy and has specifically been shown to improve or stabilise kidney function in patients with established renal disease secondary to PNH [23, 24].

Malaria

The most common pattern of renal disease is the acute kidney injury caused by *P. falciparum* (and rarely *P. vivax*) infection in adults (malarial acute renal failure, MARF). Although uncommon in native inhabitants in endemic regions, it affects 25–30 % of nonimmune non-natives who become infected [25]. The pathogenesis of MARF is multifactorial but occurs alongside severe haemolysis in approximately 70 % of cases. This may be associated with intense jaundice which, along with haemoglobinuria, leads to the dark discoloration of urine know as "black water fever". This is a severe complication of malaria, often occurring in a context of multiorgan failure and has a high mortality rate.

Glucose-6-Phosphate Dehydrogenase Deficiency

Glucose-6-phosphate dehydrogenase (G6PD) deficiency is a common X-linked genetic disorder that, like the haemoglobinopathies, has survived due to its protective nature against malaria infection. G6PD is central in the antioxidant defence of the red blood cell and hence affected individuals suffer acute haemolytic anaemia when exposed to drugs with a high redox potential or following ingestion of fava beans. Severe acute haemolysis has, on rare occasions, been associated with episodes of acute kidney injury. Table 31.2 includes a list of drugs to be avoided in patients with G6PD, though this is not exhaustive.

White Blood Cell Disorders and the Kidney

Acute kidney injury (AKI) and chronic kidney disease (CKD) are frequent accompaniments to lymphoproliferative disorders and a common cause for referral or liaison between haematologists and nephrologists. There are a myriad of pathological processes resulting in renal dysfunction in these patients and they represent a challenging and fascinating clinic group.

Table 31.2 Drugs to be avoided in patients with G6PD deficiency

Drugs unsafe for all patients with G6PD deficiency	Drugs unsafe in some patients with G6PD deficiency
Acetanilid	Aspirin in high doses
Dapsone and other sulfones	Chloroquine (acceptable in acute malaria and malaria prophylaxis)
Furazolidone	Menadione, water-soluble derivatives
Methylthioninium chloride (Methylene blue)	Probenecid
Nalidixic acid	Quinidine (acceptable in acute malaria)
Naphthalene (mothballs, henna)	Quinine (acceptable in acute malaria)
Niridazole	
Nitrofurantoin	
Phenazopyridine	
Phenylhydrazine	
Primaquine	
Quinolones	
Sulfonamides	
Toluidine blue	
Trinitrotoluene	
Uricase (rasburicase, pegloticase)	

Although there may be considerable overlaps, renal dysfunction in this setting can be broadly divided into causes secondary to toxins, sepsis and direct involvement as shown in Table 31.3

Exogenous Toxins

During the treatment of haematological malignancies, patients are inevitably exposed to a variety of medications with direct nephrotoxic effects such as antivirals (foscarnet, acyclovir, ganciclovir, cidofovir), aminoglycosides and amphotericin, and it is clearly critical to monitor renal function closely and be responsive in terms of dose adjustment in the face of rapidly changing GFRs. Some chemotherapeutic agents, classically cisplatinum, methotrexate, vincristine (via TMA) and ifosfamide, are also nephrotoxic as may be the use of ionising radiation.

The incidence of direct radiation nephritis has reduced dramatically with effective shielding of the kidneys, but when tumours (haematological and non-haematological) are located near the kidney, collateral damage is likely. This can result in acute radiation nephritis, an aggressive and progressive nephropathy, which occurs 6–12 months after radiation exposure and is associated with proteinuria, hypertension and renal impairment. Light microscopy demonstrates endothelial cell swelling, and mesangiolysis with capillary wall microaneurysmal change. Over time, the areas of mesangiolysis become collagen-filled imparting a lobular appearance to the glomeruli, and there is reduplication of the glomerular basement membrane due to subendothelial expansion.

Table 31.3 Causes of renal dysfunction secondary to WBC disorders

Causes
1. Exogenous toxins
(a) Chemotherapy
(b) Radiation nephropathy and thrombotic microangiopathy (TMA) secondary to total body irradiation (TBI)
(c) Antimicrobials
(d) Other medications such as CNIs for the treatment of GvHD, proton pump inhibitors
(e) Iodinated contrast agents
2. Endogenous toxins
(a) Tumour lysis syndrome
(b) Hypercalcaemia
(c) Systemic paraneoplastic response, e.g. secondary to IL-6 in Castleman's disease
(d) Paraproteins
(i) Light chains
(ii) Heavy chains
(iii) Cryoglobulins
3. Direct involvement of the kidney (leukaemias, lymphomas, multiple myeloma (MM), Waldenstrom's macroglobulinaemia)
(a) Obstruction
(b) Direct infiltration
(c) Vascular thrombosis
(d) Paraneoplastic vasculitis
(e) Paraneoplastic glomerulonephritis
(f) IgM capillary thrombi (Waldenstrom's and IgM MM)
4. Sepsis
(a) Systemic
(b) Direct renal infection (bacterial, viral, fungal)

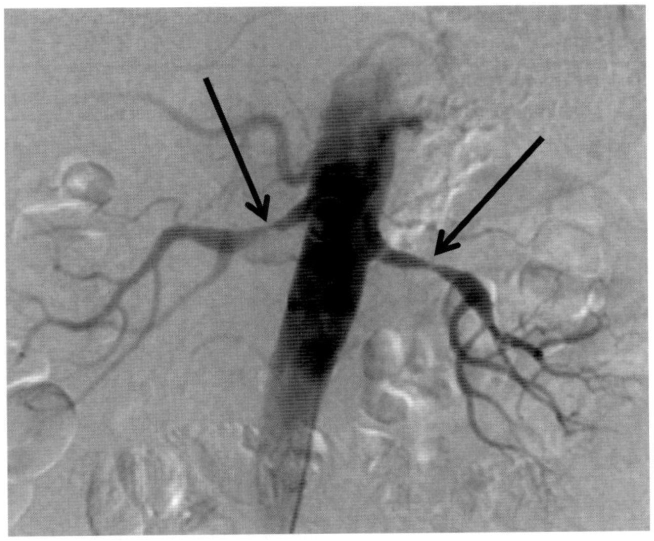

Fig. 31.3 Bilateral renal artery stenosis with poststenotic dilatation (*arrows*) occurring in a patient several years post radiation. The patient presented with recurrent episodes of severe hypertension and AKI, responding on each occasion to angioplasty

Fibrinoid necrosis of small vessel walls is seen. Acute radiation nephritis has a poor prognosis and no known effective treatment. Chronic radiation nephritis appears to be slightly more indolent and is characterised by tubulointerstitial fibrosis and CKD. Hypertension has been reported as a lone finding as has accelerated phase hypertension, with some suggestions that this may be related to radiation-induced small vessel renal artery stenosis (see Fig. 31.3). Even with effective shielding, total body irradiation (TBI) may cause renal dysfunction by provoking a chronic thrombotic microangiopathy (TMA).

Episodes of AKI are common during treatment of haematological malignancies and it is possible that this may result in subclinical CKD. In one study of 187 paediatric bone marrow transplant (BMT) patients in Sweden, renal impairment was present in 41, 31, 11 and 23 % at 1-, 3-, 7- and 10-year follow-up, respectively, with TBI being the single most important risk factor [26].

Endogenous Toxins

Tumour lysis syndrome (TLS) is an important and often preventable cause of AKI and constitutes a medical emergency. It is much more common in haematological than non-haematological malignancies. The incidence varies depending on the definition used, but approximately 10 % of patients with acute lymphocytic leukaemia (ALL) develop severe uric acid nephropathy as do roughly 5 % of patients with non-Hodgkin's lymphoma (NHL) with half these becoming anuric. Both uric acid and phosphate are thought to play a role in the AKI associated with cell lysis, and a spot urinary urate/creatinine ratio of >1 is suggestive of the diagnosis. Risk factors and clinical markers are shown in Table 31.4.

Tumour lysis syndrome may occur spontaneously in patients with a heavy burden of disease but more typically occurs 3–7 days after treatment, though severe hyperkalaemia may be present earlier. If the condition is unidentified or untreated, there is a risk of fulminant hyperkalaemia, arrhythmias, seizures and anuric renal failure with oligo-anuric patients being particularly at risk of these life-threatening complications. Appropriate treatment is supportive in conjunction with intensive monitoring. There is no evidence that alkalinisation of the urine is helpful (urate is more soluble with higher pH) possibly because xanthine, hypoxanthine and calcium phosphate are less soluble in alkaline urine. There are no trials to support early dialysis, but urate and phosphate are rapidly cleared by haemodialysis and so there is a logical argument for early renal replacement therapy (RRT). In a patient with pre-existing renal failure, it is important to anticipate metabolic mayhem and thus prepare for timely RRT.

The incidence of TLS has been dramatically reduced by prophylaxis with pre-hydration and urate reduction treatments. Allopurinol (xanthine oxidase inhibitor) inhibits the oxidation of hypoxanthine to xanthine (and thence to urate);

Hence, the challenge is to develop education, screening and management programmes for diabetes and hypertension and ensure access to subsidised medications. Guidelines specific to a resource-poor setting should be developed, and these may need to include less stringent glycaemic targets and initially focus on those with moderate to severe hypertension. In countries with limited resources, focus is often directed towards acute, symptomatic conditions; however, successful chronic disease management programmes have been reported, notably in Cuba, where the well-developed primary care system has produced some of the highest levels of attainment of target blood pressure control in the world [8].

Aetiology and Pathogenesis

Genetic Factors

While hyperglycaemia and hypertension are the two predominant aetiological factors for DN, it is clear that some persons with diabetes develop nephropathy despite good glycaemic and blood pressure control, while conversely others who have poorly controlled risk factors remain free of renal disease. It appears, therefore, that an unfortunate subset of persons with diabetes is genetically predisposed to develop nephropathy. A role for genetic susceptibility is supported by several lines of evidence.

Firstly, the proportion of persons with diabetes who develop nephropathy differs dramatically between ethnic groups. For example, the Pima Indians of North America are not only susceptible to type 2 diabetes, but 50 % of those who develop diabetes also develop nephropathy, a much higher frequency than in other ethnic groups. Secondly, diabetic nephropathy tends to cluster within families: the risk of a second sibling with diabetes developing nephropathy is much greater if the first sibling has already developed nephropathy. Furthermore, the risk of nephropathy is greater if there is a parental history of hypertension or cardiovascular disease, implying that genes which confer risk of hypertension in the general population predispose to nephropathy in people with diabetes. This may, in part, account for the close link between DN and cardiovascular disease.

Despite intensive effort, the genes that confer susceptibility to diabetic nephropathy have yet to be conclusively established; however, it is anticipated that genome-wide association studies may prove fruitful in this regard.

Glycaemic Control

While it has long been clinically apparent that those patients with diabetes who had the poorest glycaemic control were more inclined to develop a range of complications, including nephropathy, it was not until the publication of the Diabetes Control and Complications Trial (DCCT) that a causal link between poor glycaemic control and overt nephropathy [6] and the development of CKD [7] was clearly demonstrated in type 1 diabetes. Similar data for patients with type 2 diabetes were generated from the UK Prospective Diabetes Study (UKPDS) [9].

Hypertension

Tight blood pressure control is at least as important as good glycaemic control in reducing the incidence of nephropathy in patients with diabetes. Indeed, the pre-eminent role of hypertension in promoting progression to advanced diabetic kidney disease is perhaps best illustrated by an interesting experiment of nature. There are two case reports of patients with diabetes and coexisting unilateral renal artery stenosis in which there was no pathological evidence of DN in the kidney downstream of the stenosis, despite severe nephropathy in the contralateral kidney, suggesting that transmission of systemic hypertension to the diabetic glomerulus is a prerequisite for the development of advanced nephropathy. A predominant role for hypertension in preventing progressive renal failure in patients with DN has been confirmed in clinical trials such as the UKPDS study, in which tight blood pressure control was at least as effective as glycaemic control [8].

Renin-Angiotensin Aldosterone System (RAAS) Activation

The intrarenal renin-angiotensin system is activated in patients with diabetes, resulting in an increase in systemic and intraglomerular pressure, which in turn may exacerbate proteinuria. In addition, angiotensin II may directly promote inflammation and increase matrix deposition by activating cytokines such as transforming growth factor-β. Hence, there are theoretical advantages for inhibiting renin-angiotensin system activity, above and beyond lowering of blood pressure. This theory has been supported by the results of clinical trials in which the reduction in the rate of decline in renal function observed with angiotensin-converting enzyme (ACE) inhibition remains significant even after correcting for changes in blood pressure [10].

Natural History and Pathogenesis

Diabetic nephropathy is a slowly progressive disease, typically taking at least 15–20 years from the diagnosis of diabetes to reach end-stage kidney disease. The time frame may be shorter in some people with type 2 diabetes, in whom latent hyperglycaemia may have been present for some time prior to the diagnosis of diabetes. The natural history of DN may be divided into five phases as described by Mogensen (Table 32.1) [11]. The cardinal features are a triad of:

1. Progressive albuminuria: ranging from upper limit of normal through microalbuminuria to nephrotic range proteinuria.
2. Evolving hypertension: subtle abnormalities such as loss of nocturnal dipping precede and predict the onset of albuminuria. Blood pressure progressively increases and by stage 4, three or more agents are often required to achieve target.
3. Declining renal function: in type 1 diabetes, an initial hyperfiltration phase is often observed, which may predict the onset of microalbuminuria. This is followed by an insidious decline in renal function towards end-stage kidney disease.

Pathological Features

Alongside the progressive clinical hallmarks, the glomerular pathology ranges from early increases in basement membrane thickness, through increased mesangial matrix deposition, to nodular and then global glomerulosclerosis. An example of the classical Kimmelstiel-Wilson nodule is shown in Fig. 32.1a. The close relationship between diabetic nephropathy and cardiovascular disease is evident from the observation that features of small vessel injury are common, including intimal arteriolar hyalinosis (Fig. 32.1b) and glomerular fibrin caps, which are due to the insinuation of plasma proteins into the vessel wall. The above findings are highly suggestive, but not pathognomonic of DN. Indeed, such findings have also been observed in patients with severe obesity, but who are not diabetic. While much attention is focused on the glomerular findings, the degree of tubular atrophy, tubulointerstitial fibrosis and inflammation is generally a better predictor of clinical outcome [12].

Table 32.1 Stages of diabetic kidney disease

Stage	Duration diabetes (years)	Blood pressure (mmHg)	Proteinuria (albumin/creatinine ratio mg/mmol)	Renal function (ml/min/1.73 m^2)	Pathology
1.Hyperfiltration	<3	Normal	<3	>100	Glomerulomegaly
2.Silent	3–5	Loss of nocturnal dipping	<3	100	Increased basement membrane thickness
3.Microalbuminuria	5–10	Borderline increase	3–30[a]	100	Increased mesangial deposition
4.Overt nephropathy	15–20	Overt hypertension	>30 to overtly nephrotic	15–100	Mild (nodular) glomerulosclerosis and tubulointerstitial fibrosis
5.End-stage kidney disease	>20	Overt hypertension	>30 to overtly nephrotic	<15	Marked glomerulosclerosis and tubulointerstitial fibrosis

Modified from Mogensen [11]
[a]2.5–30 in females or 3.5–30 in males

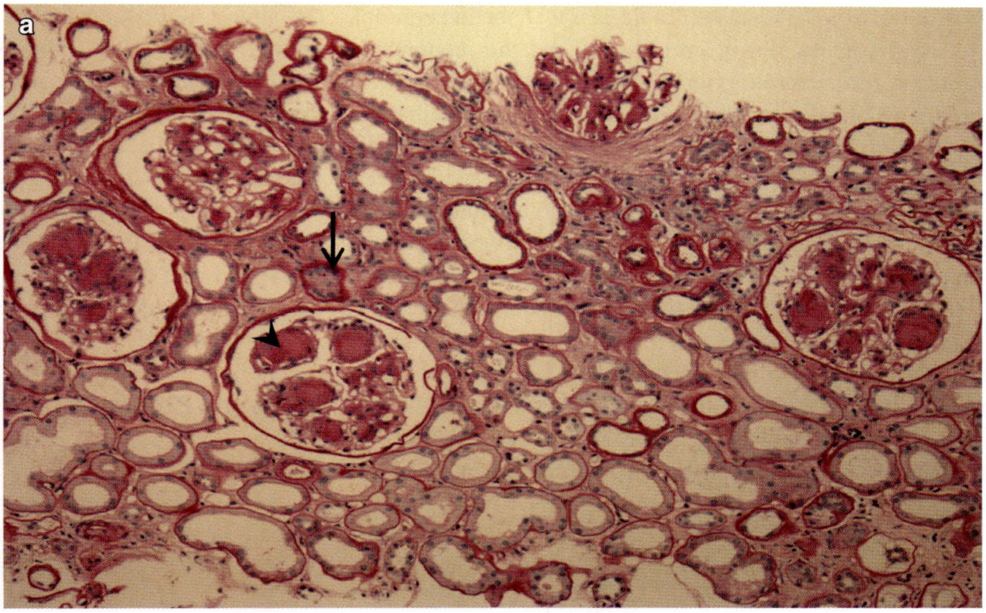

Fig. 32.1 Renal biopsy from a patient with diabetic nephropathy demonstrating (**a**) classical nodular glomerulosclerosis (Kimmelstiel-Wilson lesion, *arrowhead*), tubular atrophy and tubulointerstitial fibrosis including thickening of the tubular basement membrane (*arrow*) and (**b**) arteriolar hyalinosis (*arrow*) (Images courtesy of Dr Chris Bellamy, Consultant Pathologist, Royal Infirmary of Edinburgh)

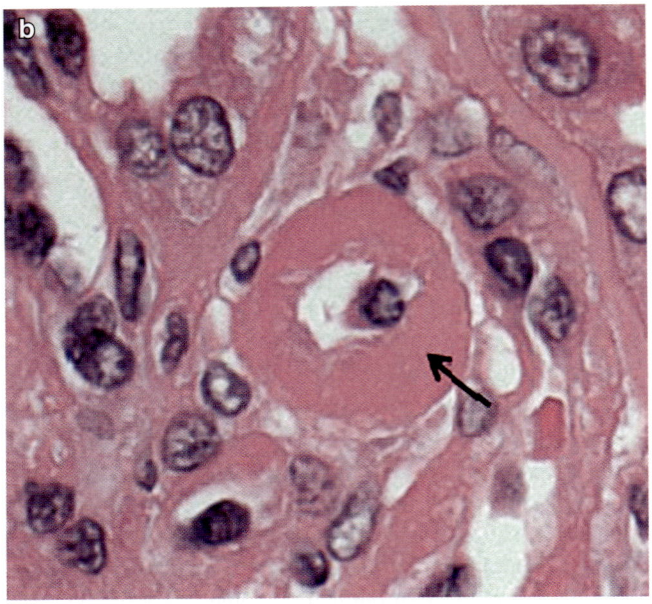

Fig. 32.1 (continued)

Diagnosis

The first clinical evidence of diabetic nephropathy is generally the onset of microalbuminuria, defined as an albumin/creatinine ratio in the range 2.5–30 mg/mmol for females and 3.5–30 mg/mmol for males in at least 2 out of 3 successive measurements. Annual screening for microalbuminuria should be performed within 5 years of the diagnosis of type 1 diabetes and from the time of diagnosis in patients with type 2 diabetes as latent diabetes may have been present for some time prior to diagnosis. Diabetic nephropathy is usually diagnosed on clinical grounds, with relatively few patients undergoing renal biopsy, which is reserved for those patients with features of atypical disease (Table 32.2). Diabetic nephropathy is classically slowly progressive, and the predominant rationale for performing renal biopsy is atypically fast progression of disease such as a sudden increase in proteinuria or a rapid decline in renal function or in those with overt nephropathy within 5 years of diagnosis of type 1 diabetes. Such features suggest the presence of another intrinsic renal disease. Retinopathy is present in up to 80 % of patients at the time of diagnosis of nephropathy; therefore, the absence of retinopathy highlights the need to consider an alternative diagnosis, but on its own, it is rarely an indication for biopsy. Similarly, microscopic haematuria may be observed in diabetic kidney disease, but again its presence suggests the need to consider alternative diagnoses. People over 50 years old who have unexplained microscopic haematuria should be referred for further urological investigation.

While microalbuminuria is classically recognised as the earliest clinically apparent feature of diabetic nephropathy, a progressive early decline in renal function, it is important to note that DN may also be observed in normoalbuminuric patients with type 1 diabetes. Furthermore, the reduction in renal function in normoalbuminuric patients may be associated with typical structural changes of diabetic nephropathy, suggesting that diabetic nephropathy, rather than an alternative diagnosis, remains the predominant mode of renal injury in these normoalbuminuric patients. In type 2 diabetes, almost 75 % of patients who have an eGFR <60 ml/min/1.73 m^2 remain normoalbuminuric [13]. Here, the absence of microalbuminuria may reflect the more heterogeneous nature of renal injury in type 2 diabetes, with a higher prevalence of nondiabetic renal disease such as hypertensive and ischaemic nephrosclerosis. These findings highlight that, in addition to screening for albuminuria, an assessment of renal function should be performed on an annual basis in patients with both type 1 and type 2 diabetes.

Table 32.2 Clinical features that may indicate the need for renal biopsy

Rapid increase in proteinuria
Rapid decline in renal function
Presence of haematuria
Absence of retinopathy
Presence of systemic symptoms

Management

Management should be aimed at reducing the rate of progression of nephropathy and the incidence of cardiovascular disease. Encouragingly, recent studies have suggested that regression of diabetic kidney disease may occur following intensive blood sugar and blood pressure control. In a study of almost 400 patients with type 1 diabetes and microalbuminuria, only 15 % progressed to overt proteinuria after 6 years' follow-up, with 40 % regressing to normoalbuminuria and the remaining 45 % exhibiting persistent microalbuminuria [14]. Factors that predicted regression included tight blood glucose and blood pressure control and low levels of lipidaemia. Perhaps more remarkably, regression of moderate glomerulosclerosis and tubulointerstitial fibrosis may be observed with prolonged normalisation of blood glucose levels following successful pancreatic transplantation.

Lifestyle Factors

All patients should be encouraged to stop smoking, lose weight and take regular exercise. Smoking exacerbates the already high risk of cardiovascular disease in patients with diabetes and kidney disease and may also synergise with poor glycaemic control to increase the rate of decline in renal function. Weight loss and exercise may assist attempts to control glycaemia but may also have independent beneficial effects on the kidney. For example, in patients with type 1 diabetes, each 10 cm increase in waist circumference is associated with a one-third greater risk of developing microalbuminuria, independent of the effects on glycaemic control. While bariatric surgery has been shown to markedly improve glycaemic control [15], no randomised controlled studies have assessed its role in preventing progression of diabetic kidney disease. Salt restriction aids blood pressure control and potentiates the anti-proteinuric effects of RAAS blockade.

Glycaemic Control

Tight glycaemic control is beneficial in reducing the risk of developing nephropathy and other microvascular complications. In people with type 1 diabetes, the DCCT trial demonstrated that a reduction in mean HbA1c from 75 (9.0 %) to 53 mmol/mol (7.0 %) for a 6-year period resulted in a 39 % reduction in the development of microalbuminuria and a 54 % reduction in the development of frank proteinuria [6]. Long-term follow-up of patients from the DCCT trial had shown that this early reduction in albuminuria translates into a subsequent reduction in the risk of CKD (eGFR <60 ml/min/1.73 m^2) [7]. The UKPDS study in type 2 diabetes demonstrated similar findings, with a reduction in mean HbA1c from 63 (7.9 %) to 53 mmol/mol (7.0 %) being associated with an absolute risk reduction of developing microalbuminuria (11 %), proteinuria (3.5 %) and a doubling in serum creatinine over 12 years (2.5 %) [12].

Long-term follow-up of patients from both the DCCT and UKPDS trials has suggested that the beneficial effect of a period of tight control, in terms of the development of complications, persists for many years. In the DCCT cohort, only 9 % of intensively treated patients had developed frank nephropathy after 30 years of type 1 diabetes, compared with 25 % who were conventionally treated [4]. In the UKPDS, after a median period of 17 years' follow-up, patients from the intensively treated cohort demonstrated a relative risk reduction for the development of microvascular disease of 24 % [16]. These findings were noted in spite of the fact that the glycaemic control in the 'intensively treated' and 'conventionally treated' cohorts from both studies converged quite quickly after the cessation of the active treatment phase of the studies. This suggests a considerable 'legacy effect' from a period of tight glycaemic control in both type 1 and type 2 diabetes, and that efforts to optimise control in the first few years after developing diabetes may well pay considerable dividends in reducing the incidence of future complications, even if control slips at a later stage.

Although there is good evidence that tight glycaemic control in both type 1 and type 2 diabetes is associated with a significantly reduced risk of developing diabetic nephropathy, the benefit of this is much less clear cut in patients with established nephropathy. Some studies, including the DCCT [6], indicate that maintaining tight glycaemic control will reduce the risk or rate of progression of nephropathy in patients who already have microalbuminuria. No randomised controlled studies have clearly indicated that intensive glycaemic control slows progression once there is overt proteinuria and a falling glomerular filtration rate. There is, however, some observational data suggesting that even in well-established chronic kidney disease, the decline in renal function may occur at a more rapid rate in those with poor glycaemic control [17]. In addition, maintaining good metabolic control may reduce the risk of development or progression of other microvascular complications of diabetes.

It appears that it is the level of glycaemia achieved, rather than the drugs used to achieve this, which is paramount. The UKPDS included cohorts treated with insulin, two different sulphonylureas and metformin. All achieved similar levels of glycaemia throughout the duration of the study, and there were no significant differences between the groups in terms of microvascular outcomes. No other studies have demonstrated a specific benefit of using one hypoglycaemic agent rather than another in terms of reducing the risk of developing diabetic renal disease, although there is limited data to indicate that pioglitazone may be more beneficial than other drugs in reducing proteinuria. Managing glycaemia in the context of chronic kidney disease does, however, present several other challenges, especially in relation to the choice of glucose-lowering drugs and dose modification.

Glucose-Lowering Drugs in Chronic Kidney Disease

Metformin

Since the publication of the UKPDS, metformin has become the most widely prescribed oral hypoglycaemic agent in patients with type 2 diabetes. This is predominantly because, in a subgroup of 342 overweight and obese patients randomised to intensive therapy with metformin, there was a reduction in all-cause mortality and in a number of major cardiovascular outcomes, including stroke, in comparison to conventional therapy. Although similar trends were seen in patients who were randomised to intensive therapy with sulphonylureas or insulin, the results in these arms of the study did not attain statistical significance. Given the fact that cardiovascular disease is the major cause of excess morbidity and mortality in people with type 2 diabetes, these findings have led to a dramatic increase in the prescription of metformin and it is now the oral hypoglycaemic of choice in overweight patients.

A major concern is that metformin and its metabolites are predominantly renally excreted and thus will accumulate in renal impairment. Furthermore, there is a well-established link between metformin and lactic acidosis, although to what extent metformin is directly causative remains a matter of some speculation. What is clear, however, is that the risk of lactic acidosis increases in the context of acute kidney injury which, in turn, is much more common in those with pre-existing chronic kidney disease.

Previously metformin was widely used by diabetologists in patients whose serum creatinine was 150–200 μmol/l, with few problems. Routine reporting of eGFR, however, led to recommendations that metformin be discontinued in stage 3 CKD. In many cases, this demonstrated just what an effective glucose-lowering agent metformin is in obese patients with type 2 diabetes. Frequently, patients who had had excellent glycaemic control on metformin alone became hyperglycaemic when this drug was stopped. Other oral agents proved less effective and usually led to significant weight gain. Insulin was often required, but despite the use of large doses due to insulin insensitivity, glycaemia remained less tightly controlled than had been achieved on metformin.

Such issues have led to a reassessment of the use of metformin in the context of CKD. There is general agreement that metformin should be avoided when the eGFR drops below 30 ml/min/1.73 m^2, but it is probably safe in most patients with an eGFR >45 ml/min/1.73 m^2. Between 30 and 45 ml/min/1.73 m^2, regular monitoring of renal biochemistry is recommended, and, if renal function is steadily declining, it is appropriate to stop metformin before the eGFR falls to <30 ml/min/1.73 m^2 [18]. Furthermore, as is recommended with ACE inhibitors and angiotensin receptor blockers, people taking metformin should temporarily discontinue the drug when a situation arises which might lead to a temporary deterioration in renal function, e.g. if the patient is suffering from vomiting or diarrhoea or is undergoing a radiological study involving the administration of contrast agents.

Sulphonylureas and Meglitinides

These drugs bind to specific, but different, receptors on the pancreatic beta cell and directly stimulate insulin secretion. As such they are inevitably associated with a risk of hypoglycaemia, and this risk increases in the context of CKD. This is partly due to accumulation of these drugs and their metabolites, as the sulphonylureas are predominantly renally excreted, with the exception of gliquidone. Longer-acting sulphonylureas, such as glibenclamide, are probably best avoided completely, and the dose of other shorter-acting agents may need to be reduced.

Meglitinides, with their shorter duration of action than sulphonylureas, have been promoted largely in relation to targeting postprandial hyperglycaemia, but have not been widely embraced, at least in the UK, due to the need for multiple daily dosing. These drugs may, however, be considered as a useful alternative to sulphonylureas in the context of CKD, especially repaglinide, which is predominantly hepatically metabolised.

Pioglitazone

Pioglitazone is now the only thiazolidinedione available in the UK. It is a peroxisome proliferator-activated receptor-gamma (PPARγ) agonist, with multiple metabolic effects, including increasing insulin sensitivity. It is metabolised by the liver and is hence potentially a useful drug in people with CKD. However, pioglitazone is associated with fluid retention and contraindicated in the presence of congestive cardiac failure. More recently identified concerns with pioglitazone relate to an increased risk of osteoporosis, especially in postmenopausal women and additionally bladder cancer.

Insulin

In addition to patients with type 1 diabetes, many patients with type 2 diabetes who develop CKD will have had diabetes for a long period of time and will already be on insulin therapy, with or without additional oral blood glucose-lowering drugs. As the liver and kidneys are the major sites of insulin clearance/degradation, the half-life of insulin is prolonged in patients with CKD, and therefore, there is a greater risk of hypoglycaemia during insulin therapy. The healthy kidney is responsible for approximately one-quarter of the body's gluconeogenesis; therefore, a reduction in gluconeogenesis in patients with CKD adds to the hypoglycaemia risk. Additionally, in patients with both type 1 and type 2 diabetes of long duration, there is an increased prevalence of loss of hypoglycaemic awareness, with a corresponding increase in the frequency of severe hypoglycaemic episodes. Hence, many patients on insulin will need to have their doses dramatically reduced as their renal function declines and some, even those with type 1 diabetes, will have very low insulin requirements. With the increased risk of hypoglycaemia, maintaining tight glycaemic control may become impractical and unsafe, and the optimal target needs to be considered on an individual patient basis.

Newer Glucose-Lowering Drugs

Glucagon-Like Peptide-1 (GLP-1) Agonists

These drugs mimic native GLP-1 and have multiple actions, including stimulation of glucose-dependent insulin secretion and inhibition of glucagon secretion. They also delay gastric emptying and increase satiety. In spite of the fact that they need to be administered by subcutaneous injection, GLP-1 agonists have become very popular amongst some diabetologists and patients with type 2 diabetes because, in addition to improving glycaemic control, they are the only glucose-lowering drugs available which promote weight loss.

The two most established drugs in this class are exenatide, which is available as twice-daily and once-weekly formulations, and liraglutide, which is administered once daily. Exenatide is predominantly excreted renally, and, as such, it is not recommended for use in patients with an eGFR <30 ml/min/1.73 m^2, and caution is advised in patients with an eGFR between 30 and 50 ml/min/1.73 m^2; this may include not titrating the drug up to its usual maximum dose. Liraglutide, by contrast, is not predominantly renally excreted; nonetheless, the current recommendation is that this drug is not used in those with stage 3 or more severe CKD as there is limited therapeutic experience in such patients. A third drug, lixisenatide, was licensed by the European Medicines Agency in early 2013. Current recommendations are that, because of lack of therapeutic experience, this drug should be used with caution in patients with a creatinine clearance between 30 and 50 ml/min/1.73 m^2 and it is not recommended in those with more severe CKD.

Dipeptidyl Peptidase-4 (DPP-4) Inhibitors

DPP-4 is the enzyme which inactivates GLP-1; therefore, DPP-4 inhibitors enhance GLP-1 levels by slowing down its degradation, but unlike the currently available GLP-1 agonists, these drugs are active orally. They are generally well tolerated and weight neutral; however, clinical experience is that they are often rather less potent glucose-lowering agents than other available drugs and our own experience has been that gastrointestinal side effects, such as nausea and vomiting may be more common with these agents in patients with CKD. Several drugs in this class are potentially useful even in patients with advanced CKD.

Vildagliptin is metabolised hepatically, but current recommendations are that it is not used in patients with moderate or severe renal disease, defined as a creatinine clearance of <50 ml/min/1.73 m^2. Sitagliptin and saxagliptin are both safe in patients with CKD, but a reduced dose is recommended. The usual sitagliptin dose of 100 mg daily should be reduced to 50 mg daily in stage 3 CKD and to 25 mg daily when the eGFR is <30 ml/min/1.73 m^2 (including patients on dialysis). The dose of saxagliptin should be reduced from 5 to 2.5 mg daily in patients with moderate or severe renal disease, again defined as a creatinine clearance of <50 ml/min. The most recently licensed drug in this class, linagliptin, is safe in all degrees of renal impairment, including end-stage renal disease, and no dose reduction is required.

Sodium-Glucose Co-transporters

Most filtered glucose is reabsorbed by the SGLT-2 co-transporter in the proximal tubules. Several drugs inhibiting the action of this co-transporter are being developed, and the first of these, dapagliflozin, has recently been licensed for use in the UK. This group of drugs act by promoting glycosuria and hence calorie loss. Early studies suggest that, while these drugs are effective in reducing HbA1c, there is a significantly increased prevalence of genital infections and a lesser risk of bacterial infections of the more proximal urinary tract, which would clearly be undesirable in the context of CKD. In addition, by promoting an osmotic diuresis, these drugs reduce intravascular fluid volume. Although a relatively modest effect, this may be more significant in the context of CKD, especially during any acute intercurrent event which might have an adverse effect on circulating volume, e.g. a bout of vomiting or diarrhoea. Furthermore, the effect of these drugs is likely to be diminished in the context of renal impairment. Dapagliflozin is not advised in patients with an eGFR of <60 ml/min/1.73 m^2, and it seems unlikely that any of these drugs will be recommended for use in patients with stage 3–5 CKD.

Blood Pressure Control

Tight blood pressure control is at least as important as glycaemic control in slowing progression of diabetic kidney disease. In the UKPDS, a reduction in blood pressure from 154/87 to 144/82 resulted in a 37 % risk reduction for microvascular events. However, in contrast to the management of hyperglycaemia, the benefit of tight blood pressure control tends to recede with time, emphasising the need for strict ongoing blood pressure control in preventing progressive DN.

In general, a reasonable target should be to reduce blood pressure to below 130/80 mmHg; however, extrapolating from the evidence obtained in nondiabetic patients from the Modification of Diet in Renal Disease Study [19], those with protein excretion of >1 g/day may benefit from a lower BP target of 125/75 mmHg. It is likely that polypharmacy will be required to achieve target blood pressure, as 29 % of patients in the tight BP control arm of the UKPDS trial required three or more antihypertensive agents [8].

n
r
s
b
ne
an
in

inc

Pregnancy and the Kidney

33

Graham W. Lipkin, Clara J. Day, Nerissa Jurawan,
Tracey A. Johnston, and Ellen M. Knox

Pregnancy in Women with Kidney Disease

Chronic kidney disease (CKD) is often clinically silent until renal function declines to less than 25 % of normal. CKD stages 1 and 2 (normal or mildly impaired renal function and abnormal albuminuria or structural kidney damage) affect roughly 3 % of women of child-bearing age, whilst stages 3–5 (GFR <60 ml/min) affect just less than 1 % of women in this age group [1]. Enhanced antenatal monitoring in pregnancy and increased complication rates offer an opportunity to identify women with hitherto unrecognised CKD in early pregnancy. Furthermore, around 20 % of women who develop severe early-onset (<30 weeks) pre-eclampsia (PET) have underlying CKD as the predisposing cause [2]. Whilst live birth outcomes have improved, pregnancies in women with CKD are at high risk for maternal and fetal morbidity and mortality. Their management is complex, and successful outcomes are optimised by collaborative antenatal care in regular joint clinics of nephrologist and maternal/fetal medicine specialist. All women with CKD contemplating pregnancy should be offered review in a joint preconception counselling clinic in order to plan pregnancy and optimise outcomes. This chapter explores maternal and fetal outcomes in women with CKD and offers guidance on optimal pregnancy management. The evidence base is limited being dominated by small, often retrospective uncontrolled studies highlighting the need to contribute to developing registry studies in this area.

G.W. Lipkin, MBChB, BSc, MD, FRCP (✉)
Department of Nephrology, Queen Elizabeth Hospital Birmingham, University Hospital Birmingham NHS Foundation Trust, Mindelsohn Way, Edgbaston, Birmingham B15 2WB, UK
e-mail: graham.lipkin@uhb.nhs.uk

C.J. Day, BMBCh, MA, PhD, FRCP
Department of Nephrology, Queen Elizabeth Hospital Birmingham, Edgbaston, Birmingham B15 2WB, UK
e-mail: clara.day@uhb.nhs.uk

N. Jurawan, MBBS,MRCP (UK)
Renal Medicine, University Hospital Birmingham, Mindelsohn Way, Edgbaston, Birmingham B15 2WB, UK
e-mail: njurawan@gmail.com

T.A. Johnston, MD, FRCOG • E.M. Knox, MBChB, MD, MRCOG
Department of Obstetrics, Birmingham Women's NHS Foundation Trust, Mindelsohn Way, Edgbaston, Birmingham B15 2TG, UK
e-mail: tracey.johnston@bwhct.nhs.uk; ellen.knox@bwhct.nhs.uk

Physiological Changes in Pregnancy

Normal pregnancy results in profound changes in renal and cardiovascular physiology. These changes are also mirrored in women with chronic kidney disease (CKD) albeit to a diminishing extent with the greater severity of CKD, reflecting reduced renal reserve, and this may underlie frequent adverse pregnancy outcomes [3–5]. It is important to recognise these changes in order to appropriately interpret the results of laboratory tests during pregnancy; the normal upper limit for serum creatinine falls to <70 umol/l, and normal serum sodium concentration falls by 5 mmol/l.

Cardiovascular Physiology in Normal Pregnancy [3]

Substantial vasodilatation leading to reduced systemic vascular resistance (SVR) occurs within 4 weeks of conception reaching a nadir at 40–50 % below baseline in the mid-second trimester which is maintained until delivery. There is a contemporaneous increase in cardiac output of 40 % (due to an increase in stroke volume in early pregnancy and increased heart rate later on). As a consequence in normal pregnancy, blood pressure (BP) falls in the first and second trimesters (sometimes allowing withdrawal of antihypertensives), returning to pre-pregnancy levels in the third trimester. There is no physiological change in cardiac ejection

M. Harber (ed.), *Practical Nephrology*,
DOI 10.1007/978-1-4471-5547-8_33, © Springer-Verlag London 2014

fraction or normal range for central venous pressure or pulmonary capillary wedge pressure during the antenatal period. In later pregnancy, inferior vena caval compression by the gravid uterus may lead to 'supine hypotension'.

Plasma and extracellular fluid volume progressively rises from conception reaching 40–50 % over baseline by 32 weeks. There is a lesser increase in red cell mass of 20–30 %, driven by enhanced renal erythropoietin production resulting in mild dilutional anaemia. A mild degree of oedema is common in normal pregnancy.

Renal Haemodynamic and Structural Changes [5]

Glomerular filtration rate (GFR) rises within 1 month of conception, peaks 40–50 % above baseline levels by the early second trimester and is sustained at this level until 1–2 weeks postpartum. Renal blood flow increases by 80 % falling off to around 60 % by term (Table 33.1 and Fig. 33.1). The rise in GFR (hyperfiltration) is mediated by elevated renal plasma flow (RPF) in the first two trimesters resulting from both pre- and post-glomerular arteriolar dilatation and not by glomerular hypertension. This may explain why multiple pregnancy in women with normal kidney function or those with CKD 1 and 2 is not associated with renal damage. However, in the third trimester, raised GFR is in addition maintained by modest increase in glomerular permeability and reduced intraglomerular oncotic pressure.

The mechanism of pregnancy-induced systemic and renal vasodilatation is incompletely understood, but the ovarian vasodilator hormone relaxin appears to mediate the upregulation of NO-dependent vasodilation via the NO-endothelin-B pathway [3].

Neither the MDRD nor the Cockcroft-Gault formulae are accurate in estimating GFR in pregnancy and should not be used. In an individual, GFR can be tracked across pregnancy by serial creatinine measurements.

Table 33.1 Physiological changes in common indices of renal function in pregnancy [5]

	Stage of pregnancy			
Measure mean (SD)	Before pregnancy	First trimester	Second trimester	Third trimester
Effective renal plasma flow (ml/min)	480 (72)	841 (144)	891 (279)	771 (175)
Glomerular filtration rate (inulin clearance)	105 (24)	162 (19)	174 (24)	165 (22)
Serum creatinine (μmol/l)	73 (10)	60 (8)	54 (10)	64 (9)
Plasma urea (mmol/l)	4.3 (0.8)	3.5 (0.7)	3.3 (0.8)	3.1 (0.7)
Plasma osmolality (mosmol/Kg)	290 (2)	280 (3)	279 (3)	279 (5)
Plasma urate (mmol/l)	246 (2)	189 (48)	214 (71)	269 (956)

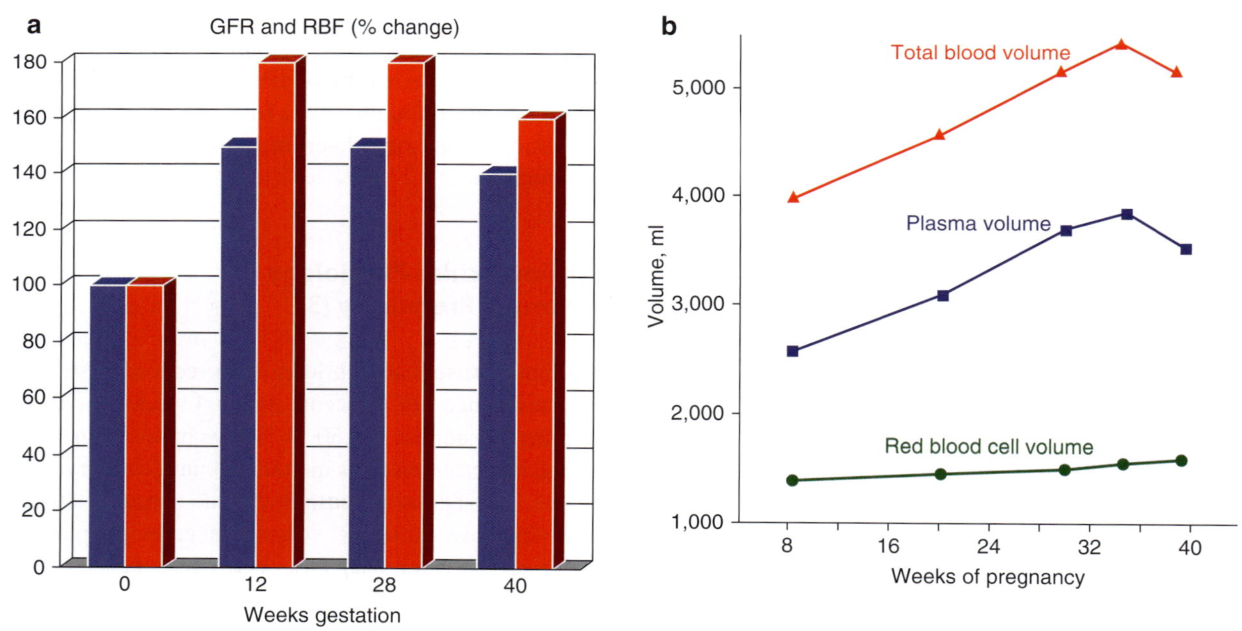

Fig. 33.1 (**a**) Renal haemodynamic (% change of GFR and renal blood flow (*RBF*) from pre-pregnancy values) and (**b**) Blood volume changes in normal pregnancy [5]

Anatomical Changes in Urinary Tract

The kidneys increase in size by 10 % in pregnancy; the minimum normal bipolar length is 10 cm. Pregnancy-related hydronephrosis and hydroureter to the level of pelvic brim are common particularly on the right side (85 %) secondary to reduction of ureteric tone and peristalsis (progesterone) and compression against the pelvic brim by the gravid uterus. In fact the dilated collecting system and ureter may hold 200–300 ml of urine resulting in urinary stasis, a potential reservoir for bacteria which may contribute to the increased risk of pyelonephritis in pregnancy. Differentiation of physiological hydronephrosis from true ureteric obstruction is difficult in pregnancy (see later). In early pregnancy, bladder wall relaxation induced by progesterone may lead to increased capacity although later in pregnancy the enlarging uterus may limit bladder volume. Urinary frequency, urgency and nocturia are common in normal pregnancy and may be associated with urge incontinence.

Tubular Changes

Electrolyte Balance

Total body sodium increases by 3–4 mmol/day resulting in a net positive balance of 900–1,000 mmol over the whole gestation (total body potassium increases by 320 mmol). Exquisite tubular control of sodium balance is achieved in pregnancy, despite the net increase of sodium filtration resulting from 50 % gestational rise in GFR. A fine balance of natriuretic factors (raised GFR, atrial natriuretic peptide and progesterone) versus antinatriuretic factors (aldosterone, deoxycorticosterone and tubuloglomerular feedback) is felt to achieve this critical task.

As a consequence of resetting of the hypothalamic osmostat, plasma osmolality falls by 10 (3) milliosmol/kg in normal pregnancy reflecting a fall in plasma sodium by 5 (2) mmol/l. This change occurs early in pregnancy and correlates closely with increased production of human chorionic gonadotrophin. Enhanced urate excretion in the first two trimesters of pregnancy leads to a fall in serum urate. In the third trimester, serum urate is restored to pre-pregnancy levels. This must be considered if urate levels are used as a maker for PET.

Acid-Base Balance

Progesterone stimulates the central respiratory centres leading to a chronic respiratory alkalosis in pregnancy. The kidney compensates leading to a fall in plasma bicarbonate level.

Pregnancy is associated with profound renal anatomical, haemodynamic, tubular and cardiovascular changes (see Fig. 33.1 and Table 33.1). These have significant implications for the outcome of pregnancy in women with CKD.

Common Themes in the Care of Pregnant Women with Chronic Kidney Disease

Preconception Counselling

This is highly desirable for all women with renal disease. It is optimally provided in a dedicated combined clinic led by an obstetrician and nephrologist. In this setting, the nephrologist and obstetrician learn to speak the same language and recognise each other's anxieties in the care of these patients. Major advances in neonatal intensive care have dramatically improved perinatal mortality over the last 40 years. Counselling should cover:

1. Contraceptive advice (see later)
2. How might pregnancy affect maternal kidney function
3. How might kidney disease affect pregnancy outcomes
4. Optimal timing of pregnancy to improve maternal/fetal outcomes
5. Pre-pregnancy modification of drug therapy to those known to be safe
6. Assessment of comorbidity, e.g. diabetes, cardiopulmonary disease, renal/bladder structure
7. General preparation for pregnancy including folic acid (400 ug daily) 3 months prior to conception until 12 weeks of pregnancy, smoking cessation and weight loss targeting an ideal BMI

Hypertension in Pregnancy

The definitions of hypertension and classification of severity are listed in Table 33.2. BP measurement should be taken in sitting position using a validated oscillometric device or manual reading to Korotkov 5 (www.nice.org.uk/nicemedia/live/11947/40115/40115.pdf). Hypertensive disorders in pregnancy affect 10 % of women and are a major cause of maternal morbidity and a leading cause of maternal death. They lead to greater perinatal morbidity and mortality by increasing the risk of preterm birth, fetal growth restriction and placental abruption [7]. Management of chronic essential or gestational hypertension is beyond the scope of this chapter, but guidelines have recently been developed by the UK National Institute for Health and Clinical Excellence (NICE CG 107) [6].

Antihypertensive Drugs

All antihypertensive drugs cross the placenta, and their half-life in pregnancy is reduced (labetalol T 1/2 is reduced to 1.7 h). Women with hypertension should receive preconception counselling and ideally be established pre-pregnancy on labetalol or nifedipine LA or be converted as soon pregnancy

Table 33.2 Definitions of hypertension and of its severity in pregnancy [6]

Definitions	Presentation (weeks)	Significant proteinuria[a]	Prevalence (%)
Chronic hypertension	<20	No	2
Gestational hypertension	>20	No	4–8
Pre-eclampsia (PET)	>20	Yes	4.1[b]/1.7[c]
PET superimposed on chronic hypertension	>20	Yes	<1
Severity of hypertension			
		Systolic BP (mmHg)	Diastolic BP (mmHg)
Mild		140–149	90–99
Moderate		150–159	100–109
Severe		>160	>110

[a]Significant proteinuria is >300 mg in a validated 24-h urine collection or urine PCR >30 mg/mmol
[b]First pregnancy
[c]Second pregnancy

Table 33.3 Antihypertensive agent use in pregnancy [7]

Drugs commonly used	**Dose**	**Comments**
Labetalol	100–400 mg PO twice to four times daily (max dose 1,200 mg/day)	First line unless contraindications, e.g. asthma
Methyldopa	250–500 mg orally two to four times daily (max dose 2 g/day)	Maternal side effects may limit dose
Nifedipine (LA)	Long-acting preparation preferred 30–120 mg/day	May aggravate pedal oedema
Drugs to be avoided	**Comments**	
Converting enzyme inhibitors (ACEi) or angiotensin receptor blockers (ARB)	Teratogenic in second and third trimester	Recent data indicates no increase in teratogenicity if stopped in first trimester. Ideally stabilise on drugs in table above preconception [8]
Atenolol	Preferential use of labetalol	May be associated with fetal growth restriction
Diuretics	Avoid in pregnancy	May limit physiological increase in plasma volume Chlorothiazide may be teratogenic [6]

is confirmed [7]. Comments on antihypertensive therapy in pregnancy are listed in Table 33.3. Recent meta-analysis comparing different agents in pregnancy identified beta blockers, predominantly labetalol to be more effective than methyldopa in controlling BP. No other differences in pregnancy outcomes were shown between agents [9].

Angiotensin-Converting Enzyme Inhibitors (See Fig. 33.2)

Outside of pregnancy, angiotensin-converting enzyme inhibitors (ACEi) or angiotensin receptor blockers (ARB) are used as first-line treatment for proteinuric CKD. However, continuation of ACEi or ARB in the second and third trimester is associated with a specific fetopathy comprising oligohydramnios, neonatal renal failure, neural tube defects and cardiac abnormalities and should be avoided [8] (Fig. 33.2). A study involving almost half a million pregnancies recorded in the Kaiser Permanente database in Northern California revealed an increased risk of congenital malformations in hypertensive women exposed to ACE inhibitors in the first trimester. However, the magnitude was the same as those receiving other antihypertensives or no BP treatment at all. It therefore appears that hypertension per se in the first trimester is associated with increased risk of birth defects with no additional adverse impact of ACEi *in the first trimester* [8].

As a rule, women with hypertension receiving ACEi who are considering pregnancy should be stabilised on antihypertensives known to be safe in pregnancy before conception (Table 33.3). Some women may take some considerable time to conceive, and those denied ACE inhibitors whilst trying for pregnancy may as a consequence suffer unnecessary renal decline which itself would have a substantial adverse effect upon pregnancy outcome. Women who have a strong indication for the use of ACE inhibitors, such as those with CKD and heavy proteinuria, may be advised to continue on the ACEi until conception. On the finding of a positive pregnancy test, they should be converted to labetalol, nifedipine long acting or methyldopa.

Outside of pregnancy, the benefit of tight BP control in patients with CKD is well established; target BP is <140/90 or <130/80 for those with significant proteinuria (http://www.nice.org.uk/nicemedia/live/12069/42119/42119.pdf). Optimal antenatal target BP in women with mild uncomplicated chronic essential or gestational hypertension is unclear. A meta-analysis of 31 RCTs failed to show improved maternal

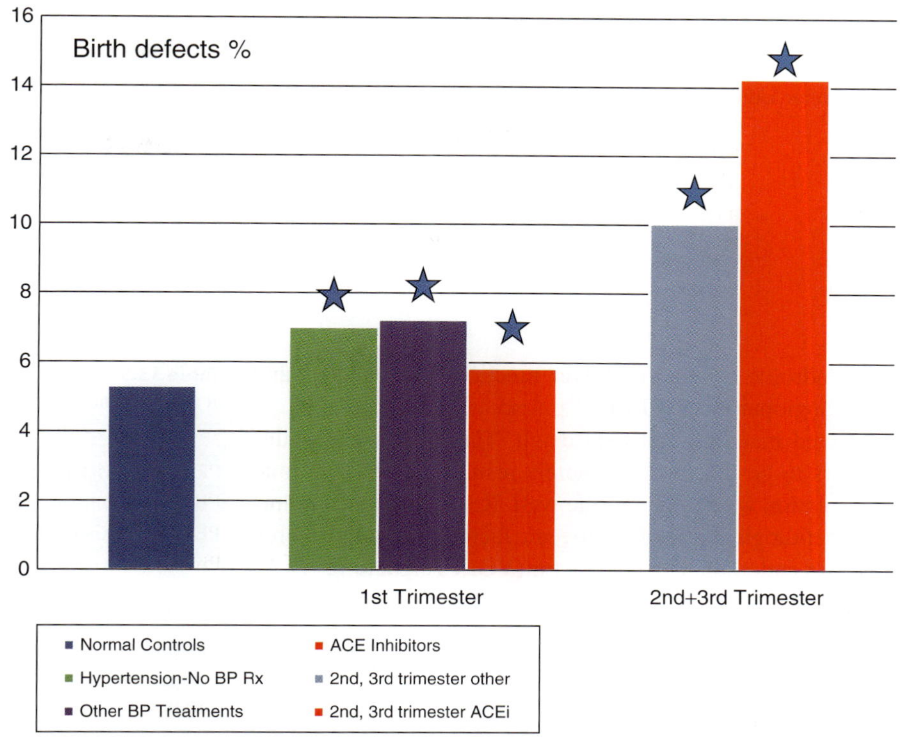

Fig. 33.2 Effect of hypertension treatment with and without ACEi in women treated with ACEi in first, second and third trimester of pregnancy (Reprinted with permission from Li et al. [8])

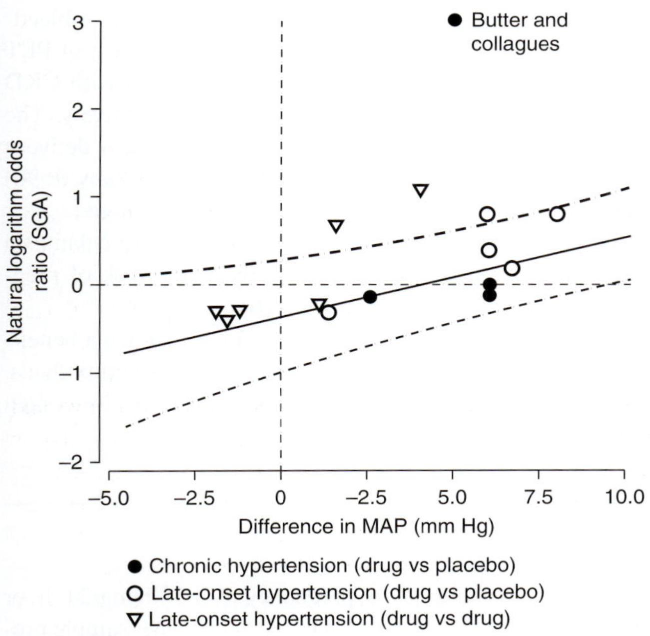

Fig. 33.3 Impact of blood pressure reduction on rate of small for gestational age babies (Reproduced with permission from von Dadelszen et al. [10])

or fetal outcomes of antihypertensive treatment in pregnant women with mild to moderate hypertension who had no evidence of CKD or end organ damage [9]. Indeed overzealous BP lowering may adversely affect fetal growth perhaps by reducing placental blood flow. A significant relationship was described between greater antihypertensive-induced falls in BP and heightened risk of growth-restricted babies in meta-analysis [10] (see Fig. 33.3). In chronic mild/moderate essential hypertension, BP target during pregnancy is <150/100. However, in the setting of renal disease, many authorities recommend lower blood pressure levels, to <140/90 [6]. The Chronic Hypertension in Pregnancy Study (CHIPS) is ongoing and may guide optimal antenatal BP targets.

Differentiation of Pre-eclampsia from Effects of Pregnancy in Women with Chronic Kidney Disease (Table 33.4)

Pre-eclampsia is functionally defined as de novo development of hypertension and proteinuria (>300 mg/day) in the second half (>20 weeks) of pregnancy. It is important to remember that whilst BP may be controlled in severe PET, the only successful treatment is delivery of the baby without which the maternal condition will deteriorate. In practice albeit rare, PET can occur without proteinuria or with proteinuria proceeding hypertension. PET is common and a potentially devastating multisystem capillary leak disorder unique to human pregnancy. Its features include the development of severe hypertension, cerebral oedema and fits (eclampsia), placenta abruption and fetal growth restriction,

Table 33.4 Distinguishing pre-eclampsia (PET) from the effects of pregnancy in women with chronic kidney disease (CKD)

	Pregnancy impact on CKD	Superimposed PET
Onset (weeks)	<20	>20
Rate of change in BP/proteinuria	Days to weeks	Hours to days
Uterine Doppler velocimetry at 24 weeks	Normal	Abnormal 'notching' sometimes
Elevated transaminase and/or low platelets	No	Sometimes
Serum urate	High	High
sFlt/PlGF ratio[a]	Normal	High
Treatment	Support/monitoring	Delivery (if severe)

[a]sFlt/PlGF soluble fms-like tyrosine kinase/placental growth factor—not in routine clinical practice

the syndrome of abnormal liver function, low platelets and microangiopathy (HELLP), pulmonary oedema and if neglected maternal and fetal death. The initiating stimulus appears to be placental ischaemia resulting from abnormal placentation within the uterine wall. Recent evidence points to an aetiological role of angiogenic factors leading to altered vascular endothelial growth factor (VGEF) signalling. There is increased expression of anti-angiogenic soluble fms-like tyrosine kinase-1 (sFlt) and reduced serum placental growth factor (PlGF) which acts via functional VGEF deficiency to cause endothelial dysfunction (hypertension) and podocyte injury (proteinuria). Abnormal sFlt and PlGF ratios may precede the clinical onset of PET by many weeks. This offers the exciting opportunity for risk prediction, early diagnosis and potential future novel therapeutic interventions.

The incidence of PET is substantially increased in patients with CKD; the severity is frequently more severe and of earlier onset. Women with CKD are frequently hypertensive and have proteinuria, both of which commonly worsen in pregnancy as a consequence of pregnancy physiology. A key element of care of these women in pregnancy is to differentiate the onset of superimposed PET from the natural response of the damaged kidney to pregnancy physiology. Discriminatory factors are listed in Table 33.3. Sonographic assessment of uterine and umbilical artery blood flow at 20–24 weeks has predictive value for PET in women with CKD in pregnancy similar that seen in the general population [11]. The ratio of plasma angiogenic factor levels (sFlt and PlGF) has recently been reported to distinguish superimposed PET from CKD changes [12]. It must be stressed that if the maternal condition is deteriorating, delivery is usually indicated. In practice, the most important discriminatory test is time: PET often progresses over hours/days, whereas pregnancy-aggravated change in CKD changes over weeks.

Prevention of Pre-eclampsia in Women with CKD and/or Hypertension

Low-Dose Aspirin (See Table 33.5)

An imbalance of vasodilator and vasoconstrictor prostaglandins contributes to abnormal placentation which led to trials of low-dose aspirin as prophylaxis for PET. Meta-analysis and systematic review of women at medium and high risk of PET treated with aspirin have shown a significant maternal and fetal benefit with no evidence of increased risk of bleeding complications [13] (Fig. 33.4). The relative risk of PET in those at high or medium risk and for women with CKD taking aspirin is RR 0.75, 0.86 and 0.63, respectively. The relative risk in women taking aspirin for preterm delivery (0.92), still birth or neonatal death (0.69), SGA baby (0.90) and placental abruption or haemorrhage is unchanged.

Table 33.5 Impact of aspirin for primary prevention of PET in women at medium and high risk and severity [13]

	Aspirin relative risk (CI)
PET—high-risk pregnancy	0.75 (0.66–0.85)
PET—medium-risk pregnancy	0.86 (0.79–0.95)
PET—pre-existing CKD	0.63 (0.38–1.06)
Preterm delivery	0.92 (0.88–0.97)
Still birth/neonatal death—high risk for PET	0.69 (0.53–0.90)
Small for gestational age	0.90 (0.83–0.98)
Postpartum haemorrhage or placental abruption	Not significant

Therefore, all women at an increased risk of pre-eclampsia should receive aspirin 75 mg from the 12th week of pregnancy up until the time of delivery [6].

No other interventions so far tested have shown a beneficial impact on prevention of PET including antioxidants, folic acid, oral magnesium, fish oils or calcium (in women with normal calcium intake).

Proteinuria

Significant proteinuria in pregnancy is >300 mg/24 h or >30 mg protein/mmol creatinine in a 'spot urine' sample protein/creatinine ratio (PCR). Women should be screened for proteinuria at each antenatal visit using *urine reagent tests assessed by an automated reagent reader device which results in far greater precision than manual readout*. Moderate proteinuria detected early in pregnancy frequently progresses to heavy proteinuria, sometimes into the nephrotic range in the third trimester even in the absence of PET (see Fig. 33.5).

Pregnancy is a thrombophilic state, and heavy proteinuria substantially increases thromboembolic risk [14]. In this setting,

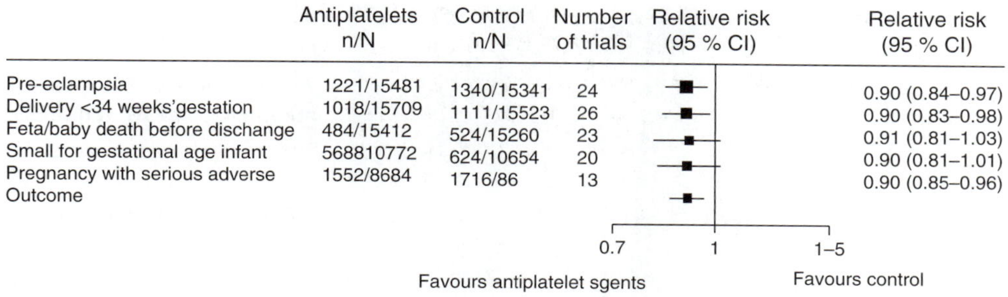

Fig. 33.4 Relative risk of pregnancy outcomes for women treated with low-dose aspirin for primary prevention of pre-eclampsia (Reproduced with permission from Askie et al. [13])

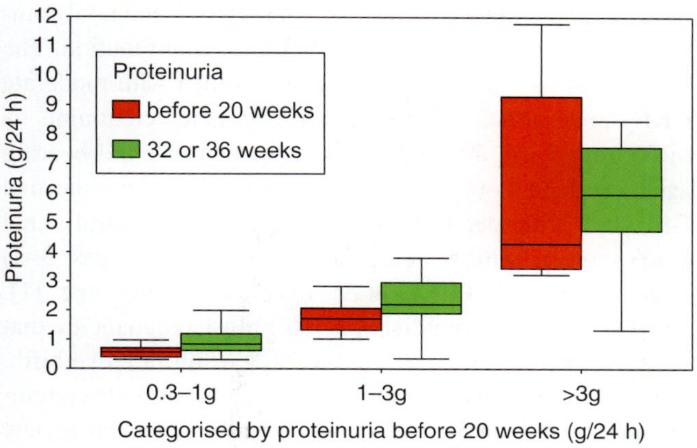

Fig. 33.5 Progression of proteinuria in women with CKD during pregnancy in the absence of PET (From UK CORD Registry)

daily S/C LMW heparin (prophylactic dose) continued until 6 weeks postpartum is recommended. The threshold level of proteinuria to initiate treatment is unclear; many authorities treat when proteinuria is >2 g/24 h (PCR >200). Monitoring anti-factor Xa activity may improve safety (samples taken 3 h after dose). A high index of suspicion for VTED should be maintained in these women during pregnancy. The risks from fetal radiation exposure from V/Q scanning are small when balanced against the risk of undiagnosed pulmonary embolism or blind treatment. Women treated with low-dose aspirin and Clexane are at high risk of symptomatic oesophageal reflux or peptic ulceration and should receive oral ranitidine which appears safe from the second trimester. Those women receiving long-term LMW heparin and/or steroids should receive calcium/D3 supplements as prophylaxis from bone mineral loss.

Urinary Tract Infection

Asymptomatic bacteruria is common (2–10 %) in normal pregnancy, and some women with CKD will have urinary tract abnormalities (e.g. renal stone disease, reflux nephropathy, bladder dysfunction, autosomal dominant polycystic kidney disease) which increase the risk further. Forty percent of women with asymptomatic bacteruria in pregnancy progress to pyelonephritis without prompt treatment which can lead to premature labour. In those with abnormal anatomy, the risk is greater. Meta-analysis demonstrates that antibiotic treatment is very effective in eradicating asymptomatic infection, prevents pyelonephritis and is associated with higher birth weight [15].

Urine should be sent for culture at each antenatal visit. Strict prophylaxis from infection is vital in those with history of recurrent UTI or abnormal urinary tract. The mainstay is bladder toilet comprising at least 3 l daily oral intake, double micturition and postcoital voiding. Those women with predisposing factors or who suffer more than one antenatal infection should also receive nocturnal prophylactic antibiotics until 6 weeks postpartum. Cephalexin 250 mg nocte is effective and well tolerated or, if allergic to beta-lactam antibiotics, nitrofurantoin 50 mg nocte (the latter should be suspended around 36 weeks due to risk of haemolytic anaemia in some babies). Where possible, quinolones or gentamicin (risk of neonatal deafness) should be avoided if safer alternatives exist based on antibiotic senilities. Co-amoxiclav used late in pregnancy may increase the risk of necrotising enterocolitis in preterm babies.

Renal Tract Obstruction Versus Physiological Hydronephrosis

Differentiation of physiological hydronephrosis from ureteric obstruction can be challenging. In general, physiological hydronephrosis is asymptomatic, whereas acute obstruction is often associated with loin pain and tenderness. Ureteric calculi are the most common cause of urinary tract obstruction in pregnancy associated with non-visible haematuria and renal colic, whilst urine in normal women rarely contains red cells. An increase in plasma creatinine from a baseline of 40 to 50 to 60 to 80 is suggestive of unilateral obstruction. Imaging techniques may be helpful in differentiating. Resistive index (RI) derived by Doppler ultrasound of a renal arcuate artery >0.7 is suggestive of obstruction if contralateral RI is <0.7 [16]. We have found magnetic resonance urography (MRU), without the use of gadolinium contrast agents, to be helpful (see Fig. 33.6) [17]. MRI is safe

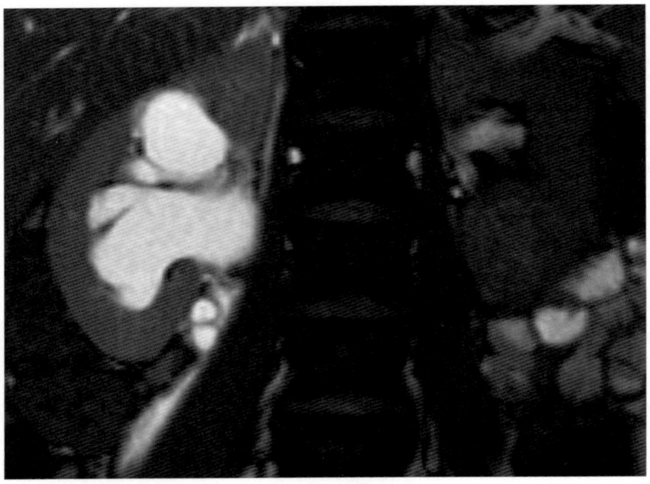

Fig. 33.6 Magnetic resonance urography (non-contrasted) in woman with physiological right renal hydronephrosis

after the first trimester of pregnancy. Although MRU does not adequately image calculi, a ureteric filling defect or a level of ureteric 'cut-off' above the pelvic brim is suggestive of a stone. Faced with a critically ill pregnant woman with tender hydronephrosis, not settling with antibiotics, obstruction should be considered likely and lead to urgent urological review. Prompt relief of obstruction either by percutaneous nephrostomy (with antibiotic cover) or retrograde stent insertion (in the mid trimester of pregnancy) can be life saving for fetus and the mother.

Drug Safety in Pregnancy

The background congenital abnormality rate in the European population is 3–5 %. Drugs that are toxic at the early embryonic development stage often result in increased rates of spontaneous miscarriage. Fetotoxic drug exposure in weeks 3–12 postconception may lead to abnormalities of organ development. Proving teratogenicity is difficult. Animal studies often fail to correspond with human experience, and even known teratogens (e.g. thalidomide) adversely affects only 20 % of exposed pregnancies.

Anaemia in Pregnancy

Women with CKD frequently fail to drive an adequate increase in red cell mass during pregnancy and may become increasingly anaemic. If required IV iron replacement appears safe, the greatest experience is with IV iron sucrose. Erythropoietin (EPO) alpha, beta and gamma does not cross the placenta and is effective (usually requiring 50–100 % dose increase) in women with CKD in pregnancy targeting hemoglobin around 100–110 g/dl. It remains unclear as to whether EPO increases the risk of worsening hypertension in pregnancy and BP requires close monitoring.

Chronic Kidney Disease in Pregnancy

Pregnancy places substantial physiological demands on the kidney which may explain why women at any stage of CKD experience a high risk of adverse maternal (sixfold) and fetal (twofold) outcomes [18]. The risk of maternal and fetal complications increases with worse baseline renal function. The gestational rise in GFR is blunted in women with moderate CKD and often absent in those where creatinine is >200 umol/l [5]. Three percent of women of child-bearing age have stage 1 or 2 CKD (mild renal impairment or normal GFR but with persistent albuminuria or structural renal abnormality), whilst moderate/severe CKD (stages 3–5) affects around 1:150 women of child-bearing age [1]. Despite the high complication rate, most pregnancies that progress beyond the first trimester will result in a live birth. The key to optimising outcome is preparation with systematic preconception counselling and regular antenatal review in combined renal/obstetric antenatal clinics comprising experienced Obstetric and Nephrology Consultants (see before).

The Evidence-Base for Guidance

Much guidance arises from 30 years of systematic literature review by John Davison and Marshall Lindheimer [5]. Recent systematic reviews, meta-analysis and ongoing registry studies including the UK Collaboration in Obstetric Renal Disease (CORD) and UK Obstetric Outcome Surveillance Studies (UKOSS) add to the knowledge base.

Role of Renal Biopsy in Pregnancy

In pregnancy, proteinuria presenting after 20 weeks is generally due to PET. Renal biopsy risks complications including fetal compromise. A recent meta-analysis of renal biopsy in pregnancy suggested increased risk of complications compared with nonpregnant patients. However, this analysis includes historic series where biopsy was performed for the diagnosis of PET [19]. Renal biopsy is technically difficult and uncomfortable for the woman after 20–24 weeks. In highly selected cases of undiagnosed, progressive kidney disease (before fetal viability, <26 weeks), early onset of nephrotic syndrome (<20 weeks) or unexplained AKI (<26 weeks), renal biopsy has a similar complication risk to

Table 33.6 Effect of pregnancy on maternal renal function in women with CKD [5]

	Loss of >25 % renal function (%)		
Pre-pregnancy serum creatinine (μmol/l)	During pregnancy	Persists postpartum	End-stage renal failure after 1 year
<125	2	0	0
125–180	40	20	2
>180	70	50	35

Based on literature 1985–2007 in pregnancies achieving at least 24 weeks [5]

the nonpregnant state. Histological diagnosis beneficially affects care in over 1/3 of cases, being safer than blind therapy [19]. Pregnant women with stable CKD and proteinuria or those presenting after 26 weeks should be observed carefully. In this situation, renal biopsy should be deferred until stable postpartum [19].

Identification of Women with CKD in Pregnancy

Routine monitoring of urinalysis and BP in pregnancy frequently identifies previously unrecognised CKD, up to 40 % in case series in pregnancy [20]. Raised urine PCR or serum creatinine >70 umol identifies kidney disease. Investigation by repeat serum creatinine, blood count, tests of soluble immunology (antinuclear antibody, complements 3 and 4, antineutrophil cytoplasmic antibody) and baseline renal ultrasound is indicated. These findings put the pregnancy at high risk for complications and thus the need for enhanced antenatal monitoring and postpartum follow-up. Neither the MDRD nor Cockcroft-Gault equations accurately predict GFR in pregnancy.

Effect of Pregnancy on Maternal Kidney Function (See Table 33.6)

Mild Renal Impairment (Stages 1–2)

Pregnancy in women with stages 1 and 2 CKD pre-pregnancy or first trimester creatinine <110 umol/l with low-level proteinuria (<1 g/24 h) and absent/well-controlled hypertension has little or no long-term adverse effect on renal function [21].

Moderate to Severe Renal Impairment (Stages 3–5)

Women with more advanced pre-pregnancy CKD are at significant risk of accelerated decline in renal function both during and following pregnancy (see Table 33.6.). In a landmark retrospective study, women who started pregnancy with moderate CKD (creatinine 124–168 μmol/l) were at a 40 % risk deteriorating renal function during pregnancy which persisted postpartum in half [22]. Two-thirds of those with severe CKD (antenatal creatinine >177 μmol/l) suffered a decline in renal function in the third trimester which persisted postpartum. A third deteriorated to the point of requiring dialysis. A prospective study confirmed adverse pregnancy outcomes of 49 women with moderate/severe pre-pregnancy CKD (mean creatinine 186 μmol/l and GFR 35 ± 12 ml/min). Mean GFR fell from 35 before to 30 ml/min after pregnancy ($p<.001$). However, the rate of decline of GFR before and after pregnancy remained the same. Those women with a pre-pregnancy GFR <40 ml/min and heavier proteinuria (>1 g/24 h) had an increased risk of accelerated deterioration in GFR post-pregnancy and progressed more rapidly to dialysis [23]. In a prospective study in 44 pregnancies of women with CKD stages 3–5, the UK CORD group confirmed a high rate of declining renal function in pregnancy (22 %), of which a third showed persistent decline in kidney function at 6 months following pregnancy. More advanced CKD pre-pregnancy and heavy proteinuria (>1 g/24 h) appeared strong predictors of an irreversible decline in renal function associated with pregnancy [5].

These studies highlight the interaction of various aspects of CKD including GFR, blood pressure and degree of proteinuria on post-pregnancy renal outcomes. More advanced CKD pre-pregnancy and heavy proteinuria (>1 g/24 h) appear strong predictors of an irreversible decline in renal function associated with pregnancy [5].

Effect of Maternal CKD on Pregnancy Outcomes (See Table 33.7)

CKD is an independent risk factor for adverse fetal and maternal outcomes in pregnancy [18, 25] even those with stage 1 CKD [4] where adverse fetal outcome was 18 versus 9 % and adverse maternal outcome 14 versus 3 % (OR 1.76 and 4.07 for CKD independent of other risk factors). Fetal factors include preterm delivery, pre-eclampsia and fetal growth restriction when compared with control pregnancies of women with normal kidney function. Adverse maternal events (gestational hypertension, pre-eclampsia, eclampsia and maternal mortality) were 5.6 times greater as compared to control pregnancies. In a prospective analysis of 267

Table 33.7 Effect of maternal CKD on pregnancy outcome [24]

Pre-pregnancy serum creatinine (umol/l)	Fetal growth restriction (%)	Preterm delivery	Pre-eclampsia	Perinatal deaths
<125	25	30	22	1
125–180	40	60	40	5
>180	65	>90	60	10

Based on literature 1985–2007 in pregnancies achieving at least 24 weeks [5]

women with CKD compared with normal controls conducted between 2000 and 2009, Piccoli demonstrated preterm delivery in 44 % (CKD) versus 5 % (normal), Caesarean section 44 % versus 25 % and need for neonatal intensive care 26 % versus 1 % [4]. Furthermore, in pregnant women with CKD, proteinuria (>1 g/24 h) and hypertension are independent risk factors for adverse pregnancy outcomes. Proteinuria >1 g/24 h increases the need for neonatal intensive care (RR of 4.2) and hypertension with preterm delivery (RR 7.2) and Caesarean section (RR 5.7) [4].

The UK CORD group, in a retrospective review of 400 consecutive pregnancies in women with CKD, demonstrated using multivariable analysis that first trimester BP >90 mmHg or treated hypertension independently increased the risk of neonatal mortality (OR 16-fold). LSCS and premature delivery were associated with CKD. As regards the interaction between hypertension and chronic kidney disease, it appeared that blood pressure was a more important factor.

How Should CKD Be Managed in Pregnancy?

See Table 33.8

All women with CKD or those identified with CKD in pregnancy should be referred promptly to an established obstetric renal clinic to plan antenatal care. Assessment of renal function, degree of proteinuria (PCR), haemoglobin, urine dip and culture, BP measurement (24 h ambulatory BP can be helpful) and baseline renal ultrasound should be performed. All women with CKD should be offered aspirin 75 mg daily. NICE recommends aspirin be started around 12 weeks as prophylaxis from pre-eclampsia although many experienced centres start earlier [6].

Monthly follow-up before 20 weeks and 2 weekly follow-up after 20 weeks (more frequent if deteriorating) are recommended. Weekly urinalysis and BP measurement in primary care after 20 weeks will identify early PET. Difficult decisions often need to be made about the timing of delivery balancing the fetal risks of premature delivery against maternal health. This requires experienced maternal medicine, nephrological and neonatal collaboration. Distinguishing the expected increase in urine protein excretion and blood pressure in the late second/third trimester of pregnancy from pre-eclampsia is key (see Comparison of Pre-Eclampsia and Physiological Change) (see Table 33.4).

Postpartum Care

Enhanced monitoring of women with CKD should continue postpartum particularly in those with deteriorating renal function of nephrotic range proteinuria in pregnancy. All women with CKD should be seen in a combined renal obstetric clinic around 4–8 weeks postpartum to assess postpartum changes, plan contraception and arrange long-term review. It can take three months for the physiological changes of pregnancy to disappear. Moreover, proteinuria, especially after severe PET, may take 6 months to return to baseline. The increased GFR of pregnancy returns to baseline 1–2 weeks postpartum leading to an expected rise in creatinine. It is vital that women newly identified with CKD in pregnancy before 20 weeks are referred for postnatal nephrological investigation and follow-up. Breastfeeding in general should be encouraged if the baby is thriving, and drugs changed to those known to have minimal breast milk excretion (see later).

Pregnancy in Women with Systemic Lupus Erythematosus [26–29]

There remains a significant risk of fetal and maternal morbidity and mortality in patients with lupus, worsened in those with nephritis. A recent meta-analysis (of what have traditionally been small retrospective case series) analysing pregnancy outcomes in women with lupus demonstrated significant associations between active lupus nephritis and maternal hypertension and premature birth. This association remained even when corrected for hypertension. Overall (renal and non-renal), the preterm delivery rate was nearly 40 %, flare rate 26 % and unsuccessful pregnancy rate 23 %.

In the pregnant woman with lupus nephritis, there are various factors to consider:

1. Fertility appears to be normal in lupus patients. As pregnancies in this group have better outcomes if planned to periods of quiescent disease with suitable changes in medication, appropriate contraception should be discussed with all women of child-bearing potential. Combined oral contraceptives are probably best avoided in this group because of increased risks of hypertension and venous thromboembolic complications.
2. Background chronic kidney disease: as with all pregnancies in women with chronic kidney disease, the degree of chronic

Table 33.8 Important points relating to specific kidney diseases during pregnancy

Condition	Possible complication needing monitoring	Key management points
Primary glomerulonephritis	Hypertension, proteinuria	Treat BP (<140/90) and monitor. If PCR >200, consider LMW heparin prophylaxis
Autosomal dominant PKD	CKD, hypertension, UTI	Discuss 50 % risk of inheritance
Reflux nephropathy	Recurrent UTIs, hypertension, CKD	Bladder toilet, prophylactic antibiotics. Screen baby for reflux
Renal calculi	Renal colic, UTI	High fluid intake, prophylactic antibiotics. MR urography may be helpful to exclude obstruction after first trimester
Diabetic nephropathy	Risk or progressive CKD, hypertension, proteinuria	Assess comorbidity, maintain tight glycaemic control pre-pregnancy, antenatal and postpartum

kidney damage caused by previous active disease is an important factor, as discussed elsewhere in this chapter.

3. Lupus activity: all case series demonstrate that maternal and fetal outcomes are worse when lupus is active at conception. This applies to renal and non-renal manifestations and emphasises the need for early and frank discussion with all female patients of child-bearing potential the importance of planning pregnancy.
4. Flares: it remains unclear whether pregnancy increases the risk of flare in the antenatal or early postnatal period. This risk is increased by any lupus activity within 6 months of conception, history of multiple flares and discontinuation of hydroxychloroquine.
5. Medication: glucocorticoids, azathioprine, hydroxychloroquine, cyclosporine and tacrolimus appear to be safe to use in pregnancy. Mycophenolate mofetil has been shown to be associated with various congenital abnormalities, particularly of the palate and face, and should be stopped at least 6 weeks prior to conception. Cyclophosphamide is associated with significant teratogenic and abortifacient effects and should not be used. Rituximab crosses the placenta and has been associated with neonatal B cell depletion and should probably be avoided in pregnancy. Antihypertensive medication may also need modification as discussed elsewhere.
6. Antiphospholipid antibodies: these have been shown consistently to increase both the rate of pregnancy loss (typically after 10 weeks) and the risk of pre-eclampsia. There appears to be a hierarchy of effect with the presence of lupus anticoagulant being associated with more adverse events than anti-cardiolipin antibodies alone. In addition, higher titres of antiphospholipid antibodies increase the risk of adverse outcomes as does a history of previous thromboembolic events or pregnancy loss.
7. Levels of anti-dsDNA antibodies and complement: women with high levels of anti-dsDNA antibodies or low complement are at greater risk of adverse pregnancy outcomes than patients with quiescent serology, but the presence of active disease with active serology gives by far the worst outcomes. It should be noted that complement levels are naturally raised in pregnancy so that trends in complement levels should be monitored in addition to absolute levels.
8. Anti Ro/SSA antibodies: these antibodies are associated with neonatal lupus and two main fetal complications:
   (a) Cutaneous neonatal lupus
   (b) Cardiac complications such as heart block (around 1–2 %) or endocardial fibroelastosis

   Higher titres of antibodies and a history of cutaneous neonatal lupus in a previous pregnancy appear to be associated with an increased risk of cardiac complications. *All lupus patients with the presence of anti Ro/SSA antibodies should undergo fetal heart monitoring weekly from 16 weeks.*
9. Other organ damage from lupus: this should also be remembered when advising with regard to future pregnancy and include pulmonary hypertension which appears to be associated with antiphospholipid syndrome and can be fatal in pregnancy even with specialist management.

Bearing in mind the above factors, ideally we recommend that all patients with lupus nephritis receive joint renal/obstetric pre-pregnancy counselling with experienced practitioners to enable tailored advice of individual risk of both maternal and fetal outcomes. In addition, this allows:

1. Discussion about lupus activity and planning therapy to achieve quiescence in preparation for pregnancy. Best outcomes result in those women with quiescent disease for >6 months on pregnancy safe drugs. Where there is uncertainty about activity of lupus nephritis, a renal biopsy is helpful as a guide.
2. Transfer from mycophenolate, cyclophosphamide or rituximab when disease is felt to be quiescent to azathioprine with a period of observation and if necessary re-biopsy prior to pregnancy.
3. In general, cessation of ACE inhibitors or angiotensin 2 receptor blockers and transfer to either labetalol or nifedipine for control of hypertension if necessary. However, with significant proteinuria, one may recommend continuation of ACEi or angiotensin receptor blockers until conception to allow anti-proteinuric benefit to continue (as discussed above).

4. Discussion around the use of folic acid for prevention of neural tube defects.
5. Discussion about the use of aspirin from the first trimester to reduce the risk of pre-eclampsia in this high-risk group. We tend to recommend from conception.
6. Discussion about the use of low molecular weight heparin; this should be used at a prophylactic level (with factor Xa monitoring):
   (a) In all cases of significant proteinuria (we use cut-off PCR or ACR of 200) whenever it develops in pregnancy
   (b) When there is a previous history of venous thromboembolic disease
   (c) When there is a history of significant pregnancy loss in the presence of antiphospholipid antibodies

   It should be used at therapeutic levels (again with factor Xa level monitoring) if the patient is currently anticoagulated with warfarin.

However, we accept that such pre-pregnancy planning can be aspirational and therefore impress into all our patients the need to present to us early if they should find themselves unexpectedly pregnant to allow for early changes in medications.

Diagnosis of Lupus Nephritis for the First Time in Pregnancy Presents Its Own Challenges

Occasionally, a patient will present with an active urinary sediment and positive lupus serology for the first time in pregnancy; indeed, the enhanced screening in pregnancy may allow detection of previously undiagnosed renal disease. We would certainly recommend a full immunology screen in any patient presenting with proteinuria prior to 20 weeks and at any stage when proteinuria is associated with haematuria or appears not to be typical for pre-eclampsia. The decision to perform a renal biopsy can then be a difficult one and have been discussed above. We would suggest that real-time, ultrasound-guided biopsy up to fetal viability can be very useful, both to confirm a renal diagnosis allowing appropriate intensity of treatment and to provide informed counselling to a woman. After viability, 'blind' treatment of assumed lupus nephritis may be required with induction of preterm delivery if significant deterioration of renal (or indeed extra-renal) parameters occurs that require treatment contraindicated in pregnancy.

Differentiation of Flare of Lupus Nephritis from Pre-eclampsia

As discussed previously, since both flare of lupus nephritis and pre-eclampsia are not uncommon in lupus patients, an ability to distinguish between the two, or indeed identify the dominating pathology when the two conditions are coexistent, is useful. This is particularly applicable when renal parameters deteriorate at a gestation when significant fetal morbidity or mortality may occur with delivery. Rapid progression in degree of proteinuria or renal impairment over days would be more likely to indicate pre-eclampsia, particularly if in association with a significant increase in blood pressure. Conversely, the presence of an active urinary sediment and leucocyturia (in the absence of infection) with an increase in serological activity of lupus would make lupus nephritis the more likely pathology. Rises in transaminases and development of thrombocytopenia can obviously occur in both conditions.

Pregnancy in Women Treated by Dialysis

Fertility in women treated by chronic dialysis is markedly reduced secondary to decreased libido and perturbations of the hypothalamic-pituitary-gonadal hormonal axis (hyperprolactinaemia occurs in 70–90 %), leading to irregular periods, anovulation or amenorrhoea. Conception on peritoneal dialysis is three times less common than on haemodialysis. However, the reported incidence has risen from 0.3 to 7 % over the last three decades and up to 16 % in a recent series of women treated by intensive nocturnal haemodialysis. Outcomes have also improved over the last three decades likely to be as a consequence of more intensive dialysis, advances in obstetric/neonatal care and reduction in therapeutic termination. Conception rates and outcomes for women who progress to dialysis during pregnancy are superior to those starting pregnancy on dialysis treatment. Nevertheless, pregnancy in women treated by dialysis is arduous, associated with high maternal and fetal morbidity, and pregnancy outcomes remain comparatively poor [30].

Diagnosis of Pregnancy

Diagnosis of early pregnancy in dialysis patients is difficult. Amenorrhoea or irregular periods are common, and urine pregnancy tests are often unreliable. Serum beta-HCG levels may be elevated in the absence of pregnancy. Trans-abdominal or the more sensitive transvaginal ultrasound is the most reliable pregnancy test in this population and allows assessment of gestation.

Pregnancy Counselling

Many women assume that it is impossible to conceive on dialysis. It is good practice to counsel women of fertile age treated by dialysis for the risks of pregnancy and routinely offer contraceptive advice (see Sect. Contraception in Women with Kidney Disease). Any woman contemplating pregnancy should be offered combined renal/obstetric preconception counselling in a unit experienced in the care of such pregnancies, and their care in pregnancy should be under the supervision of a joint renal/obstetric antenatal service. For most women, delaying pregnancy until after a successful renal transplant with much improved prospects of successful outcome is the optimum preconception advice. Pregnancy even if unsuccessful may lead to HLA sensitisation reducing opportunities for subsequent transplantation, especially spousal donation.

Pregnancy Outcomes

Peritoneal Dialysis

There are some theoretical advantages of peritoneal over haemodialysis in pregnancy including more gentle fluid, electrolyte and toxin removal, reduced hypotensive episodes and no requirement for anticoagulation. However, reported outcomes between the two treatment modalities are similar. Peritonitis has been associated with onset of spontaneous labour, and by the third trimester peritoneal space for dialysis fluid is limited even on automated nocturnal treatment often leading to reducing appetite. We do not recommend immediate switch of dialysis modality in early pregnancy but suggest formation of AV fistula early in the second trimester to enable easy conversion to haemodialysis later in pregnancy if problems are encountered [14].

Haemodialysis (See Table 33.9)

The literature is almost certainly influenced by publication bias in favour of successful outcomes and under-reporting of spontaneous miscarriage [30]. Review of older literature by Davison indicated a 50 % live birth outcome in pregnancies if dialysis was required pre-pregnancy or 75 % where dialysis was required for the first time during pregnancy [5].

An attempt at rationalisation of contemporaneous data has been made recently in a systematic review of ten heterogeneous studies of pregnancies ($n = 90$) in haemodialysis patients ($n = 78$) reported between 2000 and 2009. All incorporated joint maternal medicine/nephrologist/neonatologist care and employed an enhanced dialysis regime, 4–6 sessions/week totalling 15–40 h/week. Of these pregnancies, 10 resulted in medical termination. Outcomes appeared best in those series employing longer-hour dialysis [31]. An inverse correlation between pre-dialysis urea and successful outcome has been reported leading to a recommendation to keep pre-dialysis urea <17 mmol/l [33].

There were no reported maternal deaths. Main maternal complications include hypertension and anaemia with exact incidence of pre-eclampsia difficult to define. Most women received erythropoietin (4,500–9,000 u/week) and intravenous iron targeting Hb >9–10 g/dl. Erythropoietin dose increase of 50–100 % over pre-pregnancy dose is usually required.

Polyhydramnios is widely reported and may underlie the high rate of spontaneous premature labour precipitating delivery. It is suggested that fetal osmotic diuresis secondary to high maternal urea may be the cause. The incidence of polyhydramnios and premature labour may be reduced by better solute control achieved by more prolonged dialysis. Although difficult to be definitive, it appears that increasing hours of dialysis, whether by daily or nocturnal dialysis, are associated with better outcomes. The logistics of such therapy should be discussed with any woman undertaking pregnancy on dialysis and can be particularly difficult in those who already have caring responsibilities for other children or who remain in employment. We would recommend commencement of such dialysis therapy certainly from the second trimester and earlier if feasible.

Table 33.9 Fetal and maternal outcomes of contemporaneous series of pregnancies in women treated by haemodialysis

	Piccoli et al. (2010) ($n = 80$) [31]	Barua et al. (2008) ($n = 7$) [32]	Asamiya et al. (2009) ($n = 28$) [33]
Fetal outcome %			
Spontaneous miscarriage	6	0	14
Stillbirth/neonatal death	18	0	15
Preterm delivery (<37 weeks)	67–100 (median delivery 32 weeks)	14 (mean 36 ± 3)	92
Low birth weight/IUGR	100	28 (mean 2,418 ± 657 g)	N/A
Infant death	1	0	7
Surviving infants	76	100	64
Maternal outcomes %			
Severe hypertension/pre-eclampsia	29–63	0	39
Caesarean section delivery	33–80 (median 62 %)	28	38
Polyhydramnios	18–60 (median 38 %)	0	39

Guidelines for Management of Pregnancy in Haemodialysis Patients (Opinion Based on Literature)

1. Offer contraceptive advice and preconception counselling where indicated.
2. Intravenous iron (after first trimester) and ESA are widely used and are not associated with fetal abnormalities. Maintain haemoglobin 9.5–11 g/dl. Monitor BP closely. ESA dose increase of 50–100 % is usually required.
3. Folic acid and water-soluble vitamin supplementation is advised.
4. Dialysis dose: increase dialysis frequency to six times/week in early second trimester providing a minimum of 20 h/week, keeping pre-dialysis urea below 17 moml/l. There may be benefits in longer hours or daily nocturnal dialysis.
5. Maintain BP <140/90–130/80.
6. Avoidance of intra-dialytic hypotension with careful and regular reassessment of dry weight.
7. Anticoagulation-low molecular weight heparin does not cross the placenta and is not associated with increased antepartum haemorrhage.
8. Treatment with aspirin 75 mg daily from 12 weeks to reduce risk of pre-eclampsia.
9. Dialysate. Try to mimic pregnancy physiology. Reduce dialysate sodium to 135 mmol/l, bicarbonate to 25 mmol/l and calcium 1.25 mmol/l.
10. Regular review by an experienced obstetric renal multidisciplinary team to allow appropriate maternal and fetal monitoring and discussions with regard to optimal time of delivery.
11. Meticulous management of other comorbidities, e.g. diabetes, cardiovascular disease and immune-related conditions by experienced teams.

The long-term outcome of children born to mothers on dialysis in the long term remains unknown. The immediate risks associated with prematurity are well characterised, and there is some evidence for increased long-term cardiovascular morbidity in babies born small for gestational age. Moreover, a recent report suggests that there may be a potential risk of renal impairment in children born to dialysing mothers which is presumably multifactorial in nature [34].

In summary, pregnancy in the dialysis patient, although requiring a considerable time commitment from patient and medical staff, appears to have a better outcome than previously noted, probably related to more frequent dialysis and better maternal/neonatal care. Most women should be advised to defer pregnancy until after successful renal transplantation when maternal/fetal outlook is improved. However, pregnancy may be a reasonable option in the highly motivated, counselled patient within an experienced environment.

Registry studies of women receiving dialysis in pregnancy are ongoing and may help provide further evidence on how to best advise these women.

Pregnancy Following Renal Transplantation [35]

Renal transplantation rapidly restores fertility in women with ESKD offering for many the first opportunity to conceive with a good chance of a successful pregnancy outcome. Nevertheless, these pregnancies are complex and at high risk for fetal and maternal complications. At least 50 % of transplant pregnancies reported in the literature are unplanned. Best outcomes are most likely if early effective contraceptive advice is given on discharge post transplantation, and women considering pregnancy are advised in a joint renal/obstetric pre-pregnancy counselling clinic. Appropriate antenatal care is best provided in a joint antenatal clinic managed by nephrology and maternal medicine doctors with significant experience in this area.

The Evidence Base and Sources of Guidance

The evidence base to counsel women in guiding pregnancy management remains incomplete but has improved considerably recently. Many small single centre retrospective case series which may suffer from selection bias have recently been collated in a large meta-analysis [36]. The US National Transplant Pregnancy Registry employed voluntary submission, but three prospective registries collecting data on almost all transplants (two from UK and one from Australia/New Zealand) have recently published [35, 37, 38]. American Society of Transplantation Clinical Practice Guidelines and European Best Practice Guidelines help advise clinicians [39, 40].

The Timing of Pregnancy in Relation to Transplantation

Guidelines recommend deferring pregnancy until at least 12 months post-transplantation [41]. By this time, immunosuppressant drug doses should be at their nadir, and the risk of opportunistic infection and rejection, in particular cytomegalovirus which can affect the fetus, is remote. A recent meta-analysis however does not support a clear cut-off in the timing of conception post-pregnancy. The live birth rates for pregnancies <2 years, 3–4 years and >4 years post-transplant were 80, 76 and 75 %, respectively, whereas obstetric complications were significantly greater in earlier pregnancies [36]. In practice, it is best to wait for stable well-preserved kidney function after conversion to treatment known to be safe in pregnancy (see later).

Transplant Immunosuppression

Prednisolone crosses to the fetus but with maternal/cord blood concentration of 10:1 due to metabolism within the placenta. Daily doses of <15 mg per day have not been associated with teratogenicity or neonatal adrenal suppression. It is likely that steroids are associated with an increased risk of premature rupture of membranes and these women taking steroids are at increased risk for gestational diabetes. Glucose tolerance testing at 26 weeks is advised.

Extensive human study both in and out of transplantation has shown no association between azathioprine and congenital abnormalities. Fetal myelosuppression is extremely unlikely if the total dose is <2 mg/kg and the maternal white count maintained within the normal range [35].

The calcineurin inhibitors (CNIs) cyclosporine and tacrolimus have not been associated with an increased risk of congenital abnormalities. Babies born to women taking cyclosporine may have a lower birth weight compared to those receiving prednisolone and azathioprine alone. This is likely to relate to a higher prevalence of hypertension and worse renal function in this population. The dose of CNI required to maintain equivalent trough levels in pregnancy frequently requires dose increase, a mean dose increase of 40 % because of increased volume of distribution in adipose tissue and red cells [41]. Outcomes of pregnancies in women taking cyclosporine or tacrolimus are similar. Unsurprisingly, those treated with tacrolimus have a greater incidence of gestational diabetes mellitus (2–10 %).

There is increasing evidence that mycophenolic acid (MPA) and mycophenolate mofetil (MMF) are teratogenic. Reports in renal transplant pregnancies identify a greater than expected first trimester spontaneous miscarriage rate of 40 % (10–15 % in the general population). In addition, an embropathy comprising cleft lip and palate and ear and cerebral abnormalities is reported in a quarter of exposed pregnancies [42]. All women should be counselled for the risks of congenital abnormality at the time of transplantation and should practice secure contraception and undergo pre-pregnancy counselling if they wish to conceive. Women taking MMF or MPA should be advised to stop at least three months before planned conception (ideally six months) to enable transfer to alternative therapy, usually azathioprine and assessment of stability, before attempting conception. There is a small but definite increased risk of rejection during this period, and this must be discussed.

As yet sirolimus and everolimus have not been associated with abnormal pregnancy outcome, but their known antiproliferative and anti-VEGF action is of concern. It is too early to judge whether these drugs may be safely used in pregnancy, and at present advice should be to avoid in pregnancy where possible. The safety of biological agents including belatacept or alemtuzumab is unknown, and these drugs should be avoided in pregnancy at the present time.

Early Pregnancy Outcomes

The outcome of pregnancy in renal transplant recipients has improved over the last three decades, the live birth rate increasing from 69 to 83 % in Australian/New Zealand registry data. This is in large part due to a reduction in 'therapeutic' terminations presumably as a consequence of greater medical confidence in pregnancy outcomes [38]. The prevalence of spontaneous miscarriage (<24 weeks) is reported as 11–14 % which is equivalent to the background population rates. The rates of ectopic pregnancy, <1 %, is the same as normal controls, reassuring given pelvic transplant and the likelihood that some women have had previous peritoneal dialysis-related peritonitis.

Maternal Outcomes of Pregnancies in Renal Transplant Recipients

Pregnancies progressing beyond the first trimester have greater than 95 % chance of a successful outcome with a live birth [35]. However, maternal and fetal complications are substantially increased. Maternal outcomes are listed in Table 33.10 and provide important information to counsel transplant recipients contemplating pregnancy [35].

A significant antenatal deterioration in transplant function is seen in around a third of women. The UKOSS study

Table 33.10 Maternal outcomes of pregnancies in renal transplant recipients

	UK Obstetric Surveillance Study 2013 [37]	Meta-analysis (% (CI) 2011 [36]	UK Transplant Registry 2007 [35]
Acute rejection (%)	2	4.2	
Pre-eclampsia (%)	24	27 (25–29)	
Antenatal graft dysfunction (%)	38		30 % (>20 % rise in creatinine)
Gestational DM (%)	3	8 (6.7–9.4)	
New-onset proteinuria in the absence of PET (%)	30		
Caesarean section delivery (%)	64	57 (55–59)	72 (87 % if delivery <37 weeks)

Table 33.11 Pregnancy outcomes in renal transplant recipients

	UK Obstetric Surveillance Study [37]	Meta-analysis (CI) [36]	UK Transplant Registry 2007 [35]
Live birth (%)	91	74 (72–75)	79
Gestational age (weeks)	36 (IQR 27–43)	36 (35–36)	36.8
Preterm birth (%)	52	46 (44–48)	50
Very preterm (<32 weeks) (%)	9		
Birth weight (g)	2,483	2,420	2,316 ± 80
Low birth rate (<2,500 g) (%)	48		54
Very low birth rate (<1,500 g) (%)	9		22
Small for gestational age (%)	24		
Need for neonatal ICU (%)	30		

importantly demonstrates a significant rise in serum creatinine in the third trimester which is exaggerated in women with a poor pregnancy outcome. The cause of the rise is unexplained but is likely to result from a physiological decline in GFR rather than the adverse impact of superimposed PET.

Proteinuria develops or increases in around a third of women sometimes to near nephrotic levels.

Pregnancy Outcomes

Pregnancy outcomes are listed in Table 33.11.

As compared with the general population, the adjusted odds ratio for pre-eclampsia is 6.3 and for preterm delivery is 12.6. The majority of women are delivered by Caesarean section, 83 %, if delivery is <37 weeks. The mean gestational age at birth is 36 weeks, being remarkably consistent between different registry series and meta-analysis. Over half of births are premature (<37 weeks). As a consequence, half of babies are born with low birth weight (<2.5 kg), but around 10 % are born with very low birth weight (<1.5 kg). Intrauterine growth retardation is noted in a quarter of pregnancies. As a consequence, many babies require prolonged neonatal intensive care.

Unless otherwise contraindicated, aspirin 75 mg daily is recommended from the end of the first trimester until delivery in all women with a renal transplant in pregnancy as prophylaxis from pre-eclampsia. We recommend blood pressure targets of <140/90. Those women with nephrotic range proteinuria (>2 g/24 h or PCR >200) should in addition receive a prophylactic daily subcutaneous low molecular weight heparin which may be monitored using factor Xa activity (measured 3 h after administration).

Long-Term Effect of Pregnancy on Graft and Patient Survival

Case-control studies show no evidence of an adverse impact of pregnancy on graft and patient survival in women with preserved kidney transplant function. However, outcome in those with more significant pre-pregnancy renal dysfunction is more likely to suffer pregnancy-related decline (see Fig. 33.7).

Management of Declining Kidney Function in Pregnancy [43]

Despite immunological tolerance shown to the fetus, the reported incidence of rejection during pregnancy is similar to that in nonpregnant transplant recipients, 2–4 % [35–37]. In early pregnancy, this is associated with volume depletion and failure to absorb immunosuppression due to hyperemesis. Physiological hydronephrosis of the transplant is common in pregnancy, but ureteric obstruction by the gravid uterus is thankfully rare. Unexplained transplant dysfunction before 28 weeks should include consideration of renal biopsy as this may well be safer than blind antirejection treatment. PET may explain transplant dysfunction later in pregnancy. Any decision must be carefully considered, and the risk/benefit ratio discussed with the pregnant woman after ensuring BP control, normal coagulation and platelet count and temporary suspension of aspirin.

Factors Affecting Live Birth Rate

Risk factors for adverse pregnancy outcome (live birth or delivery >32 weeks) include:

1. Maternal age below 20 or >35 years
2. Afro-Caribbean ethnicity
3. End-stage renal failure secondary to diabetes
4. Lower pre-pregnancy renal function

The UK Transplant Registry identifies higher pre-pregnancy creatinine and systolic blood pressure at conception with adverse transplant outcome. The odds ratio for preterm birth in those women with a creatinine of <150 mmol/l at conception is 0.2 as compared to those with

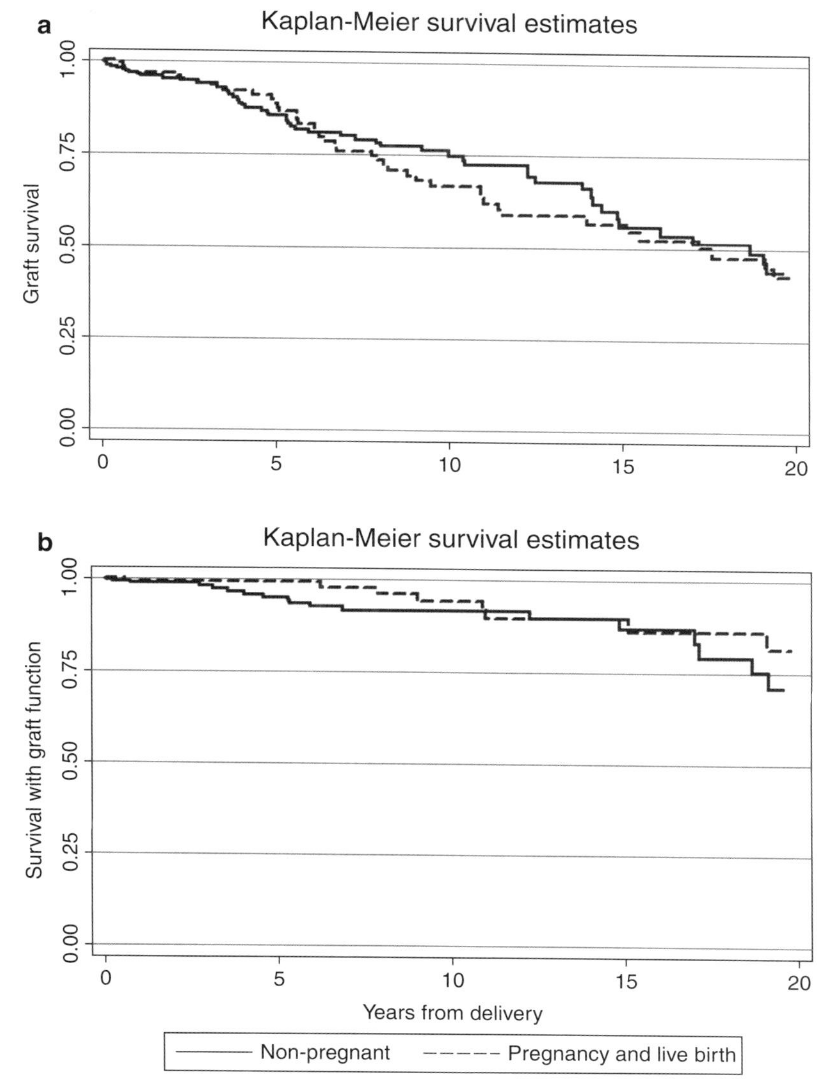

Fig. 33.7 Kaplan-Meier graft survival estimates in nulliparous and parous women with a kidney graft are shown. (**a**) Graft survival. (**b**) Patient survival (Reproduced with permission from Levidiotis et al. [38])

a serum creatinine of >150. It appears that hypertension (even when controlled) have an even greater association with preterm birth (30-fold increased risk) as compared with versus normotensive transplant recipients.

Delivery

The pelvic transplant kidney does not impair vaginal delivery nor is there evidence of damage to the transplant in the process. Instrumental delivery is indicated purely on obstetric or fetal grounds. Delivery should be 'covered' with IV steroids and IV hydration.

It is advisable for obstetricians to plan Caesarean section delivery in advance by discussion with the transplant surgeon, particularly where there may be anatomical challenges including simultaneous pancreas kidney transplantation or those with abnormal urinary drainage.

Breastfeeding

Breast milk transfer from mothers taking low-dose prednisolone or azathioprine is also safe. Azathioprine transfer in breast milk is very low and results in undetectable serum levels of the active metabolite 6-mercaptopurine in the baby. Recent data suggest low-level transfer of both cyclosporine and tacrolimus into breast milk. Cord blood levels on the day of delivery approximate maternal levels. By one week, despite breastfeeding, tacrolimus drug levels are undetectable in the baby. *With careful neonatal blood level monitoring* and following discussion with the neonatologist, it is reasonable to allow breastfeeding [44].

Most clinical studies of ARVD have considered the respective roles of revascularisation and medical therapy. The open surgical techniques pioneered in the 1950 and 1960s have been almost entirely replaced by percutaneous approaches. Percutaneous interventions were introduced in the 1980s and have evolved with improvements in technology from angioplasty alone to angioplasty and stenting, or primary stenting, which offer higher rates of long-term vessel patency. Despite these continued improvements, *no RCT has ever demonstrated superiority of an interventional approach over standard medical therapy for clinical outcomes such as progressive renal dysfunction, cardiovascular or renal events or mortality*. However, many questions remain, as the ARVD population *cannot* be considered a single homogenous group.

Prevalence

Many cases of ARVD are clinically silent, making it difficult to accurately estimate disease prevalence. Interpretation of available data is complicated both by temporal changes in availability of diagnostic tools and also by changes in attitudes towards use of these resources following publication of 'negative' RCTs such as the Angioplasty and Stenting for Renal Artery Lesions (ASTRAL) trial [4]. With these caveats considered, the most definite statement that can be made is that ARVD is not rare in the general population aged >65 years (annual incidence 0.5 %; prevalence 7 %) and is recognised as a primary cause of ESKD in a proportion of these patients (annual incidence of ESKD due to ARVD 1.3–1.7 %; prevalence 0.7–1 %) [5]. Ethnicity is not a significant factor in the development of ARVD.

Populations enriched with other vascular disease have higher rates of ARVD. Given the anatomical proximity of the abdominal aorta and the iliac vessels to the renal arteries, it is unsurprising that 20 and 40 % of patients with atheromatous disease in these respective areas have ARVD. However, the association extends to more distant vascular beds, with high rates of ARVD found in patients with carotid (10 %) and coronary (40 %) disease.

Although ARVD is a recognised cause of hypertension (and patients with ARVD are invariably hypertensive), it is often uncertain whether elevations in blood pressure are a cause or consequence of ARVD. Histological study supports the possibility that both pathological processes often coexist – renal biopsies from ARVD patients show a 50:50 split between presence of lone intrarenal atherosclerotic disease and intrarenal atherosclerotic disease with additional intrarenal hypertensive disease [6].

Screening the hypertensive population does not seem to increase identification of ARVD. Unselected screening data of hypertensive patients (>180 mmHg systolic and/or 100 mmHg diastolic) presenting to the emergency room describes an 8 % prevalence of ARVD. However higher rates of all cause RAS (including, e.g. FMD) are described when young hypertensive patients or patients with abdominal bruits are screened, with a pooled prevalence rate of 14 %. This suggests a need for more targeted investigations.

Aetiology

Despite the significant associations with other vascular pathologies, the effects of classical risk factors for development of atherosclerosis are less clear in ARVD than, e.g. coronary artery disease. Although the associations of CKD with smoking and diabetes may skew the data, single centre comparison of patients investigated for ARVD did not describe a difference in smoking rates or prevalence of diabetes mellitus between patients with normal or abnormal renal angiograms. This is despite higher rates of other vascular disease in the patients found to have ARVD [7]. The surprising lack of effect of smoking is confirmed in other data, but systematic reviews appear to suggest that increased rates of ARVD are observed in diabetic patients [8].

Given that patients with a single kidney can have an eGFR in the normal range, it is not immediately clear why unilateral RAS should lead to loss of renal function. It is most likely that renal parenchymal damage, secondary to 'flow-independent' effects of the stenosis (e.g. hypertension/micro-emboli), is the main arbiter of functional loss. In support of this, there is no correlation between degree of stenosis and level of proteinuria in ARVD, but an inverse relationship between eGFR and proteinuria. Indeed level of proteinuria is emerging as a possible marker of likelihood of improvement in eGFR following revascularisation. Even minor elevations (>0.6 g/24 h) correspond to large reductions in the chance of renal functional benefit from intervention [9].

Investigation for ARVD

As for any patient with CKD, measurement of baseline blood pressure, renal function and proteinuria should be performed. However, the key decision in the investigation for ARVD is which imaging modality is most appropriate.

Does a Patient with Asymmetrical Kidneys on Ultrasound Require Further Investigation?

Recent RCT data into the effect of revascularisation on prognosis in ARVD have at times been misinterpreted as a reason not to investigate the renal vessels where there is asymmetry of the kidneys on ultrasound. It is important to recognise that RAS is not the sole cause of differing kidney sizes, with primary renal dysplasia and reflux nephropathies typically

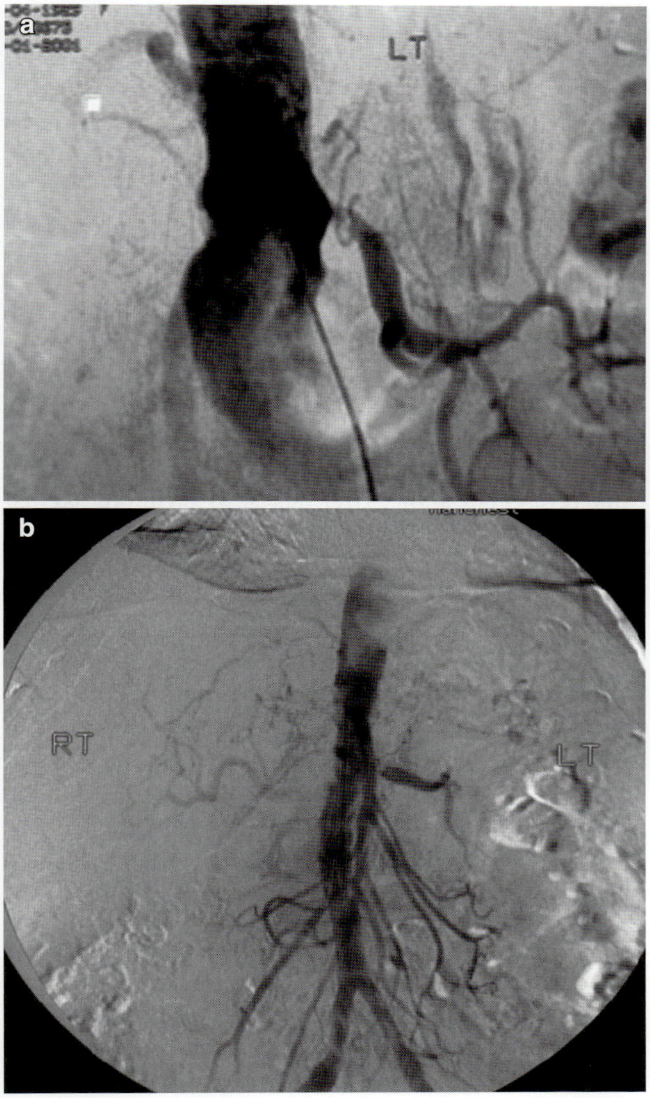

Fig. 34.4 Direct angiography in atherosclerotic renal vascular disease. (**a**) Seventy per cent left renal artery stenosis. (**b**) Right renal artery occlusion and 98 % left renal artery stenosis

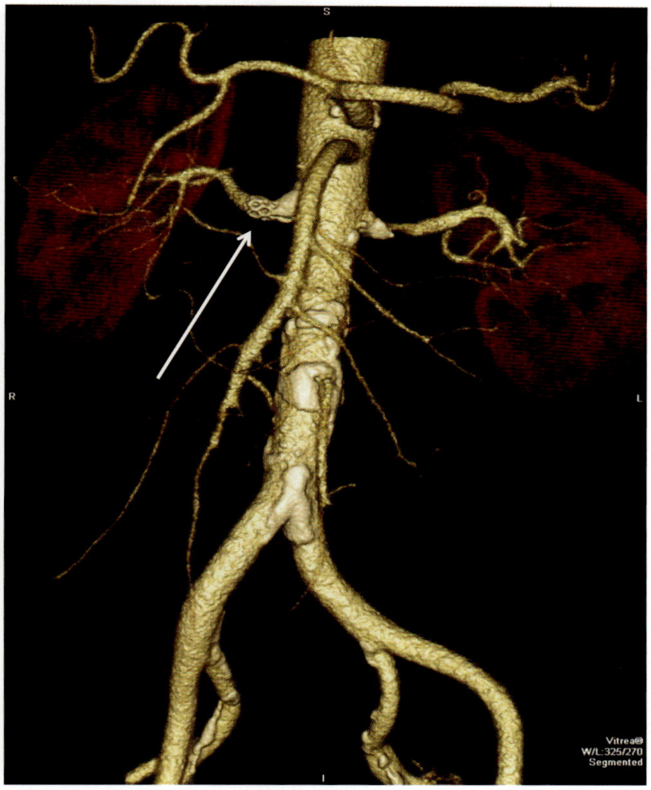

Fig. 34.5 Computed tomography angiography in atherosclerotic renal vascular disease. Reconstructed CT angiogram demonstrating patent left renal artery and patent right-sided renal artery stent (*arrow*)

resulting in asymmetric organs. As such, further investigation into the cause of renal asymmetry (and for associated complications) should be considered. Thus the decision centres around which is the best diagnostic tool?

Renal Artery Imaging

Direct angiography (Fig. 34.4) has been championed as the gold standard for diagnosis of ARVD, but it is an invasive procedure, only provides 2-D views and no functional data. As such, a variety of indirect methods have been adopted to minimise patient risk. Captopril renography has fallen into disuse; as although sensitive and specific for identification of unilateral stenoses, it is less reliable in the context of impaired renal function. Whilst local resources will play a key role in choice of investigation, duplex ultrasound (DUS), computed tomography angiography (CTA – Fig. 34.5) and magnetic resonance angiography (MRA) are all viable options to diagnose ARVD. In patients with mild to moderate (e.g. eGFR >30 ml/min) *and stable* CKD, all three investigations are comparable in terms of sensitivity and specificity and have negative predictive values in excess of 98 % [10]. Table 34.1 further compares the three techniques.

Where patients present with acute kidney injury or advanced renal dysfunction, there are often concerns that the iodinated contrast given for CTA may precipitate contrast-induced nephropathy. Although the likelihood of this is low (with online risk calculators available), the risk can act as a barrier to use of CTA. In the same settings, there is a potential risk of nephrogenic systemic fibrosis associated with the gadolinium-based contrast agents used during MRA. Therefore, in these specific settings, DUS is the most desirable test.

Cardiac Imaging

In over 95 % of patients with ARVD, an abnormality of either left ventricular function or structure can be demonstrated on transthoracic echocardiography, with risk of deterioration in all these parameters over time [11]. Baseline

Table 34.1 Diagnostic imaging techniques for atherosclerotic renovascular disease

Technique	Advantages	Disadvantages
Duplex ultrasound	Entirely non-invasive	Time consuming
	No contrast or radiation	Operator dependent
	Able to monitor disease progression	Technical failure rate >10 % (bowel gas, obesity, etc.)
Computed tomography angiography	Widely available tool	Contrast and radiation exposure Risk of contrast nephropathy
	Reproducible results	Calcified vessels can limit interpretability of images
	Most sensitive technique	Can overestimate stenosis
Magnetic resonance angiography	No risk of contrast nephropathy	Can overestimate stenosis
	No radiation	Risk of nephrogenic systemic fibrosis
	Reproducible images	

cardiac imaging is therefore an appropriate request. Currently this is of more prognostic than therapeutic benefit, although there is some limited evidence describing improvements in cardiac structure following renal artery revascularisation. Whilst published reports lack end point data, and RCT evidence is lacking, this is an area of great interest. High-quality randomised data comparing cardiac structural outcomes between medical and interventional therapy is anticipated later in 2012 [12].

Revascularisation

As of 2012, there have been five RCTs published comparing medical therapy with or without percutaneous revascularisation in ARVD. These studies (and others currently in progress) are summarised in Tables 34.2 and 34.3. A range of clinical outcome measures, rate of change in renal function and blood pressure and hard end points such as death, cardiovascular events and progression to renal replacement therapy have been assessed. No trial has shown a conclusive benefit of revascularisation over medical therapy for any outcome measure.

The first three trials published between 1998 and 2000 used angioplasty alone. Subsequently, it was established that better long-term angiographic outcomes occurred when angioplasty was coupled with bare metal stenting (PTRAS). This technique was therefore adopted for more recent trials [4, 14]. This difference in interventional technique limits direct comparison between RCTs. Small patient numbers, short follow-up periods and low rates of statin/rennin angiotensin blockade use in early trials further limit their applicability to current practice. The most recently published trial, ASTRAL, is by far the largest study (806 patients recruited worldwide compared with 140 in the next largest RCT) and has the longest follow-up period (mean >3 years). As such, much of current practice is based on data from this study. Its principal inclusion criterion was that, in a patient with anatomically significant RAS, it should be unclear whether the patient might benefit from revascularisation. Trial data was therefore skewed towards low-risk patients, who were the majority randomised in the trial. Higher-risk presentations of ARVD (who would potentially have the greatest benefit from revascularisation) were underrepresented in ASTRAL.

Stable CKD or Incidentally Diagnosed ARVD

Available evidence does not support revascularisation for patients with stable CKD. Real-world experience has duplicated trial findings, emphasising the need to focus on appropriate medical therapy for these patients. Acceptance of this finding is important to minimise risk of complications from intervention (discussed below). Whilst incidentally diagnosed ARVD could be considered to be the same as ARVD with stable CKD, specific outcome data exist for patients found to have RAS during another angiographic procedure. In line with trial data, when incidental cases of ARVD were compared between those that were revascularised versus those who were not, no difference was seen in terms of blood pressure or renal function at 12 months.

The overall lack of benefit from revascularisation when examining renal dysfunction as a primary outcome measure is almost certainly due to the slow rate of loss of renal function seen in ARVD. The annual eGFR loss associated with ageing is around 0.7 ml/min/1.73 m^2/year, with the average rate of loss in ARVD only slightly higher than this. As such, any longitudinal difference in renal function between medical and interventional groups would be subtle and require an RCT to be powered to very high patient numbers to identify a statistical difference. This raises the possibility that an interventional study would be more likely to identify differences in cardiovascular event (CVE) rates. Whilst ASTRAL showed almost identical CVE rates in each treatment group (with an annual event rate of 10 %/year), this was not the primary study end point, and other ongoing studies, most notably the Cardiovascular Outcomes in Renal Atherosclerotic Lesions trial (CORAL), have been designed to specifically answer this question.

Table 34.2 Published randomised controlled trials in atherosclerotic renovascular disease

Trial and intervention	Patient number and baseline details	Medications	Primary end points	Secondary end points	Limitations	Results
SNRASCG 1998 PCTA	55 patients 57%male Age 60 sCr 159 µmol/L BP 190/100	A2B – 0 % Statin – not documented Antiplatelet – all per protocol	Change in BP and sCr	Number of drugs to control BP	No angiotensin blockade 6-month follow-up period Small patient number	No differences between groups within follow-up period
EMMA 1998 PCTA	49 patients 73 % male Age 59 sCr 103 µmol/L BP 150/90 Minimum stenosis 60 %	A2B – unclear Statin – not documented Antiplatelet – all per protocol	Change in ABP	Complication rate Daily dose of blood pressure medications	Small patient numbers 6-month follow-up period	No difference in ABP. Reduced daily dose in PCTA group
DRASTIC 2000 PCTA [13]	106 patients 61 % male Age 60 sCr 1.25 mg/dl BP 179/104 Minimum stenosis 50 %	A2B – 22 % Statin – 39 % Antiplatelet – all in PCTA group. Unclear in medical group	Change in blood pressure at 3 and 12 months	Number of drugs to control BP Daily dose of blood pressure medications Creatinine clearance	50 % cross over from medical to interventional arm Short follow-up period	No difference in manual BP at 3 or 12 months Reduction in BP at 12 months when measured by automated device for revasc group Reduction in number of drugs for revasc group
STAR 2009 PTRAS [14]	140 patients 63 % male Age 66 sCr 149 µmol/L BP 161/82 Minimum stenosis >50 %	A2B – 56 % Statin – all per protocol Antiplatelet – all per protocol	20 % reduction in creatinine clearance	Complication rate Blood pressure change Cardiovascular events Mortality	28 % of patients randomised to PTRAS not revascularised High procedural complication rate – 3 patient deaths; 1 patient dialysis dependent	No difference in creatinine clearance or BP No cardiac event or mortality difference High complication rate in interventional group
ASTRAL 2009 PTRAS [4]	806 patients 63%male Age 70 sCr 179 µmol/L BP 150/76 Av. stenosis 75 %	A2B – 42 % Statin – 95 % Antiplatelet – 77 %	Rate of change in renal function	Blood pressure change Time to cardiovascular or renal event Mortality	No reference lab Patients felt likely to benefit from revascularisation potentially excluded	No difference between arms for any end point

Study abbreviations: *SNRASCG* The Scottish and Newcastle Renal Artery Stenosis Collaborative Group, *EMMA* The Essai Multicentrique Medicaments vs. Angioplastie Study Group, *DRASTIC* The Dutch Led Renal Artery Stenosis Intervention Cooperative Study Group, *STAR* The Stent Placement for Renal Artery Stenosis Trial, *ASTRAL* The Angioplasty and Stenting for Renal Artery Lesions Trial. Year listed is year of publication
Abbreviations: *PCTA* percutaneous renal angioplasty, *PTRAS* percutaneous renal angioplasty and stenting, *A2B* angiotensin blockade, *ABP* ambulatory blood pressure, *sCr* serum creatinine, *BP* blood pressure, *Revasc* revascularised

ARVD, with antiplatelet agents strongly considered on a case-by-case basis. These interventions have benefits in excess of blood pressure and proteinuria reduction and should be complimented by general measures to manage risk in CKD such as smoking cessation advice, good diabetic control and taking exercise.

Renin-Angiotensin Blockade

The importance of tight blood pressure control is well recognised in all cause CKD, with a widespread appreciation that blockade of the renin angiotensin aldosterone system (RAAS) provides renal benefits in excess of those delivered solely by the associated blood pressure reduction. In ARVD these agents reduce both blood pressure and risk of mortality to a greater extent than other antihypertensive agents.

Historically RAS has been considered a contraindication to RAAS blockade due to concerns over associated deterioration in renal function. However, only a minority of patients (even those with significant bilateral disease) are unable to tolerate supervised introduction of RAAS blockade [21], with any changes in eGFR reversible on withdrawal of the agent.

Second-Line Treatment of Hypertension

For ARVD patients with blood pressure not controlled by RAAS inhibition, data on second- and third-line agents is scarce. CORAL has defined thiazide diuretics as a second-line agent (replaced by loop diuretics where there is advanced renal dysfunction), with beta-blockers and calcium channel blockers third-line agents. Although no outcome data support use of diuretics in ARVD, the understanding that resistant hypertension in CKD is often due to underuse of diuretics, and especially that salt-water retention is increased by RAAS overstimulation, makes these agents a logical choice.

Support for use of beta-blockade comes from recognition of increased local sympathetic and adrenergic activity in ARVD. This local increase is associated with elevated serum noradrenaline concentrations which have been linked to both reduced eGFR and the increased cardiovascular mortality. There are some data which suggest that beta-blockade following revascularisation leads to improved renal functional outcomes and lower rates of re-stenosis. Renal artery denervation, which has been shown (in a non-ARVD population) to reduce peripheral blood pressure, may be helpful, but as yet there are no data in the ARVD population to support its use.

Statins

The evidence supporting statin therapy in ARVD has a clear narrative. Though early case reports describing regression of stenosis with statin therapy have not been duplicated, it is certain that rate of progression of stenosis is slowed. In addition, statin-treated patients (even with a normal lipid profile) have been shown to have lower rates of death and progression to dialysis [23].

Revascularised patients also benefit from treatment with statins, with a reduction in risk of death of over 80 %. Although the mechanism of benefit is not clear it is most likely achieved through a composite effect of reduced renal fibrosis, reduced left ventricular hypertrophy and the wider cardiovascular advantages of these agents.

Antiplatelet Therapy

The historical perspective of antiplatelet therapy in all forms of atheromatous disease makes an objective assessment of the role of these agents in ARVD challenging. With the coexistent burden of vascular disease in ARVD, the use of antiplatelets is easy to justify. Although the DOPPS study did not identify a benefit of aspirin therapy in dialysis-dependent patients, sub-analysis of patients with mild to moderate CKD in primary prevention studies have shown significant reduction in the rate of vascular events, albeit with a significant increase in bleeding risk [24]. Less information is available regarding alternative agents such as clopidogrel (which may have reduced pharmacological activity in CKD).

The time point for which there is definitive evidence for antiplatelet agents in ARVD is at time of intervention. The amount of micro-emboli released during stenting is significantly reduced by clopidogrel loading in combination with aspirin therapy (although the long-term functional benefits are not yet established).

A summary of the basic considerations and management for the more common clinical presentations of renovascular disease is provided in Table 34.4.

Renal Artery Embolic Disease

Cholesterol Emboli

Cholesterol embolisation occurs when cholesterol crystals are released following the rupture of an atheromatous plaque. These crystals can occlude any small vessel, precipitating a multisystem disorder. Although the true incidence and prevalence are unknown, cholesterol embolisation is typically described as a disease of the over 60s (with a male preponderance) and may account for between 5 and 10% of cases of acute kidney injury within this demographic.

Risk factors

Given the link between cholesterol embolisation and pre-existing atheromatous disease, it is unsurprising that risk factors are common between these conditions (age over 60 years, hypertension, diabetes, smoking history, Caucasian). More clinically relevant are the precipitants for embolisation, which *have* changed over time. Whilst 20–30 years ago, spontaneous plaque rupture was

Table 34.4 Example clinical scenarios

Scenario	Actions	
Patient aged <30 years presenting with hypertension	Examine for bruits Indirect angiography to investigate for FMD	Good candidate for angioplasty if angiogram shows FMD
Patient with eGFR 20 ml/min and asymmetric kidneys on ultrasound	Do not expose to gadolinium. Image renal vessels with either DUS or CTA	Consider admission for hydration for CTA
Elderly patient with chronic CKD stage 3 and renal artery stenosis	Address lifestyle factors – e.g. smoking, diabetic control	Prescribe angiotensin blockade as first-line blood pressure control. Commence statin and consider antiplatelet agent
Patient presenting with recurrent acute onset pulmonary oedema	Assess left ventricular function. If systolic function preserved, perform indirect renal angiography	If significant bilateral renal artery stenosis, consider referral for revascularisation
Patient with suspected renal artery stenosis and previously preserved renal function presenting acutely dialysis dependent	Doppler imaging of renal vessels	Refer for renal artery angioplasty and stenting
Greater than 25 % reduction in eGFR following initiation of angiotensin blockade to treat chronic heart failure	Consider volume state and concurrent nephrotoxic drugs Indirect renal angiography	If significant stenosis and no other culprit medications, consider revascularisation
Patient with uncontrolled symptoms of CHF and renal artery stenosis	Review echocardiograms regarding LVMI	If uncontrolled symptoms, increased LVMI and significant stenosis, consider revascularisation

FMD fibromuscular disease, *DUS* duplex ultrasound, *CTA* computed tomography angiography, *CHF* chronic heart failure, *LVMI* left ventricular mass index, *eGFR* estimated glomerular filtration rate, *CKD* chronic kidney disease

almost the sole cause, the greatly increased use of interventional endovascular techniques has resulted in over 75 % of contemporary cases being iatrogenic. Coronary angiography appears to carry the highest risk, with approximately 20 cases per 1,000 procedures. Additionally, anticoagulation can precipitate cholesterol emboli, although this is a rare complication [25].

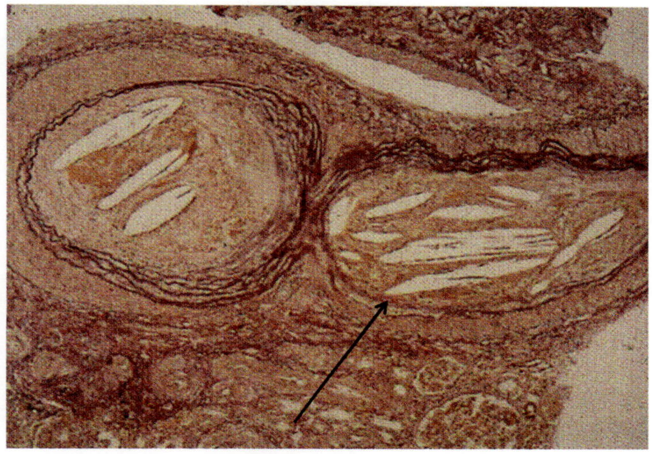

Fig. 34.6 Renal biopsy demonstrating small vessel cholesterol athero-emboli (*arrow*)

Presentation

As with vasculitis, disease presentation depends entirely on the vessels involved. Severe acute kidney injury is relatively rare, with only the minority of patients having a significant abrupt rise in serum creatinine within a few days of an interventional procedure. Mostly there is slow, progressive loss of renal function spread over a period in excess of 4 weeks. This is suggestive of two distinct pathologies – the first where a large crystal burden causes acute vascular occlusion within the kidney and a second where there is either slow sustained emboli release and/or a regional inflammatory response to emboli dispersed to the kidney.

In patients with renal involvement, the two other most commonly affected organ systems are the skin (presenting with livedo reticularis, blue toes, purpura, ulceration and gangrene) and the gastrointestinal tract (presenting with non-specific abdominal pain, bleeding, ischaemic bowel, pancreatitis). Neurological manifestations are less common and harder to define; but where retinal embolisation occurs, this should dramatically raise the index of suspicion for the diagnosis.

Diagnosis

It is highly likely that many minor or clinically asymptomatic cases of cholesterol embolisation go undetected, especially following endovascular revascularisation therapy. However, the presence of acute/subacute renal dysfunction in the context of a clear precipitant and other signs of peripheral embolisation is sufficient to confirm the diagnosis of cholesterol embolisation. Where this triad does not exist (and if retinal emboli cannot be demonstrated on fundoscopy), tissue is required to make a definitive diagnosis and exclude conditions such as small vessel vasculitis. Renal biopsy is the gold standard test (providing a positive diagnosis in over 75 % of cases – Fig. 34.6), but samples from other areas, e.g. skin, can be valuable if this is contraindicated.

Prior to biopsy, there are few serum markers of diagnostic use, but new onset proteinuria (assuming no coexisting renal disease cause) may be suggestive. A relationship between cholesterol embolisation and hypocomplementaemia is not consistently reported, and the presence of this should perhaps direct more attention to the possibility of other diagnoses such as subacute bacterial endocarditis. Of more clinical use is the presence of systemic eosinophilia, which, although transient, is commonly seen at high levels where there is cholesterol embolisation. This finding, although sensitive, is not specific and should also prompt consideration of acute interstitial nephritis if there has been a newly introduced medication.

Treatment

There is no definitive treatment for cholesterol embolisation, and between 40 and 60 % of patients suspected to have the diagnosis require acute dialysis with a significant proportion remaining dialysis dependent. Withdrawal of any clear precipitant is a vital first step. Thereafter, the mainstay of treatment is statin therapy. Although there is a lack of randomised data or a mechanistic explanation, there is good, prospective, evidence that these agents reduce risk for ESKD [26]. There is no large-scale evidence of benefit for corticosteroids and use is often limited to patients with severe multisystem disease.

Renal Artery Thromboembolism

Renal artery thromboembolism, if not immediately treated, leads to irreversible renal parenchymal damage and loss of renal function. Unfortunately, due to the non-specific nature of the symptomatology and the rarity of the condition, this is often a delayed diagnosis.

Pathology

The primary source of emboli causing renal infarction is cardiac (typically left atrial clots secondary to atrial fibrillation), although cases linked to sickle cell disease and septic emboli are reported.

Presentation and Diagnosis

Most patients are aged over 60 years and present with severe acute onset flank/abdominal pain, which can be associated with a fever and nausea and vomiting. There is no gender or racial preponderance.

Whilst the presence of new onset dipstick haematuria/proteinuria is supportive of renal thromboembolism, the key to making the diagnosis is a high index of clinical suspicion and expedient angiographic imaging (either direct angiography or CTA, as USS has very low sensitivity). When reviewing imaging it should be understood that up to 10 % of cases present with bilateral thrombi.

Treatment

The rarity of the condition makes treatment recommendations difficult. Prompt initiation of anticoagulation with i.v. heparin (followed by warfarin when stable) is the accepted first step, followed by percutaneous thrombolysis or thrombectomy as soon as possible. Renal functional prognosis is highly dependent on speed of diagnosis and treatment [27].

Renal Vein Disease

Diseases of the renal veins are rare and mainly limited to three disease presentations.

Renal Vein Thrombosis

Aetiology

In adults, renal vein thrombosis (RVT) most commonly occurs in the context of nephrotic level protein loss, typically in association with membranous nephropathy. However, associations with other glomerular diseases (e.g. lupus), malignancy (e.g. renal cell carcinoma) and hypercoagulable states (e.g. protein C & S deficiency, postpartum) are also described. Whilst the risk of all types of thromboembolic events is elevated in nephrotic states, RVT is one of, if not the most common. Why this should be the case is uncertain, but reduced renal vein pressures and increased local thrombin production secondary to glomerular injury are two proposed factors.

Diagnosis

Where RVT is acute, occlusive and bilateral, AKI will develop. However, most patients slowly develop a progressive thrombus, allowing the development of a collateral venous system. These two distinct pathologies account for the disparity in reported incidence of venous thromboembolic events in patients with membranous nephropathy when considering overt clinical presentations (less than 10 %) versus those identified by screening (50–80 %) [28].

The key symptom of an acute thrombus is loin or flank pain, typically associated with a fever, nausea and vomiting or occasionally presenting as pulmonary emboli. Leucocytosis and dipstick haematuria are common, making pyelonephritis a key differential diagnosis. Chronic thrombi are usually non-occlusive, asymptomatic and characterised by increased proteinuria and subtle alterations in renal function.

Treatment

There is no defined *gold standard* treatment strategy for renal vein thrombosis. The decision will depend mainly on local expertise and experience, but also in part on which kidney is affected (with the left kidney less likely to rupture in the setting of acute venous occlusion due to a pre-existing collateral drainage system). Thrombolysis can be considered where there are bilateral renal vein thrombi or

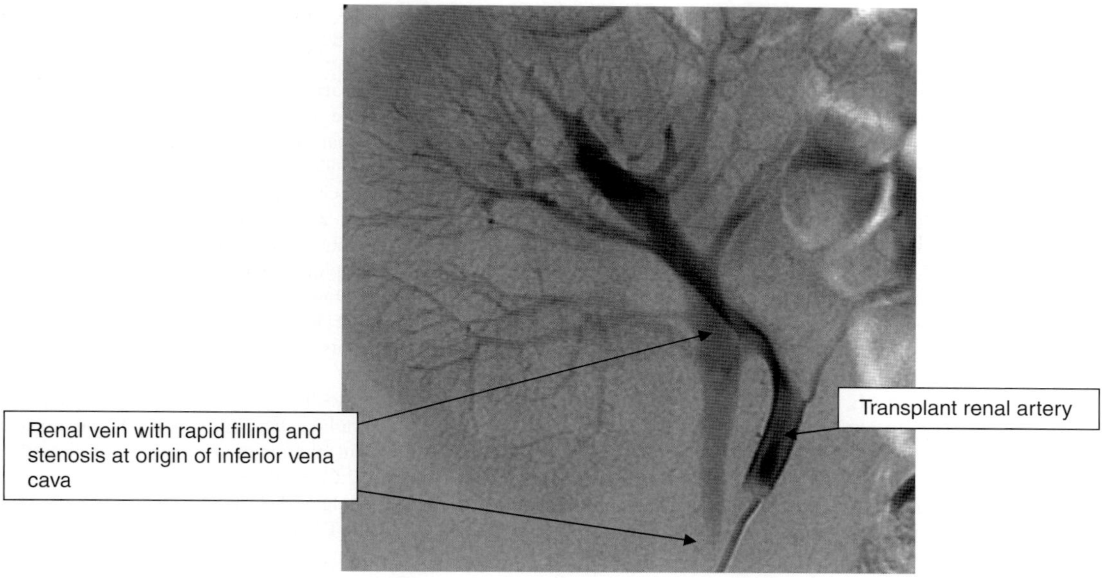

Fig. 34.7 Renal vein stenosis in a renal transplant with an arteriovenous fistula. Angiogram shows very rapid (almost simultaneous) venous return and a venous stenosis at the point of the inferior vena cava

pulmonary embolus, with medical anticoagulation (using warfarin or low molecular weight heparin) then used as chronic therapy. These agents can be utilised as first-line therapy in less severe cases. Interventional approaches including percutaneous thrombectomy, surgical venous bypass and nephrectomy are available. However, these approaches tend to be reserved for cases of extensive clot or where there is risk of capsular rupture.

Renal Vein Stenosis

Very rarely the renal vein can suffer a non-occlusive stenosis resulting in proteinuria and or reduced function. The diagnosis is easily missed and may only be picked up incidentally in the venous phase of contrast studies (see Fig. 34.7).

Left Renal Vein Entrapment Syndrome

Left renal vein entrapment (also referred to as the 'nutcracker syndrome') results from entrapment of the renal vein between the abdominal aorta and the superior mesenteric artery. The presentation can be at any age and is classically with left flank pain (which can extend to the left testicle) with non-visible or visible haematuria or orthostatic proteinuria. Diagnosis can be made either by ultrasound or computed tomography imaging.

Treatment of the 'nutcracker syndrome' is dependent on the severity of symptoms. In the most extreme cases, renal vein stenting, surgical venous bypass and autotransplantation have all been used [29].

Lymphatic Disease

Cystic dilatation of renal lymphatic channels, renal lymphangiomatosis (also called cystic lymphangioma or renal lymphangiectasia), is an exceptionally rare condition in which the renal lymphatics fail to adequately drain, resulting in structural malformations. The kidneys can enlarge to such a size that they may mimic polycystic disease or cause an obstructive uropathy. As there is minimal effect on renal function, management is normally conservative. The exception is during pregnancy in which the condition may be exacerbated to the point of requiring percutaneous drainage [30].

Internet Resources

The Fibromuscular Dysplasia Registry: http://www.fmdsa.org

Contrast nephropathy risk calculator: http://www.qxmd.com/calculate-online/nephrology/contrast-nephropathy-post-pci

References

1. Sharma S, Gupta H, Saxena A, et al. Results of renal angioplasty in nonspecific aortoarteritis (Takayasu disease). J Vasc Interv Radiol. 1998;9(3):429–35.
2. Olin JW, Sealove BA. Diagnosis, management, and future developments of fibromuscular dysplasia. J Vasc Surg. 2011;53(3):826–36.e1.
3. Trinquart L, Mounier-Vehier C, Sapoval M, Gagnon N, Plouin P-F. Efficacy of revascularization for renal artery stenosis caused by fibromuscular dysplasia: a systematic review and meta-analysis. Hypertension. 2010;56(3):525–32.
4. ASTRAL Investigators, Wheatley K, Ives N, et al. Revascularization versus medical therapy for renal-artery stenosis. N Engl J Med. 2009;361(20):1953–62.
5. Kalra PA, Guo H, Kausz AT, et al. Atherosclerotic renovascular disease in United States patients aged 67 years or older: risk factors, revascularization, and prognosis. Kidney Int. 2005;68(1):293–301.

6. Keddis M, Garovic V, Bailey K. Ischaemic nephropathy secondary to atherosclerotic renal artery stenosis: clinical and histopathological correlates. Nephrol Dial Transplant. 2010;25(11):3615–22.
7. Shurrab AE, Mamtora H, O'Donoghue D, Waldrek S, Kalra PA. Increasing the diagnostic yield of renal angiography for the diagnosis of atheromatous renovascular disease. Br J Radiol. 2001;74(879):213–8.
8. de Mast Q, Beutler JJ. The prevalence of atherosclerotic renal artery stenosis in risk groups: a systematic literature review. J Hypertens. 2009;27(7):1333–40.
9. Chrysochou C, Cheung CM, Durow M, et al. Proteinuria as a predictor of renal functional outcome after revascularization in atherosclerotic renovascular disease (ARVD). QJM. 2009;102(4):283–8.
10. Eriksson P, Mohammed AA, De Geer J, et al. Non-invasive investigations of potential renal artery stenosis in renal insufficiency. Nephrol Dial Transplant. 2010;25(11):3607–14.
11. Wright JR, Shurrab AE, Cooper A, Kalra PR, Foley RN, Kalra PA. Left ventricular morphology and function in patients with atherosclerotic renovascular disease. J Am Soc Nephrol. 2005;16(9): 2746–53.
12. Marcantoni C, Zanoli L, Rastelli S, et al. Stenting of renal artery stenosis in coronary artery disease (RAS-CAD) study: a prospective, randomized trial. J Nephrol. 2009;22(1):13–6.
13. van Jaarsveld BC, Krijnen P, Pieterman H, et al. The effect of balloon angioplasty on hypertension in atherosclerotic renal-artery stenosis. Dutch Renal Artery Stenosis Intervention Cooperative Study Group. N Engl J Med. 2000;342(14):1007–14.
14. Bax L, Woittiez A-JJ, Kouwenberg HJ, et al. Stent placement in patients with atherosclerotic renal artery stenosis and impaired renal function: a randomized trial. Ann Intern Med. 2009;150(12):840–8. W150–1.
15. Staub D, Zeller T, Trenk D, et al. Use of B-type natriuretic peptide to predict blood pressure improvement after percutaneous revascularisation for renal artery stenosis. Eur J Vasc Endovasc Surg. 2010;40(5):599–607.
16. Kanjwal K, Cooper CJ, Virmani R, et al. Predictors of embolization during protected renal artery angioplasty and stenting: role of antiplatelet therapy. Catheter Cardiovasc Interv. 2010;76(1):16–23.
17. Cooper CJ, Haller ST, Colyer W, et al. Embolic protection and platelet inhibition during renal artery stenting. Circulation. 2008;117(21):2752–60.
18. Hirsch AT, Haskal ZJ, Hertzer NR, et al. ACC/AHA Guidelines for the Management of Patients with Peripheral Arterial Disease (lower extremity, renal, mesenteric, and abdominal aortic): a collaborative report from the American Associations for Vascular Surgery/Society for Vascular Surgery, Society for cardiovascular angiography and Interventions, Society for Vascular Medicine and Biology, Society of Interventional radiology, and the ACC/AHA Task Force on Practice Guidelines (writing committee to develop guidelines for the management of patients with peripheral arterial disease) – summary of recommendations. J Vasc Interv Radiol. 2006;17(9): 1383–97. quiz1398.
19. Kane GC, Xu N, Mistrik E, Roubicek T, Stanson AW, Garovic VD. Renal artery revascularization improves heart failure control in patients with atherosclerotic renal artery stenosis. Nephrol Dial Transplant. 2010;25(3):813–20.
20. MacDowall P, Kalra PA, O'Donoghue DJ, Waldek S, Mamtora H, Brown K. Risk of morbidity from renovascular disease in elderly patients with congestive cardiac failure. Lancet. 1998;352(9121): 13–6.
21. Chrysochou C, Foley RN, Young JF, Khavandi K, Cheung CM, Kalra PA. Dispelling the myth: the use of renin-angiotensin blockade in atheromatous renovascular disease. Nephrol Dial Transplant. 2012;27(4):1403–9.
22. Cheung CM, Chrysochou C, Shurrab AE, Buckley DL, Cowie A, Kalra PA. Effects of renal volume and single-kidney glomerular filtration rate on renal functional outcome in atherosclerotic renal artery stenosis. Nephrol Dial Transplant. 2010;25(4):1133–40.
23. Silva VS, Martin LC, Franco RJS, et al. Pleiotropic effects of statins may improve outcomes in atherosclerotic renovascular disease. Am J Hypertens. 2008;21(10):1163–8.
24. Jardine MJ, Ninomiya T, Perkovic V, et al. Aspirin is beneficial in hypertensive patients with chronic kidney disease. J Am Coll Cardiol. 2010;56(12):956–65.
25. Scolari F, Ravani P. Atheroembolic renal disease. Lancet. 2010;375(9726):1650–60.
26. Scolari F, Ravani P, Gaggi R, et al. The challenge of diagnosing atheroembolic renal disease: clinical features and prognostic factors. Circulation. 2007;116(3):298–304.
27. Lopez VM, Glauser J. A case of renal artery thrombosis with renal infarction. J Emerg Trauma Shock. 2010;3(3):302.
28. Lionaki S, Derebail VK, Hogan SL, et al. Venous thromboembolism in patients with membranous nephropathy. Clin J Am Soc Nephrol. 2012;7(1):43–51.
29. Kurklinsky AK, Rooke TW. Nutcracker phenomenon and nutcracker syndrome. Mayo Clin Proc. 2010;85(6):552–9.
30. Ozmen M, Deren O, Akata D, Akhan O, Ozen H, Durukan T. Renal lymphangiomatosis during pregnancy: management with percutaneous drainage. Eur Radiol. 2001;11(1):37–40.

Urinary Tract Infection

35

Gayathri K. Rajakaruna and Mark Harber

Urinary tract infection in vulnerable groups is responsible for considerable morbidity and mortality, but even in healthy individuals, 'uncomplicated' UTIs (cystitis or pyelonephritis in a healthy woman) are responsible for a considerable health-care burden [1]. In a recent analysis, UTIs were responsible for 8.6 million visits a year in the USA, symptoms lasting an average of 6 days with 2–4 days of reduced activity and an estimated cost to the US economy of $2–4 billion per year. Patients with complicated UTIs and recurrent urosepsis in the setting of urological abnormality or transplantation are often seen by nephrologists and can represent a considerable challenge. Whether seeing a nephrologist or not, the pathway for these patients is often haphazard, without a clear structure, and patients commonly suffer care that is more disjointed than we ought to be delivering. In the setting of increasing rates of multi-resistant organisms including carbapenem resistance, this is a particularly important issue and challenge for the renal community that we need to rise to with a degree of urgency. http://www.nhs.uk/conditions/urinary-tract-infection-adults/Pages/Introduction.aspx, http://kidney.niddk.nih.gov/kudiseases/pubs/uti_ez/and http://www.nhs.uk/conditions/kidney-infection/Pages/Introduction.aspx are useful sources for patient information and recommended as a first stop.

G.K. Rajakaruna, MBBS, MRCP (UK)
Department of Nephrology, Royal Free Hospital,
Pond Street, London NW3 2QG, UK
e-mail: grajakaruna@doctors.org.uk

M. Harber, MBBS, PhD, FRCP (✉)
UCL Department of Nephrology, Royal Free London
NHS Foundation Trust, Pond Street, Hampstead,
London NW3 2QG, UK
e-mail: mark.harber@nhs.net

Diagnosis and Definition of UTI

Bacterial UTIs are classically divided into 'uncomplicated' (cystitis or acute pyelonephritis and an otherwise healthy woman) and 'complicated' (essentially everyone else, i.e. UTIs in men, pregnancy, diabetics, transplantation and anyone with an anatomically or functionally abnormal urinary tract). There is a genuine clinical utility in dividing UTIs this way in terms of patient risk and overall management. Moreover, it is also useful to divide urinary tract infection into anatomical location: balanitis, urethritis, prostatitis, cystitis and pyelonephritis, all of which can also be divided into acute or chronic.

The definition and diagnosis of UTIs are not always straightforward, for example, a poorly taken sample may be contaminated with perineal bacteria, especially if the sample is delayed, and yield a spurious result. Asymptomatic bacteriuria (ASB) is defined as the growth of bacteria from a well-taken sample in the absence of symptoms with associated pyuria. The laboratory definition of UTI derives from work in asymptomatic women with $\geq 10^5$ colony-forming units (cfu)/ml, and counts below this or 10^4 are rarely reported by laboratories; however, there is good evidence that $\geq 10^2$ cfu is an appropriate diagnostic threshold in symptomatic patients. Recent antibiotics may inhibit culture; fastidious organisms may not grow or may be overwhelmed by other organisms with standard techniques. Urinary catheters, ileostomies and urostomies will inevitably be colonised with bacteria and result in 'positive' cultures. Patients with neutropenia may have no pyuria, and there are non-infectious causes of sterile pyuria. Urethritis and vaginitis can mimic the symptoms of cystitis, and symptoms of upper and lower UTI are often minimal in the elderly and immunocompromised.

Balanitis

Acute balanitis is usually clinically obvious, but chronic balanitis, often associated with phimosis and diabetes, may not be. Recurrent short courses of antibiotics for presumed

M. Harber (ed.), *Practical Nephrology*,
DOI 10.1007/978-1-4471-5547-8_35, © Springer-Verlag London 2014

recurrent cystitis on the basis of leucocytes and positive cultures are a good way of generating multi-resistant organisms. The diagnosis is usually obvious on inspection illustrating the importance of local examination, and treatment usually involves circumcision.

Urethritis, Urethral Syndrome and Vaginitis

These conditions may be misdiagnosed as cystitis on the basis of dysuria. Symptoms more suggestive of urethritis are the predominance of dysuria, with less frequency and urgency, often more gradual onset and more common in a sexually active patient, especially with new partner(s). If urethritis is secondary to Chlamydia trachomatis, Mycoplasma genitalium or Neisseria gonorrhoeae, then it is often associated with pyuria and should be detected by urethral specimen at a sexually transmitted disease clinic visit. Culture-negative urethritis/urethral syndrome that is often not associated with pyuria is a poorly understood condition with a variety of aetiologies including autoimmune (e.g. Behcet's syndrome, GPA granulomatosis), mycobacterial, viral (e.g. adenovirus), trauma, chemical, foreign body, strictures and stones/crystalluria. Occasionally, viral infections such as herpes simplex can present with culture-negative urethritis and can respond to prophylactic acyclovir. As a chronic condition, it is often difficult to diagnose and treat; referral to a urologist or genitourinary medicine colleague with a specialist interest is worth considering.

Vaginitis is another cause for dysuria misdiagnosed as UTI, and it is important to specifically ask about vaginal discharge (absence has a good negative predictive value). Symptoms are often felt to be external, and as with urethritis frequency and urgency may be absent. Candida, gonorrhoea, chlamydia, mycoplasma and herpes simplex are all common causes.

Prostatitis

Acute prostatitis may present as a lower UTI, fever and urethral obstruction. Urine dipstick and cultures will not distinguish from cystitis, and the suspicion may only be raised following relapse of a UTI after a short course of antibiotics. The prostate is tender on palpation, and a raised prostatic-specific antigen can be a useful clue.

Chronic prostatitis may also present with relapse of UTI after antibiotics, the prostate typically less tender with less dramatic inflammatory markers than with acute prostatitis. MSU taken after prostatic massage may reveal inflammatory cells on microscopy and occasionally the organism.

For both acute and chronic prostatitis, the empiric treatment is usually fluoroquinolones for 4–6 weeks.

Interstitial Cystitis (IC) and Overactive Bladder (OAB) Complex

Interstitial cystitis and OAB form a spectrum of chronic, poorly understood conditions that can cause profound and disabling LUTS. IC is associated with mast cell infiltrate and has been associated and maybe associated with sterile pyuria, forming an important part of the differential for recurrent UTI reviewed by Moutzouris D-A [2]. From the nephrologist point of view, it is important to exclude other pathologies such as low-grade chronic infection (especially in diabetics) which can present with IC/OAB symptoms, malignancy, stones and other physiochemical causes such as radiation cystitis or ketamine-induced inflammation. A high index of suspicion is required and also early referral for cystoscopy and to a sympathetic specialist.

Epidemiology of Bacterial Cystitis and Pyelonephritis

In infancy, bacteriuria occurs in 1–2 %, more commonly in boys for the first 3 months and more likely to be associated with bacteraemia and pyelonephritis. After this time, girls are more commonly affected with a pre-school incidence of 4.5 % compared to 0.5 % in boys in whom UTI is very likely to be associated with significant congenital abnormality.

In adults, 84 % of uncomplicated UTIs occur in women with 3 % of American woman seeking medical help for this per year. 50 % of women experience at least one symptomatic UTI in their lifetime and 20–25 % of these having a recurrence within 6 months and roughly 33 % in a lifetime. For a woman, having a first-degree female relative with a history of UTI is a significant risk factor (OR ~2.5–4).

With increasing age, co-morbidity and institutionalisation, the incidence of UTI increases dramatically with the female/male ratio reducing significantly. In postmenopausal women alone, the annual risk of UTI is around 10 % with 5–15 % of women over 60 having recurrent UTIs. Instrumentation is an important and potentially modifiable risk factor; a one off urinary catheterisation carries a 1 % risk of UTI, but for hospital patients an indwelling catheter has a 10 % risk of UTI. The risk of bacteriuria secondary to indwelling catheters is strongly related to duration corresponding to 5 % risk with each day; consequently, UTIs are the most common nosocomial infection (40 %). Urinary tract infection is also very frequently in transplant recipients commonly exceeding 50 % in the first year of transplantation.

The risk factors for urinary tract infection are shown in Table 35.1 and explain much of the increase in old age and transplant recipients.

Acute uncomplicated pyelonephritis in women is roughly 3 per 1,000 person years [3] with a peak age of 15–34. The

Table 35.1 Risk factors for urinary tract infection

Risk factor	Management
Female sex	
Old age	
Sexual intercourse especially with a new partner	
Use of diaphragm and spermicides	
Previous UTIs	Consider antibiotic prophylaxis if frequent and conservative measures fail
First-degree relative with UTI	
Urological instrumentation, intermittent self-catheterisation and ureteric stents	Exclude and/or treat ASB prior to instrumentation, refresh ISC technique, minimise stent duration
Catheterisation (especially indwelling but also convene catheters)	Avoid unnecessary catheterisation and minimise catheter duration where possible
Congenital abnormality of urinary tract	
Acquired abnormality of urinary tract	
Neurogenic bladder	Consider intermittent self-catheterisation (ISC)
Stones	Where possible remove (rarely possible with nephrolithiasis or multiple stones)
Bladder diverticulum	Consider surgical repair
Rectovesical fistula	Consider surgical repair
Prolapse	Consider surgical repair
Obstruction	Restore free flow of urine, ideally avoiding foreign body
Ileal conduit	Diagnosis often difficult as urine universally infected/colonised in asymptomatic patients
Urethral strictures	Regular flow studies and post-micturition bladder volumes with urological follow-up
Prostatic enlargement	Flow studies and post-micturition bladder volumes in elderly male with UTI
Oestrogen deficiency	Consider topical (but not systemic) HRT
Renal transplant (see section on UTI in transplantation)	Very high incidence, progression to pyelonephritis common and may be asymptomatic
Pregnancy	Screening for and treating ASB, with subsequent follow-up throughout pregnancy
Diabetes	Exclude autonomic bladder, consider attempts to improve glycaemic control
Lower socioeconomic status	
Mental impairment and institutionalisation	
Insertive rectal intercourse	
Circumcision is somewhat protective	

host risk factors for acute and chronic pyelonephritis are almost identical to that of lower urinary tract infection, but diabetes stones, pregnancy and urinary tract abnormalities including transplantation are prominent. Emphysematous pyelonephritis (EPN) and xanthogranulomatous pyelonephritis (XPN) also have a very strong female predominance and a peak incidence in the sixth decade both being highly associated with diabetes (95 % of EPN) and stones [4].

Aetiopathogenesis of Urinary Tract Infection

Both lower and upper UTIs are almost exclusively the result of ascending infection of periurethral organisms, predominantly the patient's own bowel organisms with over 85 % of infections being due to gram-negative bacilli. The vast majority (75–95 %) of infections in uncomplicated upper and lower UTI are due to *Escherichia coli*. The remainder are due to other gram negatives (*Klebsiella pneumoniae*, *Proteus mirabilis*, *Citrobacter*, *Pseudomonas aeruginosa* and other Enterobacteriaceae) or gram positives (*Staphylococcus saprophyticus*, enterococci, Group B streptococci, *Staphylococcus aureus*).

It is important to note that along with increasing risk of resistance, this pattern of uropathogens significantly alters in complicated UTIs with a marked increase in other enterobacteria such as pseudomonas (especially related to catheters), Proteus (especially related to stones) and enterococci as well as gram positives such as enterococci (*Bacteroides fragilis* and *Clostridium septicum*) have been reported in EPN. *Staphylococcus aureus* infection can result from ascending infection, but particularly in the setting of APN, it is critical to exclude a haematogenous source. Multiple infections from a variety of different gut organisms suggest the possibility of an anatomical connection between the gut and

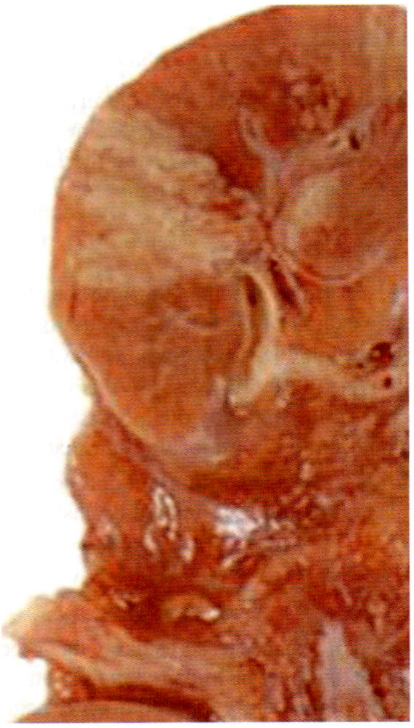

Fig. 35.2 Macroscopic section of kidney showing wedge-shaped area of infection in acute pyelonephritis

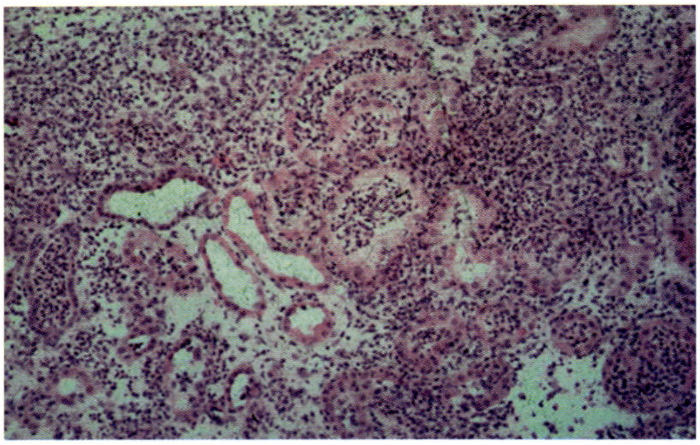

Fig. 35.3 Gross pyelonephritis at low power showing tubules full of neutrophils but also extensive inflammatory infiltrate of neutrophils, lymphocytes, macrophages and eosinophils

are highly suggestive of APN and can be very helpful if the diagnosis is uncertain (Fig. 35.4). Modest proteinuria (<1 g) and haematuria are common.

AKI is often more dependent on the degree of sepsis than the extent of renal involvement as such; renal function often appears normal in unilateral uncomplicated APN and thus if AKI present implies a severe infection and/or obstruction.

The differential diagnosis of APN includes renal arterial or venous infarction, acute nephritis, perinephric abscess, obstruction and/or stones, pneumonia or empyema and loin pain secondary to viral illness.

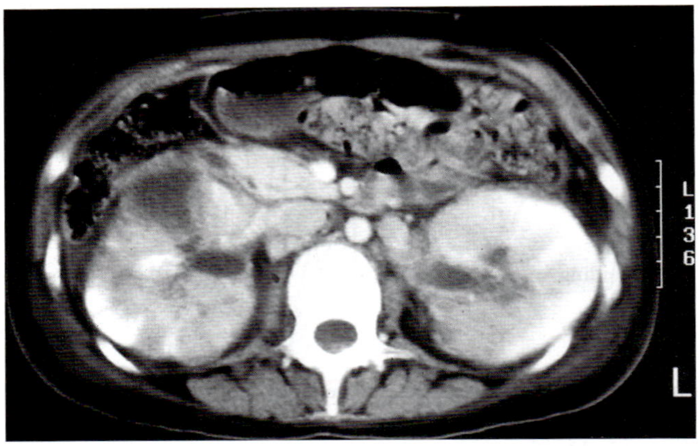

Fig. 35.4 CT KUB in a patient with acute pyelonephritis demonstrating gross swelling of the kidneys and very patchy nephrograms (Courtesy of Dr. Ian Cropley)

Only 25 % of patients with APN have positive blood cultures, but 90–95 % have positive MSU cultures. While there is an argument for treating a clear case uncomplicated cystitis without sending an MSU for culture [5], there is a strong argument for ensuring an MSU is sent before treatment of APN or any patient with a complicated/recurrent UTI as the risk of relapse, recurrence or resistance is much higher.

For uncomplicated cystitis, some would argue a first episode of uncomplicated APN imaging has a low diagnostic yield. However, for recurrent or complicated UTIs, imaging becomes increasingly critical. A plain X-ray may show calcification or gross emphysematous pyelonephritis but is insensitive and should be combined with a renal ultrasound for the initial investigation of APN [6]. Renal ultrasound is critical to rule out bladder or renal obstruction (pyonephrosis or EPN both of which are medical emergencies); it may also reveal a nephronia, diffusely enlarged kidney and renal or perirenal abscess.

However, the most sensitive imaging for pyelonephritis is contrast CT KUB (Fig. 35.4) [7] especially for identifying perinephric stranding, focal infections and stones and excluding emphysematous pyelonephritis (Fig. 35.5) or emphysematous cystitis. While MRI avoids the radiation dose of CT scanning and ionic contrast, as yet it has no diagnostic advantage over CT scanning which remains more sensitive. Functional imaging such as CT gallium and white blood cell or PET scan can sometimes identify focal or diffuse renal infection in the kidney and is worth considering in patients with PUO or recurrent UTIs (Fig. 35.6). DMSA scanning is the most sensitive method for detecting scarring, provided the patient has a reasonable GFR and the scan is at least 3 months post-APN [8]. In the context of a poor GFR, ultrasound scanning in skilled hands or CT may identify renal scarring. Establishing the presence of scarring can help make the diagnosis of APN as the cause of renal impairment in a

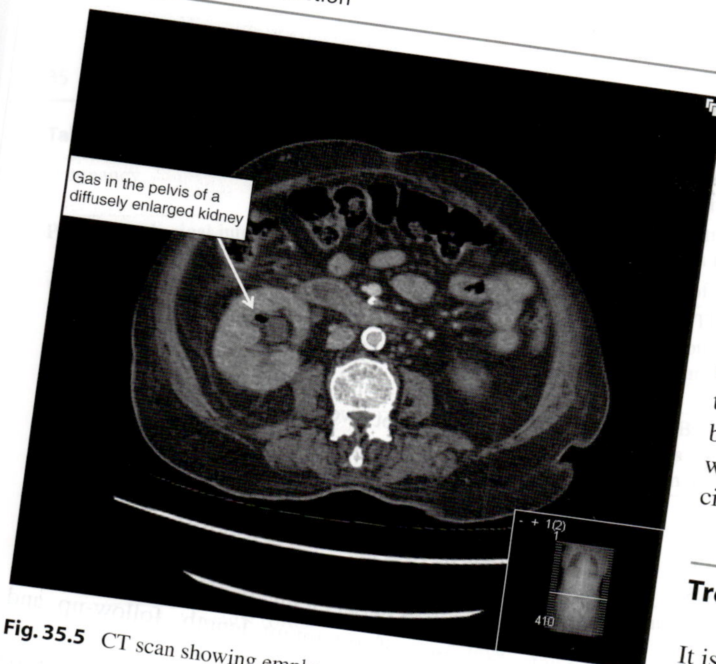

Fig. 35.5 CT scan showing emphysematous pyelonephritis

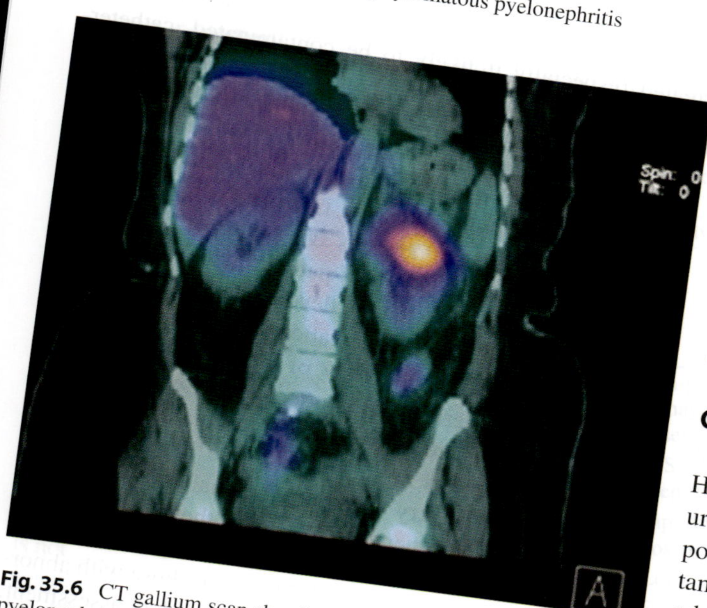

Fig. 35.6 CT gallium scan showing focal area of inflammation due to pyelonephritis in a patient being investigated for pyrexia of unknown origin (Courtesy of Dr. Ian Cropley)

new patient and is also helpful in monitoring progression in patients with recurrent upper UTI.

Pyonephrosis (obstructed and infected upper tract) and EPN deserve special mention because of their extreme risk. EPN is a severe version of APN defined by the presence of gas with rapid deterioration, septicaemia and high mortality. The vast majority of cases (90–95 %) occur in diabetics (who have a much higher rate of asymptomatic bacteriuria), up to a third of cases may be associated with obstruction (pyonephrosis) and 5–8 % can be bilateral [4]. The mortality of EPN has fallen from 78 to 13.5 % in the last four decades, and this is probably attributable to earlier diagnosis with greater access to CT scanning and the combination of broad-spectrum antibiotics plus rapid medical drainage (large-bore nephrostomy) (antibiotics alone is associated with an RR of death of 2.85) [9]. The choice between percutaneous drainage and surgical nephrectomy needs to be made on a case-by-case basis depending on the stability of the patient and the availability of experienced radiologist or surgeons; however, even if nephrectomy is appropriate, the patient can often be stabilised for this by a period of radiological drainage and antibiotics [4]. Either way, both EPN and pyonephrosis constitute medical emergencies and require a rapid and multidisciplinary approach.

Treatment of Acute UTI

It is important to ensure the correct diagnosis and differentiate a patient likely to have uncomplicated UTI from those with complicated UTI, where the risks of treatment failure or more severe disease are much higher. The advice for treatment of uncomplicated UTI is nicely summarised in a recent review [1], and antibiotic usage guidance is from the Infectious Disease Society of America [10] whose recommendations are influenced by the importance of reducing the risk of resistance and adverse side effects.

Prevention and Treatment of Uncomplicated UTI

Conservative Measures

High fluid intake, double micturition (waiting to pass further urine after completion of micturition), frequent voiding, post-coital voiding, wiping from front to back and avoiding tampons, spermicides and occlusive underwear have all been advocated to reduce the risk of UTI in women. In terms of hydration, there is theoretical advantage to a high fluid intake, principally reducing by diluting colony counts and promoting frequent voiding; however, high fluid intakes impair the ability to produce acidic, high-osmolality urine (protective) and will reduce the urinary concentrations of antibiotics and products of the innate immune system. In short, there is very little or no evidence to support any of the above interventions; however, in the face of recurrent debilitating UTIs, we advocate a pragmatic approach suggesting the following six manoeuvres:

1. Avoid the use of diaphragm or spermicides
2. >2 L fluid intake a day
3. Double micturition
4. Wiping from front to back
5. Post-coital voiding

Renal and Perinephric Abscesses

Both renal and perinephric abscesses may occur secondary to haematogenous spread or as a complication of APN, but renal abscess is more likely to be due to the former, therefore it is important to exclude a distant source. In either case, culture of *Staphylococcus aureus* or *Candida* species should provoke a fingertip search for the primary source. Both renal and perinephric abscesses may present as loin pain, fever, rigours and tenderness in the costovertebral angle or subacutely as a PUO, anaemia and a raised acute phase response. A positive urine culture is highly likely with an untreated perinephric abscess although less so with a renal abscess and commonly negative if a patient has already received a course of antibiotics for presumed APN. CT scanning is the imaging of choice and should be considered early in a patient with presumed APN not responding to treatment. Perinephric abscess is usually contained within Gerota's fascia but can infiltrate locally into the diaphragm (hiccups), lung, psoas and pelvis. Most renal abscesses respond to appropriate parental antibiotics without the need for percutaneous drainage, but the bigger the abscess, the less likely conservative management will be effective, and percutaneous (especially if culture negative) or sometimes surgical drainage should be considered if the patient is failing to respond to treatment.

Chronic Pyelonephritis

Chronic pyelonephritis (CPN) can affect the kidneys in a variety of ways, most commonly focal scarring following episodes of APN plus or minus papillary necrosis (particularly in diabetic patients) with the risk that sloughed necrotic papilla may then cause obstruction. It is also increasingly common to see patients (particularly diabetics) with progressive CKD secondary to subclinical, subacute pyelonephritis. Rarer but important presentations include xanthogranulomatous pyelonephritis (XGN) or very rarely malakoplakia. The aetiological risk factors for CPN are similar to those for APN but are frequently associated with a failure of adequate resolution secondary to an abnormal urinary tract (particularly reflux in children), recurrent infection, impaired immunity or inadequately treated infections. CPN where the infections have been resolved may be associated with salt wasting and relatively preserved urine volumes. The prevalence of ESRD secondary to CPN is not easy to determine; in the UK, it is recorded at the cause of ESRD in ~7 %, but this probably includes a whole mixture of pathologies including diabetic and reflux nephropathy.

Xanthogranulomatous Pyelonephritis (XPN)

XPN represents less than 1 % of pyelonephritis; however, we are likely to see more of it in part because of the increased diagnosis with the ready availability of CT scanning but also because the risk factors of diabetes and nephrolithiasis are increasing. XPN has been reported in all age groups but typically occurs in women with diabetes in their 60s and 70s; renal stones are extremely common (90 %, staghorn in 73 %), pyonephrosis in nearly 50 % and non-functioning kidney in a third [20, 21]. In 85 % of cases, renal tissue is replaced diffusely by yellow tissue although in 15 % the lesions are focal. The yellow tissue is made up of chronic inflammatory tissue principally lipid-filled histiocytes and multinucleate giant cells as well as neutrophils and lymphocytes. The pathogenesis seems to require obstruction with failure to eradicate chronic uropathogenic infection; whether diabetes merely predisposes to infection or handicaps the innate immune system in clearing the infection is not clear.

Patients classically present with fevers, weight loss, malaise and sometimes loin pain. Recurrent UTI infection is common or pyuria in ~60 %, and acute phase response is common as is polyclonal IgG. The non-specific nature of the symptoms means the diagnosis is often made while screening for, or confused with, malignancy and a preoperative diagnosis of XPN is made in less than 50 % of cases. CT scanning is the imaging of choice, and the identification of stones is an important clue, but MRI may be able to differentiate between XPN and renal cell cancer [21].

Treatment of diffuse XPN is supportive, antibiotics and usually nephrectomy. Renal recovery does not happen with diffuse XPN, whereas some patients with focal XPN have achieved renal salvage with removal of obstruction/stone and prolonged antibiotics. Either way, treatment requires a coordinated approach with urologists, microbiologists and radiologists, and a high index of suspicion of XPN is required in patients with diabetes, stones and either general unwellness or something funny in the kidney.

Malakoplakia

Malakoplakia is a very rare condition involving the bladder, occasionally ureters and kidneys (and very rarely other organs). It is a granulomatous condition resulting from defective lysosomal clearance of intracellular bacteria by macrophages [22]. Presentation is often non-specific and similar to XPN, i.e. fevers, recurrent UTIs, unexplained anaemia and LUTS. Like XPN, malakoplakia is often mistaken as malignancy or tuberculosis, and the diagnosis is usually made by the histopathologist rather than the clinician. The condition may respond to a very long course of quinolones, but often surgery is also required.

Recurrent UTI Service

Recurrent urinary tract infection is common in healthy females and very common in patients with abnormal uroanatomy or renal transplants. A streamlined and thoughtful pathway for such patients is probably rarer than it should be, and it is not uncommon for patients to receive multiple courses of inappropriate or inadequate antibiotics and multiple hospital admissions before receiving optimum treatment. One approach to improving the patient experience is a dedicated service for recurrent UTIs, usually, but not exclusively, led by a urologist with specialist interest. Table 35.5 gives some suggestions for referral criteria, and Table 35.6 suggests a plan for initial investigations to consider in a one-stop visit.

Table 35.5 Suggested referral criteria to recurrent UTI clinic

1. Uncomplicated recurrent lower (≥3 per year) UTI in healthy female
2. ≥2 acute pyelonephritis episodes in a woman or ≥1 in a man
3. Recurrent culture negative cystitis/urethritis
4. Complicated recurrent UTI (men, transplant recipients, augmented bladders, pregnancy, etc.)

Table 35.6 Suggested initial investigations in one-stop shop

1. Full medical history (including LUT symptom scoring, stones, past history of UTIs and family, sexual and contraceptive history. Medication including anti-cholinergics and ketamine. Fluid intake and voiding diaries and history of previous microbiology results
2. Examination to include external genitalia and perineum to exclude phimosis, epididymitis, female genital mutilation, cystocoele, rectocoele, urethrocoele and exclusion of vaginitis
3. Urine dipstick for leucocytes and nitrites (including pH)
4. MSU (liaison with microbiology to culture and identify counts as low as $10^{2 \text{ or } 3}$)
5. STD screen (chlamydia, gonorrhoeae, mycoplasma, HSV) if appropriate
6. Full blood count, ESR, urea, creatinine and electrolytes, random glucose or HbA1c if diabetic
7. Urinary flow rate and post-micturition residue
8. Flexible cystoscopy if appropriate

These tests can be obtained in a single well-organised clinic, and it is especially helpful if previous culture results are available. Following this, it may be necessary to perform a cystogram to exclude reflux or diverticula and occasionally urodynamics. Further, imaging with CT or CT gallium may be helpful to exclude upper tract abnormalities or locate a site of persisting infection.

Patient information leaflets should be available and include basic self-help advice. If avoidable or correctable causes have been treated, then well-documented trials of prophylactic antibiotics would be appropriate.

Catheter-Associated UTI (CAUTI)

CAUTI is a significant challenge for modern medicine and the most common (40 %) cause of nosocomial infection and contributes significantly to prolonged inpatient stay and morbidity. Diagnosing infection for patients with urethral and suprapubic catheters may be difficult as colonisation is extremely common and pyuria is not diagnostic (an absence of pyuria does however argue against infection) (Table 35.7). Clinically, UTI may manifest with fever and rigours but in the absence of lower urinary tract symptoms may be non-specific such as acute confusion.

Despite the limited literature, a heroic attempt has been made to produce international guidelines on the diagnosis and treatment of CAUTIs and has resulted in a useful document addressing common issues [23, 24].

Perhaps the most important issue related to catheters is whether the patient actually needs it and if so what is the minimum duration required. Institutional reform may be necessary to ensure catheters are only placed when essential; systems put in place (ideally electronic) to ensure that the need for the catheter is constantly questioned and removed as soon as safe to do so are likely to have a significant impact on the numbers of CAUTIs.

Table 35.7 Diagnosis, treatment and management of CAUTI

Catheter avoidance	Develop indications for catheterisation with mechanisms promoting pause for thought. Catheterisation for incontinence should be a last resort. Ready access to bladder ultrasound scanning may significantly reduce the need for catheterization to exclude obstruction
Reduced duration	Systems (and culture) to ensure removal of catheters at the earliest opportunity. For inpatients, the continued need for a catheter should be considered on a daily basis (as with intravenous access) ideally with an electronic alert
Drainage hygiene	Avoid disconnections of the catheter where possible and ensure catheter tubing and bag are below the level of the bladder; seems basic but stale urine flowing back into the bladder is not uncommon
Screening	There is no merit in screening asymptomatic patients with IDC; an exception to this may be pregnant patients
Antibiotic prophylaxis	There is no evidence to support single-dose antibiotics with insertion or removal of catheters unless part of a urological procedure is likely to result in bleeding
Treatment	Cultures must be sent before commencing treatment. Best guess is to treat symptomatic CAUTIs for 7 days but longer (10–14 if slow response). Once on antibiotics, change of catheter makes sense, and experience suggests this is helpful

Tuberculosis of the Urinary Tract

The global incidence of TB peaked around 2003 and had plateaued or begun to decline by 2006, but the incidence of TB in the UK and particularly in London continues to rise. Twenty to twenty-five percent of cases are extra-pulmonary tuberculosis, and genitourinary tract is the most common site at 15–20 % although isolated genitourinary TB (GUTB) occurs in just 4 % of patients.

Epidemiology

Up to 20 % of patients with pulmonary TB are thought to have urogenital involvement [25] although at autopsy evidence of TB may be present in up to 75 % of patients and urine cultures are positive in 25 % of patients with miliary TB. GUTB is twice as common in men for reasons that remain unclear. The incidence of extra-pulmonary TB is significantly higher amongst dialysis patients and patients with ESRD presumably due to impaired cell immunity. Similarly, the incidence of all forms of TB is 20–70 times higher amongst transplant patients particularly in the first year of transplantation. GUTB accounts for 7–15 % of TB cases amongst transplant recipients [25].

Pathogenesis

Genitourinary disease is mainly secondary to haematogenous dissemination although disease has been described after intravesical BCG especially in immunocompromised patients. In an immunocompetent person, tuberculous bacilli are trapped in periglomerular capillaries and are followed by granuloma formation. These are typically bilateral, cortical and adjacent to the glomeruli and can remain dormant for decades. If the patient's immune competence is disturbed, these can progress with typical tuberculous granuloma with caseating necrosis, disseminating the viable organism into the proximal tubules and loop of Henley with progression of disease to the renal medulla.

Clinical Features of GUTB

The diagnosis of renal tuberculosis is often delayed because of insidious onset and non-specific symptoms, and the interval between primary TB infection and renal involvement in the immunocompetent is usually many years. The classical symptoms of cystitis, dysuria (30 %) with sterile pyuria, weight loss and fevers should rouse clinical suspicion, but constitutional symptoms occur in less than a third of patients. Other symptoms are pretty non-specific and include back and flank pain (10–30 %), suprapubic pain, haematuria, frequency and nocturia. Calcification and fibrosis causing stricture formation (typically at the vesico-ureteric junction) in the pelvicalyceal system may result in obstruction, atrophy and auto-nephrectomy [26]. In the bladder, the chronic inflammation causes fibrosis resulting in a thick-walled non-compliant small-capacity storage unit causing secondary renal dysfunction.

Tubulointerstitial nephritis related to tuberculosis is a rare but more recognised manifestation of renal tuberculosis, which is part of the differential of granulomatous TIN although it is uncommon to identify acid fast bacilli in biopsy specimens.

Investigations

Serial early morning urine samples for culture remain the standard for identifying patients with a sensitivity of 65–90 % and a specificity of 100 % (at least three samples should be obtained). Tuberculin skin tests are positive in 90 % of normal host, but tuberculin and interferon release assays have a high false-negative rate in patients with ESRD due to impaired T cell immunity, and positive results indicated exposure to not active disease. The chest X-ray is abnormal in about 70 %. Cystoscopy and bladder biopsy may be worth considering in anyone with sterile pyuria; TB culture would need to be requested on biopsy samples. Calcification is common (>50 %) with CT scanning having the highest sensitivity. Focal hypoperfusion creating a striated nephrogram and a moth-eaten calyx secondary to papillary necrosis is characteristic; ureteric stenosis is also common.

As the parenchymal granulomata coalesce, CT can demonstrate a mass-like lesion with central low attenuation corresponding to tuberculoma with central caseous necrosis. Long-standing TB gives rise to renal parenchymal atrophy and stricture formation with thinning of cortices, multiple thin-walled cysts, progressive hydronephrosis and dystrophic calcification involving the entire kidney which is the final product of end-stage renal tuberculosis.

Ureteral involvement initially is seen as mucosal irregularity creating a sawtooth ureter appearance. Stricturing and ureteral shortening which occurs as disease advances produces corkscrew ureter with calcifications along the ureter.

Management

The aims of treatment are to render the patient non-infectious, to preserve renal function and to address any complication from GUTB infection and should be done in the context of a multidisciplinary team including urology and TB specialists.

GUTB generally responds well to treatment because of the generally low mycobacterial load. Isoniazid and rifampicin penetrate well into cavitating lesions, and a high concentration of isoniazid, rifampicin and pyrazinamide is maintained in urine. With the increasing emergence of multi-resistant TB, sensitivity testing is essential. Surgery has an important part to play in current management. This includes nephrectomy and reconstructive surgery mainly related to strictures and augmentation of the bladder for small fibrotic bladders.

Table 35.8 Predisposing factors for candiduria and *Candida* urinary tract infections

Diabetes mellitus
Renal transplantation
Extremes of age
Instrumentation of the urinary tract
Female sex
Concomitant bacteriuria
Prolonged hospitalisation
Congenital abnormalities of the urinary tract
Intensive care unit admission
Structural abnormalities of the urinary tract
Broad-spectrum antibiotics
Indwelling urinary tract devices
Bladder dysfunction
Urinary stasis
Nephrolithiasis

Fungal Urinary Tract Infections

Fungal urinary tract infections are rare in healthy community-based individuals but are more commonly found in hospitalised patients. The vast majority of these fungal UTIs are due to *Candida* species. The pathological nature of these infections is closely related to host factors, and management is dependent upon the underlying condition of the patient in particular immune competence, glycaemic control, anatomy and presence of foreign bodies (see Table 35.8). The incidence of fungal infections has increased in the context of extensive and prolonged use of broad-spectrum antibiotics, immunosuppressive medication and cytotoxic drugs.

Epidemiology

Candida species usually exist as saprophytes of the skin, oropharynx, gastrointestinal tracts and genital region and thus can contaminate as well as infect. Among normal adults, yeasts are encountered in <1 % of clean voided urine specimens but account for up to 5–10 % of positive urine culture results in tertiary care facilities, mostly in those with indwelling catheters. The incidence of infections in patients in burns units is threefold than in medical and surgical intensive care units [27]. One study in renal transplants recorded 3 % of patients having candiduria within the first 2 years. Candiduria was three times more common in women, 60 % associated with antibiotic use and 40 % with catheters [28]. Community-acquired *Candida* infections are most common amongst patients with diabetes mellitus, those who are bedridden and in patients receiving antimicrobial therapy. The microbiology of candiduria is changing globally with <50 % of urinary isolates now belonging to *Candida albicans*.

The environmental fungi such as Blastomyces, Histoplasma and Coccidioides are found primarily in soil, environment and guano. Although very serious infections, they rarely involve the renal tract, and if they do so it is invariably via haematogenous spread, usually in the profoundly immunocompromised.

Pathophysiology

Candida species can cause antegrade and retrograde infections of the urinary tract. Antegrade infections are due to haematogenous spread of the organism and may involve multiple abscesses or fungal balls and should always prompt a vigorous search for a primary site and exclusion of endocarditis. Ascending infections start from a focus of colonisation at or near the urethra. *Candida* species adhere poorly to bladder mucosa so infection is usually dependent on the presence of urinary tract obstruction, concomitant bacterial urinary sepsis or profound immune suppression.

Diagnosis of Fungal UTI

Distinguishing contamination from infection can be difficult and has significant implications although in the majority, candiduria does not represent infection. Infection is associated with typical and indistinguishable symptoms of cystitis, prostatitis, epididymo-orchitis or APN. Oliguria, stranguria, passage of particulate matter and pneumaturia in the presence of a positive urine culture result can be a feature of more severe infection such as the presence of a fungal ball. Pyuria is suggestive (except in catheterised patients), but candida is frequently a co-infection with uropathogenic bacteria in which case ruling out contamination is less straightforward and may be absent in neutropenia.

In the presence of a susceptible individual such as a critically ill patient or an immunocompromised patient, candiduria should be regarded as a marker of potential invasive candidiasis. A high index of clinical suspicion in such a scenario should follow with subsequent investigations with blood cultures, examination of the retina and skin, CXR and ECHO cardiographs to identify disseminated infection. In selected patients, a renal ultrasound should be carried out to rule out the presence of hydronephrosis/obstruction, a focal mass in the collective system. Further investigations with CT or MRI may be required to demonstrate the presence of renal abscess, fungal balls or non-functioning kidneys.

A pragmatic diagnostic approach to the finding of candiduria was expounded by Kauffman et al. [28]. In essence suggesting repeat (if absent then ignore) and if persistent in a previously healthy individual, search for predisposing condition such as diabetes, urological abnormality or catheter (which should be changed). In the absence of any obvious abnormality in a well patient, it is reasonable to monitor, but if candiduria is associated with a predisposing factor, then this should be addressed.

or raised plasma calcium, reduced plasma phosphate and reduced TMPi/GFR (this is an index of PTH-induced reduced tubular phosphate reabsorption).

Treatments

Bisphosphonates reduce hypercalciuria due to bone loss and can be used if GFR >30 mL/min. They have the advantage of also inhibiting the crystallisation of calcium salts.

It is worth noting that vitamin D itself, given as *25-OH vitamin D* (e.g. cholecalciferol) without a calcium supplement, does *not* increase hypercalciuria. Restricting dietary calcium intake is *never* recommended.

Thiazide diuretics reduce hypercalciuria by inducing a mild volume depletion which encourages proximal tubular sodium and hence calcium reabsorption. They should be used only once a primary cause of hypercalciuria has been excluded. Their tendency to cause increased urinary potassium loss results in mild potassium deficiency which can reduce the urinary excretion of citrate (a stone inhibitor). This effect can be lessened by combination with amiloride.

Hyperoxaluria

Hyperoxaluria is usually *secondary* to increased gut absorption:

- *Dietary* due to excessive intake of oxalate-rich foods, e.g. chocolate, tea, bran, nuts and also spinach and rhubarb.
- *Enteric hyperoxaluria* refers to increased intestinal absorption of oxalate due to:
  - Inappropriately low-calcium diet (sometimes, but incorrectly, advocated in hypercalciuria).
  - Malabsorption due to small intestinal or pancreatic exocrine disease or surgery, e.g. ileal resection, Roux-en-Y gastric bypass for obesity. Malabsorption increases free fatty acid availability in the colon. The excess fatty acids preferentially complex with dietary calcium, reducing the calcium available for complexing with oxalate in the colon which is the main site of oxalate absorption.
- Megadose vitamin C (rare).
- Ethylene glycol toxicity (rare).

The *primary hyperoxalurias* (see Table 36.3) are caused by autosomal recessive defects in the enzymes that metabolise glyoxylate, causing metabolism to oxalate. *Type 1* is the more common form. Normal oxalate excretion is variably defined with an upper limit of ~0.4 mmol/24 h. Primary hyperoxaluria (PH) types 1 or 2 are only suspected when excretion exceeds 0.7 mmol/24 h and usually present in childhood. However, PH *type 3* may present in adulthood, suggesting that values >0.4 mmol/24 h should also be followed up (and reviewed after dietary advice), even in the absence of a history of recurrent stones and especially if any stone analysis reports a composition of 100 % calcium oxalate. Note that only about 20 % of excreted oxalate is dietary in origin, that a low-calcium diet (never recommended in stone formers) can lead to an increase in absorption of dietary oxalate (see below) and that even small decreases in urinary oxalate can have a large impact on stone risk (due to the relatively small total daily amount of oxalate excretion).

Mechanisms of Calcium Stone Formation

The three main mechanisms have some overlap between them (Fig. 36.1):

1. *The free particle theory*. Crystals spontaneously precipitate in supersaturated urine.
2. *The fixed particle theory*. Crystals adhere to damaged tubular cell membranes.
3. *Randall's plaque theory*. Calcium phosphate is deposited in papillary interstitium, causing damage to overlying epithelium, to which calcium oxalate can then adhere.

These mechanisms are balanced by inhibitors of calcium stone formation:

1. *Citrate*. Hypocitraturia is the most easily measured and is currently the most clinically modifiable inhibitor. Citrate occurs naturally in fruit and fruit juices and is metabolised to bicarbonate. It is easily replaced orally as potassium citrate, e.g. in the management of distal renal tubular acidosis and sometimes in medullary sponge kidney.
2. *Magnesium*. Although can sometimes participate in stone formation.
3. *Pyrophosphate*. A structural analogue of bisphosphonates.
4. *Tubular proteins* such as uromodulin.

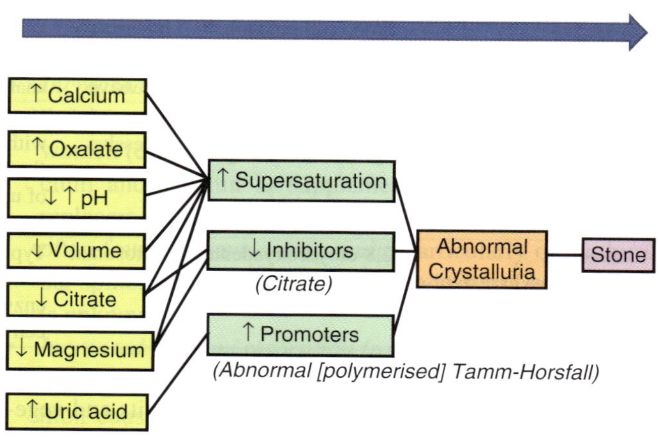

Fig. 36.1 Mechanisms of calcium stone formation

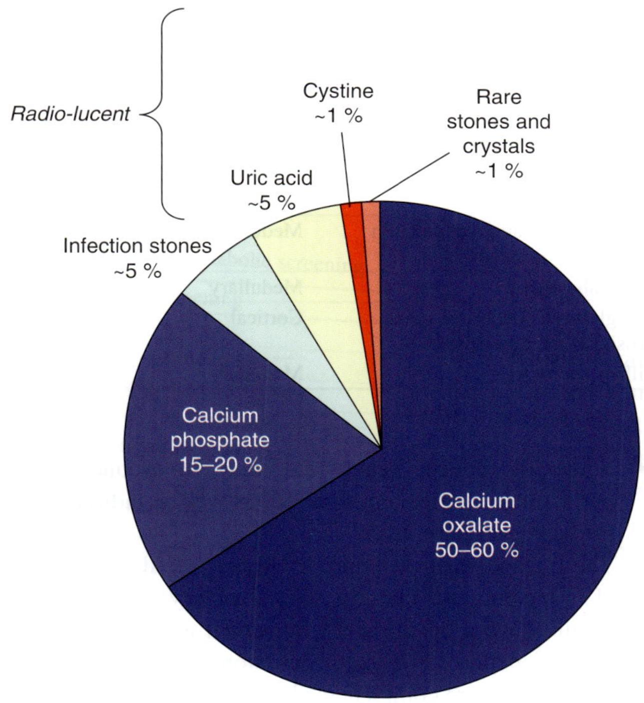

Fig. 36.2 Overall prevalence of stone types

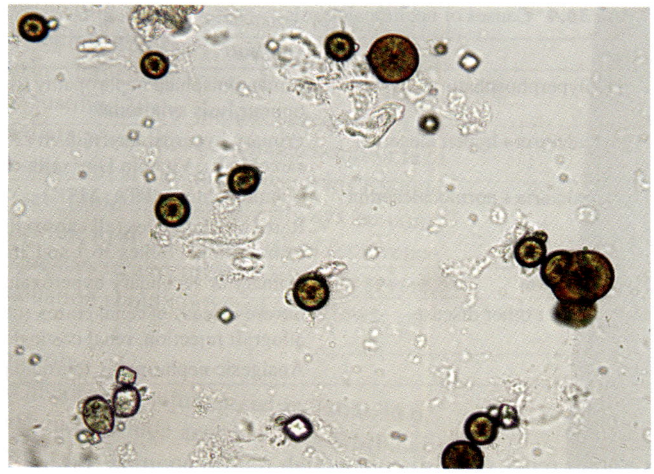

Fig. 36.3 Light microscopy of 2,8-dihydroxyadenine crystals (Kindly provided by Vidar Edvardsson, MD and Runolfur Palsson, MD, Landspitali-The National University Hospital of Iceland, and the APRT Deficiency Programme of The Rare Kidney Stone Consortium)

Stone Types

Stones are made up of 90 % mineral and the rest is water plus organic matrix. Figure 36.2 shows an overall breakdown of stone types (Fig. 36.3).

Rare stone types consist of: *xanthine, 2,8-dihydroxyadenine (APRT), silica, ammonium urate and insoluble drugs* (indinavir, acyclovir, methyldopa, triamterene, sulphonamides). Stones due to protease inhibitors such as indinavir are actually large, often pure, crystals.

Urinary pH

This is an important factor that affects solubility of many stone types and hence their formation, although calcium oxalate is pH independent. Note that pH measured on dipstick is unreliable; the most accurate assessment is by pH meter measured soon after voiding. As a guide, the normal pH range of early-morning urine sample is 5.3–6.8.

Forming at Low pH (Uric Acid, Cystine)

- Acid urine (consistently less than pH 5.3) occurs in those with *metabolic syndrome* and/or obesity, who are also more likely to have hyperuricaemia, increasing their risk of uric acid stones. Patients with *ileostomies* are also at risk of forming uric acid stones from a combination of ileal losses of bicarbonate-rich fluid, leading to low urine volumes and acid urine.
- Cystine is increasingly soluble at higher pH, but this effect is overwhelmed if urinary cystine excretion is massive.
- Some drug-induced crystals: sulphonamides, e.g. co-trimoxazole.

Forming at High pH

- Calcium phosphate (pH > 6.2) stones are suggestive of an acidification defect (deficient proton secretion in type 1 renal tubular acidosis).
- Magnesium ammonium phosphate ($MgNH_4Pi$; radio-opaque, pH > 7.0) and ammonium urate (radiolucent) stones are caused by:
  - Infection with a urea-splitting organism – urease from *Proteus*, *Klebsiella* or *Pseudomonas* species causes ammonia release.
  - Laxative abuse – this results in chronic potassium depletion and reduced urinary citrate excretion.
- Most drug-induced crystals typically form at higher pH:
  - Protease inhibitors
  - Ciprofloxacin (pH > 7.3)

Nephrocalcinosis

Nephrocalcinosis means a generalised increase in calcification of the renal parenchyma due to increased urinary excretion of calcium, phosphate or oxalate. This is distinct from

High animal protein (meat, fish and poultry) – diets high in animal protein ('high-acid ash' diets), are associated with an increased risk of stone formation due to hypercalciuria, hyperuricosuria, hypocitraturia and lower urinary pH.

High salt intake – can lead to hypercalciuria, by decreasing proximal tubular calcium reabsorption. Salt intake must be reduced before considering thiazide therapy.

High oxalate intake – foods include bran, spinach, beetroot, okra, yams, soya beans and soya products, sesame seeds, nuts, peanut butter, chocolate and tea/coffee (especially instant coffee) without milk

Calcium intake – dairy products and supplements. A common mistake is to decrease dietary calcium intake. This can lead to an increase in oxalate stone formation (due to decreased complexation in the colon) and, if sustained, to osteoporosis.

Low fresh fruit and vegetable intake – these are an important source of citrate, magnesium (inhibitors of calcium stone formation) and potassium (a promoter of urinary citrate excretion).

Further Biochemical Investigations

In addition to all the investigations mentioned above:

Spot urine in universal container– for dipstick testing as above. Also retinol binding protein if suspected proximal tubular disease (Fanconi syndrome/Dent's disease).

Twenty-four hour urine collections – accurate collections are difficult but it is essential to avoid under-/over-collection and overt/covert influences on the result (by drinking more or altering diet). Optimum collections require:

- Clear instructions to perform collections while on usual diet and fluid intake and preferably during normal weekday activity
- Avoiding collections if symptomatic urinary tract infection, known obstruction, oliguric (e.g. dialysis patient) or within 1 month of a stone episode or lithotripsy session
- At least two (and preferably three [20] 24-h collections)

Miscollection is identified by large discrepancies in creatinine excretion values between the two bottles and by obvious discrepancies between reported fluid intake and measured urine volume. Acidified (pH$<$4.0) samples prevent precipitation of calcium oxalate crystals which would cause underestimation of these metabolites. Most laboratories require separate acidic and plain collections.

Serum biochemistry – urea and electrolytes (baseline renal function), venous bicarbonate and chloride (looking for hyperchloraemic metabolic acidosis); serum calcium, magnesium, phosphate, parathyroid hormone and vitamin D; serum urate; serum glucose (features of metabolic syndrome).

Additional tests include: coeliac serology and haematinics (if malabsorption suspected or diarrhoea present) and exclusion of autoimmune causes (if dRTA suspected).

Analysis of stone or fragments – the gold standard is infrared spectroscopy with supportive wet chemistry [21], but this is often not possible or available. Clues may be obtained from:

- *Urine microscopy* – looking for presence of classic crystalluria. Some crystals are always abnormal (calcium phosphate crystals; hexagonal cystine crystals are pathognomonic of cystinuria). However calcium oxalate and urate crystals can be a feature of normal urine.
- *Radiology evidence* – Hounsfield unit (HU) density on non-contrast CT KUB can differentiate between 'soft' (e.g. urate) and 'hard' (calcium) stones. Uric acid stones have a density of around 200–400 HU, while calcium oxalate monohydrate stones may have values of >1,000 HU [22]. Plain KUB or the scout film from a CT KUB may show whether stones are radio-opaque or not and whether staghorn calculi are present.

Further Radiological Investigations

Anatomical and functional abnormalities of the urinary tract can also predispose to stone formation (see section above) or can increase the likelihood of stone complications (such as obstruction of a single functioning kidney). With the increasing use of non-contrast CT and ultrasound, anatomical abnormalities may be more readily noted.

Further Specific Investigations

After interpretation of the above results, further investigations may include:

- Urinary acidification testing
- Screening for tubular proteinuria
- Genotyping (RTA, PH, cystinuria)

Running a Medical Stone Clinic

Close clinical liaison between urologists, nephrologists and radiologists is necessary. Initially, appropriate referral criteria (see Table 36.5) must be agreed, with a mechanism for follow-up of basic screening tests previously requested in the urology clinic. There should preferably also be a system for longer-term follow-up of outcome via the urology follow-up clinic, with re-referral to a nephrologist if indicated. For most patients only two clinic visits would normally be needed: an initial visit and a review with the results of screening tests. Further review visits may be indicated for certain patients, for example, if an underlying tubular disorder is diagnosed.

Benefits of the medical stone clinic:

- Identification of high-risk patients (e.g. those with an extensive family history of stone disease, bowel surgery, known underlying metabolic disorder).
- Increase in patient empowerment and understanding – in the case of recommended lifestyle/dietary changes, patients will need to understand and maintain these recommendations long term.
- Allow a genetic diagnosis to be made (e.g. cystinuria, primary hyperoxaluria)

- Improve diagnosis of rarer stone types.
- Decide whether specific nephrological follow-up is indicated, e.g. for CKD or a tubular disorder.
- Assist urologists in determining risk (and hence follow-up arrangements) in specific cases, e.g. single functioning kidney.

Interpretation of Results and Assessment of Risk

Urinary pH

Consistently High Urinary pH

Look for:

- Renal tubular acidosis (perform urinary acidification testing)
- Recurrent urinary infection with urea-splitting bacterium
- Systemic alkalosis, e.g. chronic vomiting
- Ongoing alkali treatment

Consistently Low Urinary pH

This is an increasingly common finding, especially in obesity and metabolic syndrome. These conditions are themselves associated with an increased risk of all stone formation (see above), so it is common for acidic urine to be associated with calcium oxalate (but not calcium phosphate) stones, uric acid stones or a mixture of these types.

24-Hour Urine Collection Results

The 'normal ranges' quoted for urinary metabolites are much more variable than for serum values, reflecting the normal response of the kidneys to daily variations in intake (Table 36.7). Stone risk varies continuously with the concentration of each metabolite [24] and is affected by interactions between metabolites and by urine volume and supersaturation. Urine biochemistry must therefore be interpreted in relation to the history, clinical features and serum biochemistry.

Should urinary metabolites be measured as concentrations or total daily amounts?

There are four ways of measuring urinary metabolite excretion: as average solute concentration over 24 h (mmol/L), as total amount excreted daily (mmol/day), as a molar ratio corrected for urinary creatinine excretion, and as a fractional excretion relative to plasma concentration. The solute concentration may intuitively seem to be the most useful measure, but peak concentration (and hence supersaturation) varies greatly throughout the day. The nephron has a defined maximum excretion limit for some metabolites under normal circumstances, which is more easily expressed as a total daily amount and is subject to less variability than the concentration. Generally in UK practice, total amount excreted daily is used for all metabolites except for monitoring of patients with cystinuria, where the aim is an average cystine concentration of less than ~1 mmol/L (243 mg/L). Molar ratios, e.g. oxalate to creatinine ratio (upper limit of normal = 38 μmol/mmol), can be useful as a first-line screening test, especially where 24-h collections are not practical, e.g. young children.

Radiological Investigations

The traditional combination of the 'kidney, ureter, bladder' (KUB) radiograph and intravenous urography (IVU) has largely been replaced by the more modern imaging techniques of ultrasound (US), computed tomography (CT) and magnetic resonance imaging (MRI) (Table 36.8).

Plain Film Kidney/Ureter/Bladder (KUB) Radiograph

Even for radio-opaque stones, the sensitivity of KUB radiograph is as low as 19 % [25], limiting its usefulness in patients with acute renal colic, obese patients or those with pelvic vascular calcifications (phleboliths). A plain film KUB alone offers no information regarding urinary tract obstruction. However in patients with known radio-opaque stone disease, KUB films can be reliably used for follow-up to determine stone size, growth and clearance.

Intravenous Urography (IVU)

Usually performed in conjunction with a 'control' study (plain film KUB), the IVU was the initial investigation of choice prior to the advent of non-contrast CT. The control film is used to identify the presence of radio-opaque stones. The delayed post-intravenous contrast films demonstrate renal pelvicalyceal anatomy and the presence and level of obstruction and allow visualisation of contrast excretion into the collecting systems (e.g. allowing diagnosis of medullary sponge kidney). Example images are shown in Fig. 36.4.

Ultrasound (US)

Ultrasound is cheap, free of ionising radiation and importantly can also detect hydronephrosis but is very much operator dependent. Stones are seen as hyperechoic (bright) foci with posterior acoustic shadowing (dark area behind the stone). Colour Doppler imaging sometimes shows a rapidly changing colour complex ('twinkling artefact') behind ureteric stones.

Table 36.7 24-h urinary biochemical values and their interpretation

	'Normal' ranges (mmol/day)		Interpretation
	Male	Female	
Direct stone constituents			
Calcium	2.5–8.0 (2.5–6.0 in stone formers)	2.0–6.0	"Idiopathic" (i.e. non-hypercalcaemic) hypercalciuria may be due to (a) renal calcium leak, sometimes caused by excessive dietary sodium intake; (b) increased calcium resorption from bones; (c) increased intestinal absorption [23]. In dRTA, hypercalciuria only occurs when bicarbonate <20 mmol/L
Oxalate	0.15–0.45		Note that only 10–20 % of oxalate is dietary in origin, the rest is the urinary end product of glyoxylate metabolism. Excretion of 0.45–0.8 mmol/day suggests secondary (enteric) hyperoxaluria or type 3 primary hyperoxaluria. Excretion >0.7 mmol/day occurs in primary hyperoxaluria type 1 and 2
Urate (uric acid)	2.0–5.5	1.5–5.0	High values caused by high-purine diet (animal protein, beer), uricosuric drugs, increased protein catabolism, metabolic syndrome. Risk factor for uric acid and calcium oxalate stones. Risk of urate stones increases with higher urate excretion
Inhibitors of crystallisation			
Citrate	2.0–5.0	2.5–5.0	If very low investigate for dRTA. Low in chronic potassium depletion, e.g. high animal protein diet with little fruit/vegetables
Magnesium	2.5–8.5		Often reduced with chronic proton pump inhibitor usage, although not a directly proven stone-forming mechanism. But if increased (e.g. excess magnesium trisilicate (antacid) intake), then can contribute to stone formation
Electrolytes			
Sodium	40–220 (highly variable depending on dietary sodium intake)		High sodium excretion can cause hypercalciuria due to decreased proximal tubular calcium reabsorption. Chronic diuretic therapy in steady state does not cause high urinary sodium
Potassium	25–125		Higher excretion with diets high in fresh fruit and vegetables. Usage together with urinary sodium in calculating urine anion gap to estimate ammonium secretion
Validation of collection			
Creatinine	9–21 (very variable depending on muscle mass)		Value should be very similar between 24-h collections in an individual patient
Volume	Dependent on fluid intake		Aim for a minimum of 2 L/day in divided amounts throughout the day for all patients, although cystinurics in particular require larger volumes in order to prevent supersaturation
Other risk factors and markers			
Phosphate	13–42		If high, suggests renal phosphate wasting usually due to proximal tubular cause
Urinary pH	*See above sections on Urinary pH in "Pathophysiology" and "Interpretation"*		Average urinary pH over 24 h is more useful than spot urine pH which can be very variable (early-morning second void sample is better, but must be transported quickly to laboratory)
Urea			Sustained high excretion is suggestive of high protein intake

Variability in urine biochemistry occurs mainly due to physiological variations in day-to-day excretions but also due to under-/over-collection by the patient and differences in quality assurance between laboratories

Table 36.8 Comparison of imaging modalities and current usage in urinary tract stone disease

Imaging modality	Sensitivity for kidney stones (%)	Sensitivity for ureteric stones (%)	Specificity (%)	Modern-day usage
Plain abdominal ('KUB') radiograph	44–77	48	80–87	Follow-up of known radio-opaque stone disease
Intravenous urogram (IVU)	85	68	90	Visualisation of anatomy and exclusion of obstruction where CT is not available Diagnosis of medullary sponge kidney Diagnosis of protease inhibitor stones (or use CT urogram)
Ultrasound scan	55	73.3		Good for stones at pelviureteric and vesicoureteric junctions; less good for other ureteric stones. Use in pregnancy
CT KUB	94	97	94–96	Gold standard investigation for almost all stones. Also identifies obstruction and non-renal tract pathology
MR urogram		94	100	Alternative to ultrasound in second and third trimesters of pregnancy

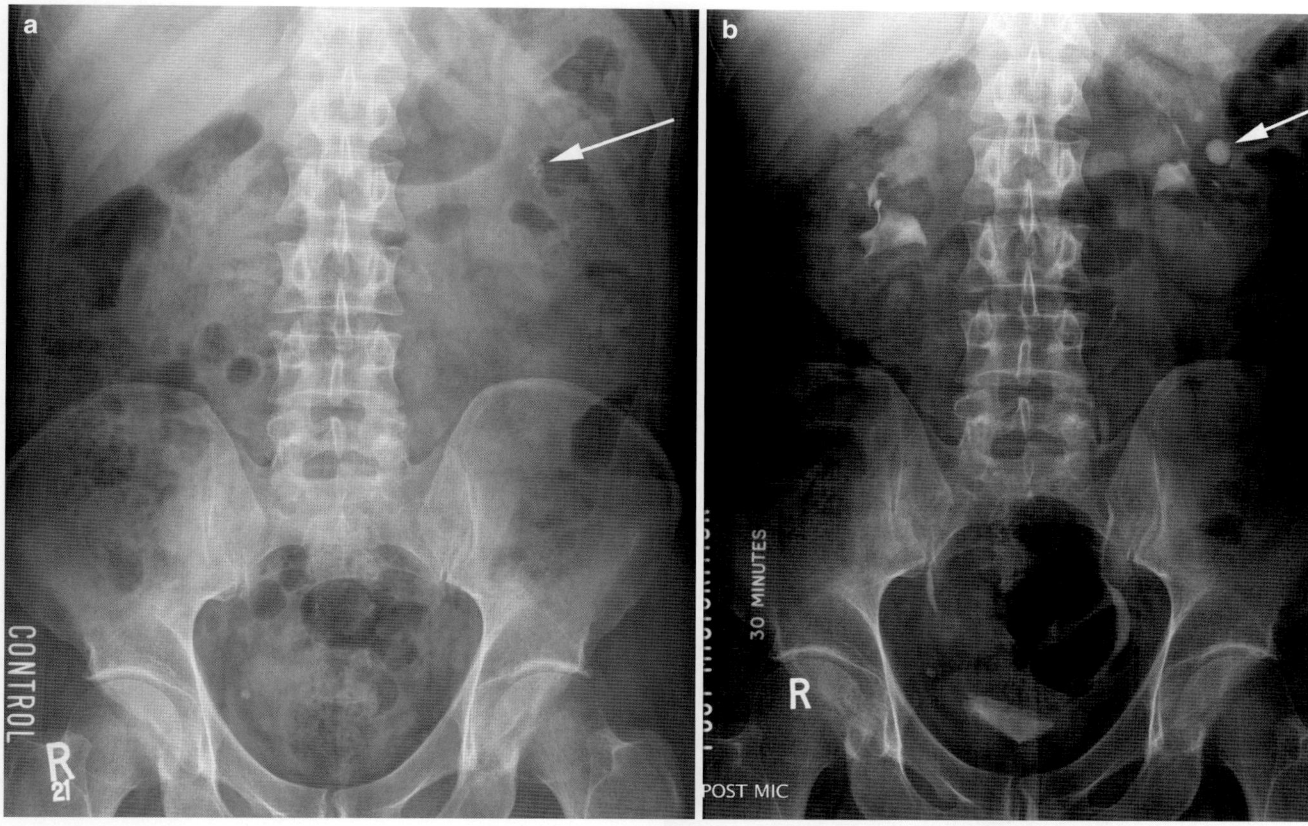

Fig. 36.4 Images from an intravenous urogram: (**a**) Pre-contrast control film shows a small cluster of stones in the left kidney (*arrowed*). (**b**) Film taken 30 min post-contrast, by which time the contrast has been excreted by the kidney into the pelvicalyceal systems and down into the bladder. The contrast outlines a rounded calyceal diverticulum in a similar position to the stones on the control film (*arrowed*), i.e. the stones lie within a calyceal diverticulum

Computerised Tomography Kidney/Ureter/Bladder (CT KUB)

CT KUB has now replaced IVU as the gold standard investigation for detecting renal and ureteric stones. There is a slightly higher radiation dose (3.5 mSv; range 2.8–4.5) compared to that from an IVU (1.5 mSv), but nowadays low-dose scanning protocols can be used in many situations, giving a radiation dose equal to or even lower than that from an IVU. However CT is used with caution in children, pregnancy and in routine frequent follow-up, in order to reduce the doses of ionising radiation in these groups (1 mSv exposure is associated with a 1 in 20,000 lifetime risk of cancer).

CT KUB has two other advantages over other modalities:

- Detection of the vast majority of 'radiolucent' stones, which are not detectable on plain KUB films. An important exception is for stones (crystals) due to protease inhibitors (antiretrovirals) which are of similar density to soft tissue (e.g. the ureter) and are therefore not detectable on non-contrast CT, although obstruction secondary to such stones may be identified.
- Diagnosis of alternative pathologies that may have a similar presentation to renal colic, such as pancreatitis, leaking aortic aneurysm, cholecystitis, biliary colic, appendicitis and diverticulitis.

Intravenous contrast may be administered in certain circumstances (the investigation is then called a CT urogram). Scanning in the urographic phase (10–15 min after injection) helps to outline the pelvicalyceal system and ureters. This may be useful to define whether a stone lies within or outside the ureter (the main cause of false positives on non-contrast CT KUB, particularly in thin subjects) and outline stones that are difficult to detect, such as protease inhibitor stones.

An example of the same stone imaged using each of these modalities is shown in Fig. 36.5.

Magnetic Resonance Urography

After ultrasound, an MR urogram is a possible alternative investigation in children and pregnant women (but not in the first trimester) to identify the level of obstruction (Fig. 36.6). T2-weighted static-fluid MR urogram does not require intravenous contrast and is useful in dilated systems. Stones are

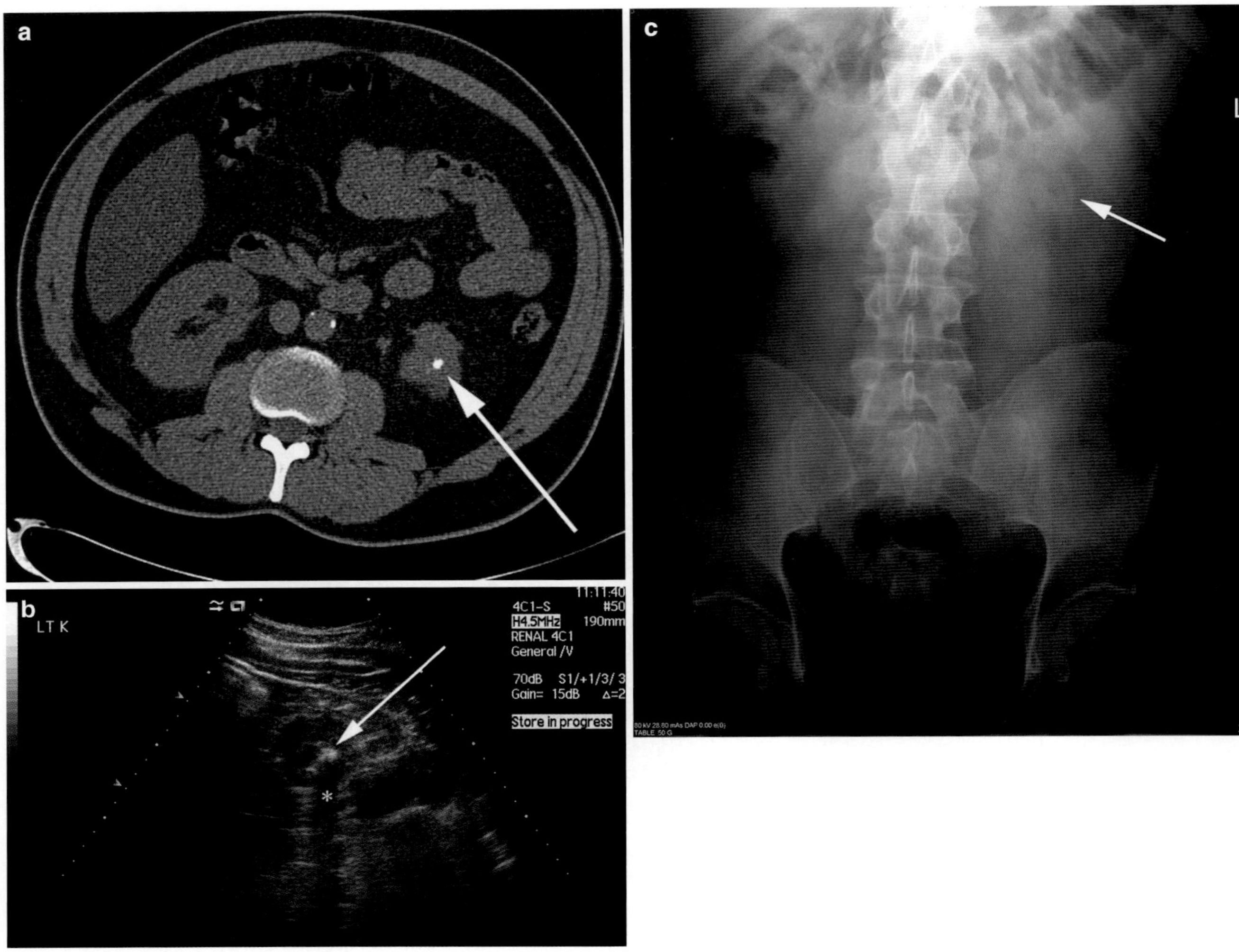

Fig. 36.5 Small left lower pole stone (*arrow*) visualised on different imaging modalities: (**a**) Axial non-contrast CT KUB is the most accurate at demonstrating the dense (i.e. white) stone. (**b**) The same stone is seen as a hyperechoic (i.e. bright) focus on ultrasound, with a posterior acoustic shadow (dark streak running vertically down underneath the stone, marked with an *asterisk*). (**c**) The stone is difficult to visualise on plain film. Overlying faeces/bowel gas and adjacent venous phleboliths can mask or mimic stones

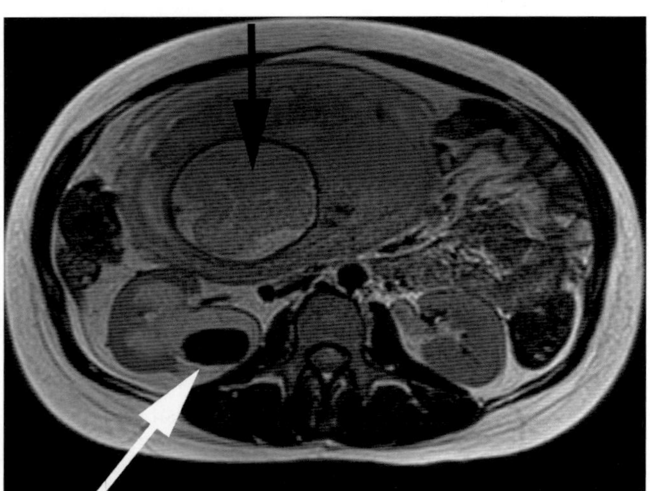

Fig. 36.6 Axial image from a non-contrast MR urogram in a pregnant patient (note that the foetal skull/brain is seen anteriorly, marked with a *black arrow*). This T2-weighted axial image shows a dilated right pelvicalyceal system with a large stone (dark in appearance and marked with a *white arrow*) in the renal pelvis

seen as areas of signal loss (black). Excretory MR urography can be performed after administering gadolinium contrast agent, similar to an IVU or CT urogram, with low GFR being a relative contraindication.

Treatment

Treatment strategies should combine treatment of the stone (medical or surgical) with preventative measures (dietary or medical) including treatment of any identified underlying cause. In general, stone-forming patients will benefit from appropriate tailored lifestyle and dietary advice, before pharmacotherapy. This advice is important even where drugs are needed (Table 36.9) as it can often improve their efficacy. Follow-up should be approximately 6 months later, with

Table 36.9 Pharmacotherapy

Drug	Action	Stone type	Suggested dose	Cautions
Thiazide diuretics	Increase tubular reabsorption of calcium leading to reduced urinary excretion; increase magnesium excretion	Calcium stones	Indapamide 2.5 mg/day; chlorthalidone 25–50 mg/day; hydrochlorothiazide 50 mg/day [26]	Dose-dependent hypokalaemia, hyperglycaemia, hyperlipidaemia and hyperuricaemia, all of which can impact on stone risk
Magnesium supplements	Works as an oxalate binder in the gut	Calcium oxalate	500 mg/day	Diarrhoea can be a problem and if severe will negate the beneficial effect
Potassium citrate	(a) Alkalinises urine; (b) citrate is itself a calcium stone inhibitor; (c) alkalinising effect increases tubular reabsorption of urinary calcium	Uric acid, cystine	20 mmol tds (either as liquid or tablets where available, e.g. *Urocit-K*, *Effercitrate*)	Over-alkalinisation promotes the formation of calcium phosphate stones, even in calcium oxalate stone formers
Sodium bicarbonate	As above, but used where potassium salts not indicated or not available	Uric acid, cystine	Standard doses	Contributes to dietary sodium load
Pyridoxine	Reduces oxalate production in type 1 primary hyperoxaluria (certain mutations only)	Calcium oxalate	300 mg/day	
Allopurinol/febuxostat	Xanthine oxidase inhibitors	Uric acid	Standard doses	Allopurinol given during very high uric acid excretion can result in xanthinuria and xanthine stones
D-Penicillamine Tiopronin (2-mercapto-propionylglycine) Captopril (but not other ACE inhibitors)	Cystine chelators which increase cystine solubility by forming a disulphide complex	Cystine	Standard doses	D-Penicillamine can cause bone marrow side effects, rash, nephrotic syndrome
Tamsulosin	α_1 (alpha-1) receptor blocker used as 'medical expulsive therapy', relaxing urinary tract smooth muscle	Any	Standard doses	Postural hypotension

repeat imaging/surgical follow-up if needed and with re-screening using 24-h urinary collections to monitor metabolic abnormalities.

Dietary

Many of the recommended interventions are consistent with general healthy eating advice and can be combined by advocating Mediterranean-style diets such as the DASH (Dietary Approaches to Stop Hypertension) diet, modified to avoid high-oxalate vegetables and nuts. Formal dietetic intervention is recommended when the patient has other diagnoses that require conflicting diets. Most of these interventions are directed towards calcium stone disease:

Fluid intake – drinking more fluid throughout the day is important (particularly in cystinuria where peak concentration is important), but this strategy is not adequate in isolation. Poor fluid intake is not by itself a cause of stones, since most people with low urine output do not suffer from stones. Trial evidence suggests that increasing urine volume to >2 L/day can reduce recurrence rates by 40–50 % [5]. Fluid is best consumed as water, as other drinks tend to contain sugar. Tea or coffee should be taken with milk (which binds oxalate).

Good calcium intake – a good intake of calcium, preferably as lower-fat dairy products such as bioactive yogurts, is beneficial in allowing enteric complexing of oxalate while maintaining bone health.

Low oxalate intake – even small reductions in dietary oxalate can lead to a significant reduction in urinary oxalate excretion and hence stone risk. This is despite dietary oxalate accounting for only 10–20 % of urinary oxalate excretion. Common oxalate-rich foods include bran, chocolate, nuts and tea/coffee (without milk). Others include spinach, rhubarb, okra, beetroot, soya beans and tofu.

Reduce dietary fat – in the short term, this increases the efficacy of calcium and oxalate binding in the colon (by reducing free fatty acids) and in the long term reduces weight gain and risk of metabolic syndrome.

Reduce animal protein intake – this will also help with uric acid stone formation. Aim for a maximum of 150 g of animal flesh per day. There is no distinction between sources of protein for stone risk.

Other measures – increasing fruit and vegetable intake increases dietary potassium, magnesium and citrate.

Dietary sodium restriction will reduce calcium excretion and is essential prior to commencing thiazide diuretic therapy.

A well-written patient information leaflet is available at http://www.guysandstthomas.nhs.uk/resources/patient-information/urology/stones/2390-diet-lifestyle-kidney-stones.pdf.

Combined Approaches for Particular Stone Types

Uric acid stone formers – low-purine-containing diet (commonest purine sources are meat, fish, seafood, pulses and beer) and alkali treatment (aim for urinary pH>6.2) with high fluid intake (aim for urine output >2.5 L/day). Add allopurinol if still forming stones.

Infection stones (calcium phosphate or magnesium ammonium phosphate) – cranberry juice is advisable since it is the only fruit juice that acidifies the urine, whereas all others alkalinise the urine. Prolonged antibiotic therapy may be needed since stones and fragments may contain organisms. Recurrent infections can sometimes be due to an obstructing stone of any type, so in this case a full metabolic screen should be performed *after* the infection has been cleared.

Cystine stones – as urinary pH becomes more alkaline, insoluble cystine is more likely to dissociate to its more soluble ion. A urinary pH of >7.5 and urine output of >3 L/day (spread throughout the day) are optimal in reducing the urinary concentration of cystine to prevent precipitation. This can be augmented by:

- Titration of fluid and alkali therapy to maintain urine cystine concentration of <1 mmol/L (preferably <0.5 mmol/L)
- If necessary, addition of a chelating agent which combines with cystine forming a soluble disulphide complex (see table above) while maintaining fluid and alkali therapy

Xanthine stones – these require dilution with large amounts of fluid and consumption of a low purine diet. Xanthine oxidase catalyses the conversion of hypoxanthine to insoluble xanthine and of xanthine to uric acid. Stones occur due to a build-up of xanthine caused by allopurinol therapy in patients with high urate production of any cause (hence stop allopurinol) or rarely due to a deficiency of endogenous xanthine oxidase.

2,8-dihydroxyadenine stones – stones formed from this metabolite are effectively treated with allopurinol.

Ammonium urate stones – in developed countries, this rare stone type is either an infection stone or a marker of laxative abuse or eating disorders. In the latter, the resulting metabolic acidosis results in an appropriate increase in urinary ammonium production to buffer the excess acid. In less developed countries, these stones may occur due to insufficient dietary phosphate resulting in increasing urinary ammonium production rather than phosphate to buffer acid.

Table 36.10 Treatment algorithm for stones in the kidney

Size of kidney stone	Position of stone within the kidney	
	Upper pole calyx or Middle pole calyx or Renal pelvis	Lower pole calyx
>2 cm	First choice: PCNL Second choice: ESWL Third choice: Flexi URS Fourth choice: Laparoscopy	First choice: PCNL Second choice: ESWL
1–2 cm	First choice: ESWL Second choice: PCNL Third choice: Flexi URS	PCNL or ESWL
<1 cm	First choice: ESWL Second choice: Flexi URS Third choice: PCNL	First choice: ESWL Second choice: Flexi URS

PCNL percutaneous nephrolithotomy, *ESWL* extracorporeal shock wave lithotripsy, *Flexi URS* flexible ureterorenoscopy

Surgical Treatment of Ureteric and Renal Stones

Stones in the Ureter

All patients with a ureteric stone should be referred for urgent urological review even if they are asymptomatic, as there is a high chance of progressing to obstruction and/or infection.

Treatment options are:

- *Direct treatment of the stone*. Lithotripsy (ESWL) is the first choice for proximal ureteric stones less than 10 mm and ureteroscopy for distal ureteric stones greater than 10 mm [17]. In all other cases, options will be determined by local expertise.
- If obstruction or infection is suspected, or if direct treatment is not possible, then *decompression of the kidney* should be performed as an interim measure, via either a percutaneous nephrostomy (under local anaesthetic) or JJ stent (a stent with two coiled ends placed in the ureter).
- *Medical expulsive therapy* with either a calcium channel blocker or alpha blocker (to relax the smooth muscle of the distal ureter and bladder trigone) is an option for lower ureteric stones. If the stone has not passed within 6 weeks, then definitive treatment is required.

Stones in the Kidney

Staghorn calculi, symptomatic stones and those causing obstruction should always be treated (Table 36.10). Increasingly, kidney stones are an incidental finding on imaging for other indications. Unlike ureteric stones, they are often asymptomatic or present subacutely with nagging back or flank pain. It is unclear whether small asymptomatic kidney stones should be observed or actively treated. A study looking at 300 men with a mean stone diameter of 10.8 mm over 3 years showed 77 % progressed and 26 % required surgical intervention [27]. All patients with kidney stones should be offered urological review to consider the benefits of treatment or to allow urological follow-up.

Types of Surgical Intervention

Extracorporeal Shock Wave Lithotripsy (ESWL)

ESWL uses acoustic energy to fragment calculi and is focused onto the stone by either ultrasound or fluoroscopy. It is performed as a day case procedure and requires minimal analgesia. Each treatment lasts between 25 and 50 min and involves 3,000 shocks delivered at a rate of between 60 and 120/min.

The resulting numerous residual stone fragments can lead to sepsis/obstruction or act as foci for the development of new stones. An alternative therapy should be considered if the stone is large, hard, in a lower calyx (poor subsequent drainage) or in the lower ureter (difficult to localise) or if the patient is obese. ESWL is contraindicated in urinary tract sepsis, obstruction and pregnancy.

Rigid Ureteroscopy and Flexible Ureterorenoscopy

These endoscopic techniques now allow the whole urinary tract to be accessed. Rigid ureteroscopy is the treatment of choice for distal ureteric stones >10 mm [17] though it can be considered for all ureteric calculi. It is more invasive with a higher risk of complications than ESWL, although it is more likely to clear the stone in a single session and offers the advantage of allowing collection of stone material for biochemical analysis.

Flexible ureterorenoscopy (often preceded by rigid ureteroscopy) can treat most stones in the kidney. Fragmentation of stones using a Holmium laser introduced via the scope is very effective even for hard stones, and the resulting fragments can then be removed via the scope, reducing the chance of distal obstruction. Post-operative stenting of the ureter is often performed, particularly where there is ureteric injury or a high risk of obstruction due to fragments or residual stones.

Percutaneous Nephrolithotomy (PCNL)

PCNL is indicated for large stones (>2 cm), stones that are difficult to access endoscopically (acutely angled lower pole or calyceal diverticulum), and where a single procedure to clear stones is preferable. A contrast imaging study allows planning of renal access, which in the UK is usually obtained by a radiologist. The tract is then dilated and a rigid nephroscope is inserted. The stone either can be grasped and removed whole or can be fragmented *in situ* prior to removal. A nephrostomy tube is usually then placed into the tract, which tamponades it and allows repeat access if needed. Complications include bleeding and occasionally sepsis. Despite formation of the tract, PCNL results in minimal damage to the renal parenchyma with an average loss of <1 % [28].

Open and Laparoscopic Stone Surgery

Only 47 open stone procedures were performed in England in 2010. Indications include failure of less invasive procedures, requirement for partial nephrectomy of a non-functioning moiety or morbid obesity.

Top Tips and Pitfalls in Assessment

Scenario	Top tips
'UTIs' diagnosed in a young man but never confirmed microbiologically	Symptoms may be due to spontaneously passed small stones. These can give dipstick abnormalities of haematuria, leucocytes and proteinuria, mimicking findings in infection
Bilateral stone disease	Suggests underlying metabolic/genetic rather than anatomical abnormality (although may coexist)
Stones with proteinuria	Differential includes infection (albuminuria), Dent's disease (low molecular weight proteinuria)
Pure oxalate stones	Screen for primary hyperoxaluria, initially by measuring 24-h urinary oxalate. 10 % present in late adulthood, so look for a family history
Unusual combinations of stone types	Ammonium urate stones are suggestive of laxative abuse [21]. Silica/calcium/magnesium stones are suggestive of antacid abuse
Stone disease in potential kidney donor	Full metabolic evaluation is helpful in determining donation decision

Acknowledgements Ben Turney DPhil, MSc, MA, FRCS (Urol), PGDipLATHE
Dariush Douraghi-Zadeh BSc, MB BS, FRCR
Navin Ramachandran BSc, MB BS, MRCP, FRCR
Darrell Allen FRCS (Urol), BSc

References

1. Worcester EM, Coe FL. Clinical practice. Calcium kidney stones. N Engl J Med. 2010;363(10):954–63. PubMed PMID: 20818905. Pubmed Central PMCID: 3192488. Epub.
2. Romero V, Akpinar H, Assimos DG. Kidney stones: a global picture of prevalence, incidence, and associated risk factors. Rev Urol. 2010;12(2-3):e86–96. PubMed PMID: 20811557. Pubmed Central PMCID: 2931286. Epub 2010/09/03. eng.
3. Turney BW, Reynard JM, Noble JG, Keoghane SR. Trends in urological stone disease. BJU Int. 2012;109(7):1082–7. PubMed PMID: 21883851. Epub 2011/09/03. eng.

4. Asplin JR. Obesity and urolithiasis. Adv Chronic Kidney Dis. 2009;16(1):11–20. PubMed PMID: 19095201. Epub 2008/12/20. eng.
5. Borghi L, Meschi T, Amato F, Briganti A, Novarini A, Giannini A. Urinary volume, water and recurrences in idiopathic calcium nephrolithiasis: a 5-year randomized prospective study. J Urol. 1996;155(3):839–43. PubMed PMID: 8583588. Epub 1996/03/01. eng.
6. Taylor EN, Fung TT, Curhan GC. DASH-style diet associates with reduced risk for kidney stones. J Am Soc Nephrol. 2009;20(10):2253–9. PubMed PMID: 19679672. Pubmed Central PMCID: 2754098. Epub 2009/08/15. eng.
7. Taylor EN, Stampfer MJ, Curhan GC. Obesity, weight gain, and the risk of kidney stones. JAMA. 2005;293(4):455–62. PubMed PMID: 15671430. Epub 2005/01/27. eng.
8. Jeong IG, Kang T, Bang JK, Park J, Kim W, Hwang SS, et al. Association between metabolic syndrome and the presence of kidney stones in a screened population. Am J Kidney Dis. 2011;58(3):383–8. PubMed PMID: 21620546. Epub 2011/05/31. eng.
9. Saigal CS, Joyce G, Timilsina AR. Direct and indirect costs of nephrolithiasis in an employed population: opportunity for disease management? Kidney Int. 2005;68(4):1808–14. PubMed PMID: 16164658. Epub 2005/09/17. eng.
10. Rule AD, Bergstralh EJ, Melton 3rd LJ, Li X, Weaver AL, Lieske JC. Kidney stones and the risk for chronic kidney disease. Clin J Am Soc Nephrol. 2009;4(4):804–11. PubMed PMID: 19339425. Pubmed Central PMCID: 2666438. Epub 2009/04/03. eng.
11. Lauderdale DS, Thisted RA, Wen M, Favus MJ. Bone mineral density and fracture among prevalent kidney stone cases in the Third National Health and Nutrition Examination Survey. J Bone Miner Res. 2001;16(10):1893–8. PubMed PMID: 11585355. Epub 2001/10/05. eng.
12. Domingos F, Serra A. Nephrolithiasis is associated with an increased prevalence of cardiovascular disease. Nephrol Dial Transplant. 2011;26(3):864–8. PubMed PMID: 20709737. Epub 2010/08/17. eng.
13. Rule AD, Roger VL, Melton 3rd LJ, Bergstralh EJ, Li X, Peyser PA, et al. Kidney stones associate with increased risk for myocardial infarction. J Am Soc Nephrol. 2010;21(10):1641–4. PubMed PMID: 20616170. Pubmed Central PMCID: 3013539. Epub 2010/07/10. eng.
14. Spivacow FR, Negri AL, del Valle EE, Calvino I, Zanchetta JR. Clinical and metabolic risk factor evaluation in young adults with kidney stones. Int Urol Nephrol. 2010;42(2):471–5. PubMed PMID: 19653114. Epub 2009/08/05. eng.
15. Wrong O. Nephrocalcinosis. In: The oxford textbook of clinical nephrology. 3rd ed. Oxford: Oxford University Press; 1998. p. 1882–905.
16. Robertson WG. Is prevention of stone recurrence financially worthwhile? Urol Res. 2006;34(2):157–61. PubMed PMID: 16456694. Epub 2006/02/04. eng.
17. Türk C, Knoll T, Petrik A, Sarica K, Straub M, Seitz C. Guidelines on urolithiasis: European Association of Urology guidelines. Arnhem, The Netherlands: 2011.
18. Johri N, Cooper B, Robertson W, Choong S, Rickards D, Unwin R. An update and practical guide to renal stone management. Nephron Clin Pract. 2010;116(3):c159–71. PubMed PMID: 20606476. Epub 2010/07/08. eng.
19. Consensus conference. Prevention and treatment of kidney stones. JAMA. 1988;260(7):977–81. PubMed PMID: 3294456. Epub 1988/08/19. eng.
20. Hess B, Hasler-Strub U, Ackermann D, Jaeger P. Metabolic evaluation of patients with recurrent idiopathic calcium nephrolithiasis. Nephrol Dial Transplant. 1997;12(7):1362–8. PubMed PMID: 9249770. Epub 1997/07/01. eng.
21. Kasidas GP, Samuell CT, Weir TB. Renal stone analysis: why and how? Ann Clin Biochem. 2004;41(Pt 2):91–7. PubMed PMID: 15025798. Epub 2004/03/18. eng.
22. Bellin MF, Renard-Penna R, Conort P, Bissery A, Meric JB, Daudon M, et al. Helical CT evaluation of the chemical composition of urinary tract calculi with a discriminant analysis of CT-attenuation values and density. Eur Radiol. 2004;14(11):2134–40. PubMed PMID: 15221262. Epub 2004/06/29. eng.
23. Sayer JA, Moochhala SH, Thomas DJ. The medical management of urolithiasis. Br J Med Surg Urol. 2010;3(3):87–95.
24. Curhan GC, Willett WC, Speizer FE, Stampfer MJ. Twenty-four-hour urine chemistries and the risk of kidney stones among women and men. Kidney Int. 2001;59(6):2290–8. PubMed PMID: 11380833. Epub 2001/05/31. eng.
25. Chan VO, Buckley O, Persaud T, Torreggiani WC. Urolithiasis: how accurate are plain radiographs? Can Assoc Radiol J. 2008;59(3):131–4. PubMed PMID: 18697719. Epub 2008/08/14. eng.
26. Reilly RF, Peixoto AJ, Desir GV. The evidence-based use of thiazide diuretics in hypertension and nephrolithiasis. Clin J Am Soc Nephrol. 2010;5(10):1893–903. PubMed PMID: 20798254. Epub 2010/08/28. eng.
27. Burgher A, Beman M, Holtzman JL, Monga M. Progression of nephrolithiasis: long-term outcomes with observation of asymptomatic calculi. J Endourol. 2004;18(6):534–9.
28. Traxer O, Smith TG, Pearle MS, Corwin T, Saboorian H, Cadeddu JA. Renal parenchymal injury after standard and mini percutaneous nephrostolithotomy. J Urol. 2001;165(5):1693–5.

37 Congenital Anomalies of the Kidneys and Urinary Tract

Angela D. Gupta, Dan Wood, and John O. Connolly

Congenital anomalies of the kidneys and urinary tract (CAKUT) encompass a broad range of developmental malformations of the kidney and the lower urinary tract. The many malformations are now detected by fetal ultrasound screening, but cases may still present for the first time in childhood with symptoms of failure to thrive or during investigation of urinary tract infection. In adults developmental abnormalities may still present with abnormal urinalysis, renal stones, hypertension or chronic kidney disease or as an incidental finding.

CAKUT are relatively common occurring in 1:500 live births and collectively represent the most common cause of chronic kidney disease (CKD) and end-stage kidney disease in childhood. Furthermore, it is likely that CAKUT are substantially under-diagnosed as a cause of CKD in young adults, and it is important that these conditions are recognized by nephrologists and urologists. With improvements in fetal screening and early urological management, the number of adults with CAKUT as a cause of CKD is likely to increase. Although the majority of CAKUT occur as isolated malformations, a significant number of patients will have familial inheritance, and many cases will occur as part of multisystem organ malformation syndromes.

Patients with CAKUT present a variety of clinical and management problems and are often cared for as part of a multidisciplinary team – involving a range of healthcare professionals. This is particularly important for young people making the transition from highly specialist paediatric care to adult follow-up.

The problems arising can be broadly categorized in three groups:

1. Congenital anomalies of the kidney without lower tract obstruction
2. Congenital anomalies causing obstruction and secondary kidney dysfunction
3. Consequences of reconstruction in patients with congenital urinary tract anomalies

Embryology and Pathophysiology of Development

Kidney malformations may both occur in isolation or accompanied by lower tract abnormalities. This association can be better appreciated when understanding the common origin of kidney and ureter during development.

Renal development begins in the third week of gestation and proceeds through an ordered series of developmental phases. At around 35 days gestation, the main precursor structures of the kidney and ureter are present. These include the mesonephric duct which gives rise to an out-pouching called the ureteric bud. The ureteric bud elongates to form the metanephric duct eventually giving rise to the ureter, collecting system and renal pelvis. The ureteric bud also grows and branches into nearby metanephric mesenchyme signalling to induce formation of nephrons. Eventually this process gives rise to the mature kidney. Nephrogenesis is complete by the 34th week of gestation although growth of the kidney continues into fetal life. At this time a rapid rise in glomerular filtration rate (GFR) is observed, doubling further in the first 2 weeks of life, indicating ongoing renal maturation. The fetal kidneys begin in the pelvis and ascend up the posterior abdominal wall. As they reach their final position, they rotate to face medially. Failure of this rotation is relatively common resulting in forward facing kidneys.

A.D. Gupta, MD
Urology, Johns Hopkins Hospital,
1800 Orleans Street, Baltimore, MD 21287, USA
e-mail: agupta45@jhmi.edu

D. Wood, PhD, FRCS (Urol)
Adolescent Urology, University College London Hospitals,
250 Euston Road, London NW1 2BU, UK
e-mail: dan.wood@uclh.nhs.uk

J.O. Connolly, PhD, FRCP (✉)
UCL Centre for Nephrology, Royal Free Hospital,
Pond Street, London NW3 2QG, UK
e-mail: johnconnolly@nhs.net

M. Harber (ed.), *Practical Nephrology*,
DOI 10.1007/978-1-4471-5547-8_37, © Springer-Verlag London 2014

Pelviureteric junction obstruction is one of the most common causes of calyceal dilatation and is associated with hydronephrosis in the absence of a dilated ureter. The abnormality is most commonly a congenital ureteric defect but occasionally may be due to extrinsic compression from crossing blood vessel or ureteric kinking. Surgical intervention is indicated with symptoms or if the anteroposterior measurement of the renal pelvis is greater than 30 mm or the ipsilateral split function is below 40 %. Many are detected on antenatal ultrasound and can be treated or monitored early in life. A few will present in later life following trauma, pyelonephritis or kidney stones. Occasionally consumption of alcohol or other fluids may precipitate symptoms.

Megaureter

A megaureter (dilated ureter) is most commonly secondary to ureteric or bladder outflow obstruction. Ureteric obstruction may be either intrinsic (e.g. stone or tumour) or extrinsic (e.g. retroperitoneal fibrosis or lymphoma). Outflow obstruction with secondary ureteric dilatation may be seen in conditions such as posterior urethral valves or neuropathic bladder. Initial reflux is likely but subsequent bladder wall thickening may result in ureteric obstruction.

Primary dilatation usually results from abnormal ureteric musculature and affected ureters may show an adynamic segment of ureteric wall. In these cases the ureter may not be obstructed and may or may not exhibit reflux – renal function may be normal. In the absence of obstruction or symptoms, a conservative approach can safely be adopted. In affected infant boys for whom UTIs are a presenting problem, circumcision is indicated to reduce the risk of further infection.

Duplex Ureters

Many patients with duplex systems never know about them – studies to determine incidence have been based on findings at autopsy. This implies that in the absence of a clinical or symptomatic problem, a conservative strategy may be appropriate. Some will have reflux; however, the rate of spontaneous resolution is far lower than those who have reflux in a singleton system.

Ectopic ureters are most commonly associated with duplex systems and arise from the upper moiety. In males they are always suprasphincteric but may insert into the posterior urethra, vas or seminal vesicle. In females they may be either suprasphincteric or sub-sphincteric in the urethra, distal vagina or intoitus. Ectopic ureters tend to be associated with a dysplastic upper pole.

A further association with this dysplasia is a ureterocele. This occurs in duplex systems affecting the ureter from the upper pole, and they are defined by a cystic dilatation of the lower part of the affected ureter. They may be confined to the bladder or extend beyond the bladder neck.

If a single ureteric bud bifurcates, a partial duplex occurs with ureters from the two renal moieties joining to form a common ureter that enters the bladder. If two ureteric buds arise, both ureters will enter the bladder separately.

Bladder and Outflow Disorders

A variety of conditions give rise to bladder abnormalities or outflow obstruction which can have long-term consequences on both bladder and kidney function and thus quality of life. Kidney damage may be due to the effects of obstruction, but many cases are associated with abnormal kidney development. Bilateral ureteric obstruction in these conditions also causes injury during development to both the kidneys and the bladder.

Posterior Urethral Valves

Posterior urethral valves (PUV) are the most common cause of congenital bladder outflow obstruction in male infants. The obstruction is created by a membrane that extends across the posterior urethra. It is most commonly suspected antenatally with bilateral hydroureteronephrosis, a thick-walled bladder and dilated posterior urethra (keyhole sign) but may present after birth with a poor stream, absence of voiding, palpable bladder or urinary sepsis. Rare adult cases with end-stage kidney disease are still reported.

Management involves immediate catheterization and confirmation of the diagnosis with a micturating cystogram (MCUG) – followed by valve resection. Some centres have reported antenatal vesico-amniotic shunting, but the long-term benefits of this remain unproven. Bladder obstruction leads to bladder compensation with muscular hypertrophy further fibrosis leads to a non-compliant bladder with thickening and 'stiffening' of the bladder wall. In later stages the bladder may decompensate functioning as a floppy reservoir with little or no contractility. A thickened bladder wall may result in ureteric obstruction – this may add to the risk of renal failure. Regardless of bladder function, low-pressure storage and good drainage are essential. For some whose bladder has decompensated, intermittent self-catheterization may be necessary. It can be difficult to persuade an adolescent man to undertake – especially if they feel otherwise asymptomatic. Continuous night-time drainage can improve hydroureteronephrosis rapidly and may help with long-term renal outcomes for this population. Once the obstruction is relieved, the management in childhood includes antibiotic prophylaxis and careful bladder management.

Prune Belly Syndrome

Prune belly syndrome occurs only in males – diagnostic features include the absence of anterior abdominal wall muscles, gross dilatation of the bladder and ureters and undescended testes. The underlying pathogenesis is probably due to defective mesenchymal development. Ureteric smooth muscle is replaced with fibrous tissue; there is an absence of the normal nerve plexus and a failure of normal prostatic differentiation

Abnormal renal development may accompany prune belly syndrome; the clinical manifestations are dependent on the degree of renal dysplasia.

There is complete absence or incomplete formation of the rectus abdominis and other muscles, which leads to the wrinkled abdominal wall of the prune infant. This gives way to a fairly smooth 'pot belly' in later life. Reconstructive surgery is not normally required.

Although true outflow obstruction is sometimes present, the gross and irregular dilation of the urinary tract that is characteristic of this syndrome is primarily caused by a developmental defect with a variable degree of smooth muscle aplasia leading to aperistaltic ureters. Urodynamics are often difficult to interpret because of gross VUR, but typically there is a low-pressure bladder. With late presentation, some patients have detrusor instability.

Differential Diagnosis

In severe cases of megacystis or megaureter with gross renal impairment (often with dysplastic kidneys), the differential diagnosis includes posterior urethral valves, renal dysplasia withor without multiple congenital defects, neuropathic bladder and nephrogenic diabetes insipidus.

Natural History

Once any outflow obstruction is dealt with, usually in infancy, the renal function should remain stable despite the frightening radiologic appearances. In those patients followed in our unit for up to 40 years, renal deterioration and hypertension have been rare. In the small number who have progressed, recurrent infection, hypertension and proteinuria have been warning signs of impending trouble.

Renal scarring should be assessed by isotopic DMSA scintigrams and renal function followed by serial isotopic GFR measurements. Lifelong attention to blood pressure, urinary tract infection and stones is necessary.

Treatment

In all children, even with good renal function, there should be a careful search for obstruction, beginning with the urethra and working up to the PUJ, but often no obstruction is found and no surgery is required. In many others, the floppy bladder is not anatomically obstructed, but bladder emptying is improvedby urethrotomy ('functional obstruction'). In infancy, there is debate about the need for reconstructive surgery. There is certainly a group of patients born with severely compromised renal function who do require reconstruction after stabilization by early diversion.

The current view is that the testes should be brought down to the scrotum in infancy. It is hoped that earlier surgery will produce proper germ cell development. There is a strong association with infertility in prune belly syndrome. Natural conception is reported but would be an exception rather than the rule.

Bladder Exstrophy

This is a rare but significant congenital anomaly which occurs in between 1 in 30,000 and 1 in 50,000 live births. The male to female ratio is 2:1. At birth the bladder opens externally and is fused with the anterior abdominal wall. In classic bladder exstrophy there is associated genital epispadias requiring reconstruction of bladder, bladder neck and in a male infant – the penis. Occasionally, the more severe condition, cloacal exstrophy, is found; this is associated with other anomalies of the bowel or kidneys and may include neuropathic damage as a result of sacral agenesis or myelomeningocele.

Surgical reconstruction is essential and has four major objectives:

1. Closure of the anterior abdominal wall
2. Reconstruction of the bladder and bladder neck achieving continence
3. Preservation of renal function
4. Genital reconstruction

Long-term outcomes are relatively good. Data from our centre examined a group of 65 patients with at least 20 years of follow-up; we found 33 % with abnormal renal ultrasounds on follow-up – for those with full data available, 7 % had a significant change in creatinine. No patient required

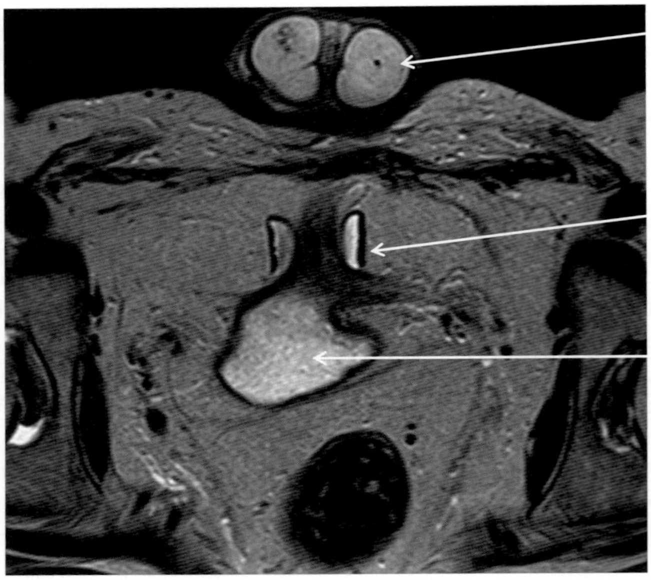

Fig. 37.2 MRI scan of the pelvis in a man with bladder exstrophy

renal replacement therapy. Only 1/3 of patients empty their bladder via the urethra with the remainder requiring a urinary diversion (see Fig. 37.2).

Neuropathic Bladders

Neuropathic bladder is usually classified into three patterns according to contractile function: hypercontractile, intermediate and acontractile.

Increased or Intermediate Bladder Contractility

The group with hypercontractility are most at risk of developing kidney damage. The bladder develops a high functional pressure as a result of neurogenic detrusor overactivity – with uncontrolled contractions against a closed sphincter (detrusor sphincter dyssynergia – upper tract damage follows as a result of a significant rise in bladder pressure). The bladder itself tends to deteriorate with hypertrophy and subsequent fibrosis.

The intermediate group tends to have poor sphincter function, and detrusor contraction will lead to incontinence. Many of these patients have no evidence of other neurological deficit.

Reduced Bladder Contractility

The majority of cases are associated with neural tube defects – the most common of which is myelomeningocele or spina bifida. Folic acid supplementation during pregnancy has reduce the incidence of these defects by 50 % in the general population. This is especially important in patients who themselves have had a neural tube defect as their risk of having an affected child is approximately 50 times higher. Bladder pressures are usually low and bladder emptying incomplete. Renal failure is not usually an issue but urinary stasis tends to lead to infection.

Other Congenital Causes of Bladder Outflow Obstruction

Recently several distinct genetic syndromes have been described in patients with severe bladder dysfunction, urodynamically consistent with a neurogenic bladder, but in whom no neurology defect can be demonstrated (Table 37.3). Urofacial or Ochoa syndrome is a rare autosomal recessive disease characterized by facial grimacing and failure of the complete bladder emptying. They are at risk of renal failure. Some but not all families have mutations of HPSE2 (heparanase 2), which is expressed in the fetal and adult central nervous system, and also in bladder smooth muscle, consistent with a role in renal tract morphology and function. A prune belly-like syndrome, or pseudo-prune, can occur as a consequence of mutation of CHRM3 (muscarinic acetylcholine receptor M3), and in boys this syndrome can be misdiagnosed as posterior urethral valves.

Management

Without careful bladder management progressive kidney damage will be seen in the first 5 years of life in 30–40 % of

Table 37.3 Bladder and outflow tract anomalies

		Diagnostic imaging
Posterior urethral valves	Mainly antenatal detection	Antenatal US and VCUG
	Accounts for around 10 % of antenatal hydronephrosis	Bilateral hydroureteronephrosis, with a thick-walled bladder and dilated posterior urethra
	All require value resection	Up to 20–30 % also develop secondary VUR diagnosed with the initial MCUG
	Can present late	
	50 % ultimately require further surgical intervention	
	Grade 3–4 postnatal hydronephrosis and relative renal function less than 40 % predict the need for requiring surgical intervention	
Bladder exstrophy/ epispadias	The condition occurs in 1 in 10,000–50,000 births. The male to female ratio is 2:1	Antenatal US
	Ectopic bladder	
	Epispadias	
	Failure of fusion pubic rami	
Prune belly syndrome	Occurs only in males	Antenatal US
	Incidence varies from 1 in 30,000 to 50,000	
	Three groups can be distinguished	
	Group I, complete urethral obstruction causes stillbirth or neonatal death (20 %)	
	Group II, acute, early presentation requires diversion and reconstruction (20 %)	
	Group III, good health and renal function exist despite urological appearances (60 %)	
Spina bifida	1–5 in 1,000 live births	Antenatal US
	Wide variation in phenotype and may present as spinal dysraphism	Prenatal testing
Neurogenic bladder	Defects in bladder contractility	US
		Voiding cystourethrogram (VCUG)

children. This can be dramatically reduced or delayed by ensuring the native or reconstructed bladder is compliant, has low pressure and provides good drainage. Clean intermittent self-catheterization plays a central role and anticholinergic medication offers additional benefit by improving bladder capacity. Children and young adults affected by a congenital urinary obstruction should have renal function and renal imaging routinely monitored into adulthood.

Multidisciplinary care is an effective way of maintaining regular, safe follow-up. Patients should have annual blood tests for estimation of GFR, urinalysis for proteinuria, blood pressure assessment and ultrasound to monitor ongoing function. Video urodynamic studies and MAG3 renography are used to assess for hydronephrosis, end filling pressures, capacity and bladder compliance. Isotopic methods to assess GFR are more accurate in those with reduced muscle mass, e.g. spina bifida.

Urinary Diversions

Ureterosigmoidostomy

Now rarely seen, in a ureterosigmoidostomy the ureters were anastomosed directly into the sigmoid colon. This technique was most commonly used in patients with bladder exstrophy. Progressive CKD; hyperchloraemic, hypokalaemic metabolic acidosis; kidney stones; infection; ureteral strictures; and increased risk for colonic carcinoma are important complications. Patients with ureterosigmoidostomy require yearly check of the anastomotic site with a flexible sigmoidoscopy.

Ileal Conduits

The ureters are directly attached to an isolated segment of ileum. The ileal conduit is free flowing with rapid urinary transit and no reservoir (see Fig. 37.3). Metabolic complications are much less common but can occur.

Enterocystoplasty and Intestinal Urinary Reservoirs

In these cases bowel is used to augment or completely replace the native bladder. A Mitrofanoff channel using appendix or small bowel may also be necessary to allow bladder drainage. This provides a continent, cutaneous channel for catheterization. Complications include infection, mucus production, kidney stones and CKD. Lifelong follow-up is needed to detect medical or surgical complications. Excess mucus production can be treated with regular bladder washouts.

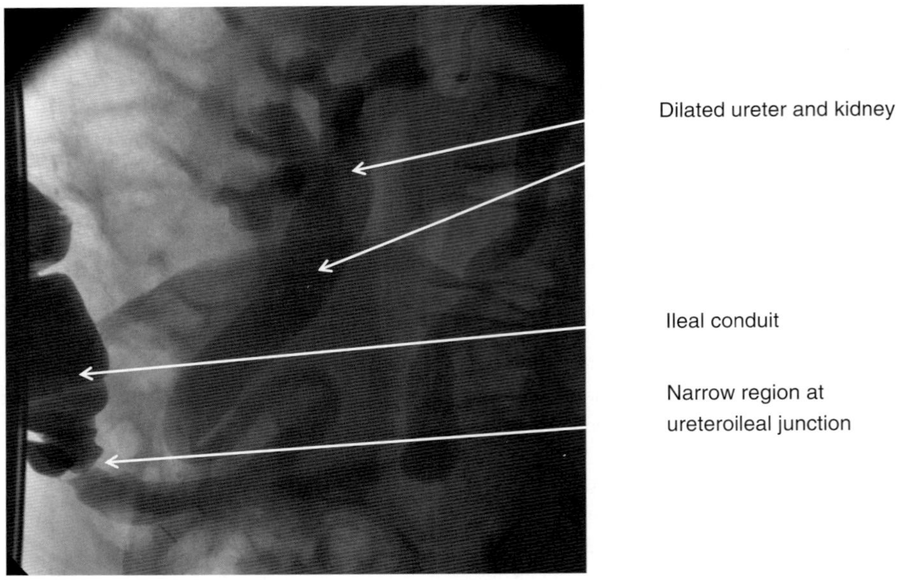

Fig. 37.3 Loopogram to examine an ileal conduit

Complications

CKD

The renal outcome of patients with CAKUT is similar whether there is primary renal dysplasia or abnormal bladder function. Predictive factors include GFR and degree of proteinuria. In young adults a GFR of less than 40 and proteinuria greater than 100 mg/mmol are poor prognostic indicators. ACE inhibitors or angiotensin receptor blockers (ARB) are preferred for patients with proteinuria and progressive renal failure.

Blood Pressure

Hypertension is common in the presence of scarred kidneys, but in patients whose renal failure is secondary to obstruction, there is significant tubular injury. This may cause problems, in particular with urinary concentration, acidification and sodium reabsorption. In these patients diuretics are often poorly tolerated because of significant polyuria or nocturia. Overfilling of the bladder can be an important cause of intermittent obstruction and should be assessed by asking the patient to complete a 24 h input and output diary.

Kidney Stones

Kidney stones may form in the presence of infected urine and are typically magnesium ammonium phosphate (struvite) or calcium phosphate. In 90 % of patients, the infecting organism is *Proteus* species. Stones are common in cystoplasties and ileal conduits (5–30 %) because of the alkaline environment. Upper tract stones must be suspected if UTIs recur or become more frequent and with the onset of severe pain or if renal function suddenly deteriorates.

Acidosis and Bone Disease

There is often a metabolic acidosis disproportionate to the degree of renal impairment. Metabolic acidosis was particularly common with ureterosigmoidostomy. It is our practice to give sufficient sodium bicarbonate to correct the plasma bicarbonate into the normal range. In addition to the typical bone disease of progressive CKD, acidosis contributes significantly to osteomalacia.

Top Tips

1. CAKUT are the most common cause of CKD in childhood and are probably under-diagnosed in young adults. Greater awareness of these conditions among adult nephrologists is needed. A careful history and investigation will improve diagnosis.
2. Up to 10 % of cases may have a genetic association and a detailed family history is always needed.
3. Proteinuria is a key prognostic indicator and probably reflects hyperfiltration injury. Treatment goals should be similar to other causes of CKD with proteinuria
4. When investigating possible renal tract obstruction, start distally, i.e. urethra, and work back towards kidneys.
5. Lifelong follow-up is usually needed. Pay particular care to metabolic complications in patients with bladder reconstructions, i.e. acidosis, stone disease and bone mineral metabolism.
6. Abnormal or reconstructed bladders may be of large capacity which can lead to functional obstruction at high volumes. In general bladder volumes

should be kept low, i.e. less than 400 ml. This can easily be assessed with 24 or 48 h recording of urine volumes together with fluid intake. Many patients will have been instructed to drink large volumes, and this childhood habit can be hard to break!

7. Patient with reconstructed bladders often have abnormal urinalysis and culture positive MSU. A careful history to corroborate symptomatic infection is essential before treating with antibiotics.

Further Reading

Lewis MA. Demography of renal disease in childhood. Semin Fetal Neonatal Med. 2008;13:118–24.

Neild GH. What do we know about chronic renal failure in young adults? Adult outcome of pediatric renal disease. Pediatr Nephrol. 2009;24:1921–8.

Neild GH, Thomson G, Nitsch D, et al. Renal outcome in adults with renal insufficiency and irregular asymmetric kidneys. BMC Nephrol. 2004;5:12–22.

Woolf AS, Jenkins D. Development of the kidney. In: Jennette JC, Olson JL, Schwartz MM, Silva FG, eds. Heptinstall's pathology of the kidney, 7th ed. Philadelphia: Lippincott-Raven. 2013.

Farrugia M-K, Woolf AS. Congenital urinary bladder outlet obstruction. Fetal Matern Med Rev. 2010;21(1):55–73.

Schedl A. Renal abnormalities and their developmental origin. Nat Rev Genet. 2007;8:791–802.

Jenkins D, Woolf AS. Uroplakins: new molecular players in the biology of urinary tract malformations. Kidney Int. 2007;71:195–200 (swap for 20).

Lee PH, Diamond DA, Duffy PG, Ransley PG. Duplex reflux: a study of 105 children. J Urol. 1991;146:657–9.

Woodhouse CR, Ransley PG, Innes WD. Prune belly syndrome: report of 47 cases. Arch Dis Child. 1982;57:856–9.

Burbige KA, Amodio J, Berdon WE, et al. Prune belly syndrome: 35 years of experience. J Urol. 1987;137:86–90. 33.

Fontaine E, Leaver R, Woodhouse CR. The effect of intestinal urinary reservoirs on renal function: a 10-year follow-up. BJU Int. 2000;86:195–8

Johnston LB, Borzyskowski M. Bladder dysfunction and neurological disability at presentation in closed spina bifida. Arch Dis Child. 1998;79:33–8.

McLorie GA, Perez MR, Csima A, Churchill BM. Determinants of hydronephrosis and renal injury in patients with myelomeningocele. J Urol. 1988;140:1289–92.

Lapides J, Diokno AC, Silber SJ, Lowe BS. Clean, intermittent self-catheterization in the treatment of urinary tract disease. J Urol. 1972;107:458–61.

Bauer SB. Neurogenic bladder: etiology and assessment. Pediatr Nephrol. 2008;23(4):541–51.

Daly SB, Urquhart JE, Hilton E, McKenzie EA, Kammerer RA, Lewis M, et al. Mutations in HPSE2 cause urofacial syndrome. Am J Hum Genet. 2010;86(6):963–9.

Weber S, Thiele H, Mir S, Toliat MR, Sozeri B, et al. Muscarinic acetylcholine receptor M3 mutation causes urinary bladder disease and a prune-belly-like syndrome. Am J Hum Genet. 2011;89(5):668–74.

Dretler SP. The pathogenesis of urinary tract calculi occurring after ileal conduit diversion. I. Clinical study. II. Conduit study. 3. Prevention. J Urol. 1973;109:204–9.

McDougal WS. Metabolic complications of urinary intestinal diversion. J Urol. 1992;147:1199–208.

Silverman SH, Woodhouse CR, Strachan JR, et al. Long-term management of patients who have had urinary diversions into colon. Br J Urol. 1986;58:634–9.

Woodhouse CR, Robertson WG. Urolithiasis in enterocystoplasties. World J Urol. 2004;22:215–21.

38 Acquired Urinary Tract Obstruction

Gillian Smith and Mark Harber

Acute and chronic urinary tract obstruction (UTO) are important causes of AKI and CKD globally, and the vast majority of such patients are managed by non-renal physicians and urologists. However, there is an important role for nephrologists in the management of AKI or CKD associated with acquired UTO, and an integrated multidisciplinary pathway for complex or sick patients is worth establishing.

Definition

There is limited data on the incidence of acquired UTO, and part of the reason for this comes from the difficulty in accurately defining cases. Absolute acute lower urinary tract obstruction is clear-cut but occurs very frequently as a merely transient phenomenon in the hospital setting; conversely many patients have some chronic post-micturition residue, the clinical relevance of which is not clear in an asymptomatic patient with normal renal function. For the upper tract, diagnosis normally relies on imaging (evidence of hydronephrosis) and a deterioration in renal function, but of course the renal reserve means it is possible to lose up to ~50 % of renal function before it becomes apparent biochemically, and Table 38.1 illustrates examples of false positives and negatives of imaging.

However UTO often predisposes to renal impairment in the absence of obstructive uropathy via urosepsis or is superimposed on other renal diseases particularly in the elderly. In practical terms the definition of obstructive nephropathy is when UTO is the primary or contributing cause of renal damage.

G. Smith, MD, FRCS(Urol)
Department of Urology,
Royal Free London NHS Foundation Trust,
Pond Street, London NW3 2QG, UK
e-mail: gilliansmith9@nhs.net

M. Harber, MBBS, PhD, FRCP (✉)
UCL Department of Nephrology,
Royal Free London NHS Foundation Trust,
Pond Street, Hampstead, London NW3 2QG, UK

Epidemiology

Acquired UTO increases with age as the predominant causes renal stones, gynaecological and urological malignancies and non-malignant causes of outflow tract increase. Globally, conditions such as schistosomiasis and tuberculosis also contribute significantly (usually from middle age onwards). Benign prostatic hyperplasia (BPH) is a common cause of bladder outflow obstruction (BOO) in ageing men; autopsy studies have demonstrated almost universal benign prostatic hyperplasia (90 %) beyond 80 years although only a proportion of these have symptoms, and it is not clear how it may have clinically relevant obstruction. As mentioned above, accurate figures for acute or chronic UTO are difficult to come by, yet it is clear that with an ageing population, UTO is responsible for a considerable and increasing healthcare burden. Moreover from the nephrologists' point of view, acquired UTO is an important treatable cause of AKI, CKD and acute or chronic CKD.

Causes

The causes of acquired UTO are multiple and can be divided up in a variety of ways, but in practical terms the most important element in terms of management is where the level of the obstruction is, i.e. upper or lower urinary tract. Table 38.2 illustrates the main causes of AUTO and divides upper and lower into intrinsic and extrinsic causes. Many of the likely causes may be suggested by the history, but when this is not obvious particularly in the setting of lower AUTO, neurological and perineal examinations are important and often neglected. It is important to note that apparent bilateral upper UTO can occur secondary to lower UTO pathology when there is (a) reflux to the native ureters or (b) when the bladder wall becomes grossly hypertrophied and occludes the distal ureters. In these circumstance patients can present with upper UTO that does not improve on catheterisation of the bladder.

M. Harber (ed.), *Practical Nephrology*,
DOI 10.1007/978-1-4471-5547-8_38, © Springer-Verlag London 2014

Table 38.1 Causes of dilated but non-obstructed and causes of obstructed but non-dilated upper tract

Common causes of dilated but non-obstructed kidney	
Pregnancy	Physiological dilatation (but potential for superimposed obstruction from gravid uterus)
Extra-renal pelvis	Very common cause of apparent dilatation but absence of dilated calyces key
Vesicoureteric reflux	Associated with (sometimes grossly) dilated ureters
Renal transplant or ileal loop	Typically mildly dilated in the setting of unrestricted reflux (may lessen post-voiding)
Megacalyces/calyx	Congenital abnormalities mimicking obstruction
Postsurgical	Post-repair of PUJ obstruction
Following removal of obstruction	Temporary persistence of dilatation after natural passage of stone or clot
Causes of obstructed but non-dilated kidney	
Malignant encasement	Most commonly in the setting of transitional cell carcinoma but can occur with any local tumour
Obstruction with AKI	Overt dilatation may not be apparent in the setting of oliguric renal failure
Micro-obstruction	AKI in the setting of crystal nephropathy, e.g. antivirals such as acyclovir (kidney may be 'bright')
Functional obstruction	High-pressure bladder, detrusor instability

Pathophysiology of Urinary Tract Obstruction

Acute obstruction has a largely functional impact on tubular function and glomerular filtration initially but if persistent interstitial inflammation with tubular apoptosis and interstitial fibrosis with nephron loss and tubular dilatation follow. Following acute UTO there is a drop in hydraulic pressure across the glomerulus and reduced filtration fraction, and renal blood flow drops significantly within a few hours with further and abrupt reduction in GFR. Urinary acidification deficits and urinary concentration deficits are common, usually only manifest when obstruction is relieved, but explain why it is possible to be polyuric in the face of partial obstruction.

These haemodynamic and tubular changes are initially fully reversible, but with ongoing obstruction, macrophage and other leucocytes infiltrate the kidney and progressive interstitial fibrosis ensues. Tubular dilatation may be seen incidentally on renal biopsy and hint at a degree of obstruction or reflux as an underlying cause. Ultimately the renal pelvis dilates further, and the surrounding renal tissue diminishes resulting in a rind of end-stage kidney around a grossly dilated pelvis. Relief of obstruction may result in hyperfiltration of remaining nephrons with glomerular enlargement and sclerosis (secondary FSGS).

Clinical Features of Urinary Tract Obstruction

The symptoms and signs of AUTO depend, to some extent, on the underlying cause, duration and completeness. The symptoms of acute lower tract obstruction are usually manifest by intensive suprapubic discomfort with the patient being clear of the diagnosis, but it may present merely as acute confusion or agitation (a simple diagnosis to make and treat). Chronic lower tract obstruction is often much more insidious with lower urinary tract symptoms of nocturia, frequency, poor stream and incontinence; lower urinary tract symptoms of prostatic hypertrophy correlate poorly with obstruction [1]; the bladder may expand to a very large capacity and may be apparent as lower abdominal swelling but equally may have a grossly hypertrophied wall without large capacity (25 % of men with lower UTO do not have a raised post-micturition volume).

Acute upper UTO may manifest as loin pain or renal colic if the cause is intraluminal such as stone or clot but is often clinically silent especially if the other kidney is healthy and unaffected. While complete bilateral upper or lower UTO results in anuria, partial obstruction can result in polyuria (see above). So while urine output is rarely a critical symptom, it does become one in a patient with a single functioning kidney especially if the other kidney was lost due to obstruction from, for example, stones.

Clinical features may also arise from the underlying pathology, e.g. back pain from retroperitoneal fibrosis, fevers with tuberculosis and malaise, anorexia and weight loss with malignancy. Chronic UTO may also present with the symptoms of advanced CKD mimicking malignancy. Urosepsis is a common presentation of an obstructed or partially obstructed system, and partial obstruction must be ruled out in a patient with recurrent urosepsis.

Examination may reveal a bladder depending on the patient's habitus; occasionally an obstructed kidney can be palpated, but examination is not a sensitive tool for diagnosing obstruction. However, in the presence of otherwise unexplained lower UTO, it is critical to ensure adequate examination of the perineum (excluding causes such as phimosis, infundibulation, prostatic enlargement,

Table 38.2 Causes of acquired obstruction

Upper tract, intrinsic	
Nephrolithiasis	Stones and occasionally crystals related to drugs (can be bilateral especially if chronic and sequential)
Blood clot	Any cause of upper tract bleeding (including biopsy)
Sloughed papilla	Any cause of papillary necrosis most commonly diabetes, sickle cell disease, analgesic nephropathy, pyelonephritis
Tumour	Benign or malignant (usually transitional cell carcinoma (TCC)) in ureter or bladder
Infection	Tuberculosis, BK virus infection in the immunosuppressed, fungal ball, schistosomiasis causing fibrotic contracted bladder (often bilateral upper tract obstruction)
Inflammatory	Vasculitis, chronic interstitial cystitis, malakoplakia
Ischaemic ureter	Loss of lower pole artery (e.g. in transplantation or ischaemic insult to lower pole in native kidneys)
Obstructed stent	Blocked especially retained stents
Upper tract, extrinsic	
Pregnancy	Physiological dilatation and obstruction from gravid uterus
Retroperitoneal	Retroperitoneal fibrosis usually bilateral (see causes), retroperitoneal tumours (e.g. lymphoma, sarcoma), radiation fibrosis, extensive haematoma
Gynaecological	Cervical cancer, ovarian or uterine malignancy, large benign gynaecological masses, endometriosis, significant prolapse
Extensive prostatic carcinoma	Spread to and involvement of ureteric orifices
Extensive peritoneal malignancy or inflammation	Crohn's disease, abscess formation, pancreatic inflammation
Vessels	Retrocaval ureter (right side)
Ligation	Inadvertent or occasionally use of native ureter in ESRD for transplanted kidney
Lower tract, intrinsic	
Intraluminal urethral mass	Stone, clot, tumour (TCC), inflammatory, infections, e.g. tuberculosis, acute non-specific urethritis
Urethral stricture	Post-instrumentation, post-radiation, post-trauma phimosis and paraphimosis, chronic non-specific urethritis (gonococcal, chlamydial), following female genital mutilation
Bladder mass	Large stone(s) or bladder haematoma
Bladder wall involvement	Bladder cancer (TCC), schistosomiasis, tuberculosis, chronic interstitial cystitis
Bladder function	Pain, immobility, confusional state, drugs (anticholinergics including some anti-dementia medication), antidepressants, cessation or non-compliance with alpha blockers
	Congenital neurological involvement, e.g. spina bifida, dysplastic bladder, acquired neurological autonomic neuropathy, e.g. diabetes, peripheral neuropathy, e.g. surgical (traumatic, tumour), or medical cord lesion, e.g. multiple sclerosis, central, e.g. cerebrovascular disease
Lower tract, extrinsic	
Prostatic enlargement	Benign prostatic hypertrophy, prostatic malignancy
Perineal malignancy	Gynaecological and pelvic malignancy
Faecal impaction	

pelvic malignancy) as well as a thorough neurological examination.

Diagnostic Tests

Bladder Ultrasound and Uroflow Studies

Portable ultrasound is sensitive, cheap and non-invasive for detecting a bladder and volumes pre- and post-micturition residual (PMR) are easy to measure. A persistent PMR is important to identify in recurrent urosepsis and may mean obstruction or detrusor failure. However, much of the data on the sensitivity and specificity of PMR and flow studies come from men with suspected bladder outflow obstruction (BOO). As mentioned above in one study, up to a quarter of men with BOO did not have a PMR, and 50 % of men with a PMR did not have obstruction [2].

Flow studies are also non-invasive, simple and a good screening test for outflow tract obstruction. Most men with BOO have reduced flow rates, and very low flow rates are a sensitive test for BOO (90 % of men with a maximum achieved flow rate (Q_{max}) of ≤10 ml/s have bladder outflow tract obstruction, but above this figure a significant proportion of men with reduced flow rates do not have BOO [2]).

While they have their limitations PMR and flow studies are simple tests easy to instil in renal clinics (avoiding the need for a second hospital visit) and may have particular merit in following patients for dynamic changes.

Table 38.3 Indications for urodynamic studies in adults

Indication	Notes
Clarification of diagnosis before invasive treatment	Urodynamic diagnosis of bladder outflow obstruction is associated with better outcomes from TURP
Incontinent patients	Failed first-line therapy Mixed storage and voiding symptoms suggesting detrusor dysfunction or bladder outflow obstruction associated with detrusor overactivity
Neurological disorders	Mismatch between symptoms and clinical assessment Neurogenic bladder dysfunction – diagnosis of poor compliance and high storage pressures with attendant risk of renal damage
Lower urinary tract symptoms/ suspected bladder outflow obstruction	Failed medical therapy Mixed symptoms, especially if marked storage symptoms Associated neurological disease Young men

Urodynamics

Urodynamics (a combination of cystometrogram and voiding pressure/flow study) is currently the definitive test for establishing the diagnosis of bladder outflow obstruction and can also be used to define other types of lower urinary tract dysfunction, for example, detrusor overactivity. Urodynamics can be combined with x-ray screening if radiological contrast medium is used to fill the bladder (videourodynamics). This technique can be useful in demonstrating anatomical aspects of storage such as capacity, reflux and diverticula. The detrusor pressure during the voiding phase helps distinguish between bladder outflow obstruction (high detrusor pressure and low flow) and detrusor dysfunction (low detrusor pressure and low flow). Detrusor overactivity manifests as spikes of high detrusor pressure during filling. For men there are nomograms to help distinguish between BOO and detrusor dysfunction [1]. The diagnosis of a poorly compliant high-pressure bladder is critical as it is likely to result in loss of renal function, and thus urodynamics can add vital information.

Cystometrography and pressure/flow studies are invasive and should only be used when the diagnosis is in doubt or where the result of the test will influence the patient's management or provide useful prognostic information. Urodynamic studies are not usually required to diagnose or institute treatment for bladder outflow obstruction in patients presenting with AKI secondary to high-pressure chronic urinary retention with upper tract dilatation. There may be a role in some patients presenting with very large residual volumes who are suspected of having atonic detrusor muscles. In these patients, urodynamic studies are sometimes useful in predicting whether outflow tract surgery (e.g. TURP) is likely to be successful in restoring voiding. General indications for urodynamic studies are listed in Table 38.3.

Bladder imaging may demonstrate a thickened trabeculated bladder wall (≥5 mm) and diverticula (Fig. 38.1)

Upper Tract Imaging

With the caveats shown in Table 38.1, radiological and nuclear medicine are required to make or exclude a diagnosis of upper tract obstruction. The diagnosis may be obvious but becomes increasingly difficult in patients with poor renal function or abnormal anatomy consistent with long-standing pelvic dilatation or encasement.

Ultrasonography

Ultrasound is sensitive for upper tract dilatation in most patients, and imaging has significant advantages in terms of availability, cost, lack of contrast or ionising radiation and ease of repeated measurements (for instance, in pregnancy). AKI guidelines generally recommend upper tract ultrasound within 24 h of unexplained AKI and within 6 h in a septic patient if pyonephrosis is suspected. A variety of enhanced US techniques may assist in the diagnosis or differentiation of obstruction [3]. Harmonic imaging (higher-frequency ultrasound) is more sensitive for identifying stones, and 3-dimensional ultrasound can generate multiplane cross-sectional imaging with enhanced definition, better characterisation and measurement of apparently dilated upper tract systems.

Computer-Assisted Tomography

A plain CT kidney, ureter, and bladder (KUB) is also sensitive at picking up pelvic obstruction, excluding extra-renal pelvis, and the modality of choice for renal stones. CT urogram has excellent spatial resolution including ureters and can demonstrate potential causes such as retroperitoneal fibrosis or malignancy (see Fig. 38.2). Late images (>2 min) may differentiate functional obstruction from dilatation.

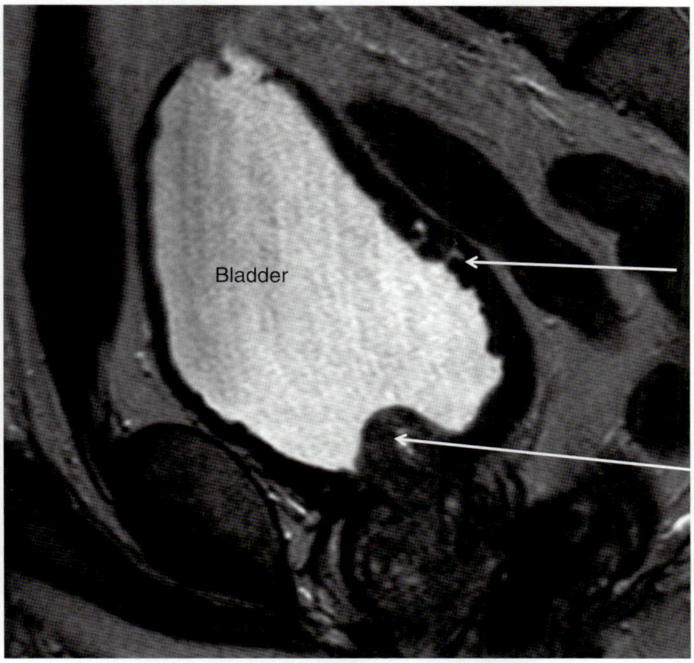

Fig. 38.1 MRI of patient with chronic lower urinary tract symptoms showing enlarged prostate and thickened bladder wall

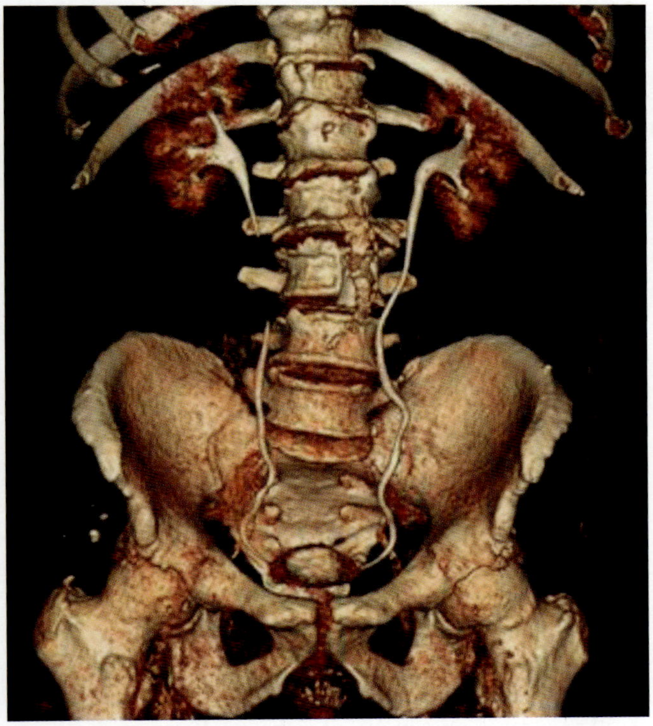

Fig. 38.2 CT urogram of an unobstructed patient showing non-dilated systems and free flow of contrast to bladder

However, there is a significant radiation dose, ionic contrast is not welcome in patients with significant dysfunction and excretion urography becomes increasingly ineffective with falling GFR.

Magnetic Resonance Imaging

MR urography is increasingly finding a place in determining the cause and functional extent of obstruction. It has excellent contrast resolution with the precontrast T2-weighted images (Fig. 38.3a, b), but also post-contrast dynamic studies are possible in combination with loop diuretics and include the potential for divided GFR as well as the detection of functional obstruction similar (but probably superior) to MAG-3 diuretic renography [4, 5].

Nuclear Medicine Renography

Dynamic renography lacks the anatomical merits of cross-sectional imaging but brings divided function and a non-contrast functional assessment to the table. The sensitivity of the renogram in obstruction is enhanced by iv loop diuretic 20 min before the injection of tracer (this is undermined by the patient routinely taking large doses of diuretics beforehand, so this is best stopped on the day). The renogram may show progressive accumulation of tracer in the obstructed kidney (see Fig. 38.4). Diuretic renography can be invaluable to exclude or identify obstruction in patients with chronically 'baggy' systems or those with encased and non-dilated upper tracts. It is also particularly useful in sequential monitoring of patients following stent removal; however, as with CT and MR urograms, sensitivity falls off sharply with poor renal function.

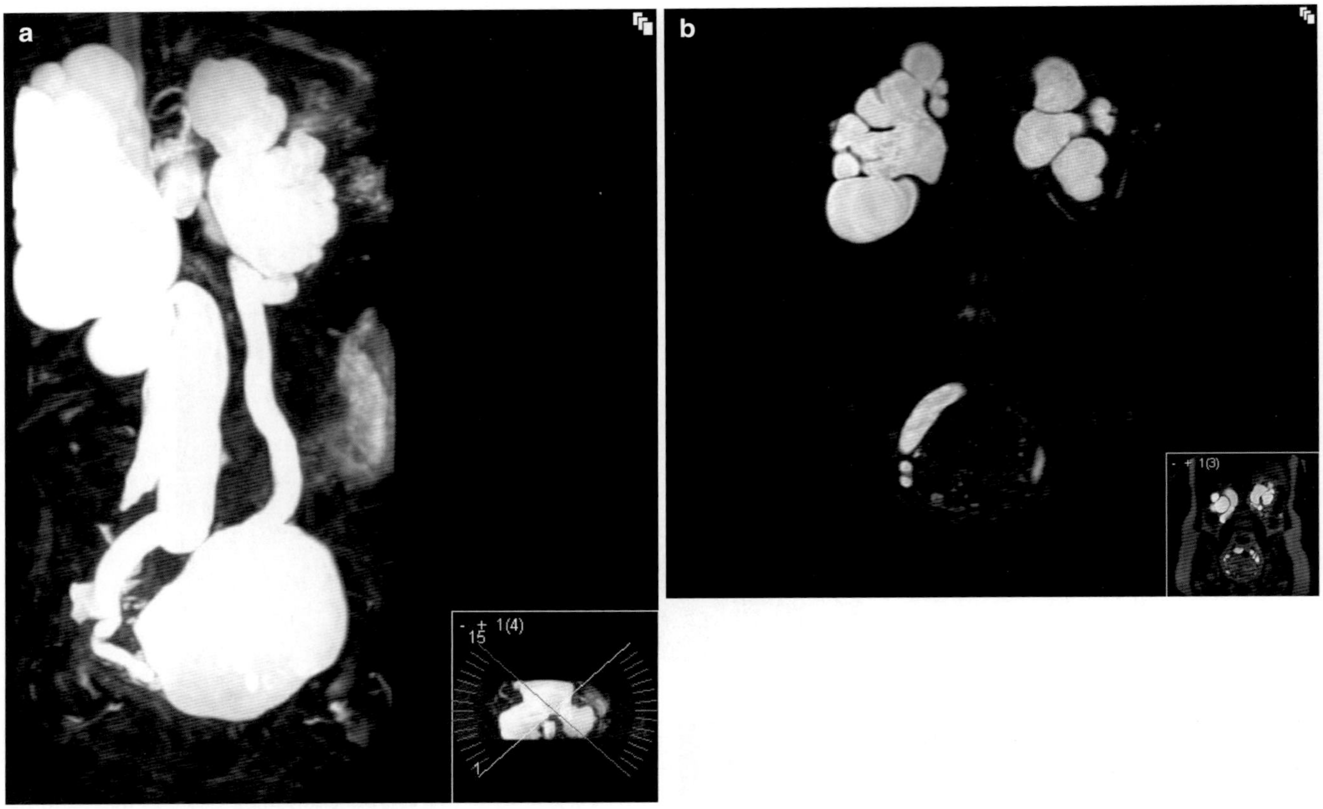

Fig. 38.3 (**a**) MR urogram in patient with bilateral congenital dilatation and obstruction. (**b**) MR urogram in a woman with bilateral vesicoureteric obstruction of unknown cause and chronic gross dilatation of both ureters and pelvicalyceal systems

Whitaker Test

This test involves antegrade pressure measurements requiring a nephrostomy with pelvic and bladder pressure measurements as fluid is instilled at 10 ml/min into the renal pelvis. A pressure differential between the pelvis and the bladder of >20 cm of water correlates with ureteropelvic or ureterovesical obstruction and can be combined with an antegrade study. The test was never intended as first line but may have merit in patients with suspected upper tract obstruction who have (a) severe renal impairment (when renogram is unlikely to be helpful), (b) an equivocal diuretic renogram and (c) intermittent obstruction particularly in the setting of chronically dilated upper tract. The test is rarely used now but may yet have a role when MRU is not available or tolerated [6, 7].

Trial of Nephrostomy or Stenting

A more pragmatic approach where there is significant doubt about drainage is to perform a nephrostomy (with antegrade study) or stent (antegrade or retrograde (with retrograde study)) and monitor renal function for days (with the former) or weeks (with the latter) (Fig. 38.5). This is not an infrequent approach to rule out obstruction and is an effective treatment if there is obstruction but is invasive and not without complications (see below) and can be falsely negative if there is acute tubular injury.

Treatment

Lower UTO

For lower urinary tract obstruction, decompression of an acutely obstructed bladder is urgent not only to relieve pain but also to prevent permanent damage to the bladder (equally important to identify and deal with treatable causes such as pain, anticholinergic medication, etc. (see Table 38.2) to avoid recurrence on removal of catheter). If catheterisation is difficult, the less experienced staff must be encouraged to escalate to the more experienced staff as it is easy to generate lifelong damage to the urethra. Ultrasound-guided suprapubic catheterisation is the alternative if urethral catheterisation is not possible.

The treatment of long-term BOO needs careful thought, and an accurate diagnosis is vital. For BPH there are a variety of options, but for severe disease then transurethral resection of the prostate, holmium laser enucleation or occasionally

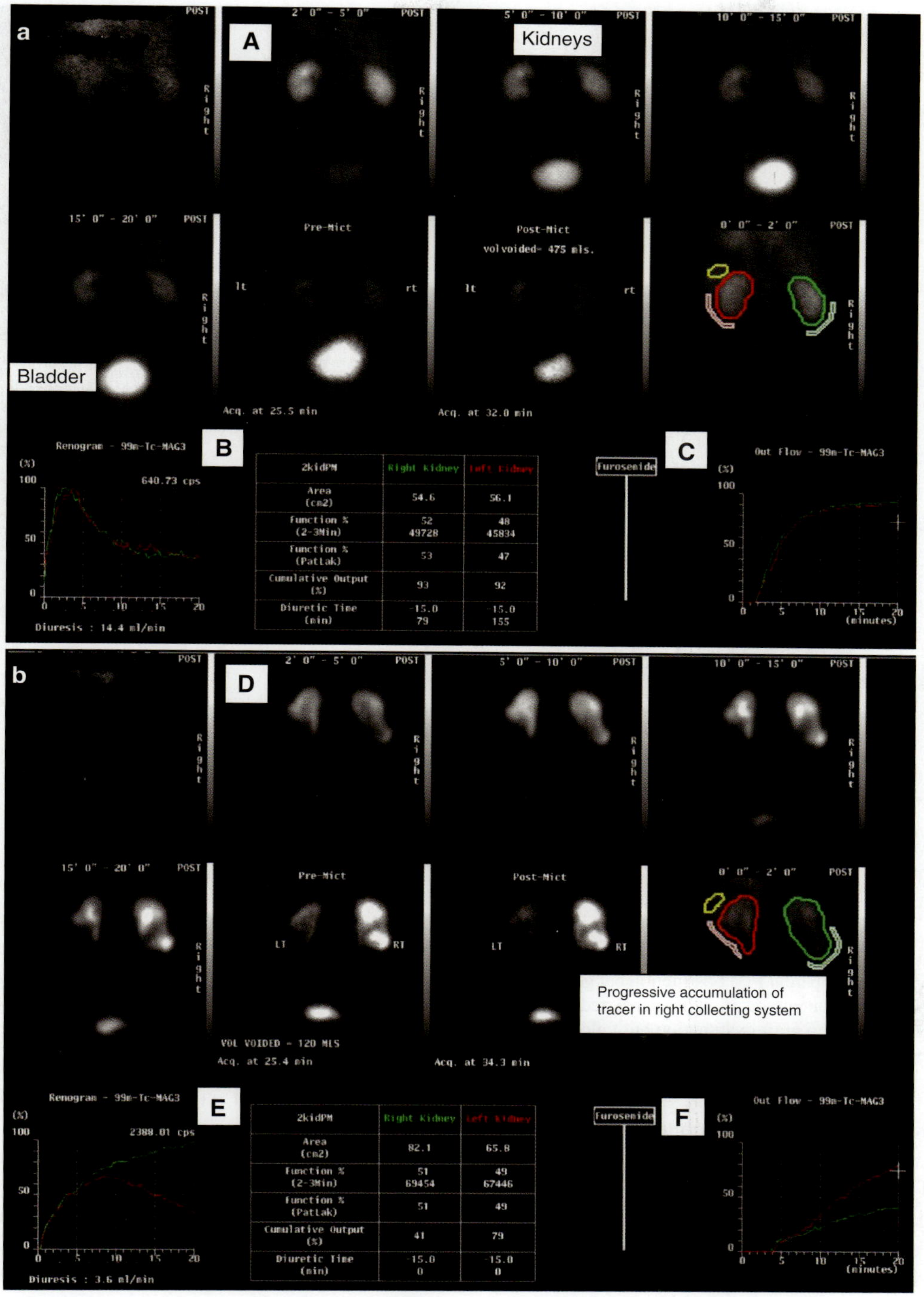

Fig. 38.4 (**a**) MAG-3 diuretic renogram in a non-obstructed individual (*A*) showing equal accumulation of tracer and equal loss of tracer from kidneys shown in renogram (*B*) with parallel outflow to bladder (*C*). (**b**) MAG-3 diuretic renogram in a patient with unilateral pelviureteric junction obstruction. (*D*) shows equal timing of nephrograms, but the right kidney continues to accumulate tracer (*E*) (nephrograms and green line on renogram) compared to the left kidney (*red line*) which excretes tracer into the bladder (*F*)

open prostatectomy are definitive treatments but are not without complications including sepsis, bleeding, sexual dysfunction and recurrence. A variety of minimally invasive surgical techniques are available but tend to have a lower success rate. Medical therapies can be very effective but require indefinite treatment. α-Blockers are usually first line (having maximal effect in 2–3 days and significantly improving the success of trial without catheter), but up to 33 % of patients do not improve, and postural hypotension is a well-recognised cause of discontinuation. Silodosin is more specific for the $\alpha 1_A$ receptor subtype predominating in the bladder neck/prostate and may be better tolerated in patients

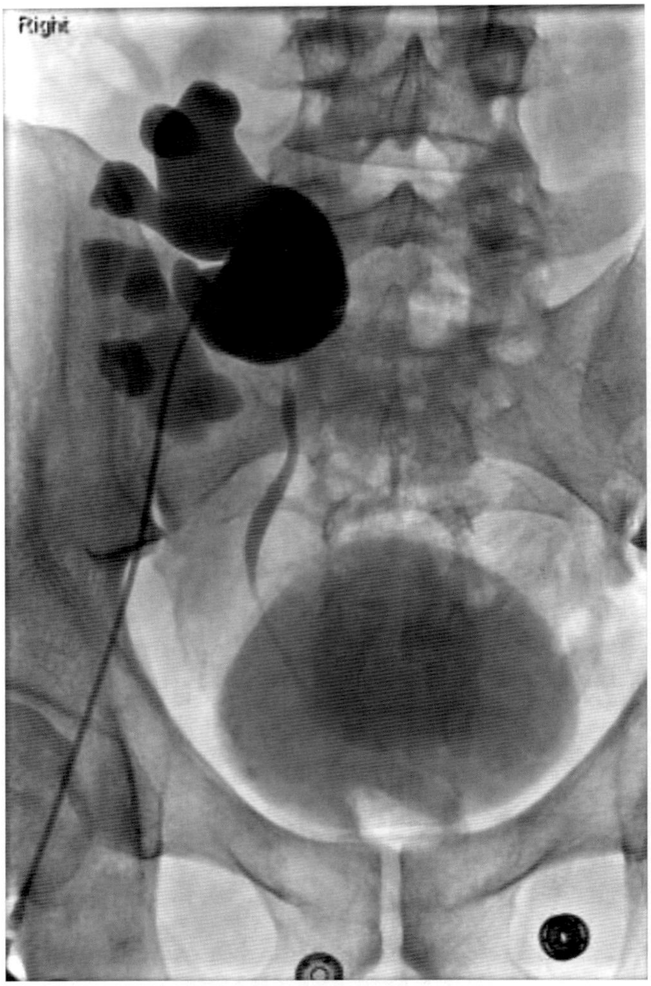

Fig. 38.5 A renal transplant with grossly dilated system but negative diuretic renogram showing apparent PUJ obstruction but good flow into the ureter and bladder. An antegrade stent was inserted to assess if obstruction was contributing to graft dysfunction but failed to improve renal function over the following month

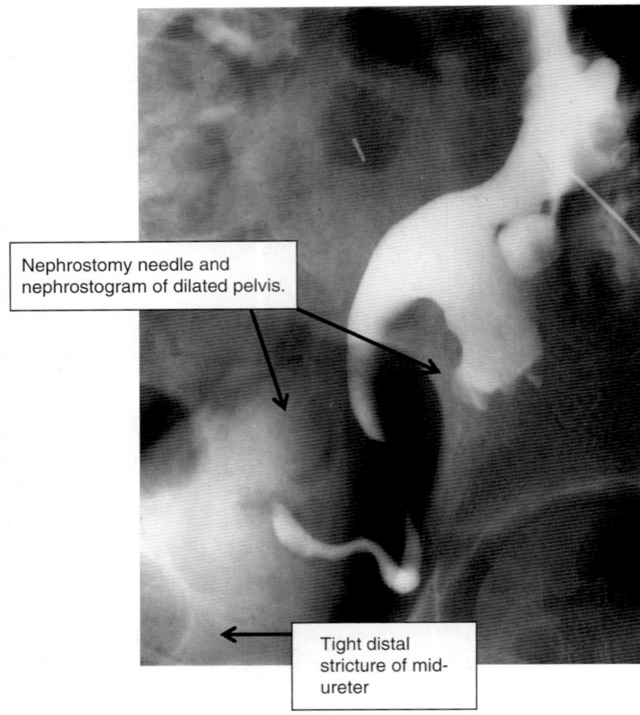

Fig. 38.6 Obstructed transplant kidney with nephrostomy and nephrostogram showing a tight stricture in the midsection of the ureter in this case secondary to mycobacterium infection with BKV and ischaemic strictures that are important differentials

with hypotension. 5-α reductase inhibitors reduce prostate size by 20–30 % (but may be 3 months before clinical benefit is evident) and can be used as monotherapy or in combination with alpha blockers but are associated with sexual dysfunction in around one in eight patients. There is significant data showing an additive benefit of combined therapy with an alpha blocker and 5 alpha reductase inhibitor. A variety of other medical and surgical approaches are in the offing but not yet proven [8]. For those without BPH the treatment depends on the diagnosis or exclusion of other causes such as urethral stricture, malignancy, detrusor dysfunction or other neurological pathologies. Ultimately the bladder needs to be effectively drained and maintained at low pressure, and options include a trial of α-blockers, intermittent self-catheterisation, indwelling urethral or suprapubic catheter or urinary diversion such as an ileal loop or urostomy.

Upper UTO

Pyonephrosis (emphysematous or otherwise) is a medical emergency and when suspected requires urgent imaging and decompression. Similarly in patients with AKI and metabolic mayhem such as hyperkalaemia, acidosis or pulmonary oedema, decompression is urgent (the alternative being dialysis followed by decompression) and the definitive treatment. In noninfected patients the time it takes for humans with complete obstruction to go from reversible to irreversible kidney dysfunction is not clear. However it seems likely given the reduction in blood flow and early infiltration of macrophages that subtle progression starts within days. Thus prolonged delay in decompressing a healthy obstructed kidney does not seem prudent for someone likely to need their kidney in the future, and as the speciality involved in managing CKD, we should encourage timely decompression. The procedure of nephrostomy is very nicely described by Uppot [9]. Figure 38.6 shows a nephrostomy and nephrostogram showing a tight stenosis of mid-ureter. In essence, nephrostomy is not risk-free with a mortality of 0.05–0.03 % and transfusion requirement in 1–3 %. Generally the sicker the patient (and the less experienced the operator), the greater the risk, so optimising the patient, operator and timing is important. Acute tubular injury, nephrostomy displacement, blockage and misplacement are common reasons for failure to drain. Flushing the nephrostomy can usually rule out blockage, and a displaced catheter is often depressingly obvious, but repeat imaging is important to ensure that the nephrostomy catheter has not perforated the urinary tract.

If possible an antegrade study is done at the time of the nephrostomy, but often clot or ureteric oedema precludes a descent study, and often a better study is achieved a day or two later. Balloon dilatation of a stricture is not universally successful [10]; strictures of less than 3 months' duration have a higher patency rate (88 %) than those >3 months (67 %) with those over a year having poor rates (15 %). Stricture length also appears to be important, greater than 2 cm having a poor long-term patency rate, and malignant strictures do predictably worse than benign ones. Ballooning is usually accompanied by stenting and the removal of stent 6–12 weeks later. Retrogrades studies can be done at the time to assess patency and the need for further stents or surgery. If clear flow and stents are removed, then given the recurrence rate patients need a mechanism for monitoring with either bloods or repeat USS or renogram; if the patient has another normal kidney, then reliance on creatinine and eGFR is probably not sufficient.

Post-obstructive Diuresis

Post-obstructive diuresis (POD) is a genuine phenomenon in part related to acquired urinary concentrating defects (including early downregulation of aquaporin channels), high levels of urea acting as an osmotic diuretic as well as appropriate excretion of accumulated salt and water and can result in a massive diuresis. Without support this can result in a collapse in intravascular volume and further AKI. Conversely stage-managed reduction in fluids is necessary to avoid perpetuating the polyuria for days. These patients are often managed by relatively junior non-renal medical staff; clear and constructive renal advice can help prevent avoidable complications and probably shorten length of stay. The first priority is to ensure adequate intravascular volume and regular reassessment followed by clear instructions for monitoring, including hourly urine output, pulse, blood pressure, accurate fluid balance and daily weights. In practical terms if the patient is euvolaemic, then ml for ml fluid replacement of urine output on an hourly basis is probably the safest approach in the short term, the choice of replacement being governed by the electrolytes although the more physiological the solution, the easier to manage. In the setting of a massive diuresis, the teams looking after the patient need to know that frequent testing of electrolytes (sodium, potassium, magnesium, calcium and bicarbonate) is critical to avoid wild excursions of electrolytes or osmolality. In particular the fractional excretion of potassium can be disproportionate because of high-sodium delivery to the distal tubule. While this is often helpful in a patient with obstruction and life-threatening hyperkalaemia, patients with significant POD can become profoundly hypokalaemic quite quickly. Large volumes can ultimately perpetuate the diuresis in part by continued washout of the countercurrent multiplier, and if the diuresis is persisting and the patient is intravascularly replete, then a gentle and carefully monitored negative fluid balance (e.g. 50 or 100 ml/h negative) needs to be introduced.

Post-obstructive Haemorrhage

Post-obstructive haematuria can occur following sudden decompression of a chronically obstructed bladder. Although macroscopic this is usually self-limiting and managed either conservatively or with irrigation. Very rarely haemorrhage can be extensive and can involve the upper tract in patients with secondary upper tract dilatation (Fig. 38.7).

Serious post-decompression bleeding is very rare, and there is no evidence that clamping the catheter periodically during decompression has any protective effect and the catheter should be left on free drainage.

Aortitis, Periaortitis and Retroperitoneal Fibrosis (RPF)

Retroperitoneal inflammation of any cause has the potential to involve the ureters and result in upper tract obstruction. A collection of diseases is increasingly recognised to cause this problem, and wider availability of ^{18}f-flurodeoxyglucose (FDP) PET scanning and identification of IgG-4-related disease are advancing the diagnosis and management of this heterogenous group. The common causes/associations of retroperitoneal fibrosis are shown in Table 38.4. It has become apparent that there is considerable overlap in some of the conditions and that a significant proportion of 'idiopathic' retroperitoneal fibrosis (70 %) and a smaller but significant proportion of aortitis and periaortitis are associated with IgG-4-related disease.

Classically RPF secondary to atherosclerotic aortitis presents in the middle-aged smoker (strong male preponderance) with extensive macrovascular disease (asbestos exposure is also a risk factor as is HLA-DRB1*03) [11] in the setting of an abdominal aortic aneurysm. However, RPF also occurs in the absence of aneurysm but in the setting of periaortitis involving vasculitis of the vasa vasorum with obliterative endarteritis or phlebitis. This is often associated with fibro-inflammatory reaction in the retroperitoneum with tissue encasing retroperitoneal structures including the ureters and left renal vein. Clinically this may present with back or

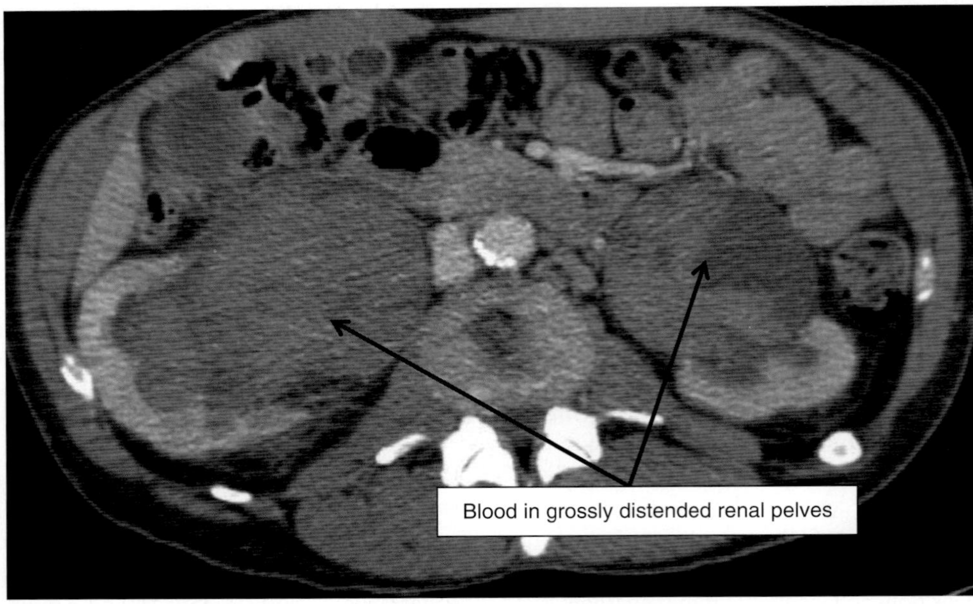

Fig. 38.7 Extensive upper tract blood clot and obstruction following urinary catheter decompression of a chronically obstructed bladder secondary to benign prostatic enlargement

Table 38.4 Causes of retroperitoneal fibrosis

Idiopathic retroperitoneal fibrosis	IgG-4-related disease associated with raised inflammatory markers, membranous glomerulonephritis, IgG-4 interstitial nephritis, others, e.g. pancreatic, biliary, ENT and orbital involvement
Secondary to aortitis	Atherosclerotic aneurysm (especially if leaking)
Periaortitis	May be IgG-4-related disease
Retroperitoneal infection	Tuberculosis
Medication	Methysergide, bromocriptine
Radiation to retroperitoneum	
Malignancy	8 % including sarcoma and lymphoma
Trauma	With haematoma

abdominal pain, fatigue, anorexia, weight loss, ureteric colic, varicocele or hydrocele with an inflammatory response (raised ESR and CRP), deep vein thrombosis and renal impairment if ureteric drainage is compromised. Renal artery involvement may occur in up to a third of cases with fibro-inflammatory tissue reaching the hilum.

'Idiopathic RPF', i.e. those with no other obvious precipitant, has an incidence of approximately 1:100,000, and 70 % of these cases are associated with IgG-4-RD. In addition, 50 % of IgG-4-related RPF cases have extraperitoneal involvement (pancreas, biliary tree, periorbital, thyroid, pericardium, skin, salivary glands, breast and meninges). The pathology of IgG-4-related RPF differs from that of other causes in that there is dense inflammatory infiltrate with a high proportion of plasma cells (35–76 % vs 0–10 % in atheroma-related RPF [12]), a significant proportion of which stain for IgG-4. Although serum levels of IgG-4 are usually hardly raised, a ratio of IgG-4 to total IgG >0.3 is indicative.

Medial deviation of the middle third of the ureters is a classic finding but has poor sensitivity, and although US is excellent for diagnosing obstruction, it is not sensitive for examining the retroperitoneum and determining the underlying cause or extra-renal involvement. Therefore cross-sectional scanning with contrast CT is probably the most helpful initial form of imaging. For those patients with evidence of periaortitis or idiopathic RPF in whom immunosuppression is planned, then ^{18}F-FDP-PET CT is both sensitive and extremely useful for monitoring response to treatment whether it be renal or extra-renal (see Fig. 38.8).

The majority of patients with RPF seen by nephrologists have developed ureteric obstruction that is usually bilateral (70 %), but renal artery and vein encasement as well as referral for management of large vessel vasculitis are also part of the case mix. The principles of management are similar and involve decompression of the kidneys (almost exclusively via nephrostomies and antegrade stenting) and correction of any critical vascular pathology. Excluding any secondary cause, such as infection or malignancy, is critical, and biopsy of the RPF tissue mass is highly desirable where and when possible (including staining for plasma cells and IgG-4). FDP-PET scanning and acute phase markers suggestive of active inflammation then a trial of immunosuppression are usually adopted. There is no consensus on this, but for 'idiopathic' or IgG-4-related RPF, medium-dose

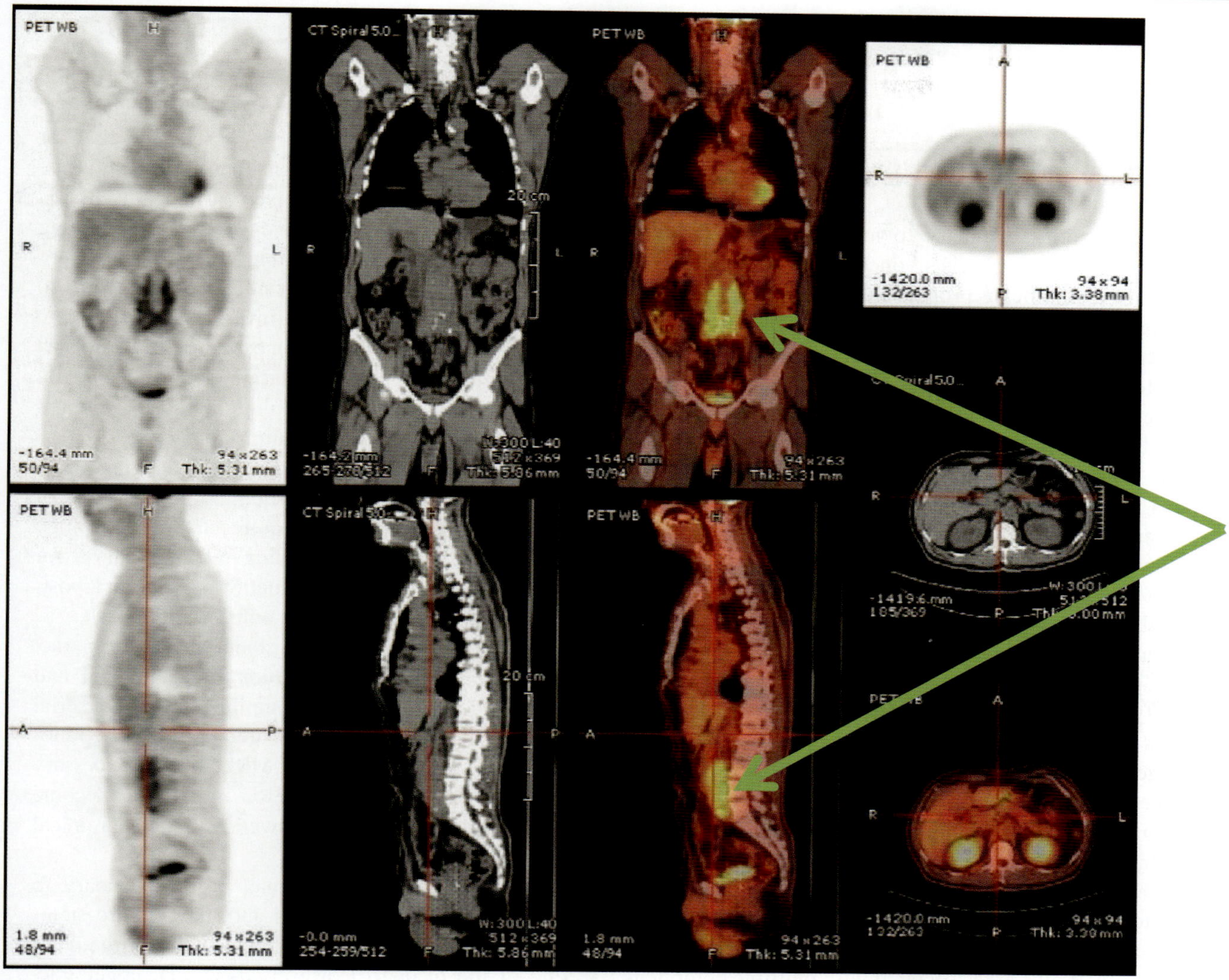

Fig. 38.8 PET CT scan in a patient with idiopathic retroperitoneal fibrosis showing an intense inflammatory process (showing *yellow*) in the prelumbar region

steroids with an antiproliferative such as azathioprine or mycophenolate mofetil are commonly adopted; symptoms, ESR/CRP and PET scan response are all useful markers of disease activity. For RPF associated with vasculitic aortitis steroids, methotrexate, azathioprine, mycophenolic acid and cyclophosphamide are all used. More recently anti-TNF monoclonal antibodies (infliximab and adalimumab) have been used with success in inflammatory aortitides such as Takayasu's aortitis [13].

The absence of an acute phase response or activity on FDP-PET scanning suggests a lack of inflammatory involvement, and immunosuppression is less likely to be helpful. Patients can be managed with retrograde stent changing, but this is not without complications, and blockade of one stent may be asymptomatic and go unnoticed resulting in permanent loss of renal function. Retrograde studies at the time of stent change may demonstrate free flow, but part of the pathology lies in the loss of ureteric peristalsis rather than occlusion or stenosis, so free flow may be falsely reassuring.

Treatment of retroperitoneal fibrosis causing ureteric obstruction is initially decompression usually with bilateral nephrostomies and antegrade stenting, establishing and treating the primary cause such as leaking aneurysm or lymphoma. In those patients with idiopathic periaortitis or retroperitoneal fibrosis in patients with FDG-PET-positive scans (whether IgG-RD disease) or an acute phase response, immunosuppression is usually with prednisolone and a steroid-sparing agent such as azathioprine [14].

If repeat imaging shows regression of the retroperitoneal mass and retrograde studies show free flow, stent removal may be justified, but a system of monitoring with US or diuretic renogram is critical. Where there is no evidence of FDG activity, acute phase response or a large burden of immunosuppression is required to maintain control, then ureterolysis with lateral or intraperitoneal transposition with omental wrap is usually definitive but can result in devascularisation of the ureter.

Malignancy

While obstruction secondary to malignancy is normally managed between urologists, oncologists and palliative care teams, a significant proportion of these patients cross the paths of nephrologists, and it is worth special mention. Ureteric obstruction secondary to malignant invasion is associated with a very poor prognosis, and survival is typically between 3 and 7 months necessitating a thoughtful and holistic approach that is not always achieved in practice. If appropriate and following a discussion of the options with the patient, their fitness and the stage of the malignancy, the first aim is to relieve the obstruction to the kidneys. Retrograde stenting is associated with a much higher (×3) rate of failure in the setting of external malignancy than with intrinsic obstruction such as stones, and this seems to be particularly bad with pelvic malignancies such as prostate, bladder and cervical malignancy (success rates of 15–21 %) compared to colorectal or breast [15]. For this reason an antegrade approach is often adopted for drainage with percutaneous nephrostomy in the first instance. Antegrade stenting is attempted either simultaneously or subsequently when the patient is more stable. The decision to decompress both kidneys depends on the stability of the patient, their prognosis, whether renal function needs to be maximised for chemotherapy and whether there is felt to be an associated sepsis. Both stenting and nephrostomy drains are associated with multiple complications and poor patient satisfaction. Long-term nephrostomy drains can become displaced (>10 %), infected (66 %) and blocked or result in excoriating urinary leaks, all of which result in high readmission and reintervention rates (Wong). Similarly ureteric stents can become misplaced, blocked or encrusted and cause irritation of the bladder (sometimes helped by oxybutynin patches) [15]. There may occasionally be a benefit of metal stents in these patients, but they are not a panacea [16]. For a small group of patients with a prognosis of several months or more, with severe symptoms or urinary leak, surgical drainage may be appropriate such as ureterostomy, ureteric reimplantation or conduit formation [17].

These are a complex group of patients facing a desperate time; an efficient, thoughtful and multidisciplinary approach is required to avoid them spending much of their remaining time in the hospital [18, 19].

Tips and Tricks

Urology MDT meetings are a good place to find patients with obstruction from stones, malignancy, retroperitoneal fibrosis or recurrent UTIs due to poor drainage. Many of these patients have or are at risk of developing CKD. Renal involvement in or discussion of the urology MDT list is an easy way of facilitating nephrological input and joined up care, if needed.

Adding post-micturition residual measurements to a formal US request is non-invasive and helpful in those with recurrent UTIs or unexplained renal impairment. Better still, it is easy to train staff to accurately measure bladder residuals in the clinic and ward setting using simple hand-held ultrasound devices.

Urologists are well practised at managing acute upper and lower tract obstruction, but a proportion of patients will have AKI that requires urgent nephrology input. Joint protocols including referral criteria for AKI in the context of obstruction, sepsis and post-obstructive diuresis are worth considering.

Where there is diagnostic doubt about upper tract obstruction, then a combination of anatomical and functional scans is often complimentary, and serial scanning (e.g. USS with measurements, isotope renogram with divided function or MRU) may be necessary to decide on intervention. MRU is likely to become increasingly valuable at answering both anatomical and functional questions.

Upper tract obstruction may occur secondary to a hypertrophied bladder wall and may require stenting until the decompressed bladder allows remodelling of the bladder. However, functional upper tract obstruction can also occur without obvious BOO in the setting of detrusor dysfunction and a high-pressure bladder; renal function may not improve with stenting unless this is identified by urodynamics and treated accordingly.

Patients with upper tract obstruction secondary to malignancy face bleak times, and it is easy for the medical professional to make this worse either by under-treating obstruction or by intervening when not appropriate. Early thoughtful discussion of the patient's wishes and needs is key and should include 'what if AKI intervenes?' for example, if blocked nephrostomies or stents occur. Monitoring of renal function can often be done by the district nurse or family practitioner without the need to drag the patient repeatedly to multiple clinics.

References

1. Nitti V. Pressure flow urodynamic studies: the gold standard for diagnosing bladder outlet obstruction. Rev Urol. 2005;7 Suppl 6:S14–21.
2. Abrams P. The diagnosis of bladder outlet obstruction: urodynamics. In: Cockett ATK, Khoury S, Aso Y, editors. Proceedings, the 3rd international consultation on BPH. Geneva: World Health Organization; 1995. p. 299–367.
3. Renjen P, Bellah R, Hellinger JC, Darge K. Advances in uroradiologic imaging in children. Radiol Clin North Am. 2012;50:207–18.
4. Perez-Brayfield MR. A prospective study comparing ultrasound, nuclear scintigraphy and dynamic contrast enhanced magnetic resonance imaging in the evaluation of hydronephrosis. J Urol. 2003;170:1330–4.
5. Grattan-Smith JD. MR urography anatomy and physiology. Pediatr Radiol. 2008;38 Suppl 2:S275–80.
6. Veenboer PW, de Jong TPVM. Antegrade pressure measurement as a diagnostic tool in modern pediatric urology. World J Urol. 2011;29:737–45.
7. Lupton EW, George NJ. The APR: 35 years on. BJU Int. 2010;105(1):94–100.
8. Parsons BA, Hashim H. Emerging treatment options for benign prostatic obstruction. Curr Urol Rep. 2011;12:247–54.
9. Uppot R. Emergent nephrostomy tube placement for acute urinary obstruction. Tech Vasc Interv Radiol. 2009;12:154–61.
10. Adamo R, Saad WEA, Brown DB. Percutaneous ureteral interventions. Tech Vasc Interv Radiol. 2009;12:205–15.
11. Uibu T, Oksa P, Auvinen A, Honkanen E, Metsarinne K, Saha H, et al. Asbestos exposure as a risk factor for retroperitoneal fibrosis. Lancet. 2004;363:1422–6.
12. Zen Y, Onodera M, Inoue D, Kitao A, Matsui O, Nohara T, et al. Retroperitoneal fibrosis: a clinicopathologic study with respect to immunoglobulin G4. Am J Surg Pathol. 2009;33:1833–9.
13. Wen D. Takayasu arteritis: diagnosis, treatment and prognosis. Int Rev Immunol. 2012;31:462–73.
14. Magrey MN, Husni ME, Kushner I, et al. Do acute-phase reactants predict response to glucocorticoid therapy in retroperitoneal fibrosis? Arthritis Rheum. 2009;61:674–9.
15. Wong LM, Cleeve LK, Milner AD, Pitman AG. Malignant ureteral obstruction: outcomes after intervention. Have things changed?. J Urol. 2007;178(1):178–83.
16. Sountoulides P, Kaplan A, Kaufmann OG, Sofikitis N. Current status for use of metal stents in the management of malignant ureteric obstruction. BJU Int. 2010;105:1066–72.
17. Woodhouse C. Supra-vesical urinary diversion and ureteric reimplantation for malignant disease. Clin Oncol. 2011;22:727–32.
18. Kouba E, Wallen EM, Pruthi RS. Management of urethral obstruction due to advanced malignancy: optimizing therapeutic and palliative outcomes. J Urol. 2008;180:444–50.
19. Liberman D, McCormack M. Renal and urologic problems: management of ureteric obstruction. Curr Opin Support Palliat Care. 2012;6:316–21.

infrequent. Sarcomatoid changes can affect most forms of RCC and, rather than a discrete entity, is indicative of an aggressive often locally infiltrative phenotype with poor prognosis.

A number of RCC that would fall within the unclassified group have been pathologically defined subsequent to the WHO classification [3]. These include those seen in patients with end-stage renal disease with tumours arising in kidneys affected by acquired cystic disease which is associated with dialysis. These tumours may exhibit combined features of clear and papillary tumours but without the typical chromosomal abnormalities affecting either clear (3p) or papillary (7p or 1q) RCC.

Staging

This is an important consideration that can dictate both treatment options and determine prognosis [4]. TNM staging is the most widely used system based on size and local extent of the primary tumour as well as the involvement of regional lymph nodes and distant metastases (Fig. 39.1). Based on the TNM 4 broad groups or stages are often considered in clinical practice.

Categorization of renal cancer based on size and invasion of primary tumour, lymph node involvement and metastates.

Primary tumour (T):

TX: Primary tumour cannot be assessed
T0: No evidence of primary tumour
T1: Tumour <7 cm in greatest dimension, limited to kidney
T1a: Tumour ≤4 cm, limited to the kidney
T1b: Tumour >4 cm but <7 cm, limited to the kidney
T2: Tumour greater than 7 cm, limited to kidney
T2a: Tumour 7–10 cm, limited to the kidney
T2b: Tumour >10 cm, limited to the kidney
T3: Tumour extends into major veins/adrenal/perinephric tissue; not beyond Gerota's fascia
T3a: Tumours with direct adrenal involvement/perinephric fat; not beyond Gerota's fascia
T3b: Tumour extends into renal vein(s) or IVC below the diaphragm
T3c: IVC involvement above diaphragm
T4: Tumour invades beyond Gerota's fascia
N: Regional lymph nodes
NX: Regional nodes cannot be assessed
N0: No regional lymph node metastasis
N1: Metastasis in a single regional lymph node
N2: Metastasis in more than one regional lymph node
M: Distant metastasis
MX: Distant metastasis cannot be assessed
M0: No distant metastasis
M1: Distant metastasis

Stages of renal cancer based on TNM categorization

Stage	TNM
I	T1, N0, M0
II	T2, N0, M0
III	T1/2, N1+, M0
	T3, N0+, M0
IV	T4, N0+, M0
	T1+, N0+, M1

Epidemiology

Kidney cancer results in approximately 2 % of all cancer deaths and is the tenth leading cause of cancer related mortality. Reported worldwide incidence rates range from 0.6 per 100,000 to 14.7 per 100,000 [5]. In western nations the incidence is approximately 10 per 100,000, with a mortality rate of 3.5 per 100,000. Most tumours present in the fifth to seventh decades of life, with a median age at diagnosis of 66 years and median age at death of 70 years. The incidence is two to three times higher in men and is slightly more common in blacks than in whites.

Over the past few decades, the incidence of renal tumours that are detected has increased although this now appears to be stabilising. It is likely that the increase purely reflects the increased availability and use of abdominal imaging for unrelated symptoms or conditions. Most RCC are detected as incidental findings, with a dramatic 'stage shift' in the modern era related to increased numbers of small T1 tumours now comprising the majority of cases. Interestingly the number of patients per head of population presenting with advanced or metastatic disease has remained essentially unchanged.

At autopsy, the incidence of renal tumours is approximately 2 %. In general, the tumours are usually solitary but may be multifocal in 6–25 % of patients. Several hereditary syndromes are associated with an increased incidence of RCC, including von Hippel-Lindau disease, hereditary papillary renal cancer and possibly tuberous sclerosis. Lesser associations have been described with cigarette smoking, obesity, diuretic use, exposure to petroleum products, chlorinated solvents, cadmium, lead, asbestos, ionising radiation, high-protein diets, hypertension and HIV infection [5]. Renal failure however has a much higher association which may be related to a number of factors. Firstly all stages of renal failure may occur with kidney cancer as a consequence of treatment. Patients requiring long-term dialysis who develop acquired renal cystic disease are at increased risk with rates three- to six-fold that of the general population [6]. Duration of haemodialysis appears a specific risk possibly due to chronic repeated exposure to high hepatocyte growth factor (HGF) levels associated with renal failure and

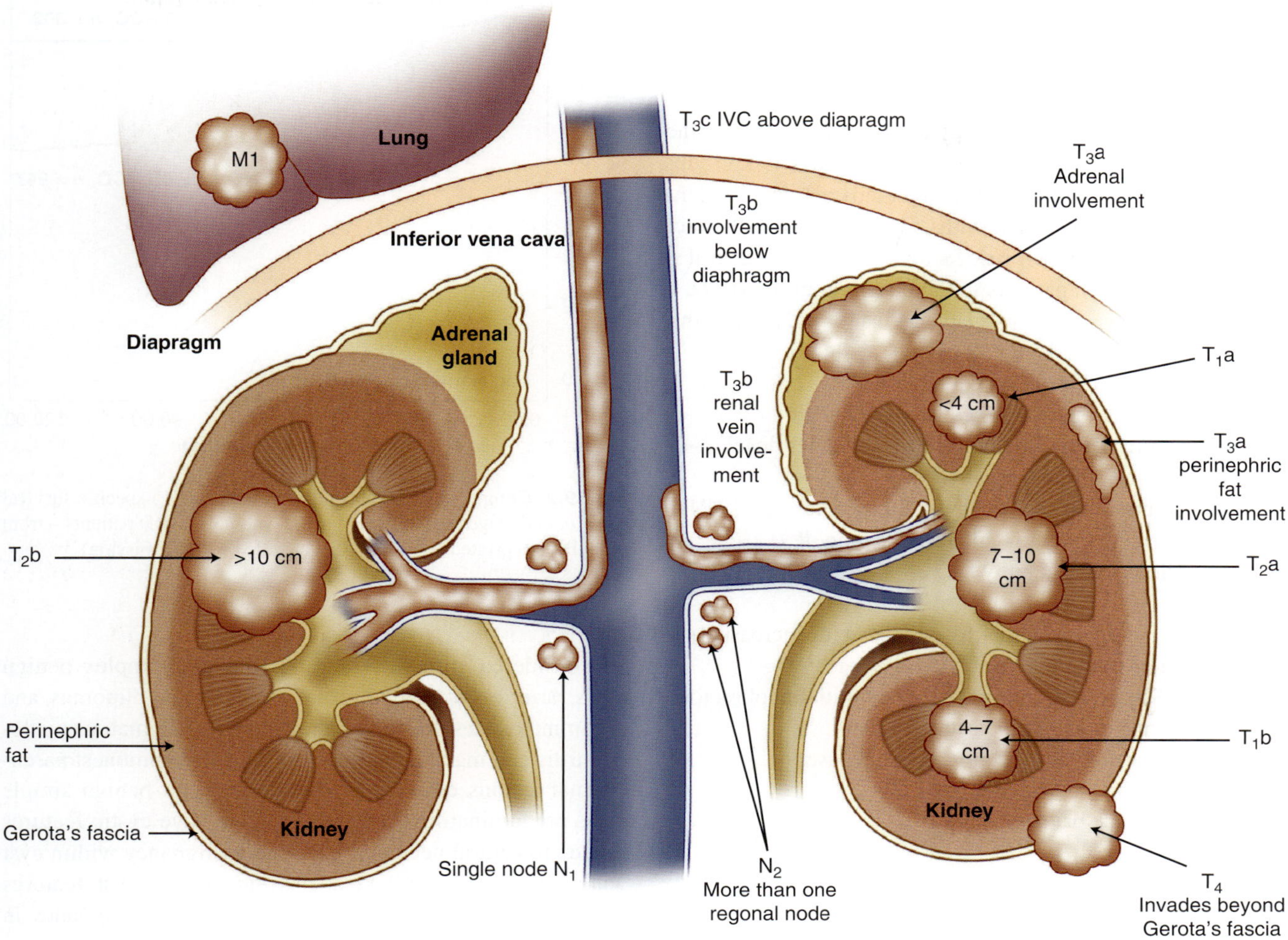

Fig. 39.1 TNM staging of renal cell cancer

elevated with heparin used with haemodialysis. HGF is the ligand for cMET – a proto-oncogene associated with papillary RCC and is found in high concentrations in cysts associated with acquired cystic disease of the kidney also seen in dialysis [7].

Prognosis

Five-Year Survival Rates for Renal Cell Carcinoma

Overall, 5-year relative survival has improved over time – rising from 51 to 67 % between 1975–1977 and 1996–2004. This change relates principally to the higher numbers of patients diagnosed with T1 tumours – many of which may not be clinically significant. Prognosis is closely linked to disease stage. For all stages co-morbidities and performance status are also independent factors that influence survival. Survival in clinical trials is invariably better than usually seen in clinical practice due to their exclusion of patients with poor performance status.

The 5-year disease-specific survival rate in patients with T1 renal carcinoma is 95 % and in those with stage T2 disease, 88 %. Patients with T3 renal carcinoma have a 5-year survival rate of 59 %, and those with T4 disease had a 5-year disease-specific survival rate of 20 %.

Nodal and distant metastases have a marked effect on prognosis. Patients with regional lymph node involvement or extracapsular extension have a survival rate of 12–25 %. Although renal vein involvement does not have a markedly negative effect on prognosis, the 5-year survival rate for patients with stage IIIB renal cell carcinoma is only 18 %. In patients with effective surgical removal of the renal vein or inferior vena caval thrombus, the 5-year survival rate is 25–50 %.

With stage IV disease, 5-year survival rates for patients with stage IV disease are low (0–20 %).

Survival Prognostic Factors: Metastatic Disease

In patients with metastatic disease, five prognostic factors have been identified for predicting survival [8]. These factors can be used to categorise patients into three risk groups. Patients in the favourable-risk group (zero risk factors) have a median survival of 20 months, and patients with intermediate risk (one or two risk factors) a median survival of 10 months, whereas patients in the poor-risk group (three or more risk factors) have a median survival of only 4 months.

Poor prognostic factors are as follows:

- Low Karnofsky performance status (<80 %)
- High serum lactate dehydrogenase (LDH) level (>1.5 times upper limit of normal ULN])
- Low haemoglobin (below lower limit of normal [LLN])
- High 'corrected' serum calcium (>10 mg/dL)
- No previous nephrectomy

The following are factors associated with increased survival in patients with metastatic disease:

- A long disease-free interval between initial nephrectomy and the appearance of metastases
- The presence of only pulmonary metastases
- Good performance status
- Removal of the primary tumour

RCC with ESRF

An association has been demonstrated between end-stage renal failure (ESRF) and RCC. RCC arising in patients with ESRF seems to exhibit many favourable clinical, pathological and outcome features compared with those diagnosed in patients from the general population [6]. Consequently the RCC-specific survival for ESRF patients is substantially better than for other patients, independent of histological subtype, as shown in Fig. 39.2. The data from this multi-institutional review whilst retrospective suggests that in most patients with ESRF, RCC, if treated, does not adversely affect their prognosis and consequently should not be viewed as a barrier to consideration of transplantation.

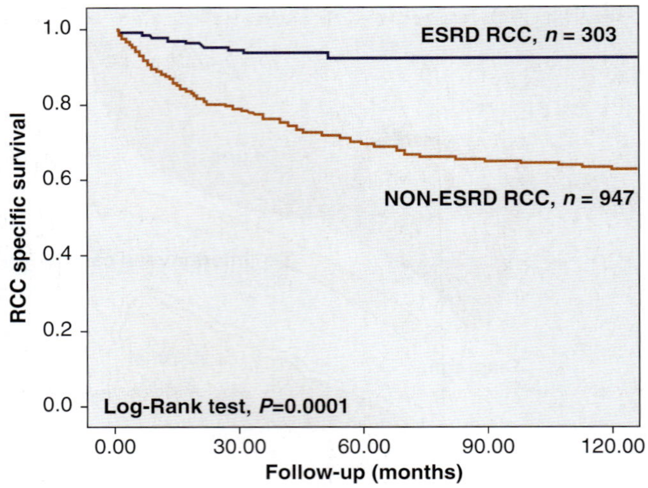

Fig. 39.2 Comparison of renal cell carcinoma (*RCC*)-specific survival time for end-stage renal disease (*ESRD*) and non-ESRD patients – from Niuzillet (Reprinted from Neuzillet et al. [6] with permission)

Diagnosis and Imaging

Diagnosis is generally based on one of several imaging modalities which may be used in combination for clarification of equivocal findings as well as staging. Typical findings are solid or complex lesions (containing solid and cystic components) demonstrating enhancement with intravascular injection of contrast agents. Other lesions which must be considered with such findings include complex benign cysts, arteriovenous malformations, angiomyolipomas and inflammatory lesions including xanthogranulomatous pyelonephritis and malakoplakia. Cysts are the commonest parenchymal lesions detected in the kidney with benign simple cysts predominating. Tumours can also have cystic features related to central necrosis as well as malignancy within cyst walls. Bosniak described a classification of cyst features that is essentially a risk stratification tool for malignancy in evaluating renal cysts [9].

Ultrasound

Renal tumours typically appear as complex parenchymal lesions. These demonstrate solid features with variable amounts of fluid, or anechoic components reflecting cystic carcinomas, necrosis or haemorrhage. Angiomyolipomas may be differentiated from RCC on ultrasound based on their uniform hyperechoic appearance with the lack of the posterior shadowing seen with calculi (Fig. 39.3). Use of Doppler is now a routine component of US imaging of renal lesions demonstrating internal blood flow. Constrast enhanced ultrasound using microbubbles is a further recent addition offering huge potential as it is able to detect microvessels (with diameters as small as 40 μm) and quantitatively assess tumour perfusion of solid tumours [10]. This remarkable resolution relates to microbubbles remaining intravascular as they are resistant to extravascular diffusion. This technique may significantly reduce the need for ionising radiation and assist in differentiating benign from malignant tumours and cysts.

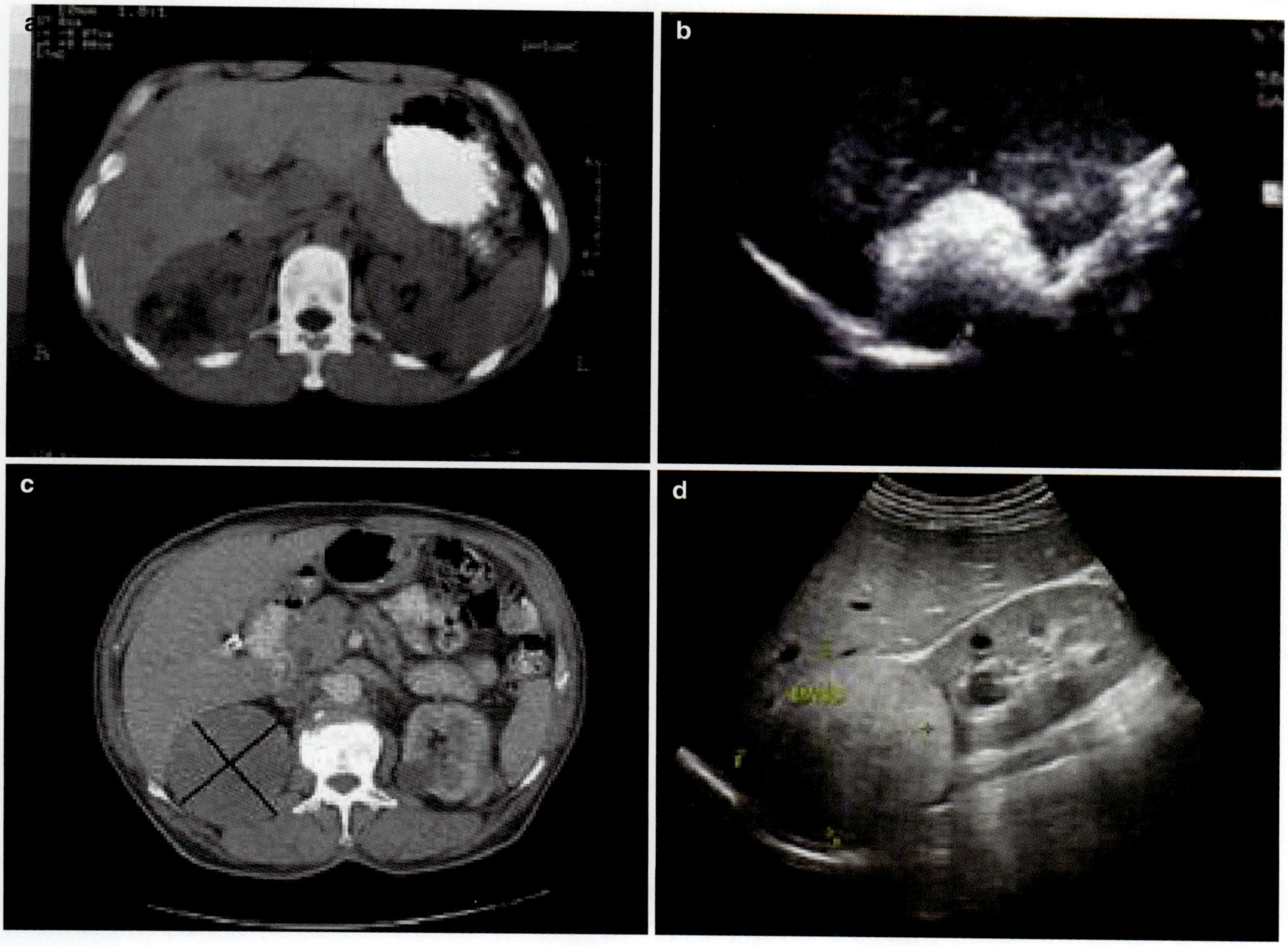

Fig. 39.3 Ultrasound and CT images of an angiomyolipoma showing typical fat density (**a**) and diffuse hyperechoic appearance (**b**) compared to RCC (**c**, **d**)

Computerised Tomography (CT)

On CT (with pre- and post-contrast and delayed scans) renal tumours appear as solid or mixed lesions which demonstrate variable enhancement with injection of iodine-based contrast media [11]. Hyperdense cysts, which reflect haemorrhage into a benign cyst may appear solid on a non-contrast CT but do not enhance with contrast. Angiomyolipomas may also appear as solid, enhancing lesions but have a substantial or significant component reflecting the features of adipose tissue (Fig. 39.2). Other benign lesions including granulomatous pyelonephritis can be more difficult to distinguish on this and also other modalities.

Magnetic Resonance Imaging (MRI)

In the assessment of renal lesions, magnetic resonance imaging (MRI) is complementary to CT imaging [11]. It has a role where intravenous contrast is problematic including contrast allergy and renal failure. It is also useful for staging purposes particularly in assessing tumour thrombus and the level of its proximal extension in the vena cava. MRI provides high inherent contrast between different forms of soft tissue. It has better contrast resolution but less spatial resolution than CT and hence not as useful for staging of the primary lesion or procedural planning of nephron-sparing interventions.

Whole-body MRI also has greater sensitivity than other modalities such as PET and bone scan in detection of bone metastases. It is also more sensitive than CT for cerebral secondary's but not as useful lung lesions.

Positron Emission Tomography (PET)

Imaging with 2-deoxy-2-[18 F]-fluoro-D-glucose (FDG) and whole-body positron emission tomography scanning has been used in assessing renal tumours but lacks sensitivity compared to other imaging modalities [10]. Newer radiotracers such as iodine-124-labelled antibody chimeric G250 (124I-cG250) which reacts with carbonic anhydrase-IX ('immuno-PET') may improve sensitivity. Whilst sensitivity may be low, its specificity is high, and a positive scan should be regarded as strongly suspicious for metastatic disease. It may be useful in the assessment of possible local recurrence which can be difficult with other modalities due to migration of other organs into the renal bed, scarring and artefacts due to surgical clips. It also provides a mechanism to examine the whole body without risk of renal functional damage or contrast allergy.

Bone Scan

This may be used to diagnose or exclude bone metastasis. These typically produce lytic lesions on plain X-ray or CT. This reflects the osteolytic activity of RCC metastases with little coexisting osteoblastic response. On nuclear imaging studies, which reflect bone turnover and specifically osteoblastic activity, metastatic lesions may not be highlighted [12]. Hence a negative scan may not exclude the possibility of bone metastasis.

Biopsy

Use of biopsy varies in clinical practice. It has a clear role in metastatic disease in patients in whom treatment is planned without or prior to nephrectomy to establish a diagnosis and histological subtype. In this context biopsy of a metastatic lesion is preferred to the primary to exclude coexisting disease such as lung carcinoma. It has also been advocated in the assessment of equivocal lesions [13]. HMB-45 (a melanocytic cell-specific monoclonal antibody) immunoreactivity is associated with AMLs but not present in any malignant parenchymal tumours. Thus it is a very specific marker to resolve radiologically indeterminate lesions where AML is suspected which occasionally occurs with tumours exhibiting diffuse hyperechoic features in US but without fat clearly being demonstrated on CT. With smaller indeterminate lesions its use is more controversial due to the negative predictive value – often as a consequence of difficulty ensuring a representative or adequate sample has been obtained.

Treatment

Localised Disease

Surgical excision has been well established as the only potentially curative modality for RCC. The changing spectrum of disease presentation, particularly with respect to small incidentally detected tumours, has resulted in the increasing utilisation of nephron-sparing surgery including minimally invasive techniques as nonsurgical ablative therapies.

Radical Nephrectomy

Radical nephrectomy (RN) that encompassed removal of the tumour-bearing kidney as well as the surrounding perinephric fat including the adrenal gland has been until recently the standard treatment option for most patients with localised tumours [14]. A number of studies have now shown that removal of the adrenal gland does not confer any survival advantage – although is usually recommended with larger upper pole tumours [14, 15]. Lymphadenectomy has also been variously advocated – although confounded by the diverse pattern of lymphatic drainage of the kidney. Published data suggests that for most renal tumours with clinically negative regional nodes, lymphadenectomy does not improve survival. In those with clinically enlarged nodes and no evidence of distant metastatic disease, however, resection of disease confirmed pathologically may confer a survival advantage [15]. Whilst some centres advocate its use, its primary utility appears as a staging tool which may be of current significance with the evolution of systemic therapies and the definition of their role in the adjuvant setting.

Tumours with renal vein and vena caval extension can also be amenable to surgical excision [16]. In the absence of metastatic disease, removal of the tumour in conjunction with the tumour thrombus may be curative. This can be undertaken in a multidisciplinary setting combining standard urological techniques with those employed in liver transplantation for removal of tumours below the diaphragm or with minimal extension above this level. With the availability of venovenous bypass, these tumours can be removed without the need for thoracic techniques. Tumours extending into the atrium, however, require a combined approach with cardiac surgery including the use of hypothermic arrest. Pre-operative embolisation has been advocated as a preliminary to surgical intervention although recent publications fail to demonstrate any increase in survival or reduction in complications.

Laparoscopic techniques were introduced in 1991 for radical nephrectomy for RCC. Its role is now well established with oncological outcomes identical to standard open techniques [17]. Laparoscopy may be limited by tumour size, volume of perinephric fat, previous surgery and other contraindications to laparoscopy.

Partial Nephrectomy

Nephron-sparing surgery with partial nephrectomy (PN) has been increasingly utilised over the past two decades [17]. This evolved from the favourable oncological outcomes reported from a number of institutions where PN was performed in the context of a solitary kidney or a functionally compromised contralateral renal unit. A further factor has been the dramatic increase in the overall proportion of stage I cases coupled with the reduction in size of T1 tumours. The size of stage I tumours decreased from a mean of 4.1 cm in 1993 to 3.6 cm in 2004 [18].

There are compelling arguments for PN over RN for many small renal tumours reflected in a progressive increase in its utilisation. Based on eGFR estimations the risk of renal impairment is less with PN compared to RN. Studies examining this are based on epidemiological data or institutional series with patients treated in a non-randomised fashion [19]. Whilst a useful tool for screening patients for chronic renal impairment, eGFR may have limitations when applied to this clinical setting [20]. A recent publication has suggested that risk factors and proteinuria are more reliable predictors of renal dysfunction following surgery [19]. The stated concern with a lower eGFR associated with RN relates to the potential impact on cardiovascular mortality. Epidemiological studies vary – from showing a higher incidence of cardiovascular deaths in patients undergoing RN compared to PN [21] to those describing no increased risk with RN [22]. Other population-based studies with large numbers of patients have also reported no statistically significant increase in either cardiovascular mortality or long-term interventions for ESRF [23, 24].

To date only a single randomised controlled trial has been reported comparing outcomes for RN and PN. The study recruited 541 patients with T1 tumours <5 cm in diameter with median follow-up over 9 years [25]. Recurrent disease was higher in the PN group although overall oncological outcomes were similar. Complications were more frequent with PN – with transfusions in 30 % – twice that reported with RN. Most importantly overall survival including cardiovascular mortality was identical in both groups. This recent publication is likely to impact on future revisions of current guidelines regarding surgery for T1 renal lesions – which have been developed in the absence of level 1 evidence.

Ablative Therapies

Several forms of energy ablative therapies have been developed as alternative options for minimally invasive nephron-sparing treatment of small primary lesions [20]. These are delivered via probes placed into renal masses either percutaneously with image-guided techniques or under direct vision via laparoscopy or open surgery.

Radiofrequency Ablation

Tumour ablation with RFA is achieved by heat generation from radiofrequency waves resulting in coagulative necrosis. It is best suited for smaller exophytic tumours (<3 cm) and has been generally delivered percutaneously.

Cryotherapy

This treatment involves placement of several probes into the renal mass with tumour destruction by repeated freezing and thawing cycles. Most studies employing this have involved vision control either laparoscopically or with open surgery although percutaneous approaches under CT guidance have been reported. For selected tumours, short- to intermediate-term oncological outcomes are similar to partial nephrectomy with an upper treatment limit of 3–3.5 cm being recommended. Complications, which include bleeding, urinary leakage and tumour persistence/recurrence, occur more commonly with larger size as well as central tumours contacting the renal sinus.

Both RFA and cryotherapy are potentially suitable for small peripheral lesions. Studies have demonstrated successful eradication of tumours based on imaging studies although most studies have only short- to intermediate-term follow-up. Both modalities however do exhibit oncological failure in 10 % or more of cases based on follow-up or investigational series where ablation was performed prior to surgical excision [15, 20]. Complications which may require additional interventions include urine leakage, bleeding, abscess formation and ureteric necrosis have been reported [20]. In cases where tumour recurrence or persistence occurs following ablative therapy retreatment has been described. Where surgical intervention is undertaken for tumour persistence or recurrence, PN may not be an option. Series reporting this scenario describe RN rather than PN as the outcome [26]. Whilst occasional series report the potential for long-term efficacy with ablative therapies, these modalities are at the present time best restricted to selected small lesions in older patients with co-morbidities for whom treatment appears necessary where surgical intervention is associated with significant risk.

Surveillance

There is now a reasonable experience in which patients with small renal tumours (<3–4 cm) have been managed expectantly with repeat imaging with a number of patients subsequently undergoing surgery or other procedure as a delayed intervention. Studies reporting this experience suggest that in the short to intermediate term, this is not associated with significant risks. A meta-analysis of series reporting observation of small solid SRM's <4 cm in diameter described 255 cases with a median tumour size of 2.48 cm and follow-up with a minimum of 2 years follow-up (mean 34 months) [27]. Overall a growth rate of 0.28 cm/year (0.09–0.86) was observed. Pathological correlation, obtained when surgery was subsequently undertaken, was available in nearly half with 92 % having histological features of RCC. Within this subset with confirmed RCC a mean growth rate of 0.4 cm/year although lesion size at presentation was not predictive of the growth rate in this group or those that did not undergo surgery. Similarly the initial size and growth rates in benign lesions were similar to those in with histological features of RCC. Only three cases of metastatic disease were described after follow-up periods of 4, 9 and 11 years.

Thus with short to intermediate periods of follow-up surveillance with selective use of surgical intervention, the risk of metastases and cancer-specific mortality appear extremely low. Consequently this is now viewed as a reasonable option for older patients or those with significant co-morbidities.

Systemic Therapy

Chemotherapy

It has been well established that kidney cancer exhibits little or no response to cytotoxic chemotherapy. This appears related to the expression of the multidrug resistance (MDR) gene – seen in tumours reflecting their origin from tubular epithelial cells. MDR encodes proteins which actively expel chemotherapeutic drugs from the cell. Efforts to bypass this mechanism have proven unsuccessful and thus standard chemotherapy has no current role in the treatment of RCC [28].

Immunotherapy

Immunotherapies

The occasional dramatic regression reported with metastatic RCC stimulated the use of various immune therapy approaches to reproduce or accentuate this response on the basis that this was an immunological phenomenon. Cytokine therapy with interferon-α (IFN-α) and interleukin-2 (IL-2), either alone or in combination, has been the most commonly used strategy and the only to have been broadly adopted in clinical practice [29]. Various immunisation strategies have also been employed although restricted to experimental settings.

Cytokines

IL-2, a polypeptide lymphokine, is the principal stimulator of T-cell growth and may activate antitumour T cells and NK cells if present. IL-2 is produced by type 1 helper T lymphocytes causing activation and proliferation of the CD4 and CD8 lymphocyte population. Following encouraging in vitro and in vivo studies, clinical use started in patients with metastatic RCC in 1984 although it has not been evaluated against standard treatments in randomised trials. A review of clinical results in 1,714 patients with metastatic RCC treated with intravenous IL-2 monotherapy indicated an overall objective response rate of 15 %. IL-2 can give response rates of up to 20 % although only 5 % of them will eventually be complete and long lasting [29].

Overall, careful patient selection is paramount for treatment with IL-2, and the best candidates for this type of therapy are patients with excellent performance status, minimal or no co-morbidities and small volume pulmonary, lymph node or soft tissue disease.

IFN-α, a glycoprotein, is a potent immune effector agent with anti-proliferative and immune-modulatory effects which can increase the expression of cell surface antigens. Its mechanism of action in RCC is not understood, but includes potentially a combination of stimulation of cell-mediated cytotoxicity including upregulation of class 1 MHC antigens on tumour cells, a direct anti-proliferative activity and effect on tumour circulation. It is administered subcutaneously. Randomised trials have demonstrated an improvement in survival of 2–3 months with thrice-weekly subcutaneous injection [29]. Response rates are low at 10–15 % and unlike therapy with IL-2 complete and lasting remissions are not seen. Similarly to IL-2, careful selection of patients with small volume disease would provide the best outcomes.

Neither IFN-α nor IL-2 is now regarded as standard of care. Their role has largely been replaced by a number of drugs with more specific activity.

Stem Cell Transplantation

Based on the principle of graft-versus-host effect, allogeneic stem cell transplantation has been used in highly selected groups of patients with encouraging results. Non-myeloablative regimes have been employed, but due to the complexity of the treatment and the high treatment related toxicity, it remains an experimental approach performed in a limited number of centres.

Immunisation

Various immunotherapy strategies have been employed using largely tumour-derived cells or tissue lysates [30]. A range of techniques have been employed including inoculation as well as ex-vivo priming of various cell groups including dendritic cells and various T-cell subsets which are then re-administered to the patient. These have not proven effective due to lack of consistent antigenic targets being developed to allow widespread use. The use of patients own tumour products as targets is also not practical outside experimental settings. Consequently these have not progressed beyond early clinical trials.

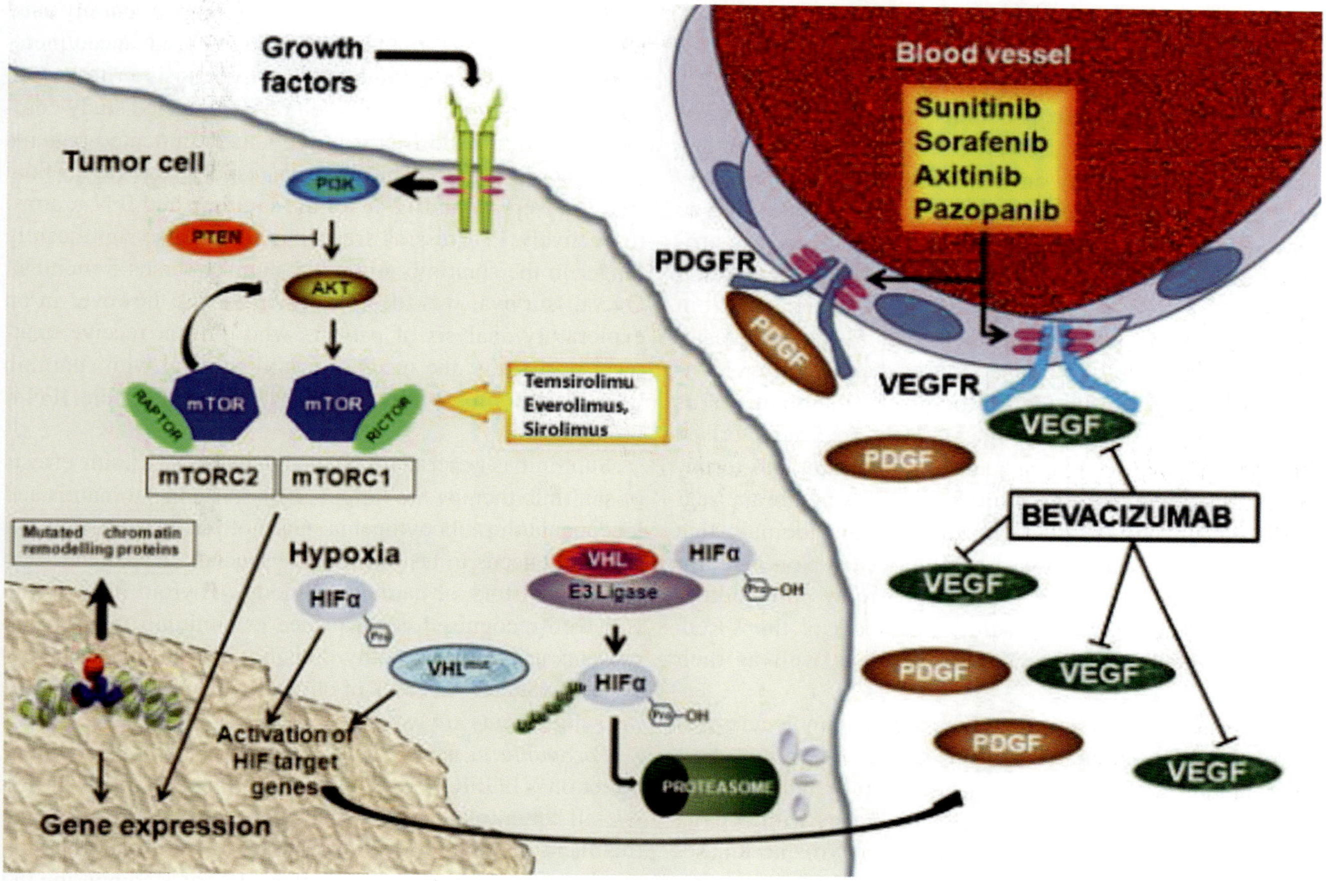

Fig. 39.4 Schematic overview of relevant pathways in clear cell RCC and targeted therapies. Under normal conditions, hypoxia inducible factor (HIF)-**α** is constitutively degraded. HIFs bind to von Hippel-Lindau (*VHL*) protein, which is part of an E3 ubiquitin ligase complex that targets the protein for proteolysis. When the VHL gene is mutated, interaction between HIF and the VHL protein is disrupted, leading to stabilisation/accumulation of HIF transcription factors. Under hypoxic conditions, the interaction between VHL and HIF is lost because specific proline residues in HIF are not hydroxylated, also leading to loss of interaction. HIF accumulation can also result from activation of mammalian target of rapamycin (*mTOR*) downstream of cellular stimuli and the PI3-K/Akt pathway. Accumulated HIF translocates into the nucleus leading to transcription of a large number of hypoxia inducible genes including vascular endothelial growth factor (*VEGF*) and platelet-derived growth factor (*PDGF*). These bind to their receptors present on the surface of endothelial cells, leading to (neo)vascularisation. The mTOR inhibitors (temsirolimus, everolimus and sirolimus) inhibit the kinase activity of the mTOR complex 1 (*mTORC1*); bevacizumab, a VEGF ligand-binding antibody, sunitinib, sorafenib, axitinib and pazopanib are small molecule inhibitors of multiple tyrosine kinase receptors including VEGF-R and PDGF-R (Reprinted with permission from Oosterwijk et al. [31])

Targeted Agents

The identification of genetic events associated with RCC and the effects on tumour cells and stromal elements, particularly angiogenesis, which are critical to progression has led to the development of a range of novel therapies specifically targeting tumour biology [31]. The various pathways associated with these new therapies are shown in Fig. 39.4.

Anti-VEGF Antibodies

Bevacizumab is a recombinant humanised monoclonal antibody which binds to VEGF-A isoforms preventing receptor activation [32]. All solid organ malignancies are dependent on neovascularisation for tumour growth and progression. This is a prominent feature of RCC and related to the dramatic upregulation of VEGF particularly in clear cell carcinoma associated with loss of pVHL, a protein which regulates VEGF production. Bevacizamides effect is thus principally on the vascular stroma, as an inhibitor of angiogenesis, with little direct effect on tumour cells. It is generally well tolerated with main toxicities being asymptomatic proteinuria (25 %) and hypertension (14 %) although thrombotic or haemorrhagic events are also noted. Bevacizumab has been used in combination with IFN-α based on a randomised phase III study that demonstrated statistically significant improvement in progression-free survival of patients with previously untreated metastatic RCC although no statistically superior overall survival [32].

Multi-targeted Receptor Kinase Inhibitors

Tyrosine Kinase Inhibitors (TKIs)

Tyrosine kinases are enzymes that catalyse the transfer of the γ-phosphate group from adenosine triphosphate to target proteins. They play an important role in diverse normal cellular regulatory processes. Tyrosine kinases can be classified as receptor protein kinases and non-receptor protein kinases. The receptor tyrosine kinases are membrane-spanning cell surface proteins that play critical roles in the transduction of extracellular signals to the cytoplasm. There are 58 receptor tyrosine kinases that have been identified, and they are divided into some 20 subfamilies as defined by receptor and/or ligand. They are characterised by immunoglobulin-like sequences in their amino-terminal extracellular domains, a lipophilic transmembrane segment and an intracellular carboxyl-terminal domain that includes the tyrosine kinase catalytic site. Non-receptor tyrosine kinases, on the other hand, relay intracellular signals. Tyrosine kinases include members of the VEGF family and other angiogenic cytokines as well as their receptors.

Tyrosine kinase inhibitors (TKIs) are small molecules that target the ATP binding site of the kinase preventing phosphorylation. As TKIs are small and generally hydrophobic, they are able to pass through cell membranes with activity and thus target receptor and non-receptor tyrosine kinases intracellular signalling pathways. There is now an increasing array of TKIs entering clinical practice – varying in the range and extent of the kinases they inhibit.

At the present time three drugs have entered clinical practice for RCC – sunitinib, sorafenib and pazopanib with others, including axitinib, currently in clinical trials [33]. The available drugs are all orally active. Due to the fact that their target profiles differ, tumour sensitivity can vary between individuals. Side effects can also vary according to their specific targets but the commonest appear to be fatigue, hypertension, oral and gut mucositis, dry skin, palmar-plantar erythrodysaesthesia [hand-foot syndrome] and altered taste [34].

Sorafenib is an oral multi-targeted TKI against VEGFR-1, 2, 3 and PDGF-R that acts on the tumour cells and tumour vasculature. Tumour cell proliferation is further inhibited by targeting the MAPK pathway at the level of Raf kinase. A multi-centre, randomised, phase III study involving 903 patients who had failed treatment with immunotherapy demonstrated improved progression-free survival with sorafenib compared to placebo. Overall survival however was not statistically significant probably due to crossover following the interim analysis. Diarrhoea, skin rash and hand-foot syndrome were the commonest side effects [32].

Sunitinib malate is another multi-targeted TKI which inhibits c-KIT, FLT-3, PDGFR-b and VEGFR-2, FGFR-1 and IGFR-1 tyrosine kinases. It is currently commonly used for the first-line treatment of patients with advanced/metastatic RCC with good/intermediate prognosis criteria [32, 33]. This is based on a multi-centre, randomised study comparing sunitinib and IFN-α in previously untreated patients with metastatic RCC. The objective response rates at the final analysis were 47 and 12 % for the sunitinib and IFN-α arms, respectively. Progression-free survival was also significantly longer in the sunitinib group [11 months versus 5 months]. Overall survival was affected by crossover; however in an exploratory analysis of patients who did not receive treatment post-study, the median overall survival with sunitinib was 28.1 months compared to 14.1 months in the IFN-α group [35].

Sunitinib is generally well tolerated. The main side effects of sunitinib therapy are fatigue, hypertension, stomatitis and leucopenia/thrombocytopenia. Cardiotoxicity, although not common, needs to be considered especially in patients with previous history of cardiac problems. Thyroid dysfunction is a well-recognised consequence of sunitinib therapy and presents usually as hypothyroidism which may affect up to 50 % of patients. In cases of clinically overt disease, thyroxine supplements are used [34].

Pazopanib, a newer oral TKI, has a selective inhibitory effect on VEGFR-1, 2, 3, c-kit as well as PDGFR-α/β. It is overall better tolerated and is an emerging agent for first-line treatment of mRCC as an alternative to sunitinib although pending results of randomised phase III trials comparing the two agents. Axitinib is a further agent with similar activity undergoing clinical evaluation.

Mammalian Target of Rapamycin Inhibitors (mTORIs)

mTOR is a serine/threonine protein kinase that together with Akt and MAPK regulates regulate cell growth, growth proliferation and angiogenesis. In RCC, through the synthesis of HIF-1, mTOR regulates the production of proteins involved in angiogenesis such as VEGF thus rendering mTOR an attractive target for development of the relevant inhibitory agents [mTORIs]. The mTORIs have evolved from sirolimus, initially noted for its immunosuppressive activity and currently employed in solid organ transplantation including renal. Three mTORIs have been used in RCC – orally administered sirolimus and everolimus and temsirolimus that is intravenously administered on a weekly basis.

Temsirolimus is an ester of sirolimus. It is a water-soluble agent and administered intravenously weekly. It is used in the first-line setting in patients with poor prognosis metastatic RCC. A large, randomised, phase III, international study which included 626 patients, mostly with poor prognosis criteria, was comprised by three arms [35]: temsirolimus, IFN-α or their combination with a lower dose of temsirolimus. The primary endpoint of the study was overall survival and temsirolimus demonstrated significantly longer overall compared to IFN-α alone [10.9 months versus 7.3 months] and combination therapy was significantly better than IFN-α alone [8.4 months versus 7.3 months]. Furthermore, temsirolimus demonstrated a better safety profile compared to the other two groups, although side effects include fatigue, stomatitis, rash, hyperglycaemia and hyperlipidaemia [34].

Everolimus, an oral second generation mTORI, is a sirolimus derivative, but unlike temsirolimus it does not convert into sirolimus in vivo. A randomised trial in patients who had failed TKI therapy with sunitinib, sorafenib or both demonstrated a statistically improved progression-free survival of 4.1 months with everolimus compared to 1.9 months with placebo [35]. As with other studies survival analysis was affected by crossover from placebo to treatment with everolimus. Analysis of patients who did not cross over however estimated survival at 14.8 months with everolimus versus 10.0 months with placebo alone. Toxicity profile is acceptable, and significant non-infectious pneumonitis – a specific mTOR-related side effect – was noted to occur in only 3 % of cases. Based on this evidence, everolimus is now used for the treatment of patients with advanced/metastatic RCC who failed TKI therapy.

Table 39.1 Suggested therapeutic options for adjuvant therapy in metastatic or advance renal cell cancer

Patient group	Systemic therapy
First line	
Good prognosis	Sunitinib/pazopanib Bevacizumab/IFN-α Interferon-a
Intermediate prognosis	Sunitinib Bevacizumab/IFN-α
Poor prognosis	Temsirolimus
Second line	
Post IFN-α	Sorafenib
Post TKI/anti-VEGF failure	Everolimus Clinical trials Best supportive care
Post mTOR failure	Clinical trials Best supportive care
Third line or beyond	
Clinical trials	
Best supportive care	

General Considerations on Systemic Therapy for Advanced/Metastatic RCC

With the continuous development of new promising agents for the management of metastatic RCC, attention shifts to the use of not only effective agents but also drugs with an improved toxicity profile. The fact that tumour resistance or intolerance to one agent in an individual may not be predictive of the effects of another is another consideration. The optimal sequence of available agents and indeed the potential for combination therapy is topical, and clinical studies are in progress addressing this issue. A suggested sequence for management based on prognosis and prior therapy is shown in the Table 39.1.

One of the more pressing and important issues in the use of systemic therapies in RCC is the development of resistance to the new targeted agents. There remains a need to identify and study in depth the pathways involved in the pathogenesis of RCC as none of the currently available agents are regarded as curative due to resistance mechanisms evolving with tumour exposure.

There are also several further considerations. Firstly these treatments rarely yield complete responses and thus are not curative. Significant improvements in survival will require ongoing basic research to identify therapies which target further mechanisms of tumour progression to be used alone or in conjunction with the current classes of drugs. Health-care economics are a further issue that will also influence their role in practice. No placebo-controlled trial has reported a health-related quality of life benefit, and the newer drugs frequently exceed the recommended guidelines for funding agencies in terms of cost-benefit or cost/quality of life year (QALY) [36].

Specific Clinical Issues

Small Renal Masses

The changing epidemiology of renal carcinoma has resulted in the commonest clinical scenario being a small incidentally detected lesion or small renal mass. This has resulted in a dramatic increase in the use of surgery and also ablative therapies to treat these lesions. Despite this the overall mortality related to RCC has not declined – suggesting that early intervention in these small lesions may represent overtreatment in many cases. Overall the options of radical nephrectomy, partial nephrectomy, tumour ablation and surveillance (with selective use of intervention for rapidly enlarging lesions) all have to be associated with similar cancer-specific survival with incidentally detected tumours <3 cm in size. Each option is associated with specific implications which may drive the choice in individual patient circumstances.

6. Neuzillet Y, Tillou X, Mathieu R, Long JA, Gigante M, Paparel P, et al. Renal cell carcinoma (RCC) in patients with end-stage renal disease exhibits many favourable clinical, pathologic, and outcome features compared with RCC in the general population. Eur Urol. 2011;60(2):366–73.
7. Konda R, Sato H, Hatafuku F, Nozawa T, Ioritani N, Fujioka T. Expression of hepatocyte growth factor and its receptor C-met in acquired renal cystic disease associated with renal cell carcinoma. J Urol. 2004;171(6 Pt 1):2166–70.
8. Manola J, Royston P, Elson P, McCormack JB, Mazumdar M, Negrier S, et al. Prognostic model for survival in patients with metastatic renal cell carcinoma: results from the international kidney cancer working group. Clin Cancer Res. 2011;17(16):5443–50.
9. Bosniak MA. The current radiological approach to renal cysts. Radiology. 1986;158(1):1–10.
10. van der Veldt AA, Meijerink MR, van den Eertwegh AJ, Boven E. Targeted therapies in renal cell cancer: recent developments in imaging. Target Oncol. 2010;5(2):95–112.
11. Gardner TA, Tirkes T, Mellon M, Koch MO. Imaging techniques for the patient with renal cell carcinoma. Semin Nephrol. 2011;31(3):245–53.
12. Sohaib SA, Cook G, Allen SD, Hughes M, Eisen T, Gore M. Comparison of whole-body MRI and bone scintigraphy in the detection of bone metastases in renal cancer. Br J Radiol. 2009;82(980):632–9.
13. Volpe A, Jewett MA. Current role, techniques and outcomes of percutaneous biopsy of renal tumors. Expert Rev Anticancer Ther. 2009;9(6):773–83.
14. Lam JS, Belldegrun AS, Pantuck AJ. Long-term outcomes of the surgical management of renal cell carcinoma. World J Urol. 2006;24(3):255–66.
15. Leveridge MJ, Jewett MA. Recent developments in kidney cancer. Can Urol Assoc J. 2011;5(3):195–203.
16. Margulis V, Master VA, Cost NG, Leibovich BC, Joniau S, Kuczyk M, et al. International consultation on urologic diseases and the European Association of Urology international consultation on locally advanced renal cell carcinoma. Eur Urol. 2011;60(4):673–83.
17. Heuer R, Gill IS, Guazzoni G, Kirkali Z, Marberger M, Richie JP, et al. A critical analysis of the actual role of minimally invasive surgery and active surveillance for kidney cancer. Eur Urol. 2010;57(2):223–32.
18. Kane CJ, Mallin K, Ritchey J, Cooperberg MR, Carroll PR. Renal cell cancer stage migration: analysis of the National Cancer Data Base. Cancer. 2008;113(1):78–83.
19. Klarenbach S, Moore RB, Chapman DW, Dong J, Braam B. Adverse renal outcomes in subjects undergoing nephrectomy for renal tumors: a population-based analysis. Eur Urol. 2011;59(3):333–9.
20. Leveridge MJ, Mattar K, Kachura J, Jewett MA. Assessing outcomes in probe ablative therapies for small renal masses. J Endourol. 2010;24(5):759–64 [Review].
21. Weight CJ, Lieser G, Larson BT, Gao T, Lane BR, Campbell SC, et al. Partial nephrectomy is associated with improved overall survival compared to radical nephrectomy in patients with unanticipated benign renal tumours. Eur Urol. 2010;58(2):293–8 [Comparative Study].
22. Zini L, Patard JJ, Capitanio U, Crepel M, de La Taille A, Tostain J, et al. Cancer-specific and non-cancer-related mortality rates in European patients with T1a and T1b renal cell carcinoma. BJU Int. 2009;103(7):894–8.
23. Miller DC, Schonlau M, Litwin MS, Lai J, Saigal CS. Renal and cardiovascular morbidity after partial or radical nephrectomy. Cancer. 2008;112(3):511–20.
24. Huang WC, Elkin EB, Levey AS, Jang TL, Russo P. Partial nephrectomy versus radical nephrectomy in patients with small renal tumors–is there a difference in mortality and cardiovascular outcomes? J Urol. 2009;181(1):55–61; discussion -2.
25. Van Poppel H, Da Pozzo L, Albrecht W, Matveev V, Bono A, Borkowski A, et al. A prospective, randomised EORTC intergroup phase 3 study comparing the oncologic outcome of elective nephron-sparing surgery and radical nephrectomy for low-stage renal cell carcinoma. Eur Urol. 2011;59(4):543–52.
26. Breda A, Anterasian C, Belldegrun A. Management and outcomes of tumor recurrence after focal ablation renal therapy. J Endourol. 2010;24(5):749–52.
27. Chawla SN, Crispen PL, Hanlon AL, Greenberg RE, Chen DY, Uzzo RG. The natural history of observed enhancing renal masses: meta-analysis and review of the world literature. J Urol. 2006;175(2):425–31.
28. Amato RJ. Chemotherapy for renal cell carcinoma. Semin Oncol. 2000;27(2):177–86.
29. Coppin C, Porzsolt F, Awa A, Kumpf J, Coldman A, Wilt T. Immunotherapy for advanced renal cell cancer. Cochrane Database Syst Rev. 2005;(1):CD001425.
30. Brookman-May S, Burger M, Wieland WF, Rossler W, May M, Denzinger S. Vaccination therapy in renal cell carcinoma: current position and future options in metastatic and localized disease. Expert Rev Vaccines. 2011;10(6):837–52.
31. Oosterwijk E, Rathmell WK, Junker K, Brannon AR, Pouliot F, Finley DS, et al. Basic research in kidney cancer. Eur Urol. 2011;60(4):622–33.
32. Escudier B. Advanced renal cell carcinoma: current and emerging management strategies. Drugs. 2007;67(9):1257–64.
33. Patard JJ, Pignot G, Escudier B, Eisen T, Bex A, Sternberg C, et al. ICUD-EAU International Consultation on Kidney Cancer 2010: treatment of metastatic disease. Eur Urol. 2011;60(4):684–90.
34. Hutson TE, Figlin RA, Kuhn JG, Motzer RJ. Targeted therapies for metastatic renal cell carcinoma: an overview of toxicity and dosing strategies. Oncologist. 2008;13(10):1084–96.
35. Coppin C, Kollmannsberger C, Le L, Porzsolt F, Wilt TJ. Targeted therapy for advanced renal cell cancer (RCC): a Cochrane systematic review of published randomised trials. BJU Int. 2011;108(10):1556–63.
36. Thompson Coon J, Hoyle M, Green C, Liu Z, Welch K, Moxham T, et al. Bevacizumab, sorafenib tosylate, sunitinib and temsirolimus for renal cell carcinoma: a systematic review and economic evaluation. Health Technol Assess. 2010;14(2):1–184, iii–iv.
37. McGuire BB, Fitzpatrick JM. The diagnosis and management of complex renal cysts. Curr Opin Urol. 2010;20(5):349–54.
38. Nicol D. Fujita S. Kidneys from patients with small renal tumours used for transplantation: outcomes and results. Curr Opin Urol. 2011;21(5):380–5. [Review]
39. Khan G, Golshayan A, Elson P, Wood L, Garcia J, Bukowski R, et al. Sunitinib and sorafenib in metastatic renal cell carcinoma patients with renal insufficiency. Ann Oncol. 2010;21(8): 1618–22.
40. Izzedine H, Etienne-Grimaldi MC, Renee N, Vignot S, Milano G. Pharmacokinetics of sunitinib in hemodialysis. Ann Oncol. 2009;20(1):190–2.
41. Bex A, Jonasch E, Kirkali Z, Mejean A, Mulders P, Oudard S, et al. Integrating surgery with targeted therapies for renal cell carcinoma: current evidence and ongoing trials. Eur Urol. 2010; 58(6):819–28.
42. Oken MM, Creech RH, Tormey DC, Horton J, Davis TE, McFadden ET, et al. Toxicity and response criteria of the Eastern Cooperative Oncology Group. Am J Clin Oncol. 1982;5(6):649–55.
43. Kurpad R, Kim W, Rathmell WK, Godley P, Whang Y, Fielding J, et al. A multidisciplinary approach to the management of urologic malignancies: does it influence diagnostic and treatment decisions? Urol Oncol. 2011;29(4):378–82.

Inherited Renal Tumour Syndromes

40

Thomas M.F. Connor and Patrick H. Maxwell

Inherited Renal Tumour Syndromes

Kidney cancer is among the most common adult malignancies [1]. The majority of cases will be detected and managed by urologists; however, in 2–3 % of all cases of RCC, there is a major inherited predisposition. These complex cases may require additional input from nephrologists and clinical geneticists [2]. The presence of characteristic tumours or extra-renal signs may point to a diagnosis of a specific RCC susceptibility syndrome. It is important to recognise that renal cancer is only one aspect of these complex multisystem disorders and that optimal patient care requires long-term follow-up and the close liaison of a broad multi-specialty team.

Kidney cancer is not a single disease, but comprises a number of histological subtypes. The Heidelberg classification system recognises five subtypes of malignant renal parenchymal neoplasm (Table 40.1).

Table 40.1 illustrates the seven genes that have been implicated in familial renal carcinoma. These genes are all implicated in two interrelated metabolic pathways. The most common cause of inherited RCC is von Hippel–Lindau (VHL) disease, which is caused by mutations in the *VHL* tumour-suppressor gene. *VHL*, *FH* and *SDHB* all impact on the cellular response to changes in oxygen tension. *FLCN*, *MET*, *TSC1* and *TSC2* are all implicated in the activity of the nutrient-sensing pathway that is centred on the mammalian target of rapamycin, mTOR.

T.M.F. Connor, MRCP, BM, BCh
UCL Division of Medicine and Centre for Nephrology, University College London, 5 University Street, London WC1E 6JF, UK
e-mail: t.connor@ucl.ac.uk

P.H. Maxwell, DPhil, FRCP, FMedSci (✉)
School of Clinical Medicine, University of Cambridge, Hills Road, 111, Cambridge CB2 0SP, UK
e-mail: regius@medschl.cam.ac.uk

Genetic Diagnosis

A comprehensive family history is an important step in the analysis of any disorder, whether or not it is known to be genetic. A family history is important because it can be critical in diagnosis, can provide information about the natural history of a disease and variation in its expression and can clarify the pattern of inheritance.

The following key points are critical in taking a good family history:

- Detail all close family and their biological relation to the index case.
- Document consanguinity.
- Include miscarriages and stillbirths.
- Document the age of disease onset in each case.
- Find out the exact histological diagnosis.
- Detail all other potentially associated conditions in other systems, such as skin lesions, deafness or pneumothorax.

A genetic disorder may be inherited from one or both parents' genes, or it may be caused by new mutations in the DNA during gametogenesis. Mutations can occur at meiosis and thus be passed on to every cell in the body, or affect just the progeny of one mutant cell (somatic mutation). In kidney cancer, the same gene, commonly the *VHL* tumour-suppressor gene, may be affected both by heritable mutations and by somatic mutations acquired during the lifetime of an individual.

Excepting translocations of chromosome 3, familial renal cancer is the result of single mutated genes. These conditions are all autosomal dominant; thus, each affected individual may have one affected parent, and there is a 50 % chance that a child will inherit the mutated gene. However, autosomal dominant conditions may have reduced or variable penetrance, which means not all individuals who inherit that mutation go on to develop the disease or express the disease in the same way.

Most cases of familial kidney cancer are caused by the loss of function of a tumour-suppressor gene. In this situation, an affected individual has one abnormal copy of the gene present in every cell in their body, but the remaining

M. Harber (ed.), *Practical Nephrology*,
DOI 10.1007/978-1-4471-5547-8_40, © Springer-Verlag London 2014

Table 40.1 Classification of renal cell tumours

Subtype	Percentage	Syndrome	Mutation
Clear cell	75–80 %	Von Hippel–Lindau disease	*VHL* (loss of function)
		Familial paraganglioma	*SDHB* (loss of function)
Papillary type 1	10–15 % (types 1 and 2)	Hereditary papillary renal carcinoma	*MET* (activating)
Papillary type 2		Hereditary leiomyomatosis and renal cancer	*FH* (loss of function)
Chromophobe ± Oncocytic	5 %	Birt–Hogg–Dubé	*FLCN* (loss of function)
Angiomyolipoma	<1 %	Tuberous sclerosis complex	*TSC1* and *TSC2* (loss of function)

copy of the gene is sufficient for cells to behave normally. It is only when a cell develops a second, 'somatic', mutation in the normal copy that a tumour begins to develop.

Many of these disorders exhibit a correlation between the position of the mutation within the causative gene and the clinical signs observed, a genotype–phenotype correlation. This is best understood for VHL disease but is also true for less common conditions, such as BHD or HLRCC. Although genotype–phenotype correlations can aid clinical decision-making, it is not usual to alter screening guidelines.

Referral Criteria

These referral criteria are designed to pick up all individuals and families who may have a genetic predisposition to develop renal tumours or cysts. Ideally all patients with known polycystic syndromes and other genetic renal cystic diseases with cancer predisposition would be managed in a specialist renal genetics clinic. The following two key principles should guide referral:

1. The most important factor determining whether screening will be informative is the presence of renal disease in a first-degree relative.
2. Referral should be based on whether establishing a genetic diagnosis would lead to productive screening of either the patient or other family members and/or affect reproductive decisions.

It is important to mention that the budget for genetic testing is usually held by the medical genetics service. This ensures that patients meeting criteria for referral will receive appropriate counselling and that cascade testing of family members can be initiated. Consequently, patients should generally be referred to medical genetics or managed in a joint clinic. It is not advisable to collect blood samples for genetic testing in the absence of this support. Our own guidelines recommend referral in the following circumstances:

- Familial renal cell carcinoma
  - Positive family history, especially first-degree relative (e.g. parent or sibling)
- Young-onset renal tumour
  - <45 years
- Multiple renal tumours
  - <55 years
  - Clear cell carcinoma
  - Chromophobe
  - Oncocytoma
- Consider in patients with single tumours but a family history of:
  - Renal tract anomaly
  - Renal cysts
  - Other renal diseases/renal failure

Von Hippel–Lindau Syndrome: VHL Disease

Introduction and Epidemiology

VHL disease (Mendelian Inheritance in Man, MIM 193300) is a dominantly inherited familial cancer syndrome. It was named after Eugene von Hippel, who described angiomas in the eye in 1904, and Arvid Lindau, who described angiomas of the cerebellum and spine in 1927 [3]. The incidence of VHL disease is approximately 1 per 36,000 live births, with similar prevalence in both genders and across all ethnic backgrounds [4]. Eighty percent of patients with VHL disease have a positive family history, but de novo *VHL* mutations and mosaicism are not uncommon.

Aetiology and Pathogenesis

VHL disease is caused by mutations in the *VHL* gene, which is located at 3p25 [5]. Mutation of the *VHL* gene is detected in nearly all VHL families and, importantly, the great majority (~90 %) of nonfamilial clear cell renal cell cancer (CCRCC) [6]. VHL functions as a classical tumour-suppressor gene. Thus, tumour tissue in patients with VHL disease shows inactivation of the remaining normal *VHL* allele, either through mutation, deletion or methylation.

The VHL protein binds to the hypoxia-inducible factor (HIF) and thereby mediates its degradation when

Table 40.2 Manifestations of VHL disease

Manifestation	Percentage of patients with VHL disease exhibiting this feature	Mean age at diagnosis	Percentage of all cases due to mutations in *VHL* (%)
CNS haemangioblastoma	Overall 60–80 % Presenting feature in 40 %	30	30
Retinal angioma	45–60 %	18	50
Renal cell cancer	70 % lifetime	45	1
Phaeochromocytoma	0–20 % depending on genotype Multifocal in 60 % Malignant in 3 %	30	10

intracellular oxygen levels are normal. HIF is a highly conserved transcription factor that mediates cellular adaptation to low levels of oxygen [7, 8]. Disruption of the VHL–HIF interaction results in the activation of HIF target genes, such as vascular endothelial growth factor (VEGF), that play a role in the growth and metastasis of primary tumours.

Clinical Features

The most frequent manifestations of VHL disease are retinal and central nervous system haemangioblastomas, CCRCC and phaeochromocytomas (Table 40.2 and Fig. 40.1). These are commonly multiple and develop at a younger age than similar sporadic tumours in the general population. Patients may also develop non-secreting neuroendocrine tumours of the pancreas, endolymphatic sac tumours (which can result in deafness), epididymal papillary cystadenoma (men) and cysts of the uterine broad ligament (women) [9]. In addition to tumours, patients develop multiple cysts of the kidney and other organs including the pancreas (Fig. 40.1) [4]. Mortality is usually due to either metastasis of RCC or complications of CNS haemangioblastomas; however, following the introduction of systematic screening for tumour development, life expectancy of VHL patients has greatly improved. There are now more than 350 distinct mutations in the VHL gene that have been linked to familial VHL disease, which demonstrates genotype and phenotype correlation [10].

The clinical phenotype is categorised on the basis of incidence of haemangioblastoma, CCRCC and phaeochromocytoma, as shown in Table 40.3. Striking aspects of the phenotype–genotype relationship are that loss-of-function alleles carry a low risk of phaeochromocytoma (type 1 disease), while some specific missense mutations predispose to phaeochromocytoma without other manifestations (type 2C disease). Significantly, mutations associated with type 2C disease do not alter the ability of VHL to regulate the hypoxia-inducible factor (HIF).

Diagnostic Criteria

The diagnosis of von Hippel–Lindau disease is based on clinical criteria or genetic testing [2]. Patients with a family history and a CNS (excluding retinal) haemangioblastoma, phaeochromocytoma or CCRCC are diagnosed with the disease. Those with no relevant family history must have either two or more CNS haemangioblastomas or one haemangioblastoma of the CNS or retina and a visceral tumour. It is important to have a strong index of suspicion in patients who do not fulfil all the criteria and consider either genetic testing or continued surveillance.

Investigations

Mutation analysis is recommended to make a definitive diagnosis. There are a number of reasons why genetic testing for VHL disease is particularly successful:

- The *VHL* gene is small and so easier and cheaper to sequence.
- It is possible to identify a mutation in virtually all families.
- Almost all genetic variations in *VHL* are implicated in disease.
- Mutations have a high penetrance.
- Clinical screening of mutation carriers prevents serious consequences.
- Preimplantation testing is entirely appropriate.

Screening for germline *VHL* mutations should also be considered in individuals with apparently sporadic cerebral and retinal haemangioblastoma since these are rare in the general population [11]. Direct sequencing is the gold standard for detecting germline *VHL* mutations and can identify the underlying abnormality in 86–100 %. 'Mutation negative' patients should be screened with techniques capable of identifying deletions, such as multiplex ligation-dependent probe amplification (MLPA), quantitative southern blotting and fluorescent in situ hybridisation (FISH).

Screening for clinical manifestations in individuals who are known to carry a *VHL* mutation should begin in infancy.

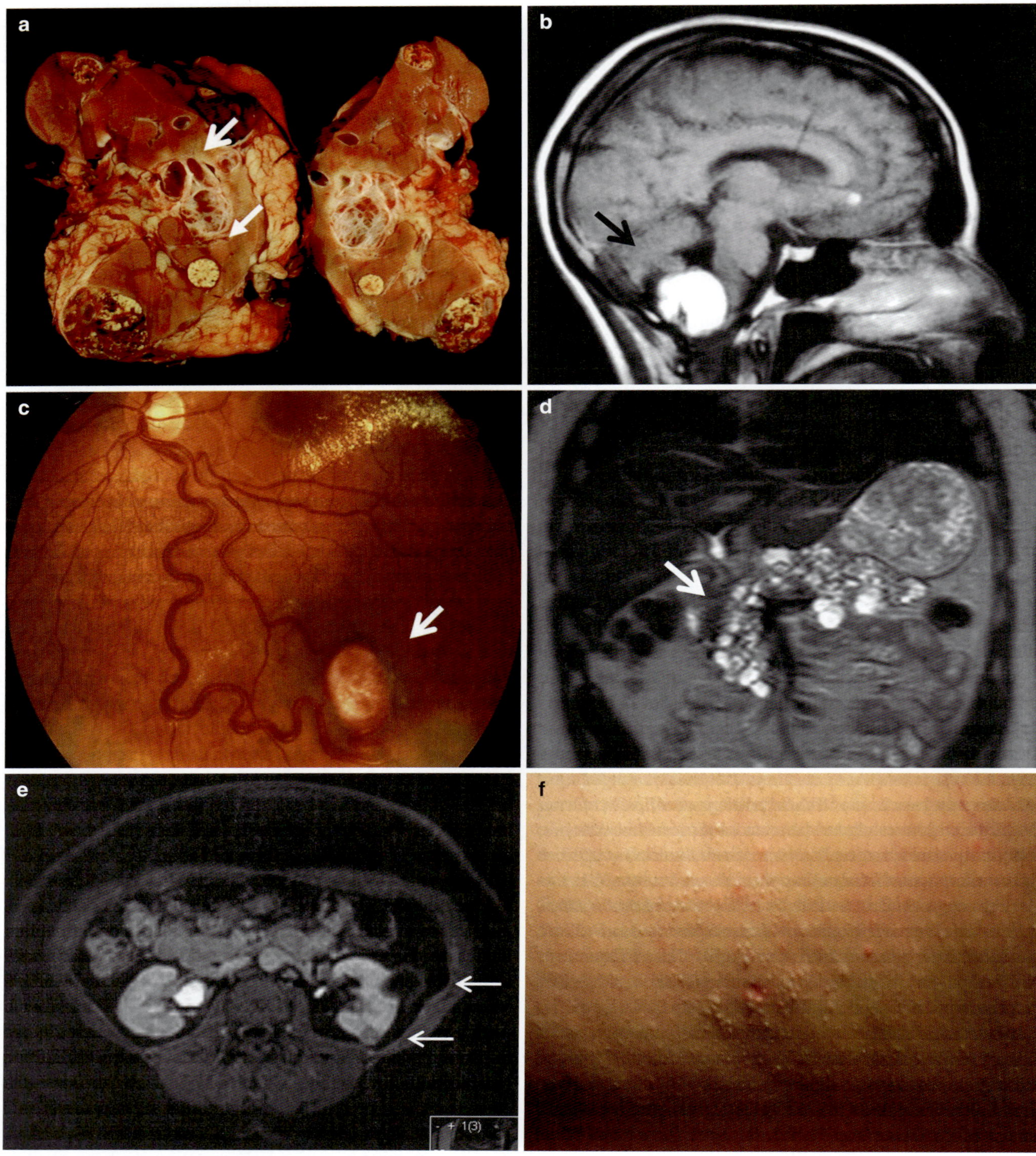

Fig. 40.1 Clinical manifestations of inherited renal tumour syndromes. (**a**) Nephrectomy specimen demonstrating multiple solid tumours (*arrowhead*) and cystic change (*arrowed*) in a patient with VHL disease. (**b**) Large cerebellar haemangioblastoma in a 35-year-old with VHL disease, *arrowed* (T1-weighted contrast-enhanced MRI). (**c**) Retinal photograph demonstrating a large retinal angioma in a patient with VHL disease (Image courtesy of Professor Sue Lightman, UCL). (**d**) Multiple areas of cystic change in the pancreas of a 33-year-old with VHL disease; note possible soft tissue enhancement *arrowed* (T1-weighted contrast-enhanced MRI). (**e**) Multiple renal cysts in a 44-year-old patient with Birt–Hogg–Dubé syndrome. Note cyst with soft tissue component, *arrowhead*, as well as simple cyst, *arrowed* (T2-weighted contrast-enhanced MRI). (**f**) Characteristic skin lesions in a patient with Birt–Hogg–Dubé syndrome

Table 40.3 Classification of VHL families on the basis of tumour risk

Category	Risk of phaeochromocytoma	Risk of haemangioblastoma	Risk of renal cell carcinoma
1	Low	High	High
2A	High	High	Low
2B	High	High	High
C	Yes	No	No

High risk tumour type observed in over 50 % affected individuals, *Low risk* tumour type observed in less than 5 % of affected individuals, *Yes* tumour type observed in all affected individuals, *No* tumour type not observed in affected individuals

Table 40.4 Recommended screening programme in VHL disease

Associated tumours	Age range of onset (years)	Screening recommendations
Retinal haemangioblastoma	1–67 (mean 25)	From 5 years to lifelong Annual ophthalmic exam
CNS haemangioblastoma	9–78 (mean 33)	From 15 years to lifelong MRI brain and spine at baseline and MRI brain every 3 years
Phaeochromocytoma	5–58 (mean 30)	From 11 years to lifelong Annual urine catecholamines or plasma metanephrines
Renal cell cancer	16–67 (mean 39)	From 15 years to lifelong Annual abdominal USS or MRI
Endolymphatic sac tumour	12–50 (mean 22)	See CNS haemangioblastoma
Pancreatic tumour	5–70 (mean 36)	See renal cell cancer
Cystadenoma	Unknown	None

Current screening recommendations are detailed in Table 40.4. Early treatment reduces both morbidity and mortality [12]. Similarly, anyone at risk of inheriting a *VHL* mutation who has not had genetic testing performed should undergo regular clinical screening to identify tumours before they result in avoidable harm.

Management Issues in VHL Disease

Clear Cell Renal Cancer

VHL patients have a 70 % risk of developing CCRCC by 60 years old [4] (Fig. 40.1a). The mean age of onset is 44 years, compared to 62 years for sporadic CCRCC in the general population, and asymptomatic tumours are frequently detected earlier (from adolescence onwards). Tumours are frequently multiple and bilateral in VHL disease, and histological examination often shows large numbers of microscopic tumour foci in apparently normal renal parenchyma. Renal cysts are also common in VHL patients and show a higher rate of malignant transformation than the simple cysts seen in the general population [9].

CCRCC probably originates from the distal renal tubule. These tumours are highly vascular, due to the overproduction of angiogenic growth factors [9]. *VHL* mutations linked to CCRCC (types 1 and 2B) show complete loss of the ability to regulate HIF consistent with HIF activation being critical in tumourigenesis. This may explain why targeted therapies that block the VEGF pathway have clinical activity as single agents in kidney cancer.

Nephron-sparing surgery is the optimum strategy for managing CCRCC in VHL disease. Many lesions are detected presymptomatically and do not require immediate intervention. Small tumours usually enlarge slowly (<2 cm/year) and can be monitored safely (typically at 6 monthly or annual intervals) until they reach 3 cm diameter [13]. Below 3 cm diameter, there is a low risk of metastasis, whereas tumours >3 cm have a 25 % risk of metastasis [14]. Surgical treatment is with partial nephrectomy or alternative techniques, such as radiofrequency ablation, and should target as many smaller lesions as feasible in order to delay the need for reoperation.

Renal replacement therapy may be required if renal function has been reduced by repeated renal surgery. Renal transplantation has been undertaken successfully, and the subsequent immunosuppression does not appear to affect the course of VHL disease [15]. It has therefore been suggested that the usual tumour-free interval until an individual is accepted on to the transplantation waiting list can be shortened to 6 months for VHL patients with tumours <3 cm [2].

Renal Cysts

Renal cysts are found in 50–75 % of patients with VHL disease (Fig. 40.1a). The cysts are usually bilateral and multiple. Kidney shape usually remains normal, with normal renal function and preserved blood pressure. Renal cysts can be either simple or complex renal cysts, which combine cystic and solid components. Complex cysts are precursors to renal cell carcinoma and require close follow-up or surgery, depending on the degree of suspicion for cancer. In contrast to ADPKD, cyst infection does not occur in VHL disease, whereas CCRCC is common (see above). Likewise, in contrast to ADPKD, pancreatic cysts can be numerous and scattered through the pancreas in VHL disease, whereas liver cysts show the opposite pattern in the two conditions.

Haemangioblastoma

Haemangioblastomas are the most common manifestations of VHL disease, occurring in up to 80 % of patients (Fig. 40.1b). They are located most commonly in the cerebellum and retina [3, 4, 9]. They are cystic tumours of lipid-filled stromal cells embedded in a capillary network. Patients with cerebellar haemangioblastoma typically present with symptoms of increased intracranial pressure and limb or truncal ataxia. Haemangioblastomas are rarely malignant, but enlargement or bleeding within the CNS can result in neurological damage and death. The removal of asymptomatic tumours is not recommended. Complex lesions benefit from surgery in units with expertise in VHL disease.

Retinal angiomas are the most common presenting feature of VHL disease and lead to visual loss in 55 % of patients with angiomas at 50 years (Fig. 40.1c). Management is directed towards identification of asymptomatic lesions and their treatment by laser photocoagulation or cryotherapy. Optic disc lesions are kept under surveillance because of the risk of optic nerve damage if they are treated.

VHL mutations are found in a third of all patients with CNS haemangioblastomas (Table 40.2) [2]. This number is even greater in those with posterior fossa or spinal lesions and in those presenting at a young age (<40 years). Over half of all patients with retinal angiomas have *VHL* mutations. It is therefore recommended that all patients with these tumours are referred for genetic testing.

Phaeochromocytoma

Seven to eighteen percent of VHL patients are afflicted with phaeochromocytomas, with a mean age of onset of 30 years [4]. Phaeochromocytomas are neoplastic intra- or extra-adrenal gland lesions that appear histologically as an expansion of large chromaffin-positive cells, derived from neural crest cells [16]. Untreated phaeochromocytomas can result in severe, episodic hypertension and stroke, malignant hypertension or death. Both intra- and extra-adrenal phaeochromocytomas can occur in VHL disease. The mechanism of phaeochromocytoma formation in VHL disease is likely to be different to that of other tumours in this syndrome and may be due to abnormal apoptosis during sympathetic neural development [16].

Up to 10 % of patients with phaeochromocytomas have germline mutations in *VHL* (Table 40.3) [2]. This proportion is higher in those with a positive family history, multifocal disease and age of onset <45 years. Given that as many as 20 % of apparently non-syndromic phaeochromocytomas have an identifiable genetic cause, it is advisable to refer these patients for consideration of genetic testing.

Novel Therapies

While surgery remains the mainstay of treatment for tumours in VHL disease, several new drug therapies have been developed. These therapies target the molecular consequences of VHL loss of function, in particular the stabilisation of HIF and consequent overproduction of secreted growth factors such as VEGF [8].

Current therapies, including monoclonal antibodies and small-molecule inhibitors, have been successfully designed to inhibit growth factor signalling [17]. The first drug used in this context was a humanised VEGF monoclonal antibody bevacizumab (Avastin). Subsequently, small-molecule inhibitors with a spectrum of activity against receptor tyrosine kinases, such as sorafenib and sunitinib, were approved by the FDA in 2005–2006. Lastly, a small molecule that targets the mTOR pathway, temsirolimus (TORISEL), has also been licensed for the treatment of metastatic CCRCC.

These agents have all shown a consistent doubling of progression-free survival over prior standard of care treatments [8]. It should be noted that the outcome of patients with metastatic RCC is poor, with median survival of only 22, 12 or 5.4 months depending on the functional criteria. Sorafenib, sunitinib and temsirolimus have shown additional overall survival benefits as well. These drugs are generally well tolerated, as demonstrated by quality of life improvement in clinical trials, and result in clinical benefit in excess of 70 % of patients treated.

Follow-Up

VHL disease is a complex multisystem disorder that requires lifelong follow-up and the close liaison of a broad multi-specialty team. Patients may have poor mobility and travel considerable distances; therefore, scans need to be closely coordinated with multidisciplinary appointments ideally on the same day with MDT discussion of management. The early diagnosis of most of the complications of VHL disease improves prognosis and reduces morbidity. All VHL patients and at-risk relatives should be entered into a comprehensive screening programme in childhood, except where VHL disease has been excluded by molecular genetic testing.

Tuberous Sclerosis Complex

Introduction and Epidemiology

Tuberous sclerosis (MIM 605284) is an autosomal dominant genetic disorder with a birth incidence of 1:6,000. It can affect virtually any organ system, and all racial and ethnic groups are affected equally. Males and females are affected equally. TSC has a highly variable phenotype, and two-thirds of cases result from sporadic genetic mutations. TSC most often presents with neurological symptoms in childhood [18, 19]. Renal lesions are the second most common finding and include multiple angiomyolipomas (80 %) and cysts (50 %), but early-onset RCCs have been reported. Renal failure is the most common cause of death for adult patients with TSC [19], and approximately 1 % of the TSC population with normal intellect requires renal replacement therapy.

Aetiology and Pathogenesis

Tuberous sclerosis (MIM 605284) is a dominantly inherited familial cancer syndrome. Molecular genetic studies have identified at least two chromosomal loci for TSC, *TSC1* on 9q37 and *TSC2* on 16p13.3. Mutations in *TSC1*, which encodes the protein hamartin, are responsible for approximately 20 % of cases. Mutations in *TSC2* account for the great majority of cases. *TSC2* encodes the protein tuberin and is adjacent to the polycystin-1 gene. Deletions of both *TSC2* and *PKD1* may account for the 2 % of individuals with TSC who develop early-onset polycystic kidney disease [18].

Hamartin and tuberin form a heterodimer that interacts with Rheb, a Ras-family GTPase, preventing it from activating mTOR signalling (via mTORC1) [18]. Thus, mutations at the *TSC1* and *TSC2* loci result in a loss of inhibition of the mTOR nutrient and energy-sensing pathway that may explain their function as a tumour suppressor. The tuberous sclerosis proteins are also involved in the formation of the primary cilium that is disturbed in many forms of renal cystic disease.

Clinical Features

TSC most often presents with neurological symptoms, and over 90 % of affected individuals have subependymal nodules and/or cortical tubers on MRI. Approximately 90 % of patients experience seizures, and virtually all subtypes of seizure have been reported [20]. About half of patients show cognitive impairment, autism or other behavioural disorders. In approximately 10 % of patients with TSC, the growth of subependymal tumours can cause hydrocephalus due to obstruction of CSF flow [18].

Renal cystic disease occurs in approximately half of patients with TSC. Renal cystic disease can be microcystic and thus undetectable by standard imaging studies. Renal cysts arise from all parts of the nephron, including the glomerulus. TSC patients may have several risk factors for acute kidney injury, including the use of certain anticonvulsant and nonsteroidal anti-inflammatory drugs as well as rhabdomyolysis and hypoxia induced by prolonged seizures [19]. Both renal cystic disease and angiomyolipomas may contribute to chronic kidney disease (CKD) [21].

Table 40.5 Diagnostic criteria for TSC [22]

Major criteria	Minor criteria
Facial angiofibroma or forehead plaque	Multiple, random dental pits
Nontraumatic ungula or periungual fibroma	Hamartomatous gastrointestinal or rectal polyps
Hypomelanotic macules (>3)	Bone cysts
Shagreen patch (connective tissue naevus)	White matter radial migration lines
Multiple retinal nodular hamartomas	Gingival fibromas
Cortical tuber(s)	Non-renal hamartomas
Subependymal nodule	Retinal achromic patch
Subependymal giant-cell astrocytoma	'Confetti' skin lesions
Cardiac rhabdomyomas	Multiple renal cysts
Lymphangioleiomyomatosis	
Renal angiomyolipoma	

Two major features or one major with two minor features indicates *definite* clinical TSC
One major feature and one minor feature indicate *probable* TSC
One major or two minor features indicate *possible* TSC

Skin lesions are present in 96 % of individuals with TSC. The most common finding is hypo-pigmented macules ('ash leaf spots'), which may require UV light (a Wood's lamp) to visualise in fair-skinned individuals. Other skin lesions that comprise the diagnostic criteria include facial angiofibromas (adenoma sebaceum), periungual fibromas and shagreen patches. Cardiac rhabdomyomas were the most frequent finding at routine antenatal ultrasound testing and are an indication for testing for TSC [20]. In all, 50–67 % children have evidence of one or more rhabdomyomas, and these may be associated with ECG abnormalities, including conduction defects and arrhythmias, and heart failure in infancy. Pulmonary involvement, specifically lymphangioleiomyomatosis (LAM), is the third most common cause of TSC-associated morbidity in approximately 35 % of female TSC patients [19]. The female preponderance is not understood. Retinal hamartomas may occur in 40 %. The most common non-retinal findings on ophthalmological examination include coloboma and papilloedema due to hydrocephalus.

Diagnostic Criteria

The diagnostic criteria for TSC are based on major and minor diagnostic features, shown in Table 40.5 [22]. Cases meeting these criteria fulfil a clinical diagnosis of TSC; the results of molecular genetic testing of the *TSC1* and *TSC2* loci are currently viewed as corroborative [18]. No single feature of TSC is diagnostic, and different manifestations of TSC appear at different developmental points from neonatal life to adulthood. Secure diagnosis usually requires assessment of all possible clinical features over a significant time period.

Investigations

Among patients meeting the clinical criteria for diagnosis of TSC, genetic testing is unable to locate the mutation in 15–20 %. Patients with an inherited mutation tend to have less severe disease, as do those with mutations in *TSC1* and those in whom no mutation is identified. TSC may arise in individuals without identifiable mutations due to mosaicism or because of a mutation in an as yet unidentified locus.

Renal ultrasound shows good sensitivity for the detection of cystic renal disease and the adipose tissue of most angiomyolipomas. However, it exhibits poor diagnostic accuracy for the detection of 'fat-poor' angiomyolipomas. The combination of fat-suppressed and non-fat-suppressed T2 signal on MRI is a very effective means of detecting both the macroscopic and microscopic adipose components of angiomyolipomas, and it is especially successful for the detection of those with minimal fat [19]. CT is a reasonable alternative where MRI is contraindicated if concern remains after ultrasound. PET scans can be helpful because angiomyolipomas are generally not PET avid.

All patients with TSC should be screened for renal involvement. All mass lesions should be referred to a urologist, and subsequent imaging will depend on the size and nature of the lesion. If no lesions are detected, repeat imaging should be performed every 3–5 years.

Management Issues in TSC

Renal Angiomyolipomas

Angiomyolipomas are the archetypal renal lesion in TSC, affecting up to 80 % of patients [19]. They typically present in childhood, increasing during adolescence and stabilising in adulthood. These lesions are benign tumours composed of abnormal vessels, immature smooth-muscle cells and fat cells. All cells in the lesion exhibit somatic mutations, which in addition to the germline mutation render the cell deficient in tuberin or hamartin.

There are two main complications of angiomyolipomas: retroperitoneal haemorrhage and progressive CKD [18, 19]. Haemorrhage occurs due to rupture of aneurisms within the disordered vasculature of these lesions. This risk is significantly elevated once they are >5 mm in diameter and is linked to greater tumour size (especially when >3 cm). Renal impairment is caused by invasion of the normal renal parenchyma by both microscopic and macroscopic lesions [21].

Angiomyolipomas tend to grow slowly in adulthood (5 % per year) and are usually asymptomatic. They may grow more rapidly and are more prone to rupture in pregnancy, so repeat imaging may be required. Given the likelihood of progressive CKD in patients with TSC, the management of these lesions should be conservative [19]. Embolisation is the current standard of care to control active bleeding or as prophylaxis in large angiomyolipomas. Corticosteroid therapy can reduce the subsequent post-embolisation syndrome. Nephron-sparing surgery or localised ablative therapy is an option for selected patients in centres with appropriate experience.

Fat-Poor Angiomyolipomas

Solid lesions in the kidney of patients with TSC are a particular concern as they are difficult to image and may be malignant. Most are fat-poor angiomyolipomas (4.5 % of all angiomyolipomas), but they can also rarely be oncocytomas or CCRCC [19]. Suspicious lesions should have repeat imaging to determine whether they are enlarging. Where diagnostic uncertainty remains, such lesions require diagnostic biopsy or nephron-sparing surgery.

Fat-poor TSC-associated angiomyolipomas can consist of a variety of cell types. Although very rare, the epithelioid type may exhibit an aggressive phenotype, with recurrence after surgery and metastasis [19, 21]. However, it is worth noting that the overall incidence of renal cell carcinoma in TSC is less than 2 %.

Hypertension

Renal cystic disease is a significant risk factor for hypertension in this population and responds well to the inhibition of the renin–angiotensin system [19]. Despite a significant burden of renal parenchymal abnormalities on imaging, renal function is often well preserved. An additional cause for hypertension is the use of adrenocorticotrophin hormone (ACTH) therapy to treat infantile spasms in some TSC patients [19]. This side effect can be ameliorated with diuretics with or without other agents.

Nephrolithiasis

Patients with TSC can be prone to nephrolithiasis both as a consequence of the disease and due to various medications used in this condition [19]. Reduced citrate excretion is the common mechanism, and nephrolithiasis can be treated with increased fluid intake and citrate supplementation where required. Direct ureteroscopic stone removal is the preferred surgical therapy for nephrolithiasis in TSC [19]. Extracorporeal shock wave lithotripsy (ESWL) may be associated with an increased risk of subcapsular haematoma formation, while percutaneous nephrolithotomy (PCNL) may be associated with an increased risk of haemorrhage due to the distorted anatomy of the kidneys in TSC.

Novel Therapies

Given that tumour cells from patients with TSC show activation of mTOR, the mTOR inhibitor sirolimus has been identified as a potential therapeutic agent [18]. Sirolimus has been shown to cause regression of renal angiomyolipomas and subependymal giant-cell tumours in patients with TSC. mTOR inhibitors are not yet in routine clinical use; however, phase 3 clinical trials are currently recruiting patients with TSC and LAM.

Follow-Up

TSC requires lifelong follow-up with regular imaging of the kidneys. Although renal angiomyolipomas are rare in the general population, only a minority of all cases are due to underlying TSC. Genetic testing is therefore not indicated in the absence of clinical criteria for TSC, in patients with angiomyolipomas. Neurological and dermatological manifestations of TSC typically present at a much younger age and cause more morbidity than do renal features. Although regular imaging may be required, involvement by a nephrologist is therefore limited prior to the development of renal impairment.

Birt–Hogg–Dubé Syndrome

Introduction and Aetiology

Birt–Hogg–Dubé (BHD) syndrome (OMIM #135150) is an autosomal dominant disease characterised by cutaneous fibrofolliculomas, pulmonary cysts, spontaneous pneumothorax and renal cancer (Fig. 40.1e) [23]. In 2001, a BHD-associated gene locus was localised to chromosome 17p11.2, and subsequently truncating germline mutations were identified in a novel gene, the *FLCN* (BHD) gene [24].

Clinical Features

BHD is probably under-diagnosed because of the wide variation in clinical presentation. Skin lesions (follicular hamartomas) are the most common manifestation, affecting 75 % of patients and usually appearing in the third decade as whitish papules on the face and neck (Fig. 40.1f). Similarly, 80 % of adult BHD patients have multiple lung cysts on CT, but the lung parenchyma generally appears normal and lung function is usually unaffected [25]. The main problem associated with these cysts is a 50-fold increased risk of pneumothorax, with 24 % prevalence of pneumothorax and a median age of 38 years. In some families, non-syndromic cystic lung disease or pneumothorax can be the only manifestation of BHD.

A quarter of patients with BHD develop RCC, which presents at an early age (mean age at diagnosis 50 years) [23, 25]. Chromophobe RCC and mixed chromophobe and oncocytic tumours are typical in BHD, although other histological subtypes can occur, including clear cell and papillary RCC. Somatic second mutations have been identified in BHD-associated renal tumours, consistent with a two-hit tumour-suppressor function; however, these were not seen in the skin tumours. BHD has also been reported in association with a range of tumours other than RCC; however, a causal relationship has not yet been proven [25].

Diagnostic Criteria

New criteria for the diagnosis of BHD have recently been proposed, taking into account the clinical variability seen with this condition (Table 40.6; after [23]).

Management Issues in BHD

Surveillance for renal tumours is indicated in BHD, although the exact risk of occurrence is uncertain and may vary between different families. There are no established guidelines; current recommendations are for annual renal MRI starting at age 20, as ultrasound is insufficiently sensitive to detect small lesions. As with other hereditary renal cancer syndromes, treatment consists of nephron-sparing surgery. It is important to determine the rate of tumour growth, although there is not yet enough evidence for the 3 cm threshold discussed earlier in relation to VHL disease.

Assessment of lung involvement by thoracic CT scan should be included at diagnosis; further investigation should be at the behest of a pulmonary physician. Treatment for pneumothorax in BHD does not differ from standard approaches. Current therapeutic options for skin involvement are limited, though the psychological burden should not be underestimated.

Table 40.6 Diagnostic criteria for BHD

Major criteria	Minor criteria
At least five fibrofolliculomas or trichodiscomas, at least one histologically confirmed, of adult onset	Multiple lung cysts: bilateral, basally located cysts with no other apparent cause, with or without spontaneous pneumothorax
Pathogenic *FLCN* germline mutation	Renal cancer: early-onset (<50 years) or multifocal or bilateral renal cancer of mixed chromophobe and oncocytic histology
	A first-degree relative with BHD

Adapted from Menko et al. [23]
Patients should fulfil one major and two minor criteria for diagnosis

Hereditary Leiomyomatosis and Renal Cancer

Introduction and Aetiology

Hereditary leiomyomatosis and renal cell cancer (HLRCC) is an autosomal dominant disorder characterised by smooth-muscle tumours of the skin and uterus and/or renal cancer (OMIM 605839). In 2001, an HLRCC-associated gene locus was localised to chromosome 1q42–44, and subsequently heterozygous germline mutations were identified in the fumarate hydratase (*FH*) gene. Inactivating mutations have since been found in approximately 180 families worldwide [26].

Clinical Features

Skin lesions are the most prominent feature of HLRCC, with multiple benign leiomyomas occurring in all men and 55 % women by the age of 35 [27]. These tumours typically cause pain, usually in response to touch and changes in temperature. Seventy-nine to one hundred percent women with *FH* mutations have uterine leiomyomas, which are larger, more numerous and of earlier onset than in the general population.

RCC develops in 20–25 % of *FH* mutation-positive patients, with a median age of diagnosis around 42 years. Most importantly, HLRCC tumours may be very aggressive and metastasise early, unlike other types of hereditary renal cancer. Renal tumours seen in HLRCC have a distinct histology, described as the type 2 papillary or collecting duct subtype.

Diagnostic Criteria

Smit et al. have listed practical criteria for the diagnosis of HLRCC (Table 40.7) [28].

Management Issues in HLRCC

Screening with annual MRI should begin at age 18. Given their aggressive nature, all renal tumours will usually be treated surgically. Preclinical data demonstrating that *FH* loss of function activates pathways that include HIF and so overlap with those in VHL disease suggests that there may be value in using similar targeted therapies; however, clinical data in this area is still scarce.

Other Causes of Familial RCC

A number of other inherited disorders may be associated with renal tumours. In the absence of a genetic diagnosis, individuals with familial non-syndromic clear cell renal cancer should be referred to a renal genetics clinic for consideration of karyotype, *VHL* and possibly *FLCN* sequence. If testing is normal, they and their first-degree relatives should receive annual ultrasound from 25 to 60 years via their GP (no published evidence).

Individuals with early-onset, non-syndromic clear cell renal cancer should have Xp11.2 TFE3 translocation carcinoma excluded. Affected family members should have their karyotype assessed. There is no clear evidence to guide whether other family members should receive screening.

Hereditary Translocation of Chromosome 3

Another rare cause of familial RCC is hereditary translocation of chromosome 3. The first to be described was a t(3;8)(p14;q24) translocation, and a further eleven cases have since been described [29]. When routine karyotype analysis identifies a chromosome 3 translocation in the context of familial RCC, this is likely to be the cause [2]. Such patients and their first-degree relatives should be screened with annual renal MRI from age 20. By contrast, the risk of developing RCC for translocation carriers in the absence of a family history is probably low, and such individuals probably do not require screening.

Hereditary Papillary Renal Carcinoma

Hereditary papillary renal carcinoma (HPRC) is a dominantly inherited familial cancer syndrome characterised by a predisposition to develop multiple, bilateral papillary renal tumours (OMIM 605074). Linkage analysis in 1997 showed that this condition was caused by activating mutations in the c-*MET* proto-oncogene on 7q34 [30]. The renal tumours in HPRC have a distinct histological appearance, characterised as type 1 papillary, and have a better prognosis than type 2 papillary

Table 40.7 Diagnostic criteria for HLRCC

Major criteria	Minor criteria
Multiple cutaneous leiomyomas (histologically confirmed)	Surgical treatment of severely symptomatic uterine leiomyomas before the age of 40
	Type 2 papillary or collecting duct renal cell carcinoma before the age of 40
	A first-degree relative who meets one of the above-mentioned criteria (leiomyomas in second-degree paternal relatives may be relevant)

Adapted from Smit et al. [28]
Fulfilling major criteria indicates HLRCC with high likelihood
HLRCC can be suspected when an individual meets ≥2 of the minor criteria

RCC [2]. Ninety-five percent of sporadic tumours with this appearance show trisomy of chromosome 7, which includes both the *MET* and hepatocyte growth factor (*HGF*) genes.

HPRC is very rare (approximate incidence one per ten million), but identification of germline MET mutations allows precise diagnosis and targeted surveillance of mutation carriers. Moreover, such molecular insights have facilitated the use of targeted oncological therapies [17].

Succinate Dehydrogenase

Germline mutations in three of the four subunits of succinate dehydrogenase (*SDHB*, *SDHC* and *SDHD*) have been associated with familial head and neck paragangliomas and sporadic and familial phaeochromocytoma [31]. Subsequently, early-onset renal tumours were also found to develop in individuals with germline *SDHB* mutations. A variety of histological subtypes of RCC may be associated with *SDHB* mutations (and less frequently *SDHD*), and the lifetime risk of RCC in *SDHB* mutation carriers was estimated to be about 15 % [32]. As with *FH* mutations, SDH inactivation results in HIF activation, which may contribute to tumour formation.

Internet Resources

Screening guidelines for VHL disease: http://www.vhl.org/handbook/vhlhb4.php#Suggested.

Patient information on VHL: http://www.vhl.org/healthcare/; http://www.vhlcg.com/80290/info.php?p=3.

Patient information on TSC: http://www.tuberous-sclerosis.org/?page_id=35; http://www.tsalliance.org/pages.aspx?content=133.

Patient information on BHD: http://www.bhdsyndrome.org/.

Patient information on HLRCC: http://hlrccinfo.org/.

References

1. Cancel Research UK. Kidney cancer – UK incidence statistics. 2011. http://www.cancerresearchuk.org/cancer-info/cancerstats/types/kidney/incidence/
2. Maher ER. Genetics of familial renal cancers. Nephron Exp Nephrol. 2011;118(1):e21–6.
3. Melmon KL, Rosen SW. Lindau's disease. Review of the literature and study of a large kindred. Am J Med. 1964;36:595–617.
4. Maher ER. Von Hippel-Lindau disease. Curr Mol Med. 2004;4(8):833–42.
5. Latif F, et al. Identification of the von Hippel-Lindau disease tumor suppressor gene. Science. 1993;260(5112):1317–20.
6. Nickerson ML, et al. Improved identification of von Hippel-Lindau gene alterations in clear cell renal tumors. Clin Cancer Res. 2008;14(15):4726–34.
7. Kaelin Jr WG, Ratcliffe PJ. Oxygen sensing by metazoans: the central role of the HIF hydroxylase pathway. Mol Cell. 2008;30(4):393–402.
8. Linehan WM, et al. Molecular diagnosis and therapy of kidney cancer. Annu Rev Med. 2010;61:329–43.
9. Kaelin WG. Von Hippel-Lindau disease. Annu Rev Pathol. 2007;2:145–73.
10. Nordstrom-O'Brien M, et al. Genetic analysis of von Hippel-Lindau disease. Hum Mutat. 2010;31(5):521–37.
11. Neumann HPH, et al. Germ-line mutations in nonsyndromic pheochromocytoma. N Engl J Med. 2002;346(19):1459–66.
12. Lonser RR, et al. von Hippel-Lindau disease. Lancet. 2003;361(9374):2059–67.
13. Walther MM, et al. Renal cancer in families with hereditary renal cancer: prospective analysis of a tumor size threshold for renal parenchymal sparing surgery. J Urol. 1999;161(5):1475–9.
14. Herring JC, et al. Parenchymal sparing surgery in patients with hereditary renal cell carcinoma: 10-year experience. J Urol. 2001;165(3):777–81.
15. Goldfarb DA, et al. Results of renal transplantation in patients with renal cell carcinoma and von Hippel-Lindau disease. Transplantation. 1997;64(12):1726–9.
16. Lee S, et al. Neuronal apoptosis linked to EglN3 prolyl hydroxylase and familial pheochromocytoma genes: developmental culling and cancer. Cancer Cell. 2005;8(2):155–67.
17. Linehan WM, Srinivasan R, Schmidt LS. The genetic basis of kidney cancer: a metabolic disease. Nat Rev Urol. 2010;7(5):277–85.
18. Crino PB, Nathanson KL, Henske EP. The tuberous sclerosis complex. N Engl J Med. 2006;355(13):1345–56.
19. Dixon BP, Hulbert JC, Bissler JJ. Tuberous sclerosis complex renal disease. Nephron Exp Nephrol. 2011;118(1):e15–20.
20. Yates JR, et al. The tuberous sclerosis 2000 study: presentation, initial assessments and implications for diagnosis and management. Arch Dis Child. 2011;96(11):1020–5.
21. Siroky BJ, Czyzyk-Krzeska MF, Bissler JJ. Renal involvement in tuberous sclerosis complex and von Hippel-Lindau disease: shared disease mechanisms? Nat Clin Pract Nephrol. 2009;5(3):143–56.
22. Roach ES, Gomez MR, Northrup H. Tuberous sclerosis complex consensus conference: revised clinical diagnostic criteria. J Child Neurol. 1998;13(12):624–8.
23. Menko FH, et al. Birt-Hogg-Dube syndrome: diagnosis and management. Lancet Oncol. 2009;10(12):1199–206.
24. Nickerson ML, et al. Mutations in a novel gene lead to kidney tumors, lung wall defects, and benign tumors of the hair follicle in patients with the Birt-Hogg-Dube syndrome. Cancer Cell. 2002;2(2):157–64.
25. Toro JR, et al. BHD mutations, clinical and molecular genetic investigations of Birt-Hogg-Dube syndrome: a new series of 50 families and a review of published reports. J Med Genet. 2008;45(6):321–31.
26. Lehtonen HJ. Hereditary leiomyomatosis and renal cell cancer: update on clinical and molecular characteristics. Fam Cancer. 2011;10(2):397–411.
27. Alam NA, et al. Clinical features of multiple cutaneous and uterine leiomyomatosis: an underdiagnosed tumor syndrome. Arch Dermatol. 2005;141(2):199–206.
28. Smit DL, et al. Hereditary leiomyomatosis and renal cell cancer in families referred for fumarate hydratase germline mutation analysis. Clin Genet. 2011;79(1):49–59.
29. Woodward ER, et al. Population-based survey of cancer risks in chromosome 3 translocation carriers. Genes Chromosomes Cancer. 2010;49(1):52–8.
30. Schmidt L, et al. Germline and somatic mutations in the tyrosine kinase domain of the MET proto-oncogene in papillary renal carcinomas. Nat Genet. 1997;16(1):68–73.
31. Baysal BE, et al. Mutations in SDHD, a mitochondrial complex II gene, in hereditary paraganglioma. Science. 2000;287(5454):848–51.
32. Ricketts CJ, et al. Tumor risks and genotype-phenotype-proteotype analysis in 358 patients with germline mutations in SDHB and SDHD. Hum Mutat. 2010;31(1):41–51.

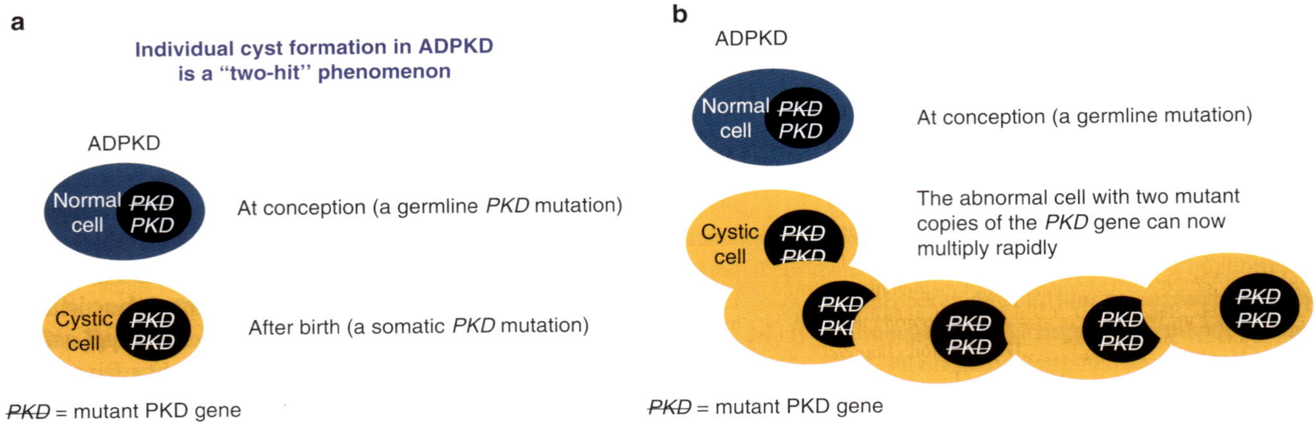

Fig. 41.1 Germline and somatic mutations of the *PKD* gene are required for kidney cyst formation. (**a**) Germline PKD mutation present at conception with subsequent somatic mutational event disrupting the 'normal' copy of the *PKD* gene. (**b**) The 'cystic' cell with mutations in both copies of the PKD gene has an altered phenotype. The 'cystic' cell has a growth advantage and proliferates resulting in development of a kidney cyst

Pathophysiology

Abnormal function of the primary cilium appears to be an integral component of the pathophysiology of ADPKD which can now be considered as one of the many ciliopathy disorders [14].

The primary cilium functions as a calcium-dependent mechanosensor, detecting urinary flow in the collecting tubules (Fig. 41.2). The integral membrane spanning proteins, polycystin-1 and polycystin-2, are located on the primary cilia of renal tubular epithelial cells. The polycystins, together with other primary cilia proteins, regulate cell-cell interactions, epithelial proliferation and downstream signalling events. Polycystins permit calcium influx from the extracellular to the intracellular compartment with alteration in gene expression in response to the flow-dependent movement (mechanosensing) of the primary cilium. Inactivating mutations in *PKD1* and *PKD2* encoding the polycystins lead to the ADPKD phenotype [8].

Several interrelated mechanisms have been proposed to account for cyst formation and growth. Firstly, the ability of the primary cilium to sense urinary flow is compromised with reduced intracellular calcium levels resulting in compensatory increases in second messengers such as cyclic AMP (cAMP) and upregulation of the mammalian target of rapamycin (mTOR) pathway that mediates cell growth and proliferation. Secondly, there is a change in the polarity of tubular cells such that the normal orientation of the mitotic spindle, that would permit tubular elongation without dilatation, is rearranged permitting tubular dilatation and the possibility of cyst formation [6, 22]. Thirdly, within cyst walls the epithelial cells proliferate consequent to the activation of the above mitogenic pathways, and the end point of this is an outpouching from the parent tubule. This outpouching is the beginning of a cyst, and once its diameter exceeds 2 mm, it will eventually lose communication with the glomerular filtrate and become a separate fluid-filled cyst. Fourthly, accumulation of fluid within the cyst is promoted by the effect of antidiuretic hormone (ADH) on the transepithelial secretion of chloride with sodium and

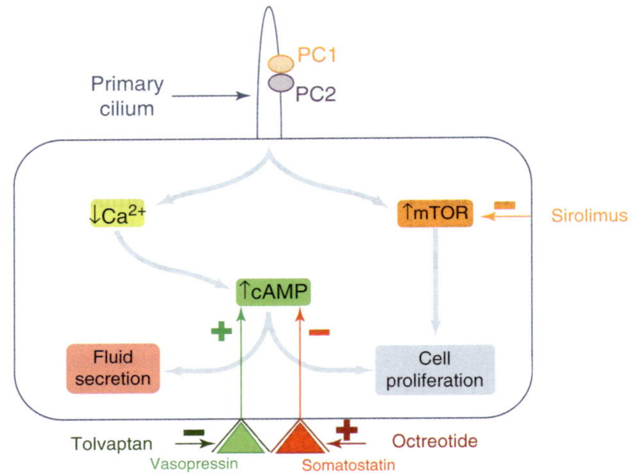

Fig. 41.2 Intracellular signalling disruption in ADPKD. Schematic of a renal tubular epithelial cell and its primary cilium. Mutations in the *PKD1* and *PKD2* genes lead to relative or absolute loss of function of the polycystin complex on the primary cilium. Reduced intracellular calcium influx occurs, and the compensatory increase in cAMP levels promotes fluid secretion and cell proliferation. Cell proliferation is also driven by upregulation of the mTOR pathway secondary to defective ciliary function. Vasopressin (antidiuretic hormone) acting through V2 receptors increases cAMP levels, while somatostatin inhibits cAMP generation. These main pathways are the targets of the therapeutic agents: sirolimus, tolvaptan and octreotide. *cAMP* cyclic adenosine monophosphate, *mTOR* mammalian target of rapamycin, *PC1* polycystin-1, *PC2* polycystin-2

water following into the cyst. The epithelia lining cells of the cyst develop a secretory phenotype, and further fluid expands the cyst. Thus pathways leading to increased intracellular cAMP levels, upregulated and disorganised cell proliferation and fluid accumulation in cysts as a result of both the action of ADH and change to a secretory phenotype have become potential therapeutic targets [4].

The net result of these processes over time is that while only a small number of tubules will generate cysts, those that do give rise to cysts that continually release cytokines and growth factors that stimulate inflammation and fibrosis. As the cyst continues to expand, adjacent structures such as blood vessels, lymphatics and tubules are physically disrupted or obstructed, and the cycle of inflammation, hypoxia and worsening tubular injury with atrophy continues [9]. The remaining glomeruli hyperfilter, but in due course enough parenchyma will have been damaged that there is a steady, irreversible decline in GFR of between 4.4 and 5.9 ml/min per year with eventual progression to ESRD [18].

Unlike the liver, in which synthetic and secretory function is usually unimpaired even in the face of massive cystic involvement, the kidney depends in great measure on the maintenance of a delicate balance between blood supply, lymphatic flow and tubular architecture in order to function. Combined with the limited regenerative capacity of the kidney vis-à-vis the liver, the importance of trying to slow progression of renal damage is readily appreciated.

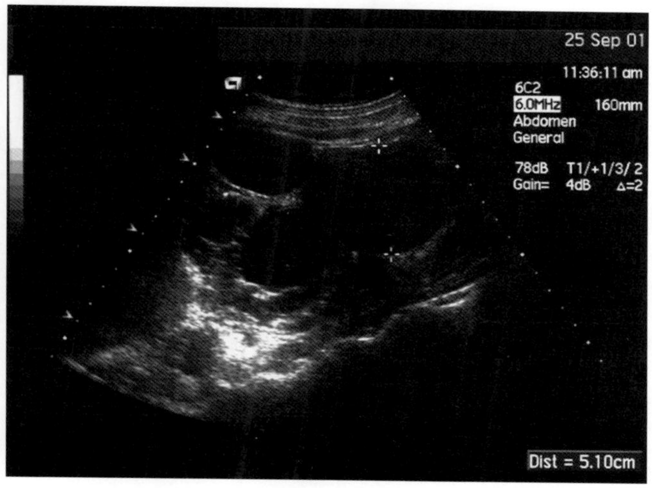

Fig. 41.3 Ultrasound scan of polycystic kidney. The scan demonstrates numerous fluid-filled renal cysts of varying diameter

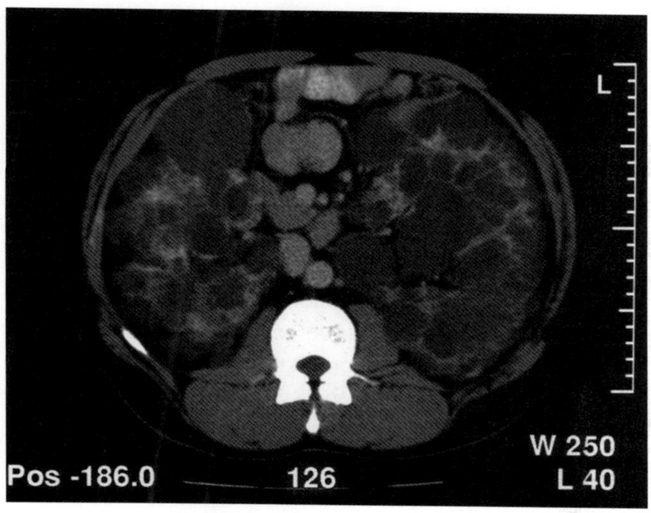

Fig. 41.4 CT scan of the abdomen. Massively enlarged polycystic kidneys occupy most of the abdominal cavity

Clinical Features

The spectrum of presentation of ADPKD is wide and includes both renal and extra-renal features.

Kidney Involvement

ADPKD may be discovered incidentally following imaging tests for other indications or following an ultrasound scan in persons with a positive family history who have requested screening (Figs. 41.3 and 41.4). Hypertension typically emerges in early adulthood and usually prior to obvious increase in kidney size on clinical examination. The hypertension is in part due to distortion of the renal microvasculature by cysts leading to activation of the renin-angiotensin-aldosterone system. Other asymptomatic findings include urinary dipstick abnormalities (non-visible haematuria, proteinuria and/or leucocytes) and as a later feature the presence of abnormal renal function (elevated serum creatinine and reduced eGFR) [10].

Renal cysts may be symptomatic resulting in loin pain secondary to infection or haemorrhage resulting in rapid cyst expansion. Visible haematuria may be secondary to cyst rupture or kidney stone disease. The cysts of PKD are not premalignant but can make the investigation and diagnosis of a coincidental renal cancer challenging, and malignancy should be considered if older patients present with new-onset haematuria.

As indicated previously development of abnormal kidney function tends to be a later feature of ADPKD although several factors are reported to be associated with an earlier decline in GFR. These include inheritance of a *PKD1* mutation versus a *PKD2* mutation (as cysts are present for longer with the *PKD1* genotype), a younger age at ADPKD diagnosis, hypertension from a younger age, male gender, hyperlipidaemia, sickle cell trait, large kidney volumes at diagnosis and visible haematuria [17]. Low birth weight may also be an independent risk factor [20]. When counselling individuals it is often helpful to determine when any affected relatives were diagnosed or required renal replacement therapy. This can help when discussing the prognosis and possible requirement or otherwise for renal replacement therapy. Unfortunately, this is not a completely reliable guide as there can be considerable variation in age at onset of ESRD, even between family members with the same documented *PKD* mutation. This heterogeneity in clinical course reflects modifying contributions from other genes as well as environmental factors which may be triggering the somatic mutational 'hits' on the normal copy of the *PKD* gene, as discussed above. At present there are no useful urinary or plasma biomarkers, other than serum creatinine, to reliably predict risk of progression in ADPKD [21].

Other Organ Involvement in ADPKD

Extra-renal features include cysts in other organs, most commonly the liver, but also in the pancreas, spleen, arachnoid membranes and seminal vesicles. There is no relationship between ADPKD and polycystic ovarian syndrome [1]. *Polycystic liver disease* (PLD) is the most common extra-renal manifestation of ADPKD (present in up to 83 % of affected individuals), and hepatic cysts can cause massive liver enlargement with abdominal pain, distension, early satiety, nausea and vomiting. It is uncommon for liver function tests (LFTs) to be abnormal due to the presence of cysts alone, and so alternative explanations such as liver cyst infection or biliary tract obstruction should be sought if a rise in LFTs is observed. Symptoms of hepatic pain, compression of the inferior vena cava or recurrent infection may require surgery [32]. Interestingly, women tend to have more severe liver cyst involvement than men, with multiparity and oestrogen exposure being recognised risk factors for PLD.

Intracranial aneurysms are perhaps the most feared extra-renal complication occurring in up to 8 % of those with PKD. A family history of intracranial haemorrhage is present in 10 %, and in those in whom an aneurysm ruptures, the median age is 39 years for those with PKD compared with 51 years for the general population. Indeed, many of the individuals with an intracranial bleed had normal renal function, and a third were normotensive at the time of aneurysm rupture. Screening for intracranial aneurysm remains controversial; definite indications for screening with MRI or CT include a personal or family history of rupture, presence of warning symptoms such as a headache or focal neurological deficit or for those in whom a loss of consciousness while working would place them or others at serious risk of harm. At present screening is not recommended outside of these scenarios unless the patient requests investigation. If an aneurysm is larger than 7–10 mm, there is an increased risk of rupture, but smaller aneurysms are generally safely managed by interval scanning [16]. Intervention for smaller, asymptomatic aneurysms is not without danger, and so the risk-benefit ratio of intervention mandates individual discussion with neurosurgical colleagues and careful explanation to patients.

Other extra-renal manifestations of PKD include an increased risk of abdominal herniae (especially in those who elect to perform peritoneal dialysis), colonic diverticula and various cardiac valvular lesions, the most common being mitral valve prolapse which occurs in up to 25 % of persons with ADPKD. Occasional case reports of thoracic aortic aneurysms have been published, and it is worth bearing this in mind if a patient presents with back pain, hypotension or chest pain for which no other obvious cause is apparent [7].

Fertility is not affected by the presence of ADPKD unless renal function is compromised. Women with normal blood pressure and renal function usually have uncomplicated pregnancies, but those with hypertension are at an increased risk of pre-eclampsia and progressive chronic kidney disease and so should receive counselling, ideally pre-conceptually, with early discussion between nephrologists and obstetricians [33]. Hypertension should be managed using drugs that are not obviously teratogenic. Male fertility can be affected by seminal or prostatic cysts.

The *psychological impact* of living with ADPKD can easily be overlooked. Some individuals may consider themselves as having an incurable illness, or may fear rapid progression to ESRD, especially if other family members required renal replacement therapy at a young age. The presence of chronic pain or discomfort from polycystic organs may contribute to depression. Uncertainty concerning the prognosis of younger family members or children can also be a source of considerable psychosocial stress, and studies are ongoing into this area [5]. Patients should be counselled about the management of chronic pain and advised not to use NSAIDs. The addition of a tricyclic antidepressant may be useful for both depression and pain.

Differential Diagnosis

Multiple kidney cysts occurring at a young age, presence of developmental malformations or the early onset of gout or type 2 diabetes should prompt consideration of alternative diagnoses to ADPKD and discussion with a clinical geneticist. Rarely individuals have a deletion of both *PKD1* and the adjacent *TSC2* gene on chromosome 16p and express the tuberous sclerosis phenotype in addition to having a much earlier onset of ADPKD in infancy [3]. Others who possess mutations in both *PKD1* and *PKD2* also display more severe disease. The main differential diagnoses for PKD are listed in Table 41.1.

Table 41.1 Renal cystic disorders

Cystic kidney disease (*and mode of inheritance*)	Incidence	Clinical features distinguishing from ADPKD	Comments
Acquired cystic disease of the kidney (*not inherited*)	5–20 % incident dialysis patients 80–100 % after 10 years on dialysis	Cysts develop as a consequence of ESRD due to causes other than ADPKD	Cysts have premalignant potential (unlike those of PKD). Individuals on dialysis with new haematuria should be investigated for RCC in cysts
Tuberous sclerosis complex (*autosomal dominant*)	1:6,000	Characteristic facial and skin signs. CNS hamartomas, developmental delay, epilepsy	Multiple renal cysts with benign angiomyolipomas which may harbour RCC. Mutations in *TSC1* and *TSC2* genes
Autosomal recessive polycystic kidney disease	1:20,000	Diagnosis in utero or infancy; hepatic fibrosis, portal hypertension	Gene defect in *PKHD1* encoding polyductin. May require liver and kidney transplantation
Von Hippel-Lindau disease (*autosomal dominant*)	1:36,000	Retinal, cerebellar, spinal and renal tumours	Mutations in *VHL* gene
Nephronophthisis (*autosomal recessive*)	1:50,000 to 1:100,000	Retinal dystrophy, blindness, oculomotor apraxia, developmental delay (10 % cases); kidneys often normal or small in size	The most common genetic cause of renal failure in children
Medullary cystic kidney disease (*autosomal dominant*)	1:100,000	Hyperuricaemia, gout, medullary cysts	Creatinine often elevated prior to the later appearance of cysts
Polycystic liver disease (*autosomal dominant*)	Unknown	Minor, if any, renal cystic involvement	Mutations in *PRKCSH* or *SEC63* genes
MODY5 (*autosomal dominant*)	Unknown	Renal cysts and diabetes syndrome. Pancreatic atrophy. May be associated with other structural genitourinary malformations	Mutations in *HNF1B* gene. Part of the maturity onset diabetes of the young (MODY) spectrum
Oral-facial-digital syndrome type 1 (*X-linked dominant*)	1:250,000	Facial, oral cavity and digital malformations with polycystic kidneys	Considered lethal in males. Mutations in *OFD1* gene

ADPKD autosomal dominant polycystic kidney disease, *RCC* renal cell carcinoma, *ESRD* end-stage renal disease, *CNS* central nervous system

Treatment of Polycystic Kidney Disease

General Principles

Identification and treatment of hypertension, dietary salt restriction, avoiding excess dietary protein intake, early introduction of statin treatment and efforts to correct disorders of bone mineral metabolism may all help to reduce progression of PKD and decrease cardiovascular morbidity. Prompt treatment of cyst infections is most effective with lipid soluble antibiotics which have better tissue penetration, e.g. ciprofloxacin or sulphamethoxazole-trimethoprim. Haematuria may be secondary to cyst rupture, but it is important to consider other diagnoses that may result in renal tract bleeding including nephrolithiasis and urological malignancy.

Hypertension

The development of hypertension is almost universal in ADPKD and is typically present when the kidneys have increased in size but before renal failure is present. Loss of normal nocturnal dipping in blood pressure occurs usually in younger adults before the emergence of more sustained hypertension. Antihypertensive treatment reduces the risk of hypertension-related complications in chronic kidney disease, but lowering blood pressure has not convincingly been demonstrated to retard progression of ADPKD. Hypertension will respond to renin-angiotensin axis blockade with ACE inhibitors or angiotensin receptor blockers (ARBs). Use of diuretics should be avoided because of experimental evidence that cyst growth is mediated by vasopressin (antidiuretic hormone). In theory, diuretic-induced intravascular volume depletion could accelerate cyst growth by increasing vasopressin levels. In contrast, maintaining a high daily oral fluid intake will suppress vasopressin release, and this strategy may be beneficial in the long-term management of ADPKD.

Preparing for Renal Replacement Therapy

ADPKD is typically slowly progressive with a predictable rate of GFR decline allowing advanced planning for renal replacement therapy (RRT). The median age of ESRD onset for persons with the more prevalent *PKD1* gene defect is 54 years of age [13]. One of the advantages of prolonged follow-up of persons with ADPKD at nephrology clinics is the ability to plan in advance the choice of RRT and optimal timing of RRT start.

Options for RRT include pre-emptive kidney transplant (living donor or listing for deceased donor transplant), haemodialysis or peritoneal dialysis. Outcomes for persons with ADPKD who are successfully transplanted are generally more favourable than for any other common cause of ESRD such as diabetes or glomerulonephritis. There is obviously no risk of recurrent disease in the renal allograft.

Practical Implications for Renal Replacement Therapy in Persons with ADPKD

The *physical size of polycystic kidneys* may be a significant clinical issue when planning for pre-emptive transplantation. Accurate measurement of kidney size, employing MRI or CT scanning, will allow the volume of each kidney to be assessed. Occasionally nephrectomy is indicated if there is persistent opiate-dependent pain, recurrent cyst infection, staghorn calculi or persistent visible haematuria resulting in anaemia. Further discussion with the transplant surgery team is necessary to establish if there will be sufficient room in the pelvis for surgical placement of a transplanted kidney (Fig. 41.5). If not, then the patient will need counselling on the requirement for polycystic kidney nephrectomy and the attendant risks of this procedure. Surgeons may elect to perform bilateral nephrectomy to ensure adequate space for transplant in either the left or right iliac fossa. Either open or laparoscopic nephrectomy is the surgical option.

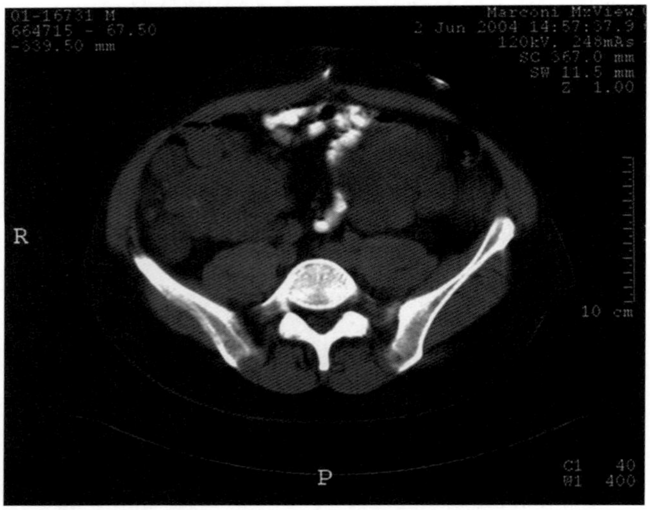

Fig. 41.5 CT scan of the pelvis. Massively enlarged polycystic kidneys extend into the pelvis. Bilateral nephrectomy was subsequently undertaken to enable this patient to have a successful renal transplant procedure

Other *indications for nephrectomy* include recurrent kidney cyst infections, persistent cyst pain and recurrent visible haematuria. The risk of kidney cancer is not increased in persons with polycystic kidney disease, but the diagnosis of cancer is challenging since symptoms of loin pain and visible haematuria are common and often reasonably attributed to ADPKD itself. Imaging of the kidneys to identify malignancy is problematic too since the renal anatomy is already grossly distorted by multiple simple and complex cysts. Occasionally an incidental renal cell carcinoma is found on careful sectioning of a polycystic kidney following nephrectomy. The finding of an incidental cancer will mean delaying transplantation until further cancer workup is completed and a disease-free interval is recorded.

Bilateral nephrectomy in ADPKD is a major procedure with considerable post-operative morbidity, and patients need to be advised concerning chest, wound and retroperitoneal infections and requirement for blood transfusion (with risk of HLA sensitisation) in the perioperative period. As the patient is anuric, they are rendered dialysis dependent, and only haemodialysis support is suitable in the post-op period. In view of these considerations, it is generally advisable to have established reliable vascular access, preferably by creating an arteriovenous fistula, prior to proceeding to nephrectomy. If a fistula has been fashioned, it may be several months before it is mature enough to be usable as vascular access. In the absence of a fistula (or arteriovenous graft), a tunnelled jugular vein catheter may be placed preoperatively. Haemodialysis support immediately post bilateral nephrectomy can be complicated by difficulties establishing an accurate dry weight. It is important to account for the weight loss related to both the removal of the large kidneys (as much as 6–8 kg) and the loss of intravascular volume if there is continued oozing of tissue fluid from the retroperitoneal site of operation into a 'third space'. Post-operative ileus with intraluminal accumulation of fluid may also occur due to intraoperative bowel mobilisation.

Recovery from bilateral nephrectomy may take several months; therefore, in planning an elective living donor transplant procedure, it is generally prudent to wait for at least 3–6 months before proceeding to transplantation.

The physical size of polycystic kidneys also has practical implications for placement of a *peritoneal dialysis* catheter and subsequent effective peritoneal dialysis therapy. Enlarged kidneys may make it difficult to ensure appropriate placement of the catheter tip in the pelvis and increase the likelihood of migration of the catheter within the abdomen. Larger volumes of peritoneal dialysate in CAPD or APD regimens are also more likely to cause patient discomfort. The addition of peritoneal dialysate fluid can exacerbate the predisposition to abdominal herniae (which are more common in persons with ADPKD). Cyst pain and cyst infection in polycystic kidneys may mimic symptoms and signs of peritonitis and

Table 41.2 Ultrasound criteria for diagnosis of ADPKD in persons with a positive family history

Age (years)	*PKD1* genotype	*PKD2* genotype	Unknown genotype
15–29	≥3 cysts[a] (94.3 %)	≥3 cysts[a] (69.5 %)	≥3 cysts[a] (81.7 %)
30–39	≥3 cysts[a] (96.6 %)	≥3 cysts[a] (94.9 %)	≥3 cysts[a] (95.5 %)
40–59	≥2 cysts in each kidney (92.6 %)	≥2 cysts in each kidney (88.8 %)	≥2 cysts in each kidney (90 %)
≥60	≥4 cysts in each kidney (100 %)	≥4 cysts in each kidney (100 %)	≥4 cysts in each kidney (100 %)

Adapted from Pei et al. [23]
All criteria have a 100 % positive predictive value
Percentage sensitivity for criteria provided for each category
[a]Unilateral or bilateral

can lead to diagnostic dilemmas if peritoneal dialysate effluent cultures are negative. Rupture of a kidney cyst can occasionally lead to visible blood staining of peritoneal fluid. Although this is an alarming symptom for patients to experience, it is usually self-limiting and settles without need for intervention. Despite these potential complications many patients will be able to tolerate peritoneal dialysis.

Assessment of a Potential Living Related Kidney Donor When There Is a Family History of ADPKD

Adult offspring of an affected parent may be considered as potential living related kidney donors. Typically the affected parent will have a *PKD1* mutation, i.e. median age of onset of ESRD in their fifties. All potential living kidney donors will have detailed kidney imaging as part of their extended clinical assessment. A CT scan or MRI (undertaken to identify number and calibre of kidney blood vessels) will be able to exclude ADPKD in potential adult donors. All potential donors should be counselled about the possibility of an ADPKD diagnosis being established before embarking on assessment.

ADPKD Diagnosis When Genotype Is Unknown

Ultrasound is the safest and most cost-effective imaging technique to establish a diagnosis of ADPKD. Molecular genotyping is rarely performed in clinical practice outside of a defined research project. If there is no prior family history of PKD, the diagnosis can be challenging particularly in younger adults who have been referred for assessment with relatively few cysts in each kidney. It is generally accepted that in adults the presence of ten or more cysts in each kidney is diagnostic of ADPKD in the absence of renal or extrarenal features of rarer cystic kidney disorders such as tuberous sclerosis complex or von Hippel-Lindau syndrome.

Age-dependent ultrasound criteria for the diagnosis of ADPKD in families with *PKD1* mutation have been in use since the 1990s [24]. These specify that a diagnosis of ADPKD is established in individuals with a *PKD1* mutation family history if the following age-dependent cyst numbers are present: 15–30 years of age with at least two unilateral or bilateral cysts, 30–59 years of age with at least two cysts in each kidney and >60 years of age with at least four cysts in each kidney. In practice, it is often uncertain whether an individual presenting with cystic kidneys has a family history of ADPKD secondary to a *PKD1* or *PKD2* mutation.

Unified age-dependent criteria for the diagnosis of ADPKD in families of unknown genotype have recently been published [23]. A diagnosis of ADPKD is established as follows: the presence of three or more cysts (unilateral or bilateral) in individuals 15–39 years of age, two or more cysts in each kidney in individuals 40–59 years of age and four or more cysts in each kidney in persons >60 years of age (Table 41.2). If a family member is being considered as a potential living kidney donor, then the diagnosis of PKD is excluded if there are two or fewer cysts in individuals >40 years of age (despite the personal history of ADPKD). A diagnosis of ADPKD is almost certainly excluded when renal cysts are absent in individuals 30–39 years of age (false-negative rate 0.7 %) [23].

Reliable Genetic Testing

Careful attention to the ADPKD patient's family history can often provide a simple and reliable means of predicting the causative mutated gene (*PKD1* or *PKD2*). The family history of renal disease severity is predictive of the *PKD* mutation. A *PKD1* mutation is highly likely (positive predictive value 100 %, sensitivity 72 %) for patients with a family member with ADPKD who developed ESRD at <55 years of age. A *PKD2* mutation is predicted for a patient with at least one affected family member who continued to have sufficient renal function or developed ESRD when they were >70 years of age (positive predictive value 100 %, sensitivity 74 %) [2].

In practice there is clinical overlap between the phenotypes associated with *PKD1* and *PKD2* mutations, e.g. a patient with ESRD in their mid-sixties may harbour either a *PKD1* or *PKD2* mutation. There can be extensive within-family variation in ADPKD with disease variability presum-

Other Cystic Kidney Diseases

42

Daniel M. McGuinness, Mark Harber, and Stephen D. Marks

Beyond ADPKD there are many other causes of renal cysts, both congenital and acquired which may present at a variety of time points through life. They can vary from simple, incidentally found cysts with no prognostic implications, to multiple large cysts that result in declining renal function and the requirement of renal replacement therapy.

The commonest renal cystic processes are simple cysts which are seen with increasing age and tend to be rare in young patients but have been reported incidentally in up to 50 % of CT imaging performed in those over the age of 40 years. They have a typical appearance of fluid-filled sacs on ultrasound imaging but are better defined with cross-sectional imaging. Cystic lesions can be categorised using the Bosniak Classification (see Chap. 38).

Acquired Cystic Kidney Disease

Acquired cystic kidney disease (ACKD) occurs in the context of chronic kidney disease (CKD) and therefore may be a concern for primary care physicians and general physicians as well as nephrologists and urologists. As it is a cystic condition associated with CKD, the kidneys are usually small to normal in size in contrast to adult polycystic kidney disease. It is characterised by the development of multiple cysts bilaterally which are usually less than 0.5 cm in diameter and are rarely greater than 2–3 cm [1]. As patients progress through successive stages of CKD and onto renal replacement therapy (RRT), the incidence of ACKD increases with a third of patients affected after 3 years of haemodialysis and occurring in up to 80 % of patients after 10 years of dialysis. Both men and women are affected equally independent of age [2]. Modality of dialysis, peritoneal or haemodialysis, appears to have no influence on the development of cysts. Plasticisers used in dialysis have been implicated in the pathogenesis of renal cyst formation but the mechanisms of the development of ACKD are not yet fully elucidated. Cysts develop in the renal tubules, and analysis of cyst fluid and epithelium suggests an origin in the proximal tubules [1]. It is thought that the process itself is driven by proto-oncogenes [3] and for this reason may explain the increased rate of renal cell carcinoma secondary to unregulated cellular proliferation (see below).

In its early stages acquired cysts are usually asymptomatic and are increasingly discovered incidentally on abdominal imaging; however, occasionally their discovery can result from the investigation of both microscopic and macroscopic haematuria, urinary tract infection, sepsis of unknown origin secondary to cyst infection, back and loin pain secondary to retroperitoneal cyst rupture, erythrocytosis or development of malignancy [1] (see Fig. 42.1). There is no association between the primary cause of renal impairment and the likelihood of development of ACKD.

Whilst the majority of ACKD runs a benign course, there is up to a 50-fold increase in the risk of development of renal cell carcinoma (RCC) compared to the general population [4]; prospective studies [5, 6] have placed its incidence at 1.7–7 % with time on dialysis (>3 years) being an important risk factor (transplantation appears to reduce risk), this incidence being much lower than the 20 % first reported in the 1970s. RCCs in ACKD are multicentric in 50 % of cases and bilateral in 9 %. It has recently become apparent that clear cell carcinoma which usually accounts for 70–80 %

D.M. McGuinness, MBBS, BSc, MRCP
UCL Centre for Nephrology, Royal Free Hospital, Pond Street, London, NW3 2QG, UK
e-mail: d.mcguinness@ucl.ac.uk

M. Harber, MBBS, PhD, FRCP
UCL Department of Nephrology, Royal Free London NHS Foundation Trust, Pond Street, Hampstead, London, NW3 2QG, UK
e-mail: mark.harber@nhs.net

S.D. Marks, MD, MSc, MRCP, DCH, FRCPCH (✉)
Department of Paediatric Nephrology, Great Ormond Street Hospital for Children NHS Foundation Trust, Great Ormond Street, London, WC1N 3JH, UK
e-mail: stephen.marks@gosh.nhs.uk

M. Harber (ed.), *Practical Nephrology*,
DOI 10.1007/978-1-4471-5547-8_42, © Springer-Verlag London 2014

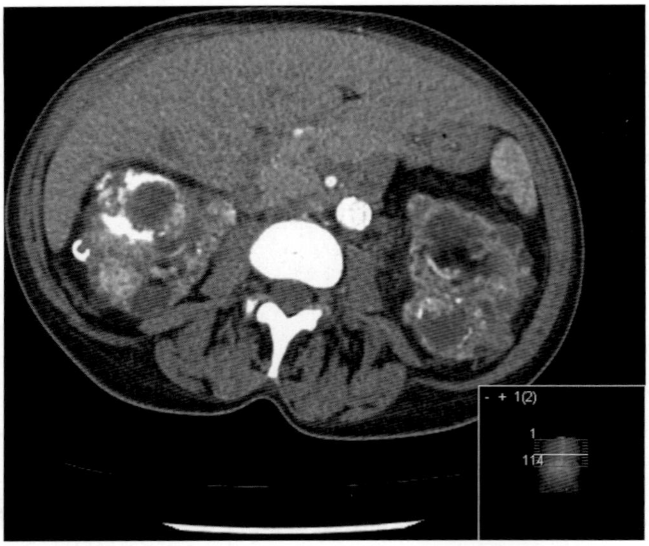

Fig. 42.1 Acquired cystic kidney disease: The CT scan of a long-standing haemodialysis patient who presented with erythropoietin resistance and haematuria. The scan shows the characteristic features of multiple complex cysts with extensive calcification

of RCCs only represents 10 % of RCC in ACKD. Sixty per cent of RCCs in ACKD appear to be due to two novel tumour types: (1) acquired cystic disease-associated RCC (ACDARCC) which appears to be unique to ACKD and (2) clear cell papillary RCC of end-stage kidney. ACDARCC tumours are often surrounded by a dense fibrous capsule and characteristically have extensive oxalate crystals within them [7]. These novel renal cancers may explain the rather surprising findings of better outcomes from RCC in patients with ESRD compared to other patients with RCC.

Renal cell carcinoma remains a clinical concern in patients with ACKD post-transplantation, and tumours may behave more aggressively in this setting, so careful monitoring must be considered in these patients [8]. Guidelines on who to screen and when have been inconsistent with some groups advocating screening 'high-risk' patients, but do not define high risk [9]. Renal ultrasound may be useful, but sensitivity for detecting small tumours is limited but this is improving with technology, and frequency of screening has not been established with some suggesting twice yearly and others recommending screening should be conducted every 2 years. For those with ACKD yearly screening seems appropriate. Due to a lack of evidence of benefits and the cost-effectiveness of screening, they were unable to recommend a particular method [9]. KDIGO guidelines from 2002 comment that ultrasound screening could be performed but found no data for the optimum frequency.

Both CT with contrast enhancement and MRI offer greater sensitivity for detecting tumours <1 cm. Despite improved sensitivity there is no data to support their routine use, and therefore decisions on local practice should be guided by consideration of the needs of the patient, potential complications of one modality and the results of previous imaging. A consensus that patients treated with dialysis for 3 years should undergo ultrasound is practical in patients with a reasonable life expectancy. If a mass is detected, then contrast-enhanced imaging should be performed yearly for surveillance unless criteria are reached for intervention [10].

Autosomal Recessive Polycystic Kidney Disease

Autosomal recessive polycystic kidney disease (ARPKD) usually manifests in childhood. Its incidence is estimated at 1:10,000 to 1:40,000 and it is seen more frequently in Caucasians [11]. This may be an underestimate however as some children will die in infancy (often secondary to pulmonary hypoplasia as a consequence of oligohydramnios) without a diagnosis. Its characteristic features are of cystic dilatations of the renal collecting ducts and congenital hepatic fibrosis. Whilst predominantly diagnosed in early childhood, often it can be asymptomatic and may not be discovered until later in childhood or adolescence.

ARPKD is the result of mutations in the PKDH1 gene located at 6p21region of chromosome 6 which encodes the transmembrane protein fibrocystin (or polyductin) [12]. It is primarily a disease of ciliary dysfunction. Evidence suggests this dysfunction results in cyst development and expansion as a consequence of its role in intracellular calcium regulation and sodium transport [13].

Around half of cases are diagnosed antenatally [14] the remainder usually diagnosed neonatally or during infancy. Prenatal ultrasound can reveal oligohydramnios in severe cases and markedly enlarged kidneys. Neonates present with large palpable flank masses and the consequences of renal disease, notably hypertension [13]. Whilst there is always hepatic involvement, this may not be clinically evident. Those who present later in life tend to do so as a consequence of hepatic disease (congenital hepatic fibrosis) and will often demonstrate the sequelae of chronic liver disease, portal hypertension and varices but may also present with deteriorating renal function, hypertension, haematuria and mild proteinuria [11]. The more severe cases may present with ultrasound features of Caroli's disease.

Whilst genetic testing is possible, in clinical practice diagnosis of ARPKD is made on clinical assessment, imaging and biochemistry. Features suggestive include:

1. Bilaterally enlarged, hyperechogenic kidneys with multiple small cysts (1–2 mm) and loss of corticomedullary differentiation and either
2. Signs or imaging compatible with hepatic fibrosis such as dilated bile ducts, evidence of portal hypertension

3. Or ARPKD in a sibling with exclusion of ADPKD in either biological parent

Detailed ultrasound and HIDA scan of children with ARPKD is normally suffice for hepatic assessment without the need for contrast-enhanced CT scanning.

Management of ARPKD is supportive with ongoing care focused on the complications of declining renal function, sepsis from pyelonephritis, infected cysts or ascending cholangitis, liver complications and eventually end-stage renal disease. Parents should be aware that further children will have a 25 % chance of being affected and a 50 % chance of being a carrier for the mutation in PKDH1 [15]. Although a parent may be a carrier as it is recessive, this would not prevent donation. Some patients may require combined liver-kidney transplant and should be jointly assessed if there is significant hepatic involvement.

Medullary Sponge Kidney

Medullary sponge kidney (MSK) is a congenital dilatation of the distal collecting tubules with subsequent enlargement of the affected pyramids; changes are confined to the medulla. It typically affects both kidneys but can also be present unilaterally or variably in different papillae [16]. It generally manifests as nephrocalcinosis and recurrent renal stones [17]; however, it may be diagnosed incidentally on radiological imaging for other indications. In an unselected radiological series, it has been observed in 0.5–1 % of cases, but occurs in up to 20 % of recurrent calcium stone formers [17]. There appears to be no male or female preponderance or racial difference in prevalence and is generally diagnosed in adulthood.

In itself MSK is symptomless, but presentations often result from its complications, most frequently renal stones and urinary tract infections. It may be associated with hemihypertrophy. There is almost universally microscopic haematuria, but macroscopic haematuria can result from urinary tract infections and stones.

Stones are predominantly calcium phosphate and calcium oxalate as a consequence of hypercalciuria, of which the mechanism is not understood. In the majority of cases, urinary acidification is inadequate with a resultant acidosis; however, this is usually incomplete and rarely does a full distal tubular renal acidosis occur.

The pathogenesis of MSK is poorly understood but appears to be congenital and is considered sporadic. To support this it has been noted to be associated with a number of congenital renal disorders as well as non-renal developmental abnormalities including hemihypertrophy, Beckwith-Wiedemann syndrome, Wilm's tumour, ADPKD, Marfan's syndrome, Ehlers-Danlos syndrome and horseshoe kidney. Given this, it is postulated that the pathogenesis lies in the renal morphogenesis, and mutations in glial cell line-derived neurotrophic factor, a protein involved in renal development, have been demonstrated in MSK [17].

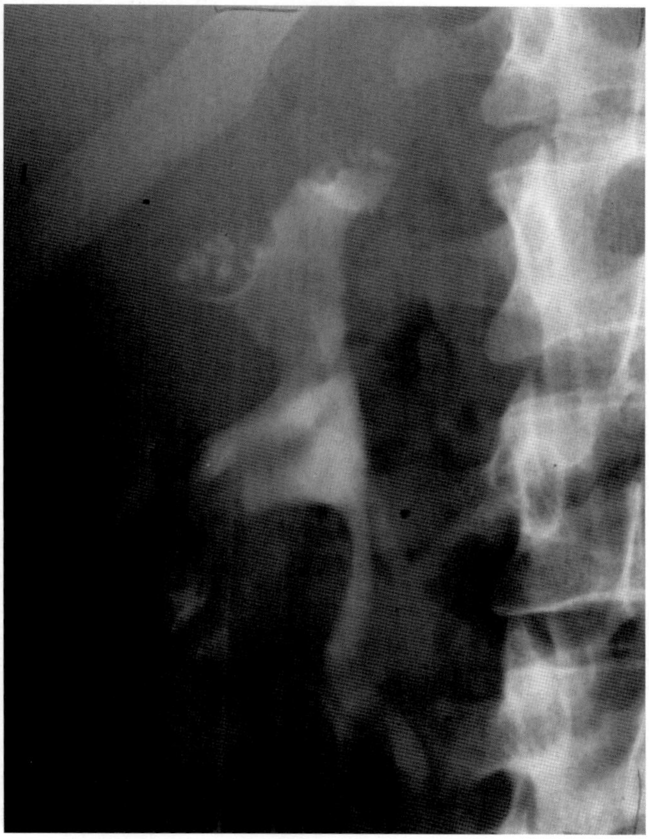

Fig. 42.2 Intravenous pyelogram in a patient with medullary sponge kidney showing the characteristic 'bunch of grapes' appearance

Diagnosis of MSK is usually made radiologically with IV urogram the gold standard. Contrast is seen collecting in dilated papillary ducts with a resultant blush in mild cases, or in more severe cases the typical 'bouquet' or 'bunch of grapes' appearance is seen (see Fig. 42.2). In a proportion of cases, nephrocalcinosis will be revealed. Unenhanced CT has replaced IV urograms in most hospitals but unfortunately has a poorer sensitivity, so making the diagnosis of MSK is one of the few reasons to request an IV urogram over a CT KUB.

There is no treatment for the condition per se, and management revolves around treating and preventing the complications, be that infective or stone related. Thiazide diuretics can be used to reduce urinary calcium excretion and decrease risk of stone formation. Given the partial distal renal tubular acidosis, some have advocated treatment with alkali citrate, with increments in dosage until 24-h collection urinary pH <7.5 demonstrating a decreased frequency of stone formation and improvement in bone mineral density [17].

Nephronophthisis

Nephronophthisis is the commonest genetic cause of end-stage renal failure in the first two decades of life. It is an autosomal recessive condition resulting from one of the NPHP genes (currently 1–11), most commonly a large deletion in exon 2 of the NPHP gene and affecting about 1 in 50,000 individuals. The mutations result in a ciliopathy, and in some cases this is associated with significant extra-renal manifestations as well as nephronophthisis (see Table 42.1) [18].

Homozygous deletion of NPHP1 gene represents the commonest known mutation (20 %) of isolated nephronophthisis, but the mutation may not be known for many affected cases where clinical diagnosis is necessary.

Histologically there is tubular basement membrane disintegration (expansion and thinning), interstitial cell infiltration with fibrosis and later tubular atrophy with cyst generation, predominantly at the corticomedullary junction [19].

The commonest form of nephronophthisis results in ESRD by 13 years of age with infantile forms and adolescent forms reaching ESRD before 4 years and 19 years of age, respectively. Initial presentation is often with polyuria and polydipsia as a result of inadequate urinary concentration and disproportionate anaemia with progressive CKD. Kidneys usually maintain a normal size in contrast to PKD or other forms of CKD. Poor growth is common in children with nephronophthisis.

Genetic screening may be diagnostic, but more often the diagnosis will be suggested by a combination of clinical features, (polyuria and polydipsia, enuresis, renal impairment, anaemia) imaging and histology. Renal ultrasound (or MRI) can aid diagnosis and demonstrate medullary cysts with loss of corticomedullary differentiation and normal- to slightly small-sized kidneys. If the diagnosis is entertained, then retinal screening is important.

Table 42.1 Syndromes and conditions associated with nephronophthisis

Senior-Loken syndrome	AR associated with retinitis pigmentosa, retinal aplasia with phenotype of Leber's amaurosis and renal dysplasia
Joubert's syndrome	AR associated with, cerebellar vermis hypoplasia, developmental delay retinal dystrophy with dysregulated eye movements, coloboma and renal dysplasia
Meckel-Gruber syndrome	AR associated with renal dysplasia, polydactyly, encephalocoele and hepatic ductal dysplasia and cysts
Cogan syndrome	AR disorder associated with liver fibrosis, hearing loss and oculomotor apraxia
Cone-shaped epiphyses	
Situs inversus	
Bronchiectasis	

Bardet-Biedl Syndrome

It is another rare (1:150,000) autosomal recessive ciliopathy associated with retinitis pigmentosa presenting with night blindness in childhood with complete blindness by 15 years. Centripetal obesity is common and can be marked; polydactyl (60–70 %), deafness, hypogonadism in males, genital abnormalities in females and learning difficulties are also common associations. Renal abnormalities occur in 50 % and are most commonly cystic dysplastic changes (including calyceal cysts), histology showing features similar to nephronophthisis, concentrating defects and progression to ESRD common in those affected.

Medullary Cystic Kidney Disease

MCKDs are autosomal dominant conditions now divided into MCKD 1 and 2, causing ESRD in adulthood. Two gene loci have been identified in MCKD, MCKD1 and MCKD2 at 1q21 and 16p12, respectively. MCKD-1 has almost identical histological characteristic to nephronophthisis and is characterised by chronic tubulointerstitial nephritis with cyst development at the corticomedullary junction.

Clinically MCKD-1 has similar features to nephronophthisis with a concentrating defect and otherwise fairly silent progressive CKD, but a median onset of ESRD much later at 62 years and no extra-renal involvement. MCKD should be considered in any patient with otherwise unexplained CKD especially if there is evidence of a family history, polyuria/polydipsia and medullary renal cysts. On imaging the kidneys are either normal sized or only slightly small with corticomedullary cysts. There is no specific treatment apart from maintaining fluid and electrolyte balance, but transplantation is curative.

MCKD-2 is associated with a defect in the uromodulin gene (UMOD) which codes for the Tamm-Horsfall protein and results in hyperuricaemia and juvenile-onset gout. The condition is similar to juvenile hyperuricaemic nephropathy, and because of the autosomal dominance, parents are often alert to the significance of gout in their children. It is not clear if urate reduction therapy slows the rate of ESRD, but it seems prudent to try this not least as a way of reducing the burden of gout. The onset of ESRD in MCKD-2 is early at about 32 years [19], and as with MCKD-1 and nephronophthisis, transplantation is curative and without recurrence.

Renal Coloboma Syndrome

It is a rare autosomal dominant condition with PAX2 mutations causing coloboma (Fig. 42.3), renal cysts and tumours (overexpression) and renal hypoplasia (underexpression).

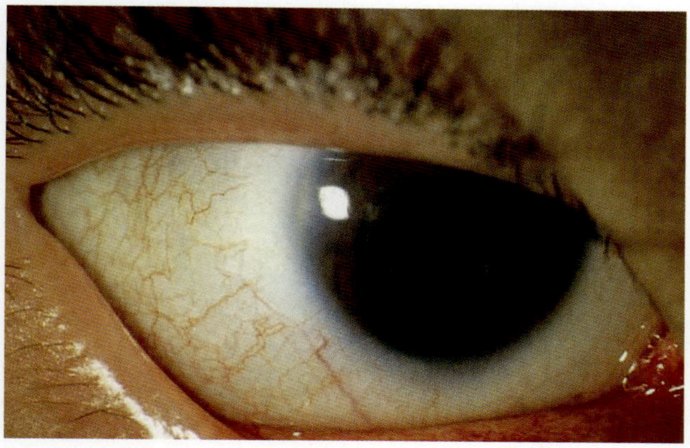

Fig. 42.3 Retinal coloboma in a patient with renal coloboma syndrome

Glomerulocystic Disease (Associated with Maturity-Onset Diabetes of the Young (MODY)

This autosomal dominant condition associated with hepatocyte nuclear factor (HNF)-1β mutations (as part of renal cysts and diabetes (RCAD) syndrome). It presents antenatally or postnatally with chronic kidney disease, hypertension and early-onset diabetes and is associated with renal magnesium wasting and hypomagnesaemia. Renal ultrasound demonstrates differing renal size with presence of glomerular cysts. A family history or history of MODY should raise suspicions.

Summary

Ciliopathies are responsible for a significant burden of ESRD with many of these cases diagnosed by paediatric nephrologists and then transitioned to adult care. In some there will be significant extra-renal manifestations, and a holistic approach to care will be needed. Some of these conditions may present in adulthood with limited clues to the cause of ESRD. A careful family history, thoughtful imaging for location of cysts and biopsy where appropriate may guide the diagnosis. Our understanding of genetics of renal conditions is improving every year; ante- and postnatal diagnosis increasingly can be confirmed using direct mutational analysis and linkage testing. Consequently genetic counselling is often possible without performing renal biopsies on patients. Even when mutational analysis is not available, it is worth considering storing DNA for the future. Ultimately, transplantation is curative of the underlying renal condition.

Resources

Contact a family. http://www.cafamily.org.uk/. Accessed 18 Mar 2012.

Information sheets for children and adolescents. http://www.gosh.nhs.uk/children/about-your-condition/; http://www.gosh.nhs.uk/teenagers/about-your-condition/. Accessed 18 Mar 2012.

Information sheets for parents. http://www.gosh.nhs.uk/medical-conditions/. Accessed 18 Mar 2012.

RaDaR: National Renal Rare Disease Registry. https://www.renalradar.org. Accessed 18 Mar 2012.

UK Genetic Testing Network. http://www.ukgtn.nhs.uk/gtn/Search+for+a+Test/Search+by+Disease+or+Gene. Accessed 18 Mar 2012.

References

1. Grantham JJ. Acquired cystic kidney disease. Kidney Int. 1991;40:143.
2. Matson MA, Cohen EP. Acquired cystic kidney disease: occurrence, prevalence, and renal cancers. Medicine (Baltimore). 1990;69(4):217–26.
3. Herrera GA. C-erb B-2 amplification in cystic renal disease. Kidney Int. 1991;40(3):509–13.
4. Truong LD. Renal neoplasm in acquired cystic kidney disease. Am J Kidney Dis. 1995;26(1):1–12.
5. Ishikawa I, Saito Y, Onouchi Z, et al. Development of acquired cystic disease and adenocarcinoma of the kidney in glomerulonephritic chronic hemodialysis patients. Clin Nephrol. 1980;14:1–6.
6. Kojima Y, Takahara S, Miyake O, Nonomura N, Morimoto A, Mori H. Renal cell carcinoma in dialysis patients: a single center experience. Int J Urol. 2006;13:1045–8.
7. Fleming S. Renal cell carcinoma in acquired cystic kidney disease. Histopathology. 2010;56(3):395–400.
8. Schwarz A. Renal cell carcinoma in transplant recipients with acquired cystic kidney disease. Clin J Am Soc Nephrol. 2007;2(4):750–6. Epub 2007 Apr 25.
9. Kasiske BL. Recommendations for the outpatient surveillance of renal transplant recipients. American Society of Transplantation. J Am Soc Nephrol. 2000;11 Suppl 15:S1–86.
10. Marple JT. Renal cancer complicating acquired cystic kidney disease. J Am Soc Nephrol. 1994;4(12):1951–6.
11. Shaikewitz ST, et al. Autosomal recessive polycystic kidney disease: issues regarding the variability of clinical presentation. J Am Soc Nephrol. 1993;3(12):1858–62.
12. Ward CJ, et al. The gene mutated in autosomal recessive polycystic kidney disease encodes a large, receptor-like protein. Nat Genet. 2002;30(3):259–69.
13. Dell KM. The spectrum of polycystic kidney disease in children. Adv Chronic Kidney Dis. 2011;18(5):339–47.
14. Guay-Woodford LM, et al. Autosomal recessive polycystic kidney disease: the clinical experience in North America. Pediatrics. 2003;111(5 Pt 1):1072–80.
15. Niaudet P. Autosomal recessive polycystic kidney disease; Orphanet encyclopedia. http://www.orpha.net/data/patho/GB/uk-ARPKD.pdf. March 2004.
16. Davison AM, et al. Oxford textbook of clinical nephrology, vol. 3. 3rd ed. Oxford/New York: Oxford University Press; 2005. Chapter 17.
17. Fabris A, et al. Medullary sponge kidney: state of the art. Nephrol Dial Transplant. 2013;28(5):1111–9.
18. Benzing T. Clinical spectrum of pathogenesis of nephronophthisis. Curr Opin Nephrol Hypertens. 2012;21(3):272–8.
19. Hildebrandt F. New insights: nephronophthisis-medullary cystic kidney disease. Pediatr Nephrol. 2001;16:168–76.

Genetic Disorders of the Glomerular Basement Membrane

43

A. Neil Turner and Eleri Williams

Basement membranes are specialised noncellular matrices, found beneath epithelial and endothelial cell layers in all organs of the body. In the kidney, the glomerular basement membrane forms part of the barrier between blood and filtrate.

Alport syndrome is the second most common genetic cause of renal failure, and thin membrane nephropathy is a common diagnosis in patients presenting with microscopic haematuria. This chapter reviews our current understanding of these conditions and other less common inherited diseases of the glomerular basement membrane (GBM).

The Glomerular Basement Membrane: Components, Structure and Function

The GBM is part of the glomerular filtration barrier and lies between two layers of cells [1]. The GBM is flanked on one side by endothelial cells that face the glomerular capillary lumen, whilst podocyte foot processes line the other side protruding into the urinary space. The GBM is thicker than other basement membranes, measuring 300–350 nm. On electron microscopy, the GBM can be seen as a strip of extracellular matrix, made up of three layers. In health, the function of the glomerular filtration barrier is to allow the passage of water and small solutes, whilst obstructing the filtration of large proteins.

All basement membranes have four major components: (1) type IV collagen, (2) laminin, (3) nidogen and (4) heparan sulphate proteoglycans. Diseases occurring as a result of type IV collagen and laminin gene mutations have been described.

A.N. Turner, PhD, FRCP (✉) • E. Williams, MB BChir MRCP
Department of Renal Medicine,
Royal Infirmary of Edinburgh,
51 Little France Crescent, Old Dalkeith Road,
Edinburgh, EH16 4SA, UK
e-mail: neil.turner@ed.ac.uk;
eleri.williams@nhslothian.scot.nhs.uk

Type IV collagen is the major component of mammalian basement membranes [1]. There are six α chains, and each molecule of type IV collagen is composed of three of these chains. A triple helical structure is common to all collagens, but type IV collagens are characterised by non-collagenous interruptions in the helical structure and retention of non-collagenous domains at each end.

The six α chains (α1(IV) to α6(IV)) are encoded by COL4A1 to COL4A6 genes which are arranged in pairs: COL4A1 and COL4A2 on chromosome 13, COL4A3 and COL4A4 on chromosome 2 and COL4A5 and COL4A6 on the X chromosome (Fig. 43.1). Each chain has a molecular weight of over 160,000, and the genes encoding them are large and complex.

The composition of the type IV molecule varies between different membranes. The α1-α2 network is common to all basement membranes. The glomerular basement membrane in adults is mainly made from the α3α4α5 network, which is also present in the eye, ear and lungs. During development, some of these type IV collagen networks change their make-up, a 'developmental switch'. This happens in the

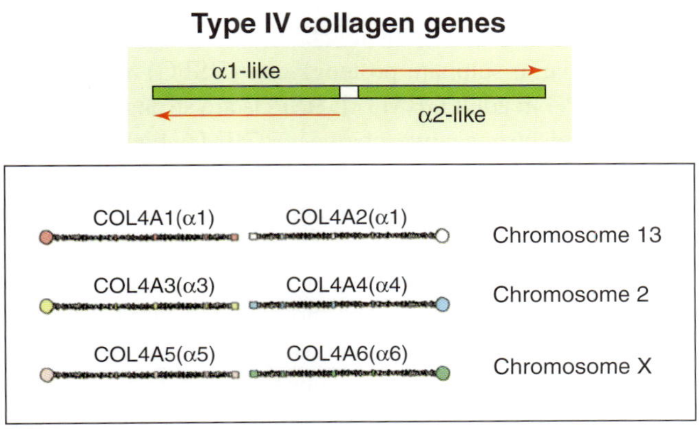

Fig. 43.1 The six type IV collagen genes and their chromosomal relationships (Reproduced with permission from Neil Turner and www.edren.org)

M. Harber (ed.), *Practical Nephrology*,
DOI 10.1007/978-1-4471-5547-8_43, © Springer-Verlag London 2014

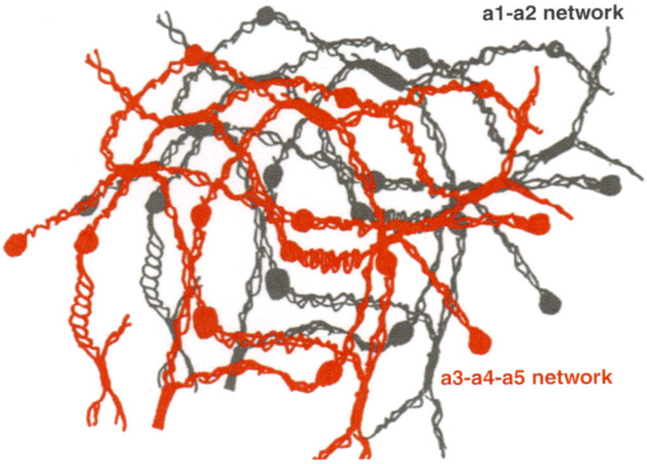

Fig. 43.2 Type IV collagen networks. The **α**3-**α**4-**α**5 is the major network in the GBM (Reproduced with permission from Neil Turner and www.edren.org)

kidney, where immature nephrons swap from the α1-α2 network to the α3α4α5 network as the capillary loops form.

Abnormal type IV collagen is the culprit in the most inherited GBM disease as we currently identify it (Fig. 43.2).

Laminins are large glycoproteins, made of one α, one β and one γ chain from the products of 5 LAMA, 4 LAMB and 3 LAMC genes. Laminin 521 (formed of the α5, β2 and γ1 chains) is the dominant component in adult GBM [1], but developmentally this shifts from 111 through 511 to a 521 network.

Laminins form a separate network in basement membranes that seems to assemble before the collagen network.

Nidogen (also known as entactin) (a universal component of basement membranes) is a dumbbell-shaped molecule with two isoforms (nidogen 1 and 2) which can bind to both laminin and collagen. NID mutations have not yet been identified in human diseases, but deletion of both isoforms is lethal perinatally in mice and associated with abnormal basement membrane development [2].

The heparan sulphate proteoglycan (HSPG) *agrin* is the major HSPG in adult GBM [3]; HSPGs are strongly anionic, giving an electronegative charge to GBM which has been thought to be functionally important. AGRN (agrin) mutations are associated with a congenital myasthenic syndrome but not renal disease [4].

Impairment of the function of the glomerular basement membrane is the prominent pathology in several diseases. Major conditions affecting the GBM are shown Table 43.1. In this chapter we will consider genetic causes.

There are two relatively common inherited disorders of the glomerular basement membrane – Alport syndrome and thin basement membrane nephropathy. There are also a handful of much rarer diseases.

Table 43.1 Diseases of the glomerular basement membrane

Inherited diseases of GBM	Acquired diseases of GBM
Alport syndrome	Anti-GBM (Goodpasture's) disease
Thin membrane nephropathy	Fibrillary nephritis – deposition
Nail-patella syndrome	Inflammatory nephritis – holes in GBM
Pierson syndrome	
HANAC	

Alport Syndrome

Alport syndrome is the best described of the hereditary GBM diseases. As the prototypical basement membrane disease, it exemplifies the many features of basement membrane pathology. In 1927 Cecil Alport described the condition that now bears his name, in a family with hereditary nephritis and deafness [5].

Epidemiology

Alport syndrome is the second only to ADPKD as most common inherited cause of renal failure. A prevalence of 1 in 5,000 in Utah was reported in the late 1980's, but in most populations the prevalence is much lower than this. Scandinavian studies found an incidence of 1 in 53,000 in Finland [6] and 1 in 17,000 in male births in southern Sweden [7]. Europe-wide, the underlying primary renal disease is Alport syndrome in approximately 1 % of patients with ESRF. In paediatric and adolescent populations, this proportion is closer to 2 % [8].

Data from the UK Renal Registry (Fig. 43.3) shows that approximately 1 % of dialysis patients in the UK have Alport syndrome as their primary renal diagnosis, a proportion that has remained stable over the last decade.

Aetiology and Pathogenesis

The underlying defect in Alport syndrome is a mutation in one of the genes encoding the α chains of the type IV collagen molecule [3]. In the most common form of the disease, X-linked Alport syndrome, the mutation arises in the gene encoding the α5 chain, COL4A5. This gene is located on the long arm of the X chromosome. Such mutations were first described in the early 1990s [9, 10] and paved the way for the discovery of hundreds of different mutations, from large deletions to small frameshift mutations. A significant proportion of patients develop the disease as a result of de novo mutations. There are no documented mutation 'hotspots', with most affected families carrying unique mutations [11].

Jais et al. [11] set out to establish the natural history of X-linked Alport syndrome and to correlate this with the

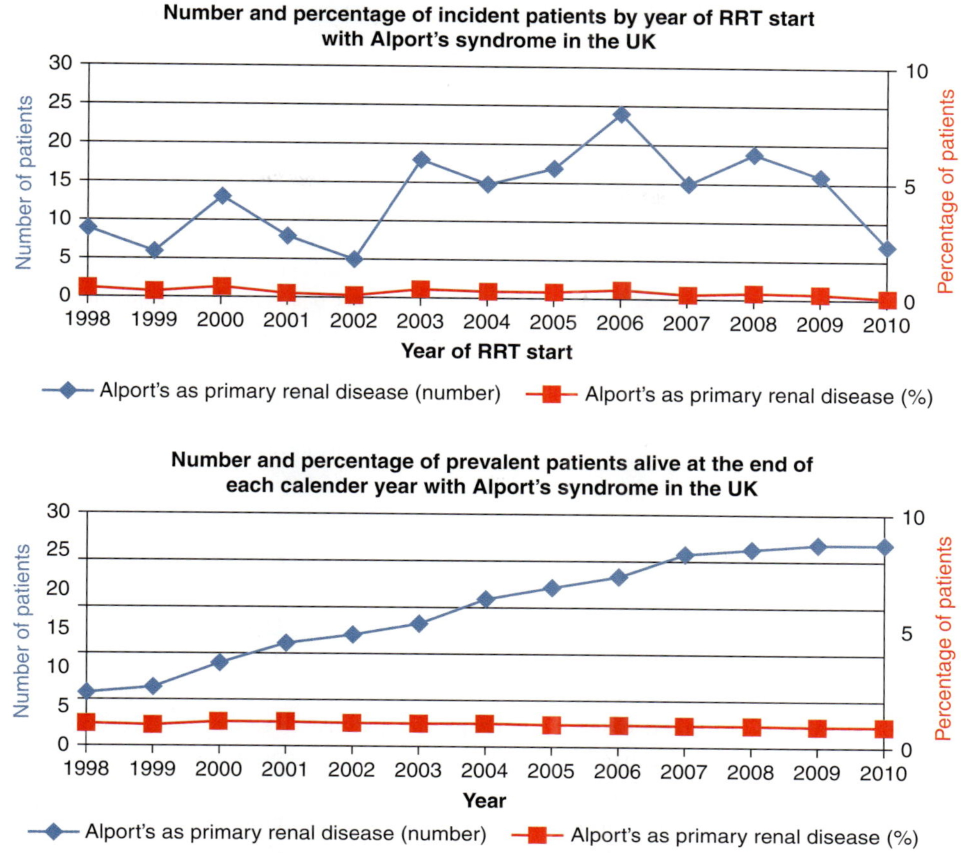

Fig. 43.3 Incidence and prevalence of Alport syndrome in UK RRT population (Data from UK Renal Registry (http://www.renalreg.com/))

type of underlying gene mutation. In a large cohort of male patients, they examined the relationship between genotypes and several phenotypes, including the rate of progression to ESRF, development of hearing loss and success of renal transplantation. Haematuria was a ubiquitous feature in this cohort. Large deletions, nonsense mutations and small frameshift mutations were associated with a higher probability of reaching end-stage disease and hearing loss by the age of 30 than missense mutations. In X-linked Alport syndrome, affected men cannot give the disease to their sons, but all of their daughters will carry the affected gene. The offspring of these female carriers, male or female, have a 1 in 2 chance of inheriting the mutant gene.

In the less common autosomal recessive form of the disease, the mutations occur in the genes encoding for the α3(IV) and α4(IV) chains, COL4A3 and COL4A4. Both of these genes map to chromosome 2 [12]. Even more rare is the autosomal dominant form of Alport syndrome, where the implicated genes are again COL4A3 and COL4A4 [13].

Clinical Features

The genetic heterogeneity of Alport syndrome is reflected in the variable clinical course of the disease. The genetic basis and corresponding clinical features of Alport syndrome are summarised in Table 43.2.

Renal Disease

Persistent haematuria is the hallmark of Alport syndrome, occurring in the first years of life. Macroscopic haematuria can occur in the context of exercise or upper respiratory tract infection. Haematuria is an invariable feature in males, and dipstick haematuria is seen in 95 % of female carriers of X-linked disease [14]. Significant proteinuria is initially absent in all genetic subtypes of the disease, but typically progresses in adulthood.

In X-linked disease, affected males all eventually develop renal failure, but the prognosis for female carriers is less certain. The clinical course in autosomal recessive Alport syndrome for both males and females is similar to that in males with X-linked Alport syndrome [12].

The rare autosomal dominant form of Alport syndrome has a more benign course. Progression to end-stage renal disease occurs later than in X-linked Alport syndrome or autosomal recessive Alport syndrome and is not inevitable [13].

Carriers and Heterozygotes

Female carriers of X-linked Alport syndrome had a significant rate of serious renal disease in Jais' study: 12 %

Table 43.2 Incidence, affected gene and clinical features of Alport syndrome

Alport syndrome			
Inheritance	Proportion of affected families	Affected gene	Clinical picture
X-linked dominant	85 %	COL4A5	Severe in male patients, progression to ESRF, high incidence of deafness No father-son transmission Variable course in females, with most never progressing to ESRF
Autosomal recessive	10–15 %	COL4A3/COL4A4	Severe form of disease in homozygotes including young women Haematuria in father of affected male Absence of severe disease in parents of patient Variable course in heterozygous carriers including (rarely) progression to ESRF
Autosomal dominant	Rare	COL4A3/COL4A4	Male to male transmission Similar severity in males and females and usually milder than in X-linked disease Progression to ESRF (if at all) aged > 50 years No ocular involvement

progressed to end-stage renal failure by the age of 40 and 30 % by the age of 60. The phenotype for heterozygous carriers of autosomal recessive Alport syndrome varies: some are asymptomatic, whilst others have haematuria. There have been reports of end-stage renal disease in such carriers. Why should they have better outcomes than female carriers of X-linked disease? Perhaps the patchy absence of α5 expression (caused by 'lyonisation'; silencing of one X chromosome) is worse than consistent underexpression. Interestingly there appears to be no correlation between the type of mutation and outcome in female carriers of X-linked disease; perhaps a 'second hit' in these patients makes more difference than the underlying mutation. The fact that autosomal mutations can occasionally cause dominantly expressed disease, albeit usually mild, suggests that there may be a gradation of mutation types and expression. However being a 'carrier' of an autosomal COL4A3 or COL4A4 mutation is associated with thin GBM nephropathy, usually characterised as a benign condition without long-term threat. It is currently wise to be slightly guarded about long-term prognosis for carriers of mutations in autosomal COL4 genes and definitely guarded about long-term prognosis for female carriers of COL4A5 mutations.

Hearing Loss

The most common extra-renal manifestation is bilateral sensorineural deafness, the severity of which is variable. High-tone loss is the earliest change. Affected children are not born deaf; hearing loss is progressive during childhood or early adult years. In X-linked disease, 79 % of males and 28 % of females are affected. Some are profoundly hearing impaired, whilst in others the auditory deficit is subclinical. Some patients have no detectable hearing problems, but have the typical renal manifestations. Males and females with autosomal Alport syndrome are affected in a similar manner to males with X-linked disease. The pathogenesis of hearing loss in Alport syndrome is not fully understood, but the 345 type IV collagen network is expressed in the cochlea [15].

Ocular

The most common eye finding is dot-and-fleck retinopathy, which does not affect visual acuity. Ocular involvement is seen in a third of males with X-linked disease; though as it is progressive, it depends on how severely affected or old the subject is when screened. Less common but much more specific is anterior lenticonus, in which the lens becomes misshapen as a consequence of thinning of the COL(IV) 345-containing lens capsule. This is typically a late change which occurs after years of renal failure. The retinopathy may be seen earlier, but it is often absent at the time the diagnosis is contemplated. It has been suggested that its appearance in a mutation-bearing parent can be helpful [9].

Ocular abnormalities have not been reported in autosomal dominant Alport syndrome [9], but retinal changes are said to be common in female carriers of X-linked disease.

Other Features

Leiomyomatosis is a rare extra-renal manifestation seen in a small proportion of patients with Alport syndrome, which occurs as a result of a large deletion involving the proximal (5′) end of the COL4A5 which extends into the proximal part of the adjacent COL4A6 gene. The oesophagus, tracheobronchial tree and female genital tract are affected [10]. As the leiomyomatosis component is dominantly expressed, female carriers are affected by it. AMEE (Alport syndrome, mental retardation, midface hypoplasia and elliptocytosis) is an even more rare contiguous gene deletion syndrome [16].

Differential Diagnosis

The principal differential diagnoses are other haematuric diseases, including TMN and IgA nephropathy or other

Table 43.3 Deafness and renal failure

Condition	Features
1. Alport syndrome	Progressive, high-tone deafness that is not present in early childhood COL4A3-5 genes
2. Branchio-oto-renal syndrome	Renal hypoplasia or malformation. Other manifestations variable and may not be obvious: some or all of deafness, preauricular pits, abnormal pinnae, sinuses in the neck from branchial fistula (or scars from operation). EYA and SIX1 and SIX5 genes involved
3. MYH9 mutations	Epstein-Fechtner syndrome; autosomal dominant renal disease probably not glomerular; with deafness, giant platelets. Epstein has no leucocyte inclusions, nor cataract formation
4. Mitochondrial DNA mutations	Look for other manifestations such as myopathy, diabetes, acidosis
5. Very small print	Other manifestations usually dominant; DIDMOAD syndrome with diabetes mellitus, diabetes insipidus, distal renal tubular acidosis with deafness, etc.
6. Coincidence	Deafness is the most common congenital abnormality

low-grade nephritis. Often, the history will go a long way in differentiating between these conditions. A family history of IgAN is uncommon, whereas a family history of deafness and ESRF makes Alport a likely diagnosis.

Other rare diseases in which deafness and renal failure occur are listed in Table 43.3.

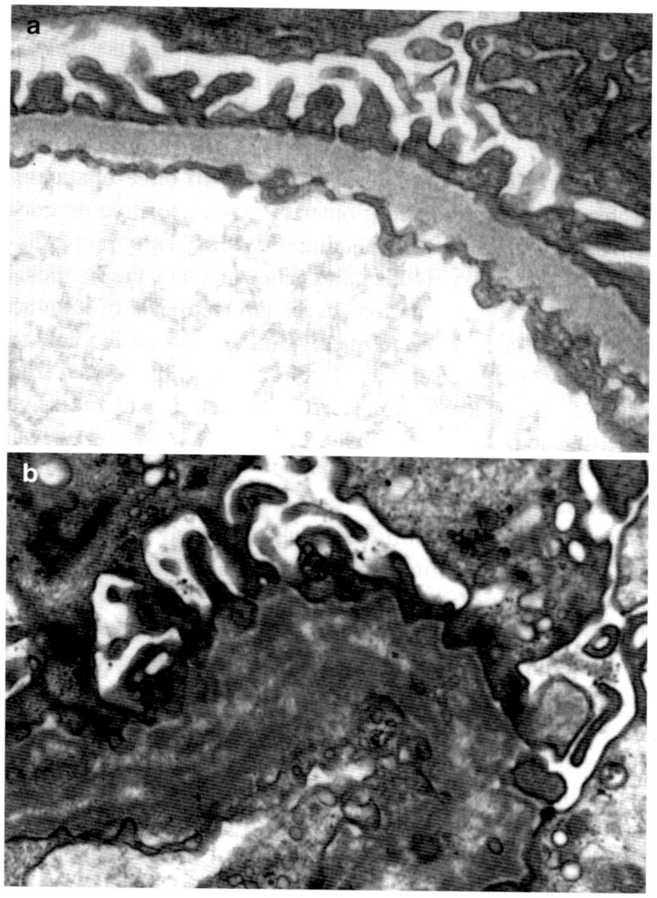

Fig. 43.4 Electron microscopy of the GBM in a normal kidney (**a**) and in Alport syndrome (**b**)

Investigations

Early diagnosis of Alport syndrome is becoming important, with increasing evidence that targeted early therapy may have beneficial outcomes in terms of disease retardation [17]. A comprehensive family history is essential as the starting point of a diagnostic approach. Diagnosing Alport syndrome with typical clinical findings and a family history can be relatively straightforward. The fact that 10–15 % of COL4A5 mutations are de novo complicates the diagnostic process.

In 1988, four criteria, of which three were necessary for definitive diagnosis, were described. These were (1) positive family history, (2) sensorineural hearing loss, (3) ocular changes and (4) typical ultrastructural changes of the GBM [18]. In reality, most patients can be given a firm diagnosis with fewer features, the most definitive of these tests being electron microscopy of the GBM. Molecular testing can now sometimes provide additional useful information. It may be valuable for diagnostic workup to include formal audiographic testing and ophthalmological referral.

Renal Biopsy

Light microscopy of glomerular tissue is mainly useful in ruling out other diagnoses in Alport syndrome. Changes seen are non-specific and in early disease may include podocyte hypertrophy and capillary wall stiffness. Later in the disease process, diffuse glomerular sclerosis is seen. Appearances of focal segmental glomerulosclerosis (FSGS) are also well described. In early disease immunofluorescence studies are negative, with presumably non-specific deposits of IgM and C3 seen in sclerosed glomeruli in more advanced disease [19].

Electron microscopy is required to demonstrate the sometimes dramatic changes in the glomerular basement membrane that occur in Alport syndrome (Fig. 43.4). Panel A shows an electron micrograph of the GBM from a normal kidney alongside a GBM from a patient with Alport syndrome. The normal architecture is destroyed, replaced by irregularly thickened GBM with multiple splits and lamellae. Not all patients exhibit such impressive ultrastructural changes, and those with earlier disease, or carriers, characteristically show thinning of the GBM. This can be the only abnormality in a significant proportion of adults with the

Table 45.1 Electrolyte content of frequently used medications in paediatric nephrology practice

Phosphate supplementation		
Joulie's solution	1 ml contains:	Na = 0.76 mmol PO_4 = 0.98 mmol
Phosphate Sandoz (soluble)	1 tab contains:	PO_4 = 16 mmol K = 3 mmol Na = 20.4 mmol
Potassium supplements		
Potassium chloride solution	1 ml contains:	K^{+1} = 1 mmol Cl^- = 1 mmol
Slow K tablets (MR-swallow whole)	1 tab contains:	K^{+1} = 8 mmol Cl^- = 8 mmol
Sando-K tablets (soluble)	1 tab contains:	K^{+1} = 12 mmol Cl^- = 8 mmol
Calcium supplementation		
Calcium Sandoz liquid	1 ml contains:	Ca^{+2} = 0.5 mmol
Sandocal 400 tablets (soluble)	1 tab contains:	Ca^{+2} = 10 mmol
Sandocal 1,000 tablets (soluble)	1 tab contains:	Ca^{+2} = 25 mmol
Magnesium supplementation		
Magnesiocard tablets	1 tab contains:	Mag = 2.5 mmol No phosphate
Magnesiocard tablets (soluble)	1 tab contains:	Mag = 7.5 mmol No phosphate
Magnesium glycerophosphate solution:	1 ml contains:	Mag = 1 mmol PO_4 = 1 mmol
Magnesium glycerophosphate	1 tablet contains:	Mag = 4 mmol PO_4 = 4 mmol
Bicarbonate supplementation		
Sodium bicarbonate solution	1 ml contains:	Na = 1 mmol Bicarb = 1 mmol
Sodium bicarbonate tablet 600 mg	1 tab contains:	Na = 7 mmol Bicarb = 7 mmol
Sodium bicarbonate capsule 500 mg	1 tab contains:	Na = 6 mmol Bicarb = 6 mmol
Citrate supplementation		
Sodium citrate mixture	1 mmol in 1 ml	
Potassium citrate mixture BP (3 g in 10 ml)	1 ml contains:	K = 2.8 mmol Citrate = 1.15 mmol (equivalent to 3.45 mmol bicarb/ml)
Albright's solution	1 l contains:	Na = 510 mmol K = 462 mmol Citrate = 636 mmol (equivalent to 1.9 mmol bicarb/ml)
	10 ml contains:	Na = 5 mmol K = 4 mmol Citrate = 6 mmol (equivalent to 1.9 mmol bicarb/ml)

Table 45.1 (continued)

Effercitrate (soluble tab)	1 tablet contains:	K = 14 mmol Citrate = 6 mmol (equivalent to 17 mmol bicarb/tab)
	i.e. 10 ml Albrights = 1 Effercitrate (except higher K^+)	
*Tricitrates oral solution (lemon flavour)	1 ml contains:	K = 1 mmol Na = 1 mmol Citrate = 0.7 mmol (equivalent to 2 mmol bicarb/ml)

*This is an unlicensed medicine made by the pharmacy manufacturing unit of Guy's and St Thomas's Hospital and can be ordered from that department (telephone 0207 118 4992) or by contacting Order Processing Service, Pharmacy Production Unit, Pharmacy Department, St Thomas's Hospital, Westminster Bridge Road, London, SE1 7EH. Fax No: 0207 188 5013

Management

General

In early life the importance of adequate correction of hydration and electrolyte imbalance is of paramount importance to improve growth. Regular review of electrolytes and phosphate supplementation is required to prevent constipation from hypokalaemia and rickets from hypophosphataemia. To maintain adequate nutritional intake, gastrostomy or nasogastric feeding is required. Growth hormone therapy is beneficial once nutritional intake is optimised. Carnitine supplementation has not been proven to have specific benefits except for restoring normal plasma concentrations. Indomethacin (1–3 mg/kg/day in two to three divided doses) is very useful in improving general wellbeing as well as reducing polyuria and may be given as a single dose at night to assist nocturia.

Cysteamine, the main drug therapy for cystinosis, is effective in circumventing the defective lysosomal cystine carrier system, thereby reducing the cystine content of the lysosomes (Figs. 45.2 and 45.3). Cysteamine bitartrate (Cystagon) is administered orally at a dose of 60–90 mg/kg/day given every 6 h [4]. NB: At commencement of therapy, the cysteamine dose must be commenced at a quarter of the final intended dose and increased gradually over the first 2–3 weeks of therapy, to avoid nausea and neurological complications. The leukocyte cystine measurements are used to gauge the compliance and adequacy of dosing. The medication is available in 50 and 150 mg capsules, and the dosage needs to be rounded into suitable multiples of these capsules for adequate administration. The usual adult dose is 500 mg taken strictly 6 hourly with regular monitoring of cystine levels. The leukocyte cystine measurements are taken as a

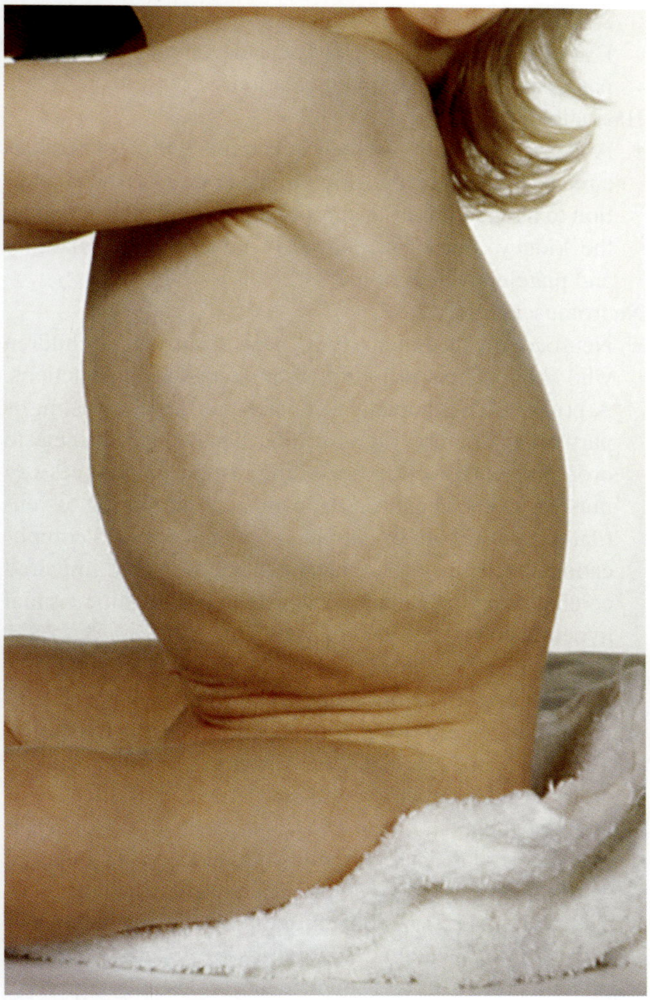

Fig. 45.1 Swollen costochondral junctions associated with rickets in cystinosis

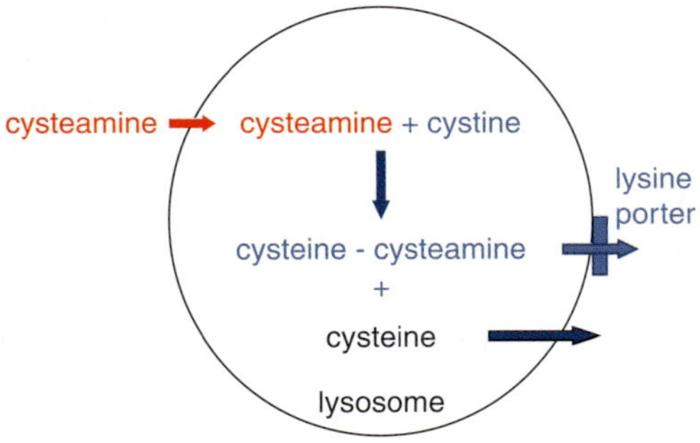

Fig. 45.2 Schematic representation of action of cysteamine in cystine transport from the lysosome

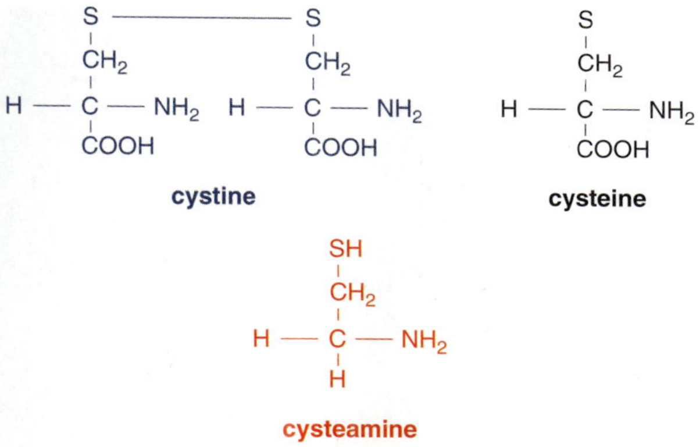

Fig. 45.3 Structural similarities between cystine and cysteamine

trough level 5½–6 h after the previous dose of medication, aiming for the white cell cystine level to be less than 2 nmol ½-cystine/mg protein. Unfortunately the sulphur component of the medication makes the cysteamine unpleasant to take and results in the odour of rotten eggs on the patient's breath and sweat, leading to compliance issues. Ten percent of patients cannot tolerate the full dose of cysteamine as many suffer nausea, vomiting and gastrointestinal upset, and thus it may be better to aim for suboptimal treatment that can at least be tolerated. Cysteamine has no effect on the Fanconi syndrome, but it does retard the rate of renal glomerular deterioration and improve linear growth in children [3]. The optimal care of patients with cystinosis requires a multiprofessional team approach with referral and advice to centres specialising in the disorder.

Management of Progression of the Disease

The progressive effects of cystinosis on organ systems and the specific management are listed below:

Renal

The early renal features are those of Fanconi syndrome. Polyuria may result in the loss of up to 6 l of dilute urine (<300 mosmol/l) per day and poses a significant problem of enuresis in children and adolescents. There is a gradual decline in creatinine clearance over years, and end-stage renal disease occurs around 10 years of age in those not receiving cysteamine treatment. The introduction of cysteamine has delayed the onset of ESRF by up to 10 years, and now many well-managed patients will reach 25 years of age before requiring kidney transplantation [5].

Pre-emptive transplantation is the treatment of choice, and both cadaveric and living related donor kidneys perform well in patients with cystinosis. Heterozygous relatives are able to donate kidneys to their offspring. Native kidneys remaining in situ can persist with renal tubular Fanconi

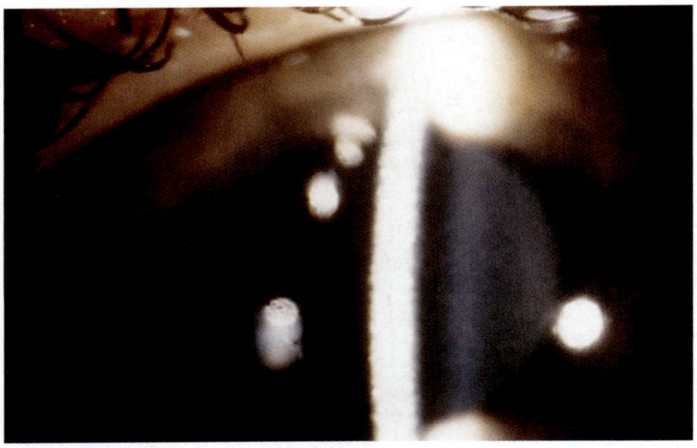

Fig. 45.4 Cystine crystals in eye

losses, and native nephrectomies may be required to control this. The donor kidney itself does not develop Fanconi syndrome. However, cystine crystals do deposit in the donor kidney through invasion of host cells with crystals noted in the interstitium but not in the tubular epithelium. Renal transplantation does not correct the systemic metabolic defect of cystinosis.

Eyes

- Cystine crystals deposit in most parts of the eye particularly the anterior chamber (Fig. 45.4). The cornea is hazy by 20 years of age and a band keratopathy can develop. Photophobia is particularly obvious in bright sunlight and dark glasses are essential for all patients. Scarring can predispose to glaucoma. Retinal damage with poor colour and night vision occurs in early adulthood. Oral cysteamine does not improve the effects in the eye, but topically administered cysteamine 0.55 % eye drops given 6–12 times per day are extremely useful. Intensive treatment with 2 hourly installation of the drops can dramatically improve photophobia within weeks. The lower strength 0.1 % cysteamine eye drops can be used but are less effective.

Endocrine Involvement

- Hypothyroidism is documented pre and post renal transplant relating initially to the loss of thyroglobulin in the urine and subsequently to deposition of crystals in the thyroid gland, such that the majority of patients are on thyroid supplements in early adulthood [6]. Primary hypogonadism is recorded in males. Infertility is common in boys but ovulatory cycles are normal in female patients with successful pregnancy outcomes noted. Diabetes post transplant is common, many patients requiring insulin treatment.

Gastrointestinal Complications

- 75 % of patients develop feeding abnormalities due to reflux dysmotility and swallowing dysfunction. Proton-pump inhibitors can be helpful. Hepatosplenomegaly is common with gradual evolution of portal hypertension. Exocrine hepatic insufficiency can develop which requires pancreatic enzyme supplementation.

Haematological

- Anaemia is commonly seen in patients with cystinosis as a result of cystine deposition in the bone marrow in addition to a reduction in erythropoietin protein production by the kidney. These patients also have hypocoagulability and platelet dysfunction.

Neuromuscular

- Neurocognitive deficits have been recorded in children who show effects primarily with visuo-spacial functions. A progressive myopathy with skeletal muscle wasting is particularly notable in adult life. This can contribute to oromotor dysfunction including dysphagia. Accessory muscles of the chest can be involved contributing to ventilatory restriction. In untreated patients cerebral complications will result in encephalopathy with impaired cerebellar and pyramidal function [6]. Idiopathic cranial hypertension is well recognised.

Cardiovascular

- Arterial hypertension is noted secondary to a renin-dependant hypertension. This together with the hypercholesterolemia of cystinosis can result in early calcification of arteries, particularly coronary.

Bone Involvement

- Bone mineral density is significantly reduced in adults and children after transplantation. The development of osteopoenia (Fig. 45.5) and bone fragility occurs irrespective of correction of metabolic mineral losses in earlier life, and calcium and vitamin D supplements are usually required.

Cysteamine treatment can provide salutary effects even when administered late to previously noncompliant patients with established complications such as severe encephalopathy. Cysteamine retards the development of serious late complications of cystinosis and ideally should be commenced immediately after birth and continued indefinitely [7, 8]. The teratogenicity of oral cysteamine has not been determined in humans. The current advice is that women planning to conceive should forgo cysteamine until after the pregnancy.

A new formulation of delayed release enteric-coated cysteamine bitartrate (PROCYSBI) has recently been shown to be as effective as the immediate release drug (Cystagon) in maintaining low leukocyte cystine levels. This may have an advantage for patient compliance although the gastrointestinal side effects with RP103 were threefold greater than with Cystagon [9]. Other therapeutic approaches are the formulation of cysteamine suppositories [10] and research consideration of bone marrow transplantation to correct the defect.

Advocacy support is available through the Cystinosis Foundation www.cystinosisfoundation.org and the Cystinosis Research Network www.cystinosis.org which provide valuable advice and support for affected families, as

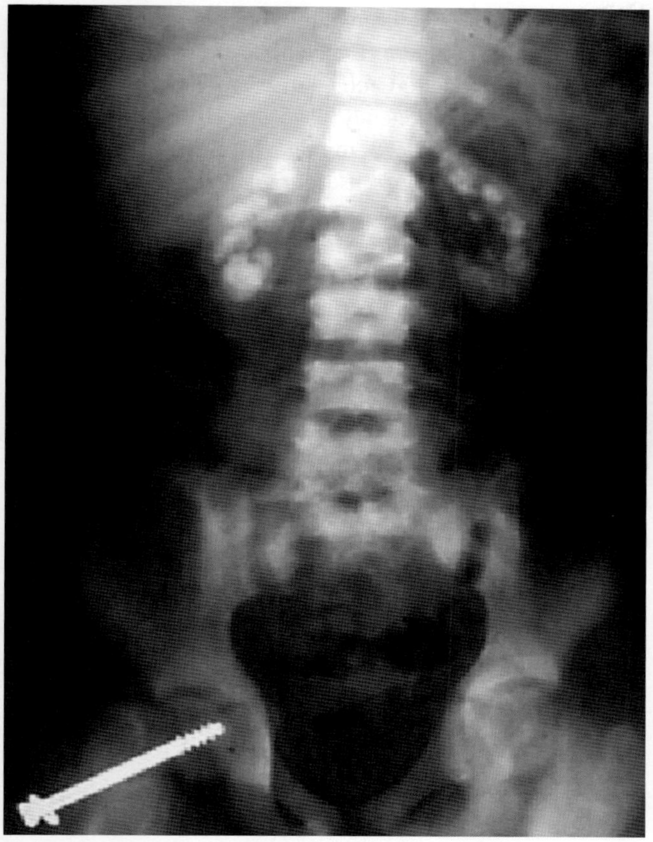

Fig. 45.5 Abdominal X-ray demonstrating marked nephrocalcinosis and severe osteopoenia associated with PH1 in a 9-year-old

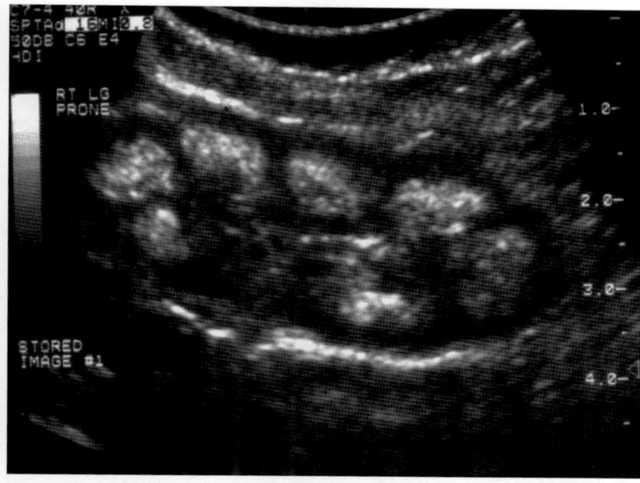

Fig. 45.6 Renal ultrasound demonstrating marked nephrocalcinosis

well as funding research. Individuals with cystinosis should be encouraged to pursue educational interests of their choice. The significant psychological difficulties experienced by this group relate to the chronic nature of the condition, multiple drug therapies, prolonged hospitalisation, missed school and often disordered family dynamics. Psychology support can be beneficial.

The Primary Hyperoxalurias

The primary hyperoxalurias are inborn errors of metabolism of which three have been described at the molecular level. Primary hyperoxaluria type 1 (PH1) is caused by mutations in the *AGXT* gene which result in dysfunction of the vitamin B6 (pyridoxine)-dependent liver-specific peroxisomal enzyme alanine/glyoxylate aminotransferase (AGT) [11]. Primary hyperoxaluria type 2 (PH2) arises from mutations in the *GRHPR* gene with subsequent dysfunction of the enzyme glyoxylate/hydroxypyruvate reductase (GRHPR) [12]. Primary hyperoxaluria type 3 (PH3) arises from mutations in the *HOGA1* gene which is believed to encode the mitochondrial enzyme 4-hydroxy-2-oxoglutarate aldolase [13].

Oxalate is derived principally from the diet and endogenous production following the metabolism of glyoxylate and ascorbic acid. Excretion is primarily via the kidney. The majority of patients presenting with hyperoxaluria do so as a result of derangement of the normal metabolic pathways. However, it is important to be aware that hyperoxaluria can occur due to hyperabsorption of ingested oxalate, as seen in patients with bowel malabsorption (e.g. inflammatory bowel disease, chronic infective diarrhoea, short-bowel syndrome or pancreatic exocrine insufficiency).

As oxalate is poorly soluble, calcium oxalate calculi will form when the urine becomes supersaturated. Bidirectional transport of oxalate has been demonstrated in proximal renal tubular cells and in intestinal epithelia with evidence to suggest a role for the *SLC26A6* gene in both enteric and renal oxalate transport. Calcium oxalate crystals form in the lumen of the renal tubules. These crystals then adhere to the tubular epithelium and are internalised into the cells with subsequent extrusion into the interstitial region where they cause an inflammatory reaction, and subsequent nephrocalcinosis (Figs. 45.6 and 45.7).

Presentation and Investigation

The primary hyperoxalurias show considerable genetic and phenotypic heterogeneity and can present in the following forms:

1. Asymptomatic
2. Occasional passage of renal stones
3. Recurrent urolithiasis
4. Recurrent urolithiasis with the development of nephrocalcinosis and eventual progressive renal failure
5. Infantile presentation with failure to thrive, early nephrocalcinosis and rapid progression to end-stage renal failure

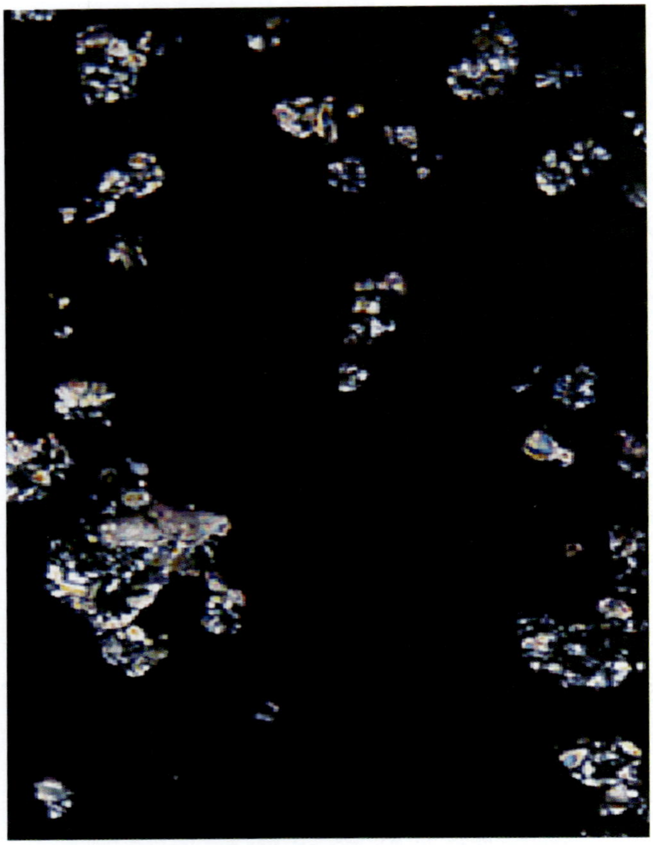

Fig. 45.7 Oxalate crystals in PH deposited in renal biopsy shown by polarised light

The investigation of any child or adult presenting with even the occasional passage of renal stones, but certainly for those presenting with nephrocalcinosis, must exclude PH as an underlying cause. In all such presentations a *fresh* urine sample must be sent for urine oxalate/creatinine ratio in the first instance. If the sample is borderline or elevated, a 24-h urine collection for oxalate excretion is required, and in some cases, three consecutive 24-h urine collections, as there is marked variability in the excretion of oxalate on a day-to-day basis. During the 24-h collection period, the urine collection must be placed into a container *acidified* with hydrochloric acid (obtained from the hospital clinical chemistry department). The plasma oxalate level may not be raised unless there is considerable nephrocalcinosis or a decline in the GFR has occurred. Note that all patients with end-stage renal failure demonstrate a raised plasma oxalate due to inadequate excretion and must be distinguished from those with true underlying metabolic disorders. Blood and urine samples collected for oxalate analysis must be sent immediately to the laboratory as any delay can result in a false elevation of the oxalate levels. In addition, patients must not be taking any form of vitamin C supplements as ascorbic acid ingestion will elevate urinary oxalate.

A urine oxalate (UOx) excretion of >0.5 mmol/1.73 m^2/day is likely to be due to a metabolic cause although some secondary cases due to Crohn's disease, short gut syndrome and pancreatic insufficiency have grossly elevated oxalate excretions >1 mmol/1.73 m^2/day. In children the urinary oxalate/creatinine ratio is useful but interpretation requires the age-related reference ranges as ratios in early life are influenced by prematurity and nutrition. Urinary glycolate excretion may be raised in PH1 but has a low diagnostic sensitivity and specificity.

All patients presenting with renal stones and/or nephrocalcinosis must also have the urine analysed for L-glyceric acid (part of a routine organic acid screen) as the hallmark of *PH2* is a high excretion of L-glyceric acid >28 mmol/mol of creatinine. For the majority of patients with PH2, this simple test is usually diagnostic with high sensitivity.

As the gene for *PH3* has been identified only recently, the patient phenotypic characteristics are still being described. The main identifying feature appears to be hypercalciuria with CaOx stones in early childhood. Other features are hyperoxaluria and mild hyperglycolic aciduria ± hyperuricosuria [13].

Genetic Testing

Once a raised urinary oxalate or glyceric acid has been identified, the patient must undergo genetic testing in order to confirm the diagnosis as well as to give an indication of prognosis. Sibling and family screening is particularly beneficial and can identify asymptomatic cases which can allow the institution of appropriate therapy before symptoms arise [14].

Conservative Management

The key aims of therapy are to prevent systemic oxalate deposition with a high fluid intake accompanied by the administration of crystallisation inhibitors. The recommendations for treatment are as follows:

1. High fluid intake is mandatory, at least 3 l/m^2/24 h. This may require the placement of a nasogastric or gastrostomy feeding tube in infants in order to guarantee adequate hydration.
2. Oral potassium citrate at a dose of 0.1–0.15 g/kg body weight per day (0.3–0.5 mmol/kg/day) to inhibit calcium oxalate crystallisation.
3. The administration of pyridoxine to any patient with proven PH1 starting at a dose of 5 mg/kg/day up to 20 mg/kg/day with the intention of decreasing the urine oxalate excretion by at least 30 %.

The alkalisation of the urine reduces calcium oxalate saturation by forming complexes with calcium and by decreasing stone production. The potassium content needs review if the patient has a significantly reduced GFR. Pyrophosphate may also inhibit calcium oxalate crystallisation, and moderate doses of phosphate, 20–30 mg/kg/day, may be administered.

Vitamin B6 is a cofactor for AGT and the administration of pyridoxine has been associated with a decrease in urine oxalate in about 30 % of *PH1* patients. Some patients are extremely responsive to vitamin B6 at small doses such as 1 mg/kg/day or even a single 5 mg daily dose. A particular subset of patients with specific gene mutations, namely p. Gly170Arg or p.Phe152Ile mutation, are more likely to respond to pharmacological doses of vitamin B6 and are predicted to have a better long-term outcome, an important reason to perform genetic mutation analysis [15].

Dietary restriction of oxalate is of limited use as the main source of oxalate is endogenous and the intestinal oxalate absorption in PH patients is lower than that of normal subjects. Some experts recommend avoiding oxalate-rich foods in the diet such as dark chocolate, strawberries, spinach and tea on a precautionary principle. Calcium intake should be normal but excessive intake of vitamin C and vitamin D should be avoided. The gut bacterium *Oxalobacter formigenes* is able to metabolise oxalate in normal subjects, but there is limited evidence of its efficacy in reducing urine oxalate excretion in PH patients.

Dialysis

Oxalate is generated at a rate of 4–7 mmol/1.73 m^2/day in contrast with clearance via conventional dialysis at a rate of 1–4 mmol/1.73 m^2/day, resulting in uncontrolled tissue accretion. Oxalate clearance on haemodialysis is greater than on peritoneal dialysis (120 ml/min on haemodialysis compared to 7 ml/min on peritoneal dialysis). Thus, standard haemodialysis programmes will result in a weekly clearance of oxalate of 6–9 mmol/1.73 m^2/week which is equivalent to 2–3 days of endogenous production of oxalate. Thus, a combination of modalities, with intermittent daily haemodialysis and overnight peritoneal dialysis, enhances the overall clearance of oxalate and attempts to reduce the rebound which occurs after haemodialysis. These combination therapies with the use of high-flux dialysers or long episodes of haemofiltration have all been advocated to improve oxalate removal [16, 17]. The aim is to prevent the requirement for dialysis and to anticipate impairment in renal function with strategic planning for organ transplantation.

Transplantation

When the GFR falls below 60 ml/min/1.73 m^2, assessment for transplantation should take place initially with isolated liver transplantation being advised if the GFR continues to fall progressively below 60 ml/min/1.73 m^2 in patients with *PH1*. The liver is the only organ responsible for glyoxylate detoxification through the enzyme AGT. Thus, liver transplantation is a cure for PH1 but the native liver must be removed in order to avoid excessive oxalate production continuing [18, 19].

Combined hepatorenal transplantation must be considered when the GFR falls below 40 ml/min/1.73 m^2 as there is a dramatic decrease in excretion of oxalate, with increase in plasma oxalate levels, resulting in systemic deposition of calcium oxalate in the heart (cardiomyopathy and conduction defects), vessel walls, skin (ulcerating lesions), nerves (peripheral neuropathy, mono neuritis multiplex), retina and joints (sinovitis). The hepatorenal transplantation can be done simultaneously with excellent success even in small infants. A sequential procedure involving hepatic transplantation first, followed by a period of dialysis, with subsequent renal transplantation months later may be considered more appropriate in certain situations. This type of approach can be useful if living related donors for split liver or kidney donation are being considered.

After combined hepatorenal transplantation, the urine oxalate can remain elevated for many years due to the slow resolubilisation of systemic calcium oxalate. These patients must still continue with a high fluid intake supported by the use of crystallisation inhibitors in order to protect the transplanted kidney from further calcium oxalate damage through stones or nephrocalcinosis [20]. The benefit of haemodialysis post transplantation is still debated and currently should be limited to patients with acute tubulonecrosis or delayed graft function [21].

Management of Urolithiasis

Surgical intervention in the management of uncomplicated urolithiasis in PH patients should be limited. Extracorporeal shock wave lithotripsy (ESWL) has now been superseded by endoscopic stone removal. This is an advantage over ESWL where in situ fragmentation can leave gravel behind with subsequent formation of new stone matrix on these residues because of the ongoing hyperoxaluria. Thus, endoscopic treatment such as semi-rigid ureterorenoscopy, flexible ureterorenoscopy and percutaneous nephrolithotomy are now procedures of choice.

PH2

The overall long-term prognosis for patients with PH2 appears to be better than for PH1 with the majority of patients presenting with urolithiasis. Nephrocalcinosis is less common but can occur in childhood and adult life [22]. End-stage renal failure tends to occur over 25 years of age. The supportive management is the same as for PH1 but there is no rationale for the use of vitamin B6. Renal transplantation has been performed in some of these patients, but the majority will have a recurrence of their condition in the transplanted kidney. Success with hepatic transplantation has not been reported.

PH3

The principles of management are the same, but in addition a role of a vegetarian diet to reduce dietary hydroxyproline is being considered.

Additional Information

Several national and international societies provide support for physicians and patients requiring more information on the primary hyperoxalurias. The European Hyperoxaluria Consortium, OxalEurope, (www.oxaleurope.org) provides contact details for clinicians and scientists, while the Oxalosis and Hyperoxaluria Foundation (www.ohf.org) is an active organisation located in the United States providing regular updates for patients internationally as well as physicians.

Methylmalonic Acidaemias

The methylmalonic acidaemias (MMA), inherited in an autosomal recessive manner, comprise a heterogeneous group of inborn errors of organic acid metabolism. Successful metabolism of branched-chain amino acids is dependent upon activity of several mitochondrial enzymes: methylmalonyl CoA racemase, methylmalonyl CoA mutase and the methylmalonyl CoA mutase cofactor cobalamin. Many different genetic defects are known to cause MMA: methylmalonyl CoA mutase deficiency (defect of the *MUT* gene), methylmalonyl CoA racemase deficiency (*MCEE*) and several defects of cobalamin metabolism CblA (*MMAA*), CblB (*MMAB*), CblD (*MMADHC*) and CblC (*MMACHC*). Enzyme deficiency leads to the accumulation of methylmalonic acid in the plasma, urine and other body fluids [23, 24].

Vitamin B_{12} nonresponsive MMA variants are the most clinically severe, characterised by recurrent episodes of decompensation, usually precipitated by intercurrent febrile illness. At present there is no satisfactory method for monitoring metabolic status in these patients. Therapy with an isocaloric low-protein diet and supplemented amino acids (which are not methylmalonate precursors) is advised by a trained dietician. With improved recognition and treatment, survival is increasing and longer-term complications including pancreatitis, chronic neurological and renal impairment are becoming more apparent [25].

Renal failure is a recognised complication of MMA which is not seen in other organic acidurias [26]. The highest incidence occurs in those with Mut 0 and CblB forms of the disease with 61 and 66 % developing chronic renal impairment over time. Renal impairment is found more commonly in those presenting early with MMA and in patients with higher urinary excretion of MMA. Progressive renal failure usually develops in adolescence or early adulthood in these groups [25, 26].

Screening for renal impairment in patients with MMA is complicated by their low muscle mass and low protein intake; thus, formal assessment of renal function and glomerular filtration rate should be performed regularly from an early age. An elevated uric acid level should be treated. The clinical manifestations of renal involvement in MMA include proximal and distal tubular dysfunction and renal tubular acidosis type 4. Renal histology demonstrates progressive tubulointerstitial nephritis with mononuclear infiltration, interstitial fibrosis and tubular atrophy. The decreased renal function is believed to be secondary to tubular damage caused by tubulointerstitial nephritis. Metabolic deterioration can be expected with worsening renal failure as methylmalonic acid is usually removed from the body by renal excretion.

Haemodialysis can improve acute metabolic decompensation [25] and is effective in clearing methylmalonic acid prior to transplantation [27]. In end-stage renal failure haemodialysis results in periodic clearance of MMA from the body associated with a reduction of hospital admissions due to metabolic decompensation. Both peritoneal and haemodialysis are effective in reducing MMA levels, even if only temporarily, and can be useful in patients with poor metabolic control but stable renal function [28]. Patients with MMA who are metabolically very brittle may benefit from a trial of renal replacement therapy, even in the absence of confirmed end-stage renal failure. The long-term options available to these patients include dialysis with subsequent transplantation, either using an isolated kidney or combined liver-kidney transplant.

The kidney is estimated to have only 18 % of the methylmalonyl CoA mutase activity of the liver, but despite this, isolated renal transplantation may offer a useful partial correction, with a significant fall in plasma methylmalonate and improved metabolic control. Maintaining strict protein restriction together with a lower incidence of infection in older children may further improve metabolic control and reduce the risk of progressive damage to the transplanted kidney.

Dysfunction of the respiratory chain and the tricarboxylic acid cycle in addition to oxidative stress has been implicated in the pathogenesis of organ damage in MMA. As the enzyme activity in the transplanted kidney is normal, intrarenal MMA metabolism should also be normal. Nevertheless, excess exogenous MMA is also believed to have a pathogenic role by inhibiting the transport of anaplerotic tricarboxylic acid cycle intermediates into renal tubular cells through the Na+-dependent dicarboxylate transporters hNAC1 and hNAC3, and the transplanted kidney may still be vulnerable to damage in the longer term.

The liver is a major site of methylmalonyl CoA mutase activity. Thus, liver transplantation for early onset of MMA has been advocated to prevent recurrent metabolic decompensation and avoid subsequent neurodevelopmental complications [29]. Successful liver transplantation requires careful perioperative management but offers consistent protection from metabolic decompensation and dietary derestriction in the majority of patients. Longer-term outcomes following transplantation may vary, with several case reports describing acute and chronic neurological complications and progressive renal failure despite successful grafting [30].

Combined liver-kidney transplantation offers the potential of reducing plasma methylmalonic acid by up to 95–97 % with improved urinary excretion, but unfortunately neurological damage may progress [31], accompanied by high morbidity and mortality [29].

The management of chronic renal impairment secondary to MMA continues to evolve. Although experience is limited, isolated renal transplantation in suitable patients is a viable alternative to liver or combined liver-kidney transplantation as it appears to have similar salutary effects on metabolic stability with a lower risk of morbidity and mortality.

Acknowledgements The author would like to thank Drs Anupam Chakrapani and Joanna C Clothier for their input.

References

1. Town M, Jean G, Cherqui S, Attard M, Forestier L, Whitmore SA, Callen DF, Gribouval O, Broyer M, Bates GP, van't Hoff W, Antignac C. A novel gene encoding an integral membrane protein is mutated in nephropathic cystinosis. Nat Genet. 1998;18(4):319–24.
2. Kalatzis V, Antignac C. Cystinosis: from gene to disease. Nephrol Dial Transplant. 2002;17(11):1883–6.
3. Gahl WA, Thoene JG, Schneider JA. Cystinosis. N Engl J Med. 2002;347:111–21.
4. Levtchenko EN, van Dael CM, de Graaf-Hess AC, Wilmer MJ, van den Heuvel LP, Monnens LA, Blom HJ. Strict cysteamine dose regimen is required to prevent nocturnal cystine accumulation in cystinosis. Ped Nephrol. 2006;21(1):110–3.
5. Markello TC, Bernardini IM, Gahl WA. Improved renal function in children with cystinosis treated with cysteamine. N Engl J Med. 1993;328(16):1157–62.
6. Geelen JM, Monnens LA, Levtchenko EN. Follow-up and treatment of adults with cystinosis in the Netherlands. Nephrol Dial Transplant. 2002;17(10):1766–70.
7. Brodin-Sartorius A, Tete MJ, Niaudet P, Antignac C, et al. Cysteamine therapy delays the progression of nephropathic cystinosis in late adolescents and adults. Kidney Int. 2012;81:179–89.
8. Cherqui S. Cysteamine therapy: a treatment for cystinosis, not a cure. Kidney Int. 2012;81:127–31.
9. Langman CB, Greenbaum LA, Sarwal M, Grimm P, Niaudet P, et al. A randomised controlled crossover trial with delayed-release cysteamine bitartrate in nephropathic cystinosis: effectiveness on white blood cell cystine levels and comparison of safety. Clin J Am Soc Nephrol. 2012;7(7):1112–20.
10. Buchan B, Kay G, Matthews KH, Cairns D. Suppository formulation as a potential treatment for nephropathic cystinosis. J Pharm Sci. 2012;101(10):3729–38.
11. Purdue PE, Takada Y, Danpure CJ. Identification of mutations associated with peroxisome-to-mitochondrion mistargeting of alanine/glyoxylate aminotransferase in primary hyperoxaluria type 1. J Cell Biol. 1990;111:2341–51.
12. Cregeen DP, Williams EL, Hulton SA, Rumsby G. Molecular analysis of the glyoxylate reductase (GRHPR) gene and description of mutations underlying primary hyperoxaluria type 2. Human Mutation, Mutation in Brief [Online Journal]. 2003. http://www.interscience.wiley.com/humanmutation/pdf/mutation/671.pdf
13. Belostotsky R, Seboun E, Idelson GH, Milliner DS, Becker-Cohen R, Rinat C, Monico CG, Feinstein S, Ben-Shalom E, Magen D, Weissman I, Charon C, Frishberg Y. Mutations in DHDPSL are responsible for primary hyperoxaluria type III. Am J Hum Genet. 2010;87:392–9.
14. Rumsby G. An overview of the role of genotyping in the diagnosis of the primary hyperoxalurias. Urol Res. 2005;33:318–20.
15. Williams EL, Acquaviva C, Amoroso A, Chevalier F, Coulter-Mackie M, Monico CM, Giachino D, Owen EP, Robbiano A, Salido E, Waterham H, Rumsby G. Primary hyperoxaluria type 1: update and additional mutation analysis of the AGXT gene. Hum Mutat. 2009;30:910–7.
16. Illies F, Bonzel KE, Wingen AM, Latta K, Hoyer PF. Clearance and removal of oxalate in children on intensified dialysis for primary hyperoxaluria type 1. Kidney Int. 2006;70:1642–8.
17. Hoppe B, Graf D, Offner G, Latta K, Byrd DJ, Michalk D, Brodehl J. Oxalate elimination via haemodialysis or peritoneal dialysis in children with chronic renal failure. Pediatr Nephrol. 1996;10:488–92.
18. Perera MT, Sharif K, Lloyd C, Foster K, Hulton SA, Mirza DF, McKiernan PJ. Pre-emptive liver transplantation for primary hyperoxaluria (PH1) arrests long-term renal function deterioration. Nephrol Dial Transplant. 2011;26:354–9.
19. Cochat P, Fargue S, Harambat J. Primary hyperoxaluria type 1: strategy for organ transplantation. Curr Opin Organ Transplant. 2010;15:590–3.
20. Hoppe B, Latta K, von Schnakenburg C, Kemper MJ. Primary hyperoxaluria – the German experience. Am J Nephrol. 2005;25:276–81.
21. Harps E, Brinkert F, Ganschow R, Briem-Richter A, van Husen M, Schmidtke S, Nashan B, Fischer L, Kemper MJ. Immediate postoperative intensive care treatment for pediatric combined liver-kidney transplantation: outcome and prognostic factors. Transplantation. 2011;91:1127–31.
22. Johnson SA, Rumsby G, Cregreen D, Hulton SA. Primary hyperoxaluria type 2 in children. Pediatr Nephrol. 2002;17(8):597–601.
23. Ogier de Baulny H, Saudubray JM. Branched chain organic acidurias. Semin Neonatol. 2002;7:65–74.
24. Fowler B, Leonard JV, Baumgartner MR. Cause of and diagnostic approach to methylmalonic acidurias. J Inherit Metab Dis. 2008;31:350–60.
25. Ogier de Baulny H, Benoist JF, Rigal O, Touati G, Rabier D, Saudubray JM. Methylmalonic and proprionic acidaemias: management and outcome. J Inherit Metab Dis. 2005;28:415–23.
26. Hörster F, Hoffmann GF. Pathophysiology, diagnosis, and treatment of methylmalonic aciduria-recent advances and new challenges. Pediatr Nephrol. 2004;19:1071–4.

27. Van't Hoff WG, McKiernan PJ, Surtees RAH, Leonard JV. Liver transplantation for methylmalonic acidaemia. Eur J Pediatr. 1999;158:S70–4.
28. Paik KH, Lee JE, Jin D-K. Successful dialysis in a boy with methylmalonic academia. Pediatr Nephrol. 2004;19:1180–1.
29. Morioka D, Kasahara M, Horikawa R, Yokoyama S, Fukuda A, Nakagawa A. Efficacy of living donor liver transplantation for patients with methylmalonic academia. Am J Transplant. 2007;7:2782–7.
30. Leonard JV, Walter JH, McKiernan PJ. The management of organic acidaemias: the role of transplantation. J Inherit Metab Dis. 2001;24:309–11.
31. McGuire PJ, Lim-Melia E, Diaz GA, Raymond K, Larkin A, Wasserstein MP, Sansaricq C. Combined liver-kidney transplantation for management of methylmalonic aciduria: a case report and review of the literature. Mol Genet Metab. 2008;93:22–9.

Supplementary Reading

Brodin-Sartorius A, Tete M-J, Niaudet P et al. Cysteamine therapy delays the progression of nephropathic cystinosis in late adolescence and adults. Kid Int. 2012;81:179–89

Cochat P, Hulton SA, Acquaviva C, Danpure CJ, Daudon M, De Marchi M, Fargue S, Groothoff JW, Harambat J, Hoppe B, Jamieson N, Kemper MJ, Mandrile G, Marangella M, Picca S, Rumsby G, Salido E, Straub M, van Woerden CS, on behalf of OxalEurope. Primary hyperoxaluria type 1: indications for screening and guidance for diagnosis and treatment. Nephrol Dial Transplant. 2012;27:1729–36.

Dermatology in Kidney Disease

46

Ferina Ismail

A wide variety of skin conditions arise in patients with chronic kidney disease (CKD). These are sometimes related to the underlying pathologic process causing the renal disease but are also frequently associated with the uraemic state itself. Cutaneous examination of patients with CKD has shown an almost 100 % prevalence of skin disorders in dialysis populations [1], with a marked impact on quality of life [2]. In addition, there is over a 100-fold increase in the incidence of certain types of skin cancer in renal transplant recipients, placing a significant burden on healthcare resources as well as causing significant morbidity and in some cases mortality [3]. Early recognition of these skin problems can therefore avert such complications, making a basic knowledge of the dermatological conditions arising in the setting of renal disease extremely valuable to practising nephrologists.

The cutaneous manifestations of renal disease may be broadly divided into three general categories including (1) skin manifestations of diseases associated with chronic kidney disease (Table 46.1), (2) skin manifestations of diseases associated with renal involvement (Table 46.2) and (3) skin conditions associated with renal transplantation.

Skin Conditions Associated with Chronic Kidney Disease

Examination of the skin and nails can reveal abnormalities in patients with end-stage renal disease that precede dialysis or kidney transplantation. Chronic renal failure, regardless of its cause, often produces xerosis, pruritus, hyperpigmentation and nail changes. Although the majority of dermatological conditions in CKD are relatively benign, a few skin diseases have the potential to cause serious morbidity and mortality, and it is these conditions which are discussed in more detail (Table 46.1).

Uraemic Pruritus

With improvements in dialysis and the development of biocompatible dialysis membranes, the prevalence of uraemic pruritus (UP) has declined in the past decade. Despite this however, a significant proportion of haemodialysis patients still report itching [4] which can have a significant effect on quality of life as it causes considerable discomfort, anxiety, depression and sleeping disorders. In addition, UP is increasingly recognised as an indicator of increased mortality risk in patients with CKD [5].

UP is characterised by daily bouts of itching that tend to worsen at night and may prevent sleep. The itch may be generalised or localised to one area, most often the back, abdomen, head and arms. The skin may appear normal or dry (xerosis), associated with signs of chronic scratching including excoriations, superimposed infections, nodular prurigo, eczema and lichenification. The first step in treatment is optimising dialysis efficacy. It makes sense to try and control calcium phosphate and PTH, although the evidence base that this improves pruritus is very limited. Dry skin can be managed by applying regular emollients and the use of soap substitutes. Phototherapy using UVB may be used for severe uraemic pruritus. Oral antihistamines and systemic steroids are generally not effective.

The pathophysiology of UP is complex with several theories postulated. Increased understanding of the nervous pathways has allowed novel agents to be tested. For example, opioid receptor agonists (e.g. nalfurafine) have been shown to be effective in patients with CKD [6]. Other agents reserved for more resistant forms of UP include gabapentin and thalidomide. Kidney transplantation usually results in resolution of uraemic pruritus.

F. Ismail, BSc, MBBS, MRCP, PhD
Department of Dermatology,
Royal Free London NHS Foundation Trust,
Pond Street, London NW3 2QG, UK
e-mail: ferina.ismail@nhs.net

M. Harber (ed.), *Practical Nephrology*,
DOI 10.1007/978-1-4471-5547-8_46, © Springer-Verlag London 2014

Calciphylaxis

Calciphylaxis or calcific uraemic arteriolopathy is a painful necrotising disorder which is potentially life threatening. It is associated with an estimated 1-year survival rate of 45 %, with death predominantly due to infectious complications. Its incidence is estimated to be around 4 % in patients on dialysis and less than 1 % in patients with CKD. Risk factors for the development of calciphylaxis include obesity, diabetes, female sex, white ethnicity, time on renal replacement therapy and the use of warfarin [7]. Other factors reported to be associated with calciphylaxis include the use of vitamin D analogues, calcium-containing phosphate binders and glucocorticosteroids.

Clinical presentation is characterised by progressive cutaneous ulceration on a background of livedo reticularis-like skin changes (Fig. 46.1). There is a predilection for sites with large amounts of subcutaneous fat such as the abdomen, buttocks and thighs, with the evolution of painful subcutaneous purpuric plaques which subsequently develop in to necrotic ulcers often covered by eschars. Prompt recognition and diagnosis enables timely initiation of therapy leading to improved prognosis. A skin biopsy is preferable though the histological features are not pathognomonic. Calciphylaxis should be differentiated from warfarin induced skin necrosis, vasculitis and pyoderma gangrenosum.

Management involves optimising dialysis, often increasing the frequency of sessions, diligent wound care, as well as normalising biochemical abnormalities including parathyroidectomy in the presence of raised PTH levels. Cinacalcet may be effective for control of patients with secondary hyperparathyroidism. Sodium thiosulphate during dialysis at a dose of 5–25 g i.v. has also shown to be effective, and works by chelating calcium from soft tissue, and may need to be continued for a period of weeks to months, in association with the above measures [8].

Table 46.1 Skin conditions associated with chronic kidney disease (those highlighted in bold discussed further in text)

Uraemic pruritus
Calciphylaxis
Nephrogenic systemic fibrosis
Acquired perforating dermatosis
Porphyria cutanea tarda
Hyperpigmentation
Xerosis
Cutaneous infections (bacterial/fungal/viral)
Purpura
Alopecia
Nail changes

Nephrogenic Systemic Fibrosis

Nephrogenic systemic fibrosis (NSF) is a scleroderma-like condition that occurs in patients with CKD and is characterised by skin thickening and fibrosis, as well as systemic involvement of major organs such as the heart and lungs Major clinical criteria include symmetrically distributed indurated plaques and nodules, particularly on the upper and lower limbs, associated with joint contractures and restriction of movement. There is often red/brown discolouration of the skin with orange-peel thickening (peau d'orange) Mean age of onset is 46 years, with equal sex incidence. Exposure to gadolinium-based contrast media is associated with the development of NSF in patients with CKD [9], with a very variable interval of signs of NSF, ranging from 2 days to 18 months post-gadolinium exposure. Diagnosis is confirmed by skin biopsy which demonstrates thickened collagen and proliferation of CD34+ spindle cells.

There is currently no effective treatment for NSF, and prevention by avoidance of, or limited exposure to, gadolinium in patients with CKD (see chapter on imaging) is key [10]. Various therapeutic options have been reported including

Table 46.2 Skin manifestations of diseases associated with renal involvement

Systemic disorder	Skin manifestations
Diabetes mellitus	Necrobiosis lipoidica, perforating dermatosis, eruptive xanthomas
Systemic lupus erythematosus (SLE)	Photosensitivity, malar erythema, cutaneous LE lesions, diffuse alopecia, vasculitis
Henoch-Schönlein purpura	Palpable purpura
Wegener granulomatosis/ polyarteritis nodosa (PAN)	Palpable purpura, subcutaneous nodules, livedo reticularis, ulcers
Systemic sclerosis	Acral or diffuse sclerosis, CREST syndrome, Raynaud's phenomenon
Amyloidosis	Purpura, xanthomatous papules, scleroderma-like changes
Anderson-Fabry disease	Angiokeratomas
HIV	Eosinophilic folliculitis, Kaposi's sarcoma
Cholesterol emboli	Livedo reticularis, petechiae, purpura
Hepatitis C	Purpura, porphyria cutanea tarda, lichen planus, cutaneous PAN
Tuberous sclerosis	Facial angiofibromas, ash-leaf macule, shagreen patch, periungual fibromas

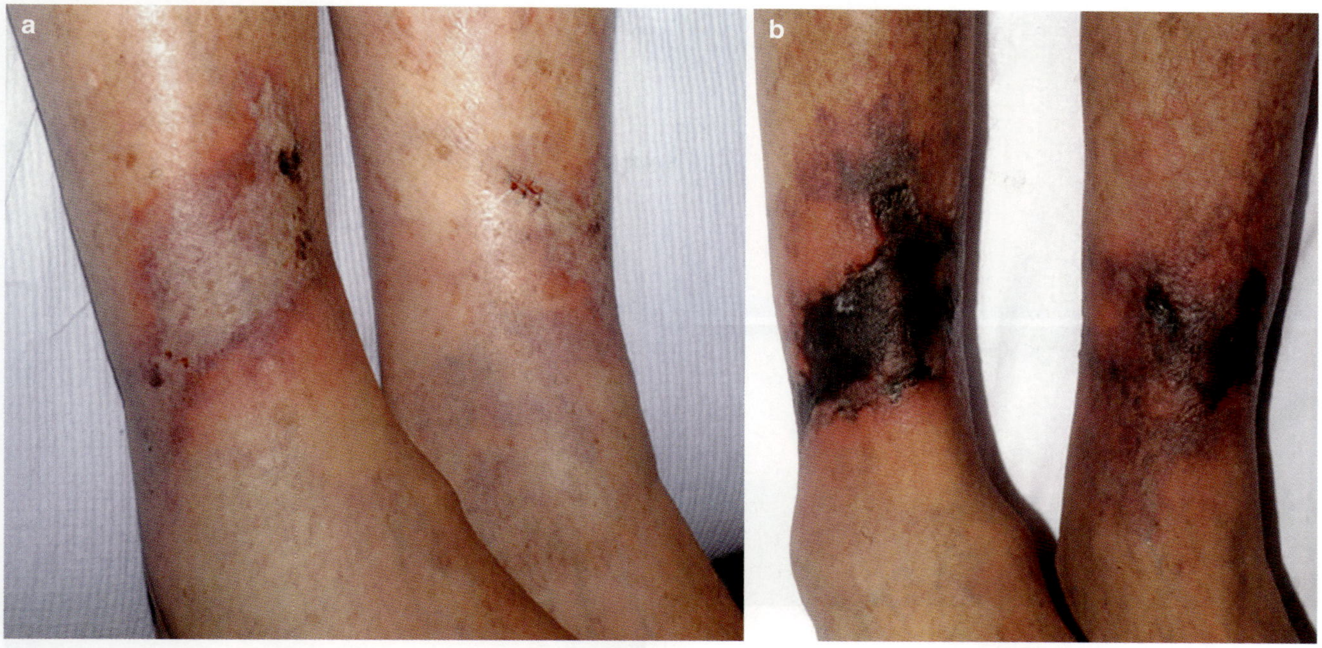

Fig. 46.1 Calciphylaxis 1 week apart

phototherapy, imatinib, extracorporeal photopheresis and sodium thiosulphate. There is no reported clinical benefit of "prophylactic" haemodialysis for the prevention of NSF in patients receiving gadolinium-enhanced scans. Measures directed towards preventing contractures and maintaining mobility includes physiotherapy and deep tissue massage.

Acquired Perforating Dermatosis

Acquired perforating dermatosis (APD), or Kyrle disease, occurs in approximately 10 % of HD patients, with a strong association with diabetes mellitus. APD is also linked with other medical conditions such as hepatitis, thyroid disease, malignancies and HIV. It is characterised by papules with a central hyperkeratotic plug, mainly localised to the trunk, proximal extremities, scalp and face (Fig. 46.2). Lesions are often pruritic and difficult to treat. Often the clinical presentation is typical though histological findings include the presence of epidermal invaginations with a central keratotic plug. Treatment options include emollients, potent topical steroids, topical or systemic retinoids and UVB phototherapy.

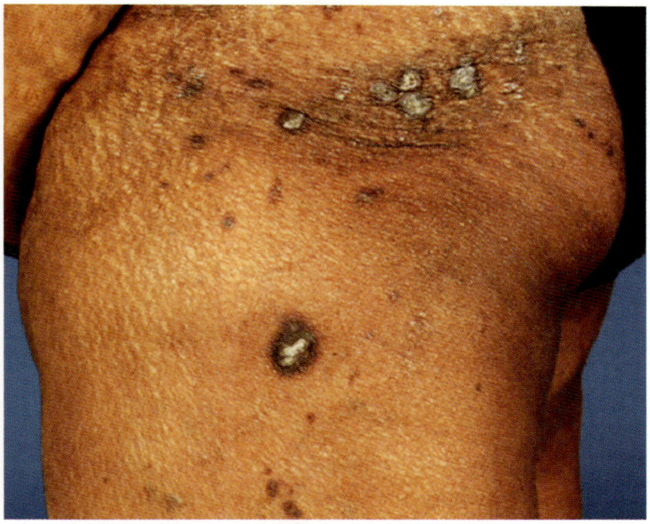

Fig. 46.2 Perforating dermatosis

Porphyria

The porphyrias are a group of inherited or acquired disorders of the enzymes involved in the haem biosynthetic pathway. Porphyria cutanea tarda (PCT) is associated with end-stage renal disease and HD, and commonly presents as bullae on the dorsal aspects of the hands and sun-exposed sites, which often heal with scarring (Fig. 46.3). This is frequently accompanied by facial hyperpigmentation and hypertrichosis. The sporadic form of PCT occurs in approximately 5 % of patients on dialysis and can be precipitated by alcohol, oestrogens, hepatitis B or C infections or HIV. Pseudoporphyria is a condition clinically and histologically identical to PCT but characterised by normal serum and urine porphyrin levels. It is triggered by medications, e.g. amiodarone, tetracyclines and naproxen. Photoprotection is

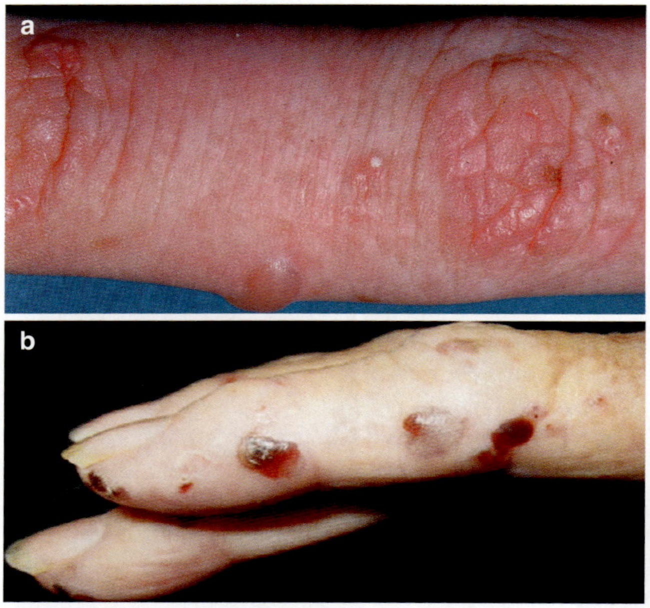

Fig. 46.3 Porphyria cutanea tarda

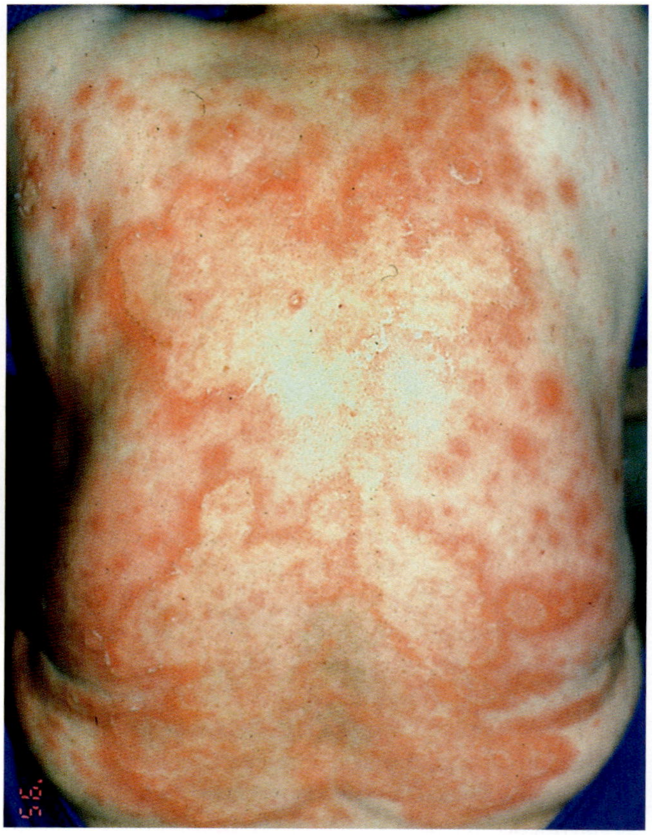

Fig. 46.4 Subacute cutaneous lupus erythematosus

the mainstay of managing such patients via the use of sunscreens and clothing.

Skin Manifestations of Diseases Associated with Renal Involvement

Lupus Erythematosus

The various clinical types of cutaneous lupus erythematosus (CLE) may be subdivided according to the risk of systemic involvement and clinical outcome. With the advent of immunological testing, groups such as subacute cutaneous lupus have been described [11], and the role of drugs in the development of lupus has also been identified. Broadly speaking, CLE may be classified into three subsets: (1) chronic CLE (CCLE), of which the most common manifestation is that of discoid lupus (DLE); (2) acute CLE (ACLE); and (3) subacute CLE (SCLE). Significant systemic involvement occurs in up to 28 % of patients with CCLE with a higher proportion of patients with SCLE (Fig. 46.4) having the diagnostic criteria for systemic lupus but with mild systemic disease. Severe renal disease is uncommon [12, 13]. Mucocutaneous abnormalities occur in around 85 % of patients with SLE. Clinically, chronic discoid lesions tend to lead to scarring with more acute and subacute lesions resolving with pigmentary change. Ordinary histology is poor at differentiating between the subtypes of CLE with direct immunofluorescence positive in ~80 % of involved skin. Potent topical steroids are usually the mainstay of treatment of skin lesions, along with photoprotection (SPF 50+ with UVA protection) and hydroxychloroquine. Patients with CLE require accurate clinico-pathological correlation, not least to attempt to answer the question of the progression of cutaneous disease to systemic disease.

Cutaneous Vasculitis and Renal Disease

Vasculitides can be classified based on the size of the vessel affected. Small-vessel vasculitides include Henoch-Schönlein purpura (HSP) and ANCA-associated vasculitis. 90 % of cases of HSP affect children and renal involvement may not be apparent at initial diagnosis (Fig. 46.5). Although occurring rarely in adults, the sequelae of disease tend to be more severe with more significant renal impairment. ANCA-associated vasculitis includes Wegener's granulomatosis with skin disease occurring in 14–77 % of patients and is associated with a higher frequency of renal involvement [14, 15]. Cutaneous lesions include palpable purpura most commonly on the lower legs, subcutaneous nodules and ulcers. Polyarteritis nodosa (PAN) is a medium and small-vessel disease which may be systemic or solely cutaneous. Skin lesions occur in 25–50 % of patients with systemic PAN and include livedoid changes (Fig. 46.6) and ulceration attributed

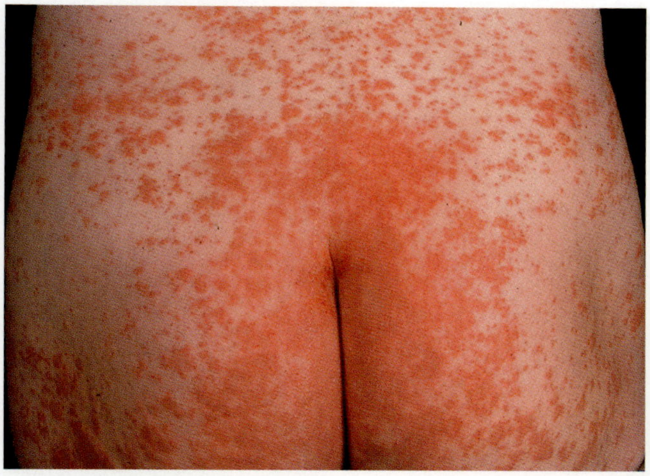

Fig. 46.5 Henoch-Schönlein purpura

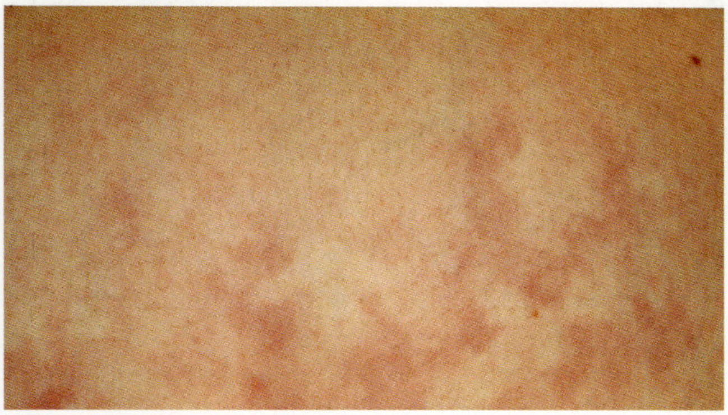

Fig. 46.6 Livedoid changes of PAN

to a necrotising vasculitis, with subcutaneous nodules formed by aneurysms of superficial blood vessels. Renal involvement occurs in 25–60 % of systemic PAN and is a poor prognostic indicator.

Systemic Sclerosis

The clinical separation of scleroderma into limited and diffuse is based on whether truncal skin or proximal parts of the extremities are involved (diffuse), or the induration is limited to the face and distal extremities (limited) [16]. In general diffuse disease carries a worse prognosis however, overlap does exist between the two subtypes. Patients with limited disease tend to have features of CREST syndrome (calcinosis, Raynaud's phenomenon, oesophageal involvement, sclerodactyly, telangiectasia). With sclerosis of the skin, there is often symmetric cutaneous induration and thickening caused by progressive accumulation of excess collagen, frequently associated with itching (Fig. 46.7). This is often

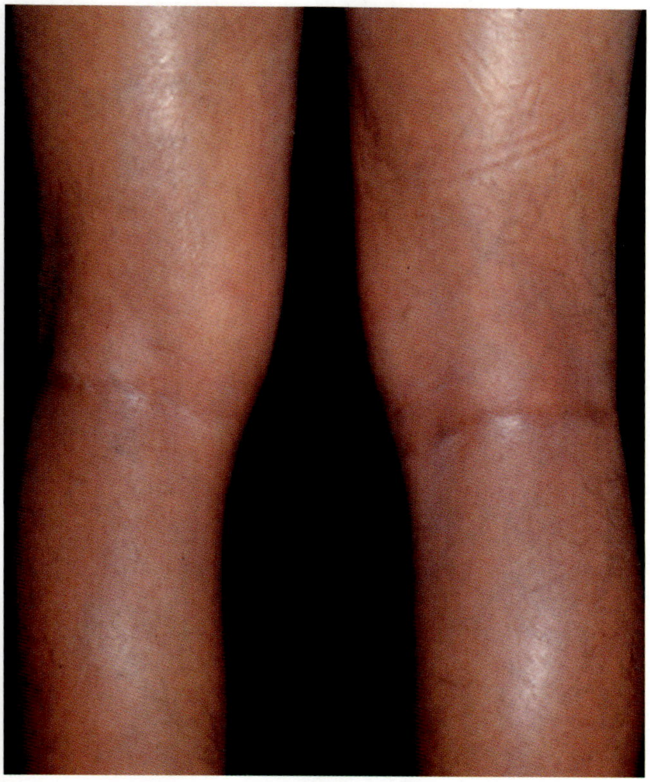

Fig. 46.7 Systemic sclerosis

coupled with diffuse facial hyperpigmentation, as well as localised areas of complete pigment loss with sparing of the perifollicular skin. Telangiectasias are most common in patients with CREST syndrome, particularly on the palms and lips. Capillary abnormalities in the proximal nail fold are present in over 90 % of patients, characterised by capillary loss alternating with dilated loops, which can be visualised with a dermatoscope. First-line agents for cutaneous disease include the use of either potent topical steroids or topical tacrolimus ointment, with the addition of either mycophenolate mofetil or methotrexate. These may be helpful particularly for localised and early stage disease. Phototherapy, particularly UVA, may also be used, as well as exercises and physiotherapy to maintain mobility.

Amyloidosis

In amyloidosis normally soluble plasma proteins are deposited in the extracellular space in an abnormal insoluble fibrillar form. Amyloidosis may be a systemic condition or solely localised to the skin. Cutaneous manifestations are common in systemic amyloidosis, particularly the AL type and are reported in up to 40 % of patients [17]. The lesions usually reflect capillary infiltration and fragility with petechiae and purpura (Fig. 46.8). Xanthomatous papules are frequent and

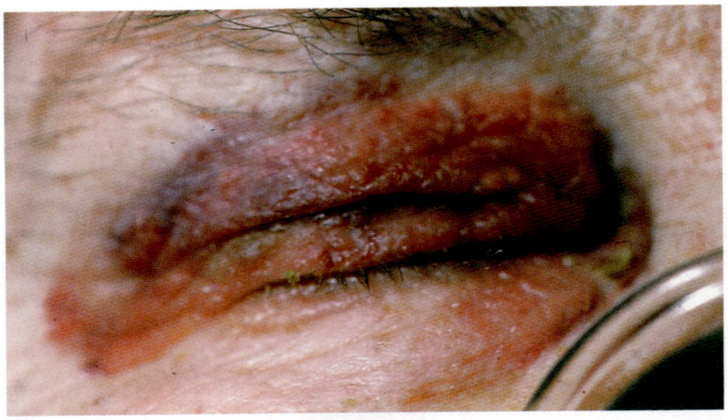

Fig. 46.8 Purpura associated with amyloidosis

other cutaneous lesions include hyperpigmented keratotic lesions, scleroderma-like changes, alopecia and nail dystrophy. Bullous amyloidosis has also been described. Generalised infiltration of cutaneous tissues frequently causes the appearance of skin thickening with loss of facial wrinkles, and can limit mouth opening.

Anderson-Fabry Disease

Anderson-Fabry disease is an X-linked lysosomal storage disorder arising from mutations in the GAL A gene. Deficiency of the enzyme galactosidase A results in the accumulation of globotriaosylceramide (Gb3) within cellular lysosomes throughout the body. The cutaneous hallmark of Fabry disease is angiokeratoma which is present in approximately 70 % of males and 39 % of females. Sites of predilection include the bathing trunk area and genitals in males and the trunk in females (Fig. 46.9). Lips, oral mucosa, umbilicus and extremities may also be affected [18]. Patients with angiokeratoma have higher overall disease severity scores than those without cutaneous vascular lesions. A proportion of Fabry patients also have characteristic facial features including prominent supraorbital ridges, periorbital puffiness, eyelid ptosis, bushy eyebrows, widened nasal bridge, fuller lips and prognathism [19]. Other less well-recognised cutaneous manifestations are sweating abnormalities, lower limb oedema, lymphoedema and Raynaud's phenomenon.

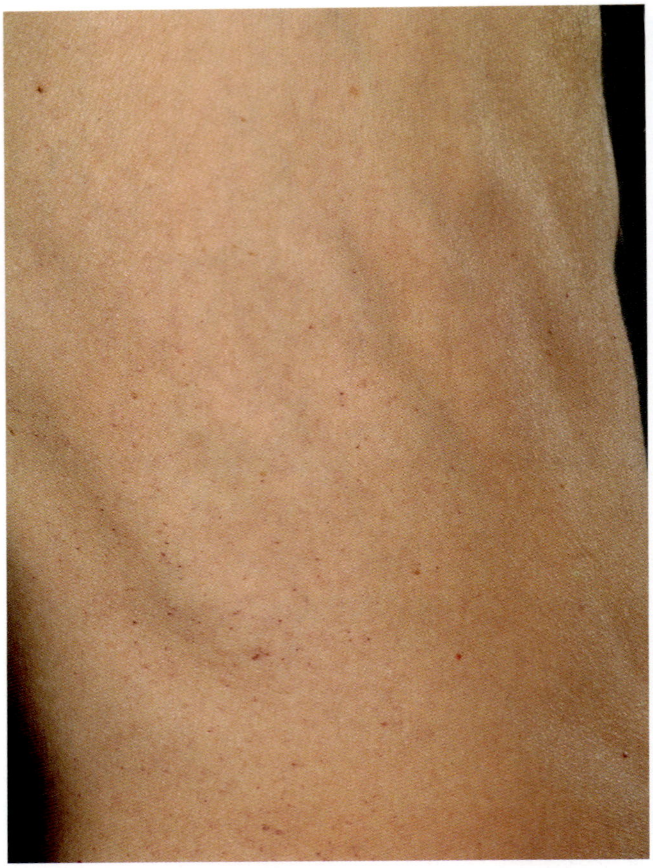

Fig. 46.9 Fabry disease

HIV

Patients with HIV are prone to a variety of skin manifestations which can be attributed to an increased susceptibility to various types of infection, e.g. bacterial, viral and fungal, as well as to inflammatory dermatoses and cutaneous malignancies. HIV-associated skin disease also includes eosinophilic folliculitis which is characterised by recurrent episodes of follicular papulopustules which are often itchy. The lesions predominantly occur on the scalp, face and upper trunk and are observed in an HIV-infected patient with a CD4 count of less than 300 cells/mm^3. Histologically eosinophils are present around the follicular epithelium. Treatment of the underlying HIV infection with a rise in the CD4+ cell count may lead to resolution of the lesions. Other treatment options include topical steroids, UVB phototherapy, oral antibiotics, itraconazole and isotretinoin. (Kaposi's sarcoma will be discussed in the renal transplantation and skin disease section.)

Skin Conditions Associated with Renal Transplantation

Various cutaneous manifestations arise in renal transplant recipients (RTRs) which are mainly attributable to post-transplant immunosuppression. The dermatological complications of immunosuppressive therapy can broadly be divided into drug-specific dermatoses and skin conditions

Table 46.3 Skin conditions associated with renal transplantation

Drug-specific dermatoses	Skin manifestations of immunosuppression			Miscellaneous
Hypertrichosis (Cyclosporin)	*Infection*	*Pre-malignant*	*Malignant*	Skin tags
Gingival hypertrophy (Cyclosporin)	Viral warts	Actinic keratoses	Squamous cell carcinoma	Melanocytic naevi
Acne (Steroids/sirolimus)	Fungal infections (e.g. onychomycosis, pityriasis versicolor)	Bowen's disease	Basal cell carcinoma	Seborrhoeic dermatitis
Sebaceous gland hyperplasia (Cyclosporin)	Folliculitis		Melanoma	Seborrhoeic keratoses
Cushingoid features (Steroids)	HSV/VZV		Merkel cell carcinoma Kaposi sarcoma	

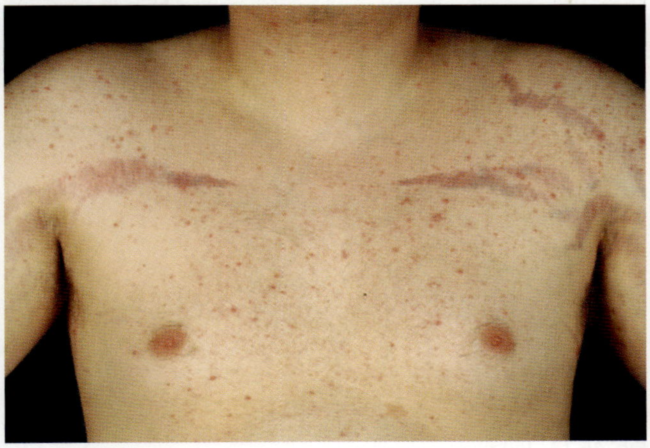

Fig. 46.10 Steroid induced acne and striae

associated with the immunosuppressed state itself, namely infection and malignancy (Table 46.3). There is also a group of miscellaneous skin conditions which are not directly related to the immunosuppression or drugs but observed more frequently in the transplant population. Skin conditions are a significant problem in renal transplant patients with their frequency in one study reported to be 95 % [20], with a major impact on quality of life [2].

Drug-Specific Dermatoses in Transplantation

The well-documented drug-specific skin manifestations are listed in Table 46.3. Acne (Fig. 46.10) in RTRs can often be severe and disfiguring and as such it is important to treat lesions promptly in order to minimise the subsequent risk of scarring. First-line agents for patients with mild to moderate acne include topical agents such as benzoyl peroxide and topical antibiotics such as erythromycin or clindamycin. Use of oil-free or water-based moisturisers and cosmetics should also be recommended. More severe cases of acne may warrant treatment with systemic agents, under the supervision of both dermatologists and nephrologists. These include oral tetracyclines for a minimum of 2–3 months, in combination with suitable topical treatment, or if this fails, then the use of the oral retinoid isotretinoin. The latter may only be prescribed by a dermatologist with close monitoring of lipids and liver function, as well as enrolling women of childbearing age into a pregnancy prevention programme due to its teratogenicity. Most courses of isotretinoin last for 4 months but may often be longer depending on the dose used and how well it is tolerated. Any scope for reducing the dose of the offending agents (particularly steroids) should also be considered.

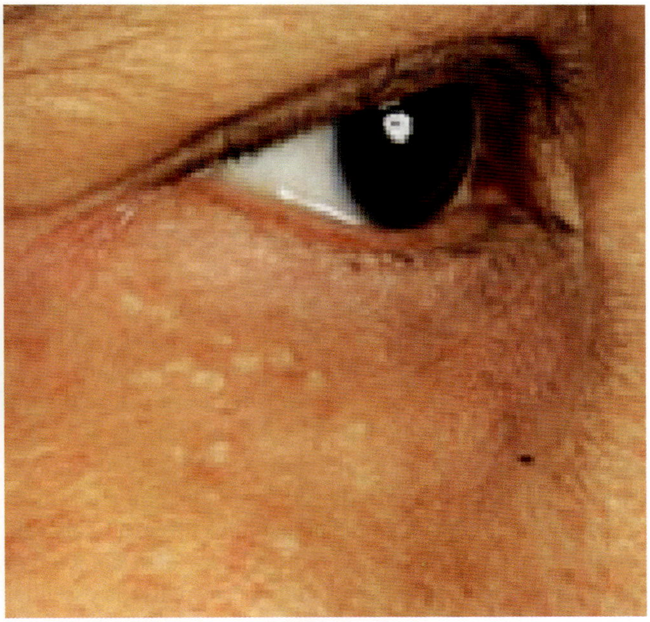

Fig. 46.11 Sebaceous gland hyperplasia

Sebaceous gland hyperplasia can often be disfiguring for patients and may be treated with gentle cautery, though lesions often recur (Fig. 46.11).

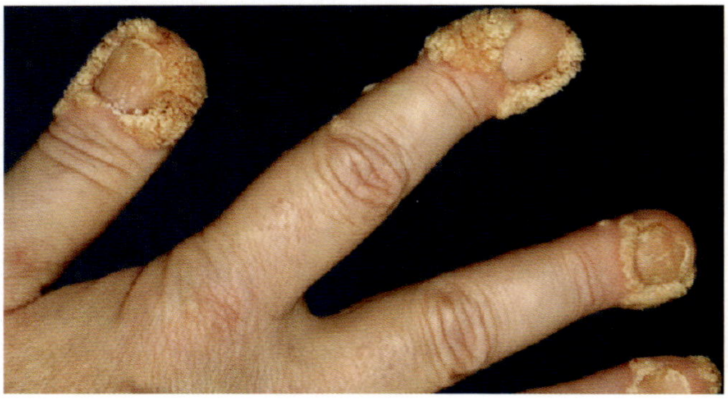

Fig. 46.12 Viral warts

Skin Infections in Solid Organ Transplantation

Infectious lesions arising in transplant recipients most commonly include human papillomavirus (HPV)-related viral warts. They are often numerous and recalcitrant to treatment (Fig. 46.12). Conventional treatments include cryotherapy and salicylic acid (SA) with up to 50 % SA used on plantar warts. Other therapeutic options include curettage and cautery, topical sensitisation with diphencyprone, photodynamic therapy, laser and systemic retinoids (acitretin). A reduction in immunosuppression where possible may be curative. No treatment is also an option, and indications for treatment will depend on the level of discomfort, cosmetic embarrassment and risk of malignancy. Molecular studies reveal a likely role for HPV infection in skin carcinogenesis, as a cofactor in association with UV [21]. An immune response is essential for clearance, and immunocompromised individuals may never show wart clearance.

Pityriasis versicolor has been shown to be a common fungal infection in transplant recipients and is characterised by flat, scaly, hyper- or hypopigmented patches which predominantly occur on the trunk (Fig. 46.13). The mainstay of treatment is with topical antifungal agents such as ketoconazole shampoo which may be used as a wash. More resistant cases may be treated with oral itraconazole, again in liaison with the nephrologist. Fungal nail infections (onychomycosis) also frequently occur, particularly affecting the large toenails, and are notoriously difficult to treat. Again, if asymptomatic, no treatment is acceptable since they are rarely more than a cosmetic problem. If treatment is desired, application of a nail lacquer (e.g. amorolfine) may be suggested. Systemic antifungals such as terbinafine are generally avoided since prolonged courses are required which are ultimately often unsuccessful in adequately treating fungal nail infections.

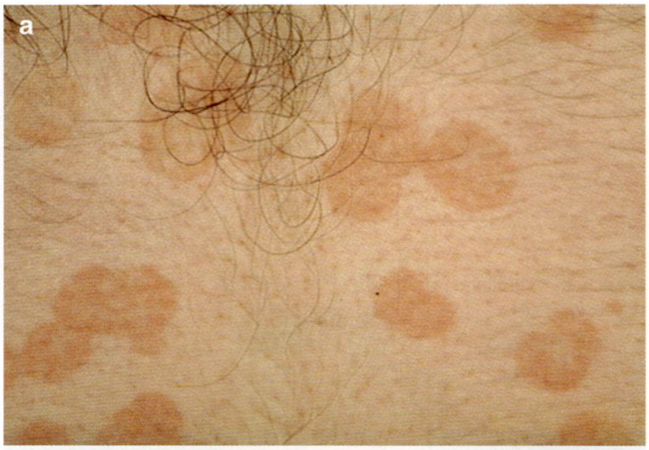

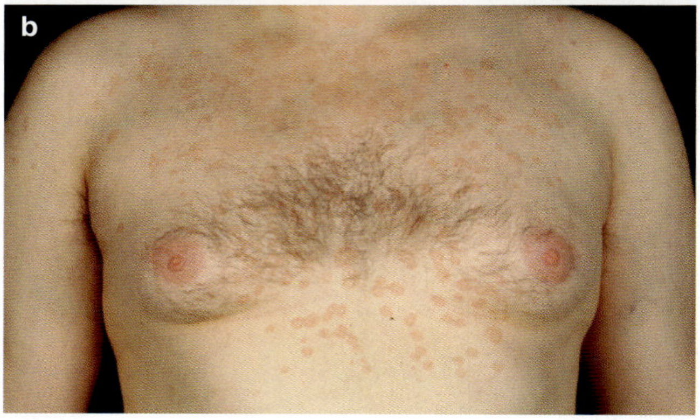

Fig. 46.13 Pityriasis versicolor

Premalignant and Malignant Skin Conditions

RTRs are at significant increased risk of cutaneous malignancy compared to the general population. Non-melanoma skin cancers (NMSC), in particular squamous cell carcinoma (SCC) and basal cell carcinoma (BCC), are by far the most common, affecting more than half of organ transplant recipients during their long-term course [3]. NMSCs in RTRs not only place a significant burden on healthcare resources but also cause significant morbidity for individuals as rates are over 100 times that of the general population and tumours are often multiple and more aggressive [3]. Studies have shown that after a first cutaneous SCC, multiple subsequent skin cancers develop in 60–80 % of RTRs within 3 years [22]. It is predicted that NMSC incidence will continue to escalate relentlessly as a clinical problem in RTRs as an inevitable consequence of continuing improvements in long-term graft survival. Immunosuppression and HPV have been implicated as possible cofactors in transplant skin carcinogenesis, but cumulative exposure to ultraviolet radiation remains the dominant risk factor [23]. Sunscreen use has been shown to significantly reduce the incidence of cutaneous SCC in immunocompetent individuals with the incidence of SCC lower in the sunscreen group than in the no daily sunscreen group (1,115 vs 1,832 per 100,000; 0.61 [0.46–0.81]), which is the only robust RCT for cutaneous SCC prevention [24]. Primary and secondary prevention campaigns have accordingly emphasised the importance of photoprotection and self-surveillance. Where possible, a reduction in immunosuppression should be considered as a means of attempting to reduce the incidence and subsequent complications of such tumours.

Many precancerous conditions can be treated by non-surgical means, for example, by spraying liquid nitrogen (cryotherapy), applying a topical agent such as 5-fluorouracil or 5 % imiquimod as well as photodynamic therapy (PDT). Most skin cancers themselves can be removed by a minor surgical procedure performed under a local anaesthetic, which is often curative. Aggressive margin control is required and as such Mohs micrographic surgery is often the treatment of choice for difficult BCCs and SCCs on the face. This is a scar-minimising surgical technique which enables microscopic examination of all the surgical margins at the time of surgery, thus ensuring complete removal of the tumour whilst sparing as much normal skin as possible. Since most skin cancers arise on sun-exposed sites, e.g. the face, prompt diagnosis potentially minimises the extent of surgery and subsequent scarring. More importantly, rapid treatment reduces the risk of possible tumour spread with certain types of skin cancer.

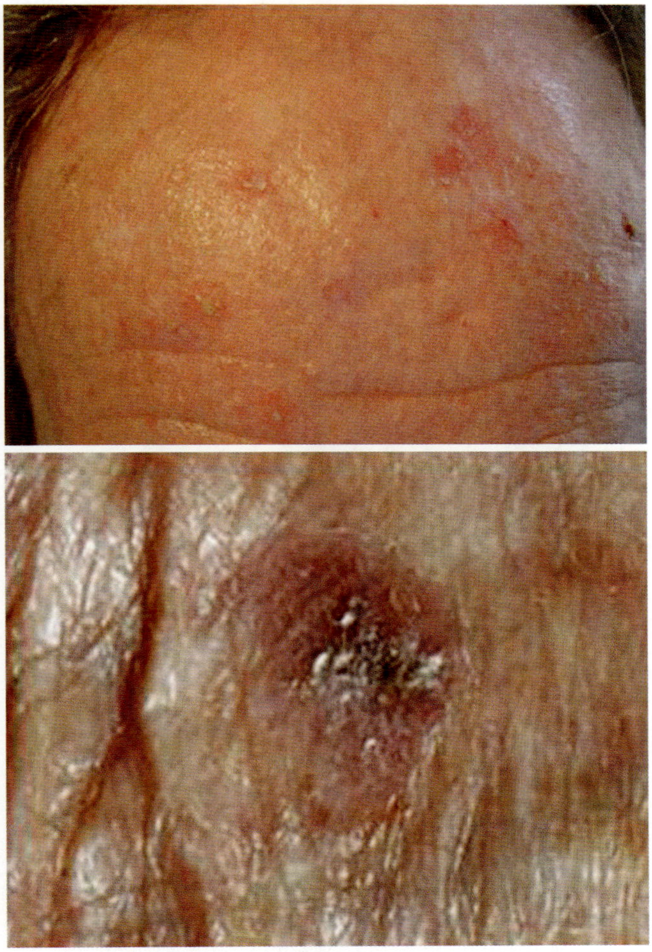

Fig. 46.14 Actinic keratoses

Actinic Keratoses (Solar Keratoses)

These are precancerous skin lesions which are characterised by pink/red scaly patches, on sun-exposed sites. The most commonly affected areas are the face and backs of the hands, with confluent areas of involvement known as field change (Fig. 46.14). There is a lack of evidence to suggest that treating AK/field change actually prevents progression to SCC though currently it is standard practice to do so.

Basal Cell Carcinomas (BCC or rodent ulcers)

These are slow growing, often pearly-pink lesions that typically arise on sun-exposed sites (Fig. 46.15). They seldom if ever spread; however, if left untreated they can erode the skin, eventually leading to ulceration and local invasion. Surgical removal is the mainstay of treatment though other options include local radiotherapy as well as cryotherapy, topical agents and PDT for certain superficial subtypes of BCC.

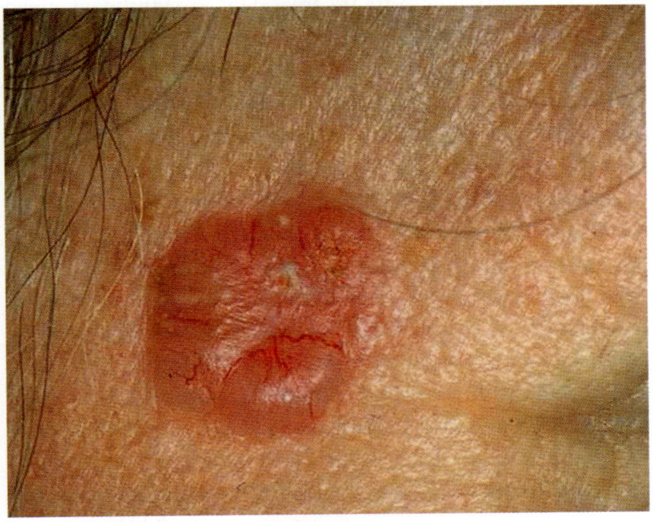

Fig. 46.15 Basal cell carcinoma

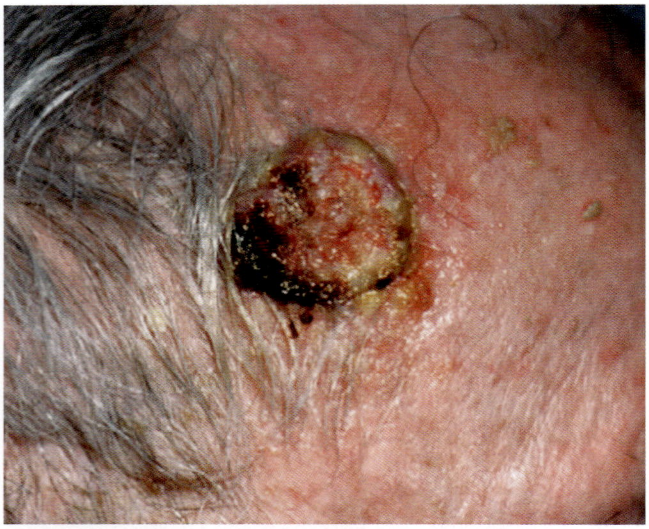

Fig. 46.16 Cutaneous squamous cell carcinoma

Squamous Cell Carcinoma (SCC)

SCCs frequently appear as a scaly crusted area of skin, with a red, inflamed base and are often ulcerated (Fig. 46.16). A painful enlarging lump is suspicious for SCC, predominantly occurring on sun-exposed sites, particularly on the ears, lips and backs of the hands. This is the most frequent type of skin cancer in organ transplant patients and if left untreated, has the potential to metastasise, with a 7 % metastatic risk overall. SCCs are generally best treated by surgical removal. Chemoprevention with the systemic retinoid acitretin has been reported to lead to a significant reduction in SCC development in RTRs and is often used in high-risk individuals with >1 cutaneous SCC. In a retrospective study of 28 RTRs receiving continuous retinoid treatment, a significant mean reduction of 1.46 SCCs occurred in the first year of treatment, 2.24 SCCs by the second year and 2.14 SCCs in year 3. This reduction was sustained, but nonsignificant, at years 4 and later, indicating a loss of efficacy in the chemopreventive properties of acitretin. In addition, a "rebound" phenomenon is also recognised whereby interruption of acitretin treatment leads to a relapse in tumour development [25]. There is now strong evidence to suggest that switching from calcineurin inhibitors to sirolimus in RTRs with at least one previous cutaneous SCC is associated with a lower risk of subsequent skin cancers. The number of SCCs was lower by a factor of 3.4 in the sirolimus group than in the calcineurin-inhibitor group. Survival free of cutaneous squamous cell carcinoma was significantly longer in the sirolimus group than in the calcineurin-inhibitor group, with a relative risk in the sirolimus group of 0.56. There were however a much higher rate of adverse events in patients converted to sirolimus [26].

Melanoma

Melanomas are much rarer than BCCs and SCCs, with an 8–10-fold increased risk in RTRs, though are potentially more aggressive if not detected early. A multicentre European study reported a worse prognosis for stage II disease compared with the general population [27]. They are usually an irregular brown or black lesion, which may start in a preexisting mole or appear on previously normal skin. Any change in a mole, or any new mole occurring for the first time after the age of 30, should be urgently assessed by a dermatologist with a view to surgical excision.

Merkel Cell Carcinoma

Merkel cell carcinoma (MCC) is a rare yet aggressive skin tumour occurring more commonly in RTRs, in whom it has a significantly worse prognosis. They present as solitary red nodules, often on sun-exposed sites and are highly aggressive, metastasising early. They are of neuroendocrine origin and thought to be of viral aetiology with a relatively new virus, the Merkel cell polyomavirus (MCPyV), having been identified in a significant proportion of such tumours [28]. Management is predominantly surgical with the use of adjuvant radiotherapy for local disease. Metastatic MCC may involve the need for transplant-directed dosage adjustment of chemotherapeutic agents in association with possible modification of immunosuppression. Further research on the role of MCPyV may offer hope for more targeted approaches to MCC treatment and prevention.

Kaposi's Sarcoma

The incidence of Kaposi's sarcoma (KS) among recipients of solid organs is greater than 100 times the rate in the general population, with clinical presentation in transplant patients often confined to the skin. KS is especially prevalent in Mediterranean and African populations and is caused by HHV8. The main approach to managing transplant-associated Kaposi's sarcoma is to reduce or even discontinue immunosuppressive therapy, which usually causes skin lesions to regress, although it carries a risk of acute rejection of the graft. KS generally recurs when immunosuppressive therapy is reintroduced or after a second transplantation. In a study of 15 renal transplant recipients, it was found that sirolimus inhibits the progression of dermal KS when given at the usual immunosuppressive doses, with remission induced in all 15 subjects within 3 months [29].

Specialist Transplant Skin Clinics

The need for post-transplant skin cancer surveillance has been recognised in many international expert consensus guidelines. In the UK, the National Institute for Health and Clinical Excellence recommend surveillance in dedicated dermatology clinics [30] and it has been shown that such clinics significantly improve compliance with sun protection and skin cancer awareness [31]. Other guidelines in Europe and the USA also advise specialist full skin examination of RTRs every 6–12 months; however, these recommendations do not take account of individual risk nor the needs of practising clinicians with limited resources. The effectiveness and cost-benefit of skin surveillance in RTRs is unknown and as such, a surveillance model for skin cancer in RTRs has been proposed by Harwood et al. [32], based on a 22-year prospective study of more than 1,000 patients. They define surveillance intervals that enable close follow-up of higher-risk individuals with routine follow-up of those at much lower risk. This risk stratification is based upon a number of patient characteristics including skin phototype, age at transplantation, sunburn history and history of confirmed skin cancer. This is of practical use to those setting up transplant skin clinics, facilitating targeted surveillance and active management to those who need it most.

Any such service should involve a multidisciplinary approach with close interaction between dermatologists, transplant clinicians, plastic surgeons/dermatology surgeons, medical/clinical oncologists, pathologists, clinical nurse specialists and primary care physicians. The relationship between dermatologists and transplant clinicians enables discussion of potential revision of immunosuppression in high-risk individuals as well as the potential need for systemic agents to be introduced. The role of a specialist nurse should also be highlighted, in particular facilitating urgent access for patients, as well as undertaking nurse-led surveillance clinics and patient education in relation to photoprotection and skin cancer awareness. Preferably, primary prevention of skin cancers should be emphasised from the outset, i.e. to all patients on transplant waiting lists.

Further information for transplant patients, as well as patients awaiting an organ transplant, can be obtained via the British Association of Dermatologists websitehttp://www.bad.org.uk/site/792/default.aspx

Other useful websites include:

British Society for Skin Care in Immunocompromised Individuals (BSSCII)http://www.bad.org.uk/site/1434/default.aspx

Skin Care in Organ Transplant Patients Europe (SCOPE)http://www.scopenetwork.org/index.htm

International Transplant Skin Cancer Collaborative (ITSCC)http://www.itscc.org/

After Transplantation – Reduce Incidence of Skin Cancer (AT-RISC Alliance)http://at-risc.org/Home.aspx

Acknowledgements Professor Catherine Harwood and Dr Cate Orteu kindly provided many of the clinical photographs and contributed to sections “Skin Conditions Associated with Renal Transplantation” and “Skin Manifestations of Diseases Associated with Renal Involvement” of this chapter, respectively.

References

1. Udayakumar P, Balasubramanian S, Ramalingam KS, Lakshmi C, Srinivas CR, Mathew AC. Cutaneous manifestations in patients with chronic renal failure on haemodialysis. Indian J Dermatol Venereol Leprol. 2006;72(2):119–25.
2. Moloney FJ, Keane S, O’Kelly P, Conlon PJ, Murphy GM. The impact of skin disease on renal transplantation on quality of life. Br J Dermatol. 2005;153(3):574–8.
3. Euvrard S, Kanitakis J, Claudy A. Skin cancers after organ transplantation. N Engl J Med. 2003;348(17):1681–91.
4. Patel TS, Freedman BI, Yosipovitch G. An update on pruritus associated with CKD. Am J Kidney Dis. 2007;50(1):11–20.
5. Narita I, Alchi B, Omori K, Sato F, Ajiro J, Saga D, Kondo D, Skatsume M, Maruyama S, Kazama JJ, Akazawa K, Gejyo F. Aetiology and prognostic significance of severe uraemic pruritus in chronic haemodialysis patients. Kidney Int. 2006;69:1626–32.
6. Wikström B, Gellert R, Ladefoged SD, Danda Y, Akai M, Ide K, Ogasawara M, Kawashima Y, Ueno K, Mori A, Ueno Y. Kappa-opioid system in uremic pruritus: multicenter, randomized, double-blind, placebo-controlled clinical studies. J Am Soc Nephrol. 2005;16(12):3742–7.
7. Weenig RH, Sewell LD, Davis MD, McCarthy JT, Pittelkow MR. Calciphylaxis: natural history, risk factor analysis and outcome. J Am Acad Dermatol. 2007;56(4):569–79.
8. Hayden MR, Goldsmith DJ. Sodium thiosulfate: new hope for the treatment of calciphylaxis. Semin Dial. 2010;23:258–62.
9. Broome DR. Nephrogenic systemic fibrosis associated with gadolinium based contrast agents: a summary of the medical literature reporting. Eur J Radiol. 2008;66(2):230–4.
10. The Royal College of Radiologists – Gadolinium-based contrast media and Nephrogenic Systemic Fibrosis (2007). http://www.rcr.ac.uk/docs/radiology/pdf/BFCR0714_Gadolinium_NSF_guidanceNov07.pdf
11. Sontheimer RD. Subacute cutaneous lupus erythematosus: 25-year evolution of a prototypic subset (subphenotype) of lupus erythematosus defined by characteristic cutaneous, pathological, immunological, and genetic findings. Autoimmun Rev. 2005;4(5):253–63.
12. Gronhagen CM, Fored CM, Granath F, Nyberg F. Cutaneous lupus erythematosus and the association with systemic lupus erythematosus: a population-based cohort of 1088 patients in Sweden. Br J Dermatol. 2011;164:1335–41.
13. Chong BF, Song J, Olsen NJ. Determining risk factors for developing systemic lupus erythematosus in patients with discoid lupus erythematosus. Br J Dermatol. 2012;166:29–35.
14. Walsh JS, Gross DJ. Wegener’s granulomatosis involving the skin. Cutis. 1999;64(3):183–6.
15. Frances C, Du LT, Piette JC, et al. Wegener’s granulomatosis. Dermatological manifestations in 75 cases with clinicopathologic correlation. Arch Dermatol. 1994;130(7):861–7.

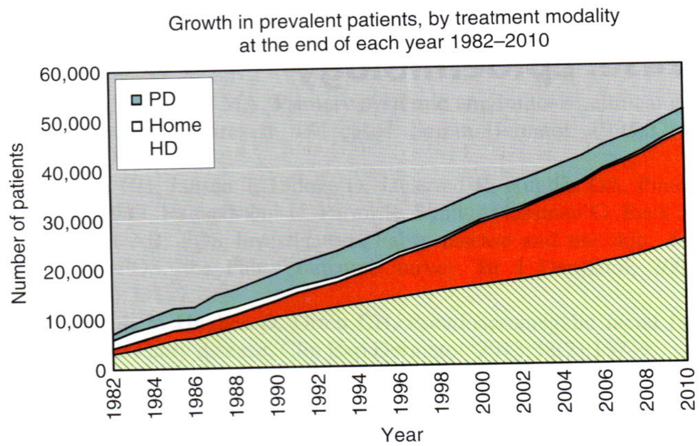

Fig. 47.2 Growth in prevalent patients, by treatment modality, at the end of each year 1982–2010

Table 47.1 CKD staging according to the National Kidney Foundation and Kidney Disease Outcomes Quality Initiative (NKF-KDOQI)

Stage 1	'Kidney damage'; normal or raised glomerular filtration rate, abnormalities of urine tests or imaging
Stage 2	Glomerular filtration rate 60–89 ml/min per 1.73 m^2 with abnormalities of urine tests or imaging
Stage 3[a]	3A glomerular filtration rate 4,559 ml/min per 1.73 m^2
	3B glomerular filtration rate 30–44 ml/min per 1.73 m^2
Stage 4	Glomerular filtration rate 15–29 ml/min per 1.73 m^2
Stage 5[b]	Glomerular filtration rate <15 ml/min per 1.73 m^2

[a]Stage 3 is sometimes subclassified into two groups, 3A and 3B: 3A defines a lower-risk group with eGFR of 45–59; 3B defines a higher-risk group with eGFR of 30–44

[b]Stage 5 is sometimes demarcated with a suffix based on treatment regimes, e.g. 5D for those treated with dialysis

incidence in a given population depends therefore on a series of assumptions with regard to the referral and availability of RRT, people with CKD stage 5 being started on dialysis, reversibility of the kidney problem, the survival in the first 90 days of the dialysis (*numerator*) and the coverage (*denominator*).

Most renal registries in developed countries have reported alarming increases in RRT over the past years, particularly in those aged over 65 years, but there remains doubt to what extent additional referral of patients previously deemed 'unsuitable' may play a role. Whether very elderly patients or patients with other chronic conditions such as HIV, malignancy or severe cardiovascular disease are referred to RRT depends to a large extent on national legislation with respect to life-prolonging therapy in the face of chronic disease and the degree of renal knowledge and ethical opinions of treating doctors. There is also a concern that if government freely funds RRT as has happened in the USA, there is less development of palliative care services and some argue less emphasis on preventive therapy of earlier CKD. Moreover, there is evidence, that even if there is in theory a free access for everybody to RRT care, the actual number of facilities that are available will drive substantive socioeconomic differentials amongst patients offered RRT.

Using the CKD Definition in Populations to Define CKD Incidence and Prevalence

It is perhaps easier to discuss first how we define prevalence of chronic kidney disease (CKD). The term CKD covers a number of primary disease processes that result in structural and/or functional kidney abnormalities persisting for at least 3 months. Abnormal urinalysis with proteinuria and/or haematuria or abnormal kidney structure/histology, with or without a decreased glomerular filtration rate (GFR less than 60 ml/min per 1.73 m^2) are the defining presentations.

Expert groups have subdivided CKD into five stages according to the measured GFR (Table 47.1) reflecting their idea that CKD progresses slowly through these stages before a minority reach end-stage renal disease (ESRD). The expert groups thought that such a CKD staging system has two important advantages: firstly, it suggests that if CKD is detected at an early stage, intervention may prevent or slow progression to more advanced stages, and, secondly, it reflects the observation that as GFR declines the risk for the patient and associated complications change. Thus, staging allows for structuring therapy and prioritising interventions for the management of CKD.

When the initial NKF-KDOQI CKD staging was proposed, it was not very evidence based. Nevertheless, it was an important and useful first step as it initiated a flurry of epidemiological studies that tried to refute or support the proposed CKD staging system [2]. The interesting aspect is that the prominent expert groups were very successful of getting the NKF-KDOQI staging system implemented into clinical policy without at the time any clear indication that the application of the staging system directly relates to the incidence of RRT in populations [3].

In practice the largest group of patients to come to clinical attention with CKD are those with reduced GFR (stage 3–5), many of whom have multiple contributing causes – although in reality for most the cause is unknown. The vast majority of these patients are not the classic 'nephrology' patients that you see in kidney clinics – most are frail elderly people which would have been traditionally managed by general pratictioners and geriatricians. The biggest problem of the NKF-KDOQI system is that it is not reflecting the true risk of who actually progresses to RRT and who actually has a treatable kidney problem. There are many patients with earlier CKD particularly with proteinuria/albuminuria and maintained renal function that merit relatively more attention in practice because there is a greater potential to prevent progression, and all epidemiological data suggest that proteinuria/albuminuria are far stronger prognostic markers for RRT onset than a low eGFR on its own [3, 4].

The incidence of CKD is much harder to ascertain than the incidence of RRT. This may initially seem counterintuitive, as many people assume that creatinine or a urine dipstick test is done in most people at one point in their life. In order to measure 'incidence of CKD', i.e. true new CKD cases in a perfect epidemiological cohort study, one would need to exclude those with CKD at baseline from our follow-up study. Saving money by asking people whether they have CKD will not work, as most lay people do not know that they have CKD. The follow-up requires remeasuring kidney function at regular time points on every participant. The current study design assumes a perfect measurement of CKD, but as we discuss below, this is not feasible. In order to have enough observations to understand the risk factors for ending up on RRT, the study would be of enormous size – for a million population in the UK, we would get about 100 incident RRT cases per year, so the cost of a proper research study just to define CKD incidence, and how this relates to RRT incidence, is prohibitive. There is no universal screening for kidney disease in the general population at pre-specified time points in life and the use of routine data is therefore challenging and relies on some untestable assumptions.

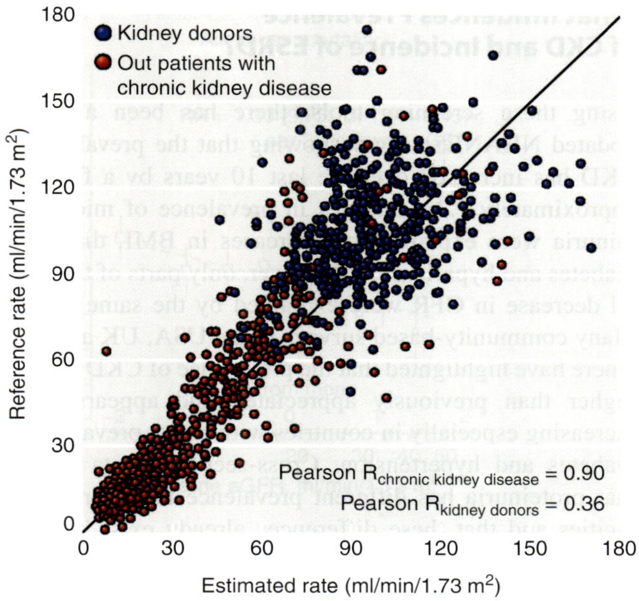

Fig. 47.3 Comparison of gold-standard GFR measurement (*Y* axis) against eGFR. If the estimation formula was very precise, then we would anticipate to see only little variation around the *black line*. As is evident from the figure, the precision of estimation increases with lower eGFR (Reprinted with permission from Giles et al. [18])

Measuring Estimated GFR

Due to the nonlinear (exponential) relationship between serum creatinine and GFR, an elevated serum creatinine is a relatively late marker for loss of renal function. Serum creatinine only rises above the reference range when ~50 % of kidney function has been lost. The traditional indirect measure of GFR in clinical practice was the 24 h creatinine clearance. These 24 h urine collections are subject to substantial measurement error and not feasible in large studies. NHANES III was the first population-based survey that assessed renal impairment using a serum creatinine-based formula that had been validated for the US population [5]. Formula-based estimated GFR (eGFR) measurements, using serum creatinine values, are now established in routine clinical practice and have been modified and incorporated into clinical practice guidelines [6]. The typical eGFR formula requires simple input data such as the age, gender and ethnicity, in addition to serum creatinine. Because creatinine is a product of the endogenous muscle metabolism, these calculations assume the presence of a stable muscle mass. Average muscle mass in a population is largely a function of age and gender and to a smaller extent height and weight. An investigation in standardisation of creatinine assays showed that the type of assay plays a role for an estimated GFR >60 ml/min per 1.73 m^2. US recommendations advise practitioners to repeat their renal assessment after 3 months – this was however not done in NHANES due to considerations of practicability and cost.

It is important to appreciate that each of the available eGFR formulae has its own biases, e.g. the MDRD formula is biased for women, and not validated in older-age groups [7]. The CKDEPI formula is thought to perform better in Western populations [8] but does not appear to work in less well-nourished populations in other parts of the world. The measurement error around an eGFR measurement ranges from ±20 ml/min relative to the gold-standard GFR measurement (worse errors when eGFR is >60 ml/min), and so any survey using eGFR data will be imprecise by default (Fig. 47.3). Moreover, most epidemiologic studies only use a single time point eGFR, and this means that all the associations that have been found are to some degree affected by non-differential misclassification. Non-differential misclassification means that the observed associations for eGFR and urine spot urine or dipstick measurements in all the research studies will underestimate the true degree of risk associations.

Overall, despite above criticisms – in comparison with pure serum creatinine measurements and 24 h collections of urine, serum creatinine-based GFR estimates and urinary albumin/creatinine or protein/creatinine ratios seem to perform well as screening tools for the presence of kidney disease.

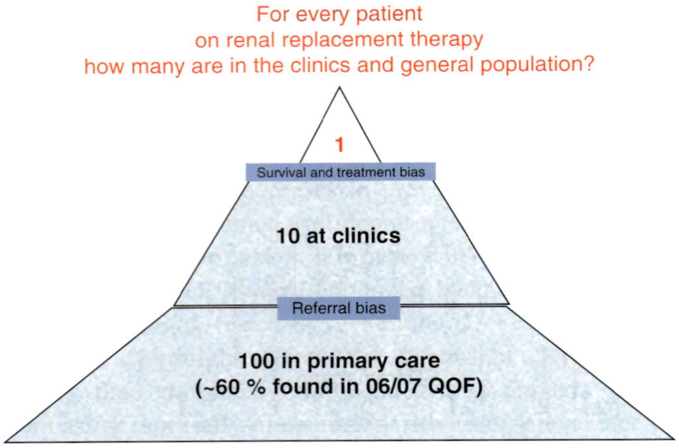

Fig. 47.6 CKD-ESRD spectrum: understanding biases in CKD and ESRD data due to referral and survival or treatment biases

reach ESRD. Overall there are many more patients with in primary care than seen by a nephrologist in secondary or tertiary care (Fig. 47.6). This means that a renal physician's perspective of 'late referral' may in parts be true, but certainly there are plenty of people out in the community who had many other problems apart from the kidney problem.

CKD is now recognised as a contributory factor worldwide for cardiovascular disease (CVD). The high cardiovascular risk of CKD patients is however a possible argument for screening. After all, according to the World Health Organization, coronary heart disease is now the leading cause of death worldwide and more than 60 % of the global burden of coronary heart disease is present in low- to middle-income countries. From the epidemiologic studies, it appears that a large proportion of people with CKD have to do with lifelong exposure to an adverse lifestyle, in particular, obesity. Hence, targeting common cardiovascular risk factors such as smoking, obesity, diabetes and hypertension is likely to prevent CKD and renal failure development. Depending on the health system and the pay for performance structures, it may well be that the cardiovascular risk or diabetes management may well be better done by other specialities.

A complicating factor impeding CKD screening is the low awareness of primary care physicians of the importance of CKD as a cardiovascular risk factor. In a study based on primary care data across over 300 general practices in Italy, ICD-9-codes for CKD were reported in 2.5 % of the cohort compared to an age-adjusted eGFR-based CKD diagnosis of 9.3 % [15]. This is relevant to studies of CKD where the patients may be ascertained based on some other factor (such as diabetes or symptoms) rather than the biochemical definition of CKD by eGFR measurement. Interestingly, amongst patients with decreased kidney function (by GFR), primary care practitioners correctly diagnosed CKD (with ICD codes) in only 15.2 % of such patients. Furthermore, specific diagnoses of CKD, such as diabetic nephropathy and hypertensive nephropathy, were rarely reported (0.1 and 0.5 %, respectively) despite a high prevalence of diabetes (11.1 %) and hypertension (34.1 %) in the group of patients with eGFR <60 ml/min per 1.73 m^2. There has been a global initiative to educate primary care practitioners on the appropriate interpretation of serum creatinine and the utility of estimated GFR in the early detection of CKD patients. In the UK, there is evidence that this approach is reaping benefits with CKD patients referred earlier to renal services (with higher GFRs at time of referral) and a lower proportion of patients starting dialysis in an unplanned fashion. The only 'disadvantage' of this earlier recognition is that many more older patients with nonprogressive CKD are being assessed at hospital clinics. However, these older people with known CKD are at a high risk of AKI and medication side effects and therefore benefit from medication review. In Canada, there is now evidence that the reporting of estimated GFR has substantially increased referral to specialists and should in time improve the outlook for these patients.

Defining an Underlying Cause of CKD: Considerations and Causes Not to Miss

Individuals born in developing countries may have a smaller renal reserve to start with as a result of the high prevalence of poor maternal health and malnutrition during pregnancy.

For instance, data from Pakistan suggest that blood pressures in South Asian children are higher when compared to white children living in the USA, with also a relatively high prevalence of proteinuria. Data from the UK show convincingly that people who have low birth weight and who gain weight in early adulthood will have a lower eGFR than people who are overweight in middle or older age [16]. In short, some patients are preconditioned to reduced GFR and superimposition of secondary causes such as hypertension, diabetes or even AKI such as post-streptococcal glomerulonephritis may result in a higher risk of CKD. This temporal delay in having kidney disease related to diabetes may in parts be also a function of ethnicity. For example, South Asian diabetic patients seem to have a two to four times faster progression to renal disease when compared to Dutch diabetic countrymen.

Within the UK, recorded primary causes of ESRD include in 20 % diabetic nephropathy, in probably more than 15 % severe CVD unrelated to diabetes, in 8 % polycystic kidney disease and in autoimmune diseases, as for example glomerulonephritis or systemic lupus erythematosus (SLE), 30 %. In registries worldwide, 20–25 % of ESRD diagnoses are recorded as unknown partly because patients may present with small kidneys that it is not appropriate or possible to biopsy. This leads to selective missing data in any registry study; moreover, there is evidence that doctors make their diagnosis of this disease dependent on the known ethnicity of a patient. The same case report is twice as likely to be assigned the diagnosis hypertensive renal disease by a nephrologist if the ethnicity of a patient is recorded to be black – ethnicity however was randomly assigned to the case report by the investigator as either black or white [17]. This is an important issue; it is clearly important to know the extent and impact of diseases that result in ESRD, and accurate reporting of diagnoses to registries needs to be improved. Moreover, there are undoubtedly new renal diseases waiting to be discovered in the CKD population as illustrated by the recent discovery of C5 nephropathy in the Cypriot dialysis population.

Ideally the primary cause of CKD would be established in every patient but a substantial percentage (20–30 %) of registry returns worldwide have 'CKD unknown cause' as the reason for ESRD. There are many reasons for this, not least that renal biopsies are considerably more dangerous in advanced CKD and the histology of advanced CKD may not be diagnostic of the primary cause, so the risk benefit is not in favour of histological diagnosis. However, there are advantages to the patient in honing down the differential diagnosis in terms of (a) the possibility of an inheritable condition, (b) recurrent disease and (c) potential ongoing treatment for systemic conditions.

Table 47.2 shows some conditions worth considering in the patient first presenting with CKD in whom the diagnosis is not clear (obstruction and other obvious causes excluded) and a biopsy either non-diagnostic or inappropriate. This is not a comprehensive list, nor are most of these tests

Table 47.2 Some causes of ESRD to consider (beyond the obvious) with non-invasive tests that may make or suggest the diagnosis

Genetic causes	
Nephronophthisis	AR, urinary concentrating defect, *medullary cysts, screening NPHP1* (and others) childhood and adolescent CKD
MCKD1	AD, urinary concentrating defect (polyuria), preserved renal size
MCKD2	AD, *gout in adolescence, high urate*
RCAD	AD HNF1B *type 2 diabetes in youth* (MODY)
Thin basement membrane nephropathy	AD haematuria and family history, *genotyping: COL4A3/4/5*
CFHR5 nephropathy	AD *haematuria and macroscopic haematuria (in Cypriots)*
Branchio-oto-renal	AD *pre-auricular pits, deafness, branchial clefts*
Alport's syndrome	X-linked (and AR) *deafness* (but not always), haematuria, retinal signs
Anderson-Fabry	X-linked angiokeratomas, eye and heart signs, pain, *white blood cell alpha- galactosidase urine for 'Maltese cross'*
Nail patella syndrome	AD *X-ray of pelvis (iliac horns), absent patellae and dystrophic nails (especially thumbs)*
Nephrocalcinosis and ESRD	
Primary hyperoxalosis	Nephrocalcinosis, *oxalate levels, mutation analysis* AGAT
Adenine phosphoribosyl transferase deficiency	Nephrocalcinosis, AR, *APRT enzyme level, stone analysis*
Dent's disease	Nephrocalcinosis, X-linked, tubular proteinuria *proximal tubulopathy*
Cystinosis	Nephrocalcinosis, AR, corneal crystals (photophobia), proximal tubulopathy
Infections	
Tuberculosis	Sterile pyuria, early morning urines for TB culture, QuantiFERON assay, X-ray for calcinosis
Chronic pyelonephritis	Especially in diabetics, recurrent UTIs, *scarring* on DMSA (if function good enough) or USS/CT
Xanthogranulomatous pyelonephritis	Diabetes and stones (often staghorn) and abnormal kidney on CT or MRI, pyuria, recurrent UTIs
HIV, hepatitis B and C	Serology and viral load, large bright kidneys suggests HIVAN, polyclonal gammopathy, hypocomplementaemia
Schistosomiasis	Obstructed system and or *small high-pressure bladder, serology, early morning urine for ova, cystoscopy and biopsy*
Tubulointerstitial nephritis	
Heavy metal toxicity	Anaemia, rashes, *proximal tubular disorder/Fanconi syndrome, blood, urine or hair analysis (Ar, Cd, Pb)*
Lithium	Polyuria, nephrogenic diabetes insipidus
Analgesic nephropathy	*CT scan small, irregular kidneys with papillary calcification*
Balkan/aristolochic acid nephropathy	Endemic region, exposure to herbal remedies with aristolochic acid
IgG-4-related disease	'Autoimmune' pancreatitis, sialadenitis, aortitis, retroperitoneal fibrosis, elevated IgG-4 ratio

(continued)

Table 47.2 (continued)

Sjögren's syndrome	*Dry eyes and mouth, sterile pyuria, anti SS-A and SS-B (anti-Ro and anti-La) antibodies*, polyclonal gammopathy
Sarcoid	Raised serum ACEI, sterile pyuria, hypercalcaemia (especially with vitamin D supplements), positive gallium scan
Sickle cell nephropathy	HbSS or HbSC, *papillary necrosis*
Glomerular disease (significant protein or blood, dysmorphic RBC on microscopy)	
IgA	Raised serum IgA may be a clue, ethnicity, history of chronic microscopic haematuria or episodes of synpharyngitic macroscopic haematuria
FSGS primary	Usually history of oedema, frothy urine relatively rapid course (NPHS1, NPHS2, NPHS3, other genetic screening available)
FSGS secondary	Low birth weight, reduced nephron-mass (e.g. subtotal nephrectomy) history of renal dysplasia, obesity, body building (anabolic steroids), sickle cell disease, HIV, CMV, parvovirus, congenital heart disease (cyanotic), heroin, interferons, lithium, pamidronate
Membranous primary	*Anti-phospholipase A2 receptor antibody*
Membranous secondary	Hepatitis B, C, HIV, syphilis, schistosomiasis, filariasis, leprosy, malignancy, Rheumatological conditions, medications
MPGN primary and C3 glomerulopathies	Dense deposit disease: low C3, *partial lipodystrophy, Drusen* and retinal atrophy, *Anti-C3Nef (80 %)* CFHR5 nephropathy: Cypriot ancestry, family history, synpharyngitic macroscopic haematuria
MPGN secondary	Hepatitis B, C, HIV, schistosomiasis, *cryoglobulinaemia, hypocomplementaemia, positive rheumatoid factor*, rheumatological conditions (SLE, rheumatoid, Sjögren's syndrome)
Light chain related disease	*Igs, protein electrophoresis, Bence Jones proteinuria, serum-free light chains* (abnormal ratio), skeletal survey, bone marrow biopsy
Amyloid	Usually *heavy proteinuria and normal-sized kidneys, macroglossia, abdominal fat or rectal biopsy*. Causes of AA amyloid, i.e. chronic infection or chronic inflammatory disease, history of IV or subcutaneous drug abuse, causes of AL amyloid (see above), serum *amyloid-P scan*
Systemic lupus erythematosus	Clinical features, *low complement, raised antinuclear antibody, double-stranded DNA antibody*, polyclonal gammopathy
Vasculitis	Extrarenal clinical features, raised inflammatory markers, *ANCA (MPO or PR3 positive)*
Goodpasture's syndrome	Always presents acutely but results in ESRD if diagnosis missed, *Anti-GBM antibodies*
Episode(s) of AKI	
Documented or presumed episodes of AKI	Severity of AKI (1–3, especially need for renal replacement), length and number of AKI, cancer therapy, major surgery, (especially cardiac bypass or cross-clamping aorta/renal vessels), cardiac or liver disease, non-renal transplant, episodes of sepsis, haemolytic uraemic syndrome, episodes of nephrotoxic drugs including chemotherapy. Obtaining previous creatinines from previous hospital admissions invaluable
Miscellaneous	
Diabetes	Proteinuria (evidence of progressive increase) and normal-sized kidneys, retinopathy, 20-year history for type 1 diabetes, other end-organ disease history
Radiation nephritis	Unequal-sized kidneys (if only one irradiated), low-grade TMA
Arterial/venous insufficiency	Unequal size, US/MRA-V of renal vessels, cholesterol emboli: episodes of low complement, eosinophilia, vascular intervention
Impaired drainage	Chronic obstruction usually obvious on imaging but dysfunctional high-pressure bladder may not be obvious, *history of enuresis*, UTIs or *posterior urethral valves*. Abnormal neurology, *thick bladder wall*, upper tract dilatation, high detrusor pressure on urodynamics
Cardiorenal syndrome	Evidence of right or left heart failure (systolic or diastolic dysfunction), often low blood pressure and 'saw-toothed' pattern to creatinine
Hepatorenal syndrome	Exclusion of other causes in patient with cirrhosis

appropriate in most patients, but some in the right setting can be diagnostic or very suggestive of the underlying disease.

Summary

CKD is common and has profound implications in terms of cardiovascular risk and mortality as well as the risk of progressive renal disease and risk of ACKD. There is very little understanding of the epidemiology of CKD progression in the older general population. Robust systems for identifying and screening at-risk populations to prevent medication side effects, especially in the setting of acute illness, and higher awareness of proteinuria being a marker for progression to dialysis are likely to result in reducing the risk for these patients.

References

1. Feest TG, Harrison P. Simulation model for planning renal services. BMJ. 1992;305(6860):1018.
2. Levey AS, Stevens LA, Coresh J. Conceptual model of CKD: applications and implications. Am J Kidney Dis. 2009;53(3 Suppl 3):S4–16.
3. Hallan SI, Orth SR. The KDOQI 2002 classification of chronic kidney disease: for whom the bell tolls. Nephrol Dial Transplant. 2010;25(9):2832–6.
4. Levey AS, de Jong PE, Coresh J, El Nahas M, Astor BC, Matsushita K, et al. The definition, classification, and prognosis of chronic kidney disease: a KDIGO Controversies Conference report. Kidney Int. 2011;80(1):17–28.
5. Coresh J, Astor BC, Greene T, Eknoyan G, Levey AS. Prevalence of chronic kidney disease and decreased kidney function in the adult US population: Third National Health and Nutrition Examination Survey. Am J Kidney Dis. 2003;41(1):1–12.
6. Levey AS, Bosch JP, Lewis JB, Greene T, Rogers N, Roth D. A more accurate method to estimate glomerular filtration rate from serum creatinine: a new prediction equation. Modification of Diet in Renal Disease Study Group. Ann Intern Med. 1999;130(6):461–70.
7. Froissart M, Rossert J, Jacquot C, Paillard M, Houillier P. Predictive performance of the modification of diet in renal disease and Cockcroft-Gault equations for estimating renal function. J Am Soc Nephrol. 2005;16(3):763–73.
8. Matsushita K, Mahmoodi BK, Woodward M, Emberson JR, Jafar TH, Jee SH, et al. Comparison of risk prediction using the CKD-EPI equation and the MDRD study equation for estimated glomerular filtration rate. JAMA. 2012;307(18):1941–51.
9. Hallan SI, Coresh J, Astor BC, Asberg A, Powe NR, Romundstad S, et al. International comparison of the relationship of chronic kidney disease prevalence and ESRD risk. J Am Soc Nephrol. 2006;17(8):2275–84.
10. Group TEIS. Geographic, ethnic, age-related and temporal variation in the incidence of end-stage renal disease in Europe, Canada and the Asia-Pacific region, 1998–2002. Nephrol Dial Transplant. 2002;21(8):2178–83.
11. Matsushita K, Ballew SH, Astor BC, Jong PE, Gansevoort RT, Hemmelgarn BR, et al. Cohort profile: the chronic kidney disease prognosis consortium. Int J Epidemiol. 2013;42(6):1660–8. doi:10.1093/ije/dys173.
12. Xue JL, Daniels F, Star RA, Kimmel PL, Eggers PW, Molitoris BA, Himmelfarb J, Collins AJ. Incidence and mortality of acute renal failure in Medicare beneficiaries, 1992 to 2001. J Am Soc Nephrol. 2006;17(4):1135–42.
13. Prescott GJ, Metcalfe W, Baharani J, Khan IH, Simpson K, Smith WC, MacLeod AM. A prospective national study of acute renal failure treated with RRT: incidence, aetiology and outcomes. Nephrol Dial Transplant. 2007;22(9):2513–9.
14. Coca SG, Yusuf B, Shlipak MG, Garg AX, Parikh CR. Long-term risk of mortality and other adverse outcomes after acute kidney injury: a systematic review and meta-analysis. Am J Kidney Dis. 2009;53(6):961–73. doi:10.1053/j.ajkd.2008.11.034.
15. Minutolo R, De Nicola L, Mazzaglia G, Postorino M, Cricelli C, Mantovani LG, Conte G, Cianciaruso B. Detection and awareness of moderate to advanced CKD by primary care practitioners: a cross-sectional study from Italy. Am J Kidney Dis. 2008;52(3):444–53. doi:10.1053/j.ajkd.2008.03.002.
16. Silverwood RJ, Pierce M, Hardy R, Sattar N, Whincup P, Ferro C, Savage C, Kuh D, Nitsch D. Low birth weight, later renal function, and the roles of adulthood blood pressure, diabetes, and obesity in a British birth cohort. Kidney Int. 2013;84(6):1262–70. doi:10.1038/ki.2013.223.
17. Perneger TV, Whelton PK, Klag MJ, Rossiter KA. Diagnosis of hypertensive end-stage renal disease: effect of patient's race. Am J Epidemiol. 1995;141(1):10–5.
18. Giles PD, Fitzmaurice DA. Formula estimation of glomerular filtration rate: have we gone wrong. BMJ. 2007;334(7605):1198–200.
19. Kidney Disease: Improving Global Outcomes (KDIGO) CKD Work Group. KDIGO 2012 clinical practice guideline for evaluation and management of chronic kidney disease. Kidney Int. 2013;3(Suppl):1–150.
20. Landray MJ, Wheeler DC, Lip GY, Newman DJ, Blann AD, McGlynn FJ, Ball S, Townend JN, Baigent C. Inflammation, endothelial dysfunction, and platelet activation in patients with chronic kidney disease: the chronic renal impairment in Birmingham (CRIB) study. Am J Kidney Dis. 2004;43(2):244–53.

Chronic Kidney Disease: Management

48

Charles R.V. Tomson and Shona Methven

This chapter aims to provide a pragmatic approach to the management of patients with CKD. First, we must correctly identify those with CKD, impart the information to the patient in an informative and appropriate way and then offer strategies to ameliorate the complications of CKD and prevent progression of the kidney disease.

Ascertainment of CKD

The diagnosis of CKD relies upon the accurate measurement of excretory kidney function and proteinuria, both of which have some pitfalls. Given that kidney disease is predominantly asymptomatic (in the early stages at least), healthcare providers must ensure that they correctly identify those with CKD in order to offer optimal care to those with CKD and reassure those who do not.

Measurement of Glomerular Filtration Rate in the Management of CKD

It is seldom necessary to measure glomerular filtration rate directly in routine clinical practice, but there are exceptions:

1. To reassure patients with high muscle bulk, a high serum creatinine concentration and a low *estimated* GFR that excretory kidney function is normal
2. When considering use of drug treatments using renally cleared drugs with a narrow therapeutic index, e.g. cytotoxic chemotherapy
3. In assessing excretory kidney function prior to live kidney donation

Measurement of GFR can be performed using isotopic methods (such as ^{125}I-iothalamate) or using contrast media (such as iohexol). Alternatively creatinine clearance may be measured using 24-h urine collection and a serum creatinine measurement taken during the collection period. However, creatinine clearance overestimates GFR as a result of tubular creatinine secretion (approximately 15 % in normal renal function, rising to 50 % in advanced CKD). This can be corrected by the concurrent administration of a drug that blocks tubular creatinine secretion such as 48 h pretreatment with full-dose cimetidine.

Quantification of Proteinuria

Proteinuria is the cardinal feature of renal disease; therefore, the accurate identification and quantification of proteinuria is paramount in the management of patients with CKD.

Proteinuria may be glomerular (predominantly albuminuria), tubular (as a result of the failure of tubular reabsorption of filtered low-molecular-weight proteins) or overflow (such as excess light chain excretion in myeloma which overwhelms the normal tubular reabsorptive capacity). Quantification of urinary protein using a total protein assay will take account of all of these varying proteins; however, measuring albuminuria will only give an indication of glomerular disease. The measurement of albumin is generally favoured in the biochemistry community as it is quantified using an immunoassay which has technical advantages over the less precise physicochemical assays used for total protein. It has also been said that albuminuria is the better test at low levels (<0.5 g/day total proteinuria equivalent) as the noise/signal ratio (with physiological proteins being the noise and the albuminuria being the signal) is superior. However, the early studies of diabetic nephropathy (from which this received wisdom emanated) did not measure total proteinuria, so no head-to-head comparison was made. This

C.R.V. Tomson, MA, BMBCh, FRCP, DM (Oxon) (✉)
Department of Renal Medicine, Southmead Hospital, Bristol BS10 5NB, UK
e-mail: charlie.tomson@nbt.nhs.uk

S. Methven, BSc (Med Sci) (Hons), MD, MRCP(UK)
Academic Renal Unit, University of Bristol, Southmead Hospital, Westbury-on-Trym, Bristol BS10 5NB, UK
e-mail: sm12266@bristol.ac.uk

M. Harber (ed.), *Practical Nephrology*,
DOI 10.1007/978-1-4471-5547-8_48, © Springer-Verlag London 2014

Metabolic Acidosis

Metabolic acidosis is common in stage 4–5 CKD and is associated with multiple metabolic derangements including muscle wasting and loss of bone density and also with increased tubular ammoniagenesis, which may cause tubular damage and contribute to progressive loss of GFR. Several studies now support the hypothesis that correction of metabolic acidosis by sodium bicarbonate supplementation improves nutritional status and slows progression, and the KDIGO CKD guidelines suggest that patients with CKD and a serum bicarbonate concentration of <22 mmol/l should be treated to maintain serum bicarbonate within the normal range [3]. Larger studies are awaited.

There is good evidence that increased intake of sodium in the form of sodium bicarbonate does *not* result in volume expansion or worsening of hypertension amongst patients with CKD; these effects are only seen with increased sodium chloride intake. Although this has been known for more than 30 years [31, 32], the precise physiological explanation remains unclear but must relate in some way to renal chloride handling.

Hyperkalaemia

Hyperkalaemia is a common problem in CKD, particularly diabetics who may have an element of type 4 renal tubular acidosis (hyporeninaemic hypoaldosteronism) but also patients treated with RAAS blockade. Managed badly, this can result in multiple admissions with hyperkalaemia often with inappropriate doses of insulin and dextrose, stop-starting of important drugs and increased levels of anxiety. Careful, thorough culture-specific dietary advice is valuable in patients with persistent problems and patient information leaflets should be readily available for those with minor hyperkalaemia. Correction of chronic acidosis (see above) and addition of diuretics are often very helpful medium-term solutions. In type 4 RTA, the renin production is suppressed by real or apparent volume expansion, and the addition of a thiazide diuretic (in full dose) can combat this and concurrently improve the hyperkalaemia. In those with recurrent hyperkalaemia who are taking RAAS blockade, a careful review of the balance of risk and benefit is required, once other reversible causes have been dealt with. Clear guidelines on acceptable and not-acceptable hyperkalaemia need to be available for those encountering patients with CKD, and education on this front is an important task for nephrologists.

Dyslipidaemia

A meta-analysis of statins and albuminuria found that they may have a beneficial effect on pathological albuminuria, but the quality of the evidence was poor [33]. Treating dyslipidaemia in CKD, using an HMG Co-A reductase inhibitor (statin), with or without a selective cholesterol absorption inhibitor (e.g. ezetimibe), has not been shown to retard the progression of CKD in the study of heart and renal protection (SHARP) and the protection against nephropathy in diabetes with atorvastatin (PANDA) studies, respectively [34, 35]. The role of these drugs in cardiovascular risk reduction in CKD is discussed elsewhere.

Other Drug Therapy

It is important for prescribers to recognise impaired excretory renal function for two reasons; firstly, to avoid drug accumulation in renally cleared drugs (such as excess bleeding with low-molecular-weight heparins when eGFR <30 ml/min/1.73 m^2) and to avoid renal toxicity at inappropriate doses (such as gentamicin). A calculated creatinine clearance is often preferred to eGFR for drug dosing purposes because it is not normalised to body surface area.

Fibrates

Most fibrates, with the possible exception of gemfibrozil, can cause a reversible increase in urea and creatinine concentration. In some patients, a progressive rise over time has also been demonstrated. Studies in people with normal kidney function have not demonstrated an effect of fibrates on isotopically measured GFR, but no such studies have been done in patients with CKD. Very few patients with CKD 3–5 were included in the FIELD and ACCORD studies. One study suggests that fibrates increase the rate of release of creatinine from muscle; this would explain a rise in creatinine, but not a progressive rise over time, nor a rise in serum urea concentration. In patients with CKD, it is probably safe to ignore a small, stepwise increase in serum creatinine concentration following the initiation of fibrate therapy, particularly if the serum urea concentration is unchanged; however, if there is a progressive rise in creatinine over time, particularly if accompanied by a rise in urea, the drug should be stopped.

Trimethoprim and Cimetidine

Trimethoprim and cimetidine inhibit the tubular secretion of creatinine. The use of trimethoprim in a patient with CKD can result in a marked rise (20–50 %) in serum creatinine concentration and fall in *estimated* GFR, without any change in true GFR. A clinician who does not understand what is happening may think that the patient has acute kidney injury and arrange unnecessary admission, invasive investigations, etc. Although no systematic studies have been reported, in our experience the serum creatinine can remain above baseline for at least 14 days after completion of a course of full-dose trimethoprim. Trimethoprim also reduces renal potassium excretion (through an amiloride-like action), and clinically apparent hyperkalaemia may be observed. This is of particular importance in patients with CKD and/or taking other drugs associated with hyperkalaemia (such as RAAS blockade) and the balance of risk versus benefit should be considered before prescribing trimethoprim in this context.

The effect is dose-dependent: high doses used for treatment of Pneumocystis infection, for instance, are much more likely to cause hyperkalaemia.

Nonsteroidal Anti-inflammatory Drugs (NSAIDs)

NSAIDs inhibit the action of vasodilator prostaglandins that play a major role in maintaining GFR, particularly in the presence of pre-existing CKD. Therefore, all NSAIDs can cause salt and water retention, a fall in GFR and hyperkalaemia. These effects are amplified amongst patients with effective or true hypovolaemia, those on RAAS blockade and in sepsis. These drugs must be used with great care in patients with CKD, who should be warned not to buy NSAIDs over the counter. However, an absolute 'ban' on prescription of these drugs in all patients with CKD is neither practicable nor justified. In some patients with severe osteoarthritis, for instance, in whom paracetamol is ineffective and opiate-based analgesics cause unacceptable adverse effects, it is reasonable to prescribe NSAIDs even in the presence of CKD4 *so long as* kidney function, blood pressure and fluid status are monitored carefully and regularly.

NSAIDs can also cause minimal change nephrotic syndrome and interstitial nephritis, but these are idiosyncratic reactions and may be drug-specific.

Aminoglycosides

As part of the drive to reduce hospital acquired infections, such as *Clostridium difficile* infection, there has been a switch from broad spectrum antibiotics to aminoglycoside antibiotics (especially gentamicin), with some hospitals seeing gentamicin prescribing doubling [36]. If monitored appropriately and dose alterations are made in light of changing renal function, gentamicin can be administered safely to patients with CKD. This requires multidisciplinary working between medical, nursing and pharmacy colleagues. Nephrotoxicity has not been shown to occur with single doses given as prophylaxis.

Clinical Management of CKD: Preparation for End-Stage Renal Failure

Multidisciplinary Education Programmes

Initiating renal replacement therapy (RRT) is a major life change, with practical, social, psychological and financial consequences as well as physical consequences. Physicians who focus solely on the physical consequences (e.g. treatment of anaemia, acidosis, hypertension and phosphate retention) are therefore missing the 'bigger picture' – and, when patients do not always adhere to complex drug treatments, may blame the patient for 'poor compliance' when in reality, the patient is struggling to cope with other aspects of their life and accords low priority to drug treatments that might affect their health some time into the future (think of Maslow's hierarchy of needs – food is a basic need but a low-potassium, low-phosphate, fluid-restricted diabetic diet accompanied by the correct timing of insulin therapy before the meal and a phosphate binder afterwards is a need of a different magnitude. It requires a complex interplay of financial resources, strict dietary modification, memory, eyesight, manual dexterity, time, organisation *and* patient motivation).

While there is no reason in principle why doctors should not be trained, and given time, to address the 'nonbiological' aspects of coping with CKD and RRT, they are an expensive resource, and there is evidence that the most cost-effective way of preparing patients with CKD for major decisions about RRT is to provide a multidisciplinary clinic. Patients may meet other patients in small groups, including patients who have experienced various RRT modalities, nursing staff with expertise in patient education, psychologists, dietitians and others. Several observational studies have found that patients who have attended a multidisciplinary clinic are better informed and better prepared for RRT than similar patients attending conventional medical clinics. A nonrandomised comparison of a formal education programme ('RightStart') with standard care found improved morbidity and mortality over the first year after starting RRT [37]. A randomised trial in Canada amongst relatively low-risk patients with CKD not previously known to nephrologists found no clear evidence that multidisciplinary care slowed progression or improved management of complications compared to care by primary care physicians [38] but proved cost-effective largely due to a lower number of days in hospital; patients receiving multidisciplinary care reported a higher quality of life [39].

Identification and Workup of Patients Suitable for Transplantation

This is an important area and often delivered in an inconsistent manner. For most young patients, preemptive transplantation, ideally with a live donor transplant, is the treatment of choice when approaching ESRD. There are caveats and conditions around this but early assessment and education of appropriately selected patients is important. Strategies to avoid blood transfusion and advice on contraception in women of childbearing age are very important to avoid sensitisation.

Shared Decision-Making: Patient Decision Aids

Patients with CKD will be faced with numerous 'medical' decisions over the course of their life with CKD – some of

Table 48.3 Examples of preference-sensitive decisions in CKD care

Clinical scenario	Options
Stable stage 3B CKD	Phosphate binder treatment Aspirin as primary prevention
Stable stage 4 CKD	Fistula construction (if HD would be preferred treatment option) vs wait and see if function declines
Young active patient with CKD: renal anaemia, Hb 9.5, adequate iron stores	Correction with ESA – target range 10–12 Correction with ESA – target range 12–13
Progressive CKD, currently stage 4	Conservative care or RRT Home-based or hospital-based RRT Pre-emptive transplant listing HD or PD (assuming not transplanted)
Plan for kidney transplantation	Perfectly matched ideal donor HLA mismatched donor (specify acceptable degree of mismatch) 'Marginal' donor

which are listed in Table 48.3. For some decisions, the choice is straightforward, because of strong evidence that the outcomes are better with one choice than with the other. In guidelines using the GRADE classification, these options will be given as level 1 recommendations and will normally be supported by level A or B evidence. However, many other options are based on weaker evidence, will be given as level 2 suggestions, and will normally have level C or D evidence in support. The definition of a 'suggestion' for patients is 'The majority of people in your situation would want the recommended course of action, but many would not'. For clinicians, the definition reads 'Different choices will be appropriate for different patients. Each patient needs help to arrive at a management decision consistent with her or his values and preferences'.

Achieving high-quality shared decisions with patients about aspects of CKD care is morally the right thing to do, but there are also important pragmatic reasons. Patients who feel 'ownership' of the decision are more likely to implement it – improving adherence to treatment. Patients who are 'activated' to take control over their own treatment will require less support, in the medium term, than those who are the passive recipients of patriarchal, 'doctor knows best' care.

Achieving shared decision-making in practice is culturally disruptive both for caregivers and for patients. Doctors, for instance, have more knowledge about the risks and benefits of the various options than patients can possibly have; patients used to conventional medical care may well reply 'you're the doctor, you should know what's best for me'. Accepting these attitudes means that patients will probably spend more time researching their next holiday than they will researching their medical options. One way of facilitating shared decision-making is to encourage patients to participate in their own 'kidney care plan'. An example of this is shown in the Appendix and can be modified for local bias and individual needs. The version shown is popular with patients and acts as prompt to ensure that the patient is encouraged to voice their wishes.

'Crashlanding'

Despite all of the efforts, described above, to identify patients with deteriorating renal function, there are still a significant proportion of patients who commence RRT within 3 months of first nephrology consultation (known as 'crashlanding'). This is particularly challenging for the patient, family and nephrologist. It may be as a result of an unavoidable acute irreversible deterioration (such as anti-GBM disease), or late presentation or late referral. Hospital haemodialysis often becomes the default option for this group of patients, but with appropriate multidisciplinary input, other forms of RRT can still be successfully adopted.

Increasingly patients are also referred with AKI on a background of CKD, often frail, elderly patients with only scant available information on patient preference and functional status. A decision about the benefits of providing acute renal replacement therapy must be made relatively promptly, frequently out-of-hours. These patients deserve careful and thoughtful assessment, and a decision to withhold or commence renal replacement therapy should be made at a senior level.

Conclusion

The recognition of CKD has changed dramatically over the past 15 years with the introduction of eGFR reporting and the introduction of schemes such as the UK Quality and Outcomes Framework. It is no longer a collection of rare diseases looked after by specialists in hospital clinics; it is a common condition predominantly managed in primary care with appropriate support and input from nephrologists. Our current management strategies reflect these changes with greater emphasis on risk stratification, avoidance of AKI and financial incentives to attain blood pressure targets. It is a rapidly evolving field with many exciting developments on the horizon for us and our patients.

Appendix

My Kidney Care Plan

Name ....

Hospital number ....

Welcome to the Chronic Kidney Disease (CKD) Service (designed by Katy Gerrard)

This is **your** care plan; it will help all members of your healthcare team (including your GP) to care for you. Hopefully it will also help you understand and get involved in your kidney problems and plans for treatment.

Please bring it with you to every appointment and also if you get admitted to hospital or go to your GP.

The chronic kidney disease team is a group of renal specialists who help manage people with kidney problems. As well as running clinics at the Royal Free Hospital, we also run clinics at Barnet Hospital, Mary Rankin (St. Pancras) and North Middlesex Hospital.

Your nurses are:

....

Your consultant is: ....

....

The specialist nurses and doctors in this team work alongside dieticians, social workers, psychologists, your primary care team (GP surgery) and of course you and your family/carers to manage your kidney problems.

We can help with many aspects of kidney problems in our clinic, including:

- Further monitoring and stabilisation of your kidney function
- Management of any associated symptoms or complications you may have
- Anaemia (blood count) management
- General health and wellbeing promotion
- Preparation for dialysis
- Assessing whether you are physically fit enough for a kidney transplant
- Conservative management if you choose not to have dialysis

We are happy to discuss any/all of the above issues with you and also any other matters you are concerned about. You will still continue to see a renal doctor (specialist) regularly.

All your other day-to-day health problems will still be managed by your general practitioner (GP). We recommend that you take this care plan with you when you attend your GP surgery.

If you need to contact us about any *kidney-related* problems then you can call us on .... (office hours). We might not be able to answer your call straight away as we run clinics every day, but we will return your call as soon as we can. **If the problem is urgent, then please contact your GP or go straight to your nearest Accident and Emergency.**

Lifestyle

There are many things you can do to try and keep yourself healthy:

- We recommend that you follow a balanced healthy diet and do not eat salty foods or add extra salt to your food.
- Some patients need to follow specific diets like low potassium or low phosphate; we will advise you, if you are one of these patients – you can use this section of your folder to insert relevant diet sheets. We also have dieticians who you will be able to see. If you want to contact the dieticians, please call ext 31719.
- It is beneficial to take regular exercise as your condition allows.
- If you smoke, we strongly advise that you stop as it will damage your kidneys further. Your GP will be able to provide help for you to stop smoking.
- We recommend that you do not drink too much alcohol; this is no more than 14 units for women and 21 for men per week.
- It is advisable to be a healthy weight; we will recommend what weight is ideal for you.
- High blood pressure (BP) damages kidneys further, so it is very important that you make sure your BP is well controlled. We will advise you what your BP should be.
- If you are diabetic, it is vital that your diabetes is well controlled as high blood sugars will damage the kidneys further; your healthcare team can help you with this.
- It is advisable that blood is taken from the veins in your hands; if this is not possible, then your dominant arm can be used; this is in case we need to make a fistula for dialysis.

Transition Clinics

- There are various models of transitioning of patients which are as follows:
  - Paediatric service to adult service
  - Paediatric service to transition clinic to adult service
  - Paediatric service to adolescent service to young adult service to general adult service

The children's clinic may take place in a small, playful, child-friendly environment in a central children's teaching hospital, whereas the adult clinics tend to take place in a different geographical location in a larger, more impersonal, quieter yet busier, individual-focused setting in a regional adult or local district general hospital. Consequently clinic attendance results in young adults being surrounded by much older patients whose disease experience may be very different from their own. Classically adult clinic appointments result in patients being less likely to see the same medical staff at each visit with shorter consultations and less readily available support and advice from staff as there is usually an increased number of medical and nursing staff (who may not have come across their medical condition previously).

An ideal transition clinic should conform to the requirements or wishes of young adults with:

- Adequate consultation with professionals and patients
- Flexibility in the timing of transition
- A period of preparation for the young person and family
- Information transfer
- Monitoring of attendance until the young person is established in the appropriate adult-oriented service
- A cohort of young adults in the clinic at the same time
- Being seen by the same medical and nursing staff

The ideal immediate post-transfer scenario would consist of a special young adult clinic within the adult unit and run by the same core key personnel each time.

The American Society of Adolescent Medicine recommended that services in any health-care setting should be appropriate for both the chronological age of the patient and development attained. Patient surveys of adolescent patients with chronic conditions suggest that the ideal transition age is around 17–20.

Non-adherence

Non-adherence with treatment is a significant and difficult issue throughout medicine, in all age groups. Normal adolescence is marked by rebelling, risk-taking behaviour which may involve experimentation of drugs and a sense of being invincible. Experience rather bitterly tells us that there is no magic solution to this, but it is obviously critically important that young adults are educated and understand the causes of their renal condition and the importance of medications (especially immunosuppressive medications for renal transplant recipients) to improve concordance to therapy. Renal transplant recipients of all ages need to be clear that non-adherence to immunosuppressive medications likely results in renal allograft loss and the requirement for dialysis. Poorly planned transition from paediatric to adult-oriented health services may be a factor in medication non-adherence and missed clinics, thus well-planned transition may improve clinical, educational and social outcomes for young people (Fig. 49.1). The timing of transition can be very important and should take into account chronological age/maturity, adolescent readiness and medical and psychosocial stability.

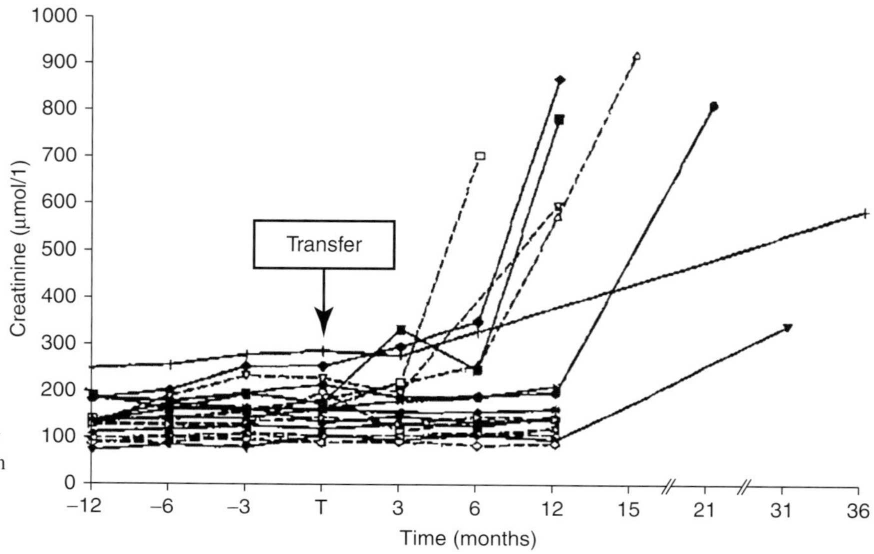

Fig. 49.1 Decline of renal allograft function after transfer from paediatric to adult nephrology services (Reprinted with permission from Watson et al. Non-compliance and transfer from paediatric to adult transplant unit. Pediatr Nephrol. 2000;14:469–72)

With the above in mind, it is worth setting up an education programme for the transition process to enable the young patient to acquire the necessary knowledge and skills to function in an adult service, largely independent of parents and staff, before they are transferred.

For patients of all ages, it is extremely important for the successor nephrologist to know of recent episodes of non-adherence, what was thought to have precipitated them and whether the patient has learned from this and moved on or remains at high risk of further non-adherence. If the underlying precipitant is not identified and/or resolved, then review by an empathetic clinical psychologist may be helpful. It is worth considering that quite a lot of non-adherence, at any age, is related not to rebellion but to more mundane issues such as language barriers, financial woes, significant social responsibilities or just chaotic lifestyles. Until these are identified and the patient given robust strategies for overcoming them, they remain at high risk.

Transitioning Models

There are several different models of transition in young adults with renal disease, but each model should involve a multidisciplinary team of physicians, surgeons, nurse specialists, pharmacists and allied health professionals, including the psychosocial team. All members of the multidisciplinary team should be trained in managing adolescents and involved in the transition process.

The simplest model is a dedicated clinic provided within the adult setting without a combined paediatric-adult clinic and with no direct input or continuity from paediatric services; the success of this model is dependent on a good coordinated transition process between the two services, such as meetings between the paediatric and adult clinic staff to plan coordinated care and the involvement of nurse specialists (who can escort young people to the adult clinics if required).

Ongoing continuity can be provided where both paediatric and adult professionals provide ongoing care in a joint clinic from adolescence to adulthood allowing patients to benefit both from experts in paediatric diseases and the appropriate management of more pertinent adult issues, such as sexual health, fertility issues and cardiovascular disease, and the duration of joint care can be individualised for each patient. This model is used in the transitioning of adolescent renal transplant recipients where the joint clinic lasts for around 2 years (Fig. 49.2). During the preparatory phase of transitioning, patients attend a special joint transition clinic at 3–4-month intervals in addition to both regular and adolescent clinic appointments.

The transition clinic allows the development of a relationship and trust between the patient and adult team during the pre-transfer period and enables a joint decision on timing of transfer and, if necessary, access to a buddy scheme to foster peer support.

Other transitioning models particularly used in North America include a generic transition team located within a children's hospital and consisting of one or two dedicated nurse specialists who coordinate transitions for all patients in different specialities.

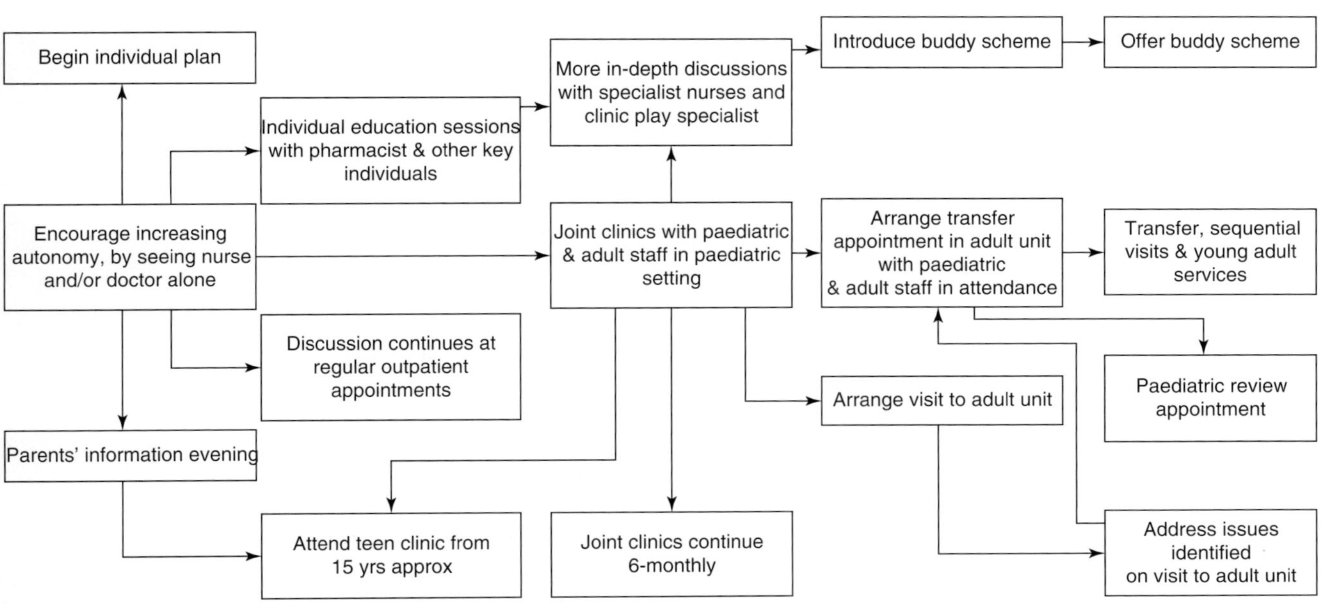

Fig. 49.2 Model of care for transitioning adolescents with renal disease

Barriers to Successful Paediatric Transition

There are various barriers to successful transition which can be overcome by careful preparation during the transitioning process (see Table 49.1). Joint transition clinics are particularly useful in identifying issues and smoothing out these difficulties.

Adult Transition/Transfer

For the most part adults with CKD are well versed in their condition and need little guidance or joint clinics in transferring to another unit. However, almost all renal patients have an involved history, results, often extensive imaging and histopathology slides. Much of this is, or may be, invaluable to their next nephrologist for the patient's continued management, avoidance of pointlessly repeating investigations and for the review of diagnosis and progression. Yet imaging, histology and anti-HLA screens, for example, are rarely spontaneously transferred with a patient. Subsequently requesting such data is often an inefficient, slow and occasionally fruitless exercise and is something as a community that nephrologists should consider improving.

While most adults may not need a formal transition, most units will have a few patients who have significant physical, mental health or learning problems that provoke considerable anxiety when moving to a new unit. It should not be too difficult to identify these patients and consider ways of smoothing their transition of care.

Summary

Careful transition of paediatric (and adult patients) is critically important and a minimum standard of professional care. Every adult nephrology unit should construct their own transitional care pathways in collaboration with local paediatric units and facilitate continuity of care with ongoing educational and social programmes.

The duration of the preparatory phase and the timing of transition should be flexible and geared to the individual needs of the young adult looking specifically at chronological and developmental ages, maturity, medical stability and psychosocial issues.

For both adult and adolescent transition, units need to establish clear lines of communication as well as a robust system for transfer of relevant radiology, histopathology, surgical notes, specialist reports and sequential laboratory data.

Finally, most of us do not routinely canvass first impressions of patients about the quality of their welcome and the efficiency of the service they have just joined, but occasionally this can be a very salutary experience and an opportunity to significantly improve the patient experience.

Table 49.1 Barriers to successful transition

1. Barriers from young adults
(a) Fear of the unknown
(b) Reluctant to leave friends and health care personnel
(c) Ongoing dependence on parents or guardians or other adults
(d) Lack of maturity compared to peers
(e) Concordance issues
2. Barriers from parents
(a) Overprotective and used to taking the lead in the paediatric setting
(b) Reluctant to leave familiar staff and clinic surroundings
(c) Resist attempts by the adult service to enhance the self-advocacy of their child if not adequately prepared
(d) May have become aware of lack of confidence in adult staff by other health professionals
3. Barriers from paediatric nephrologists
(a) Attachment to patient
(b) Lack of confidence in adult staff if aware of differences in the attitudes and priorities of adult services
4. Barriers from adult nephrologists
(a) Lack of confidence in managing adolescents
(b) Lack of training in child and adolescent development and the impact of chronic disease
(c) Concern regarding different dynamics of consultation (such as unused to presence of parents)
5. Barriers from care delivery system
(a) Time and financial constraints such as lack of funding and limited psychosocial resources in adult renal units
(b) Shorter adult consultation times
(c) Different locations with difficult transition of medical files

Resources

1. Adolescent transition care: guidance for nursing staff. http://www.rcn.org.uk/__data/assets/pdf_file/0011/78617/002313.pdf. Accessed 18 Mar 2012.
2. Bridging the gaps: health care for adolescents. http://www.rcpch.ac.uk/sites/default/files/bridging_the_gaps.pdf. Accessed 18 Mar 2012.
3. Dobbels F, Van-Damme-Lombarert R, Van haecke J, De Geest S. Growing pains, non-adherence with the immunosuppressive regimen in adolescent transplant recipients. Pediatr Transplant. 2005;9:381–90.
4. e-Learning for healthcare: adolescent health. http://e-lfh.org.uk/projects/ah/index.html. Accessed 18 Mar 2012.
5. Lost in transition: moving young people between child and adult health services. http://www.rcn.org.uk/__data/assets/pdf_file/ 0010/157879/003227.pdf. Accessed 18 March 2012.
6. Milford DV, Fisher D, Marks SD. Adolescent transfer to adult renal units. Br J Renal Med. 2008;13:30–1.
7. National service framework for children, young people and maternity services website. http://www.dh.gov.uk/en/Publicationsandstatistics/ Publications/PublicationsPolicyAndGuidance/DH_4089114. Accessed 18 Mar 2012.
8. Transition: getting it right for young people. http://www.dh.gov.uk/en/Publicationsandstatistics/Publications/PublicationsPolicyAndGuidance/DH_4132145. Accessed 18 Mar 2012.
9. You're Welcome Quality Criteria. Making health services young people friendly. http://eazysecure12a.net/nya.org.uk/dynamic_files/yourewelcome/Self%20Assessment%20Toolkit.pdf. Accessed 18 Mar 2012.
10. Harden PN, Walsh G, Bandler N, Bradley S, Lonsdale D, Taylor J, Marks SD. Bridging the gap: an integrated paediatric to adult clinical service for young adults with kidney failure. BMJ 2012; 344: e3718.

Iron Supplementation: Oral Versus Intravenous?

Oral iron supplementation is simple and cheap to administer, with a cost of only a few pence per week. Unfortunately, in many CKD patients, iron absorption is impaired due to hepcidin upregulation, and this renders oral iron supplementation ineffective. Although hepcidin levels progressively increase with worsening kidney function, it is largely in late-stage 3 onwards that they reach a level when oral iron is most likely to be ineffective.

Table 50.2 Markers of iron status

Marker	Characteristics
Serum ferritin	Reasonable marker of iron stores, but artificially elevated in the presence of inflammation or liver disease
Transferrin saturation (TSAT)	Subject to considerable diurnal variation; widely used in the USA
Hypochromic red cells	Several studies suggest that this is the most sensitive/specific marker of iron deficiency, but requires to be performed on a fresh blood sample and requires specific automated blood count analysers which are not widely available
Reticulocyte haemoglobin content (CHr)	Also a fairly sensitive/specific marker of iron deficiency, but requires specific automated blood count analysers which are not widely available
MCV, MCH, MCHC	Abnormalities of these red cell indices will only occur in long-standing iron deficiency, and therefore not a sensitive marker of iron status
Serum transferrin receptor	Used outside the nephrology setting, but not helpful in patients receiving ESA therapy since this parameter will increase in either iron deficiency or enhanced erythropoiesis
Erythrocyte zinc protoporphyrin levels	Largely a research investigation with no practical applicability
Serum hepcidin levels	A novel biomarker of iron status which remains experimental
Bone marrow	Useful investigation, but invasive and not practical for repeat assessments

Iron requirements in haemodialysis patients are almost universally too great for oral iron supplementation to keep pace with the demand, and this patient population is usually treated with intravenous iron [2]. Non-dialysis CKD patients, those on peritoneal dialysis and kidney transplant recipients may receive oral iron first, although the other problem with this mode of administration is a high incidence of gastrointestinal side effects due to a local Fenton reaction at the site of the gastric or colonic mucosa. Compliance with oral iron supplementation is often poor due to these side effects. Finally, many drugs may interfere with iron absorption such as proton pump inhibitors (e.g. omeprazole), phosphate binders and certain antibiotics such as ciprofloxacin. Certain foodstuffs and tea may also impair dietary iron absorption.

If oral iron supplements are used, then the first choice is often ferrous sulphate. Attempts to reduce gastrointestinal side effects include taking iron supplements with meals, but this will also reduce their absorption. Other iron salts such as ferrous fumarate or ferrous succinate are sometimes reported as being better tolerated. The reason for this is that they contain lower amounts of elemental iron.

Intravenous iron is used widely in the CKD setting. Not only does this guarantee a readily available supply of iron, but it is extremely easy to administer to a haemodialysis population who already have vascular access in situ. Thus, intravenous iron is usually administered on dialysis.

There are several IV iron preparations available (Table 50.3). All of these have a core containing the iron salt, surrounded by a carbohydrate shell to allow the slow release of the iron (Fig. 50.1). The older iron preparations such as iron dextran carried a small but definite risk of anaphylaxis due to preformed dextran antibodies. This has also been found to be more prevalent with high-molecular-weight iron

Table 50.3 Requirements for a test dose and dosing schedule for various IV iron preparations licensed in the USA and Europe, as per the product label

IV iron preparation	Country/region	Test dose required	Dosing schedule
Iron dextran – HMW (Dexferrum®)	USA	Yes	100 mg bolus injection or slow IV infusion of up to 20 mg/kg
Iron dextran – LMW (INFeD®)	USA	Yes	100 mg bolus injection or slow IV infusion of up to 20 mg/kg
Iron dextran – LMW (Cosmofer®)	Europe	No	100 mg bolus injection or slow IV infusion of up to 20 mg/kg
Iron sucrose (Venofer®)	USA	No	100–200 mg bolus over 5–10 min respectively
Iron sucrose (Venofer®)	Europe	No	100–200 mg bolus over 5–10 min respectively
Ferric gluconate (Ferrlecit®)	USA, Germany, Italy	No	62.5–12.5 mg bolus over 5–10 min
Ferumoxytol (Feraheme®)	USA	No	510 mg bolus over 17 s
Ferumoxytol (Rienso®)	Europe	No	510 mg bolus over 17 s
Ferric carboxymaltose (Ferinject®)	Europe	No	500 mg bolus over 6 min 1 g infusion over 15 min (max 20 mg/kg)
Iron isomaltoside (Monofer®)	Europe	No	500 mg bolus over 30 min 1 g infusion over 60 min (max 20 mg/kg)

HMW high molecular weight, *LMW* low molecular weight

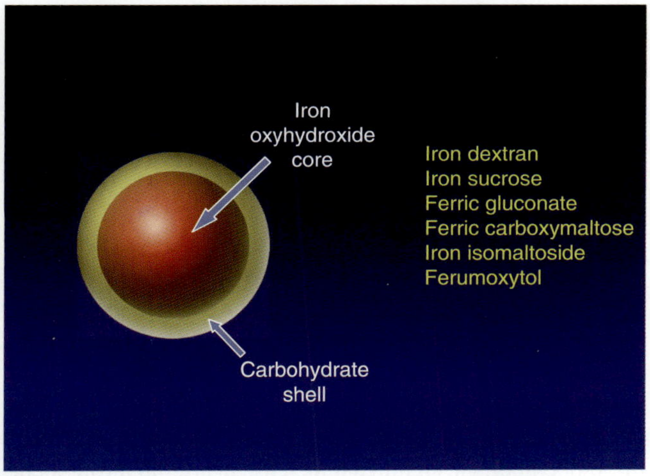

Fig. 50.1 IV iron preparations

dextran compared to low-molecular-weight iron dextran compounds.

Iron sucrose has been around for many years and is tried and tested in millions of doses worldwide. The dose usually administered is 100 or 200 mg, since tolerance at higher doses is reduced. Iron gluconate is not licensed or marketed in the UK, but is used widely in the USA, Italy and Germany.

There are three new IV iron preparations recently licensed in Europe. These include ferric carboxymaltose (Ferinject®), iron isomaltoside (Monofer®) and ferumoxytol (Feraheme® in the US; Rienso® in Europe). These newer IV preparations may be administered in a larger dose over a shorter period of time and do not require a test dose. There may be lower levels of free iron and oxidative stress with these newer preparations, although clinical and hard outcome data are lacking.

In some countries, such as France and Spain, iron sucrose 'similars' are marketed. It is clear, however, that these products are very different from the iron sucrose originator (Venofer®), with different levels of oxidative stress and also different efficacy.

The choice of IV iron preparation depends on the patient population to be treated. Thus, iron sucrose (Venofer®) is often the IV iron of choice for haemodialysis patients (mainly due to cost), with boluses of 100 or 200 mg being administered once a month or once weekly depending on iron requirements. Various sets of guidelines suggest that the optimum serum ferritin level for haemodialysis patients is between 200 and 500 ug/l and the transferrin saturation level should be maintained above 20 %. If hypochromic red cells can be measured, then this should be maintained below 10 %.

For non-dialysis patients, the choice of IV iron is a balance between patient convenience versus cost. Traditionally, many such patients received repeated boluses of IV iron sucrose, 200 mg at a time, but often three separate visits were required to administer the required amount of IV iron. The newer IV iron preparations allow larger doses to be administered at a single visit, and thus doses of 500 or 1,000 mg can be given as either a slow bolus injection or a fairly rapid IV infusion. Although the newer IV irons are slightly more costly, this is balanced by savings on repeated outpatient visits and transport costs.

Reactions to IV Iron

Over the years, IV iron administration has been notorious for causing immediate hypersensitivity-type anaphylactoid reactions. As previously mentioned, the iron dextran-containing preparation caused type-I anaphylactic reactions, which resulted in several fatalities. The modern-day intravenous iron preparations do not usually induce anaphylactic reactions, but may (not uncommonly) cause a hypotensive episode, characterised by sudden onset of dizziness and light-headedness and associated with a fall in blood pressure. This usually responds to lying the patient supine, and there is usually no need to give antiallergenic treatment such as adrenaline or steroids. The reaction is usually self-limiting after periods of a few minutes up to half an hour. Admission to hospital is not usually necessary.

These reactions to IV iron are rare but can be frightening for both the patient and the healthcare professional, and appropriate debriefing for the patient is important as they are likely to be dependent on further IV iron.

ESA Therapy

Erythropoiesis-stimulating agents remain the cornerstone of CKD anaemia management. They were introduced in 1990, and they transformed the management of anaemia in dialysis patients, many of whom were transfusion-dependent and iron overloaded.

Epoetins

The first generation of ESAs were the recombinant human erythropoietins, epoetin alfa (Eprex®) and epoetin beta (NeoRecormon®). Both products are fairly short-acting, with a plasma half-life of between 6 and 8 h, and this requires them to be administered by intravenous or subcutaneous injection two or three times weekly. Following the expiration of the patent for these products, several biosimilar epoetins have recently appeared on the market, including epoetin zeta (Retacrit®) and biosimilar epoetin alfa (Binocrit®). Another recombinant human erythropoietin (epoetin theta, Eporatio®) has also recently been licensed.

Darbepoetin Alfa

The main difference between darbepoetin alfa (*Aranesp*®) and the epoetins is the presence of an additional two N-linked carbohydrate chains to enhance the metabolic stability of the molecule in vivo. Thus, the intravenous half-life of darbepoetin alfa is approximately 25 h, while the subcutaneous half-life is between 48 and 70 h. This property allows less frequent dosing, and this product is effective once weekly or once every 2 weeks. Moreover, in some patients, once-monthly dosing is possible.

Methoxypolyethylene Glycol-Epoetin Beta

Methoxypolyethylene glycol-epoetin beta (CERA, Mircera®) was created by attaching a pegylation chain to the epoetin beta molecule. This considerably prolonged the circulating half-life of the molecule to around 130 h, which allows once-monthly administration. This is particularly useful in non-dialysis patients.

Peginesatide

In March 2012, peginesatide was licensed as an ESA in the USA (Omontys®). Peginesatide is an EPO-mimetic peptide that has no structural homology with erythropoietin, but shares the same biological and functional properties as the native or recombinant protein. Thus, it simulates erythropoiesis by binding to the erythropoietin receptor and evoking the same intracellular signalling cascade. Four large Phase 3 clinical trials of this product were conducted (PEARL 1 and 2, EMERALD 1 and 2) [10, 11], allowing a cumulative exposure in approximately 2,600 patients. As described above, in contrast to the other licensed ESAs, peginesatide does not cross-react with anti-erythropoietin antibodies, and thus this molecule may be used to 'rescue' patients who have developed an antibody-mediated pure red cell aplasia with the other ESAs [6]. In March 2013, following several severe reactions to peginesatide (including a few fatalities), however, the product was voluntarily recalled by the manufacturer, and at the time of going to press, is no longer available.

The practical issues with the use of all ESAs are the trigger haemoglobin concentration for introducing therapy, the target haemoglobin range for treatment and the management of a poor response to ESA therapy.

Trigger Haemoglobin Concentration

Three previous randomised controlled trials (US Normal Hematocrit Trial [12], CREATE study [13] and CHOIR study [14]) all suggested potential safety concerns with the use of ESA therapy to normalise the haemoglobin concentration. This was followed by a more definitive result from the TREAT study [15], which was a randomised double-blind, placebo-controlled trial in over 4,000 non-dialysis diabetic CKD patients. The results of this trial compared various outcomes in two groups of patients, the first group being randomised to target a haemoglobin of 13 g/dl, while the second group received placebo, being rescued only if their haemoglobin fell below 9 g/dl. Targeting a higher haemoglobin concentration showed a significant reduction in the use of blood transfusions, but only a fairly modest improvement in quality of life. Against this was a significant increase in a number of adverse events, such as a doubling of stroke risk, doubling of venous thromboembolism, significant increase in arterial thromboembolism and a more than tenfold increase in cancer-related mortality in the subpopulation of patients previously diagnosed with a malignancy (Fig. 50.2). The results from this study suggest that for CKD patients, ESA therapy should be introduced somewhere around 9–10 g/dl, with the aim of preventing patients falling below 9 g/dl. This trigger haemoglobin concentration is somewhat lower than was previously recommended in both US and European clinical practice guidelines. Because of concerns about increasing tumour growth and worsening the risk of venous thromboembolism, ESA therapy should be used with caution in all patients with cancer, and the benefit to risk ratio should be carefully evaluated.

Target Haemoglobin

The results of the TREAT study have also impacted on the target haemoglobin concentration. Whereas previously, guidelines had suggested targeting a haemoglobin concentration of between 11 and 12 g/dl, this has now been reduced to around 10–12 g/dl. Indeed, the recently published KDIGO Anemia Guideline suggests an upper limit of 11.5 g/dl [16] (see below).

Poor Response to ESA Therapy

There are two types of poor response to ESAs. The first is a failure to show an increase in haemoglobin concentration despite repeated increases in ESA dose. The second is characterised by a loss of response to treatment, again despite increased ESA doses. Both of these conditions require a careful systematic approach.

The causes of hyporesponsiveness to ESA therapy are several (Table 50.4). Investigating a patient who is showing hyporesponsiveness to ESA therapy demands a stepwise approach (Fig. 50.3). If the patient is self-injecting, compliance with therapy should be questioned and confirmed. The reticulocyte count may give a clue as to whether there is a

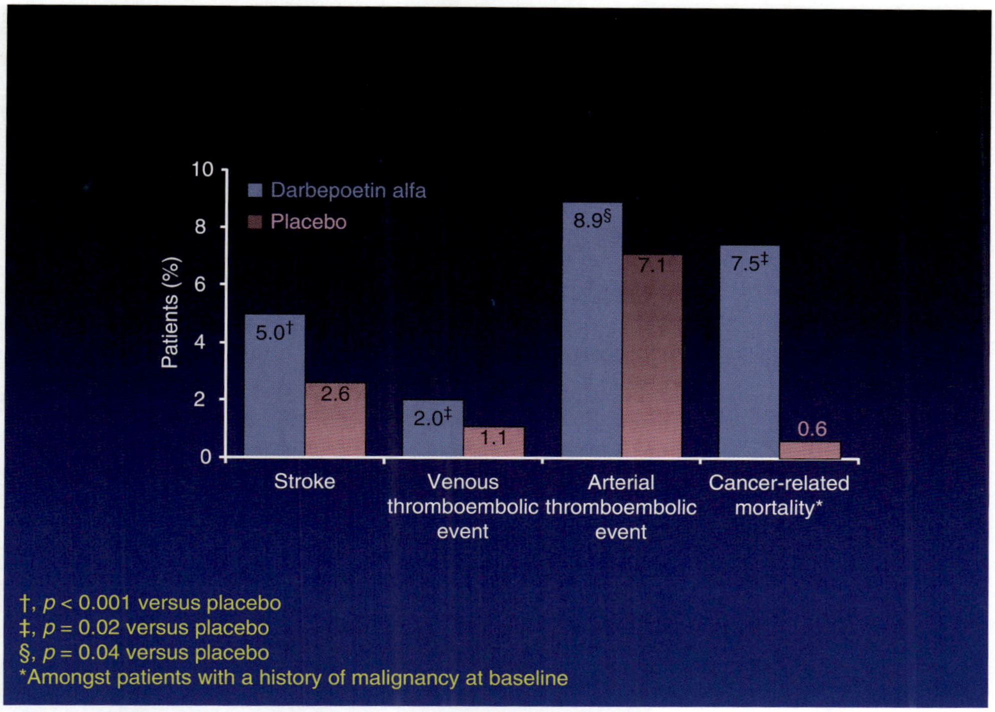

Fig. 50.2 Safety concerns in the TREAT study (Created with the use of data obtained from Pfeffer et al. [15]. Copyright © 2009 Massachusetts Medical Society)

Table 50.4 Causes of hyporesponsiveness to erythropoiesis-stimulating agent therapy

Common	Iron deficiency
	Infection/inflammation
	Underdialysis
Less common	Blood loss
	Hyperparathyroidism
	Aluminium toxicity
	Vitamin B_{12}/folate deficiency
	Haemolysis
	Bone marrow disorders
	Haemoglobinopathies
	Angiotensin-converting enzyme inhibitors
	Carnitine deficiency
	Obesity (in subcutaneous administration)
	Anti-EPO antibodies (pure red cell aplasia)

primary problem with erythropoiesis or whether the bone marrow is already working overtime but the red cell survival is reduced as a result of bleeding or haemolysis.

The possibility of either absolute or functional iron deficiency should be entertained, and a trial of IV iron may be helpful. A raised CRP may suggest active infection or inflammation, and this should be vigorously investigated. Occult conditions such as tuberculosis or malignancy may prove hard to elucidate. An increase in dialysis prescription and/or a change from conventional haemodialysis to haemodiafiltration may be of benefit. Screening for B_{12} or folate deficiency, blood loss or haemolysis may be indicated. A sharp fall in haemoglobin coupled with a very low reticulocyte count should alert the physician to the very rare condition of antibody-mediated pure red cell aplasia. Bone marrow examination may be required to exclude some haematological conditions such as myelodysplastic syndrome. A higher reticulocyte count makes it more likely that bleeding or haemolysis is the cause, and a full haemolytic screen and possible G-I investigations may be indicated.

Whereas previously, physicians were happy to continue escalating the dose of ESA therapy, recent randomised controlled trials have suggested possible harm in using high doses in EPO-resistant patients. It is not clear whether the poor outcomes in this situation are due to the high doses of ESA therapy per se or whether this simply represents a 'sicker' group of patients. Nevertheless, repeated dose escalation is no longer advised, and a maximum dose of epoetin of around 15,000 units per week in divided doses seems reasonable. This translates into a weekly dose of approximately 75 ug of darbepoetin alfa or a monthly dose of approximately 300 ug of methoxypolyethylene glycol-epoetin beta.

Blood Transfusions

Prior to 1990, red cell transfusions were very frequently used in chronic haemodialysis patients. The advent of erythropoietin therapy led to a dramatic reduction in the incidence of transfusions, the Annual Report of the US Renal Data System (USRDS) in 2009 indicating a halving of blood transfusions

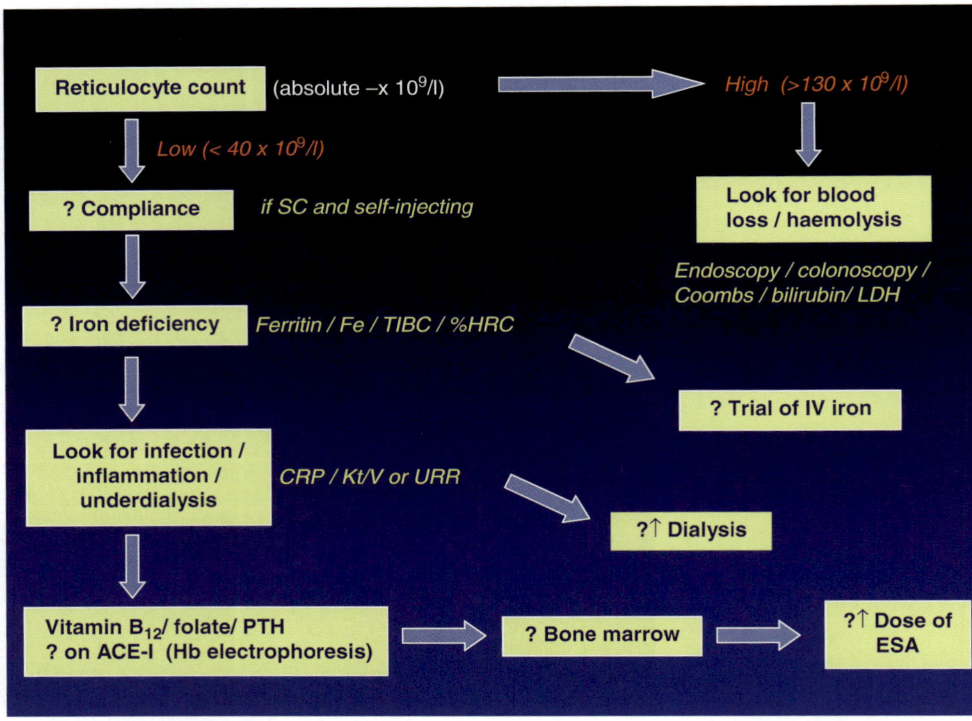

Fig. 50.3 Investigation of hyporesponsiveness to erythropoiesis-stimulating agent therapy. *ACEI* angiotensin-converting-enzyme inhibitors, *CRP* C-reactive protein, *ESA* erythropoiesis-stimulating agent, *Hb* haemoglobin, *PTH* parathyroid hormone, *URR* urea reduction ratio

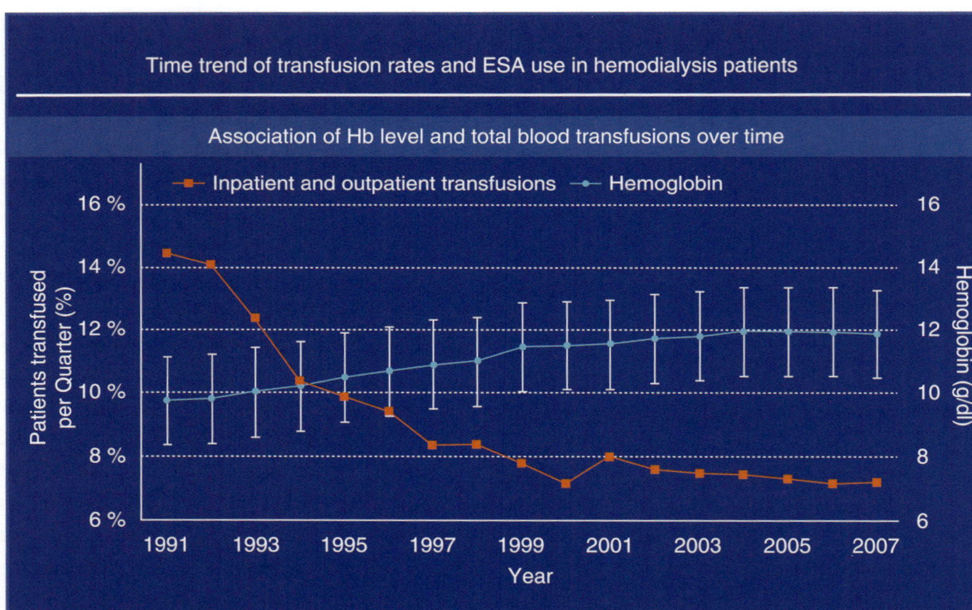

Fig. 50.4 Reduction in blood transfusions following the introduction of erythropoietin as a therapeutic agent [17] (Created with the use of data from US Renal Data System [17]. The data reported here have been supplied by the US Renal Data System (USRDS). The interpretation and reporting of these data are the responsibility of the author(s) and in no way should be seen as an official policy or interpretation of the US governments)

from around 14 % to around 7 % over the first decade of ESA use [17] (Fig. 50.4).

Given the safety concerns associated with ESA therapy, however, it is likely that the use of red cell transfusions will once again increase. The major concerns associated with blood transfusion use are the fairly rare occurrence of transmission of infectious agents and some rare but life-threatening transfusion reactions, such as transfusion-related lung injury and transfusion-related acute circulatory overload, but the main concern with blood transfusion use in CKD patients is the risk of HLA sensitisation [18].

Recent data from the USRDS confirm that this remains a problem, and HLA sensitisation is associated with a longer waiting time for kidney transplantation, reduced likelihood of receiving a kidney transplant and poor graft outcomes if transplanted. Thus, every attempt should be made to avoid blood transfusions where possible, particularly in younger patients.

The current 'catchphrase' in renal anaemia management is *individualisation of treatment*, and the balance between the use of ESA therapy and blood transfusions is a good example of this. For example, patients resistant to ESA therapy who are elderly and have no chance of receiving a kidney transplant should have a lower threshold for using red cell transfusions compared to a young patient who is keen to receive a transplant.

Blood transfusions may be used in either the acute or the chronic setting. Their use in an acute haemorrhagic state or immediately prior to any urgent surgical procedure is understandable.

Elective transfusion for chronic anaemia in the absence of active bleeding, however, is more controversial. A randomised controlled trial of two trigger haemoglobins for blood transfusion in the critical care setting (7 g/dl versus 10 g/dl) showed no benefit in transfusing patients when their haemoglobin fell below 10 g/dl [19], and this has resulted in a significant reduction in the trigger haemoglobin for transfusion to around 7–8 g/dl. Even in the cardiac setting, when patients may be suffering from acute coronary syndrome, the use of blood transfusion above a haemoglobin of 8 g/dl has been critically questioned.

Thus, in the absence of acute bleeding, there is little indication to transfuse a patient above 7–8 g/dl unless a surgical procedure is planned in which significant blood loss might be expected.

Guidelines on Anaemia Management in CKD

Ever since ESA therapy was introduced, clinical practice guidelines on the management of anaemia in CKD patients have been devised in various parts of the world. Thus, US, European, UK (NICE), Australian, Canadian and Japanese anaemia guidelines have all been published over the last two decades (Table 50.5). The guidelines have discussed most of the issues outlined in this chapter, focusing mainly on ESA and iron management, and there has been an evolution of recommendations over time. Since 2010, the work group of the KDIGO Anemia Guideline has reviewed the latest evidence on the management of anaemia in CKD patients, and their final report was published in August 2012 [16]. Subsequent to the KDIGO Anemia Guideline publication, the European Renal Best Practice group published a report of the latest recommendations [20]. Finally, following publication of the TREAT study, the UK NICE group revised their anaemia guideline with regard to trigger and target haemoglobin only [21]. No review of iron management was conducted at this review, but the main features of the NICE anaemia guideline (published in February 2011) were a trigger haemoglobin of 11 g/dl for the use of ESA therapy and a target (aspirational) haemoglobin range of 10–12 g/dl.

Table 50.5 Clinical practice guidelines on the management of anaemia in chronic kidney disease

Region	Guideline	Year of publication
USA	National Kidney Foundation [23]	1997
Europe	European Best Practice Guidelines [24]	1999
Canada	Canadian Guidelines on Anemia [25]	1999
USA	National Kidney Foundation [26]	2001
Europe	Revised European Best Practice Guidelines [27]	2004
Japan	Japanese Guidelines on Anemia [28]	2004
Australasia	Caring for Australasians with Renal Impairment [29]	2005
UK	National Institute for Health and Clinical Excellence [30]	2006
USA	KDOQI Clinical Practice Guideline and Clinical Practice Recommendations for Anemia in Chronic Kidney Disease: 2007 Update of Hemoglobin Target [31]	2007
Europe	European Best Practice Guidelines [32]	2010
UK	National Institute for Health and Clinical Excellence (update) [33]	2011
Global	KDIGO Clinical Practice Guideline for Anemia in Chronic Kidney Disease [34]	2012
Europe	European Renal Best Practice position statement [35]	2013

Conclusions

Anaemia management in chronic kidney disease has seen many changes over the last few decades. Prior to 1990, the mainstay of treatment was blood transfusions and/or iron supplementation. The introduction of ESA therapy in 1990 led to a dramatic reduction in the use of red cell transfusions, and at the same time iron supplementation was instituted more widely in order to maximise the response to ESAs (as well as to keep the doses and costs as low as possible). The results from the TREAT study have strongly influenced the latest thoughts regarding anaemia management, and although ESA therapy is still of critical importance in this condition, a more conservative approach has since been recommended. Finally, other strategies for treating anaemia in CKD are currently being researched [22], including stabilisation of hypoxia-inducible factor by prolyl-hydroxylase inhibitors as well as hepcidin modulation strategies. It is too early to say what the role of these new scientific developments will have in the management of CKD anaemia, but they are certainly of academic interest and worthy of further investigation.

Do's and Don'ts in Renal Anaemia Management

Do's

- Do use IV iron first whenever possible, *esp. if ferritin <100 ug/l.*
- Do start ESA therapy when Hb 9–10 rather than 10–11.
- Do aim for target Hb 10–12 g/dl.
- Do consider benefit to risk ratio in CKD patients with previous stroke or cancer.

Don'ts

- Do *not* escalate ESA dose in patients responding poorly to treatment.
- Do not administer IV iron to patients with active infection.

References

1. Caro J, Brown S, Miller O, et al. Erythropoietin levels in uremic nephric and anephric patients. J Lab Clin Med. 1979;93:449–58.
2. Macdougall IC. Monitoring of iron status and iron supplementation in patients treated with erythropoietin. Curr Opin Nephrol Hypertens. 1994;3:620–5.
3. Macdougall IC, Obrador GT, El Nahas M. How important is transfusion avoidance in 2013? Nephrol Dial Transplant. 2013;28: 1092–9.
4. Astor BC, Muntner P, Levin A, et al. Association of kidney function with anemia: the Third National Health and Nutrition Examination Survey (1988–1994). Arch Intern Med. 2002;162:1401–8.
5. Rossert J, Casadevall N, Eckardt KU. Anti-erythropoietin antibodies and pure red cell aplasia. J Am Soc Nephrol. 2004;15: 398–406.
6. Macdougall IC, Rossert J, Casadevall N, Stead RB, Duliege AM, Froissart M, Eckardt KU. A peptide-based erythropoietin-receptor agonist for pure red-cell aplasia. N Engl J Med. 2009;361: 1848–55.
7. Ganz T. Hepcidin and iron regulation, 10 years later. Blood. 2011;117:4425–33.
8. Tessitore N, Solero GP, Lippi G, Bassi A, Faccini GB, Bedogna V, Gammaro L, Brocco G, Restivo G, Bernich P, Lupo A, Maschio G. The role of iron status markers in predicting response to intravenous iron in haemodialysis patients on maintenance erythropoietin. Nephrol Dial Transplant. 2001;16:1416–23.
9. Tessitore N, Girelli D, Campostrini N, Bedogna V, Pietro Solero G, Castagna A, Melilli E, Mantovani W, De Matteis G, Olivieri O, Poli A, Lupo A. Hepcidin is not useful as a biomarker for iron needs in haemodialysis patients on maintenance erythropoiesis-stimulating agents. Nephrol Dial Transplant. 2010;25:3996–4002.
10. Macdougall IC, Provenzano R, Sharma A, Spinowitz BS, Schmidt RJ, Pergola PE, Zabaneh RI, Tong-Starksen S, Mayo MR, Tang H, Polu KR, Duliege AM, Fishbane S, PEARL Study Groups. Peginesatide for anemia in patients with chronic kidney disease not receiving dialysis. N Engl J Med. 2013;368:320–32.
11. Fishbane S, Schiller B, Locatelli F, Covic AC, Provenzano R, Wiecek A, Levin NW, Kaplan M, Macdougall IC, Francisco C, Mayo MR, Polu KR, Duliege AM, Besarab A, EMERALD Study Groups. Peginesatide in patients with anemia undergoing hemodialysis. N Engl J Med. 2013;368:307–19.
12. Besarab A, Bolton WK, Browne JK, Egrie JC, Nissenson AR, Okamoto DM, Schwab SJ, Goodkin DA. The effects of normal as compared with low hematocrit values in patients with cardiac disease who are receiving hemodialysis and epoetin. N Engl J Med. 1998;339:584–90.
13. Drüeke TB, Locatelli F, Clyne N, Eckardt KU, Macdougall IC, Tsakiris D, Burger HU, Scherhag A, CREATE Investigators. Normalization of hemoglobin level in patients with chronic kidney disease and anemia. N Engl J Med. 2006;355:2071–84.
14. Singh AK, Szczech L, Tang KL, Barnhart H, Sapp S, Wolfson M, Reddan D, CHOIR Investigators. Correction of anemia with epoetin alfa in chronic kidney disease. N Engl J Med. 2006;355:2085–98.
15. Pfeffer MA, Burdmann EA, Chen CY, Cooper ME, de Zeeuw D, Eckardt KU, Feyzi JM, Ivanovich P, Kewalramani R, Levey AS, Lewis EF, McGill JB, McMurray JJ, Parfrey P, Parving HH, Remuzzi G, Singh AK, Solomon SD, Toto R, TREAT Investigators. A trial of darbepoetin alfa in type 2 diabetes and chronic kidney disease. N Engl J Med. 2009;361:2019–32.
16. National Kidney Foundation. KDIGO clinical practice guideline for anemia in chronic kidney disease. Kidney Int Suppl. 2012; 2:v-335.
17. US Renal Data System. USRDS 2009 Annual Data Report: atlas of chronic kidney disease and end-stage renal disease in the United States. National Institutes of Health, National Institute of Diabetes and Digestive and Kidney Diseases, Bethesda; 2009.
18. Obrador GT, Macdougall IC. Effect of red cell transfusions on future kidney transplantation. Clin J Am Soc Nephrol. 2013;8:852–60.
19. Hébert PC, Wells G, Blajchman MA, Marshall J, Martin C, Pagliarello G, Tweeddale M, Schweitzer I, Yetisir E. A multicenter, randomized, controlled clinical trial of transfusion requirements in critical care. Transfusion Requirements in Critical Care Investigators, Canadian Critical Care Trials Group. N Engl J Med. 1999;340:409–17.
20. Locatelli F, Bárány P, Covic A, De Francisco A, Del Vecchio L, Goldsmith D, Hörl W, London G, Vanholder R, Van Biesen W, on behalf of the ERA-EDTA ERBP Advisory Board. Kidney disease: improving global outcomes guidelines on anaemia management in chronic kidney disease: a European renal best practice position statement. Nephrol Dial Transplant. 2013;28:1346–59.
21. National Institute for Health and Clinical Excellence (NICE). Anaemia management in people with chronic kidney disease. http://guidance.nice.org.uk/CG114. Updated November 2012. Accessed 26 May 2013.
22. Macdougall IC. New anemia therapies: translating novel strategies from bench to bedside. Am J Kidney Dis. 2012;59:444–51.
23. National Kidney Foundation. DOQI clinical practice guidelines for the treatment of anemia of chronic renal failure. Am J Kidney Dis. 1997;30(4 Suppl 3):S192–240.
24. European Best Practice Guidelines. Nephrol Dial Transplant. 1999;14(Suppl 2):61–5.
25. Canadian Guidelines on Anemia. J Am Soc Nephrol. 1999;10(Suppl 13):S292–6.
26. National Kidney Foundation. KDOQI clinical practice guidelines for anemia of chronic kidney disease: update 2000. Am J Kidney Dis. 2001;37((Suppl 1):S182–238.
27. Revised European Best Practice Guidelines. Nephrol Dial Transplant. 2004;19(Suppl 2):ii1–47.
28. Japanese Guidelines on Anemia. Ther Apher Dial. 2004;8:443–59.
29. Caring for Australasians with Renal Impairment. Nephrology (Carlton). 2005;10(Suppl 4):S108–15.
30. National Institute for Health and Clinical Excellence. 2006. http://www.nice.org.uk/CG039.

31. KDOQI. KDOQI clinical practice guideline and clinical practice recommendations for anemia in chronic kidney disease: 2007 update of hemoglobin target. Am J Kidney Dis. 2007;50: 471–530.
32. European Best Practice Guidelines (position statement only; no new evidence review). Nephrol Dial Transplant. 2010;25: 2846–2850.
33. National Institute for Health and Clinical Excellence. 2011. http://guidance.nice.org.uk/CG114.
34. KDIGO Clinical Practice Guideline for Anemia in Chronic Kidney Disease. 2012. http://www.kdigo.org/clinical_practice_guidelines/pdf/KDIGO-Anemia%20GL.pdf.
35. Locatelli F, Bárány P, Covic A, De Francisco A, Del Vecchio L, Goldsmith D, Hörl W, London G, Vanholder R, Van Biesen W; ERA-EDTA ERBP Advisory Board. Kidney Disease: Improving Global Outcomes guidelines on anaemia management in chronic kidney disease: a European Renal Best Practice position statement. Nephrol Dial Transplant 2013;28:1346–1359.

Chronic Kidney Disease: Mineral and Bone Disorder (CKD-MBD)

51

Richard S. Fish and John Cunningham

Definition

Chronic kidney disease mineral and bone disorder (CKD-MBD) is defined as a systemic disorder of mineral and bone metabolism due to CKD comprising either one or a combination of the following:

- Abnormalities of calcium, phosphorus, PTH or vitamin D metabolism
- Abnormalities in bone turnover, mineralization, volume, linear growth or strength
- Vascular or other soft tissue calcification

Clinical manifestations are very variable between subjects and are not entirely predictable from any given set of biochemical results. As such treatment strategies should be individualized.

Pathophysiology and Clinical Correlates

Normal mineral metabolism involves the integrated actions of the kidney, parathyroid glands, GI tract and bone. These organs act in linked fashion to maintain calcium and phosphate balance and skeletal integrity (see Fig. 51.1). CKD results in a number of disturbances to this system ultimately resulting in CKD-BMD (Fig. 51.2).

R.S. Fish, MRCP, BMBS, BMedSci (Hons) (✉)
UCL Centre for Nephrology, UCL Medical School,
Royal Free Campus, Rowland Hill Street, London NW3 2PF, UK
e-mail: rsfish@doctors.org.uk

J. Cunningham, DM, FRCP
UCL Centre for Nephrology, University College London Medical School, Rowland Hill Street, London NW3 2PF, UK
e-mail: drjohncunningham@gmail.com

M. Harber (ed.), *Practical Nephrology*,
DOI 10.1007/978-1-4471-5547-8_51, © Springer-Verlag London 2014

Biochemical Features

Failure of phosphate excretion and renal calcitriol production underlie many of the changes seen in early and late CKD. At early stages of CKD changes in serum phosphate are minimized by adaptive increases of the phosphaturic hormones PTH and FGF-23 such that appropriate phosphate balance is initially maintained. Hyperphosphataemia is not usually present before the GFR drops below 30 ml/min (see Fig. 51.3), at which point the adaptive responses can become overwhelmed.

PTH

Decreased calcitriol and calcium and increased phosphate all increase synthesis and release of PTH. PTH promotes calcium and phosphate resorption from bone, inhibits the sodium-phosphate cotransporter in the proximal tubule (promoting phosphate excretion) and by stimulating calcitriol production indirectly increases intestinal calcium and phosphate absorption. Sustained stimulation of the parathyroid glands results in hyperplasia and clonal proliferation of parathyroid cells which express fewer receptors for both vitamin D and calcium. PTH secretion may become uncontrolled with resulting hypercalcaemia representing the transition from secondary (appropriate) to tertiary (inappropriate) hyperparathyroidism. Gross elevation of PTH is catabolic to bone and has been implicated in cardiac fibrosis, left ventricular hypertrophy, hypertension, neuropathy and impotence. Bone marrow fibrosis as a result of hyperparathyroidism contributes to erythropoietin-stimulating agent (ESA) resistance.

Vitamin D

25-Hydroxyvitamin D (calcidiol), generated in the liver from its precursor, vitamin D, is terminally activated by 25-hydroxyvitamin D-1a-hydroxylase (CYP27B1) to produce 1,25-dihydroxyvitamin D (calcitriol). The bulk of the hormonal form is synthesized in the kidney where production is stimulated by PTH and inhibited by FGF-23 and

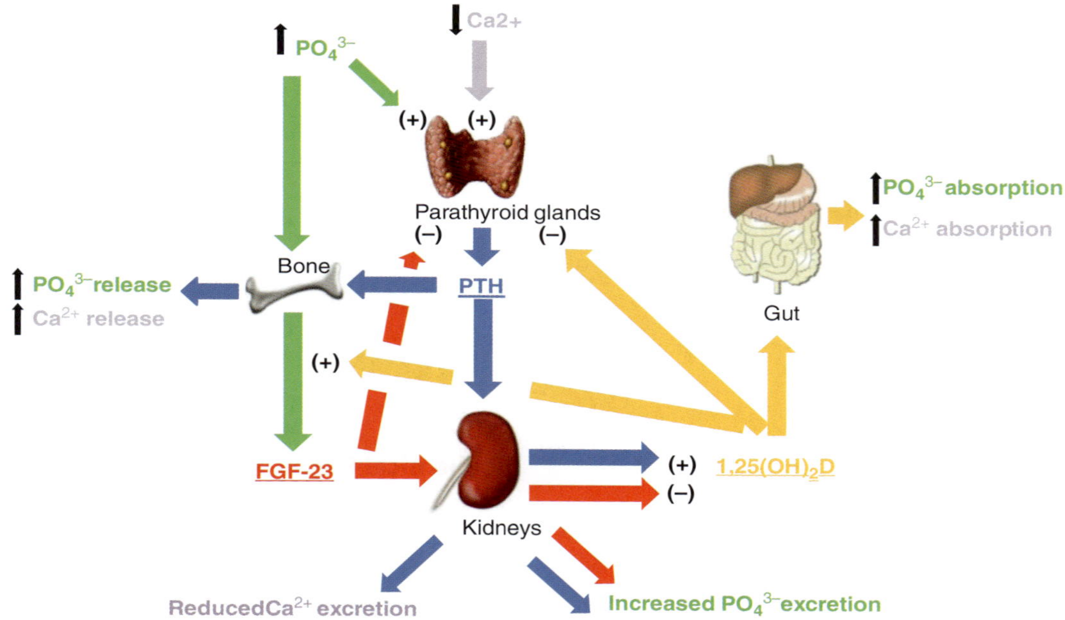

Fig. 51.1 Normal mineral metabolism. The actions of PTH (*blue arrows*) are to (1) increase phosphate and calcium release from bone, (2) enhance renal calcitriol production, (3) increase renal tubular calcium reabsorption and (4) increase renal phosphate excretion. PTH release is stimulated by decreases in serum calcium or calcitriol or a rise in serum phosphate. The actions of calcitriol (*orange arrows*) are to (1) increase intestinal calcium and phosphate absorption, (2) inhibit PTH release and (3) enhance FGF-23 release. Calcitriol production is stimulated by PTH and inhibited by FGF-23. The actions of FGF-23 (*red arrows*) are to (1) enhance renal phosphate excretion, (2) inhibit renal calcitriol production and (3) inhibit PTH release. FGF-23 production and release is stimulated by increased phosphate and calcitriol

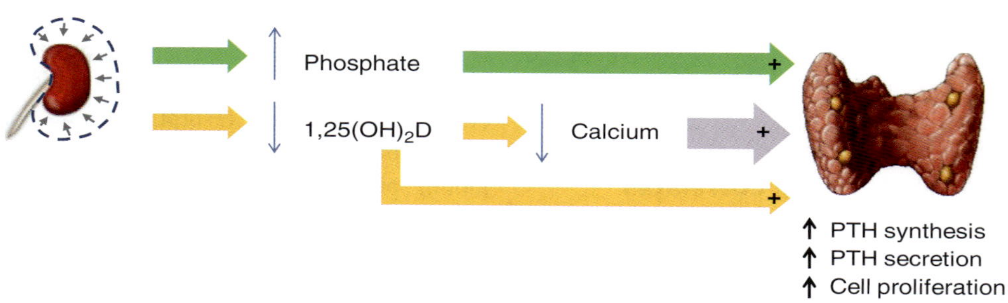

Fig. 51.2 Effects of advanced CKD on mineral metabolism. As glomerular filtration rate (GFR) declines, phosphate accumulates and calcitriol production decreases with a consequent fall in calcium. These three effects all stimulate PTH synthesis and release. In addition prolonged stimulation results in clonal proliferation of parathyroid cells which express fewer receptors for both vitamin D and calcium. Ultimately the gland becomes unresponsive to these downregulators – tertiary hyperparathyroidism

phosphate. Acting through the vitamin D receptor (VDR), circulating calcitriol acts to promote intestinal and renal absorption of calcium and phosphate and to inhibit PTH. Osteoblast activity is augmented and enhances bone remodelling and mineralization. A number of novel roles have been recently described for vitamin D and are discussed below.

FGF-23

FGF-23 is a hormone produced by osteocytes and induces phosphaturia by downregulation of proximal tubular sodium-phosphate cotransporters. In addition, FGF-23 decreases serum calcitriol by suppressing synthesis by renal 1a-hydroxylase (CYP27B1) and stimulating catabolism by 24-hydroxylase (CYP24A1). FGF-23 also negatively regulates PTH. Increased levels of FGF-23 associate with comorbidities including vascular calcification, left ventricular hypertrophy, endothelial dysfunction and progression of renal disease. Moreover, serum FGF-23 correlates strongly with mortality risk in both CKD and dialysis populations, and in this respect FGF-23 is emerging as a powerful biomarker, and possible mediator, of adverse clinical outcomes in these groups.

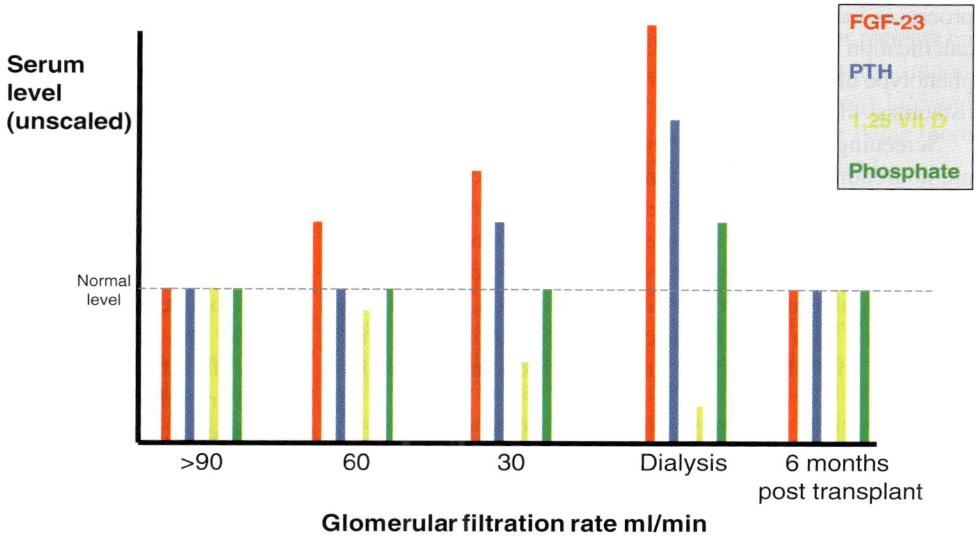

Fig. 51.3 Changes in CKD-BMD-associated biochemical parameters as CKD progresses and following transplantation. FGF-23 begins to increase at very early stages of CKD with PTH beginning to climb somewhat later. These two adaptive responses keep serum phosphate levels within the normal range until GFR drops well below 30 ml/min. 1,25 vitamin D begins to fall at a GFR of around 60 ml/min. These changes are corrected with kidney transplantation

Renal Bone Disease

The risk of fracture is elevated about fivefold in dialysis patients with the mortality rates following a fracture at least double than that seen in the general population.

Renal osteodystrophy comprises alterations of bone morphology in patients with CKD and defines the skeletal component of the systemic disorder of CKD-MBD. It is only quantifiable reliably by bone histology, though bone biopsy is seldom done due to the invasive nature of the procedure and the expertise required for interpretation. Biochemical markers, especially PTH and bone-specific alkaline phosphatase (bALP), are used as surrogates for histology.

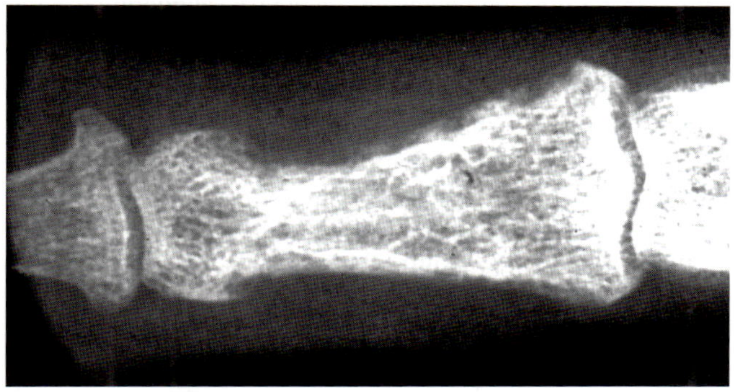

Fig. 51.4 Middle phalanx of a patient with secondary hyperparathyroidism showing subperiosteal reabsorption

High Turnover (Hyperparathyroid) Bone Disease

This is characterized by a PTH-driven increase in the activity of osteoblasts (direct) and osteoclasts (indirect) with disordered bone formation, accelerated resorption and evidence of fibrosis on bone biopsy. PTH and bALP are raised. Serum calcium concentrations are variable.

Overt symptoms are not usually apparent until disease is very advanced, at which point potential manifestations include bone pain and deformity, proximal muscle weakness and pruritus secondary to cutaneous mineral deposits. Hyperparathyroid bone disease does lead to a marked increase in fracture rates, and children with hyperparathyroid bone disease exhibit marked growth failure. Typical radiological features include subperiosteal reabsorption, often seen best in the middle phalanges (see Fig. 51.4).

Adynamic Bone Disease (ABD)

ABD is characterized by decreased bone cell activity, and typical biochemical findings include a raised calcium (adynamic bone buffers calcium poorly) and phosphate, with low-normal PTH and bALP. Clinical symptoms are often absent, as are positive radiological findings. Fracture rates are increased and fractures heal poorly. ABD associates with vascular calcification and high osteopenia risk post transplantation.

Vascular Calcification (VC)

VC occurs frequently in patients at all stages of CKD and its severity correlates with survival. Medial calcification of vessels predominates in CKD (compared to intimal disease which is the usual finding in the general population), which leads to arterial stiffening, an increase in afterload and subsequently left ventricular hypertrophy. In addition, calcification can make transplantation and vascular access for dialysis problematic and is probably involved in the development of calciphylaxis (see below). VC involves overlapping and integrated

Surgery requires localization of the parathyroid glands preoperatively and identification of any ectopic tissue. This can be achieved by nuclear medicine scans such as those using methoxyisobutyl isonitrile (MIBI). Subtotal parathyroidectomy is usually preferred over a total procedure. As with thyroid surgery, preoperative assessment by an ear, nose and throat clinician will depend on the local policy.

Unopposed bone uptake of calcium ('hungry bone syndrome') in the early postoperative phase is the most frequently seen complication and is highest in patients with severe disease. High doses of active vitamin D (e.g. 5 ug alfacalcidol) are administered for 5 days pre-procedure and decrease, but do not eliminate, the risk of postoperative hypocalcaemia. Intravenous calcium is needed in severe cases.

Following the procedure, careful monitoring of calcium is vital. A typical protocol would be to check blood calcium immediately after the operation, then 4 hourly for the first 24 h and 12 hourly for 2 days. A combination of oral calcium and active vitamin D (e.g. at least 2 g calcium and 2 ug alfacalcidol as starting doses) should be employed, with dose adjustments as appropriate. Calcium and vitamin D requirements decrease over time and can be titrated down in the outpatient clinic.

Severe hypocalcaemia (<1.8 mmol/l) postoperatively, or symptoms of hypocalcaemia, necessitates intravenous (iv) therapy. An initial 10 ml of 10 % calcium gluconate (which contains 2.25 mmol calcium) over 2–3 min through a large vein (extravasation can lead to tissue necrosis), repeated if necessary, can be followed by an infusion of 50 ml of 10 % calcium gluconate (10 mmol of calcium) in 500 ml of either 5 % dextrose or 0.9 % saline initially at 2 mmol/h with adjustments as required. Two hourly clinical assessment and serum calcium measurement is appropriate during iv calcium infusion, and continuous cardiac monitoring is needed.

The other main postoperative complication is bleeding which can cause airway compression and compromise. This is a dangerous scenario necessitating immediate anaesthetic assistance.

Additional Considerations and Controversies

Native Vitamin D Therapy

Experimentally, vitamin D has been shown to protect against left ventricular hypertrophy, hypertension and renal fibrosis and to have regulatory functions in the immune system and tumourogenesis. It is now clear that the VDR is ubiquitous. Both autocrine and paracrine effects are demonstrable, in addition to classic endocrine effects of calcitriol, and it may therefore be appropriate to replace both 1,25 hydroxyvitamin D and its precursor 25 hydroxyvitamin D in patients with CKD. Below 75 nmol/l is considered to represent insufficiency, but no definitive guidelines exist in relation to replacement of native vitamin D. A typical regime would be cholecalciferol 20,000 units taken orally once a week. Side effects are minimal and no significant alterations in calcium or phosphate are seen. Elevated PTH in vitamin D insufficient patients falls with therapy in those with mild to moderate, but not more advanced, CKD.

Calciphylaxis

Calciphylaxis or calcific uraemic arteriolopathy (CUA) is a relatively rare and often fatal complication of CKD-MBD. It is part of the spectrum of vascular calcification in advanced CKD, most often seen in the dialysis population. Initial presentation is with superficial, violaceous, painful, hyperaesthetic or pruritic skin lesions. Secondary infection and overwhelming sepsis can ensue. The most commonly affected areas are the thighs, buttocks and abdomen, although distal lesions are also seen.

The differential diagnosis is relatively wide and includes atheroembolic phenomena, severe ischaemic lesions and vasculitides. The definitive diagnostic investigation for calciphylaxis is a skin biopsy.

The most promising treatment is sodium thiosulphate. This leads to calcium exchange for sodium and results in the highly soluble compound calcium thiosulphate. Experience with its use is limited at present although increasing. A typical dosing regime would be 25 g iv over 1 h immediately following haemodialysis for patients receiving thrice weekly haemodialysis. The experience in peritoneal dialysis patients and non-dialysis patients is extremely limited. Metabolic acidosis may complicate therapy and necessitate dose adjustment or termination of therapy. Anecdotal evidence also exists for emergency parathyroidectomy, cinacalcet, intensive dialysis and bisphosphonates. It is often exquisitely painful and therefore regular review of analgesia is important. A referral to a pain specialist may be necessary.

Bone Mineral Density and Fracture Prophylaxis

Dual-energy X-ray absorptiometry (DXA) is the conventional tool used to assess fracture risk and define bone mineral density (BMD) in the general population, but is unreliable in CKD 4-5D though has some utility in early and moderate CKD. In patients with CKD stages 1–3, BMD assessment and treatment can proceed in the same way as those from the non-CKD population. Bisphosphonates and denosumab are safe and effective in these patients.

Patients with CKD stages 3–5D represent a more difficult cohort. Their bone disease is more heterogenous and although treatment could be guided by bone biopsy, this is not always possible. There are no data concerning the safety of bisphosphonates in this patient group and their use cannot routinely be advised.

The Transplant Patient

A well-functioning graft will lead to normalization of calcium and phosphate, enhanced vitamin D production and an improved PTH profile. These advantages are somewhat countered by increased bone turnover and a decrease in bone mineral density (particularly during the first 6 months post transplant). Risk factors for this include an abnormal skeletal substrate from previous dialysis, steroid use and treatment with calcineurin inhibitors. Many transplant centres in the UK are now adopting 'steroid sparing' protocols to address this and other complications of glucocorticoids.

The lifetime risk of sustaining at least one fracture is significant in transplant recipients and is not effectively predicted by DXA scans. Early bone loss in these patients is preventable with bisphosphonates, but these agents are not proven to reduce fracture.

Avascular Necrosis

This debilitating condition has previously complicated up to 1 % of transplant per year and is caused by ischaemic injury to bone parenchyma, particularly the femoral head. Steroid use is the biggest risk factor with others including a longer dialysis vintage, hyperparathyroidism, weight gain and trauma. Presentation is frequently with severe hip pain, especially on weight bearing. MRI is the investigation of choice to detect early disease. Plain X-rays are often normal initially. Steroids should be withdrawn if possible. The role for bisphosphonates is not certain. Orthopaedic surgery is usually required, with decompression procedures initially and ultimately joint replacement.

Tips and Tricks

1. When measuring PTH in the context of CKD, remember mild elevations (to within KDIGO guidelines) can be adaptive and may be beneficial.
2. A combination of diet, dialysis and binders is most efficacious for phosphate management, whereas active vitamin D and calcimimetics are most suitable for lowering PTH. Activated vitamin D therapy should not be introduced before phosphate controlling measures are in place.
3. Peri-parathyroidectomy management should be handled by a multidisciplinary team including physicians, endocrine and ENT surgeons, anaesthetists and radiologists. Preloading with calcium is essential (see text).
4. Risk factors for developing calciphylaxis include diabetes, obesity, Caucasian race, female gender and malnutrition.

Resources for Patients

'Phosphorus and your CKD diet': available from the National Kidney Foundation at http://www.kidney.org.

Information from the UK National Kidney Federation concerning CKD-BMD available at: http://www.kidney.org.uk/Medical-Info/Calcium-Phosphate/index.html.

Kidney Research UK factsheet on renal bone disease available at: http://www.kidneyresearchuk.org/health/factsheets/ckd-and-issues/bone-disease-in-chronic.php.

Suggested Further Reading

British Renal Association guidelines for managing CKD-BMD. Available at: www.renal.org.

Cunningham J, Zehnder D. New vitamin D analogs and changing therapeutic paradigms. Kidney Int. 2011;79:702–7.

Cunningham J, Locatelli F, Rodriguez M. Secondary hyperparathyroidism: pathogenesis, disease progression, and therapeutic options. Clin J Am Soc Nephrol. 2011;6:913–21.

Hruska K, Mathew S, Lund R, Fang Y, Sugatani T. Cardiovascular risk factors in chronic kidney disease: does phosphate qualify? Kidney Int Suppl. 2011;121:S9–13.

Hsu CY. FGF-23 and outcomes research – when physiology meets epidemiology. N Engl J Med. 2008;359:640–2.

KDIGO guidelines on CKD-BMD. Available at: www.kdigo.org.

Miller PD. Diagnosis and treatment of osteoporosis in chronic renal disease. Semin Nephrol. 2009;29:144–55.

Moe SM, Chen NX. Mechanisms of vascular calcification in chronic kidney disease. J Am Soc Nephrol. 2008;19:213–6.

Ott SM. Bisphosphonate safety and efficacy in chronic kidney disease. Kidney Int. 2012;82:833–5.

Ross EA. Evolution of treatment strategies for calciphylaxis. Am J Nephrol. 2011;34:460–7.

52 Chronic Kidney Disease: Cardiovascular Complications

Ben Caplin and David C. Wheeler

Diseases of the cardiovascular system, presenting as sudden death, myocardial infarction, stroke, heart failure, and gangrene are particularly common in patients with chronic kidney disease (CKD) and substantially limit their quality of life and life expectancy [1]. Whether established treatment strategies that have proven to be successful in other high-risk groups have similar benefits in the context of CKD is not clear, partly because these patients are often excluded from large clinical trials. Furthermore, the underlying pathophysiology of cardiovascular disease (CVD) may change as kidney function declines, so additional or alternative approaches to management may be appropriate. Thus, the management of cardiovascular disease remains a huge and often poorly accomplished challenge for health-care professionals looking after patients with CKD.

Epidemiology and Pathophysiology of CVD in CKD

Both reduced kidney function and proteinuria are associated with cardiovascular mortality [2] (Fig. 52.1). In a comprehensive population-based study, the risk of a cardiovascular event was 1.4 and 3.4 times greater in patients with CKD stage 3a and Stage 5, respectively [3]. Furthermore, outcomes for CKD patients suffering cardiovascular events are worse than for those with normal kidney function [4]. Thus, cardiovascular events represent the most important avoidable cause of morbidity and mortality in patients with impaired kidney function.

B. Caplin, BSc (Hons), MBChB, PhD (✉) • D.C. Wheeler, MD, FRCP
Centre for Nephrology, UCL Medical School,
Royal Free Campus, Rowland Hill Street, London NW3 2PF, UK
e-mail: b.caplin@ucl.ac.uk; d.wheeler@ucl.ac.uk

The Association Between CKD and CVD

The interrelationship between CVD and CKD is complex (Fig. 52.2). Firstly, there may be a vascular component to progressive kidney disease. Many cardiovascular risk factors including hypertension, smoking and diabetes have also been linked to progression of CKD, suggesting that kidney and cardiovascular disease may share common pathogenic mechanisms [5].

Secondly, in another clinical scenario ('cardio-renal syndrome'), patients with cardiac failure, but without primary kidney disease, develop a reduction of GFR resulting from hypoperfusion of the kidney, due to reduced arterial pressure or central venous congestion (or both). Although often coexisting with widespread atherosclerosis, this cardio-renal syndrome can occur in patients without atherosclerotic arterial disease, for example, in the context of advanced congenital heart disease or non-ischaemic cardiomyopathies [6].

Finally, chronic kidney disease per se, or its complications, for example, hyperphosphataemia, may also play an important causal role in the development of cardiovascular diseases. Impaired kidney function and/or proteinuria have been implicated in the pathogenesis of a wide range of cardiovascular syndromes including heart failure, sudden cardiac death and stroke [7]. Furthermore, a causal role for the kidney in cardiovascular disease is supported by the stepwise increase in the risk of adverse cardiac events with worsening of kidney function and the reduction in risk following successful kidney transplantation.

Therefore, cardiovascular disease and CKD often coexist and may be causally linked. As in individuals with normal kidney function, optimal management of cardiovascular disease in CKD patients requires risk stratification and attention to the management of risk factors. At the present time, it is unclear whether alternative strategies that target "non traditional" risk factors associated with CKD, such as hyperphosphataemia or hyperparathyroidism, are worthwhile.

M. Harber (ed.), *Practical Nephrology*,
DOI 10.1007/978-1-4471-5547-8_52, © Springer-Verlag London 2014

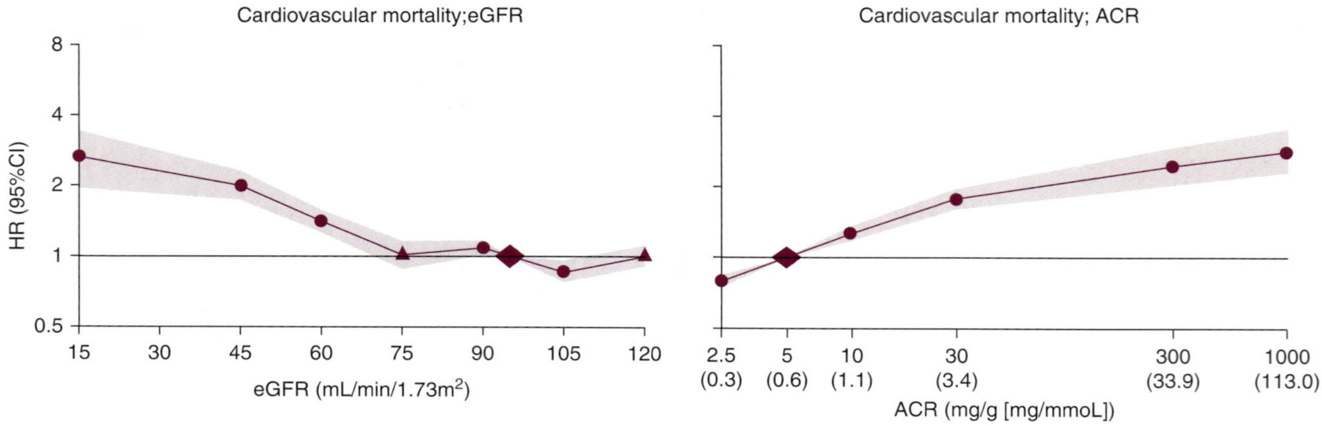

Fig. 52.1 Association between cardiovascular mortality and both estimated glomerular filtration rate and albumin:creatinine ratio. Hazard ratios (with 95 % confidence intervals, *shaded areas*) are adjusted for each other, age, sex, ethnic origin, history of cardiovascular disease, systolic blood pressure, diabetes, smoking and total cholesterol (Reproduced from Matsushita et al. [2] with permission)

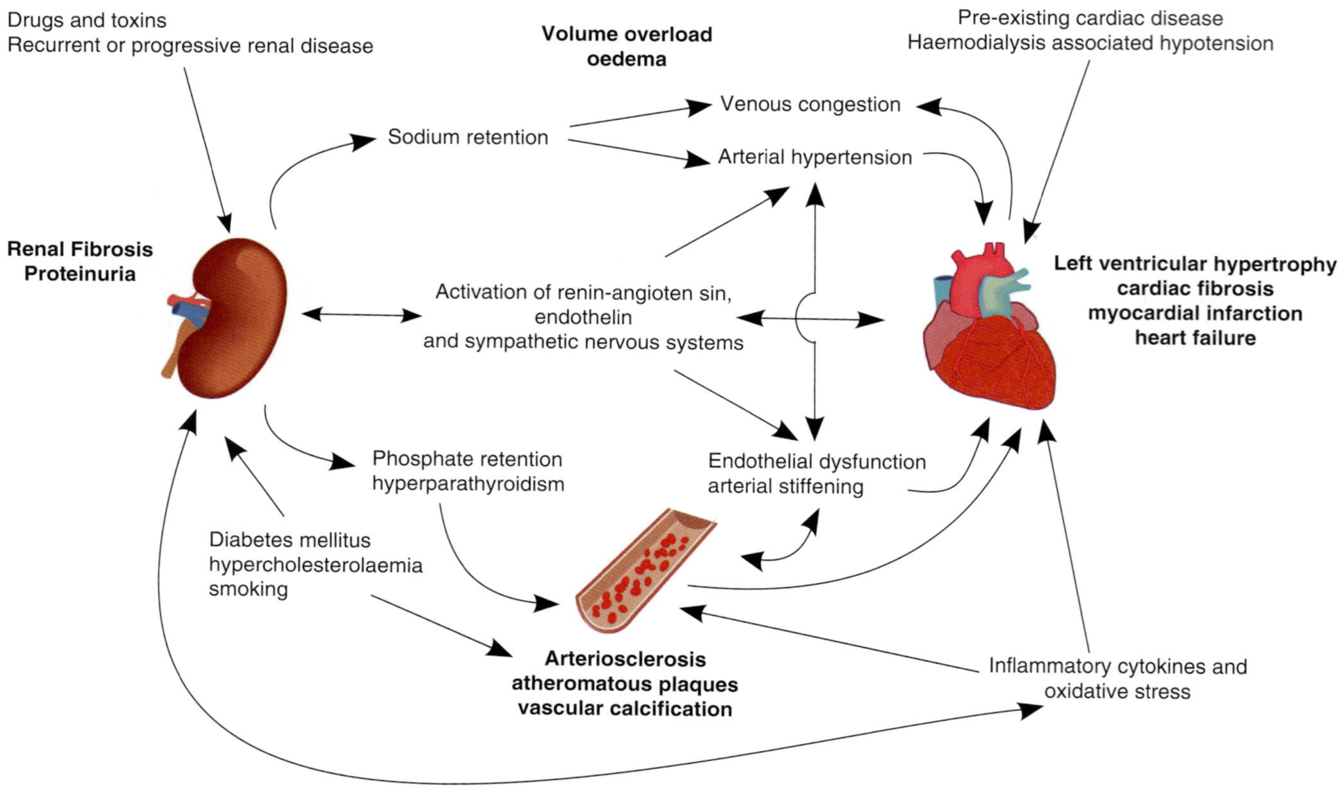

Fig. 52.2 Mechanisms of CV disease in CKD

Atherosclerotic and Non-atherosclerotic Disease in the CKD Population

Atherosclerosis

The high co-prevalence of shared risk factors such as diabetes mellitus means that atherosclerosis is an important cause of cardiovascular disease in patients with kidney disease [5]. The process of plaque formation, rupture and vessel occlusion is likely to be similar in those with and without CKD. Furthermore, atherosclerosis is a systemic disease, meaning that plaque formation in the arterial supply to one organ (e.g. in the coronary arteries) (Fig. 52.3d) is likely to reflect coexistent disease in the arterial supply to other organs (e.g. in the renal, carotid or femoral arteries).

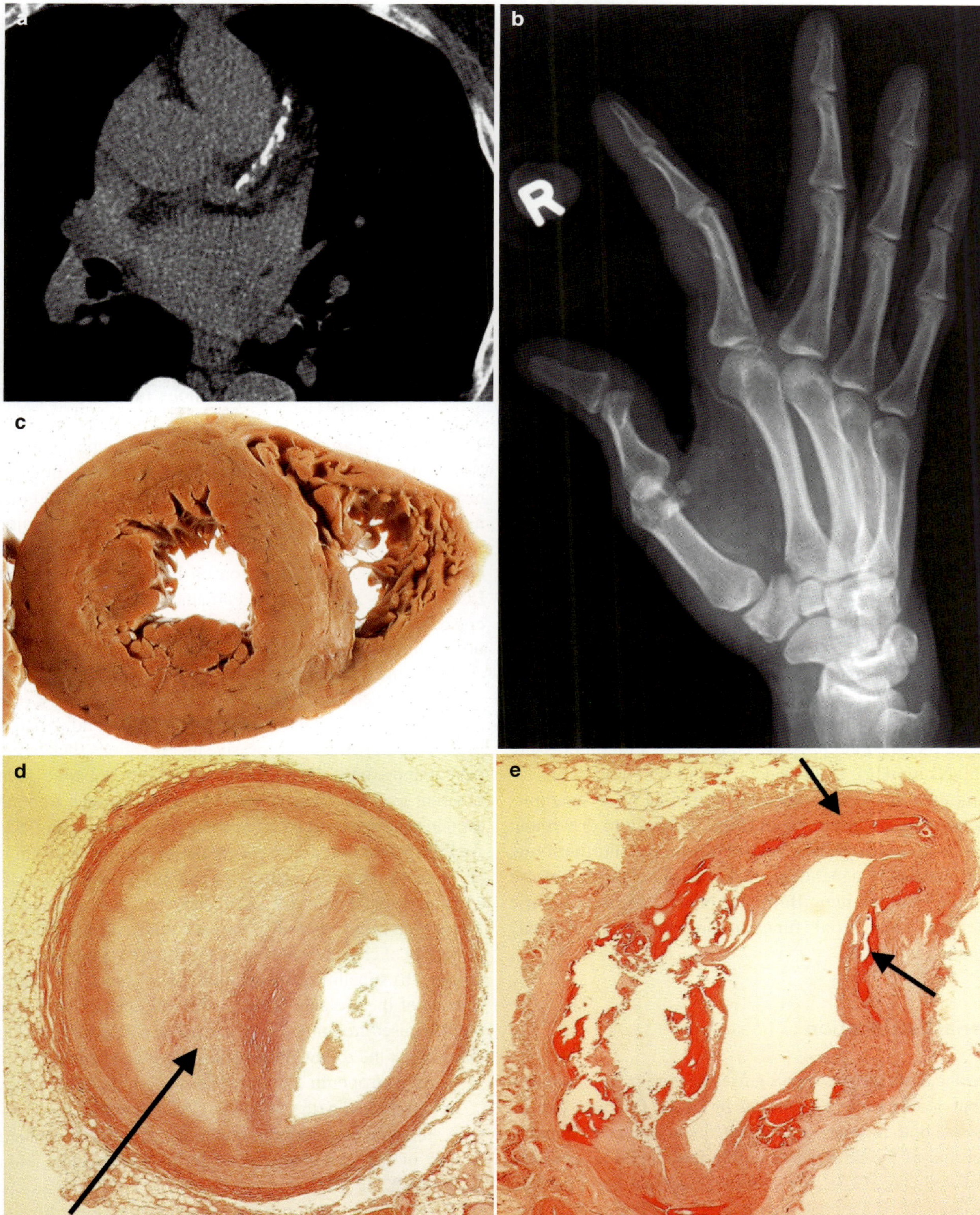

Fig. 52.3 Vascular changes in CKD patients. (**a**) An electron beam CT scan of the heart in a patient with CKD demonstrating calcium in the left anterior descending coronary artery. (**b**) Plain x-ray of the hand in a patient on haemodialysis showing calcification of the deep branches of the radial artery as well as osteopaenia of the small bones of the hand. (**c**) Postmortem specimen of the heart from a patient with CKD demonstrating left ventricular wall thickening (Courtesy Dr Paul Bass, Consultant Pathologist, Royal Free London). (**d**) Histological section of a diseased atherosclerotic artery showing obstructive lipid-filled subintimal plaque (*arrow*; ×300, H&E). (**e**) Histological section of aterio-sclerotic artery demonstrating arterial wall thickening and medial calcification (*arrows*; ×300 H&E) (**d**, **e**: Courtesy Professor Mary Sheppard, Department of Cardiovascular Pathology, St George's University of London)

Left Ventricular Disease

Echocardiographic studies suggest that a large proportion of patients with CKD have structural heart disease, rising from 30 % of patients with CKD stage 2 to 75 % in those with stage 4 [8]. This is usually manifest as left ventricular hypertrophy (Fig. 52.3c). Although coronary artery occlusion will cause segmental infarction as in those with normal kidney function, there may also be ultrastuructural abnormalities of the heart, such as myocardial fibrosis, in those with abnormal kidney function. Whether these changes reflect the consequences of ischaemia secondary to coronary microvascular disease or a specific effect of metabolites that accumulate in CKD remains unclear. In addition, there is now compelling evidence that hypotension during haemodialysis may contribute to recurrent cardiac ischaemia providing another mechanism to drive structural damage to the heart [9].

Arterial Stiffening

The compliance of the arterial tree lessens with normal ageing, but this process is accelerated in patients with CKD. Complaint arteries improve perfusion throughout the cardiac cycle by accommodating the maximal pressure during systole and maintaining blood flow during diastole. Arterial stiffening may be manifest by a widened pulse pressure, meaning that although the systolic pressure may be high, the diastolic pressure is low (e.g. a blood pressure of 160/60 mmHg). Both structural and functional changes are thought to lead to arterial stiffening. For example, thickening of the arterial wall (Fig. 52.3e), with or without calcification, will reduce vessel elasticity. Furthermore, vasodilatation is dependent on basal nitric oxide release from the endothelium. Both the bioavailability of nitric oxide and endothelial function are abnormal in CKD patients.

Arterial Calcification

Arterial calcification is a recognised feature of atherosclerosis, but is particularly common in CKD. Calcium can be deposited both in atherosclerotic plaques (which are found in the intima of the artery) and within the medial layer of the vessel wall (Fig. 52.3a, b, e). Medial calcification in particular is likely to be associated with arterial stiffening. It is generally accepted that deposition of calcium in soft tissues is one feature of the CKD-bone mineral disorder and may be exacerbated by treatment strategies aimed at preventing secondary hyperparathyroidism.

Approach to Cardiovascular Syndromes in Patients with Kidney Disease

Cardiac Ischaemia

Aetiology and Clinical Presentation

Although anginal symptoms may be experienced by patients with CKD, the high prevalence of underlying vascular disease, diabetes and other comorbidities may make the presentation of ischaemic cardiac disease atypical. For example, syncope, arrhythmia, sudden onset of symptoms of left ventricular failure or even isolated hypotension should prompt further investigation to detect underlying coronary ischaemia.

Patients on haemodialysis may also be exposed to asymptomatic chronic myocardial ischaemia. As discussed above, there are well-documented reductions in cardiac perfusion during dialysis in response to removal of circulating volume. This may be particularly damaging in patients with non-compliant arteries and limited left ventricular functional reserve and can in turn cause myocardial stunning and hibernation, leading to progression of chronic myocardial injury.

Patients with CKD who sustain a myocardial infarction may present with ST elevation on ECG; however, atypical ECG changes are common. Patients with multiple previous episodes of cardiac ischaemia may have signs of previous infarction on ECG and the consequences of any new ischaemia on the tracing may not be obvious.

Raised levels of troponin T (cTnT) and troponin I (cTnI) are thought to reflect myocardial injury and are now routinely used to select patients for invasive investigations such as coronary angiography. However, patients with impaired kidney function may have raised blood levels of cardiac troponins, even in the absence of an acute coronary syndrome (Fig. 52.4). As kidney function declines, circulating cardiac troponin levels increase, with the majority of patients having raised cTnT and a substantial minority a cTnI above the normal range [10]. These high levels of cardiac troponins have been attributed to (a) failure of clearance of troponin breakdown products via the kidney, (b) subclinical myocardial injury and (c) noncardiac sources of the proteins. This presents difficulties when interpreting raised troponin levels in patients with chronic kidney disease, but the following generalisations can be made:

- Elevated troponin T and troponin I concentrations should be interpreted with caution in CKD patients.
- A single measurement cannot be used to stratify a patient's risk in the same way as in those with normal kidney function.
- Troponins predict poor outcomes including cardiovascular death in patients with CKD. The higher the troponin, the greater the risk of death.
- An acute rise in cardiac troponin (>20 % above baseline) is likely to reflect an acute myocardial injury.

Fig. 52.4 Troponin levels in patients with CKD but without acute coronary syndrome. Distribution of highly sensitive troponin I (**a**) and highly sensitive troponin T (**b**) in 148 subjects with CKD and 288 healthy controls (Reprinted with permission from DeFilippi et al. [10])

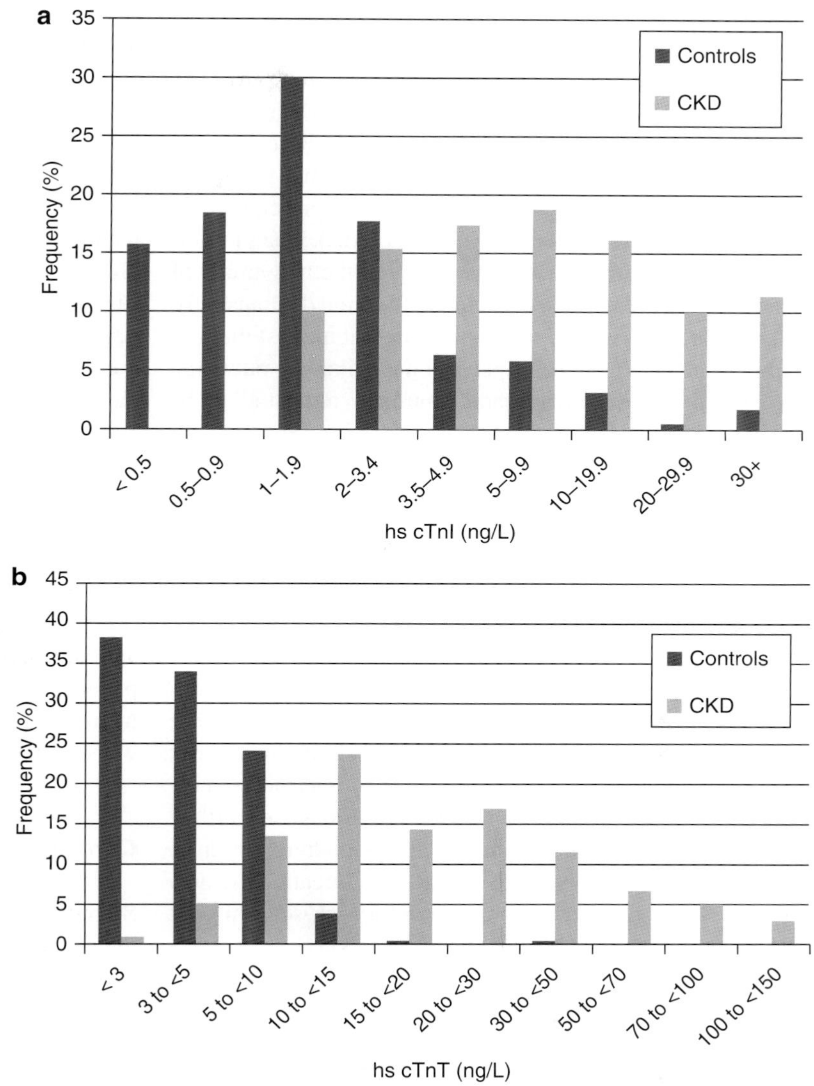

In patients receiving haemodialysis, the dialysis process itself may influence troponin levels, but the magnitude of this effect may dependent on the type of dialysis membrane used [11].

Diagnostic Imaging

Angiography remains the investigation of choice for detecting athero-occlusive disease of the coronary and peripheral vessels. Other imaging modalities such as CT angiography and cardiac MRI are rapidly evolving and may soon become the standard approach for visualisation of arterial plaque. Coronary CT also allows assessment of the vessel wall, so the overall degree of coronary calcification can also be quantified. These three imaging modalities require contrast administration with the associated risks. Iodinated radiocontrast used in digital subtraction and CT angiography can lead to acute kidney injury. This is generally mild and reversible if adequate precautions are taken before the procedure (hydration, omission of ACE-I/diuretics), although the potential to damage residual kidney function in patients approaching dialysis must be taken into account when making a decision to proceed with these investigations.

Given that myocardial disease may occur in the absence of occlusive plaque, cardiac functional studies can be useful in patients with advanced CKD. Possible approaches include myocardial perfusion scanning or stress echocardiography, and there is evidence that the latter of these two approaches can provide useful prognostic information [12]. However, the appropriate management of patients with abnormal cardiac functional scans, who do not have stenosis of the coronary arteries on angiography, remains unclear.

Treatment

Emergency Reperfusion

There have been no randomised controlled trials to date assessing cardiac reperfusion strategies in CKD. In patients without impaired kidney function, primary percutaneous coronary angioplasty (PTCA) improves outcomes following ST-segment elevation myocardial infarction (or acute coronary syndromes with evidence of myocardial injury) compared to conservative treatment. Although the magnitude of this benefit may be reduced as kidney function declines [13], reperfusion is considered first-line treatment in most dialysis centres, and the benefits of reperfusion are likely to outweigh any risk to the kidney from radiocontrast in almost all clinical scenarios.

Where PTCA is not available, thrombolysis using t-PA or streptokinase is an alternative approach to reperfusion. There is no reason to assume that patients with renal impairment should not benefit from thrombolysis. However, it should be remembered that patients receiving dialysis are generally at higher risk of bleeding than those with normal kidney function.

As discussed above, the haemodialysis procedure itself can lead to reductions in myocardial perfusion. Haemodialysis should be avoided during and immediately following acute coronary ischaemia unless there are absolute indications such as hyperkalaemia or fluid overload. Furthermore, in the period immediately following an acute coronary event, the haemodialysis prescription should be modified to maximise cardiovascular stability with short daily treatments, low blood flow, minimal ultrafiltration and a high-sodium concentration in the dialysis fluid (see Chap. 59).

Delayed/Elective Intervention

The appropriate clinical approach to the management of a CKD patient with stable symptoms and documented coronary stenosis remains uncertain. Although PTCA appears relatively safe in patients with moderate CKD, as in patients with normal kidney function, there have been no studies showing a positive impact on clinical outcomes when compared to maximising medical therapy in this group [14].

In subgroup analyses of CKD patients entered into trials comparing PTCA to surgical bypass grafting, no differences in mortality between these two approaches have been shown, although revascularisation rates are lower following surgery [15]. However, the risks of major surgery are high in patients with additional comorbidities, and postoperative death is more frequent in dialysis patients. Therefore, the choice as to whether to proceed to PTCA or to refer for CABG should be determined by clinical judgement in the absence of good quality evidence.

Medical Therapy

Anticoagulant treatment is routinely administered to patients presenting with acute coronary syndromes. There is no reason to assume that these agents will be less effective in patients with CKD. There is an increased risk of bleeding among patients with CKD stages 4–5, and in addition, the low-molecular-weight heparins accumulate in patients with advanced kidney disease.

Antiplatelet agents such as clopidogrel and glycoprotein IIa/IIIb inhibitors have not been shown to benefit patients with CKD when added to aspirin in the context of acute coronary syndromes. Data from post hoc analyses of large trials suggest that addition of these agents does not reduce the incidence of further cardiovascular events or death, but increases the risk of serious bleeding [16]. Therefore, optimal medical therapy in the secondary prevention of ischaemic heart disease consists of aspirin in addition to renin-angiotensin system inhibition, beta-blockade and aggressive lipid management. As there is no evidence indicating that beta-blockade or drugs targeting of the renin-angiotensin system are any less effective in patients with CKD, given the increased prevalence of IHD, the number of patients needed to treat to gain benefit is likely to be smaller. However, observational studies suggest that despite this likely benefit, patients with CKD do not receive such aggressive medical management following acute coronary syndromes as patients with normal kidney function [17].

Cardiovascular Causes of Shortness of Breath

Symptoms and signs of pulmonary oedema may present diagnostic difficulty in CKD patients who can develop sodium and water overload due to a failure of natriuresis, independently of left ventricular dysfunction. Additionally, CKD patients with left ventricular failure secondary to structural abnormalities, such as LV hypertrophy, or ischaemic damage (due to coronary artery occlusion or microvascular disease) will also develop secondary salt and water retention. More rarely, a disruption of cardiac rhythm can precipitate pulmonary oedema. Given the high prevalence of coexistent CKD and CVD, most patients present with a combination of left ventricular dysfunction and failure of natriuresis.

Chest x-ray will usually show evidence of engorged pulmonary vessels (and the ECG may reveal a left ventricular strain pattern). The polypeptide n-terminal pro-brain natriuretic peptide (nt-proBNP) is a highly sensitive marker of cardiac stretch and left ventricular failure in patients with a normal GFR. nt-proBNP is cleared by the kidney and levels are significantly higher in CKD, with a stepwise increase as GFR falls, but whether additional mechanisms (reflecting the burden of cardiac pathology) are also responsible for the higher levels observed in patients with CKD is controversial. Therefore, although nt-proBNP levels correlate with LV dysfunction in patients with mild and moderate CKD, the upper limit of normal for the assay should be increased in this group of patients. Levels of nt-proBNP are highest in dialysis patients and do not necessarily show an independent association with LV dysfunction in this group [18] although serial measurements may provide useful additional information as to changes in total body salt and water overload. As in the case of troponin, the dialysis procedure may influence circulating concentrations of this marker, and whatever the mechanisms of elevation in patients with CKD, higher levels of nt-proBNP predict adverse outcomes.

Echocardiography is a useful non-invasive investigation in CKD patients with pulmonary oedema. Evidence of reduced left ventricular ejection fraction suggests underlying cardiac dysfunction. However, abnormal left ventricular geometry is common in CKD patients as a result of chronic pressure and volume overload, cardiac ischaemia and fibrosis. Assessment of left ventricular function is further complicated in patients receiving haemodialysis by the effects of changes in volume status and the potential for myocardial stunning. Thus, the timing of the investigation with reference to the dialysis session may be an important factor in interpreting the result. Based on these considerations, assessment of the extent of left ventricular failure in a dialysis-dependent patient can only be made reliably once intravascular volume status has been optimised.

Acute Treatment

As in the patient with normal kidney function, the treatment of acute pulmonary oedema in CKD includes maintaining gas exchange and venodilation, followed by salt and water removal. Nitrates remain the mainstay of venodilatory therapy in all patients, and intravenous therapy allows minute-by-minute titration according to arterial blood pressure.

Loop diuretics, which have both natriuretic and vasodilatory effects when given intravenously, are also useful in CKD patients, except in those who are anuric. Higher doses of loop diuretics are often required when GFR is reduced as compared to when kidney function is normal and these large doses (e.g. 500 mg of frusemide/furosemide) are best given by continuous infusion over a 24-h period as rapid injection of large doses of these drugs can cause deafness. Additional blockade of sodium reabsorption in the distal nephron with thiazide or potassium-sparing diuretics will lead to additional natriuresis. However, very careful monitoring is required when using this combined approach, which can lead to rapid intravascular volume depletion with associated organ dysfunction. In addition, acidosis and hyperkalaemia often complicate the use of potassium-sparing diuretics in those with CKD.

In patients who are dialysis dependent or acutely oliguric, ultrafiltration may be required and should be initiated in a timely fashion. In the acute setting and in situations where the metabolic disturbance is limited, isolated ultrafiltration without dialysis will improve cardiovascular stability and may be the treatment of choice. Furthermore, where diagnostic doubt exists as to the aetiology of the shortness of breath in a dialysis patient, a therapeutic trial of ultrafiltration may be useful. Removal of as little as 500 mL of ultrafiltrate can acutely improve symptoms if due to pulmonary oedema.

Prevention of recurrent pulmonary oedema usually requires attention to both cardiac and renal factors. Management of fluid overload in non-dialysis-dependent CKD patients includes salt restriction and diuretic therapy, sometimes requiring combinations of loop and thiazide or potassium-sparing agents. Care must be taken to avoid over-diuresis, progressive prerenal dysfunction and biochemical deterioration. Regular review of volume status and blood biochemistry along with patient education and daily home monitoring of weight are important strategies. Ultimately, failure of volume control in a CKD patient may be the primary indication for initiating long-term RRT.

Both ACE inhibitors and beta-blockers are likely to have a valuable role in the management of left ventricular failure in CKD, with beneficial effects on cardiac remodelling and clinical outcomes. The roles of spironolactone and newer aldosterone antagonists have not been adequately defined in patients with impaired kidney function.

Arrhythmia and Sudden Death

Atrial fibrillation is the commonest cardiac rhythm disturbance in CKD patients. Episodes of atrial fibrillation are not uncommon during haemodialysis and often resolve spontaneously. Other cardiac rhythm disturbances are less common and less extensively studied, but may also present with syncope or other consequences of hypotension.

Furthermore, approximately a quarter of patients on dialysis die suddenly from unascertained causes, and it is estimated that in approximately 20 % of these cases, the underlying cause is an arrhythmia. Patients with mild and moderate CKD are also at increased risk of sudden death, with the magnitude of this risk associated with GFR, independent of other known risk factors. Thus, patients with CKD stage 3–5 have twice the risk of sudden cardiac death as individuals with normal kidney function [19]. Patients with CKD have numerous risk factors for cardiac conduction disturbances as described above. Furthermore, they are often exposed to substantial electrolyte disturbances, and in the case of haemodialysis, rapid shifts in ions (such as potassium) occur over very short time periods. In these patients, low-potassium dialysate, as well as both high and low predialysis serum potassium, have been associated with an excess risk of mortality [20, 21].

Patients with CKD often take multiple medications, so review of the prescription is important in any patient suspected of having an arrhythmia. The role of cardiac monitoring using either the Holter system or implantable recording devices has not been systematically studied in CKD patients, but given the high relative risk of arrhythmias, these techniques are probably underutilised, especially for patients with syncope and hypotension. Thyroid function should also be checked in patients presenting with tachy- or bradyarrhythmias.

Treatment

Beta-blockade currently represents the first-line treatment for rate control in atrial fibrillation. There are no trials of catheter-based ablation techniques for the treatment of AF in patients with CKD. Anticoagulation in the primary prevention of AF-associated stroke is discussed in detail below.

As with other arrhythmias, electrolyte disturbance should be corrected where possible and exacerbating drugs withdrawn. Investigations to exclude occult coronary ischaemia should be considered. A role of implantable defibrillators in CKD patients has yet to be established.

Noncardiac Athero-Occlusive Disorders

Aetiology and Clinical Presentation

Both stroke and peripheral arterial disease are more common in CKD patients than in age- and gender-matched controls, and as discussed above, the arteries of these patients may be structurally and functionally abnormal. As well as an increased prevalence of atherosclerotic disease, increased vascular stiffness leads to reduced peripheral perfusion, and calcification of arteries may impact on the success of revascularisation strategies (both angioplasty and bypass).

The standard investigation for occlusive carotid stenosis and peripheral vascular disease is digital subtraction angiography. In obtaining consent, the patient must be aware of the risk of radiocontrast induced nephropathy, and pre-procedure precautions should be taken.

Treatment

Secondary prevention strategies for noncardiac atherosclerotic events include aggressive control of risk factors, for example, blood pressure and cholesterol lowering. Risk factor modification is discussed in detail below, but certain invasive interventions require specific attention.

Thrombolysis for Stroke

Thrombolysis for acute stroke in patients with normal kidney function presenting within 4½ h is currently a routine part of clinical practice. No evidence for increased risk of bleeding has been observed in patients with moderate CKD, although the benefits of thrombolytic therapy in this group have not been specifically addressed. As discussed in the section on coronary reperfusion above, the increased risk of bleeding complications must be considered when offering thrombolytic therapy to patients receiving dialysis. No randomised controlled trials of thrombolysis for acute stroke in patients receiving haemodialysis have been published, and opinion on the appropriateness of this treatment remains divided.

Carotid Endarterectomy for Prevention of Stroke

The benefits of endarterectomy in those with symptomatic high-grade carotid stenosis appear to extend to patients with impaired kidney function, with the number needed to treat to avoid further events being lower in those with CKD not receiving dialysis. The magnitude of risks and benefits has not been defined in those patients with ESRD.

Dialysis Around Acute Stroke

Haemodialysis leads to brain swelling, with documented changes in brain volume of around 3 % attributable to the procedure [22]. Therefore, most physicians would attempt to avoid haemodialysis immediately after acute brain injury unless there was an absolute life-threatening indication such as hyperkalaemia or pulmonary oedema. Dialysis prescriptions should be designed to maximise stability as described in Chap. 59, and systemic anticoagulation should be avoided, particularly in those with intracerebral haemorrhage or when the nature of the stroke has not been determined.

Outcomes of Interventions for Critical Limb Ischaemia

As with all other atherosclerotic disease, outcomes for patients with limb ischaemia caused by peripheral vascular disease worsen with declining kidney function. Patients on dialysis have some of the highest rates of amputation and other complications from peripheral vascular disease with over 13 % of incident haemodialysis patients going on to experience lower-limb amputation in one American cohort study [23]. As with other forms of vascular disease, aggressive risk-factor management should be pursued, but there are currently no evidence-based medical therapies for critical limb ischaemia. Furthermore, there are no randomised controlled trials investigating different interventional management strategies and decisions regarding angioplasty, bypass and amputation must be made on an individual patient basis. Involvement of the multidisciplinary team is critical in such decision making, which should involve close liaison between vascular, infectious diseases and nephrology teams.

Prevention of Cardiovascular Complications in Patients with Kidney Disease

Traditional Vascular Risk Factors and Treatment

Blood Pressure

Control of blood pressure has been shown to reduce the risk of both cardiovascular events and retard progression of kidney dysfunction in patients with CKD. The optimal level of blood pressure control has been debated, but current guidelines recommend a systolic pressure of ≤140 mmHg and diastolic pressure of ≤90 mmHg, except in patients with urinary protein excretion greater than 30 mg/day (i.e. microalbumiuria and macroalbuminuria) when this target should be reduced to ≤130/80 mmHg, regardless of the presence or absence of diabetes.

Salt Restriction

Blood pressure control can be more difficult in patients with moderate to severe CKD and is complicated by a degree of salt and water overload. Salt restriction, which can improve blood pressure in those with normal kidney function, may have an even more important role in those with renal dysfunction. Reducing salt intake in patients with CKD is therefore critical for control of blood pressure, proteinuria and oedema. There is evidence that patients with CKD have a reduced taste sensation for salt. Importantly, salt restriction, even of relatively short duration (1 week), leads to an increased sensitivity to salt [24]. This means that patients can be reassured that although their food may taste bland during the initial period following salt restriction, gustatory sensation will normalise with time. In controlled trials in subjects with CKD, randomisation to salt restriction, targeting 50 mMol Na^{2+}/day (~3 g salt), results in a similar or greater reduction in BP than the addition of another class of antihypertensive medication, even though in reality patients generally only manage to reduce their intake to around 100 mMol Na^{2+} /day [25, 26] (Fig. 52.5).

Renin-Angiotensin Blockade

Inhibitors of the renin-angiotensin system are effective antihypertensive agents. These agents have additional cardiovascular benefits as well as the potential to reduce proteinuria and retard rate of decline of kidney function, possibly independent of blood pressure lowering. Although there is currently no clear evidence to support the use of one class of these agents over another nor evidence supporting

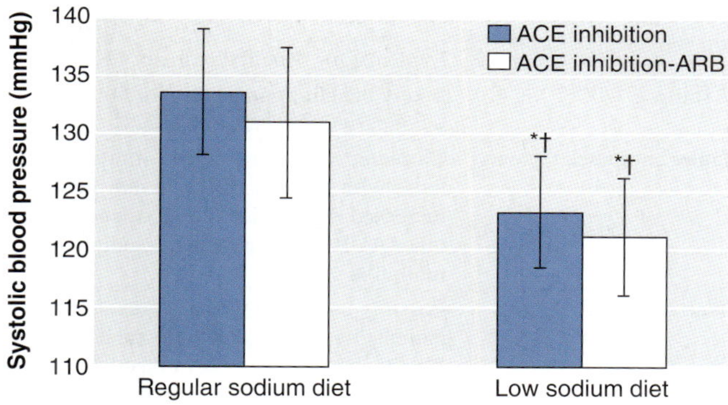

Fig. 52.5 Impact of sodium intake on blood pressure. 52 patients with nondiabetic nephropathy taking an ACE inhibitor received four phases of treatment: ARB or placebo in addition to either regular or a low-sodium diet, each for 6 weeks. Sodium restriction led to a greater reduction in SBP than addition of an ARB (Reproduced from Slagman et al. [25] with permission)

combination treatment, patients with CKD or proteinuria should receive one of these agents unless there are strong contraindications (such as a history of angioneurotic oedema associated with ACE inhibitors).

The nature of action of ACE inhibitors and angiotensin receptor blockers means that the initiation of treatment is often associated with a reduction in GFR. Biochemical tests should be repeated 1–2 weeks following initiation or a dose increase, and although there will often be a small rise in serum creatinine, this reflects the underlying beneficial mechanism of action of these agents and should not lead to discontinuation of treatment. A serum creatinine rise reflecting a drop in GFR of up to 25 % is generally accepted, assuming that there is a subsequent stabilisation. Hyperkalaemia can also complicate the use of these agents, and dietary potassium restriction will often be needed in those with a low eGFR. Severe hyperkalaemia may necessitate withdrawal of these agents.

A further challenge in blood pressure control relates to the increase in arterial stiffness seen in many CKD patients. The correct therapeutic approach to a high systolic BP in association with a low diastolic BP is unclear. The risk of reducing cardiac perfusion, which occurs largely in diastole, must be balanced by attempts to reach target systolic blood pressures with serial escalation of antihypertensive therapy.

In summary, hypertension in patients with CKD is a difficult clinical problem. Dietetic input along with a regimen of multiple antihypertensive agents, including a diuretic, may be required to control blood pressure in an individual patient (Table 52.1). Patient education, along with home monitoring, may be particularly beneficial in some patients, improving adherence and preventing overtreatment.

Table 52.1 Cardiovascular medication in CKD

	Evidence for benefits/harms in CKD	Practical use in CKD
Aspirin	Likely benefit in prevention of both primary and secondary CV events in CKD	No dose adjustment necessary
Other antiplatelet agents	Clopidogrel appears to be of limited in benefit/efficacy in those with reduced GFR and may be associated with increased risk of bleeding. Evidence base is poor for other ADP receptor blockers and glycoprotein IIa/IIIb inhibitors	Several glycoprotein IIa/IIIb inhibitors require dose adjustment in patients with reduced GFR
Warfarin	Possibly useful for primary prevention of stroke in patients with atrial fibrillation and moderate CKD. Significant increase risk of bleeding observed and doubt as to overall benefit when used as primary prevention of stroke in patients receiving haemodialysis	No specific dose alteration required but care with drug interactions required
Heparins	Reduce early ischaemic events in acute coronary syndromes. LMWH accumulates in renal impairment. Increased bleeding seen with use of enoxaparin in CKD	Dose reduction of LMWH in CKD. Factor Xa monitoring or unfractionated heparin may be preferred in severe renal impairment
Oral factor Xa inhibitors	May be a useful alternative to heparins and warfarin, but further data are needed	May require dose reduction in CKD
Renin-angiotensin blockade (ACE-I/A2 blockers/renin inhibitors)	Possible cardiovascular benefits, both in primary and secondary prevention and probable benefit in slowing of decline in kidney function. No clear evidence for combined use of ACE, ARB or renin inhibitors	Monitoring of biochemistry required following commencement or dose increases. Hyperkalaemia can occur and may require dose adjustment or withdrawal. Stable increases in serum creatinine of 20–30 % are generally thought to be acceptable
Beta-blockers	Possible benefit in patients with heart failure and CKD and in secondary prevention post-MI. Can be used for rate control in atrial fibrillation	Most agents dosed as in normal renal function but may need to commence at low doses
Diuretics	Thiazide diuretics are useful antihypertensive agents in mild and moderate CKD. Addition of loop diuretics to other antihypertensive therapy is a useful therapeutic strategy in moderate to severe CKD. High doses of loop diuretics for the treatment of oedema may be required in advanced CKD	Thiazides may become less effective as GFR falls. Combination therapy with loop and thiazide diuretics recommended in CKD stage 4 and 5. Hyperkalaemia and acidosis may complicate the use of potassium-sparing diuretics in CKD
Calcium channel blockers	Similar benefit in terms of primary prevention of cardiovascular events as compared to ACE inhibitors and diuretics in hypertensive patients with CKD. Dihydropyridines may exacerbate proteinuria	No specific dose adjustments
Digoxin	Can be used for rate control in atrial fibrillation	Standard loading dose, but low maintenance doses required in CKD. Risk of accumulation and toxicity so monitoring levels is essential. Not removed in haemodialysis patients
Cholesterol-lowering agents	Proven benefits of statin plus ezetimibe combination in primary prevention of atherosclerotic CV disease in stages 3–5 CKD. Probable benefit in patients receiving haemodialysis and following kidney transplantation	No evidence for increased statin toxicity in CKD when used in low doses, even when used in combination with ezetimibe. Fibrates should be avoided in patients with stages 4–5 CKD. High doses of statins best avoided because of the potential for muscle injury

Cholesterol

Typical patterns of dyslipidaemia vary with different causes and stages of CKD (Table 52.2). However, treatment with cholesterol-lowering agents leads to a substantial reduction in cardiovascular events in patients with stages 3–5 CKD. In the Study of Heart and Renal Protection (SHARP), the largest prospective randomised controlled study in subjects with CKD (including dialysis patients), patients receiving simvastatin 20 mg with ezetemibe 10 mg (rather than placebo) suffered almost one-fifth fewer cardiovascular events over the approximately 5-year follow-up period with no safety concerns (Fig. 52.6) [27].

Evidence as to whether cholesterol reduction reduces the risk of cardiovascular disease specifically in patients with CKD stage 5 is less clear. In two randomised trials recruiting dialysis patients, statin therapy did not result in a clear reduction in cardiovascular events [28, 29]. In the SHARP trial, a reduction in atherosclerotic cardiovascular events was observed in dialysis patients on active treatment, roughly consistent with the achieved reduction in LDL cholesterol, which was less in dialysis than in non-dialysis patients due to poor compliance [27]. Based on data from an extended follow-up of patients in a trial comparing fluvastatin to placebo, which demonstrated a 20 % reduction in cardiac events over

Table 52.2 Patterns and management of dyslipidaemia in patients with kidney disease

Syndrome	Typical pattern of dyslipidaemia	Management
Nephrotic syndrome	Hypercholesterolaemia due to elevated LDL	Treat underlying glomerular disease if possible Reduce proteinuria with ACEi and/or ARB Prescribe statin
Chronic kidney disease stages 1–2	Lipid profile usually normal in the absence of proteinuria	Regardless of starting cholesterol, consider statin to reduce risk of CV disease
Chronic kidney disease stages 3–5	Hypertriglyceridaemia with low HDL due to reduced clearance of triglyceride-rich VLDL and chylomicrons. Cholesterol usually normal	Benefits of reducing triglycerides with fibrates unproven Focus on reducing CV risk by lowering cholesterol with statins Avoid maximum doses of statin by adding Ezetimibe

LDL low-density lipoprotein, *VLDL* very low-density lipoprotein, *HDL* high-density lipoprotein, *CV* cardiovascular

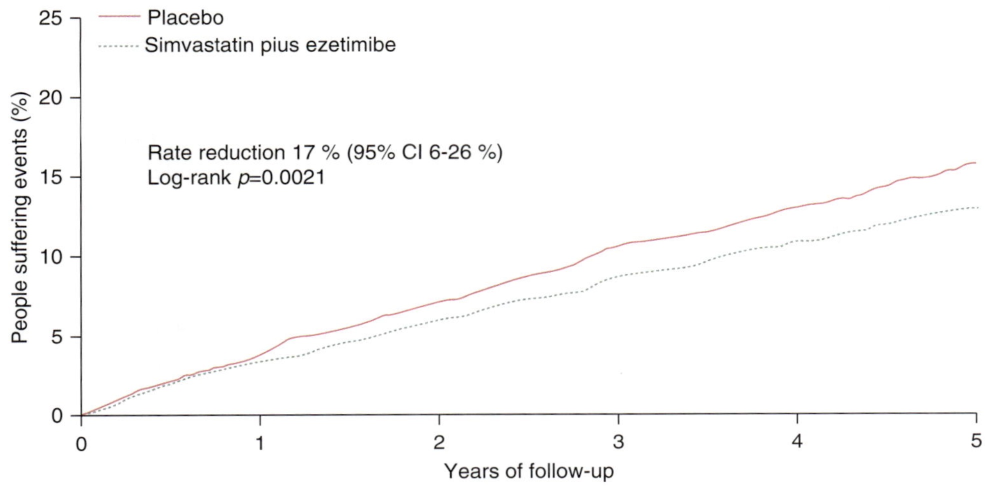

Fig. 52.6 Risk of cardiovascular events in CKD subjects randomised to simvastatin/ezetimibe combination or placebo (Reproduced from Baigent et al. [27] with permission)

approximately 6½ years [30], most clinicians use statins in kidney transplant recipients, particularly when LDL cholesterol levels are elevated.

Cigarette Smoking

Smoking is associated with an approximate 50 % increased risk of new cardiovascular events in dialysis patients [31]. Therefore, reductions in cardiovascular events, slowing of progressive loss of kidney function as well as fewer cases of respiratory and malignant disease would be predicted with smoking cessation. So all patients who smoke should be encouraged to give up and offered appropriate support to do so as required. Care should be taken with pharmacological adjuncts that assist smoking cessation and dose reductions may be required in advanced CKD.

Diabetes

Tight glycaemic control has been shown to reduce cardiovascular complications in the context of diabetes, with the effects lasting many years beyond the intervention. Therefore, adequate control of blood glucose must be integral to strategies aimed at preventing cardiovascular events in patients with CKD. The optimal level of blood glucose control still needs to be properly defined in patients receiving renal replacement therapy, with observational studies suggesting that both high and a very low HbA1c are associated with adverse outcomes.

Antiplatelet Agents

Aspirin reduces the risk of future cardiovascular events, and there is some evidence that this benefits extends to patients with impaired kidney function. In a subgroup analysis of the Hypertension Optimal Treatment, randomisation to aspirin was associated with an estimated reduction of 20 major cardiovascular events but 7.5 more major bleeding episodes per 1,000 patient years [32]. Therefore, although the exact groups who will benefit have not been well defined and although the risk of bleeding in CKD may be increased, aspirin can be used for both primary and secondary prevention of cardiovascular events in CKD. Evidence for the use of alternative antiplatelet agents such as clopidogrel for primary prevention of cardiovascular events in patients with CKD is lacking [16].

Prevention of Stroke in Chronic Atrial Fibrillation

In patients with normal kidney function, atrial fibrillation and other risk factors for stroke, anticoagulation is indicated with warfarin currently being the best evidence-based therapy. In patients with CKD, benefits have also been observed [33], with warfarin prescription associated with a 24 % relative risk reduction. However, in patients receiving haemodialysis, warfarin treatment has been associated with a doubling in risk of intracerebral haemorrhage [34], so the risks of treatment may well outweigh the benefits in this group. Although aspirin therapy may be indicated for prevention of cardiac events in this group, it does not appear to be associated with a reduced risk of stroke.

Interventions for Kidney-Related Risk Factors

Proteinuria

Proteinuria is an independent risk factor for cardiovascular events, even in patients with preserved kidney function (Fig. 52.1). Approaches aimed to reduce blood pressure, such as salt restriction and renin-angiotensin blockade, will also reduce proteinuria.

Nephrotic Syndrome

As well as being prone to venous thromboembolism (discussed in Chap. 1), patients with nephrotic syndrome are also at greater risk of cardiovascular events such as stroke or coronary heart disease, with an estimated fivefold increased risk of myocardial infarction compared to the general population [35]. Reduction in cardiovascular risk in the context of proteinuria relies on achieving remission or even partial remission where possible. Although no good evidence is available, control of other risk factors such as hypercholesterolaemia and hypertension may also help reduce the risk of vascular events. The routine use of aspirin would seem appropriate although there is no evidence base for this. Formal anticoagulation is also used in severely hypoalbuminaemic patients as prophylaxis against venous thromboembolism, and whether this has a role in preventing arterial disease is unclear.

Decline in GFR

As a lower GFR is associated with an increased risk of cardiovascular disease, prevention of loss of kidney function should lead to an amelioration of the accompanying cardiovascular risk. Treatment of the underlying kidney disorder, e.g. with immunosuppression, may reduce the chances of a decline in GFR. Furthermore, general measures that reduce blood pressure and proteinuria may lower the risk of GFR decline as well as impacting directly on cardiovascular risk.

Bone Mineral Disorder/Hyperphosphataemia

Derangements in mineral metabolism occur even in patients with stage 3 CKD as part of the bone mineral disorder (see Chap. 3). Although increases in calcium and phosphate are associated with increased risk of cardiovascular events, whether this relationship is directly causal and the degree to which different treatment strategies alter this risk remain open to question.

Medications Used in Renal Medicine

Several medications used in the treatment of kidney disease have adverse cardiovascular profiles. Most commonly used in patients with kidney transplants, calcineurin inhibitors are known to impact on cardiovascular risk factors. Ciclosporin use is associated with an increase in blood pressure and tacrolimus with an increased risk of diabetes. Similarly, corticosteroids can lead to insulin resistance, weight gain and hypertension. Other drugs that modify cardiovascular risk factors include sirolimus (lipid abnormalities) and antiretrovirals used in HIV treatment (lipid abnormalities and effects of mitochondrial function).

Evidence for Other Proposed Kidney-Associated Risk Factors

A number of circulating markers that potentially contribute to vascular disease in the context of CKD have been identified. These include homocysteine, uric acid, reactive oxygen species, fibroblast growth factor-23 and endogenous inhibitors of nitric oxide synthesis. Although levels of all of these substances are associated with both reduced kidney function and cardiovascular events, evidence for a causal role remains inconclusive to date.

There have been a number of small, unblinded studies showing benefits associated with targeting these nontraditional risk factors; however, the results from larger high-quality controlled trials targeting these potential mediators have not been encouraging. For example, in the case of homocysteine, there are a number of studies reporting that increases are independently associated with future cardiovascular events in CKD [36], and there is also a simple therapeutic intervention, folic acid, which has been shown to reduce levels. However, evidence from several good quality randomised trials now demonstrates that treatment with folic acid does not reduce the risk of cardiovascular events in CKD patients [37]. Therefore, although there are several proposed novel mediators of cardiovascular risk in CKD, the gap between exploratory studies and evidence-based intervention remains.

References

1. McCullough PA, Li S, Jurkovitz CT, et al. Chronic kidney disease, prevalence of premature cardiovascular disease, and relationship to short-term mortality. Am Heart J. 2008;156:277–83.
2. Matsushita K, van der Velde M, Astor BC, et al. Association of estimated glomerular filtration rate and albuminuria with all-cause and cardiovascular mortality in general population cohorts: a collaborative meta-analysis. Lancet. 2010;375:2073–81.
3. Go AS, Chertow GM, Fan D, et al. Chronic kidney disease and the risks of death, cardiovascular events, and hospitalization. N Engl J Med. 2004;351:1296–305.
4. Herzog CA, Ma JZ, Collins AJ. Poor long-term survival after acute myocardial infarction among patients on long-term dialysis. N Engl J Med. 1998;339:799–805.
5. Whaley-Connell AT, Sowers JR, Stevens LA, et al. CKD in the United States: Kidney Early Evaluation Program (KEEP) and National Health and Nutrition Examination Survey (NHANES) 1999–2004. Am J Kidney Dis. 2008;51:S13–20.
6. Ronco C, Cicoira M, McCullough PA. Cardiorenal syndrome type 1: pathophysiological crosstalk leading to combined heart and kidney dysfunction in the setting of acutely decompensated heart failure. J Am Coll Cardiol. 2012;60:1031–42.
7. Sarnak MJ, Levey AS. Cardiovascular disease and chronic renal disease: a new paradigm. Am J Kidney Dis. 2000;35:S117–31.
8. Park M, Hsu CY, Li Y, et al. Associations between kidney function and subclinical cardiac abnormalities in CKD. J Am Soc Nephrol. 2012;23:1725–34.
9. McIntyre CW, Burton JO, Selby NM, et al. Hemodialysis-induced cardiac dysfunction is associated with an acute reduction in global and segmental myocardial blood flow. Clin J Am Soc Nephrol. 2008;3:19–26.
10. Defilippi C, Seliger SL, Kelley W, et al. Interpreting cardiac troponin results from high-sensitivity assays in chronic kidney disease without acute coronary syndrome. Clin Chem. 2012;58:1342–51.
11. Lippi G, Tessitore N, Montagnana M, et al. Influence of sampling time and ultrafiltration coefficient of the dialysis membrane on cardiac troponin I and T. Arch Pathol Lab Med. 2008;132:72–6.
12. Bergeron S, Hillis GS, Haugen EN, et al. Prognostic value of dobutamine stress echocardiography in patients with chronic kidney disease. Am Heart J. 2007;153:385–91.
13. Szummer K, Lundman P, Jacobson SH, et al. Influence of renal function on the effects of early revascularization in non-ST-elevation myocardial infarction: data from the Swedish Web-System for Enhancement and Development of Evidence-Based Care in Heart Disease Evaluated According to Recommended Therapies (SWEDEHEART). Circulation. 2009;120:851–8.
14. Sedlis SP, Jurkovitz CT, Hartigan PM, et al. Optimal medical therapy with or without percutaneous coronary intervention for patients with stable coronary artery disease and chronic kidney disease. Am J Cardiol. 2009;104:1647–53.
15. Ix JH, Mercado N, Shlipak MG, et al. Association of chronic kidney disease with clinical outcomes after coronary revascularization: the Arterial Revascularization Therapies Study (ARTS). Am Heart J. 2005;149:512–9.
16. Palmer SC, Di Micco L, Razavian M, et al. Effects of antiplatelet therapy on mortality and cardiovascular and bleeding outcomes in persons with chronic kidney disease: a systematic review and meta-analysis. Ann Intern Med. 2012;156:445–59.
17. Fox CS, Muntner P, Chen AY, et al. Use of evidence-based therapies in short-term outcomes of ST-segment elevation myocardial infarction and non-ST-segment elevation myocardial infarction in patients with chronic kidney disease: a report from the National Cardiovascular Data Acute Coronary Treatment and Intervention Outcomes Network registry. Circulation. 2010;121:357–65.
18. Booth J, Pinney J, Davenport A. N-terminal proBNP–marker of cardiac dysfunction, fluid overload, or malnutrition in hemodialysis patients? Clin J Am Soc Nephrol. 2010;5:1036–40.
19. Pun PH, Smarz TR, Honeycutt EF, et al. Chronic kidney disease is associated with increased risk of sudden cardiac death among patients with coronary artery disease. Kidney Int. 2009;76:652–8.
20. Pun PH, Lehrich RW, Honeycutt EF, et al. Modifiable risk factors associated with sudden cardiac arrest within hemodialysis clinics. Kidney Int. 2011;79:218–27.
21. Foley RN, Gilbertson DT, Murray T, et al. Long interdialytic interval and mortality among patients receiving hemodialysis. N Engl J Med. 2011;365:1099–107.
22. Walters RJ, Fox NC, Crum WR, et al. Haemodialysis and cerebral oedema. Nephron. 2001;87:143–7.
23. Plantinga LC, Fink NE, Coresh J, et al. Peripheral vascular disease-related procedures in dialysis patients: predictors and prognosis. Clin J Am Soc Nephrol. 2009;4:1637–45.
24. Kusaba T, Mori Y, Masami O, et al. Sodium restriction improves the gustatory threshold for salty taste in patients with chronic kidney disease. Kidney Int. 2009;76:638–43.
25. Slagman MC, Waanders F, Hemmelder MH, et al. Moderate dietary sodium restriction added to angiotensin converting enzyme inhibition compared with dual blockade in lowering proteinuria and blood pressure: randomised controlled trial. BMJ. 2011;343:d4366.
26. Vogt L, Waanders F, Boomsma F, et al. Effects of dietary sodium and hydrochlorothiazide on the antiproteinuric efficacy of losartan. J Am Soc Nephrol. 2008;19:999–1007.
27. Baigent C, Landray MJ, Reith C, et al. The effects of lowering LDL cholesterol with simvastatin plus ezetimibe in patients with chronic kidney disease (Study of Heart and Renal Protection): a randomised placebo-controlled trial. Lancet. 2011;377:2181–92.
28. Fellstrom BC, Jardine AG, Schmieder RE, et al. Rosuvastatin and cardiovascular events in patients undergoing hemodialysis. N Engl J Med. 2009;360:1395–407.
29. Wanner C, Krane V, Marz W, et al. Atorvastatin in patients with type 2 diabetes mellitus undergoing hemodialysis. N Engl J Med. 2005;353:238–48.
30. Holdaas H, Fellstrom B, Cole E, et al. Long-term cardiac outcomes in renal transplant recipients receiving fluvastatin: the ALERT extension study. Am J Transplant. 2005;5:2929–36.
31. Foley RN, Herzog CA, Collins AJ. Smoking and cardiovascular outcomes in dialysis patients: the United States Renal Data System Wave 2 study. Kidney Int. 2003;63:1462–7.
32. Jardine MJ, Ninomiya T, Perkovic V, et al. Aspirin is beneficial in hypertensive patients with chronic kidney disease: a post-hoc subgroup analysis of a randomized controlled trial. J Am Coll Cardiol. 2010;56:956–65.
33. Olesen JB, Lip GY, Kamper AL, et al. Stroke and bleeding in atrial fibrillation with chronic kidney disease. N Engl J Med. 2012;367:625–35.
34. Winkelmayer WC, Liu J, Setoguchi S, et al. Effectiveness and safety of warfarin initiation in older hemodialysis patients with incident atrial fibrillation. Clin J Am Soc Nephrol. 2011;6:2662–8.
35. Mahmoodi BK, ten Kate MK, Waanders F, et al. High absolute risks and predictors of venous and arterial thromboembolic events in patients with nephrotic syndrome: results from a large retrospective cohort study. Circulation. 2008;117:224–30.
36. Moustapha A, Naso A, Nahlawi M, et al. Prospective study of hyperhomocysteinemia as an adverse cardiovascular risk factor in end-stage renal disease. Circulation. 1998;97:138–41.
37. Jardine MJ, Kang A, Zoungas S, et al. The effect of folic acid based homocysteine lowering on cardiovascular events in people with kidney disease: systematic review and meta-analysis. BMJ. 2012;344:e3533.

Coagulation in Kidney Disease

53

Duncan Brian and Pratima Chowdary

Patients with renal impairment are paradoxically at an increased risk of both bleeding and venous and arterial thromboembolism. These complications are seen frequently, and assessment of the balance between bleeding and prothrombotic tendency in individual patients can be challenging. This is compounded by the lack of evidence-based guidelines or consensus recommendations for appropriate investigations and management.

Normal Coagulation

Haemostasis is triggered by tissue injury, and magnitude of response is appropriate to severity of injury (Fig. 53.1). Primary haemostasis is characterised initially by platelet adhesion to subendothelial tissues following tissue trauma. This is facilitated by circulating von Willebrand factor (vWF) anchoring to collagen in subendothelial tissues and glycoprotein Ib (GPIb) receptors on platelet surface. Subsequent platelet activation is brought about by interaction of subendothelial collagen with glycoprotein VI (GPVI) platelet receptors, reinforced by action of thrombin on platelet protease-activated receptors (PAR4) receptors. Platelet activation results in the release of platelet alpha and dense granules including adenosine diphosphate (ADP) and thromboxane A2 generation, all which are necessary for platelet recruitment and aggregate formation. Aggregate formation is mediated by platelet glycoprotein IIb/IIIa (GPIIb/IIIa) receptors on adjacent platelets interacting with each other through fibrinogen.

Secondary haemostasis is characterised by thrombin generation and fibrin clot formation and is brought about by exposure of tissue factor (TF) following tissue trauma. TF is a transmembrane glycoprotein that acts as the cell surface receptor for factor VIIa. It is expressed constitutively in fibroblasts and smooth muscle cells around blood vessels, and expression can be induced in monocytes and endothelial cells. Thrombin generation requires a phospholipid (PL) surface and calcium. In the initiation phase, formation of extrinsic tenase complex (factor VIIa.TF.PL.Ca++) results in generation of small quantities of Xa leading to thrombin formation. This small amount of thrombin is necessary for priming the amplification pathway to facilitate explosive thrombin generation crucial for fibrin clot formation. The priming of the amplification pathway is achieved through activation of cofactors V and VIII, activation of platelet membrane with exposure of phospholipids and activation of factors IX and XI. Two complexes are assembled in the amplification pathway, intrinsic tenase (IXa.VIIIa.PL.Ca++) acting on factor X to generate Xa and prothrombinase complex (Xa.Va.PL.Ca++) acting on prothrombin to generate thrombin. This thrombin converts soluble fibrinogen molecules to insoluble fibrin meshwork that traps red cells and white cells.

Natural anticoagulants ensure control of thrombin generation spatially and temporally, and they include tissue factor pathway inhibitor (TFPI), antithrombin (AT) and protein C and S and thrombomodulin. TFPI is a rapid and potent inhibitor of initiation through the formation of an inactive quaternary complex with FVIIa.TF.Xa. Activated serine proteases, including IXa, XIa, VIIa, Xa and thrombin, are inhibited irreversibly by AT, the principal physiological inhibitor. Its primary targets are Xa and thrombin, and interaction with heparin-like glycosaminoglycans (GAGs) increases its activity 2,000- to 10,000-fold. Endogenous GAGs key to this are heparan sulphate and dermatan sulphate which are expressed on the surface of the endothelial cells at the level of microcirculation. Cofactors Va and VIIIa are inactivated by the activated protein C with protein S as a cofactor, and activation of protein C by thrombin requires the former bound to endothelial protein C receptor and the latter to thrombomodulin on the endothelial surfaces.

D. Brian, MBBS, MRCS, MRCP (Lond)
P. Chowdary, MBBS, FRCPath (✉)
Katharine Dormandy Haemophilia Centre and Thrombosis Unit, Royal Free London NHS Foundation Trust, Pond Street, London NW3 2QG, UK
e-mail: duncanbrian@nhs.net; p.chowdary@nhs.net

M. Harber (ed.), *Practical Nephrology*,
DOI 10.1007/978-1-4471-5547-8_53, © Springer-Verlag London 2014

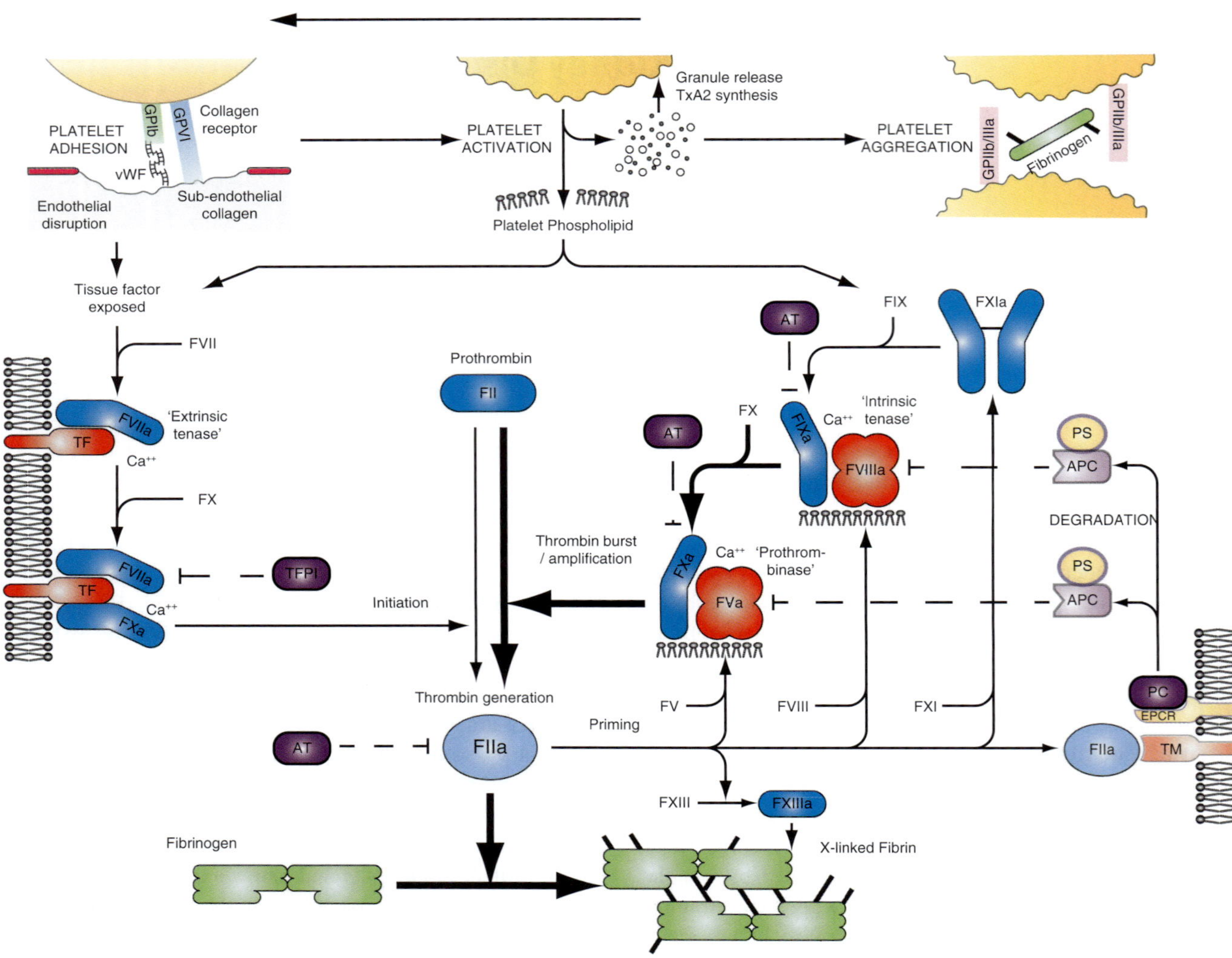

Fig. 53.1 Diagram of normal haemostasis. *GPIb* glycoprotein Ib, *GPVI* glycoprotein VI, *vWF* von Willebrand factor, *TxA2* thromboxane A2, *GPIIb/IIIa* glycoprotein IIb/IIIa, *TF* tissue factor, *AT* antithrombin, *TM* thrombomodulin, *EPCR* extracellular protein C receptor, *PC* protein C, *APC* activated protein C, *PS* protein S. Primary haemostasis is characterised by vWF and collagen-mediated adhesion at sites of trauma and subsequent platelet activation, which results in further platelet recruitment and provides phospholipid for subsequent factor activation. Secondary haemostasis begins with exposed tissue factor leading to formation of the extrinsic tenase which activates factor X hence initiating thrombin generation. Thrombin primes activation of the intrinsic factors V, VIII and XI resulting in formation of prothrombinase which leads to a thrombin burst and rapidly amplified thrombin generation. Thrombin converts soluble fibrinogen into insoluble fibrin which is then cross-linked by activated factor XIII. Fibrinogen also leads to platelet aggregation while thrombin also stimulates platelet activation via PAR4 receptors (not shown). Thrombin activates protein C via thrombomodulin. Activated protein C, with protein S, negatively regulates thrombin generation. Only the principal anticoagulant proteins TFPI, antithrombin, protein C and S are shown (see text for further detail)

Bleeding Diathesis and the Renal Patient

Uraemia, in both acute and chronic renal failure, causes a bleeding tendency mediated by platelet and endothelial dysfunction. The clinical manifestations are indistinguishable from other causes of platelet dysfunction and may occur in up to 50 % of patients with renal failure to varying degrees.

Pathophysiology of Bleeding Diathesis

The development of bleeding tendency is multifactorial, and abnormalities are seen at all stages of primary haemostasis including platelet adhesion, secretion and aggregation, and some important mechanisms are elaborated in Table 53.1 [1, 2]. It is believed that the uraemic substances present in the plasma mediate these abnormalities.

Clinical Presentation

The most common observation is prolonged venipuncture site bleeding with frequent easy bruising and mucocutaneous bleeding (epistaxis, gastrointestinal bleeding, menorrhagia, haematuria). Other symptoms include procedure- or trauma-related bleeding and rarely spontaneous retroperitoneal or

Table 53.1 Pathophysiology of bleeding diathesis

Site	Mechanism
Endothelium	↑ nitric oxide(NO) due to ↓ red cell scavenging and ↑ prostacyclin – result in abnormal platelet adhesion
	Anaemia – ↓ platelet interaction with vessel walls
Platelets	↓ platelet activation due to ↓ TxA_2 production and abnormal intracellular Ca^{2+} mobilisation
	↓ platelet aggregation due to ↓ ADP, epinephrine and serotonin pool in the platelets
	GPIIb/IIIa receptors show ↓ affinity for both vWF and fibrinogen
Clotting factors	↓ vWF activity with abnormal platelet adhesion at high shear

intracranial haemorrhages. Haemarthroses and spontaneous intramuscular haematomas are uncommon. Haemorrhagic pericardial and pleural effusions can still occur in poorly dialysed patients or those with advanced chronic renal failure. The use of antiplatelet and anticoagulant agents for comorbid conditions further contributes to the increased incidence of bleeding complication. Gastrointestinal (GI) and intracranial haemorrhage (ICH) in particular remain significant causes of morbidity and excess mortality in patients with renal failure.

Mucosal bleeding commonly presents as increased physiological blood loss from the GI tract, which in normal subjects is about 1 ml/day and can be as high as 4–6 ml/day in uraemic patients [3]. US data suggest that peptic ulcer disease constitutes only a third of the upper GI bleeding [4, 5] and that erosive gastritis, oesophagitis, vascular ectasia and angiodysplasia are relatively common. Capsule endoscopy in haemodialysis patients with obscure GI bleeding has shown erosions in the jejunum and vascular lesions in the ileum [6]. It is believed that platelet dysfunction contributes to this excessive bleeding, although the mechanism is not well elucidated.

Patients with uraemia have a higher prevalence of haemorrhagic cerebral events, and a cohort study in the UK has shown a 20-fold increase in subdural haematomas compared to the general population and an associated poorer outcome [7]. A retrospective cohort study of patients undergoing coronary artery bypass grafting showed that patients with renal impairment had significantly higher 30-day mortality and post-operative bleeding and ventilatory complications [8].

A systematic review attempted to identify risk factors for symptomatic bleeding in native kidney biopsy with automated biopsy device under real-time ultrasonographic guidance [9]. The review spanned 31 years and included 9,474 biopsies, and the rate of macroscopic haematuria was 3.5 %, red cell transfusion was 0.9 % and angiographic intervention was 0.6 %. Hemorrhagic risk was higher with a 14-guage needle compared to smaller biopsy needles, in female patients, in patients with elevated serum creatinine or decreased haemoglobin or when performed as part of workup for acute kidney injury. Mean systolic blood pressure above 130 mmHg and age over 40 were also associated with higher transfusion rates. In a single-centre retrospective review, where risk factors were controlled with bed rest for 24 h, desmopressin injections, red cell transfusions for prolonged bleeding time and antihypertensives for hypertension, incidence of post-biopsy haematoma was 33.4 %, and major complications (blood transfusion, nephrectomy and angiography) were seen in 1.2 % of patients [10]. The same investigators in a randomised controlled trial in patients with normal renal function have shown that pre-biopsy administration of desmopressin decreased bleeding and haematoma size [11].

Investigation of Platelet Dysfunction

Investigations for platelet dysfunction include global assays, i.e. bleeding time and PFA-100 (Platelet Function Analyser-100®, Dade Behring), and more specific platelet function tests, i.e. platelet aggregation studies, assays of granule content.

Investigations in uraemic patients in the pre-dialysis era revealed prolonged bleeding time and impaired platelet aggregation to a range of agonists including ADP, epinephrine and collagen. Impaired platelet aggregation response did not however differentiate patients with clinically significant bleeding from non-bleeding patients. However, the absolute prolongation of bleeding time between the two groups was statistically significant which correlated with inhibition of collagen-induced platelet aggregation [12]. Skin bleeding time is an unreliable assay for assessing bleeding risk and is not recommended for routine use.

The PFA-100® is a global in vitro platelet assay used to assess platelet-dependent primary haemostasis. The test measures the time required for flowing whole blood to occlude a collagen and adenosine diphosphate (CADP) or a collagen and epinephrine (CEPI)-coated cartridge. A prolonged closure time is seen in patients with platelet dysfunction and von Willebrand disease. In patients with mild inherited platelet dysfunction, the sensitivity and specificity of prolonged closure time in the PFA-100® assay is not of the same order as abnormalities seen in platelet aggregation assays. In a prospective study of haemodialysis patients and control population, abnormalities of PFA-100®, platelet aggregation and skin bleeding time were seen, respectively, in 60, 40 and 20 % of haemodialysis patients and 0, 10 and 3 % of control population [13]. Although the test appears sensitive for acquired platelet dysfunction, it has not been validated in outcome studies to predict increased risk of procedure-related or spontaneous bleeding.

Therapy for Uraemic Bleeding

Management of the uraemic bleeding tendency is in part dictated by the clinical presentation. Broadly, treatments are aimed at long-term prevention of spontaneous bleeding, prevention of procedure-related bleeding or management of active bleeding [1] (Table 53.2).

In the setting of acute renal failure and in preparation for procedures such as renal biopsy, the treatment and prevention of bleeding complications continues to be challenging. There is no consensus on the investigation and risk stratification of patients, bleeding tendency for procedures nor are there any consensus guidelines on the role of desmopressin for prevention and management of procedural-related bleeding. Conjugated oestrogens have a role in the management of obscure GI bleeding where responses have been seen. It is important to appreciate that most of the suggested interventions correct bleeding diathesis partially, and procedures must be performed with appropriate risk assessment. In management of patients with active bleeding, intervention with cryoprecipitate must be considered earlier rather than later, and aggressive resuscitation and early intervention are key to improving outcomes.

Venous and Vascular Access Thrombosis

Thrombotic complications are common in patients with chronic renal disease and present as arterial events, venous thromboembolism (VTE) or problems related to vascular access for haemodialysis. There are multiple reasons for the excess of arterial events including accelerated atherosclerosis, hypertension, loss of normal vessel elasticity and vascular calcification and are covered in Chap. 52.

The risk of VTE is increased across the spectrum of chronic kidney disease, including patients with mild renal impairment and nephrotic syndrome. Data extracted from US administrative databases confirms the excess risk presenting as a 1.3-fold increased risk in very early CKD (stages I and II) and 2.3-fold increased risk in stage III and IV CKD patients [14]. Haemostatic changes described include elevated procoagulants, impaired natural anticoagulant pathways and a decrease in fibrinolytic activity. These are described in Table 53.3 [15].

Nephrotic Syndrome

Thromboembolic disease is an important complication in patients with nephrotic syndrome, presenting with both arterial thromboembolic (ATE) and venous thromboembolic events. Venous thromboembolic complications in nephrotic syndrome include deep venous thrombosis, pulmonary embolism, cerebral vein thrombosis and, in particular, renal vein thrombosis with asymptomatic events being common. The prevalence of thrombosis is in part related to the underlying aetiology and is highest in patients with membranous glomerulonephritis, affecting a third of patients in a review of published case series [16]. A retrospective study of patients with nephrotic syndrome over a 10-year period revealed that the risk of thromboembolic events was highest in the first 6 months, with an event rate of 9.85 % for VTE and 5.52 % for ATE, and during follow-up annual incidence of objectively verified symptomatic thromboembolic events was 1.02 % for VTE and 1.48 % for ATE [17]. Thrombosis in some studies has been linked to the presence of hypoalbuminaemia, which may be a surrogate marker for coagulation changes. There is a suggestion that the magnitude of changes in procoagulant factors may be higher in patients with nephrotic syndrome and a change specific to this syndrome is low AT due to loss from the circulation. The low AT levels do not preclude treatment with low molecular weight heparin, and there is no consensus on the role of prophylactic anticoagulation in this group of patients. Decisions need to be individualised, and the following risk factors have been suggested as indicators for prophylactic anticoagulation: personal and family history, severity of the hypoalbuminaemia (<20–25 g/l), magnitude of proteinuria (>10 g/24 h), presence of membranous nephropathy and risk factors for bleeding precluding the use of prophylactic anticoagulation [18, 19]. Symptomatic events are best treated initially with heparin followed by warfarin, continued as long as the underlying risk is present.

Vascular Access Thrombosis

A common complication seen in patients on haemodialysis, this presents as arteriovenous (AV) fistulae thrombosis, AV graft thrombosis or thrombosis of a central venous catheter. Recurrent events can compromise a haemodialysis programme and contribute to increasing costs related to thrombolysis and redo procedures. The thrombotic episodes are in part related to stenosis caused by fibromuscular and intimal hyperplasia, and the role of hypercoagulability is poorly defined. In a case-control study evaluating the importance of thrombophilia defects, an association between thrombophilia and access thrombosis was noted with an adjusted OR of 2.4, and for each additional defect the odds of access thrombosis increased significantly [20]. In patients with more than one episode of venous access thrombosis, screening for thrombophilia could be justified but there are no prospective studies on the prophylactic use of anticoagulation to prevent access thrombosis in this context. A Cochrane review on the use of antiplatelet and anticoagulants in vascular access thrombosis suggested a potential benefit with aspirin and dipyridamole and no benefit with warfarin [21].

Table 53.2 Therapeutic interventions for uraemic bleeding

Therapy/agent	Mechanism of action	Onset/duration	Dose	Clinical scenarios	Limitations
Haemodialysis	Removal of toxins that impair platelet function	Partial correction of platelet dysfunction after dialysis, and effect is present as long as patient is dialysed	Not clear but good control of urea probably a reasonable surrogate	Prevention of bleeding prior to procedures	The anticoagulant used may on occasions contribute to bleeding
Peritoneal dialysis	As above	Correction of platelet dysfunction appears better when compared to haemodialysis	Continuous	As above	
Red cells	Target haematocrit of >30 %, anaemia decreases platelet-vessel wall interaction	Post transfusion		Ongoing bleeding, prior to surgery or biopsy	Volume/potassium overload
EPO	Glycoprotein (R), increases haematocrit thus platelet-wall interactions, increases number of reticulated platelets	7 days[a] 90 days[b]	50–100 units/kg SC/IV three times per week	Long-term prophylaxis	Slow onset. Can cause thrombosis
Conjugated oestrogens (e.g., Premarin)	Steroid hormone mixture, decreases L-arginine (NO precursor) potentially increasing TxA2 and ADP[c]	With IV preparation effect seen in 6 h and with oral preparation after a few days. Lasts several days	0.6 mg/kg/day IV or 50 mg/day PO for 5 days	Short-term prophylaxis	Hot flushes, hypertension, liver dysfunction
Desmopressin (DDAVP®)	ADH analogue, V2 agonist (S) stimulates the release of stored ultralarge vWF multimers and FVIII from the endothelial cells	1 h/24 h. It is believed that the vWF multimers released contribute to platelet aggregation	Different preparation for IV, SC or intranasal use. 0.3 mcg/kg, repeat every 24 h	Pre-procedure	The effect decreases with repeat dosing, and fluid retention is a risk. NB risk of ACS in patients with IHD: *give slowly!*
Cryoprecipitate	Has vWF, fibrinogen, fibronectin (P)	15 min	10 units or 2 adult doses	In acute bleeding or pre-procedure	Correction seen in only 50 % of patients
Tranexamic acid	Lysine analogue (S), inhibits fibrin/plasmin(ogen) interaction and acts as an antifibrinolytic agent by improving clot stability	1 h/6 h (upto 24 hours in severe renal impairment)	Oral or IV, dose needs to be adjusted in renal disease	With procedures and during active bleeding	Clot obstruction, drug accumulation, oral formulation not available in the USA
rFVIIa (NovoSeven®)	Recombinant activated FVII (R), direct activation of extrinsic pathway	15 min/2–3 h	90 mcg/kg IV bolus, consider repeat at 2 h[d]	In acute bleeding as last resort	Thrombosis risk, benefit outside haemophilia unclear
Prothrombin complex conc. (Beriplex®)	FII, FVII, FIX, FX, proteins C and S (P), replacement of plasma vitamin K-dependent clotting factors	15 min/6–8 h	20–30 units/kg[e,f] IV slow bolus, consider repeat 6–8 h per INR	In acute bleeding/pre-procedure when on warfarin	Plasma derived, for warfarin reversal
Vitamin K (phytomenadione)	Fat-soluble vitamin (S), optimise production of vitamin K-dependent clotting factors	Onset within 6–12 h after IV dose	Major bleed 5 mg IV slow bolus; minor bleed 1 mg IV or 2 mg PO	For longer-term warfarin reversal or if deficient	Not immediate

Key: S synthetic, *R* recombinant, *P* plasma derived, *V2* vasopressin receptor type 2, *vWF* von Willebrand factor, *FVII* factor VII, *FVIII* factor VIII, *FIX* factor XI, *FX* factor X, *FII* prothrombin, *AT* antithrombin, *NO* nitric oxide

[a]Effect on platelets

[b]Effect on haematocrit

[c]Oestrogens also decrease AT and protein S levels and increase FVII concentrations; these effects may also contribute to the therapeutic effect in uraemic bleeding

[d]In discussion with a haematologist, up to four doses may be given

[e]If warfarin reversal longer than 4–6 h is required, vitamin K should be administered concomitantly in discussion with a haematologist

[f]FFP at 15 ml/kg may be given if PCC is not available

Table 53.3 Pathophysiology of thrombotic tendency

Site	Mechanism
Endothelium	Endothelial cell and monocyte activation
	↓ thrombomodulin leads to ↓ protein C activity
Platelets	↑ platelet activation by uraemia/haemodialysis membranes
	↑ thrombin generation, ↑ CRP/inflammatory cytokines
Clotting factors	↑ fibrinogen, FVII, FVIII and vWF
	↑ markers of coagulation activation, including D-dimers, thrombin-antithrombin complexes
	↑ lipoprotein(a) causes impaired fibrinolysis
	↓ antithrombin (AT) in nephrotic syndrome

A randomised controlled trial published in 2008 evaluating the use of clopidogrel demonstrated a reduced frequency of early thrombosis in new arteriovenous fistulae without any increase in the proportion of fistulae that became suitable for dialysis [22].

Anticoagulants in Renal Disease: Heparins, Warfarin and New Oral Anticoagulants

The indication for anticoagulant use is similar to general population, and indications specific to this group include anticoagulation for haemodialysis and recurrent vascular access thrombosis.

Warfarin is most commonly used in the context of atrial fibrillation, and a retrospective review of Danish registries showed that patients with non-end-stage and end-stage kidney disease had an increased risk of stroke and systemic embolism (hazard ratio of 1.49, 1.83, respectively) compared to patients without renal disease. Further, major bleeding was twice that seen in patients without renal disease with an event rate per 100 person-yrs of 3.54 and 8.66 in patients with normal renal function and non-end-stage kidney disease, respectively. Warfarin use was associated with a decreased risk of events in all groups of patients and an increased risk of bleeding (hazard ratio of 1.3) when compared to patients with normal renal function [23].

Therapeutic anticoagulation for patients with renal impairment in the acute situation can be achieved either with intravenous unfractionated heparin (UFH) or low molecular weight heparin (LMWH). It is often suggested that UFH should be used preferentially as it does not accumulate in patients with renal failure, but the disadvantages of unpredictable response and regular venipuncture for monitoring should be not be overlooked. Subcutaneous administration may avoid the wide fluctuations in APTT ratios but has the same disadvantages, and there are no algorithms for dose adjustment to achieve therapeutic range rapidly. LMWHs accumulate in renal impairment especially when used in therapeutic doses, and this is associated with a bleeding tendency. In addition to the dose of LMWH, the type of LMWH determines the degree of accumulation with enoxaparin accumulating more than dalteparin and both more than tinzaparin. Therapeutic anticoagulation with LMWH requires initial dose reduction followed by monitoring of 4 hr peak anti-Xa levels every day to once every 3 days with doses adjusted until stable levels are achieved [24]. For patients with severe renal impairment or who are unstable, the balance between UFH and LMWH is in part related to venous access for sampling and the lab facilities for Xa monitoring and timely reporting.

In patients requiring prophylactic doses, accumulation has been seen with enoxaparin in patients with severe renal impairment (CrCl <30 ml/min) but not with mild or moderate renal impairment, and similar level of accumulation is not seen with prophylactic tinzaparin or dalteparin. In patients with mild to moderate renal impairment, LMWH can be used safely for thromboprophylaxis, and monitoring is probably indicated only when enoxaparin is used for extended periods of time.

The new oral anticoagulant agents licensed for use include a thrombin inhibitor, dabigatran (Pradaxa®), and anti-Xa inhibitors, rivaroxaban (Xarelto®) and apixaban (Eliquis®). The indications include management of venous thromboembolism, prevention of VTE post-orthopaedic surgery and non-valvular AF. Although there is a decreased risk of bleeding when compared to warfarin because of renal excretion, decisions need to be individualised in patients with renal impairment. Dabigatran is renally excreted, greater than three quarters, and caution needs to be exercised in patients with moderate renal impairment, with appropriate dose adjustments, and further it is contraindicated in patients with severe renal impairment or on dialysis. Rivaroxaban in contrast is mostly metabolised in liver, but a third is renally cleared, and it is not recommended in severe renal impairment and patients on dialysis. In patients with mild to moderate renal impairment, caution needs to be exercised, and currently a dose reduction is not recommended. Apixaban similarly is mostly metabolised with a quarter renally cleared and is not recommended in severe renal impairment and patients on dialysis. Dose reductions are indicated in patients with age ≥80 years, body weight ≤60 kg or serum creatinine ≥133 μmol/l.

Antiplatelet Therapy

The cardiovascular benefit of antiplatelets other than aspirin in renal disease, including clopidogrel and glycoprotein IIb/IIIa inhibitors including abciximab, eptifibatide and tirofiban, is the subject of considerable debate. Heterogeneous definitions of bleeding outcomes and trial durations limit the clinical relevance of currently available evidence. A recent systematic review and meta-analysis suggested that the addition of glycoprotein IIb/IIIa inhibitors or clopidogrel in CKD patients with acute coronary syndromes or undergoing percutaneous coronary revascularisation procedures appears to increase major bleeding with little or no effect on myocardial infarction, death or coronary revascularisation; further the authors were of the opinion that evidence was of poor quality with no risk stratification by the severity of renal dysfunction [25]. As platelet dysfunction is in part related to the severity of renal disease, one would expect that use of glycoprotein IIb/IIIa inhibitors is to be associated with a higher risk in patients on haemodialysis.

Heparin-Induced Thrombocytopenia (HIT)

HIT is an immune-mediated adverse drug reaction, comprising thrombocytopenia with or without thrombosis, following an immunising exposure to heparin. Diagnostic criteria include detection of platelet-activating HIT antibodies in the blood during the acute event [26]. Until recently, the term 'HIT type II', was used to distinguish HIT from the innocuous entity of heparin-associated platelet aggregation, a non-immune and self-limiting process resulting in mild thrombocytopenia in around 10 % of patients treated with unfractionated heparin within 48–72 h. This phenomenon, in contrast to HIT is self-limiting and not associated with thrombosis or increased mortality.

Pathophysiology of HIT

The antibodies responsible for HIT are platelet-activating IgG antibodies, against platelet factor 4 (PF4)/heparin complexes. PF4 is a chemokine that promotes coagulation when released from platelet alpha granules. An important physiologic function is the binding and neutralisation of heparin and heparin-like substances on vessel endothelium helping prevent activation of AT and thus facilitating haemostasis [27]. Plasma concentrations rise significantly following platelet activation or heparin infusion, and heparin binding results in formation of PF4/heparin macromolecular complexes, with exposure of cryptic epitopes that become targets for HIT-antibody binding [28]. PF4/heparin/HIT-antibody complexes can form on the surface of platelets or bind to platelets after formation via their Fcγ receptor IIa. The receptor cross-linking causes platelet activation, resulting in platelet granule release (including further PF4), membrane activation and microparticle formation, leading to platelet aggregation and thrombus formation [29]. HIT antibodies also activate endothelial cells and monocytes, additionally causing tissue factor expression, thrombin generation and fibrin clot formation (see Fig. 53.1).

Symptomatic HIT: Clinical Presentation

Thrombocytopenia, with or without thrombosis is the classic manifestation of HIT. The thrombocytopenia typically develops between 5 and 14 days after starting treatment with heparin but may occur within 1 day if there has been prior exposure to heparin in the last 100 days [30]. A 50 % decrease in platelet count from baseline is a more sensitive clinical marker of HIT compared to a conventional definition of thrombocytopenia. Although the median nadir is 60×10^9/l, the platelet count in some cases may not fall below 100×10^9/l, and counts below 20×10^9/l are seen in fewer than 10 % of cases. Resolution of thrombocytopenia occurs over 1–2 weeks following heparin cessation.

Despite thrombocytopenia, bleeding tendency is very uncommon due to the platelet activation resulting from HIT. Indeed thrombosis occurs in over 50 % of patients diagnosed with HIT, usually with the onset of thrombocytopenia, or on the day of platelet fall of >50 % from baseline. Importantly prophylactic platelet transfusion in HIT is not indicated, and risk and benefit need to be evaluated according to individual circumstances. Venous thrombotic events are more prevalent than arterial events and can present either in limbs or in the viscera.

Rare presentations of HIT include skin necrosis at heparin injection sites, initially presenting as small erythematous painful nodules. A further uncommon and potentially fatal complication is venous limb gangrene, seen with warfarin use very early in disease process. The onset of gangrene coincides with high INRs related to a sudden fall in both factor VII and protein C, resulting in a transient prothrombotic effect before the eventual decrease in factor II and X responsible for the antithrombotic effect. For this reason *warfarin and other vitamin K antagonists are contraindicated in the treatment of HIT until the resolution of thrombocytopenia.*

Other presentations have been described including an acute systemic reaction 5–30 min after UFH bolus, presenting with fever and chills, with or without cardiorespiratory compromise or arrest [31, 32]. Various mechanisms have been postulated, but these are thought to be distinct from heparin-related anaphylactic reactions.

Natural History of HIT (Iceberg Model)

Prospective and retrospective studies have now shown that symptomatic HIT is the tip of an iceberg (Table 53.4): asymptomatic seroconversion is seen in up to 20 % of general medical patients receiving heparin, including those undergoing acute haemodialysis [33]. Essentially, a proportion of patients develop antibodies that are detectable by sensitive enzyme immunoassays (EIA), but only some of these antibodies tend to

Table 53.4 The spectrum of clinical and subclinical HIT (iceberg model)

HIT with thrombosis (HIT-T)	0.03% to 1.5%
Heparin induced thrombocytopenia (HIT)	0.1% to 5%
HIT abs detected by activation assays	0.1% to 20%
HIT abs detected by EIA	1.5% to 50%
Heparin exposure	100%

Table 53.5 The 4Ts (thrombocytopenia, timing, thrombosis and other causes) pretest probability score

Score	2	1	0
Thrombocytopenia	>50 % fall in platelets or lowest count >20 × 10⁹/l	30–50 % fall in platelets or lowest count 10–19 × 10⁹/l	<30 % fall in platelets or nadir <10 × 10⁹/l
Timing	Days 5–10 or ≤1 day if heparin exposure within the last 30 days	>10 days or unclear or ≤1 day if exposed in last 31–100 days	Within 1 day with no recent exposure
Thrombosis	New proven thrombosis, skin necrosis or acute systemic reaction	Progressive, recurrent or silent thrombosis; erythematous skin lesions	None
OTher cause of platelet fall	None evident	Possible	Definite

Interpretation of pretest probability: score 6–8 (high), 4–5 (moderate), 0–3 (low)

be platelet activating as demonstrated by the functional serotonin release assay (SRA). Only a proportion go on to develop thrombocytopenia with and without thrombosis. Incidence of HIT depends upon underlying medical condition as well as the type of heparin administered. Prospective studies show that frequency of HIT is higher in surgical patients compared to medical patients. Heparin-related risk factors include source of UFH (bovine > porcine, the latter now the most common) duration of exposure >5 days. LMWHs are in general associated with a 5- to 10-fold lower risk for HIT compared to UFH.

HIT with thrombosis (HIT-T)	0.03–1.5 %
Heparin-induced thrombocytopenia (HIT)	0.1–5 %
HIT abs detected by activation assays	0.1–20 %
HIT abs detected by EIA	1.5–50 %
Heparin exposure	100 %

HIT Prevalence in Haemodialysis Patients

In patients on haemodialysis a recent review of aggregated data showed positive EIAs in 8.1 % of the 1,450 patients exposed to UFH and in 1.8 % of 218 patients dialysed with LMWH [34]. EIA positivity at the end of 6 months in a prospective cohort study was 10.3 % when UFH was used for haemodialysis [35]. Besides thrombocytopenia, studies have suggested that HIT antibodies in the haemodialysis population may contribute to frequent clotting of the extracorporeal circuit or an increase in the number of failed arteriovenous fistulae.

Diagnosis

As thrombocytopenia is common in patients on dialysis or receiving heparin, laboratory testing is required to confirm the diagnosis of HIT where clinical probability is moderate or high. Crucially, antibodies are transient for few weeks to months, and it is essential that testing should be performed using acute serum or plasma.

Standard tests fall into two categories: functional assays including ^{14}C-serotonin release assay (SRA) and heparin-induced platelet activation assay (HIPA) which detect antibodies that induce heparin-dependent platelet activation, and immunologic assays (EIAs) which identify circulating anti-PF4/heparin antibodies, irrespective of their capacity to activate platelets [36]. Functional assays are more specific than EIAs but are cumbersome and require expertise. EIAs are widely available and highly sensitive with almost 100 % negative predictive value, whereas their specificity is around 50 %, resulting in a poor positive predictive value, although this is improved with the use of IgG-specific EIAs.

Because of the low specificity of the EIA and the risk of bleeding with alternative anticoagulants if used empirically, the clinical criteria remain important when electing to perform testing and interpreting results. Various scoring systems have been developed including 'the 4Ts' proposed by Warkentin for estimating the pretest probability of HIT [36] (Table 53.5). Where the pretest probability score is 3 or less, testing is generally not indicated [37]. However this scoring system has not been validated in all patient groups [38].

Treatment

Treatment of HIT requires immediate withdrawal of all heparin, including heparin-containing flushes and catheters. Heparin cessation alone is not sufficient to prevent thrombosis. Historical series of untreated patients document a thrombosis risk of 5–10 % per day in the first couple of days after discontinuation of heparin therapy, and a 30-day cumulative risk of new thromboembolism as high as 50 % [39]. Initiation of non-heparin parenteral anticoagulant is the standard of

Table 53.6 HIT treatment agents for renal patients [34, 40]

Agent	Class/source	Monitoring	Route and dose	Elimination and clearance (half-life)
Danaparoid[a]	AT-dependent inhibition of Xa and thrombin, heparinoid	Anti-Xa 0.5–0.8 U/ml, daily monitoring until steady state is reached	IV bolus (2,500 units), <55 kg (1,250 units) and 3,750 units if >90 kg. IV infusion 400 units/h for the first 4 h then 200 units/h; adjust to anti-Xa levels	Renal, t1/2 of anti-Xa activity is about 24 h and in renal impairment can increase up to 4 days
Lepirudin[b]	DTI, irreversible recombinant	APTT 1.5–2.5× baseline or ECT, monitor 4 hourly until steady sate is achieved and thereafter daily	IV bolus (avoid unless life/limb threat)[c], IV infusion – Cr 140–400 umol/l (0.01 mg/kg/h) Cr >400 = 0.005 mg/kg/h	Renal and t1/2 is 80 min and can increase up to 13 days in renal impairment and development of anti-lepirudin antibodies that increase the t/12. Dialysed, generally by high-flux polysulfone but not low flux
Bivalirudin	DTI, reversible synthetic	APTT 1.5–2.5× baseline or ECT, monitor as above	IV bolus – none, IV infusion, 0.15 mg/kg/h, reduce in severe renal impairment	Enzymatic cleavage and renal elimination, t1/2 is 25 min–3.5 h in patients requiring dialysis
Argatroban[d]	DTI, reversible synthetic	APTT 1.5–3.0× baseline, monitor 2 hourly until steady state is achieved and regularly thereafter	IV bolus – none or 250 mcg IV infusion – 2 μg/kg/min, decrease further if post-surgery or if there is multiple organ failure	Hepatobiliary (40–50 min) with some increase in t ½ with renal impairment. Dialysed −20 % increase
Fondaparinux, dabigatran, rivaroxaban[e]	AT-dependent selective Xa inhibitor, synthetic	Anti-Xa levels, aim for therapeutic range, daily monitoring until steady state is achieved	SC, not approved for HIT Contraindicated in CrCl <30. <50 kg: 5.0 mg SC, 50–100 kg: 7.5 mg SC, >100 kg: 10 mg SC once daily	Renal – 17 h in normal adults, increasing to 29 h in moderate and 72 h in severe renal impairment

AT antithrombin, *DTI* direct thrombin inhibitor, *ECT* ecarin clotting time
[a]Danaparoid – not available in the USA since 2002
[b]Lepirudin – discontinued worldwide in 2012; however, experience may be helpful in guiding use of similar agents such as hirudin RB, available in Africa and Asia
[c]Significant risk of anaphylactoid reaction and bleeding risk with reduced clearance
[d]Not available in the UK
[e]Not approved for treatment of HIT

care, and several such anticoagulants are available for the treatment of HIT (Table 53.6). Oral vitamin K agonists are contraindicated in acute HIT due to risk of necrosis/gangrene, as is platelet transfusion.

Parenteral anticoagulants are continued until full recovery of platelet counts when conversion to warfarin may be performed. *An overlap of 5 days or longer of warfarin with non-heparin anticoagulation is required during conversion, until the INR is in the target range for greater than 2 days*, in order to prevent further thrombosis associated with the initial pro-coagulant state on commencing warfarin. The optimal duration of anticoagulation is unclear, although in general 3–6 months is appropriate depending on other risk factors.

Dialysis in Patients with HIT

When patients develop acute HIT, alternate anticoagulation regimens including lepirudin, danaparoid or fondaparinux can be utilised for the haemodialysis. Other possibilities include regional citrate anticoagulation or prostaglandins. The antibody positivity declines with time, and retesting should be done every few months until the test becomes negative. Once the antibodies disappear, recurrence is uncommon, and re-challenge with heparin is not unreasonable although caution needs to be exercised and patients monitored closely [34].

References

1. Hedges SJ, Dehoney SB, Hooper JS, Amanzadeh J, Busti AJ. Evidence-based treatment recommendations for uremic bleeding. Nat Clin Pract Nephrol. 2007;3(3):138–53. doi:10.1038/ncpneph0421.
2. Noris M, Remuzzi G. Uremic bleeding: closing the circle after 30 years of controversies?. Blood. 1999;94(8):2569–74. Retrieved from http://www.ncbi.nlm.nih.gov/pubmed/10515859.
3. Sohal AS, Gangji AS, Crowther MA, Treleaven D. Uremic bleeding: pathophysiology and clinical risk factors. Thromb Res. 2006;118(3):417–22. doi:10.1016/j.thromres.2005.03.032.
4. Sood P, Kumar G, Nanchal R, Sakhuja A, Ahmad S, Ali M, et al. Chronic kidney disease and end-stage renal disease predict higher

risk of mortality in patients with primary upper gastrointestinal bleeding. Am J Nephrol. 2012;35(3):216–24. doi:10.1159/000336107.
5. Yang J-Y, Lee T-C, Montez-Rath ME, Paik J, Chertow GM, Desai M, et al. Trends in acute nonvariceal upper gastrointestinal bleeding in dialysis patients. J Am Soc Nephrol. 2012;23(3):495–506. doi:10.1681/ASN.2011070658.
6. Ohmori T, Konishi H, Nakamura S, Shiratori K. Abnormalities of the small intestine detected by capsule endoscopy in hemodialysis patients. Intern Med. 2012;51(12):1455–60. doi:10.2169/internalmedicine.51.7190.
7. Power A, Hamady M, Singh S, Ashby D, Taube D, Duncan N. High but stable incidence of subdural haematoma in haemodialysis–a single-centre study. Nephrol Dial Transplant. 2010;25(7):2272–5. doi:10.1093/ndt/gfq013.
8. Anderson RJ, O'brien M, MaWhinney S, VillaNueva CB, Moritz TE, Sethi GK, et al. Renal failure predisposes patients to adverse outcome after coronary artery bypass surgery. VA Cooperative Study #5. Kidney Int. 1999;55(3):1057–62. doi:10.1046/j.1523-1755.1999.0550031057.x.
9. Corapi KM, Chen JLT, Balk EM, Gordon CE. Bleeding complications of native kidney biopsy: a systematic review and meta-analysis. Am J Kidney Dis. 2012;60(1):62–73. doi:10.1053/j.ajkd.2012.02.330.
10. Manno C, Strippoli GFM, Arnesano L, Bonifati C, Campobasso N, Gesualdo L, et al. Predictors of bleeding complications in percutaneous ultrasound-guided renal biopsy. Kidney Int. 2004;66(4):1570–7. doi:10.1111/j.1523-1755.2004.00922.x.
11. Manno C, Bonifati C, Torres DD, Campobasso N, Schena FP. Desmopressin acetate in percutaneous ultrasound-guided kidney biopsy: a randomized controlled trial. Am J Kidney Dis. 2011;57(6):850–5. doi:10.1053/j.ajkd.2010.12.019.
12. Steiner RW, Coggins C, Carvalho AC. Bleeding time in uremia: a useful test to assess clinical bleeding. Am J Hematol. 1979;7(2):107–17. Retrieved from http://www.ncbi.nlm.nih.gov/pubmed/539588.
13. Zupan IP, Sabovic M, Salobir B, Ponikvar JB, Cernelc P. Utility of in vitro closure time test for evaluating platelet-related primary hemostasis in dialysis patients. Am J Kidney Dis. 2003;42(4):746–51. doi:10.1053/S0272-6386(03)00913-2.
14. Warkentin TE, Chong BH, Greinacher A. Heparin-induced thrombocytopenia: towards consensus. Thromb Haemost. 1998;79(1):1–7. Retrieved from http://www.ncbi.nlm.nih.gov/pubmed/9459312.
15. Pavord S, Myers B. Bleeding and thrombotic complications of kidney disease. Blood Rev. 2011;25(6):271–8. doi:10.1016/j.blre.2011.07.001.
16. Singhal R, Brimble KS. Thromboembolic complications in the nephrotic syndrome: pathophysiology and clinical management. Thromb Res. 2006;118(3):397–407. doi:10.1016/j.thromres.2005.03.030.
17. Mahmoodi BK, Ten Kate MK, Waanders F, Veeger NJGM, Brouwer J-LP, Vogt L, et al. High absolute risks and predictors of venous and arterial thromboembolic events in patients with nephrotic syndrome: results from a large retrospective cohort study. Circulation. 2008;117(2):224–30. doi:10.1161/CIRCULATIONAHA.107.716951.
18. Barratt J, Topham P, Harris K, editors. Nephrotic syndrome. In: Oxford desk reference: nephrology. 1st ed. Oxford, UK: Oxford University Press; 2009. p. 84.
19. Glassock RJ. Prophylactic anticoagulation in nephrotic syndrome: a clinical conundrum. J Am Soc Nephrol. 2007;18(8):2221–5. doi:10.1681/ASN.2006111300.
20. Knoll GA, Wells PS, Young D, Perkins SL, Pilkey RM, Clinch JJ, et al. Thrombophilia and the risk for hemodialysis vascular access thrombosis. J Am Soc Nephrol. 2005;16(4):1108–14. doi:10.1681/ASN.2004110999.
21. Osborn G, Escofet X, Da Silva A. Medical adjuvant treatment to increase patency of arteriovenous fistulae and grafts. Cochrane Database Syst Rev (Online). 2008;(4):CD002786. doi:10.1002/14651858.CD002786.pub2.
22. Dember LM, Beck GJ, Allon M, Delmez JA, Dixon BS, Greenberg A, et al. Effect of clopidogrel on early failure of arteriovenous fistulas for hemodialysis: a randomized controlled trial. JAMA. 2008;299(18):2164–71. doi:10.1001/jama.299.18.2164.
23. Olesen JB, Lip GYH, Kamper A-L, Hommel K, Køber L, Lane DA, et al. Stroke and bleeding in atrial fibrillation with chronic kidney disease. N Engl J Med. 2012;367(7):625–35. doi:10.1056/NEJMoa1105594.
24. Schmid P, Fischer AG, Wuillemin WA. Low-molecular-weight heparin in patients with renal insufficiency. Swiss Med Wkly. 2009;139(31–32):438–52. smw-11284.
25. Palmer SC, Di Micco L, Razavian M, Craig JC, Perkovic V, Pellegrini F, et al. Effects of antiplatelet therapy on mortality and cardiovascular and bleeding outcomes in persons with chronic kidney disease: a systematic review and meta-analysis. Ann Intern Med. 2012;156(6):445–59. doi:10.1059/0003-4819-156-6-201203200-00007.
26. Wattanakit K, Cushman M. Chronic kidney disease and venous thromboembolism: epidemiology and mechanisms. Curr Opin Pulm Med. 2009;15(5):408–12. doi:10.1097/MCP.0b013e32832ee371.
27. Sandset PM. CXCL4-platelet factor 4, heparin-induced thrombocytopenia and cancer. Thromb Res. 2012;129(Suppl):S97–100. doi:10.1016/S0049-3848(12)70026-9.
28. Amiral J, Bridey F, Dreyfus M, Vissoc AM, Fressinaud E, Wolf M, Meyer D. Platelet factor 4 complexed to heparin is the target for antibodies generated in heparin-induced thrombocytopenia. Thromb Haemost. 1992;68(1):95–6. Retrieved from http://www.ncbi.nlm.nih.gov/pubmed/1514184.
29. Kelton JG, Warkentin TE. Heparin-induced thrombocytopenia: a historical perspective. Blood. 2008;112(7):2607–16. doi:10.1182/blood-2008-02-078014.
30. Warkentin TE. How I diagnose and manage HIT. Hematology Am Soc Hematol Educ Program. 2011;2011:143–9. doi:10.1182/asheducation-2011.1.143.
31. Warkentin TE. Hemodialysis-associated acute systemic reactions and heparin-induced thrombocytopenia. Thromb Res. 2012;129(4):405–6. doi:10.1016/j.thromres.2011.11.004.
32. Davenport A. Sudden collapse during haemodialysis due to immune-mediated heparin-induced thrombocytopaenia. Nephrol Dial Transplant. 2006;21(6):1721–4. doi:10.1093/ndt/gfl124.
33. Arepally GM, Ortel TL. Clinical practice. Heparin-induced thrombocytopenia. N Engl J Med. 2006;355(8):809–17.
34. Syed S, Reilly RF. Heparin-induced thrombocytopenia: a renal perspective. Nat Rev Nephrol. 2009;5(9):501–11. doi:10.1038/nrneph.2009.125.
35. Asmis LM, Segal JB, Plantinga LC, Fink NE, Kerman JS, Kickler TS, et al. Heparin-induced antibodies and cardiovascular risk in patients on dialysis. Thromb Haemost. 2008;100(3):498–504. doi:10.1160/TH08-03-0144.
36. Warkentin TE, Greinacher A, Gruel Y, Aster RH, Chong BH. Laboratory testing for heparin-induced thrombocytopenia: a conceptual framework and implications for diagnosis. J Thromb Haemost. 2011;9(12):2498–500. doi:10.1111/j.1538-7836.2011.04536.x.
37. Cuker A, Cines DB. How I treat heparin-induced thrombocytopenia. Blood. 2012;119(10):2209–18. doi:10.1182/blood-2011-11-376293.
38. Pouplard C, Gueret P, Fouassier M, Ternisien C, Trossaert M, Régina S, et al. Prospective evaluation of the "4Ts" score and particle gel immunoassay specific to heparin/PF4 for the diagnosis of heparin-induced thrombocytopenia. J Thromb Haemost. 2007;5(7):1373–9.
39. Warkentin TE, Kelton JG. A 14-year study of heparin-induced thrombocytopenia. The Am J Med. 1996;101(5):502–7. Retrieved from http://www.sciencedirect.com/science/article/pii/S0002934396002586.
40. Linkins L-A, Dans AL, Moores LK, Bona R, Davidson BL, Schulman S, et al. Treatment and prevention of heparin-induced thrombocytopenia: Antithrombotic Therapy and Prevention of Thrombosis, 9th ed: American College of Chest Physicians Evidence-Based Clinical Practice Guidelines. Chest. 2012;141(2 Suppl):e495S–530. doi:10.1378/chest.11-2303.

Symptom Control and Palliative Care in Advanced CKD

54

Fliss E.M. Murtagh and Sara N. Davison

As CKD advances and life expectancy reduces, the priorities and preferences of patients change. Many patients and families place increasing priority on quality of life, symptom control, and psychological and social concerns [1]. It is important therefore that renal professionals adjust the goals of care to match these changing preferences and priorities.

Most patients with advanced CKD needing palliative care are older people, with high levels of co-morbidity; they have variable and often complex needs, with symptoms which are often unaddressed. Although detailed evidence about palliative needs and interventions is limited, the symptom burden in ESKD is high [2, 3] and the psychological and social impacts are known to be considerable [4], with extensive demands on patient and family, and complex transitions to be negotiated. Communication, especially in relation to dialysis decision-making and advance planning, is key [5], yet presents many challenges.

Providing high-quality palliative and supportive care to patients with advanced CKD has the potential to markedly improve patient outcomes, but has not always received sufficient attention. It needs a systematic approach, relevant training and dedicated resources.

F.E.M. Murtagh, PhD, MRCGP, MBBS (✉)
Department of Palliative Care, Policy and Rehabilitation, King's College London, Cicely Saunders Institute, Bessemer Rd, London SE5 9RJ, UK
e-mail: fliss.murtagh@kcl.ac.uk

S.N. Davison, MD, MSc
Department of Medicine, University of Alberta, 11-107 Clinical Sciences Building, 11350-83 Ave, Edmonton, AB T6G 2P4, Canada
e-mail: sara.davison@ualberta.ca

Which Renal Patients Need Palliative and Supportive Care?

Patients whose palliative and supportive care needs should be considered are those with Stage 5 CKD who:

- Decline renal replacement therapy (dialysis or transplant) through their own preference
- Are advised against renal replacement therapy because the burden of frequent dialysis is felt to outweigh likely survival and quality-of-life benefits (a complex and difficult decision likely to apply more frequently to those with most adverse prognoses)
- Have been on dialysis but are now withdrawing or about to withdraw from dialysis
- Are on dialysis but with a poor prognosis, often because of co-morbid conditions (especially cardiac disease)

Palliative and Supportive Care Assessment

Palliative and supportive care assessment requires a holistic and patient-centred approach. It includes detailed assessment of:

- Preferences for communication, involvement in decisions and place of care
- Physical symptoms
- Psychological symptoms and emotional well-being
- Social and occupational well-being
- Family well-being
- Planning ahead as the illness advances, in order to maximise influence over quality of life and place of death, in accordance with preferences

Detailed guidance has been published in the UK (see Internet Resources) to guide professionals on the depth and range of palliative and supportive care assessment that is required if excellent care is to be achieved. Once these needs have been identified and fully assessed, appropriate interventions should then be implemented. As well as symptom management, and other targeted interventions, co-ordination of care across providers is also important.

M. Harber (ed.), *Practical Nephrology*,
DOI 10.1007/978-1-4471-5547-8_54, © Springer-Verlag London 2014

Symptom Management

Excellent symptom management is important for advanced CKD patients and their families. These patients are among the most symptomatic of any chronic disease group [6]; good control of symptoms is important. Renal replacement therapy may generally improve symptoms, but it will not always abolish symptoms and may sometimes contribute to them.

Symptom Prevalence

Recently, evidence on the epidemiology of symptoms has increased, and the prevalence and severity of individual symptoms is better understood. Prevalence depends in part on the stage of CKD, whether a patient is receiving dialysis or not, and the nature and extent of co-morbid conditions. Figure 54.1 presents an overview of the prevalence of different symptoms, according to whether the patient is receiving dialysis or not and including those who are withdrawing from dialysis.

This illustrates how prevalent individual symptoms are, but multiple symptoms often interact [7] and persist over time [8]. Pain and nausea, for instance, are more burdensome for a patient who is not sleeping well with restless legs, or with low mood.

Symptom Assessment

Symptoms are not assessed routinely or well by renal professionals and are frequently under-recognised [3, 9]. Patients do not always raise their symptoms for discussion spontaneously, partly because their symptoms are often from co-morbid conditions and not the kidney disease itself and partly because professionals tend to focus more on biochemical markers and renal management.

Routine and proactive assessment of symptoms is therefore important. An appropriate, clinically relevant and valid symptom score should be used systematically for all patients at regular intervals, or at least triggered by a change in health status. There are three global symptom scores in regular use which have been adapted and validated specifically for use in those with renal disease:

- The renal version of the Palliative (or Patient) Outcome Scale – symptom module (POSs renal) [10] – developed in the UK
- The Modified Edmonton Symptom Assessment Scale (ESAS) [11] – developed in Canada
- The Dialysis Symptom Index (DSI) [12] – developed in the USA

All are patient-completed symptom scores which ask about the presence and severity of a range of symptoms common in renal disease, and they can be downloaded for use from the relevant websites (see Internet Resources).

Symptom Management

Once symptoms are clearly identified, they need active management. It is important to consider non-pharmacological management, especially for symptoms such as itch which have high psychological and social impact, but this chapter focuses predominantly on pharmacological management.

The aim of symptom management is to control or ameliorate symptoms whilst avoiding drug toxicity. The use of medication in advanced CKD is challenging because of the pharmacokinetic impact of renal disease. The evidence presented here applies to Stages 4 or 5 CKD, when eGFR is $\leq$30 ml/min/1.73 m^2. At these levels of renal impairment, drug metabolism is significantly altered, and the risk of toxicity from accumulation of renally excreted drugs is very high.

For those still receiving dialysis, the effects of dialysis on the drug should be considered too. Removal of a drug from the systemic circulation during dialysis is dependent on the following:

- The molecular size of the drug
- The water solubility of the drug
- The degree of protein binding of the drug
- Dialysis-related factors (such as frequency, duration, type of dialysis, type of dialyser membrane)

An up-to-date review of the effects of dialysis on drugs should be used for guidance on the effect of dialysis on medications, e.g. dialysis of drugs (updated annually) (see Internet Resources).

Pain

Recent evidence shows that pain is common among dialysis patients [3], those managed without dialysis [13] and those withdrawing from dialysis [14]. Pain should be addressed using the World Health Organisation (WHO) recommendations, including the WHO ladder (a three-step model to achieve effective pain relief – see Fig. 54.2).

This has been used effectively in kidney disease [15] and improves pain among renal patients. In severe pain, it may be appropriate to move from Step 1 to Step 3, without using Step 2.

Which Opioids to Use?

Of the Step 2 opioids, codeine and dihydrocodeine should generally not be used in CKD 4 or 5. This is because of the evidence on adverse effects, including accumulation and toxicity [16]. Tramadol is a better option, but is still

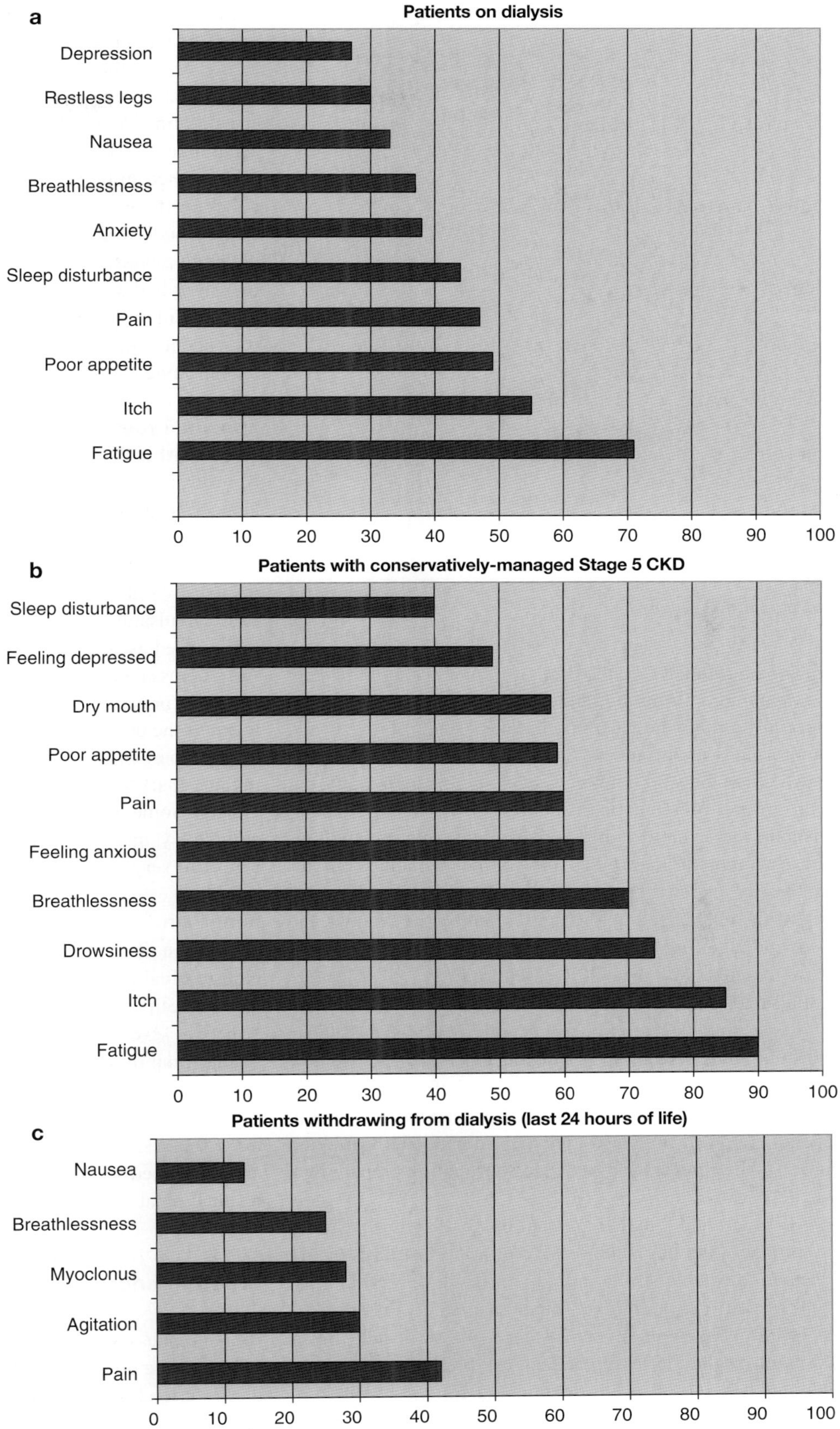

Fig. 54.1 Proportion (%) of patients with common symptoms in renal disease. (**a**) Patients on dialysis. (**b**) Patients with conservatively managed Stage 5 CKD. (**c**) Patients withdrawing from dialysis (last 24 h of life)

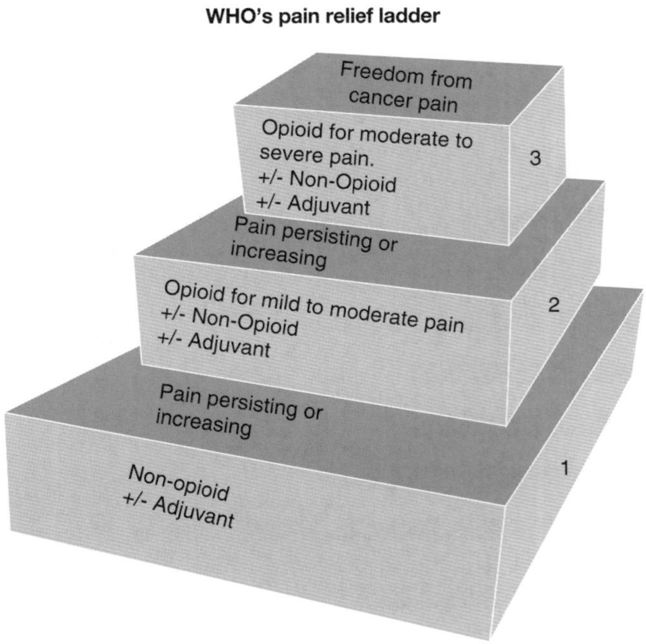

Fig. 54.2 WHO analgesic ladder (Reprinted from WHO's Pain Relief Ladder [25] with permission)

problematic. In CKD 5, the dose of tramadol should be kept to a maximum 50 mg bd, and adverse effects are common, especially among the older population, so careful review and monitoring is important.

All of the Step 3 opioids can cause significant toxicity, but some are less problematic than others. Most undergo metabolism in the liver to either active or inactive metabolites. These compounds (as well as some of the unchanged opioid) are usually excreted by the kidneys. If a significant proportion of the unchanged opioid is excreted by the kidneys and the metabolites are active, then the opioid is highly likely to cause toxicity when the eGFR <30 ml/min.

Full details are available in several reviews [17–20], but all Step 3 opioids should be used cautiously, with both dose reduction and increase in the dosing interval. Early review and regular monitoring should be undertaken, since accumulation and subsequent adverse effects can occur quickly (within hours). It is also strongly recommended to avoid the longer-acting preparations and use short-acting preparations whenever possible.

Alfentanil and fentanyl are cautiously recommended and are probably the best opioids to use in the last days of life when an injectable strong opioid is needed. Several clinical and practical considerations (other than safety) need to be taken into consideration; for instance, the short half-life of alfentanil makes it less practical for break-through pain, although it is appropriate for continuous infusion.

Transdermal fentanyl patches are useful earlier in the disease trajectory, but professionals unfamiliar with these should recognise that even lowest strength patches represent a significant opioid dose, and careful titration of immediate-acting oral opioids is usually needed before commencing them. Transdermal fentanyl can be used, provided there is careful titration of dose and early regular review to watch for accumulation. Transdermal buprenorphine is increasingly widely used clinically, without reports of adverse effects, although the evidence to support this remains limited. For oral immediate-acting preparations, oxycodone, hydromorphone and buprenorphine all have very limited evidence to indicate whether they are safe or not, although buprenorphine is increasingly used clinically, and both hydromorphone and oxycodone are likely to be a better choice than morphine or diamorphine.

Specific Types of Pain

Neuropathic Pain

Neuropathic (nerve) pain is unlikely to respond to opioids alone. Certain Step 3 opioids may be more useful than others in neuropathic pain. For instance, methadone may be appropriate but should only be prescribed by someone experienced in its use (usually pain or palliative care specialists). Anticonvulsants and antidepressants in low dose are commonly used as adjuvant medication to improve pain control. Antidepressants can be used in CKD 4 and 5, but it is better to avoid longer-acting preparations, reduce the dose and/or increase the dosing interval. Anticonvulsants are more problematic, particularly gabapentin and pregabalin which accumulate markedly in renal impairment to cause adverse effects. Some clinicians avoid gabapentin and pregabalin completely in CKD 5 without dialysis, whilst other clinicians use very small doses with careful monitoring.

Bone Pain

Bone pain is also unlikely to respond to opioids alone. Nonsteroidal anti-inflammatory drugs (NSAIDs) are likely to be beneficial for bone pain, but carry high risk of adverse effects in severe renal impairment, including risk of loss of any residual renal function. This consideration may be critical and prevent use of NSAIDs completely, but each case should be reviewed by an experienced clinician in order to make the best judgement. Sometimes, short-course NSAIDs are prescribed as a considered risk in the absence of any residual renal function or towards the very end of life.

Breathlessness

Breathlessness or dyspnoea in the patient with advanced CKD may be due to anaemia, pulmonary oedema (related to fluid overload or to coexisting cardiovascular disease), or co-morbidity (cardiac or respiratory disease). It is important to identify the underlying cause, since treating this is almost always the most appropriate and effective first line of management. Diuretic use and fluid restriction may or may not be appropriate, depending on the clinical circumstances. Optimising anaemia management can be helpful although the correlation between symptoms and degree of anaemia is unclear. If treatment of the underlying cause has been exhausted, then the situation may arise (particularly in far advanced disease or close to the end of life) where symptomatic measures to relieve breathlessness are required.

General measures, such as sitting upright rather than lying (which maximises vital capacity), using a fan or stream of cool air which can provide effective symptom relief, inhaled oxygen if hypoxia is confirmed or suspected and a calm, settled environment, are important. Physiotherapy and occupational therapy can help to maximise mobility and provide appropriate aids to improve function constrained by breathlessness. Breathlessness is very commonly associated with anxiety, often in an escalating cycle (anxiety causing worsening dyspnoea, which triggers worsening anxiety, and so on). Appropriate information, education and support of patient and family are therefore critical.

As prognosis worsens, general and non-pharmacological measures will have less to offer, and pharmacological measures become more appropriate. This applies only when treatment of the underlying cause of breathlessness has been exhausted. Untreated moderate or severe dyspnoea towards end of life is very distressing and should be treated as actively as pain or any other distressing symptom. Breathlessness is an increasingly important and dominant symptom in renal patients towards the end of life, so it is important to plan with the patient who has had one or more episode of acute breathlessness (or steadily increasing breathlessness over time) how they would like to be treated if they become more symptomatic in the future. Not all patients will, for instance, choose to be admitted for maximal treatment with intravenous diuretics in the last days or weeks of life.

Pharmacological treatments directed specifically at breathlessness include opioids and benzodiazepines (especially if there is moderate or severe associated anxiety). Low-dose opioids are helpful in relieving breathlessness near the end of life in end-stage cardiac and respiratory disease [21], and clinical experience suggests that this is also true for patients with kidney disease.

Step 3 opioids can be used to control breathlessness (following the pain guidelines) but note that doses should be much smaller (25–50 % of those for pain), and if not effective, titration should be more careful and slower. Towards the last few days of life, if small doses are not at least partly effective, combining an opioid such as fentanyl with low-dose midazolam may bring relief where either alone is only partially effective. This is often a better strategy than increasing the dose, since adverse effects quickly increase as doses rise.

Benzodiazepines are useful when there is coexisting anxiety (as there often is), but again need to be used with considerable care and in reduced doses. Shorter-acting benzodiazepines are recommended, such as lorazepam 0.5–1 mg orally or sublingually qds (if used sublingually, it has a quicker onset of action and may more readily restore a sense of control to the frightened and anxious patient). If the patient is in the last days of life, midazolam (at 25 % of normal dose if eGFR <10) can be given subcutaneously and titrated according to effect. Midazolam can be given every 2–4 h, although CKD patients are sensitive to its effects and do not usually need frequent or large doses. A starting dose of 1.25 or 2.5 mg is common. If more than one or two doses are required, a subcutaneous infusion over 24 h is most practical.

Constipation

Constipation is common among patients with CKD. The causes can be multifactorial, including fluid restriction, reduced mobility, medication (i.e. aluminium or calcium phosphate binders, iron supplements, and opioids), poor dietary intake, reduced muscle tone through debility and dietary restriction of high potassium fruits and vegetables (reduced fibre content of food ingested).

Management requires detailed assessment, treatment of reversible causes where appropriate/possible, acute management to overcome current constipation (including rectal measures). Action to prevent further recurrence includes improving mobility and ensuring adequate dietary intake, and including sufficient fibre and fluid (within the constraints of any reduced fluid intake). Laxatives, such as softeners or osmotic laxatives, and stimulant laxatives can be used, and often a combination of softener or osmotic laxative with a stimulant is required. Laxatives which contain magnesium, citrate or phosphate should be avoided in end-stage kidney disease. Polyethylene glycol is not ideal for renal patients because it requires high concurrent fluid intake and also contains potassium, but it may be useful short term for constipation which does not respond to other measures.

Nausea and Vomiting

Nausea and vomiting are extremely unpleasant symptoms. They may frequently be multifactorial. Assessment requires a thorough history including establishing the history and pattern of both nausea and vomiting separately. The relationship between the two should also be established, as well as the frequency and volume of vomits, whether there is associated constipation, and a detailed medication history. Profound nausea and/or repeated vomiting will prevent absorption of any medications taken orally, and alternative routes (such as sublingual, rectal or subcutaneous routes) need to be considered, at least until nausea and vomiting is controlled.

The first step is to identify the specific cause where possible, since treatment specifically directed to the cause is most likely to succeed. If medication or toxins are causing nausea, then nausea is usually persistent and unremitting, and sometimes unaccompanied by vomiting. Uraemia and a variety of drugs (including opioids, anticonvulsants, antibiotics and antidepressants) can cause this kind of persistent nausea. Gastroparesis or delayed gastric emptying (which may be caused by drugs such as opioids, as well as occurring secondary to diabetes mellitus, for instance) usually presents with a history of postprandial nausea or vomiting of undigested food which relieves nausea. Bloating, epigastric fullness, flatulence, hiccough or heartburn may accompany this. Nausea related to gastritis is often associated with heartburn, dyspepsia or epigastric pain. Constipation may exacerbate nausea and vomiting.

If gastroparesis or delayed gastric emptying is suspected, then metoclopramide or domperidone (which both increase gastric motility) are preferred. Metoclopramide needs 50 % dose reduction in CKD 4 and 5, and there is increased risk of adverse effects such as dystonia in renal patients. If uraemia is a suspected cause, then haloperidol or possibly a 5HT3 (a serotonin receptor subtype) antagonist may be the best choice. The dose of haloperidol should be reduced, as there is increased cerebral sensitivity in renal failure. 5HT3 antagonists often cause moderate or severe constipation – this should be anticipated by co-prescribing of laxatives when appropriate. Drug-induced nausea can be relieved by stopping the causative drug. When this is not feasible, haloperidol is often effective. Gastritis (high risk in uraemia) may sometimes contribute to nausea and should be actively treated with a proton pump inhibitor to help control related nausea. Towards the end of life, levomepromazine (a 'broad-spectrum' antiemetic which works on several of the relevant receptors) in low dose can be effective to control nausea and vomiting, but higher doses can be very sedative.

Pruritus or Itch

The cause of itch has not yet been fully elucidated. Given the complexity in understanding the causes of pruritus in CKD, it is not surprising that it can be a difficult symptom to manage, with a variety of different treatments proposed, each of limited effectiveness.

The first step in management is to optimise renal management; high phosphate may contribute to pruritus, so attention to reducing phosphate levels may be important – consider dietary advice and the use of phosphate binders. Hyperparathyroidism may also be a contributory factor and should be considered. Dry skin (especially in older people) may both cause and contribute to pruritus and so should be treated actively; liberal emollients should be used if dry skin is present. Older people living alone may find it hard to apply emollients easily; spray applications are often helpful in this instance. Preventive measures, such as nail care (keeping nails short), and keeping cool (light clothing and tepid baths or showers) are useful concurrent measures.

It is hard to recommend specific pharmacological measures given the lack of clear evidence to support any one management over another. UVB light has good supporting evidence, but may not be readily available. Gabapentin does have some supporting evidence, although it can be difficult to use gabapentin unless a patient is on dialysis (without dialysis to remove it, in CKD 5 gabapentin accumulates rapidly and causes adverse effects such as drowsiness or sedation, so doses need to be very small and carefully monitored). Mirtazapine has had some evidence to suggest it is effective [22], with reduced dose in renal impairment. Antihistamines are widely used, but there is little supporting evidence, and it may be most helpful to use a sedating antihistamine (such as chlorpheniramine) at night, in order to help patients sleep better.

Restless Legs

Restless legs syndrome (RLS) is characterised by the urge to move the legs, uncomfortable sensations in the legs and worsening of symptoms at rest, especially during the night. The formal International Restless Legs Syndrome Study Group (IRLSSG) criteria for diagnosis are:

- Urge to move the legs, usually with unpleasant sensations in the legs
- Worse during periods of rest or inactivity like resting or sitting
- Partial or total relief by physical activity
- Worse symptoms in the evening or night rather than the day

The exact cause for restless legs is not understood as yet; it is widely accepted, however, that the dopaminergic system in the central nervous system is somehow disrupted. There is limited evidence in uraemic RLS that iron deficiency, low parathyroid hormone, hyperphosphataemia and psychological factors may all play a role. Treatment should involve correction of these factors and reduction of potential exacerbating agents, such as caffeine, alcohol, nicotine and certain drugs (sedative antihistamines, metoclopramide, tricyclic antidepressants, calcium antagonists, selective serotonin uptake inhibitors, lithium and dopamine antagonists).

There is very limited evidence about treatment of restless legs in people with CKD and much of the evidence is extrapolated from idiopathic restless legs. Gabapentin or pregabalin can be used with those receiving dialysis and are often effective. Dopamine agonists (pergolide or pramipexole) are also effective, although nausea is common, especially with pergolide, as are other adverse effects such as dreams or nightmares. There is also uncertainty about the long term use of dopamine agonists, because of an association with restrictive cardiac disease and pulmonary fibrosis. Co-careldopa can be used for restless legs and is effective at low dose. However, augmentation (return of the symptom, often at a worse level) is very problematic (80 % will eventually experience augmentation with co-careldopa). Augmentation does occur with dopamine agonists, although much less so than with co-careldopa. Clonazepam is also used, and can be useful, although associated with drowsiness. In treating restless legs, the choice of drug management should be tailored to the individual and will depend on presence of other symptoms, age and tolerance of side effects, and whether the patient is receiving dialysis or not.

Symptom Management at the End of Life

Traditionally, it was believed that a uraemic death was relatively symptom-free, but the evidence does not support this. Where studies have specifically reviewed end-of-life symptoms, it appears that although some renal patients have peaceful and symptom-free death, a significant minority experience severe or distressing symptoms [23, 24]. Pain, breathlessness, nausea, retained respiratory tract secretions and terminal agitation can all be problematic.

These symptoms can be relatively well controlled in the majority of patients. Agitation usually responds to low doses of anxiolytics, such as midazolam. Retained respiratory tract secretions can be improved (although not always resolved) by glycopyrronium or hyoscine, and treatment is optimal if commenced early. Pain or breathlessness can be effectively managed with opioid medication, and often only low doses are required. If a patient was on regular strong opioids orally and can no longer take oral medication, then convert the total daily dose of strong opioid to the equivalent for subcutaneous fentanyl or alfentanil over 24 h and start a subcutaneous infusion.

Summary

Detailed and thorough holistic assessment of the palliative and supportive needs of those with advanced CKD and deteriorating health is important.

Symptom burden is high in this population, and there is evidence of under-prescribing and under-management. In those managed without dialysis or in those withdrawing from dialysis, symptoms (whether caused by renal disease or more commonly by co-morbid conditions) therefore need careful attention if optimal quality of care is to be achieved.

Symptom assessment should be an integral part of clinical assessment, alongside routine review of renal status and biochemical markers. Use of a formal, validated symptom assessment tool will help this, and subsequent symptom management needs careful attention to detail and regular review. Towards end of life, anticipatory prescribing (prescribing in advance of symptoms) is also recommended to ensure distressing symptoms are minimised.

Internet Resources

How to assess palliative and supportive care needs in advanced CKD:

1. NHS end of life care programme [homepage on the Internet]. Leicester: National Health Service; updated 2013 18 July. Available from: http://webarchive.nationalarchives.gov.uk/20130718121128/. http://endoflifecare.nhs.uk. Cited 14 Jan 2014.
2. End of life care in advanced kidney disease: a framework for implementation. NHS Kidney Care [homepage on the Internet]. London: National Health Service; 2009 June 1. Available from: http://www.ncpc.org.uk/sites/default/files/EndOfLifeCareInAdvancedKidneyDisease.pdf. Cited 14 Jan 2014.
3. Getting it right: end of life care in advanced kidney disease. NHS Kidney Care [homepage on the Internet]. London: National Health Service; 2012 March 1. Available from: http://webarchive.nationalarchives.gov.uk/20130504185629/. http://kidneycare.nhs.uk/document.php?o=470. Cited 14 Jan 2014.

Symptom Measures

4. Palliative care outcome scale [homepage on the Internet]. London: Cicely Saunders Institute, King's College London; updated 2012 May 14. Available from: http://pos-pal.org/index.php. Cited 14 Jan 2014.
5. Edmonton Symptom Assessment System: Numerical Scale. Alberta Health Services, April 2002. Available from: http://www.albertahealthservices.ca/ps-1022201-narp-tools-esas.pdf. Cited 14 Jan 2014.

Prescribing Resources

6. Dialysis of drugs 2013. Renal Pharmacy Consultants [homepage on the Internet]. Michigan: Renal Pharmacy Consultants, LLC; updated 2013. Available from: http://renalpharmacyconsultants.com/assets/2013dodbooklet.pdf. Cited 14 Jan 2014.

References

1. Steinhauser KE, Christakis NA, Clipp EC, McNeilly M, McIntyre L, Tulsky JA. Factors considered important at the end of life by patients, family, physicians, and other care providers. JAMA. 2000;284(19):2476–82. Epub 2000/11/14.

2. Murtagh FE, Addington-Hall J, Higginson IJ. The prevalence of symptoms in end-stage renal disease: a systematic review. Adv Chronic Kidney Dis. 2007;14(1):82–99. Epub 2007/01/04.
3. Davison SN. Pain in hemodialysis patients: prevalence, cause, severity, and management. Am J Kidney Dis. 2003;42(6):1239–47. Epub 2003/12/05.
4. Murtagh FE, Addington-Hall J, Edmonds P, Donohoe P, Carey I, Jenkins K, et al. Symptoms in the month before death for stage 5 chronic kidney disease patients managed without dialysis. J Pain Symptom Manage. 2010;40(3):342–52.
5. Davison SN, Torgunrud C. The creation of an advance care planning process for patients with ESRD. Am J Kidney Dis. 2007;49(1):27–36.
6. Murtagh FEM, Weisbord S. Symptoms in renal disease: their epidemiology, assessment and management. In: Chambers EJ, Germain M, Brown E, editors. Supportive care for the renal patient. 2nd ed. Oxford: Oxford University Press; 2010.
7. Weisbord SD, Fried LF, Arnold RM, Fine MJ, Levenson DJ, Peterson RA, et al. Prevalence, severity, and importance of physical and emotional symptoms in chronic hemodialysis patients. J Am Soc Nephrol. 2005;16(8):2487–94.
8. Davison SN, Jhangri GS, Johnson JA. Longitudinal validation of a modified Edmonton symptom assessment system (ESAS) in haemodialysis patients. Nephrol Dial Transplant. 2006;21(11):3189–95.
9. Weisbord SD, Fried L, Mor MK, Resnick AL, Unruh ML, Palevsky PM, et al. Renal provider recognition of symptoms in patients on maintenance hemodialysis. Clin J Am Soc Nephrol. 2007;2:960–7.
10. Murphy EL, Murtagh FE, Carey I, Sheerin NS. Understanding symptoms in patients with advanced chronic kidney disease managed without dialysis: use of a short patient-completed assessment tool. Nephron Clin Pract. 2009;111(1):c74–80. Epub 2008/12/18.
11. Davison SN, Jhangri GS, Johnson JA. Cross-sectional validity of a modified Edmonton symptom assessment system in dialysis patients: a simple assessment of symptom burden. Kidney Int. 2006;69(9):1621–5. Epub 2006/05/05.
12. Weisbord SD, Fried LF, Arnold RM, Rotondi AJ, Fine MJ, Levenson DJ, et al. Development of a symptom assessment instrument for chronic hemodialysis patients: the Dialysis Symptom Index. J Pain Symptom Manage. 2004;27(3):226–40. Epub 2004/03/11.
13. Murtagh FE, Addington-Hall JM, Edmonds PM, Donohoe P, Carey I, Jenkins K, et al. Symptoms in advanced renal disease: a cross-sectional survey of symptom prevalence in stage 5 chronic kidney disease managed without dialysis. J Palliat Med. 2007;10(6):1266–76. Epub 2007/12/22.
14. Germain MJ, Cohen LM, Davison SN. Withholding and withdrawal from dialysis: what we know about how our patients die. Semin Dial. 2007;20(3):195–9. Epub 2007/06/09.
15. Barakzoy AS, Moss AH. Efficacy of the world health organization analgesic ladder to treat pain in end-stage renal disease. J Am Soc Nephrol. 2006;17(11):3198–203.
16. Davies G, Kingswood C, Street M. Pharmacokinetics of opioids in renal dysfunction. Clin Pharmacokinet. 1996;31(6):410–22.
17. Murtagh FE, Chai MO, Donohoe P, Edmonds PM, Higginson IJ. The use of opioid analgesia in end-stage renal disease patients managed without dialysis: recommendations for practice. J Pain Palliat Care Pharmacother. 2007;21(2):5–16. Epub 2007/09/12.
18. Dean M. Opioids in renal failure and dialysis patients. J Pain Symptom Manage. 2004;28(5):497–504. Epub 2004/10/27.
19. Broadbent A, Khor K, Heaney A. Palliation and chronic renal failure: opoid and other palliative medications – dosage guidelines. Prog Palliat Care. 2003;11(4):183–90.
20. Mercadante S, Arcuri E. Opioids and renal function. J Pain. 2004;5(1):2–19.
21. Jennings AL, Davies AN, Higgins JP, Broadley K. Opioids for the palliation of breathlessness in terminal illness. Cochrane Database Syst Rev. 2001;(4):CD002066. Epub 2001/11/01.
22. Davis MP, Frandsen JL, Walsh D, Andresen S, Taylor S. Mirtazapine for pruritus. J Pain Symptom Manage. 2003;25(3):288–91. Epub 2003/03/05.
23. Cohen LM, Germain MJ. Measuring quality of dying in end-stage renal disease. Semin Dial. 2004;17(5):376–9. Epub 2004/10/06.
24. Cohen LM, McCue JD, Germain M, Kjellstrand CM. Dialysis discontinuation. A 'good' death? Arch Intern Med. 1995;155(1):42–7.
25. WHO's Pain Relief Ladder. Available from: http://www.who.int/cancer/palliative/painladder/en/. Cited 14 Jan 2014.

Nutrition and Kidney Disease

55

Peter Choi and Jessica Stevenson

The relationship between nutrition and kidney disease is complex but has a major influence on patient experience and outcomes. The bidirectional interaction can be considered as either the effect of declining GFR on nutritional status or the effect of primary nutritional dysfunction on kidney function: The former is stereotyped by the common appearance of anorexia and wasting in uraemic patients; the latter is represented by the role of obesity in development of CKD.

This chapter will briefly discuss:

- Nutritional deficiency in kidney disease
- The difficulties of nutritional assessment in kidney disease
- Evidence supporting nutritional therapies in kidney disease
- Dietary guidelines for CKD patients
- Obesity and kidney disease
- Specific nutritional situations including anorexia nervosa, transplantation

Nutritional Deficiency in Kidney Disease

Protein-Energy Wasting (PEW)

Nutritional homeostasis in health is a highly regulated system to ensure optimal delivery and utilisation of essential dietary components. A principal requirement is energy balance, which is regulated by a complex system of circulating peptides such as leptin and ghrelin, with these peripheral appetite signals being centrally integrated within the hypothalamus to determine effector eating behaviours. Higher cognitive function also affects appetite, but overall energy balance is tightly regulated to maintain stable weight. Protein balance is also strictly regulated. Tissue proteins are maintained in a dynamic equilibrium with a pool of amino acids, available for new protein synthesis. A minimal dietary intake of protein is required to replace lost amino acids, and deficient dietary intake will result in proteolysis of tissue protein, notably from skeletal muscle, in order to replenish amino acid levels.

Protein-energy wasting (PEW) is common in CKD, with a severity and frequency, which increases with declining GFR. Anorexia and weight loss are common symptoms of severe CKD and represent an indication for initiation of renal replacement therapy. Almost 75 % of patients have evidence of PEW when dialysis is commenced, and despite an increase in appetite associated with the initiation of dialysis, between 20 and 70 % of prevalent maintenance dialysis patients still have evidence of PEW. Certain patient populations, including the elderly, socially isolated, diabetic patients and patients with cardiovascular comorbidity, are especially at-risk of protein-energy deficiency. Protein-energy wasting is also prominent in health-care systems which emphasise protein restriction as a treatment to retard progression of CKD.

Epidemiological studies have suggested complex associations between protein-energy status and patient outcome, which may be different in specific patient populations. Much attention has focused on the survival advantage of increasing nutritional status in populations with end-stage kidney disease, to the extent that levels of obesity which confer poor survival in the general population are apparently protective in dialysis populations. The strength of association requires that nutritional condition should always be taken into account in observational studies of survival on dialysis. It is self-evident that the appearance of wasting should confer poor prognosis in dialysis patients. However, it is unclear whether higher BMI is itself protective or exerts a statistical effect via the association of higher BMI with either increased muscle mass or increased amounts of metabolically protective brown fat. It is not recommended that dialysis patients seek obese body habitus as a response to these data.

The pathophysiology of PEW is complex (Fig. 55.1). Anorexia arises in kidney disease because of the retention of

P. Choi, MBBChir, PhD, FRCP (UK) (✉)
Department of Nephrology, John Hunter Hospital, Lookout Road, New Lambton Heights, NSW 2305, Australia
e-mail: Peter.choi@hnehealth.nsw.gov.au

J. Stevenson
Nutrition and Dietetics Department, John Hunter Hospital, 2 Lookout Road, New Lambton, NSW 2305, Australia
e-mail: Jessica.Stevenson@hnehealth.nsw.gov.au

M. Harber (ed.), *Practical Nephrology*,
DOI 10.1007/978-1-4471-5547-8_55,

Table 55.1 Dietary advice in CKD

	Aims of dietary prescription	Energy	Protein	Potassium	Phosphate	Sodium	Fluid
Stage 1–3	Slow progression of CKD. Control BP and diabetes and maintain healthy weight	30–35 kcal/kg IBW/day <60 years 30 kcal/kg IBW/day >60 years	0.75–1 g/kg IBW/day	Target range 3.5–5 mmol/L *Nil dietary restriction*	Target range 0.75–1.4 mmol/L *Nil dietary restriction*	No added salt 1,800–2,500 mg/day 80–110 mmol/day	Nil restriction *Unless otherwise medically indicated*
Stage 4–5	Optimise nutritional status, minimise uraemic symptoms and support slowing the progression of CKD and electrolyte management	30–35 kcal/kg IBW/day <60 years 30 kcal/kg IBW/day >60 years	0.75–1 g/kg IBW/day	Target range 3.5–5 mmol/L *Dietary restriction as required*	Target range 0.75–1.4 mmol/L *Dietary restriction as required*	No added salt 1,800–2,500 mg/day 80–110 mmol/day	Nil restriction *Unless otherwise medically indicated*
Haemodialysis	Optimise nutritional status, electrolyte management and fluid status	30–35 kcal/kg IBW/day <60 years 30 kcal/kg IBW/day >60 years	1–1.2 g/kg/day Acutely unwell At least 1.2 g/kg IBW/day	Target range 4–6 mmol/L Dietary restriction 1 mmol/kg/day	Target range 1.1–1.8 mmol/L Dietary restriction 800–1,000 mg/day	No added salt 1,800–2,500 mg/day 80–110 mmol/day	500 mL + daily urine output
Peritoneal Dialysis	Optimise nutritional status, manage electrolytes and fluid balance.	30–35 kcal/kg IBW/day <60 years 30 kcal/kg IBW/day >60 years *To include glucose from PD bags*	1.2–1.4 g/kg IBW/day Peritonitis 1.5 g/kg IBW/day Acutely unwell At least 1.3 g/kg	Target range 3.5–5 mmol/L Dietary restriction Not often needed As per biochemistry	Target range 1.1–1.8 mmol/L Dietary restriction 800–1,000 mg/day	No added salt 1,800–2,500 mg/day 80–110 mmol/day	800 mL + daily urine output
Conservative management	Optimise nutritional status, reduce uraemic symptoms and manage electrolytes and fluid balance and support slowing progression of CKD	30–35 kcal/kg IBW/day <60 years 30 kcal/kg IBW/day >60 years	0.75 g/kg/day	Target range 3.5–5 mmol/L *Dietary restriction as required*	Target range 0.75–1.4 mmol/L *Dietary restriction as required*	No added salt 1,800–2,500 mg/day 80–110 mmol/day	As per urine output and fluid balance
Transplant – acutely	Optimise nutritional status, manage electrolytes and fluid balance. Promote safe food hygiene practices	30–35 kcal/kg IBW/day <60 years 30 kcal/kg IBW/day >60 years	1.3–1.5 g/kg IBW/day *Increased requirements due to surgery and high dose steroids*	Target range 3.5–5 mmol/L	Target range 0.75–1.4 mmol/L *May need supplementation/high phosphate diet until within normal range*	No added salt 1,800–2,500 mg/day 80–110 mmol/day	As per urine output and fluid balance
Transplant – long term	Promote BP and diabetes control and weight management. Promote safe food hygiene practices	30–35 kcal/kg IBW/day <60 years 30 kcal/kg IBW/day >60 years	0.75–1 g/kg IBW/day	Target range 3.5–5 mmol/L	Target range 0.75–1.4 mmol/L	No added salt 1,800–2,500 mg/day 80–110 mmol/day	Nil restriction *Unless otherwise medically indicated*

Acute Kidney Injury	Optimise nutritional status, manage electrolytes and fluid balance	25–35 kcal/kg *Must take into account both specific metabolic disturbances associated with the kidney injury and also the underlying disease process*	Maximum of 1.7 g/kg IBW/day	As per biochemistry *To avoid hypokalaemia and hyperkalaemia*	As per biochemistry	No added salt 1,800–2,500 mg/day 80–110 mmol/day	As per urine output and fluid balance

Modified protein

In the pre-dialysis patient, moderate protein intake is encouraged to help reduce uraemic symptoms and slow the progression of CKD, whilst maintaining good nutritional status. Once on dialysis, protein requirements are increased to compensate for losses through dialysis (approximately 10 g per dialysis session) and to maintain good nutritional status. It is recommended that throughout all stages of CKD, patients include at least 50 % high biological value protein sources to ensure adequate amino acids.

Protein-rich foods which should be included:

- Fresh meats (e.g. chicken, beef, lamb, turkey, pork)
- Dairy products – need to limit amount due to phosphate and potassium content (e.g. milk, yoghurt, custard, cheese)
- Nuts and seeds
- Tofu and Quorn
- Legumes and lentils
- Egg (particularly egg whites)

Low-potassium diet

As kidney function declines, most people need to limit potassium-rich foods to avoid complications. A trained dietitian should review patients regularly and provide individualised advice based on biochemistry. Some general advice for lowering potassium intake includes:

- Limit fruit to 2 serves daily (avoid potassium-rich fruits including banana, dried fruit, fruit juice, avocado)
- Reduce potassium in vegetables through preparation and cooking methods (e.g. peeling and boiling)
- Limit high-potassium vegetables, including: potato, cassava, green banana, yam, spinach, mushrooms, tomato and concentrated tomato products (e.g. tomato paste/puree)
- Other high-potassium foods: chocolate, chocolate spread (e.g. *Nutella*), golden syrup, nuts, seeds, nut butters (e.g. peanut butter), potato-based snacks, cereals with dried fruit and nuts, coconut milk, evaporated milk, condensed milk

Low-phosphate diet

High serum phosphate levels are correlated with poor bone health, calcification of tissues and blood vessels and poor outcomes. Phosphate is predominantly found in animal-based foods and is now commonly used as an additive in many processed foods. A trained dietician should review patients regularly and provide individualised advice based on biochemistry. Those foods which are high in phosphate and may need to be avoided include:

- Offal and organ meats
- Hard cheeses (e.g. cheddar, parmesan) and processed cheeses
- Prawns and shellfish
- Fish with edible bones
- Cola drinks
- Nuts and seeds
- Bran-based cereals

Note: It is important that in addition to adhering to a low-phosphate diet, patients are educated about their phosphate-binding medication. It is important that if this medication is prescribed, patients understand when and how this should be taken

No-added-salt diet

A low-salt diet is recommended to help reduce blood pressure, reduce proteinuria, assist with fluid management and reduce excessive thirst. Patients with CKD should be encouraged to reduce their sodium intake (unless otherwise medically indicated). Some general tips for reducing sodium intake:

- Avoid adding salt to cooking and at table
- Avoid processed meats (e.g. salami, bacon, ham), dried/smoked foods (e.g. fish) and canned foods

(continued)

Table 56.2 Approximate GFR for renal replacement modalities

Renal replacement therapy	Typical theoretical GFR achieved during therapy (ml/min)
Intermittent haemodialysis	150–200 during dialysis (0–10 between dialysis periods)
Continuous arteriovenous haemofiltration (CAVH)	10–15
Continuous venovenous haemodiafiltration (CVVH)	15–25
Continuous arteriovenous haemodiafiltration (CAVHD)	20
Continuous venovenous haemodiafiltration (CVVHD)	30–40
Continuous ambulatory peritoneal dialysis (CAPD) (4 exchanges daily)	5–10

Data from Industry Submission, Renal National Service Framework (Acute Renal Failure) October 2003

However, there are websites that can perform the calculation within seconds, and as a result of the Renal NSF, most laboratories in the UK now routinely report MDRD eGFR both in primary and secondary care.

Elimination of Drugs by Haemodialysis/Filtration and Peritoneal Dialysis

The same principles of drug elimination apply to dialysis and filtration membranes as to native kidneys. Drug removal follows first-order kinetics, and the amount of drug removed is determined by plasma concentration, the sieving coefficient or permeability of the membrane, the molecular weight of the drug and the extent to which it is bound to plasma proteins.

Newer "high-flux" dialysis membranes can remove larger molecules and are particularly useful when trying to remove middle molecules including β_2 microglobulin responsible for dialysis amyloid. Haemofilters remove molecules smaller than inulin (average molecular weight 5,200 Da). This difference is especially important as most drugs which are not protein bound are removed by haemodialysis including most antibiotics, but drugs such as vancomycin (1,800 Da), amphotericin (960 Da) and erythromycin (734 Da) behave differently in haemodialysis, "high-flux" haemodialysis and haemofiltration. Just as in the native kidney, water-soluble drugs are more readily filtered than fat soluble ones. When deciding on drug dosing regimens for patients on renal replacement therapy (RRT), it is essential to ascertain which mode of RRT the patient is receiving. This is because the different modalities all have differing solute clearance rates, which has major implications for drug dosing to ensure the patient is neither overdosed nor underdosed (see Table 56.2).

The plasma concentration of a drug is determined by its volume of distribution and tissue binding characteristics. Digoxin, phenytoin and antidepressants, for example, have large volumes of distribution with only very low plasma concentrations and are therefore hardly influenced by dialysis or filtration. Conversely, gentamicin has a very small Vd and negligible protein binding, so is removed extremely efficiently by dialysis.

Table 56.3 Antibiotics that still achieve therapeutic levels when given three times a week on haemodialysis

1. Vancomycin
2. Gentamicin
3. Amikacin
4. Meropenem
5. Ceftazidime
6. Temocillin
7. Teicoplanin
8. Ertapenem

Drugs are eliminated much less efficiently by the peritoneal membrane than by synthetic dialysis or filtration membranes. This poor permeability is used to advantage in treating peritonitis in peritoneal dialysis (PD) patients where antibiotics are injected into the peritoneal fluid.

There is one small advantage of ESRD in that reduced dosing of some antibiotics means that some patients can be easily managed with three times a week administration of antibiotics on haemodialysis, thus facilitating early discharge or avoiding daily outpatient administration of antibiotics (see Table 56.3).

Handy Hints for Prescribing for Patients with Renal Impairment

- A number of published tables that provide dosing guidelines exist to assist in dose modification (www.globalrph.com/renaldosing2.htm). Individualisation of therapy should be based on pharmacokinetic principles whenever possible [8].
- Most texts use creatinine clearance (as calculated using Cockcroft and Gault) as an estimation of GRF for recommending doses [6].

- For most drugs there is a broad creatinine clearance range for guidance on dosage and so in practice the variations of measurement will not change the recommendations [7] but it is important to consider the implications of under and over dosing for patients with GFR levels which are borderline.
- If non-renal clearance accounts for elimination of more than 50 % of a drug, then no adjustments need be made to dose or frequency of administration.
- Dosages of toxic drugs which are mainly excreted in active form by the kidney (i.e. as unchanged drug or active metabolites) may need to be modified to avoid accumulation.
- In renal failure, potentially toxic drugs should only be used if there is a specific indication for their use and if therapy can be monitored appropriately.
- If dose adjustment is required, then dose, dose interval or both can be adjusted to achieve the desired therapeutic profile.
- If dose amendment is required, then dose, dose interval or both can be adjusted to achieve the desired therapeutic effect. For example, with antibiotics, particular peak concentrations are required for optimal bacteriocidal or bacteriostatic effects, so typically the normal dose given less frequently is prescribed. Conversely, with digoxin, a steady plasma concentration is desirable, so the dosing interval remains at 24 h, and the dose is reduced.
- If the drug is unaffected by renal impairment, it may be used in usual doses and the patients should be monitored for signs of increased sensitivity to the effects of the drug or to the side effects.
- Drugs that require therapeutic levels quickly may require a loading dose as the time taken to reach steady state will be prolonged for drugs where the metabolism and excretion is slowed in renal impairment.
- Supplementary doses for RRT – some texts quote supplementary doses to be given after intermittent RRT. They will only be important for drugs with a low Vd and a narrow therapeutic range which are cleared efficiently by dialysis. In practice, it is better to adjust the timings of doses so that the next dose falls after the RRT session rather than add in extra doses.
- A number of sources are now available to provide drug dosing guidelines for the adjustment of doses for the severity of renal impairment or stage of chronic kidney disease (CKD).
- Electronic prescribing systems may assist in the use of medications in AKI and such systems have been developed in University Hospitals Birmingham Foundation Trust and Vanderbilt University Hospital, USA.

Prescribing in Acute Kidney Injury

From a drugs perspective, it is essential in AKI to review all the medications that a patient is taking, including those for co-morbidities.

- Temporarily, or permanently, withdraw drugs that affect kidney haemodynamics especially NSAIDs and drugs blocking the renin-angiotensin system.
- Stop any nephrotoxic drugs and avoid prescribing nephrotoxic therapy.
- Review drugs that may have adverse effects in patients with AKI, for example, antihypertensives, metformin, statins and any drugs which may exacerbate hyperkalaemia.
- Ensure drug dosing is appropriate for the level of renal impairment or the type of renal replacement therapy used.

Caution should be taken with drug dosing in AKI. The use of eGFR and Cockcroft and Gault is unreliable in AKI as serum creatinine levels are regularly changing and their rate of change might not reflect current renal function. However, the daily assessment of renal function using eGFR or GFR may be an appropriate estimation for drug dosing, as long as the patient's prescription is reviewed each day.

In addition, review doses of medications as AKI resolves. This may happen quickly in a patient with dehydration where fluids are given to resolve the cause of AKI. Underdosing of drugs such as antibiotics may have an adverse impact on the management of sepsis, and doses of low molecular weight heparins may need to be increased in VTE prophylaxis.

It is also worth bearing in mind that drugs are very commonly the primary or contributing cause of AKI (see Table 56.4); an obsessional medication history (prescribed and over the counter) with start dates, courses, dose increments and potential drug interactions is important and may involve contacting prescribers such as the patients family practitioner.

Summary

Drug dosing in patients with impaired renal function is a complex area. It is important to have an understanding of how drug handling may be altered in renal impairment and RRT and on the limitations of the calculations used to estimate renal impairment in order to help make informed decisions on drug doses. Where possible, textbooks on drug dosing in renal impairment should be consulted and in addition, liaise with pharmacists with a special interest in the field who have clinical experience with these patients. In all cases once a drug regimen has been prescribed, monitor the patient for efficacy, side effects and signs of toxicity.

Table 56.4 Medication well documented to cause renal injury

Drugs that can cause glomerulonephritis		
Allopurinol	Captopril	
Dapsone	Gold	
Halothane	Hydralazine	
NSAIDs	Penicillamine	
Penicillins	Phenindione	
Probenecid	Rifampicin	
Sulphonamides	Procainamide	
Tolbutamide	Psoralen	
Thiazide diuretics	Levamisole	
Drugs that can cause acute tubular injury		
Aciclovir	Furosemide	
Aminoglycosides	Gold	
Amphotericin	Ifosfamide	
Cephalosporins	Lithium	
Cisplatin	Mannitol	
Contrast media	NSAIDs	
Ciclosporin	Paracetamol	
Ethylene glycol	Tacrolimus	
Foscarnet	Vancomycin	
Drugs that can cause interstitial nephritis		
Allopurinol	Erythromycin	Phenobarbitone
Aminosalicylates	Furosemide	Phenytoin
Amlodipine	Gentamicin	Proton pump inhibitors
Azathioprine	Gold	Quinolones
Bumetanide	Interferon	Ranitidine
Carbamazepine	Isoniazid	Rifampicin
Cephalosporins	Lithium	Sulfonamides
Cimetidine	Mesalazine	Thiazides
Cotrimoxazole	NSAIDs	Vancomycin
Diltiazem	Penicillins	

References

1. Gabardi S, Abramson S. Drug dosing in chronic kidney disease. Med Clin North Am. 2005;89(3):649–87.
2. Cockwell P, Stringer S, Marriott J. Acute kidney injury. In: Walker R, editor. Clinical pharmacy and therapeutics. 5th ed. London: Churchill Livingstone; 2011. p. 255–71.
3. Dhillon S, Kostrzewski A. Clinical pharmacokinetics. London: Pharmaceutical Press; 2006. p. 53–78.
4. Matzke GR, Frye RF. Drug administration in patients with renal insufficiency: minimising renal and extrarenal toxicity. Drug Saf. 1997;16(3):205–31.
5. Aronson JK. Drugs and renal insufficiency. Medicine. 2007;35: 396–9.
6. Bauer L. Creatinine clearance versus glomerular filtration rate for the use of renal drug dosing in patients with kidney dysfunction. Pharmacotherapy. 2005;25(9):1286–7.
7. Thompson CA. Better renal-function estimates not expected to alter drug dosing right away. Am J Health Syst Pharm. 2005;62(23):2442–4.
8. Vidal L, Shavit M, Fraser A, et al. Systematic comparison of four sources of drug information regarding adjustment of dose for renal function. Br Med J. 2005;331:263–6.

57 Prevention of Infection in Kidney Patients

Sophie Collier and Susan Hopkins

Renal patients are particularly vulnerable to infection. They are relatively immunocompromised and undergo numerous invasive procedures, which put them at risk of infection. They receive multiple antibiotics, which select out resistant organisms and attend healthcare environments on a frequent basis, allowing ample opportunity for multidrug-resistant organisms to spread. Many patients are on immunosuppressive agents to treat their underlying renal disease or following a kidney transplant.

In 2009, infection was the second most frequent prevalent cause of death in those undergoing renal replacement therapy with dialysis and the most frequent cause of death in those with a renal transplant. In renal patients mortality associated with sepsis is 50 times higher than the general population and accounts for 30 % of hospital admissions [1].

It is particular telling and alarming that the first reports of both vancomycin-resistant enterococci (VRE) and vancomycin-resistant *Staphylococcus aureus* (VRSA) came from renal patients. As our antibiotic armamentarium diminishes, one of our most important weapons against infection is now prevention.

This chapter will discuss in the following elements in prevention of infections in renal patients:

1. Core principles of infection prevention and control
2. Specific important organisms including multidrug-resistant organisms (MDRO)
3. Access-related infections
4. Prevention of other important healthcare-associated infections
5. Preventing the spread of blood-borne viruses
6. Vaccine-preventable diseases (including travel health)

S. Collier, BMBCH, MA, MRCP, FRCPath (✉)
Department of Microbiology, Royal Free London NHS Foundation Trust, Royal Free Hospital, Pond Street, London NW3 2QG, UK
e-mail: sophiecollier@nhs.net

S. Hopkins, BA, MBBCh, BAO, MSC, FRCPI, FRCP
Department of Infectious Diseases and Clinical Microbiology, Royal Free London NHS Foundation Trust, Pond St, London NW3 2QG, UK
e-mail: susanhopkins@nhs.net

M. Harber (ed.), *Practical Nephrology*,
DOI 10.1007/978-1-4471-5547-8_57,

Core Principles of Infection Prevention and Control

The prevention of infection is core to the provision of any healthcare. The following are essential to prevent infections in the healthcare environment:

1. Hand hygiene
2. Personal protective equipment (PPE)
3. Sharps disposal
4. Cleaning and decontamination
5. Surveillance and feedback
6. Education of healthcare workers and patients
7. Early and prompt recognition and treatment of infection
8. Isolation of patients with potential or confirmed significant cross-transmissible pathogens

In the UK, healthcare workers (HCW) are required by law to have appropriate supplies of hand decontamination, PPE and sharps disposal.

Hand Hygiene

Despite advances in healthcare delivery and technology, *the single most effective method to prevent onward transmission of infection in healthcare settings is hand hygiene*. The WHO is promoting the 5 moments – before patient contact, before an aseptic task, after body fluid exposure, after patient contact and after contact with patient surroundings – of hand hygiene worldwide and have reviewed the evidence extensively in a recent publication [2]. Resources to help develop hospital and unit campaigns are located at http://www.npsa.nhs.uk/cleanyourhands/ and http://www.who.int/gpsc/5may/en/.

Normal human skin is colonised with multiple bacteria, and the bacterial counts on the hands of HCW have been estimated at 4×10^4 CFU/cm^3: Transient organisms – for example, *Staphylococcus aureus*, gram-negative bacilli or yeasts – are most frequently acquired by direct contact with patients or healthcare environment and are very amenable to

diseases prior to immunosuppressants [45]. In those with autoimmune disease, it has been shown to reduce infection risk by 51 % and postherpetic neuralgia by 66 % 3 years postvaccination. Varicella zoster immunoglobulin (VZIG) should be considered in immunosuppressed patients who are exposed to cases of zoster infection – both chickenpox and shingles – from 48 h prior to rash developing until crusting of vesicles. VZIG use does not preclude infection and therefore if these patients develop early signs of infection, they should be given empirical antivirals. Immunoglobulin use alters the normal immune response to vaccine and therefore use of vaccines should be delayed until 3 months after immunoglobulin administration [45]. Our practice is not to suspend patients on the waiting list post-VZV vaccination, but to give acyclovir if transplanted within 2 weeks of vaccination.

Tuberculosis

Up to 10 % of patients with latent TB infection (LTBI) develop reactivation of the disease. The use of immunomodulatory drugs in rheumatological or autoimmune diseases allows reactivation of LTBI to occur, through dysregulation of the granulomatous process.

Prior to starting immunosuppressive therapy, individuals should be assessed for active and latent TB. An accurate history of previous TB exposure, diagnosis or treatment should be taken and a clinical examination performed to look for signs of active TB, particularly lymphadenopathy. A chest X-ray should be performed to determine whether there are radiological appearances of active or old TB. If there are signs of active TB, referral to a TB specialist physician is recommended.

For those with no TB history and no active TB on chest radiograph, further tests should be performed. The current UK guidelines recommend the use of blood interferon gamma release assays (IGRA) to diagnose LTBI in immunocompromised patients, as they appear to be more sensitive in this population [46]. IGRAs are in vitro blood tests using antigens that detect a T cell response to TB antigens by releasing measured interferon gamma.

Positive IGRA tests require prompt treatment for LTBI in those due to undergo immunosuppressive treatment if the risk of treatment (mainly hepatotoxicity) is less than the risk of reactivation. Those deemed at high risk of hepatotoxicity should be monitored 3–4 monthly and warned of TB symptoms. Standard LTBI therapy is 3 months of combination rifampicin and isoniazid or alternatively 6 months of isoniazid monotherapy [46].

Vaccination against TB uses a live attenuated vaccine derived from *Mycobacterium bovis* that confers up to 70–80 % protection depending on individual response [46]. It is generally not recommended over the age of 16 years, and as it is a live vaccine is also contraindicated in individuals on immunosuppressive therapy.

Patient Education

Patients and their carers should receive education about hand hygiene and when to use different types of hand decontamination and their role.

Patients should be educated on the ability to challenge their HCW – in a recent study, only 16 % of patients (independent of MRSA status) tried to ask medical personnel to wash hands during their last stay in hospital. However, when doctors and nurses invited patients to challenge, it increased those challenging 2.5-fold.

Patients should be given written and verbal information about care of all devices (CVC, PD, etc.) when it is inserted. When patients regularly attend for dialysis with wet or soiled dressings, further education is a key part of preventing exit site infections and CRBSIs.

PD patients need to fully understand how to use an aseptic technique when they connect up their dialysis fluid. Published studies have demonstrated how the training programme can influence rates of exit site infections and peritonitis [28].

Summary

Infections are frequent and life threatening in renal patients and excellent infection control measures are paramount in looking after these patients. Simple, proven measures can reduce the risk of infections in these patients and these should be performed on all patients at all times.

References

1. Sarnak MJ, Jaber BL. Mortality caused by sepsis in patients with end-stage renal disease compared with the general population. Kidney Int. 2000;58(4):1758–64.
2. WHO guidelines on hand hygiene in health care. 2009. http://whqlibdoc.who.int/publications/2009/9789241597906_eng.pdf.
3. Shahid NS, et al. Hand washing with soap reduces diarrhoea and spread of bacterial pathogens in a Bangladesh village. J Diarrhoeal Dis Res. 1996;14(2):85–9.
4. Luby SP, et al. Effect of intensive handwashing promotion on childhood diarrhea in high-risk communities in Pakistan: a randomized controlled trial. JAMA. 2004;291(21):2547–54.
5. Cardoso CL, et al. Effectiveness of hand-cleansing agents for removing Acinetobacter baumannii strain from contaminated hands. Am J Infect Control. 1999;27(4):327–31.
6. Gordin FM, et al. Reduction in nosocomial transmission of drug-resistant bacteria after introduction of an alcohol-based handrub. Infect Control Hosp Epidemiol. 2005;26(7):650–3.
7. Pratt RJ, et al. The epic project: developing national evidence-based guidelines for preventing healthcare associated infections. Phase I: guidelines for preventing hospital-acquired infections. Department of Health (England). J Hosp Infect. 2001;47(Suppl):S3–82.

8. Public Health Laboratory Service AIDS and STD Centre. Occupational transmission of HIV. London; 1999.
9. Haley RW, et al. Update from the SENIC project. Hospital infection control: recent progress and opportunities under prospective payment. Am J Infect Control. 1985;13(3):97–108.
10. Piraino B, et al. Peritoneal dialysis-related infections recommendations: 2005 update. Perit Dial Int. 2005;25(2):107–31.
11. Engemann JJ, et al. Clinical outcomes and costs due to Staphylococcus aureus bacteremia among patients receiving long-term hemodialysis. Infect Control Hosp Epidemiol. 2005;26(6): 534–9.
12. Simor AE. Staphylococcal decolonisation: an effective strategy for prevention of infection? Lancet Infect Dis. 2011;11(12):952–62.
13. Tacconelli E, et al. Mupirocin prophylaxis to prevent Staphylococcus aureus infection in patients undergoing dialysis: a meta-analysis. Clin Infect Dis. 2003;37(12):1629–38.
14. Fluck R, Kumwenda M. Renal association guidelines – vascular access for haemodialysis; 2011. www.renal.org/guidelines/modules/vascular-access-for-haemodialysis.
15. Woodrow G, Davies S. Clinical practice guidelines: peritoneal dialysis. UK Renal Association; 2010. www.renal.org/guidelines/modules/peritoneal-dialysis-in-ckd.
16. Clostridium difficile infection: how to deal with the problem. 2008. www.hpa.org.uk/webc/hpawebfile/hpaweb_c/1232006607827.
17. Cornely OA, et al. Fidaxomicin versus vancomycin for infection with Clostridium difficile in Europe, Canada, and the USA: a double-blind, non-inferiority, randomised controlled trial. Lancet Infect Dis. 2012;12(4):281–9.
18. Louie TJ, et al. Fidaxomicin versus vancomycin for Clostridium difficile infection. N Engl J Med. 2011;364(5):422–31.
19. Klevens RM, et al. Dialysis Surveillance Report: National Healthcare Safety Network (NHSN)-data summary for 2006. Semin Dial. 2008;21(1):24–8.
20. Hannah EL, et al. Outbreak of hemodialysis vascular access site infections related to malfunctioning permanent tunneled catheters: making the case for active infection surveillance. Infect Control Hosp Epidemiol. 2002;23(9):538–41.
21. O'Grady N, Alexander M, Burns L, Dellinger E, Garland J, O'Heard S, Lipsett P, Masur H, Mermel L, Pearson M, Raad I, Randolph A, Rupp M, Saint S. The Healthcare Infection Control Practices Advisory Committee (HICPAC). Guidelines for the preventions of intravascular catheter-related infections. Clin Infect Dis. 2011;52(9):e162–93.
22. Chatzinikolaou I, et al. Antibiotic-coated hemodialysis catheters for the prevention of vascular catheter-related infections: a prospective, randomized study. Am J Med. 2003;115(5):352–7.
23. Chaiyakunapruk N, et al. Chlorhexidine compared with povidone-iodine solution for vascular catheter-site care: a meta-analysis. Ann Intern Med. 2002;136(11):792–801.
24. NKF KDOQI Guidelines: clinical practice guidelines for vascular access. 2006. www.kidney.org/PROFESSIONALS/kdoqi/guideline...PD.../index.htm.
25. Lok CE, Mokrzycki MH. Prevention and management of catheter-related infection in hemodialysis patients. Kidney Int. 2011;79(6):587–98.
26. Lok CE, et al. Hemodialysis infection prevention with polysporin ointment. J Am Soc Nephrol. 2003;14(1):169–79.
27. Yahav D, et al. Antimicrobial lock solutions for the prevention of infections associated with intravascular catheters in patients undergoing hemodialysis: systematic review and meta-analysis of randomized, controlled trials. Clin Infect Dis. 2008;47(1):83–93.
28. Piraino B, et al. ISPD position statement on reducing the risks of peritoneal dialysis-related infections. Perit Dial Int. 2011;31(6): 614–30.
29. Figueiredo A, et al. Clinical practice guidelines for peritoneal access. Perit Dial Int. 2010;30(4):424–9.
30. Dombros N, et al. European best practice guidelines for peritoneal dialysis. 3 Peritoneal access. Nephrol Dial Transplant. 2005;20 Suppl 9:ix8–12.
31. Strippoli GF, et al. Catheter-related interventions to prevent peritonitis in peritoneal dialysis: a systematic review of randomized, controlled trials. J Am Soc Nephrol. 2004;15(10):2735–46.
32. Nessim SJ, Bargman JM, Jassal SV. Relationship between double-cuff versus single-cuff peritoneal dialysis catheters and risk of peritonitis. Nephrol Dial Transplant. 2010;25(7):2310–4.
33. Bernardini J, et al. Randomized, double-blind trial of antibiotic exit site cream for prevention of exit site infection in peritoneal dialysis patients. J Am Soc Nephrol. 2005;16(2):539–45.
34. Churchill DN, et al. Canadian hemodialysis morbidity study. Am J Kidney Dis. 1992;19(3):214–34.
35. Englesbe MJ, et al. Single center review of femoral arteriovenous grafts for hemodialysis. World J Surg. 2006;30(2):171–5.
36. Zibari GB, et al. Preoperative vancomycin prophylaxis decreases incidence of postoperative hemodialysis vascular access infections. Am J Kidney Dis. 1997;30(3):343–8.
37. van Loon MM, et al. Buttonhole needling of haemodialysis arteriovenous fistulae results in less complications and interventions compared to the rope-ladder technique. Nephrol Dial Transplant. 2010;25(1):225–30.
38. Nesrallah GE, et al. Staphylococcus aureus bacteremia and buttonhole cannulation: long-term safety and efficacy of mupirocin prophylaxis. Clin J Am Soc Nephrol. 2010;5(6):1047–53.
39. Report of the Rosenheim Advisory Group. Hepatitis and the treatment of chronic renal failure. London: Department of Health and Social Security; 1972.
40. Department of Health (UK). Good practice guidelines for renal dialysis/transplantation units: prevention and control of blood-borne virus infection. London: Department of Health (UK); 2002.
41. Kidney Disease: Improving Global Outcomes (KDIGO). KDIGO clinical practice guidelines for the prevention, diagnosis, evaluation, and treatment of hepatitis C in chronic kidney disease. Kidney Int Suppl. 2008;73(109):S1–99.
42. Canadian Society of Nephrology guidelines for prevention of blood borne infections in dialysis units. CANNT J. 2007. www.thefreelibrary.com.
43. Jadoul M, Cornu C, van Ypersele de Strihou C. Universal precautions prevent hepatitis C virus transmission: a 54 month follow-up of the Belgian Multicenter Study. The Universitaires Cliniques St-Luc (UCL) Collaborative Group. Kidney Int. 1998;53(4): 1022–5.
44. Department of Health (UK). Good practice guidelines for renal dialysis/transplantation units, prevention & control of blood-borne virus infection. Addendum guidelines for dialysis away from base. London: Department of Health (UK); 2010.
45. Department of Health. Immunisation against infectious disease – 'The Green Book' – 2006 updated edition. 2nd ed. London: Department of Health (UK); 2007.
46. NICE guideline: clinical diagnosis and management of tuberculosis, and measures for its prevention and control. 2011. www.nice.org.uk/nicemedia/live/13422/53642/53642.pdf.

58 Setting Up and Running a Haemodialysis Service

Roger N. Greenwood and Hugh Feidhlim Woods

The task of setting up a haemodialysis (HD) service will provide different challenges in different countries. In some countries, all haemodialysis centres operate under a publicly funded healthcare system; in others the facilities operate as private providers, and in others there is a mixed economy. Most commonly, however, there will be a fixed amount of money allocated from the health service budget to renal services, the majority of 'renal' spending usually being on haemodialysis. In most countries, there are tariff systems in place whereby a fixed reward is paid to the HD provider for each session, with the agreement that up to 3 sessions weekly will be remunerated. There are other approaches to funding, but generally the fiscal environment is tight wherever maintenance HD is established or services are developing. The challenge is to optimise the patient experience while ensuring adherence to accepted standards of care and patient safety. This requires the HD service to extend way beyond the delivery of the dialysis session itself.

Good clinical governance requires clear lines of accountability and responsibility for the medical care of each patient and agreed pathways for transfer to inpatient care services in the event of intercurrent illness. On average, haemodialysis patients are hospitalised for approximately 14 days each year. Access to healthcare professionals other than nephrologists and dialysis nurses is required; these include dietetics, counselling, social work, pharmacy and technical support. Wherever patients are being prepared for long-term HD treatment and wherever HD patients are hospitalised, 24/7 access to vascular surgery and interventional radiology and an 'acute HD' team are required. Since the establishment of a new HD service will normally be within an existing network of medical facilities, these requirements can usually be met. The HD provider needs to have developed protocols, not only for the dialysis procedure but also for dealing with intercurrent medical problems and both intra- and inter-dialytic events.

This chapter will discuss the main design features and components of care of a modern haemodialysis unit. The important subjects of staff recruitment, education and training are addressed. Finally the components of clinical governance are detailed.

The Haemodialysis Facility

Location and Layout

A useful question at the outset is whether the HD unit should be a place for being sick or a place to get well; the latter should be the aim. Regular haemodialysis for end-stage renal failure has typically scored poorly on quality of life measures compared to living with other long-term medical conditions. Thrice weekly treatment, travelling time and often post-dialysis fatigue add to the burden of chronic kidney disease and comorbid medical conditions. Careful attention to location and design is therefore very important and can positively contribute to the patient experience.

Capacity

Facility size is an important consideration. This has to be carefully judged in terms of local demographics, predicted demand for haemodialysis, the ability of payers to finance growth and, most importantly, the potential to recruit staff locally and the training resources available to achieve the desired skill mix.

Typically, in a large city, there may be a mixture of large central renal facilities (exceeding 25 stations) and a number of smaller 'local' HD units (c. 8–20 stations). As an example, a possible facility mix in a city such as Kuala Lumpur is illustrated in Fig. 58.1.

R.N. Greenwood, MSc, ACGI, MD, FRCP (✉)
Renal Unit, Lister Hospital, East and North Herts NHS Trust, Stevenage SG1 4AB, UK
e-mail: roger.greenwood@nhs.net

H.F. Woods, MBBCh, BAO, MRCP(UK)
Fresenius Medical Care Asia Pacific, Hong Kong, SAR (China)
e-mail: feidhlim.woods@gmail.com

M. Harber (ed.), *Practical Nephrology*,
DOI 10.1007/978-1-4471-5547-8_58, © Springer-Verlag London 2014

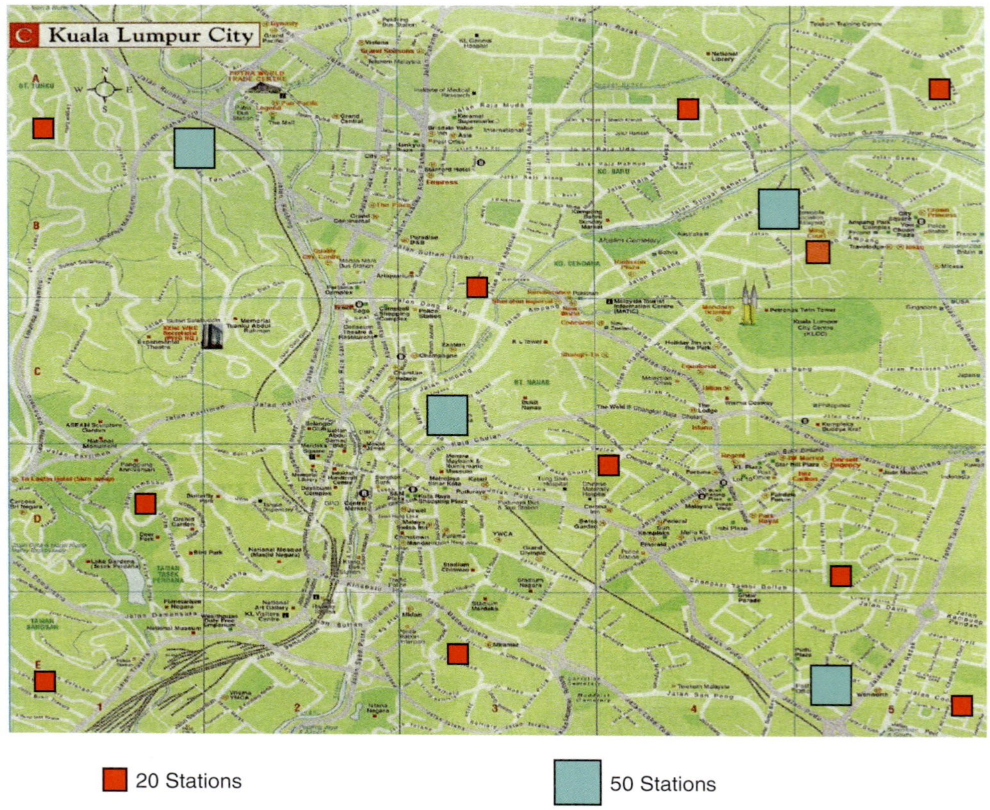

Fig. 58.1 Possible facility mix in a city such as Kuala Lumpur. In a typical large city, there may be a mixture of large central facilities (c. 50 stations) and a number of smaller 'local' HD units (c. 12–20 stations)

A large central unit has the following:

Advantages	Disadvantages
Cost efficiency (overhead)	Large patient pool
Larger staff pool	Less individualised care
	Geography and distance

A small centre has the following:

Advantages	Disadvantages
Nearer to client's community base	Higher cost overhead
Small patient pool	Small staff pool
More individualised care	Less staffing flexibility

Location

Perhaps the most important preliminary consideration is whether to have the new HD facility 'in-hospital' or 'free-standing'. The latter refers to a location at some distance from a major hospital or nephrology inpatient centre.

Hospital siting has the following pros and cons:

Advantages	Disadvantages
Flow of new patients in a familiar and reassuring environment	Shared cost of large overhead
Access to other health and administrative services	Geography and distance
Access to a wide pool of healthcare professionals	

A free-standing unit has the following:

Advantages	Disadvantages
Nearer to client's community base	Remote from other services
Customised design	Remote from other health professionals
Economy – less overheads	

Functional and Safety Factors

The occupational health and safety (OHS) of staff is an important consideration. Indeed the provider of the service is probably liable under law. The same applies to the physical risk of injury not only to staff but also to visitors, family members and carers. Security against trespass has to be considered as does the security and reliability of utilities which includes power, telephone and IT communications and water supply. All staff members should be properly trained in disaster planning in anticipation of power outage, flood and earthquake. The focus is on continuity of the service and/or transfer of patients to a safe environment.

Access to the Unit

Ideally the haemodialysis unit should be on a recognised public transport route while, at the same time, protected against the hazards of local traffic. Set down of patients will be by either private car or taxi or from ambulance and should be within

Table 58.1 Facilities required in a haemodialysis unit

1. Main entrance, cover waiting area and reception
2. Male and female WC (including disabled facility), changing room and lockers
3. Doctors' consulting room and facilities for outpatient attendances
4. The main treatment area
5. Nursing office and meeting/education room
6. Staff room incorporating pantry, fridge, microwave cooker, easy chairs and table
7. Clean utility area for blood sample processing, pharmacy stores and dispensing
8. Dirty utility for all clinical waste collection, packaging and disposal
9. Cleaners room
10. Water treatment plant room
11. Dialysis machine prepare and 'run-up' room
12. Technical workshop
13. Power distribution cupboard incorporating IT connections
14. Main store and subsidiary store(s)

100 m of the unit. Car parking should ideally be secured for both staff and patients. HD centres are best placed on the ground floor of any building. Failing this, lifts should be able to take a wheelchair and also a stretcher in rarer emergency situations. Access points to the unit should be adequately signposted and illuminated day and night and preferably security controlled by CCTV. Adequate lighting around the facility and on connecting pathways further helps to ensure staff safety at nighttime.

Functional Areas

A typical HD centre will need the functional areas shown in Table 58.1:

Patient and staff traffic flows have to be given particular consideration in the design of a HD centre. The design should be patient centred to provide maximum convenience and a comfortable personal environment during the dialysis process. At the same time, staff should be able to work efficiently, bearing in mind that infection control and attention to hygiene in between patient interactions have assumed much greater importance in recent years. The ergonomic design is now an area of specialised expertise, and professional help should be sought at all stages.

Safety

All avoidable risk factors which could cause physical injury to patients and visitors should be identified. The dimensions of communication areas such as corridors must be adequate to allow access/egress for delivery carts, wheelchairs and stretchers.

Occupational health and safety of workers is of paramount importance. All staff should be immunised against hepatitis B infection. Protocols must be in place to ensure prompt treatment for needlestick injuries.

Water Treatment

The main components of a typical water treatment plant are shown in Fig. 58.2. The design should ensure the reduction of the concentrations of metals, other chemicals and bacteria to agreed standards which now exist in most countries. Even in the modern era, poor design and poor maintenance can have severe consequences in dialysis where typically a patient is exposed to 120 L or more of aqueous solution per treatment.

Pretreatment storage should have adequate capacity for one complete dialysis shift. Source water passed through course filters to remove particulate matter. It is then softened to reduce the calcium load using a resin coated with sodium ions which are exchanged for calcium and magnesium ions. Activated carbon filters (preferably two in series) then adsorb substances which are not removed by a softening such as endotoxins, chloramines and chlorine. The water then passes through at least one (preferable two) reverse osmosis (RO) units. The name, RO, derives from the flow direction of product water which is in the reverse direction to the osmotic gradient. It is achieved by pumping water at high pressure through a tight membrane. The tiny pore size of these membranes provides an absolute barrier for molecules larger than 100–300 Da. Finally, post-RO water is subject to ultraviolet (UV) irradiation to ensure final breakdown of dying bacteria. This is usually necessary if treated water is stored. Ensuring that ultrapure water is delivered to the individual dialysis stations is probably the first duty of care for a haemodialysis facility.

Treatment Area and Patient Stations

The main treatment area is made up of individual HD stations separated by privacy curtains. Each facility should have a number of side rooms where patients can be isolated. There are various medical reasons for this, a common one being the need to isolate patients who have recently returned from dialysing in a region with a high prevalence of blood-borne virus infections. One isolation room to four general HD stations is a comfortable ratio.

A typical HD station layout is shown in Fig. 58.3. Ten square metres should be allowed for each station. Ideally the HD machine could be plugged into service panels which house circulating water and drainage points.

Within the patients' reach should be controls for audiovisual entertainment with individual headsets in consideration of neighbour patients. Digital channels should be available, and Wi-Fi should also be freely available for patient use (Fig. 58.4).

Patient's individual choices vary greatly. Some wish to use the four-hour dialysis session (typical) for rest, or alternatively the time can be used constructively; this can include exercise during the dialysis session. Dialysis stations should be equipped

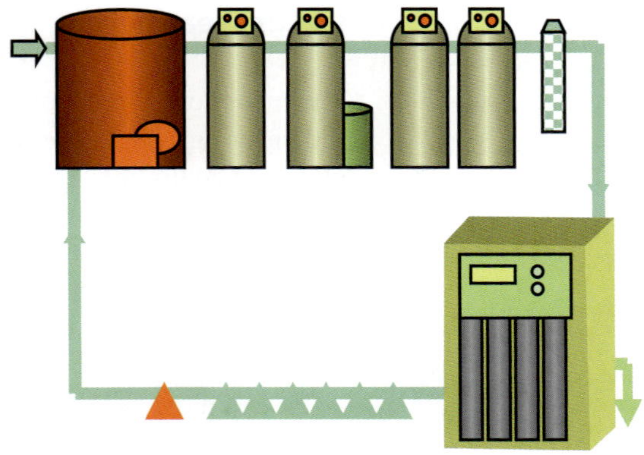

AAMI standards for chemicals

Contaminant	Maximum concentration (mg/L)
Calcium	2 (0.1 mEq/L)
Magnesium	4 (0.3 mEq/L)
Potassium	8 (0.2 mEq/L)
Sodium	70 (3.0 mEq/L)
Antimony	0.006
Arsenic	0.005
Barium	0.10
Beryllium	0.0004
Cadmium	0.001
Chromium	0.014
Cyanide	0.02
Lead	0.005
Mercury	0.0002
Selenium	0.09
Silver	0.005
Aluminum	0.01
Chloramines	0.10
Free Chlorine	0.50
Copper	0.10
Fluoride	0.20
Nitrate (as N)	2.0
Sulfate	100
Thallium	0.002
Zinc	0.10

Microbiological quality standard

Standard (ISO and others)
- **Bacterial growth**
  <100 CFU /mL (nutrient poor media)
- **Endotoxin**
  LAL < 0.25 u/mL

Ultrapure (required for convective therapies)
- **Bacterial growth**
  <1 CFU /mL
- **Endotoxin**
  LAL < 0.003 u/mL

Fig. 58.2 The typical layout of a water treatment and distribution system. The basis of treatment of water for HD in most clinics is a process called reverse osmosis (*RO*) which is capable of achieving extremely low levels of almost all potentially toxic solutes found in tap water. Before being treated with reverse osmosis, tap water needs pretreatment. In brief, the media filter just after the water tank removes large particulate matter from tap water. The softener is the means for removing calcium and other hard salts from the water: it does this by exchanging sodium ions for the hard ions and therefore requires a source of high-concentration sodium provided from the brine tank. Charcoal filtration removes chlorine, chloramines and various organics from water: since the risk to the patient of chlorine or chloramine exposure is potentially fatal, commonly two carbon filters are placed in series. Screen filtration removes small particulate matter including any carbon particles released from the carbon tanks. The pretreated water undergoes RO, and in this process about ½ the water inflow is rejected to the drain. The RO-treated water, called the permeate, is then distributed to the dialysis unit machines (and reuse unit if present). In ideal design, the distribution loop of pipes is a closed system so that unused permeate returns to the water reservoir or to some other point in the circuit

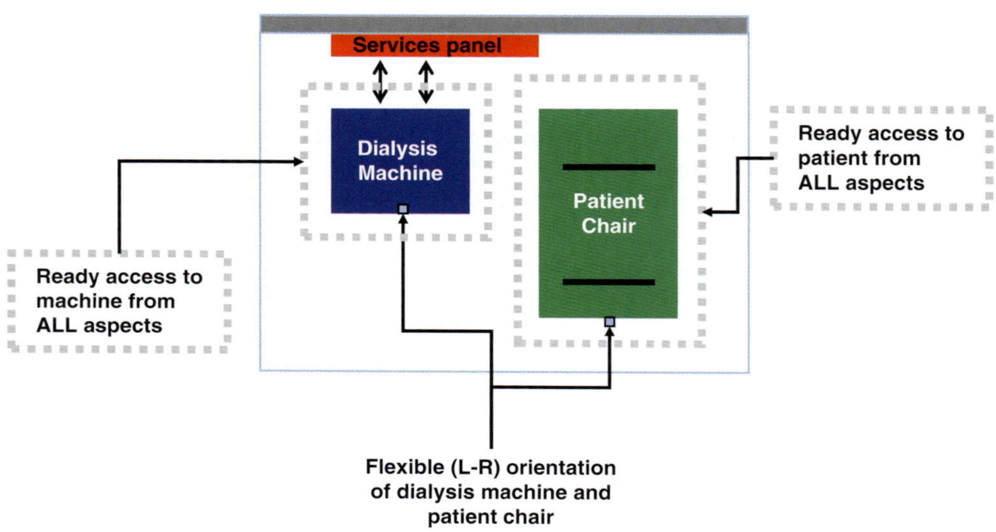

Fig. 58.3 A typical HD station layout. Ten square metres should be allowed for each station. Ideally the HD machine could be plugged into service panels which house circulating water and drainage points

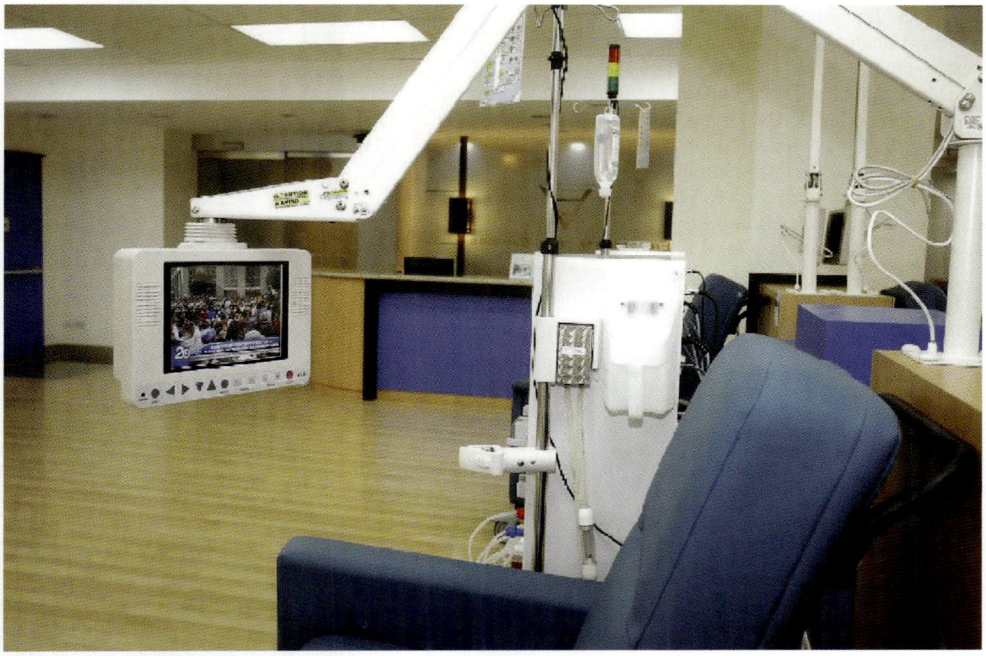

Fig. 58.4 Personal AV system. Within the patients' reach should be controls for audiovisual entertainment with individual headsets in consideration of neighbour patients. Digital channels should be available and Wi-Fi should also be freely available for patient use

with chairs which allow the connection of pedalling machines (cycles). This is a convenient exercise source when movement of the upper limbs may be somewhat restricted by vascular access.

Chairs or beds? Chairs are generally preferred to beds for the following reasons:

Beds	Chairs
Wrong message "I am sick"	Correct message "I am awake and active"
Immobile	Mobile and flexible
Cumbersome	Adjustable posture
Too low (OHS)	Easily cleaned between treatments
Difficult to clean	

Haemodialysis Machines

While the basic principles of HD have changed little since the 1960s, the technologies employed, the reliability and the software 'intelligence' of dialysis machines have improved greatly. There are a number of internationally recognised manufacturers each with its own branding regarding appearance and functionality. However, all will meet international safety standards for Class 2 medical devices. Most will be volumetric or flowmetric controlled to allow prescription of fluid removal (ultrafiltration) during the dialysis session. Most will employ bicarbonate buffer dialysis fluid, and the machines will be designed in a fail-safe manner regarding correctness of temperature and dialysis fluid conductivity (a surrogate for sodium concentration). Dialysis fluid will be switched into bypass in the event of failure to supply it within strict preset parameters.

A significant advance in membrane technology took place 25 years ago, and much more porous membranes can now be produced. As a result of mass production, the costs of each individual dialyser have reduced such that for each individual session the costs of disposables are often less than staffing costs. One of the opportunities provided by porous membranes is the ability to add convection to the basic diffusive process of dialysis so producing a broader spectrum of molecular removal. This process known as haemodiafiltration (HDF) has gained popularity particularly in Europe and the Far East. Nowadays, there is very little cost differential if any between HDF and diffusive dialysis.

Infection Control

Infection control has to take centre stage in the design of the HD unit. Integrated hand wash stations need to be placed strategically around the unit to make it easy for staff to access them easily between interventions. Hands-free technology with careful attention to the materials used for services is essential nowadays (Fig. 58.5). Discipline applied to hygiene and handwashing can have a dramatic impact on the overall performance of a HD centre from the infection control point of view, and embedding a culture that no nosocomial infection is acceptable, is critical.

Haemodialysis Schedule

Over the last two decades, there has been a convergence of practice such that the great majority of patients worldwide have three

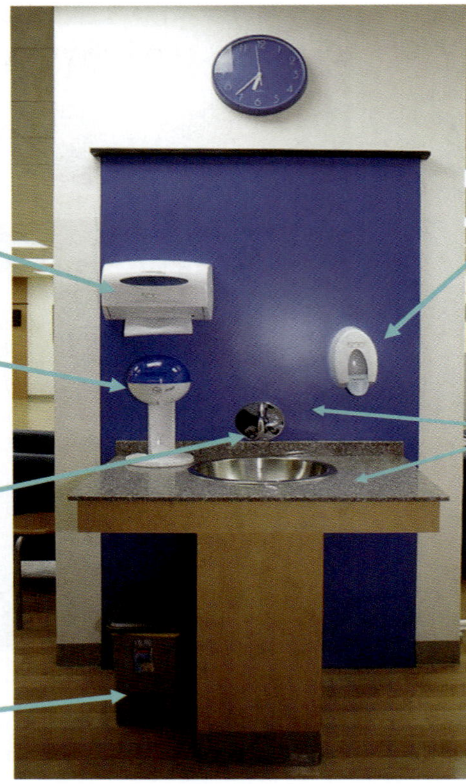

Fig. 58.5 Integrated handwash system. Infection control has to take centre stage in the design of the HD unit. Integrated handwash stations need to be placed strategically around the unit to make it easy for staff to access them easily between interventions. Hands-free technology with careful attention to the materials used for services is essential nowadays

sessions of dialysis weekly for approximately 4 h as the basis of their care. All measures of adequacy are derived around thrice weekly treatment. In recent years, evidence has emerged that there is an increased risk of hospitalisation after the 2-day break which is inherent in this schedule [1]. More frequent dialysis can abolish this risk, and the Frequent Haemodialysis Network (FHN) study [2] showed cardiac risk benefits in 'daily' dialysis but the optimum prescription if not yet clear [3]. Frequent dialysis in-centre is costly, and as a result there has been a resurgence of interest in self-care 'home' dialysis to allow more patients the opportunity to improve their health prospects by more frequent sessions. There has also been a recognition that patient involvement in their own care has psychological benefits. It may be prudent therefore to include an area in the renal centre for training in self-care for patients motivated to become self-sufficient with a view to making the transition to 'home dialysis'. Adjustments in staff skill mix may be required to facilitate self-care training. In a number of centres, upwards of 15 % haemodialysis patients are now self-caring and accessing 'extended dialysis'.

Staffing

Among all medical specialties, it was probably when maintenance haemodialysis for end-stage renal failure became established in the 1960s that true multi-professional working started to happen. Nurses and managers started working shoulder to shoulder with doctors and later with other health professionals to support the complex requirements of patients with this disease. Team working survives as the critical component in the matrix of skills required in a haemodialysis unit.

Within the multi-professional team in the HD centre, there should be clear leadership and accountability. The aim should be to provide a service which is patient centred with emphasis on continuous quality improvement and continuing professional development of the staff.

Direct Patient Care Staff

Direct patient care (DPC) staff initiate, oversee and disconnect patients from the HD treatment. Up to four patients per one DPC staff member would be a typical ratio. The following groups are represented:

1. Registered nurses – RNs
2. Clinical support workers – CSW
3. Patient care technicians
4. Dialysis assistants

Registered Nurses

RNs to CSW ratio varies across countries, some being able to staff their facilities with 100 % RNs. RN duties (Fig. 58.6) include:

- Patient assessment and documentation
- Dialysis prescription – dose, UF and drugs
- Connection including anticoagulation

- Patient assessment and intervention during HD
- Identify significant adverse events
- Discharge documentation

Clinical Support Workers

CSW duties include:

- Prescription – dose, UF and drugs
- Connection including anticoagulation
- Patient assessment and intervention during HD
- Identify significant adverse events
- Discharge documentation
- Machine setup
- Safety checks
- Some of RN duties according to competencies

In addition to the duties listed above, direct patient care staff have wider responsibilities including quality assurance and administration (Fig. 58.7). The lead nurse will typically have to deal with the staff rota, sickness, the use of bank and agency nurses but will also have to have budgetary accountability and will oversee capacity, new referrals and transfers in and out of the unit. Registered nurses typically will have weekly quality assurance meetings with nephrologists and will also be involved in transport issues and arranging holidays for patients to other units.

RN duties include:

- Patient assessment and documentation
- Dialysis prescription – dose, UF, drugs
- Connection including anticoagulation
- Patient assessment, interventions during HD
- Identify significant adverse events
- Disconnection
- Discharge documentation

CSW duties include:

- Machine set-up
- Safety checks
- Re-use
- Some of RN duties according to competencies

Fig. 58.6 Direct patient care staff initiate, oversee and disconnect patients from the HD treatment. Figure shows registered nurses (*RNs*) and clinical support worker (*CSW*) duties

Equipment Technicians

Technicians may be employed directly by the HD provider or outsourced. A pool of technicians may support a group of facilities rather than being assigned to one clinic and would typically need one full-time equipment technician per 150 patients. In some countries, technical clinical support workers assist with machine setup, tear down, inventory, stores and other duties. Technicians' responsibilities include:

1. Machine maintenance/repair
2. Water treatment plant – chemical and microbiological surveillance
3. Equipment procurement
4. Supplies/storage
5. Health and safety

Indirect Patient Care Staff (Fig. 58.8)

Dieticians

Ideally should be 0.75 WTE per 100 HD patients. The role of the dietician typically extends into pre-dialysis clinics and inpatient care. Duties include general surveillance, intradialytic nutrition and overseeing bone mineral metabolism.

Social Work/Counsellor

Depression and relationship problems are common in HD patients as are issues regarding housing and finance. As the dialysis population ages and becomes generally more frail, withdrawal from dialysis and other end-of-life issues are assuming greater and greater importance. One may typically

Lead Nurse, duties include:

- Staff roster
- Sickness
- Use of bank and agency nurses
- Budgetary accountability
- Capacity, new referrals, transfers in/out

RN, duties include:

- Weekly QA meeting with nephrologist (15 patients discussed)
    - *Mineral bone metabolism, review binders, vitamin D, cinacalcet*
    - *Anaemia management*
    - *Dialysis prescription, solute and volume control, residual renal fn*
    - *Vascular access status*
    - *Transplant status*
- Transport
- Holiday dialysis

Fig. 58.7 In addition, direct patient care staff have wider responsibilities including quality assurance and administration. The lead nurse will typically have to deal with the staff rota, sickness, the use of bank and agency nurses but will also have to have budgetary accountability and will oversee capacity, new referrals and transfers in and out of the unit. Registered nurses typically will have weekly quality assurance meetings with nephrologists and will also be involved in transport issues and arranging holidays for patients to other units

Dieticians
- 0.75 FTE for 100 patients
- Role extends into pre-dialysis clinic and in-patient care
- General suveillance, intradialytic nutrition, bone-mineral metabolism

Social Work, Counselling
- 0.5 FTE for 100 patients
- Depression, relationship problems
- Housing, financial issues
- Withdrawal from dialysis
- End-of-life issues

Clinical Educators (usually RNs)
- 0.5 FTE for 100 patients
- Procedures and protocols –disseminate good practice
- Training new staff
- Clinical governance

Vascular Access Co-ordinator
- 1 FTE per 300 HD patients
- Liason between surgeons, nephrologists and RNs

Fig. 58.8 Indirect patient care staff ratios, roles and duties

expect 0.5 WTE social work and counselling personnel per 100 HD patients.

Clinical Educators (Usually RNs)

This group of staff produce procedures and protocols, and their duty includes dissemination of good practice. Their central role is training new staff and involvement in clinical governance. A typical expectation is 0.5 FTE clinical educators for 100 HD patients.

Vascular Access Coordinator

Establishing and maintaining good vascular access are critical to successful rehabilitation on HD. It is a highly specialised area, and it has been common place for a liaison person to work between the HD patients, the dialysis facility and the vascular surgeons and radiologists who are involved in this work. One might see 1 WTE per 300 HD patients.

Clinical Governance

Scope of Clinical Governance

Outcome measures and data sharing are part and parcel of the modern era.

This is a central responsibility of the whole multi-professional team in the HD centre. It involves all staff, and it should assume a central place in timetabling activities. The components of clinical governance are summarised in Fig. 58.9. The whole process is ideally lead by a team representing the major disciplines. The lead clinician and lead nurse must be involved, and there should also be representation of management and allied health professionals. Clinical audit involves the critical appraisal of data which is gathered in any area of dialysis practice.

- Clinical governance team, responsible for cascading information
  - *Lead Clinician*
  - *Lead Nurse*
  - *Lead Manager*
  - *Allied Health Professional*
- Clinical audit
  - *Monthly presentations: all team members invited*
  - *Programme reviewed 6 monthly*
  - *Attendance record for yearly appraisal*
- Clinical effectiveness
  - *Performance against guidelines*
  - *Data submission to national registry*
  - *Check patient pathways fit for purpose*
- Risk management
  - *Risk register review and prioritisation*
  - *Key staff trained to perform risk assessments*
  - *Infection control/manual handling/agression/fire*
- Serious untoward incidents – Root cause analysis
- Complaints and complements
- Status of staff education and development
- Patient and public involvement

Fig. 58.9 The components of clinical governance. Clinical governance is a central responsibility of the whole multi-professional team in the HD centre. It involves all staff, and it should assume a central place in timetabling activities

Appraisal Process

An important component of clinical governance is the appraisal process. It is important that each HD staff member knows his or her line manager and that there is a yearly review of competence and career progression which would include a review of objectives from the previous year, identifying gaps in knowledge and reviewing attendance at education and audit meetings. Training needs should be identified, and agree objectives and milestones for the coming year should be agreed. This is essentially a contract between the appraiser and appraisee.

Clinical Guidelines

Development

The National Kidney Foundation (NKF) in the United States responded to the poor outcomes in haemodialysis in the 1980s and early 1990s by embarking on the ground-breaking 'Dialysis Outcomes Quality Initiative'. The DOQI guidelines were published in 1997. The interest in standard setting through guidelines was extended to include other aspects of chronic kidney disease through KDIGO [4]. Similar initiatives took place in many countries with the result that expected standards are widely available and provide a useful backdrop to maintaining the quality of haemodialysis care in day-to-day practice.

Comparative Audit

The audit cycle includes comparison of performance against known guidelines, identifying areas for improvement and documentation of progress made. There would be key topics which would be repeatedly audited. One good example of this would be review of infection rates within the unit and route cause analysis of serious infective episodes. Different professional groups can usefully be invited to present their findings to colleagues. A snapshot of the 'rolling' monthly audit programme at the Lister Renal Unit is illustrated in Fig. 58.10 together with the reporting of *Staph. aureus* bacteraemias (Fig. 58.11).

The audit process can usefully benchmark the HD unit's performance against neighbouring facilities or renal centres within the same group. Comparative audit is an effective tool in identifying shortcomings and in motivating improvement in team performance.

Protocols and Procedures

It has become a necessary part of medical practice to carry out interventions according to clearly written protocols and procedures. Any new haemodialysis service needs to have these in place, visible and easily referenced by all staff.

Presentations by MDT members:

- Care of tunelled lines, line locks
- Usefulness on sodium profiling
- Review transition from unfractionated to LMW heaparin
- Review of bacteraemias in HD patients
- Early experience with cinacalcet for PTH control, revue budget
- Evaluation of button-hole needling technique
- Audit of patient dependency in HD patients
- Hepatitis vaccination programme
- Eating during HD
- Water quality – outcomes and review sampling protocols
- Privacy and dignity in the HD unit

Fig. 58.10 A snapshot of the 'rolling' monthly audit programme at the Lister Renal Unit

National and International Benchmarks

Many countries now have well-established 'renal' registries with high levels of participation and data submission by renal centres. Deviations from the norm of many measurable outcomes can be identified so allowing comparative audit and learning. Easily downloaded biochemical and haematological measures often comprise the bulk of the data, but useful variations of uptake onto the different forms of dialysis, hospitalisation and transplant rates also appear.

While there had been a convergence in the practice of regular HD worldwide with most patients being prescribed between 3.5- and 4-h treatments thrice weekly, there remain large differences in patient survival and other outcomes. Some may be explained by differences in genetic/environmental susceptibility to harm associated with ESRF much of this is likely to result from practice differences. This was the starting point for the hugely successful Dialysis Outcomes and Practice Patterns Study (DOPPS) coordinated by the University of Michigan since the late 1990s. Data from renal centres in 15 countries constitutes a huge and impressive learning resource from which both local and national policy changes have resulted over the years. DOPPS has primarily focussed in in-centre haemodialysis.

Concluding Remarks

Emerging as a new practical means of maintaining life after the onset of ESRD in a few affluent countries in the 1960s, maintenance haemodialysis is now practiced worldwide. It remains an expensive undertaking, but its success ensures that it is included in the planning of many health services including those in emerging countries. Much experience has been accumulated about the design and quality requirements

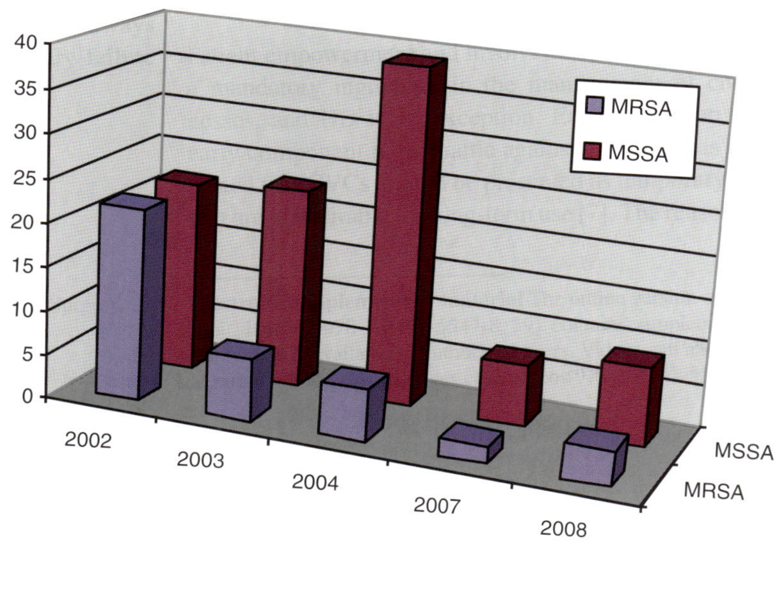

Fig. 58.11 Reporting of *Staphylococcus aureus* bacteraemias at the Lister Renal Unit between 2002 and 2008

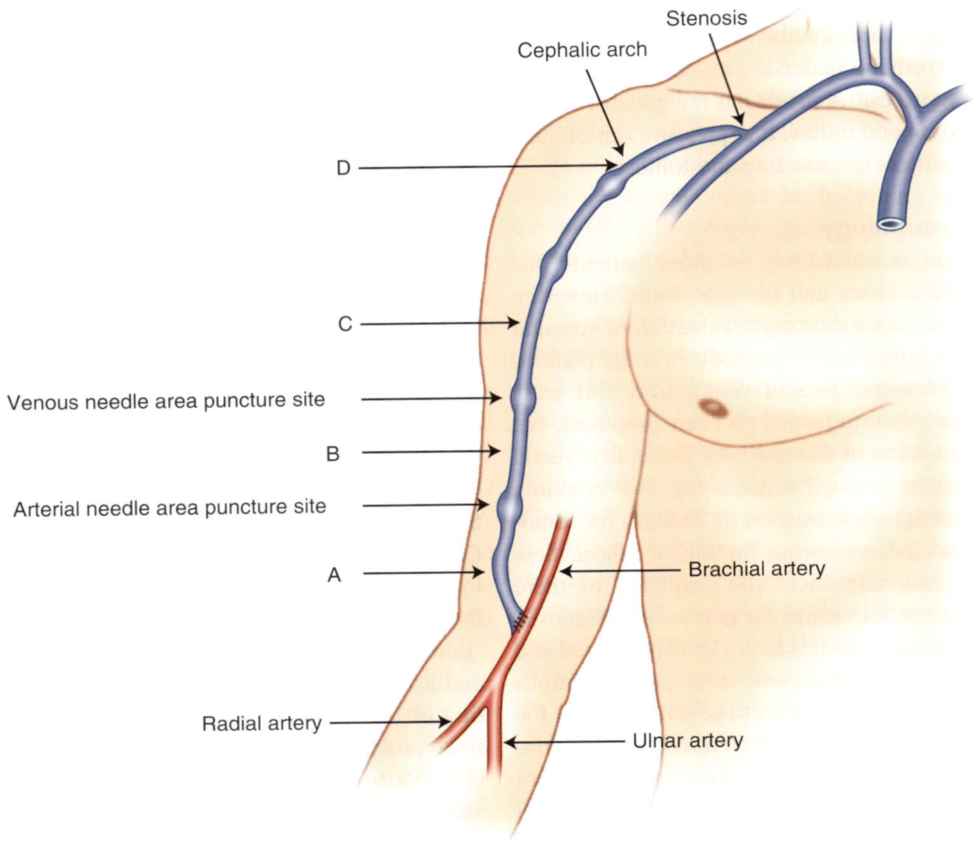

Fig. 59.2 Anatomy of an AVF including needling sites and a cephalic arch stenosis

safety factors notwithstanding, it may be prudent to delay RRT until definitive access can be obtained [12]. PD can be a very useful tool in the battle to avoid CVCs, even in those patients that present at a late stage of their CKD, and should be a consideration at all stages of the RRT patient journey. Lastly, AVG may be a useful method of obtaining definitive vascular access, even in those requiring urgent HD initiation.

It would be ideal if acute PD could be offered to patients who present with advanced CKD requiring urgent RRT. This is probably most frequently achieved following HD via a temporary line, after which PD catheter insertion is carried out as a local anaesthetic (LA) or general anaesthetic (GA) procedure. Immediacy of use is essential, and the preferred approach is either percutaneous medical or laparoscopic insertion. The pneumoperitoneum required for laparoscopic insertion will predictably place a higher demand on the anaesthesia team. The technique requires the PD catheter to be placed through an 8 mm trocar that has been passed obliquely through the abdominal wall as well as following a long pre-peritoneal course. This affords a seal which will allow low-volume exchanges to commence immediately. Patients that cannot have a GA, if not too obese, can have the procedure done under LA, and this requires some practical surgical attention to detail to maximise the likelihood of this being immediately usable.

Late-presenting patients not suitable for acute PD will have either a CVC or an AVG for immediate dialysis, which very much depends upon unit policy, and appropriately trained personnel.

The common upper limb sites for AVG are the forearm loop and the straight brachio-axillary graft (BAG) – options 1.6a and 1.6b respectively, in Fig. 59.1. The majority of cases need either a GA or a regional anaesthetic (RA) in the form of either an axillary or supraclavicular arm block. Even after RA block, placement of a brachio-axillary graft often requires local top-up LA infiltration to anaesthetise the proximal incision which is unavoidably made through the territory of the intercostobrachial nerve. A forearm loop has the advantage that it may be undertaken under RA.

Graft technology is moving on rapidly. It is a general belief that an AVG cannot be utilised for 2 weeks, following which the haemostatic rind will have formed appropriately

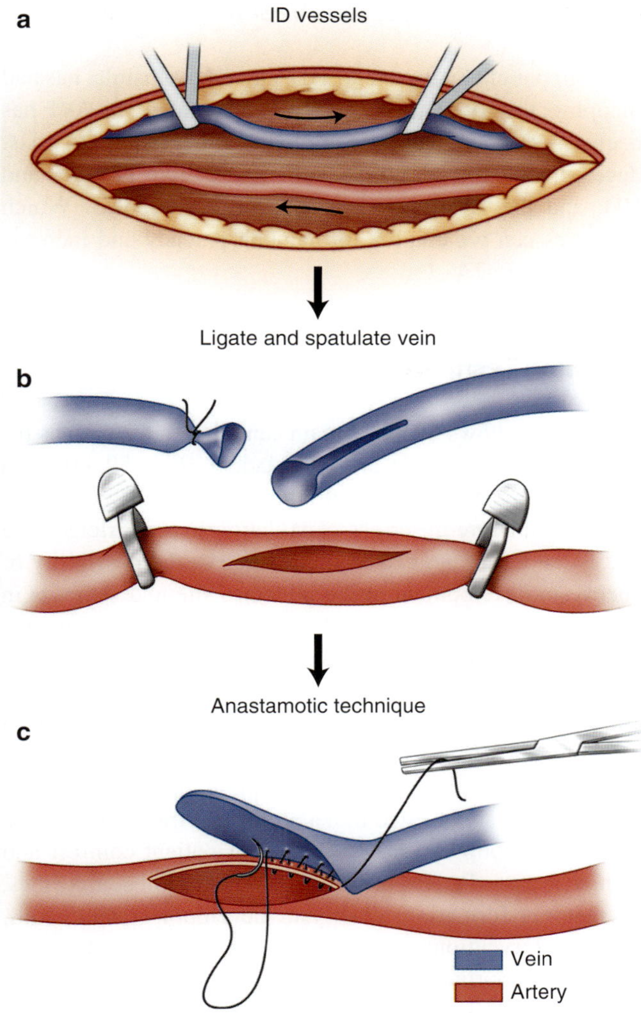

Fig. 59.3 Surgical techniques during AVF creation

and the post-operative subcutaneous oedema will have resolved thereby permitting palpation of the graft. However, it is the surgical author's practice to use AVG immediately, encouraging very oblique cannulation with ultrasound guidance to ensure that there are no failed puncture attempts, i.e. only two punctures per dialysis session. Great care is required post decannulation to press exactly over the point at which the needle enters the graft. This practice will reduce the number of patients requiring a temporary CVC when presenting with an unsalvageable access.

Surgeons anastomosing a forearm loop graft onto a vein at the antecubital fossa do so in the hope that the vein will then arterialise. This could be a cephalic vein, basilic vein or as a last resort one of the brachial artery vena comitans as listed in Fig. 59.1 (option 1.6a). Future thrombosis/failure and unsuccessful salvage of the forearm graft may then permit the immediate anastomosis of the previously arterialised downstream vein onto the brachial artery, and the fistula may be needled immediately. Similarly if the graft has been anastomosed to the deeper veins, these can be superficialised, joined to the brachial artery and in some cases needled immediately. In cases with only a short distance of arterialisation, possibly as a result of multiple tributaries, alternative access will be needed whilst further maturation takes place.

Leg loops are associated with a much higher risk of infection because they are being needled below the level of both the waste as well as the waist. The key word of caution for any surgeon putting these in is to assume that a proportion of leg loops will need to be taken out. For this reason, it is always important to anastomose them to the superficial femoral artery (SFA) rather than the common femoral artery (CFA). This means that if entire graft removal is mandated for early sepsis, ligation of a mycotic superficial femoral artery can be effected, with lower likelihood of limb loss than would be associated with ligation of the more proximal common femoral artery above the origin of the profunda femoris.

Patients who require new vascular access mandating anaesthetic input will by definition be well advanced in their access career. The factors that contribute to traditional native AV access failure will also be those that make anaesthesia challenging. Nephrologists should always plan ahead and wherever possible ensure that the HD patient is as biochemically stable and as euvolaemic as possible in a timely fashion. New access attempts are probably best performed electively wherever possible. Communicating with your anaesthetists and surgeons is vital.

Assisted Patency

Primary failure of an autogenous AVF, defined as an access that never provided reliable HD postsurgical creation, occurs in up to 50 % of cases [4]. Access which is patent but unusable for successful HD (non-functional) is frustrating for patients, surgeons and nephrologists alike, but measures can be undertaken to maximise success rates, thereby ensuring durable AVFs are ready for cannulation at an appropriate time for HD initiation.

Primary patency is often defined as the time interval between access placement and intervention to maintain or re-establish patency following failure or thrombosis. Assisted patency is the use of endovascular/surgical measures to maintain patency prior to thrombosis, and secondary patency can be defined as the interval from the access creation until access abandonment [13]. The increase in blood flow that characterises a developing AVF is often apparent in the first 2 weeks, and inadequate AVF maturation often relates to insufficient arterial inflow or non-ligated side branches [14]. The American Vascular Surgery guidelines recommend monitoring of new access at 4 weeks to ensure patency and appropriate maturation, and if not, then intervention should be considered [15]. This requires an individualised approach but usually includes (1) duplex scanning, (2) radiological angioplasty or (3) surgical intervention such as revision using one of the techniques in this chapter or a very simple tributary ligation. Following this algorithm, 92 % of non-functional access became usable [16].

In addition, if the access is too deep (>1 cm), it is also rendered non-functional. In our experience, access needs to be clinically assessed within 48 h post-operatively and is then assessed at weekly intervals, often with the adjunct of portable ultrasound to assess vessel diameter and depth. If the access is not maturing successfully, fistulography is performed with a view to correcting inflow/outflow stenoses if present and technically feasible. Other potential corrective measures are discussed first at a multidisciplinary team meeting.

First Use

The optimal timing of the initial AVF cannulation is not known. Traditionally, an experienced dialysis nurse/nephrologist assessed a fistula and deemed it to be suitable for first use if it was sufficiently palpable and had a relatively straight venous segment of sufficient length (10 cm) for two needles, an adequate diameter for needle insertion (>4 mm) and a uniform thrill to palpation [17]. It became common practice to delay cannulation to allow AVF to mature further. However, as discussed, AVFs that are going to mature usually do so within the first 2–4 weeks, failure is often due to anatomical reasons, and watchful, hopeful waiting is often not going to alter maturation by itself.

There is often a major concern that inappropriate cannulation may predispose to access failure due to thrombosis or extrinsic compression from haematoma/infection. However, the DOPPS study demonstrated that early cannulation (<4 weeks) in Japanese units was not associated with access failure [18].

If early cannulation is deemed desirable, factors such as clinical examination, vessel diameter and depth are all considered. Only experienced dialysis nurses, often with the use of ultrasound, will cannulate at an early stage in our unit, and the ensuing HD session will take place with reduced blood pump speeds and measures to prevent intradialytic hypotension in order to reduce the thrombosis risk.

Although there is no 'right answer', there is a clear mandate that cannulation before 6 weeks may be both successful and advantageous particularly if the patient is receiving HD via a CVC. Reducing exposure to CVC complications will always be beneficial.

Maintaining the Current Vascular Access

So, your patient has opted for HD, agreed to a fistula, has had mapping; the AV anastomosis has been created; the AVF has been assessed and has had radiological intervention to assist development; the AVF is of sufficient calibre to withstand HD; and the AVF has been successfully needled. Which measures can we employ to maintain patency and increase AVF longevity?

Needling Technique

Figure 59.4 shows the three main cannulation techniques for vascular access. These are rope ladder (Fig. 59.4a), area puncture (Fig. 59.4b) and buttonholing (Fig. 59.4c).

Area puncture describes cannulation in a restricted area and is the least favoured technique due to the possibility of aneurysm development at the puncture site and stenoses in adjacent areas. The rope-ladder technique (needling is progressively moved up and down the length of the fistula) is widespread across the UK and has been utilised since the 1980s with the intention of reducing aneurysm development.

Buttonholing, a technique only applied to AVF, in which blunt needles are inserted into a preformed tract, has become increasingly popular due to reports of patient comfort and technical ease. Patient cannulation anxiety, bleeding times, haematoma formation, aneurysm development and radiological interventions were all reduced in buttonholed AVF [19]. It is important to note that the incidence of infection in buttonholed AVF may be higher and meticulous aseptic procedures are required. It is also important to note that AVG should only be cannulated by the rope ladder technique in order to avoid weakening the AVG integrity.

Monitoring - the Physical Examination

Vascular access monitoring and surveillance are common components of any strategy to minimise thrombosis and thereby maintain AVF/G patency and are often used interchangeably. However, monitoring is the evaluation of the vascular access by physical examination to detect signs that suggest the presence of dysfunction, and surveillance is the periodic evaluation of the vascular access by using tests that may involve special instrumentation and for which an abnormal test result suggests the presence of dysfunction [11].

Physical examination is an extremely important component of vascular access care [20]. As previously discussed, the development of successful access can often be predicted from the physical examination by experienced dialysis nurses [17]. So, how should a fistula be examined?

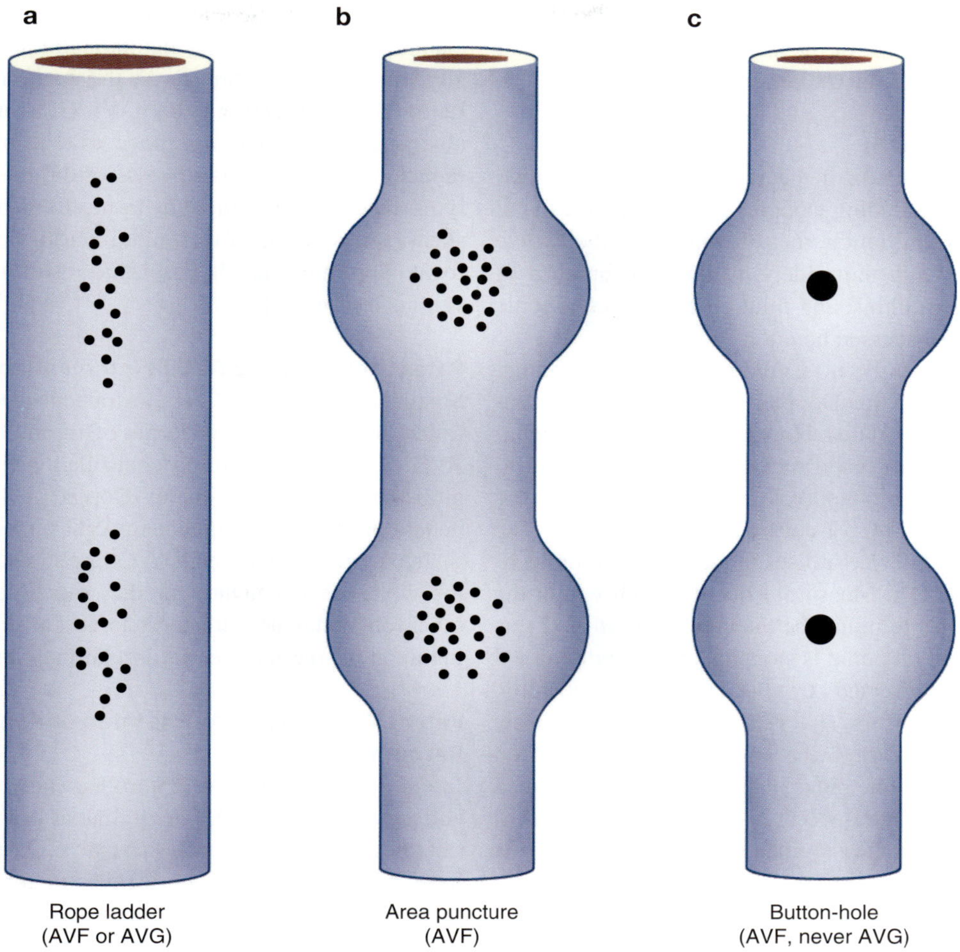

Fig. 59.4 Access cannulation techniques: (**a**) rope ladder (**b**) area puncture (**c**) button-hole

A normal mature AVF has a soft pulse and is easily compressible. There is a palpable thrill and/or audible bruit throughout the length of the fistula as well as throughout the cardiac cycle. When the extremity is elevated, the AVF will usually partially collapse.

With inflow stenosis, the access may be flat and collapse excessively upon elevation. There may also be palpable stenoses in the juxta-anastomotic area. The thrill may be weak, the bruit may be high pitched, or the pulse may be weak or difficult to compress in the juxta-anastomotic or cannulation areas.

In contrast, an outflow stenosis is recognised with the following features: (1) arm swelling, (2) no partial vein collapse upon arm elevation, (3) palpation of stenotic segments in the venous region beyond the cannulation area and (4) abnormal thrill/bruit/pulse (weak and/or discontinuous bruit with only a systolic component or a weak or resistant pulse that is difficult to compress) in the venous region beyond the cannulation area [20].

With experience, it is therefore possible to use physical examination as the first step in the identification of inflow/outflow dysfunction, which when combined with a full fistula history will inform the clinician as to whether a radiological or a surgical solution is required.

Surveillance

There is considerable controversy regarding access surveillance. The basic tenet is that the longevity of thrombosed but rescued access is shorter than the long-term patency of a patent, yet stenosed access that undergoes angioplasty [11]. It is therefore proposed that surveillance would allow the detection of subclinical stenoses with haemodynamic significance, thereby leading to judicious endovascular intervention, resulting in fewer incidences of thrombosis and therefore greater access longevity.

Interventions to remedy subclinical stenoses, either through surgical or endovascular means, are associated with patient morbidity, require experienced vascular surgeons or interventional radiologists and can be expensive. Therefore, we will now discuss some of the techniques, advantages and disadvantages of access surveillance.

Intra-access Flow (QA)

There are several methods of measuring intra-access blood flow (QA, ml/min) including Doppler ultrasound, ultrasound dilution, haematocrit dilution, thermal dilution and effective ionic dialysance. Only the widely available techniques of Doppler ultrasound, ultrasound dilution and effective ionic dialysance will be discussed here.

Vessel diameter can be measured with duplex scanning, and when combined with Doppler-derived velocity, intra-access flow can be calculated. However, it should be emphasised that Doppler ultrasound measurements are subject to operator error, turbulent blood flow and variability in the cross-sectional area of the vascular access.

The Transonic™ device utilises ultrasound dilution techniques to measure QA. Measurements are taken within the first hour of dialysis to minimise the effects of reduced cardiac output. The blood pump is stopped, and the arterial and venous lines are reversed from their normal position. Photometric flow sensors attached to an electronic flow metre are then clipped onto the reversed lines. The blood pump is restarted, a saline bolus is injected into the reversed venous line, and the intra-access blood flow is calculated. The error of duplicate measurements in the same patient is small, but the technique requires dedicated, expensive equipment and interrupts the delivered HD therapy [20, 21].

Ionic dialysance techniques can be used to measure QA. Access recirculation results in a dilution of the urea content of the dialyser arterial line and is inversely proportional to QA. It has since been validated that needle reversal, without injection of diluents, can measure QA by observing the effect on dialysate urea concentrations, a technique known as effective ionic dialysance (EID) [22]. This has been successfully validated against the Transonic™ device and has the advantage of being cheap, reproducible, non-operator dependent and easily performed in a busy dialysis unit.

Is Access Surveillance Useful?

Access guidelines recommend monthly measurement of access flow in AVF and AVG. Angiography is recommended if intra-access flow in AVF decreased to <500 ml/min or >20 % from baseline or if AVG flow <650 ml/min or >20 % from baseline [23].

The question remains, does access surveillance ultimately result in reduced access thrombosis and increased access longevity or just predict angiographically identified stenoses with attendant morbidity and over-zealous intervention? The data is conflicting, often based on non-randomised studies using different access surveillance techniques in a mixture of fistulas and grafts.

Early and late access failure is often due to different anatomical reasons. Early fistula maturation failure is usually due to inflow stenosis at the juxta-anastomotic site. Late failure of autogenous AVF/G is usually, but not always, due to the appearance of outflow stenoses that reduce flow and increase the risk of thrombosis. The underlying mechanism is thought to be the marked increase in shear stress in the thin-walled outflow vein, triggering focal fibromuscular hyperplasia resulting in a fibrotic venous lesion [24].

Patent Yet Stenosed AVG: Is Intervention Useful?

Small studies initially demonstrated successful outcomes following angioplasty in terms of thrombosis reduction in AVG [25], but randomised controlled trials utilising either ultrasound dilution or duplex Doppler US did not show a benefit of access surveillance in AVG survival [26].

In our practice, although AVGs are subject to surveillance, the QA does not always predict subclinical stenosis, and other functional measurements are just as important in deciding upon the merits of endovascular intervention.

Patent Yet Stenosed AVF: Is Intervention Recommended?

In contrast, a prospective controlled study by Tessitore and colleagues utilising UDT and clinical examination in AVF did show increased access survival [27], and other studies have demonstrated that corrective treatment to haemodynamically significant stenoses improved patency and reduced thrombosis [28]. Although not a randomised controlled trial, a clinically relevant 5-year controlled cohort study in 197 mature AVF analysed the efficacy of clinical monitoring, QA surveillance and elective stenosis repair. AVF loss and access-related costs were significantly reduced, but these effects were only observed in the first 3 years after fistula maturation [29].

Intervention in all access without good cause to suggest access dysfunction does not appear to be recommended. Analysis of >40,000 patients with an AVG or AVF did not demonstrate an overall benefit at 12 months of routine access surveillance/angioplasty repair. However, in those patients with low QA or new access, angioplasty (as opposed to non-intervention) did improve access survival [30].

If a Subclinical Stenosis Is Suspected: What Next?

Once access dysfunction is suspected, the next step is often but not always an endovascular intervention. Informed consent is essential, and the risks of discomfort, bruising, contrast reactions (including effect on residual renal function), infection and vessel rupture should all be explained.

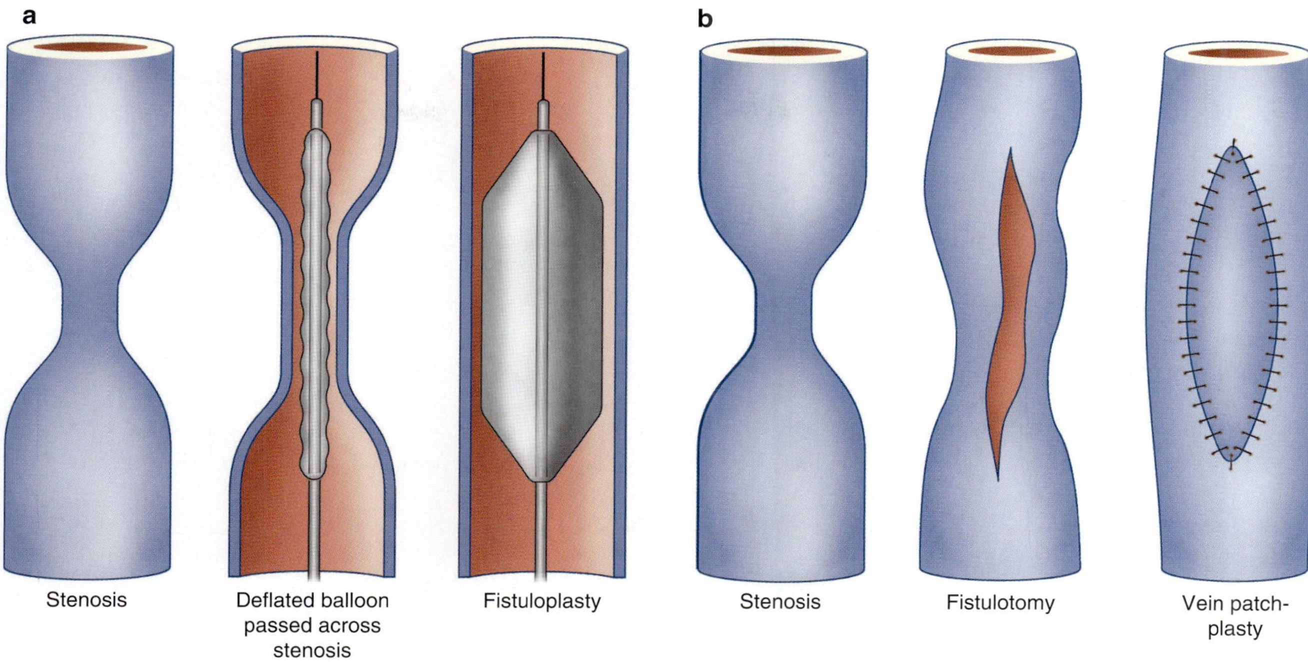

Fig. 59.5 (**a**) Fistuloplasty (**b**) surgical techniques to manage AVF stenoses

Complication rates are low; studies report vessel rupture and free perforation in <1 %. The surgical author suspects the incidence is higher having surgically explored a number of AVF following failed intervention and discovered defects in the fistula wall.

Percutaneous Fistuloplasty

A pathogenic stenosis is often defined as one which reduces the vessel diameter by >50 % thereby reducing the cross-sectional area by 75 %, the critical point at which blood flow is dramatically reduced [21]. Fistuloplasty is undertaken in a stepwise manner under aseptic conditions (Fig. 59.5a). The vascular access is entered percutaneously, the stenosis is identified with angiography, and conventional angioplasty balloons are inflated to dilate the stenosis. High inflation pressures are often required to overcome the fibrotic nature of the stenosis. After fistuloplasty, the remainder of the outflow and the central veins are imaged with venography. Surveillance tests should return to baseline following radiological intervention.

Other Endovascular Techniques to Maintain Access Patency

Newer technologies including cutting, high pressure and drug-eluting balloons are providing vascular radiologists with alternative tools to treat stenoses, but there is a lack of evidence to define their exact role in the treatment algorithm. They are often reserved for resistant lesions because of the increased likelihood of vessel rupture [31].

Bare-metal stents (BMS) should probably only be used in the treatment of resistant venous stenoses. A covered stent may be required to control an angioplasty-induced rupture. Stent placement for early recurrent stenosis (<6 months) in AVF and AVG doubled the interval between interventions. Stent grafts (a metal stent with PTFE covering the internal and/or external surface) may be very useful for failing or thrombosed access with resistant stenoses [32] or recurrent cephalic arch stenoses. However, there are risks to consider including stent migration/shortening/fracturing and the induction of intimal hyperplasia leading to recurrent stenosis.

Surgical Techniques to Maintain Patency

Peripheral stenoses that recur despite sequential fistuloplasties need a different approach. This can be with either a surgical patch fistuloplasty – also termed a patch venoplasty (Fig. 59.5b) – or a more complex surgical solution in the form of either a bypass (jump graft Fig. 59.6a) or re-routing (Fig. 59.6b). A good example of the latter is the cephalic vein 'turndown' for cephalic arch stenosis in which the fistula is divided upstream from the cephalic arch and anastomosed onto the axillary, brachial or basilic vein providing a low-resistance path back to the right atrium (Fig. 59.6b).

Juxta-anastomotic Stenosis

In radiocephalic AVF, 55–75 % of stenoses occur in the area just beyond the anastomosis (juxta-anastomotic) as shown in Fig. 59.7a. In native elbow AVFs, (brachiocephalic and

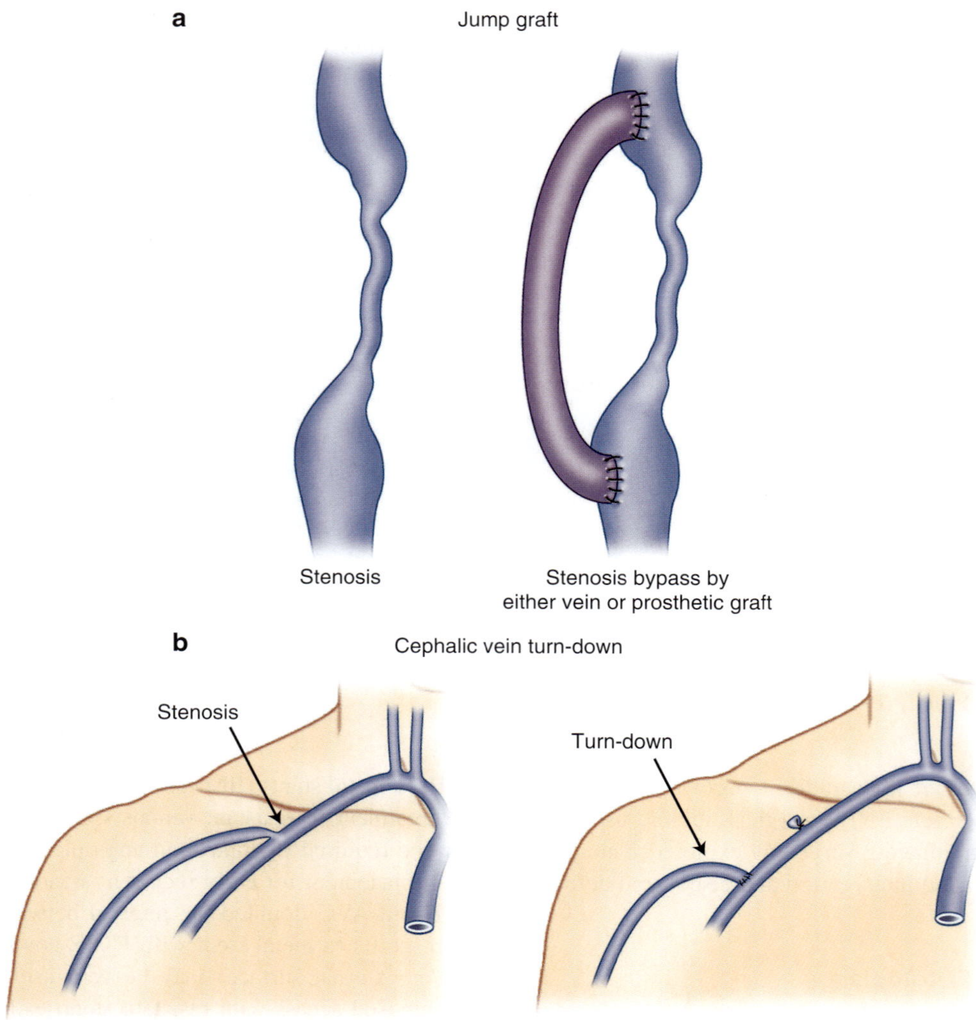

Fig. 59.6 Further surgical techniques to manage AVF complications: (**a**) jump graft (**b**) cephalic vein turn-down

brachiobasilic), 45 % of stenoses are juxta-anastomotic, and the remainder tend to be at the junction between the superficial and deep veins. In AVG, 85 % of the stenoses are found in the venous outflow region 2 cm downstream from the venous landing site of the prosthetic graft (Fig. 59.7d). Changes in the flow pattern as well as wall compliance mismatch are attributed to the cause of stenoses in these regions. Many of these can be treated in the first instance with fistuloplasty (Fig. 59.5a); however, a proportion of these will recur or be resistant to endovascular treatment and so should be treated with open surgery in the form of vein patch plasty (Figs. 59.5b and 59.7b) or proximalisation of the anastomosis (Fig. 59.7c).

No comparative studies exist between the endovascular and open treatments. If the puncture stretch is short, an endovascular approach is a justifiable first choice.

Access Monitoring and Surveillance: A Summary

To conclude, there is emerging data to support a tailored radiological/surgical intervention programme in individualised patients in order to maintain access patency and longevity. Our key recommendation is that all the available information is utilised in the decision to perform angioplasty in patent, yet failing access. This includes the physical examination; information on needling difficulties, i.e. difficult needle insertion; elevated venous/arterial pressures; and flow rates as well as information from surveillance tests. Recurrent lesions, particularly if recurring at a rapid rate, should be discussed in a multidisciplinary meeting, ideally with vascular interventional radiologists, nephrologists and vascular surgeons in order to ascertain a treatment plan that is individualised for the patient, their dialysis vintage, previous access attempts and anticipated access longevity.

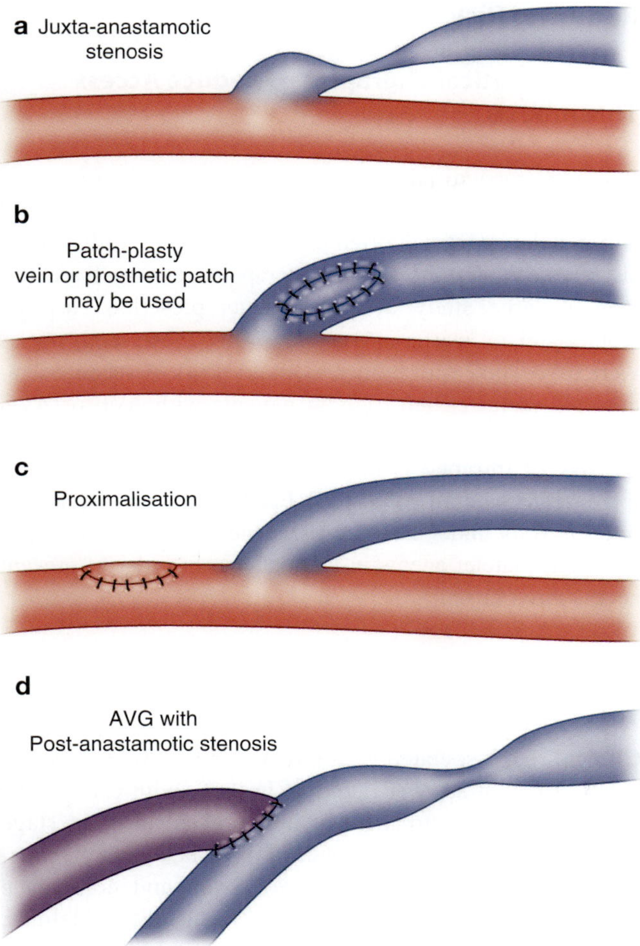

Fig. 59.7 Surgical techniques to manage juxta-anastomotic stenoses (**a**) a stenosed AVF (**b**) utilising native venous or prosthetic patch techniques (**c**) proximalising the venous circulation (**d**) an AVG with a post-anastomotic stenosis

Thrombosed Access

Unfortunately, despite physical examination and surveillance, thrombosis, either predictable or unpredictable, will still occur. The steps to attempt to rescue thrombosed access are as follows.

Recognition and Patient Safety

Thrombosed access is usually recognised by either the patient (no longer aware of a 'buzz' in their access) or by the dialysis unit staff (no thrill or bruit; clinical detection of thrombus or inability to cannulate the access). If patients are encouraged to check their access is buzzing on a daily basis, then it is wise to suggest that it is done in the morning rather than the evening! This will increase the likelihood that the access can be salvaged on the same day. Prompt action is required to prevent access and patient-related harm.

The first consideration is patient safety; the degree of fluid overload and the presence of hyperkalaemia should be identified, and if necessary, placement of a temporary CVC may be required for HD prior to attempted salvage. In addition, it is prudent to ascertain the presence of any thrombocytopenia and coagulopathy. Informed consent should be obtained for endovascular thrombectomy as well as angioplasty. The additional complications include risk of distal arterial thrombus if the anastomosis is involved and of pulmonary embolus (PE) (0–7 % reported). Most vascular radiologists and surgeons would accept that many patients undergoing radiological de-clotting of a fistula will have multiple subclinical, asymptomatic PEs. Particularly in those patients with poor cardiopulmonary reserve, it may be prudent to consider the potential impact of thromboembolism, but the literature and our experience appear to support the benefits of access salvage in the majority of cases.

Contraindications

Contraindications to thrombectomy are few. Immature AVFs that have never been cannulated are relatively poor candidates for de-clotting due to technical and anatomical factors and should be assessed on a case-by-case basis. Local infection may preclude thrombectomy due to the risks of sepsis from infected thrombi entering the circulation, but it is important to note that thrombosis frequently presents with localised erythema, pain and tenderness, and a senior opinion should be obtained in these circumstances. These signs and symptoms are almost always the result of a chemical phlebitis due to thrombosis rather than a bacterial, infective process.

Large aneurysms (in which thrombus extraction is technically more difficult and less likely to be complete) and huge clot burden (>100 ml) are relative contraindications due to the high risk of PE [32]. Other centres quote contraindications that include the presence of a right-to-left intracardiac shunt, pulmonary hypertension or surgical revision <30 days before intervention. Chronic thrombus is often hard on palpation, likely to be organised thrombus and less amenable to successful rescue thrombectomy. Ideally, access salvage should be attempted within 48 hours of thrombosis.

AVG thrombectomy has a higher success rate due to the absence of aneurysmal segments, and the synthetic graft material allows a more aggressive technical approach. The decision to attempt percutaneous thrombectomy rests between the patient, nephrologist, interventional radiologist and the surgeon.

Thrombectomy-Treatment Techniques

Techniques are highly dependent upon individual operators and centres, patient circumstances and equipment availability. The procedure is usually performed with patients fully monitored (pulse oximetry, blood pressure and continuous electrocardiography). Prophylactic antibiotics may or may not be required. Percutaneous thrombectomy involves three stages. Firstly, thrombus is removed, sometimes with a mechanical device; secondly, the cause of the thrombus, usually an outflow stenosis, is dealt with; and lastly, a fistulogram is performed from the arteriovenous anastomosis to the superior vena cava. Success rates vary according to the mechanical device that is utilised and the case mix that is attempted, but access patency is reported to be >80, >60 and >40 % at 30 days, 3 and 6 months, respectively. Other complications include puncture site haematomas, vessel dissection or rupture, infection and contrast reactions [32]. Some centres do not use mechanical devices but hope that once flow is re-established, autolysis occurs. If not, surgical thrombectomy should be considered. Intravenous heparin is a useful tool to clear residual thrombosis, and some centres recommend HD post-radiological thrombectomy [32]. These decisions should be individualised and undertaken by a senior clinician as the data is limited. Some centres routinely warfarinise patients for 6–12 months post-salvage of a thrombosed fistula.

Thrombolysis

Thrombolytic drugs alone have reduced in popularity as single agents for thrombosed access since the introduction of mechanical thrombectomy but remain a useful tool when combined with mechanical devices in maximising thrombus clearance and reducing procedural times [32, 33]. Urokinase and tissue plasminogen activator (tPA) can be used for infusion thrombolysis. Antegrade vascular access is obtained as close to the arteriovenous anastomosis as possible, and the thrombolytic drug is infused directly into the vascular access via a multiple side-hole catheter. Doses and infusion times vary (3–20 h). Usual contraindications to thrombolytic agents apply.

It is still not clear if a radiological or a surgical approach is best to deal with the thrombosed AVF or AVG. Clinical practice varies within each renal unit, and access to either experienced vascular radiologists or vascular surgeons probably dictates the preferred approach. It is likely that a combined approach is probably best with each patient undergoing fistulography in a combined theatre and angiography suite.

Maintaining vascular access is time-consuming but rewarding. However, it is important to accept that long-term patency is not guaranteed despite radiological/surgical intervention. In these circumstances, planning for new access whilst utilising the existing, failing access may be beneficial in some individualised patients in order to avoid CVCs. There is insufficient evidence to suggest any further generalisations.

Reducing Risk

Pharmaceutical Therapies to Reduce Access Thrombosis

It is well recognised that access thrombosis is associated with morbidity and hospitalisations. Anticoagulants and anti-platelet agents are often prescribed to prevent thrombosis, but the data supporting this therapeutic approach are limited. A large study of HD patients prescribed aspirin, clopidogrel or warfarin concluded that these medications were associated with higher mortality [34]. A recent meta-analysis evaluated ten trials in patients with AVF or AVG thrombosis and concluded that anti-platelet agents reduced the risk of thrombosis in AVF (but not AVG) without an increase in bleeding events [35]. Further trials are required in order to fully understand the risk/benefit ratio of anticoagulants/anti-platelet agents in HD patients in order to prevent access thrombosis.

Infection

Clinical risk associated with infected definitive access still exists, albeit at a lower rate than in those with CVCs. The usual approach is to identify infection at an early stage (erythema, tenderness, presence of pyrexia, etc. in the presence of negative blood cultures), swab and commence empirical antibiotic therapy as per local unit guidelines, which are then tailored to positive microbiology specimens. Prompt treatment is recommended as metastatic spread from AVF can still occur. The presence of aneurysms, infected thrombi or localised abscess formation may all increase the risk of AVF rupture, and early vascular surgical assessment is suggested as AVF ligation may be required [2].

As discussed previously, buttonholing may be advantageous but does appear to confer an elevated risk of infection. Meticulous care is required during cannulation, and infectious complications can be reduced following dialysis staff education [36]. Some centres use topical mupirocin ointment over buttonholes although data supporting this approach are limited.

Superficial AVG infection should be swabbed and treated promptly with broad-spectrum antibiotic therapy and then treatment should be tailored to the causative organism. More extensive AVG infection can lead to bacteraemia, sepsis and death, and a combined antibiotic and surgical approach is often required for complete resolution. Subclinical infection is a difficult problem, occurring in abandoned and non-functioning grafts. It may present with erythropoietin resistance or elevated C-reactive protein and may require specialist radiological imaging in order to identify the source

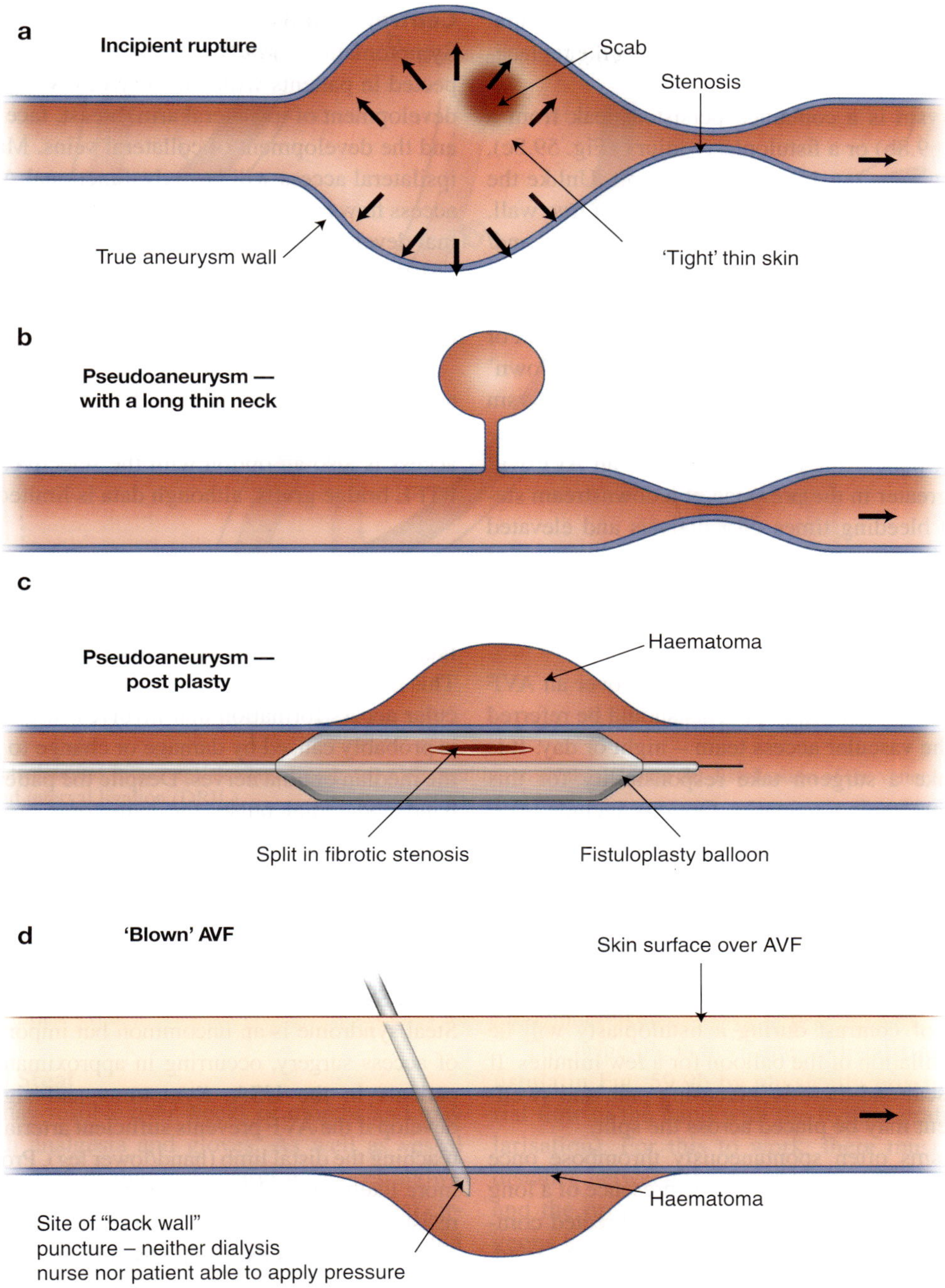

Fig. 59.8 Other AVF complications: (**a**) Incipient rupture in a true aneurysm (**b**) pseudoaneurysm post HD cannulation (**c**) pseudoaneurysm following fistuloplasty (**d**) haematoma formation following inadvertent puncture of the posterior aspect of the AVF wall

of the infection. AVG removal may be needed but can be difficult for technical reasons.

Mechanical Issues

The development of complications in an established AVF or AVG is predictable, and their management reflects an understanding of the basic rules of physics.

True Aneurysms, Pseudoaneurysms, Bleeding and Ruptures

A true aneurysm represents dilatation of all the layers of the arterial wall. This may occur in a patient with poorly controlled blood pressure with other vascular risk factors. Generalised thinning and stretching of the AVF wall will, according to Laplace's law, continue to result in further expansion (Fig. 59.8a). Usually, a pseudoaneurysm or false aneurysm will only form as a result of a downstream stenosis

radiologists and surgeons are essential components in the maintenance of vascular access.

Important Learning Points

- 'Fistulas first, lines last' culture should resonate throughout the dialysis unit.
- Patient education regarding vascular access including the risk/benefits of AVF versus CVCs should begin at an early stage.
- Patients should be referred for vascular access in a timely fashion.
- It is recommended that AVFs are placed in the forearm if anatomically and technically possible.
- Once definitive access is created, monitoring is essential, and failing to mature AVF should be considered for endovascular intervention or surgical revision.
- AVF should be monitored and subject to surveillance. The suspicion of failing access should prompt consideration of endovascular intervention with angioplasty.
- Insufficient data exists to recommend agents for preventing access-related thrombosis.
- Reducing vascular access morbidity is time-consuming but rewarding and is associated with a reduction in hospitalisations and mortality. Definitive vascular access provision requires communication and co-ordination amongst patients, dialysis unit staff, nephrologists, vascular radiologists, vascular surgeons and anaesthetists.

Acknowledgements With grateful thanks to Dr. Pete Bungay and Carolyn James for their help with preparing the manuscript, to our dedicated vascular access team for their ongoing hard work and attention to detail and to our dialysis patients and staff for their participation in the pursuit of definitive vascular access.

References

1. Lacson Jr E, Wang W, Lazarus JM, Hakim RM. Change in vascular access and mortality in maintenance hemodialysis patients. Am J Kidney Dis. 2009;54(5):912–21.
2. Fluck R, Kumwenda M. Renal association clinical practice guideline on vascular access for haemodialysis. Nephron Clin Pract. 2011;118 Suppl 1:c225–40.
3. Pisoni RL, Young EW, Dykstra DM, Greenwood RN, Hecking E, Gillespie B, Wolfe RA, Goodkin DA, Held PJ. Vascular access use in Europe and the united states: results from the DOPPS. Kidney Int. 2002;61(1):305–16.
4. Allon M, Robbin ML. Increasing arteriovenous fistulas in hemodialysis patients: problems and solutions. Kidney Int. 2002;62(4): 1109–24.
5. Lok CE, Allon M, Moist L, Oliver MJ, Shah H, Zimmerman D. Risk equation determining unsuccessful cannulation events and failure to maturation in arteriovenous fistulas (REDUCE FTM I). J Am Soc Nephrol. 2006;17(11):3204–12.
6. Jennings WC, Landis L, Taubman KE, Parker DE. Creating functional autogenous vascular access in older patients. J Vasc Surg. 2011;53(3):713–9.
7. Rehman R, Schmidt RJ, Moss AH. Ethical and legal obligation to avoid long-term tunneled catheter access. Clin J Am Soc Nephrol. 2009;4(2):456–60.
8. Xi W, Harwood L, Diamant MJ, Brown JB, Gallo K, Sontrop JM, MacNab JJ, Moist LM. Patient attitudes towards the arteriovenous fistula: a qualitative study on vascular access decision making. Nephrol Dial Transplant. 2011;26(10):3302–8.
9. Guo A, Mujais S. Patient and technique survival on peritoneal dialysis in the United States: evaluation in large incident cohorts. Kidney Int Suppl. 2003;88:S3–12.
10. Wasse H, Speckman RA, McClellan WM. Arteriovenous fistula use is associated with lower cardiovascular mortality compared with catheter use among ESRD patients. Semin Dial. 2008;21(5): 483–9.
11. [No authors listed] III. NKF-K/DOQI Clinical Practice Guidelines for Vascular Access: update 2000. Am J Kidney Dis. 2001;37(Suppl 1):S137–81.
12. Cooper BA, Branley P, Bulfone L, Collins JF, Craig JC, Fraenkel MB, Harris A, Johnson DW, Kesselhut J, Li JJ, Luxton G, Pilmore A, Tiller DJ, Harris DC, Pollock CA, ; IDEAL study. A randomized, controlled trial of early versus late initiation of dialysis. N Engl J Med. 2010;363(7):609–19.
13. Huijbregts HJ, Bots ML, Wittens CH, Schrama YC, Moll FL, Blankestijn PJ, ; CIMINO study group. Hemodialysis arteriovenous fistula patency revisited: results of a prospective, multicenter initiative. Clin J Am Soc Nephrol. 2008;3(3):714–9.
14. Beathard GA, Settle SM, Shields MW. Salvage of the nonfunctioning arteriovenous fistula. Am J Kidney Dis. 1999;33(5):910–6.
15. Sidawy AN, Spergel LM, Besarab A, Allon M, Jennings WC, Padberg Jr FT, Murad MH, Montori VM, O'Hare AM, Calligaro KD, Macsata RA, Lumsden AB, Ascher E, ; Society for Vascular Surgery. The Society for Vascular Surgery: clinical practice guidelines for the surgical placement and maintenance of arteriovenous hemodialysis access. J Vasc Surg. 2008;48(5 Suppl):2S–5.
16. Beathard GA, Arnold P, Jackson J, Litchfield T, ; Physician Operators Forum of RMS Lifeline. Aggressive treatment of early fistula failure. Kidney Int. 2003;64(4):1487–94.
17. Robbin ML, Chamberlain NE, Lockhart ME, Gallichio MH, Young CJ, Deierhoi MH, Allon M. Hemodialysis arteriovenous fistula maturity: US evaluation. Radiology. 2002;225(1):59–64.
18. Saran R, Dykstra DM, Pisoni RL, Akiba T, Akizawa T, Canaud B, Chen K, Piera L, Saito A, Young EW. Timing of first cannulation and vascular access failure in haemodialysis: an analysis of practice patterns at dialysis facilities in the DOPPS. Nephrol Dial Transplant. 2004;19(9):2334–40.
19. van Loon MM, Goovaerts T, Kessels AG, van der Sande FM, Tordoir JH. Buttonhole needling of haemodialysis arteriovenous fistulae results in less complications and interventions compared to the rope-ladder technique. Nephrol Dial Transplant. 2010;25(1):225–30.
20. Tessitore N, Bedogna V, Melilli E, Millardi D, Mansueto G, Lipari G, Mantovani W, Baggio E, Poli A, Lupo A. In search of an optimal bedside screening program for arteriovenous fistula stenosis. Clin J Am Soc Nephrol. 2011;6(4):819–26.
21. Vesely TM. Optimizing function and treatment of hemodialysis grafts and fistulae. Semin Intervent Radiol. 2004;21(2):95–103.
22. Mercadal L, Hamani A, Béné B, Petitclerc T. Determination of access blood flow from ionic dialysance: theory and validation. Kidney Int. 1999;56(4):1560–5.

23. Vascular Access 2006 Work Group. Clinical practice guidelines for vascular access. Am J Kidney Dis. 2006;48 Suppl 1:S176–247.
24. Swedberg SH, Brown BG, Sigley R, Wight TN, Gordon D, Nicholls SC. Intimal fibromuscular hyperplasia at the venous anastomosis of PTFE grafts in hemodialysis patients. Clinical, immunocytochemical, light and electron microscopic assessment. Circulation. 1989;80(6):1726–36.
25. Martin LG, MacDonald MJ, Kikeri D, Cotsonis GA, Harker LA, Lumsden AB. Prophylactic angioplasty reduces thrombosis in virgin ePTFE arteriovenous dialysis grafts with greater than 50% stenosis: subset analysis of a prospectively randomized study. J Vasc Interv Radiol. 1999;10(4):389–96.
26. Moist LM, Churchill DN, House AA, Millward SF, Elliott JE, Kribs SW, DeYoung WJ, Blythe L, Stitt LW, Lindsay RM. Regular monitoring of access flow compared with monitoring of venous pressure fails to improve graft survival. J Am Soc Nephrol. 2003;14(10):2645–53.
27. Tessitore N, Mansueto G, Bedogna V, Lipari G, Poli A, Gammaro L, Baggio E, Morana G, Loschiavo C, Laudon A, Oldrizzi L, Maschio G. A prospective controlled trial on effect of percutaneous transluminal angioplasty on functioning arteriovenous fistulae survival. J Am Soc Nephrol. 2003;14(6):1623–7.
28. Tonelli M, Jindal K, Hirsch D, Taylor S, Kane C, Henbrey S. Screening for subclinical stenosis in native vessel arteriovenous fistulae. J Am Soc Nephrol. 2001;12(8):1729–33.
29. Tessitore N, Bedogna V, Poli A, Mantovani W, Lipari G, Baggio E, Mansueto G, Lupo A. Adding access blood flow surveillance to clinical monitoring reduces thrombosis rates and costs, and improves fistula patency in the short term: a controlled cohort study. Nephrol Dial Transplant. 2008;23(11):3578–84.
30. Chan KE, Pflederer TA, Steele DJ, Lilly MP, Ikizler TA, Maddux FW, Hakim RM. Access survival amongst hemodialysis patients referred for preventive angiography and percutaneous transluminal angioplasty. Clin J Am Soc Nephrol. 2011;6(11):2669–80.
31. Bittl JA. Venous rupture during percutaneous treatment of hemodialysis fistulas and grafts. Catheter Cardiovasc Interv. 2009;74(7):1097–101.
32. Bent CL, Rajan DK, Tan K, Simons ME, Jaskolka J, Kachura J, Beecroft R, Sniderman KW. Effectiveness of stent-graft placement for salvage of dysfunctional arteriovenous hemodialysis fistulas. J Vasc Interv Radiol. 2010;21(4):496–502.
33. Bent CL, Sahni VA, Matson MB. The radiological management of the thrombosed arteriovenous dialysis fistula. Clin Radiol. 2011;66(1):1–12.
34. Chan KE, Lazarus JM, Thadhani R, Hakim RM. Anticoagulant and antiplatelet usage associates with mortality among hemodialysis patients. J Am Soc Nephrol. 2009;20(4):872–81.
35. Coleman CI, Tuttle LA, Teevan C, Baker WL, White CM, Reinhart KM. Antiplatelet agents for the prevention of arteriovenous fistula and graft thrombosis: a meta analysis. Int J Clin Pract. 2010;64(9):1239–44.
36. Labriola L, Crott R, Desmet C, André G, Jadoul M. Infectious complications following conversion to buttonhole cannulation of native arteriovenous fistulas: a quality improvement report. Am J Kidney Dis. 2011;57(3):442–8.
37. Shah R, Vachharajani TJ, Agarwal AK. Aneurysmal dilatation of dialysis arteriovenous access. Open Urol Nephrol J. 2013;6:1–5.
38. Kundu S. Central venous obstruction management. Semin Interv Radiol. 2009;26(2):115–21.

Vascular Access: Fistulae and Grafts

60

Madhu Kalyan Potluri, Dominic Yu,
Justin Michael Harris, and Jennifer M. Cross

Registry data suggests that approximately 20 % of patients present to renal services with dialysis-dependent renal failure without the opportunity to create timely native AV access. Many studies have drawn attention to the potentially serious complications associated with central venous dialysis catheters (CVC) [1]. These include the risk of thrombosis and infection septicaemia, deep-seated metastasis infection and central venous stenosis [2, 3]. Dialysis using a catheter is also associated with a lower survival than that with definitive AV access. In addition, CVC access is associated with lower blood flow rates compared with fistulae or grafts [4, 5] and shorter access survival [6–9]. Thus, all patients who commence dialysis therapy in the absence of definitive access (fistula, graft, peritoneal dialysis catheter) without significant parallel co-morbidity should be considered for peritoneal dialysis (NICE guidance 2002). Many patients can use peritoneal dialysis to bridge them to the creation of a native AVF particularly with the recent provision of a separate tariff for assisted peritoneal dialysis. If PD can't be provided and you anticipate dialysis will be required for >1 week, then a tunnelled CVC should be considered to reduce infection risk.

Haemodialysis catheters come in two basic forms: tunnelled and non-tunnelled or temporary. They are made of silicone and polyurethane with a polyester cuff designed to promote tissue in growth to both fix and seal the catheter in the tunnel. A variety of coatings are now available on the surface of catheters designed to reduce infective complications and reduce clotting of lines including heparin, rifampicin, minocycline and silver or copper nanoparticles. All catheters have at least two ports, traditionally marked with a red and blue hub. The blue or venous port terminates at least 2 cm proximal and pulls blood from the patient, and the red or arterial port terminates distally and is used for the return of blood to the patient. The distance between the ends reduces direct return of blood between these two ports (recirculation). How long a catheter continues to function adequately with an effective blood pump of at least 300 ml min is highly variable. The vast majority of dialysis catheters require some sort of intervention to maintain flow over a 12-month period, and almost all of line failures relate to infection.

National Kidney Federation (UK) Patient information leaflet (PIL) for central venous catheters: http://www.kidney.org.uk/Medical-Info/haemodialysis/dialysis-line-insertion.html

Preparation for Line Insertion

Patients should be prepared for line insertion with education describing the procedure they are about to undergo specifically discussing possible complications both short and long term including pain, haematoma, rarely pneumothorax or haemothorax. DOH guidance suggests that this information should be delivered by an individual who is trained in line insertion. The NKF patient information leaflet is a useful resource (see link above). All line insertion

M.K. Potluri, MBChB, BSc MedSci, MRCP (UK) (✉)
Renal Department, Royal Free Hospital,
Pond Street, Hampstead, London NW3 2QG, UK
e-mail: madhupotluri@nhs.net

D. Yu, MBBS, MRCPI, FRCR
Department of Radiology,
Royal Free London NHS Foundation Trust,
Pond Street, London NW3 2QG, UK
e-mail: dominic.yu@nhs.net

J.M. Harris, BSc(Hons), MBBS, FRCR
Department of Radiology, Conquest Hospital, The Ridge,
St Leonards-on-Sea, Hastings, East Sussex TN37 7RD, UK
e-mail: justin.harris@esht.nhs.uk

J.M. Cross, MBChB, FRCP, PhD
Department of Nephrology,
UCL Centre For Nephrology, Royal Free Hospital Foundation Trust,
Pond Street, London NW3 2QG, UK
e-mail: jennifer.cross@nhs.net

M. Harber (ed.), *Practical Nephrology*,
DOI 10.1007/978-1-4471-5547-8_60, © Springer-Verlag London 2014

should be performed using strict aseptic technique with an assistant under direct vision using screening or ultrasound guidance to avoid insertion complication [1]. Prophylaxis with antibiotics is not recommended for line insertion. A record of all line insertion should be made in the patient's medical record.

Catheter Selection

Tunnelled dialysis catheters (Table 60.1) have demanding requirements that exceed all other CVC including delivering volume flow of 300–400 ml/min at moderate pressure gradients without obstructing, minimising trauma to the vein, resisting occlusion by biofilm/clot/lumen collapse or kinking, prevention of infection, resistance to antiseptic agent deformation and radiopacity for site confirmation.

There are many commercially available tunnelled dialysis catheters and a similar number of publications extolling the virtues of one catheter over another, but these data are conflicting. There is little compelling evidence that one dialysis catheter has significant advantage over others as evidenced by the variety that are currently in use in units around the world. In your choice of dialysis catheter, you should consider whether its length is appropriate for the anatomical position (18 cm right internal jugular, 22 cm left internal jugular, to achieve a tip position at the confluence of the jugular and the right atrium 28 cm femoral to achieve a tip position in the distal inferior vena cava). The longer, the narrower, and the greater the bends in the path of a catheter, the lower the volume flow achieved. Invariably right-sided internal jugular lines have better volume flows than left for those reasons. The true blood flow rate displayed on the dialysis blood pump is generally lower than the actual blood flow rate achieved partly because of negative pressure exerted as blood is sucked through using the rolling pump system that partially deforms the flexible catheter. This effect may reduce the actual volume flow by as much as 25 %, thus reducing dialysis efficiency. An elevated haematocrit will also have the effect of reducing effective volume flow by increasing viscosity and thus resistance to flow. Commercial line packs vary in the technical ease of insertion and the equipment that is included in the line pack. Many lines include features that may reduce infection rates (coating/nano-impregnation of silver or copper), features that reduce biofilm formation, antimicrobial hubs and the presence of subcutaneous cuffs [10]. Most catheters for chronic dialysis, both single and dual lumen, have side holes in addition to end holes. The position of the catheter holes is relevant to line flow rate and catheter dysfunction related to the formation of clots in addition to the migration of line locks and the development of biofilm for a review of the factors affecting line performance (for a review on the subject) [11].

Table 60.1 Tunnelled dialysis catheters

Split-Cath III™ (*Medcomp*): dual-lumen catheter with end and side ports
HemoSplit™(*Bard Access Systems*): pre-curved dual-lumen catheter with end and side ports
Tesio twin catheter (*Medcomp*): two separate catheters, with end and side ports
Permcath™ (*Quinton Instruments*): dual-lumen catheter with end ports

Choosing a Tunnelled CVC Position (KDOQI Vascular Access Guidelines 2006) [1]

Insertion positions are described in descending order of preference:

1. *The right internal jugular vein* is the optimal position for insertion of a tunnelled CVC catheter as there is a straight anatomical run from this position to the SVC/atrial confluence where the catheter tip should sit. This position minimises the risk of central vein stenosis (10 %) [12].
2. *The left internal jugular vein* has a serpiginous course, and catheter tips commonly lie against the wall of the innominate vein/SVC which can intermittently occlude side and end ports resulting in poor dialysis flow rates; in addition, this position is also associated with higher rates of central vein stenosis and thrombosis [13].
3. *The femoral vein catheter insertion* is easily accessible, and a 28 cm line ought to be used to try and place the tip in the distal IVC as the calibre of the vessel increases as you ascend. Flow problems encountered in the first week of insertion in this position are commonly related to inadequate line length. Femoral tunnelled CVC are more likely to become infected (19.8 % risk of bacteraemia [14]), and the risk of gram-negative/gut-related organisms is increased because of the proximity to the groin. During hip flexion/walking, femoral catheters kink/dislodge, and they have a higher failure rate in this position with an overall patency rate of approximately 2 months. Unwitnessed bleeding from end ports is a greater risk in femoral catheters as a result of the relatively hidden position, and DVT is common on the side of the catheter [15].
4. *Translumbar vein catheter insertion* should only be performed by specialist interventionalists. It is not a routine site of insertion as it is technically demanding, has a high early failure rate, is associated with a poor flow and the risk of thrombosis extending to the IVC and has an increased risk of infection compared with upper body access [16].
5. *Transhepatic vein catheter insertion* should only be considered in a specialist centre where there is experience of this technique in this patient group. The technique utilises the hepatic venous sinus to gain entry to the venous drainage vessels to the IVC but requires a needle and Seldinger

wire to be inserted through the liver tissue which is not uncommonly associated with significant bleeding. In a small series of transhepatic line insertion, 29 % experienced a complication including intraperitoneal haemorrhage, catheter migration and catheter thrombosis [17].

6. *Intra-atrial catheter insertion* involves the direct insertion of a CVC under general anaesthesia into right atrium [18]. This technique is rarely used and should not be considered in centres that have not used this access in the past.
7. *Subclavian catheter insertion* access is associated with highest rate of stenotic complication at 50 % and should be avoided where possible [19].

In the setting of acute kidney injury, intensive care units and multi-organ failure related to sepsis syndrome, you may require short-term vascular access. This should be placed with full aseptic technique and does not require antibiotic prophylaxis.

The femoral vein is most commonly used for temporary access, and bleeding complications are less likely in this site; however, large unnoticed bleeds occur with insertion sites above the inguinal ligament where blood tracks back and upwards into the retroperitoneum and are not outwardly visible and may only become evident when the patient is hypotensive/shocked or develops an unexplained ileus. For an average adult, a femoral catheter should be a minimum length of 25 cm to ensure tip lies in the distal inferior vena cava [20].

This risk of infection which is more likely to be with a gram-negative organism rises exponentially after a period of 5 days of temporary access at the femoral site. In prescribing dialysis therapy, you should consider dialysing daily and replacing with a permanent catheter if practicable. Alternatively, femoral temporary catheters should be removed electively at day 5, and careful consideration should be given to prophylactic heparin to avoid deep vein thrombosis which is increased in hospital patients and still further in those with femoral access. Thereafter, right internal jugular and left internal jugular are used, and the external jugular and subclavian routes should be avoided.

Catheter Insertion Procedure (See Video 60.1)

Catheters are inserted using the Seldinger technique of needle followed by a curve-ended guidewire. Insert link for Justins DVD of catheter insertion. The straight end of the guidewire should not be used to guide the catheter as it is associated with an increased risk of mediastinal trauma and atrial puncture than the curved wire tip which is designed for the purpose and is much softer. The catheter tip should be at least at the caval/atrial junction to ensure adequate blood flow. Positioning the line tip deep within the atria may be associated with irritation of the mitral valve and result in atrial and ventricular tachyarrhythmias. Temporary dialysis catheters tend to be more rigid than tunnelled catheters and are associated with an increased risk of vein and atrial trauma so atrial placement of temporary catheters should therefore be avoided.

The position of all lines inserted into the thorax should be checked by screening or chest X-ray prior to use to ensure that the line has been correctly inserted into the vein and advanced adequately, to confirm there are no kinks and exclude haemo- or pneumothorax or pneumomediastinum, all of which are rare but accepted complications of line insertion. Though tunnelled lines are fixed in position by the subcutaneous cuff and two hub stitches initially, line tip retraction is common when patients move from the horizontal to the vertical position immediately after insertion, and a perfect tip position while supine may require advancement when vertical making a CXR or fluoroscopic imaging while standing invaluable so this can be corrected before line use. If a line has inadvertently been placed in an arterial position, do not use the line and do not remove the line without consulting a surgeon who may be required to control bleeding after line removal. The cause of a newly placed catheter failing to deliver adequate flow in the first week is usually related to a mal position, too short, too long, proximity of side holes against a vein wall with 'sucking' or a clot in the lumen because of inadequate locking at the time of placement or after use. Dialysis catheters tend to 'prove' or harden after insertion in the first 48 h, and not uncommonly the line may have a poor volume flow during the first dialysis session only to settle subsequently with no specific intervention. Distinguishing these catheter problems is not possible without a chest X-ray.

Complications of Catheter Insertion (See Video on Complications)

The large bore of dialysis catheters and the coagulopathy associated with renal failure increase the probability, and potential consequences of trauma to the vein, inadvertent arterial puncture, massive extravasation of blood and mediastinal or right atrial perforation are greater. These risks are associated with the introducer, wire, tissue expander and line itself. If an introducer needle is placed in an artery, this should be obvious in all but the most shocked and hypoxic patients, but processing a sample for blood gas analysis if there is doubt can be helpful. The needle should be removed and direct finger pressure placed on the access site for 10 min. Insertion of access into the external jugular vein rather than the internal increases the probability of lacerating the subclavian vein particularly with the more rigid temporary catheters because of the 90° angle of incidence at the confluence and should thus generally be avoided. Unwitting insertion of a line into an artery can result in massive neck, thoracic, or retroperitoneal bleeding. In such an event, the catheter should not be used or locked, and a vascular surgeon should be consulted before removal as bleeding is often a greater issue after removal than at the time of insertion. Any CVC insertion can result in a haemothorax, and the development of a new ipsilateral pleural effusion soon after line placement with SOB ought to alert you to the possibility of a haemothorax from a catheter malplacement and a communication into the mediastinum. Finally, air embolus though rare is more common during insertion of dialysis catheters because of their greater calibre. This can be avoided by placing the line with patient in a head-down position, ensuring that during the line insertion the clamps on the ports are sealed, asking the patient to slowly breathe out during line insertion and passage of the introducer sheath. Finally, during difficult CVC insertion where multiple attempts have been made to site the line, it is possible to cannulate both the artery and vein creating an artificial communication between the two resulting in a fistulous communication. This can result in a bruit over the area and aneurysmal dilatation of the vessel. This can usually be rectified using occlusion devices such as amplatz wires, onyx or thrombin instillation. Occasionally, a formal surgical procedure may be required.

Catheter Locks

At the end of each dialysis session, both arterial and venous ports are locked with an anticoagulant/antimicrobial which is designed to prevent thrombus or fibrin formation [1].

The ideal lock solution should prevent line occlusion, not migrate from the line lumen to the systemic circulation, and resist planktonic organisms and sessile organisms existing in a biofilm.

It is important, given its frequent use that it is safe, relatively low in cost and simple to use. Currently, there are a variety of catheter locks (citrate, taurolidine, low-dose gentamicin, heparin), but there is insufficient data to compare different strategies for optimal approach, and therefore, larger randomised controlled trials in haemodialysis population are required.

In the interdialytic period, inevitably some of the anticoagulant is lost in equilibrium with blood; this is greatest with dense locking agents such as 46 % citrate. This equilibration occurs soon after the line lock is placed [21]. The anticoagulant lost is replaced by blood and its clotting factors potentially resulting in thrombosis of the catheter tip and catheter dysfunction eventually culminating in occlusion [1].

If the catheter is in the superior vena cava, this increases risk of fibrin deposition and tip thrombosis. Line manipulation may be possible to place the line tip caval/atrial junction or beyond into right atrium [22]. There is little evidence to suggest that using thrombolytics as a lock contributes to medium-term resolution of a dysfunctional catheter as the thrombolytic effect is limited to the interior of the lumen and will not disrupt either biofilm or external ball valve clot, and therefore, its expense in regular use cannot be justified.

Table 60.2 Exclusion criteria for t-PA infusion

Bleeding diathesis
History of active peptic ulceration (<3 months)
CVA/TIA
Recent haemorrhage or surgery (<7 days)
Untreated proliferative diabetic retinopathy

The current practice in our centre is to use a 46 % concentrated citrate solution as a lock and to salvage occluded catheters using alteplase (t-PA) (Table 60.2) 8 mg as an online infusion via the heparin infusion device into the venous trap before the kidney which has the advantage of low relative cost, a longer duration of action and greater efficacy compared with other agents [23, 24].

Techniques for fibrin or thrombus removal that have gone out of favour recently are the endoluminal catheter brush [25]. This device can be inserted, gently up to tip of catheter and slightly beyond. On gentle withdrawal, any fibrin may be dislodged enough to improve blood flow through the catheter [25].

Failure of the measures, described so far, to restore adequate blood flow should prompt review of the need for line exchange. Exchange in the same position over a wire can result in the new line following the path of the previously established fibrin sheath and may result in a rapid return of line dysfunction. The general experiences of other salvage techniques such as line stripping or thrombectomy have been largely unsuccessful and are associated with an increased risk of infection and are not commonly practised in our institution. There is little evidence that anticoagulation with coumarin-based agents is the mechanism of obstruction in infrequently simple thrombin-mediated clot production, and there is substantial evidence of an augmented bleeding risk in dialysis-dependent patients and the practice is not recommended.

Catheter Complications

Catheters are associated with various complications due to long-term use (>3 weeks), such as catheter-related bacteraemia, occlusion secondary to fibrin or thrombus, central vein stenosis or catheter extrusion.

The frequency and severity of complications are dependent on the frequency of catheter insertions and duration of dwell time.

Catheter Occlusion [1]

Catheters may be occluded in various ways [1]:

1. Intraluminal occlusion by thrombus which may cause partial or complete occlusion and usually results from failure to completely exclude blood from the lumen at the time of locking (wrong lock volume, failure to flush with online fluid or saline prior to lock, failure to fully clamp lines prior to lock, ingress of blood as a result of interdialytic lock migration).
2. Catheter tip thrombus of fibrin at tip may cause complete occlusion or act like a ball valve.
3. Fibrin sheath (sleeve): fibrin adheres to external surface of catheter and thrombus trapped between sheath and catheter tip.
4. Fibrin tail (fibrin flap): fibrin adheres to CVC end causing 'ball valve' effect.
5. Mechanical bend or kink which can be identified on a chest X-ray and is often an early cause of catheter malfunction
6. Catheter migration which is common in obese individuals or those with large abdomens or chests.

Catheter dysfunction as a result of partial or complete occlusion is common. In general this is manifest as poor blood flow, increased line arterial or venous pressure, deteriorating clearance and increased recirculation (see Table 60.3). Luminal clots can often be managed if identified early by a high-pressure flush using a very small syringe (small surface area plunger means that the small fluid volume is ejected with greater force and can be more effective in dislodging a small luminal clot than a 20 ml syringe). First, check that the line has not moved or been kinked, since insertion, by inspecting the line, looking for an externalised cuff. Perform a chest X-ray to confirm there are no kinks and identify the position of the line tip. If these are in place, then it is likely that the line has developed a clot or a biofilm. Thrombosis of a dialysis catheter can either be within the lumen of the line, encircling the external surface of the line, mural and adherent to the wall of the vessel or a ball of clot adherent to the tip acting as a ball valve occluding the line during aspiration. Clots on lines are probably much more common than we realise and often give rise to no clinically evident problems. The incidence of pulmonary embolus as a result of line thrombosis appears low, and the greater risk is associated with an infected clot which may result in mycotic pulmonary emboli. Clots can be delineated using Doppler ultrasound in many cases or echocardiography in the case of the right atrial clots or using digital subtraction angiography. Management of an incidentally identified large ball clot (>2 cm) in the right atrium attached to the line tip while investigating line dysfunction is unclear from the literature. A reasonable approach is to remove the line and consider the risk benefit ratio of systemic anticoagulation for 6 months and repeat echocardiography to monitor the size and stability of the thombus at an interval of 1 week. The safety and efficacy of thrombolytics in this setting is unclear. In the setting of a significant bleeding risk, some patients have been managed with thrombectomy rather than anticoagulation.

Table 60.3 Signs of catheter dysfunction [1]

Signs
Blood flow rate <300 ml/min
Arterial pressure <–250 mmHg
Venous pressure >250 mmHg
Conductance <1.2 (ratio of blood pump flow to the value of prepump pressure)
URR <65 % or KT/V <1.2
Unable to aspirate blood freely (late sign)
Frequent pressure alarms (not responsive to patient repositioning or catheter flushing)

A biofilm often forms in and around the catheter starting at the hub and progressing down the length of the line. Biofilm is produced by the interaction of microbial glycocalyx with fibrin, fibronectin and extracellular polysaccharides [1]. This does not usually happen overnight, and nursing staff have often identified these problems for days or weeks before the line fails completely so it typically affects the more proximal venous/blue lumen before the arterial/red giving rise to the observation that the lines had to be 'reversed' on dialysis sessions for a period prior to failure of line volume flow. If you suspect a biofilm or clot/thrombus, then this can be disrupted using a thrombolytic. You can either infuse the thrombolytic systemically in 20 ml of saline throughout the dialysis session using the heparin syringe driver. Alternatively, arrange for a day case admission to administer the drug down each lumen over 4 h. Both appear to be efficacious and safe [26].

Thrombolytics are contraindicated in patients with a bleeding diathesis, recent haemorrhagic stroke, recent surgery, proliferative retinopathy or malignant hypertension.

Catheter Infection

Line infection is the most common and potentially most important complication of a long-term dialysis catheter. Catheter-related infection is one of the commonest reasons for access loss.

Catheters may be colonised by bacteria soon after insertion [27], and bacteria commonly colonise the catheter hub, and colonisation of the catheter or the relatively immunologically shielded catheter biofilm results in apparent bacterial resistance to systemic antimicrobial therapy [28].

At the first sign of a local exit site infection characterised by redness, tenderness and discharge, the wound should be swabbed, and empiric flucloxacillin 500 mg PO QDS should be given for 10 days. If MRSA is positive, then IV vancomycin as per local policy should be given for three sessions according to levels (15–20). Antibiotics should be modified in light of culture results.

Exit site infection if treated late or inadequately can progress to involve the tunnel. This is associated with neovascularisation of the tunnel wall which may be detected with ultrasound scan and is a reliable sign of tunnel infection and precedes abscess formation. The presence of a tunnel infection requires parenteral antibiotics (such as vancomycin or gentamicin with levels). Line removal should be considered if this has not settled after 14 days of antibiotics or if it recurs after cessation of antibiotics or if the organism at the exit site is a pseudomonas or yeast or other slime former with a predilection for plastic [1].

Although bacteraemia may result from the progression of an exit site infection, to involve the tunnel and progress to systemic bacteraemia with circulating organisms, line-related bacteraemia occurs in their absence. The commonest organisms identified are skin commensals such as coagulase-negative staphylococci (CNS) and strep viridans. In a dialysis patient with a line in situ who has no obvious chest or abdominal complaint, then it is reasonable to assume that fever even in the absence of an exit site or tunnel infection represents systemic bacteraemia related to the line. The exit site should be swabbed, blood cultures and CRP taken, and empiric antibiotic should be administered according to the likely culprit. We use flucloxacillin 1 g QDS and gentamicin (MRSA negative) and vancomycin and gentamicin (MRSA +ve). Line removal is essential in the event of S. aureus, Candida albicans and pseudomonas species as the line is unlikely to be cleared and will act as a reservoir of organisms. The longer the line is left in situ, the greater the risk of metastatic deep-seated infective complications. In an uncomplicated infection with an indolent organism, parenteral treatment should continue for a minimum of 14 days. If the CRP fails to fall or there is persistent bacteraemia in the face of sensitive antibiotics, it suggests either that there is a deep-seated infection (discitis, endocarditis, osteomyelitis, paraspinal, psoas or other abscess are the most common) or that the catheter is colonised and should be replaced. Investigations should be tailored to the clinical situation. Deep-seated infection often declares itself. Ask patients if they have back pain, are breathless or have other sites of pain to focus the hunt for deep-seated infection, and remember to identify any old PTFE access still in situ. Investigations to consider are CXR, TTE, complement, rheumatoid factor, MRI back which is much more sensitive than plain X-ray or CT in detecting discitis.

Central Vein Stenosis

Endothelial injury occurs with recurrent short-term central venous catheter placements [29, 30], over time the vein wall thickens and is invaded by smooth muscle cells, and collagen accumulates with overlying thrombus [31].

Central vein stenosis is defined as 50 % narrowing of the diameter of the vessel and is more common in patients of African or Caribbean origin [31]

Most frequently, it can cause massive head and neck swelling and upper limb or breast oedema rendering the subsequent creation of definitive access in the upper body difficult.

Additional symptoms or signs may include [31]:

- Pleural effusion [32]
- Venous collateral formation (upper chest, neck, shoulder, and upper arm) [31]
- Increased risk of infection [31]
- Thrombosis of AVF [15]
- Increasing length of time to establish haemostasis post dialysis (possible central or peripheral venous stenosis)
- Headaches
- Nose bleeds

Central vein stenosis is most prevalent at these sites in descending order:

- Subclavian vein (up to 50 % [19] due to direct injury to vein due to anatomical curvature of the junction between subclavian, innominate and superior vena cava [6])
- Left internal jugular vein (due to complex anatomy with several angulations in its course and due to overlying structures such as brachiocephalic artery and aorta which can cause extrinsic compression, this route is not preferred [31])
- Right internal jugular vein (approximately 10 % [12, 13])

Stenosis can be functional due to the catheter itself contributing to the reduction of lumen diameter, and removal can resolve symptoms; this is often temporary however.

Investigations

If symptoms of superior vena cava obstruction become apparent and/or swelling of unilateral arm, then the patient should undergo a magnetic resonance venogram to confirm the diagnosis if this is available (Fig. 60.1a). Ultrasound scan is usually unhelpful as the views of the deep thoracic great veins are impaired by the overlying anterior thoracic cage. However, a normal polyphasic atrial waveform on the duplex excludes the possibility of central venous stenosis of greater than 80 % [33].

Fluroscopic venography is useful if an interventional procedure with venoplasty is planned (Fig. 60.1b–e). In general, the use of venous stents is discouraged as they frequently obstruct with clot, and if a line is required through them, the incidence of SVC stent colonisation is high.

Management of Central Vein Stenosis

Not all >50 % stenotic lesions [31] require intervention. Only consider intervention if the patient is symptomatic or dialysis adequacy is impaired [31, 34].

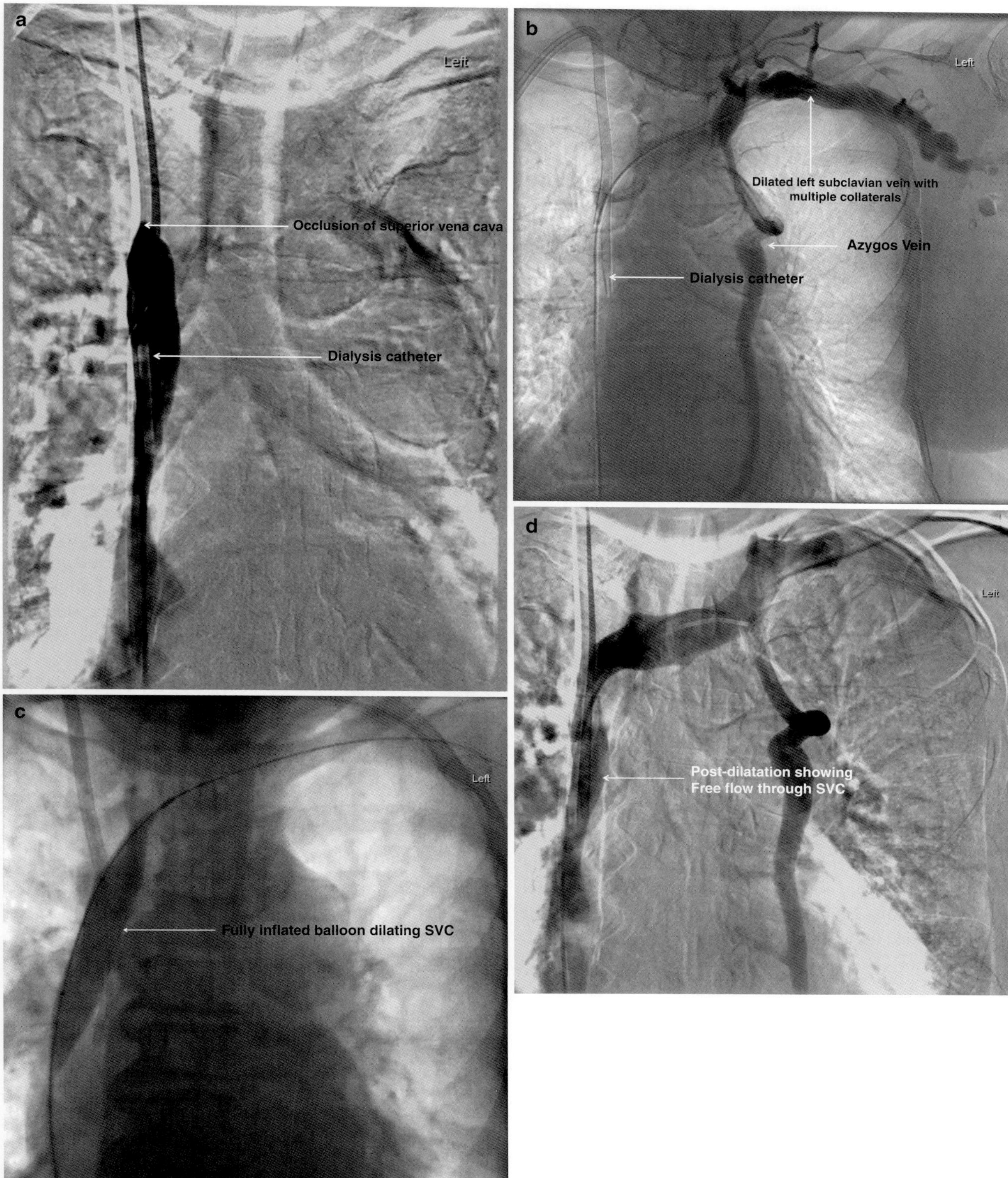

Fig. 60.1 (**a**) Central venogram from the femoral route showing complete occlusion of the superior vena cava (SVC) in patient with a right internal jugular dialysis line complaining of marked facial swelling and headaches worse on wakening; (**b**) guidewire and catheter having crossed the obstruction radiocontrast dye fails to pass into the SVC but outlines the grossly enlarged azygous vein; (**c**) dilatation by 10 mm balloon across SVC stenosis; (**d**) post-dilatation flow through SVC with symptomatic relief; (**e**) MRV in a patient with SVC stenosis and failed attempts at internal jugular line insertion

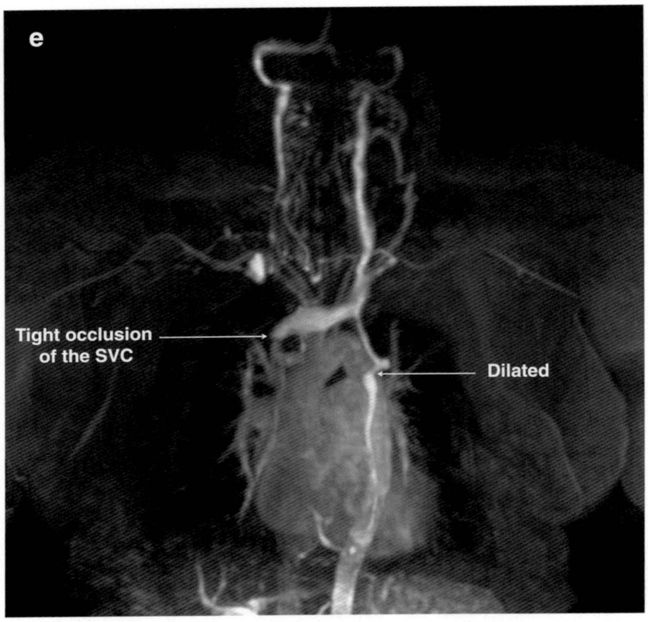

Fig. 60.1 (continued)

Lesions commonly progress and the management is percutaneous central venoplasty without stent [1, 31]. These lesions tend to be recurrent and repeat percutaneous venoplasty is required between 3 and 6 monthly [35, 36]

In 2006, the KDOQI guidelines recommended that stent placement should be considered if there is acute elastic recoil of the vein (which had greater than 50 % stenosis) after angioplasty [31] or if there is recurrent stenosis within a 3-month period post-angioplasty [31].

Surgery is reserved as last resort for recurrent stenosis or severe head and neck oedema with respiratory embarrassment. This approach requires bypassing the occluded segment to the atrium [37] or ipsilateral femoral vein via tunnelled subcutaneous graft [38]. Additionally as a final measure, if the patient has ipsilateral arteriovenous fistula, it can be occluded to rapidly relieve symptoms [31].

Removal of a Haemodialysis Catheters

Removal of a venous dialysis catheter may be necessary because definitive access has been created and reliably used for 14 days, of line-associated sepsis, a tunnel infection or an exit site infection that has failed to resolve despite 10–14 days of an appropriate antibiotic or finally a proximal line leak. In the setting of *S. aureus* bacteraemia, the removal of the catheter is an emergency and should be achieved without delay to reduce the risk of metastatic seeding.

This procedure may be undertaken in a treatment room in a ward area rather than in a theatre setting (see Video 60.2). New CVC that have been in place for less than a month or in which a tunnel infection is present may simply be removed by gentle pulling as the cuff may not be adherent to surrounding tissues. If any resistance is met, then a formal skin incision with cuff exposure and dissection as demonstrated in the attached video clip will be required. The critical point is to be aware at all times identifying, occluding and keeping hold of the proximal line portion preferably with a pair or arterial clamps during removal to avoid retraction of the open line inside the patient risking air embolus, haemorrhage and line loss into circulation all of which are recorded.

Dialysis Catheter Repair

Catheter may become extruded and is defined as cuff being visible outside of tunnel and commonly occurs because the cuff or tunnel has been colonised with bacteria or there is a low-grade tunnel infection. Unfortunately, this cannot be repaired, and attempts to replace the catheter in the tunnel are likely to be associated with a tunnel infection and potentially an episode of septicaemia. Patients with an extruded cuff should receive a single dose of parenteral antibiotics (flucloxacillin/vancomycin and gentamicin), they can dialyse through the line and arrangement should be made to remove the line and replace with a new catheter ideally in a new tunnel. Catheters may be damaged, cracked or split or dilated and leak which may only become evident when the catheter is in use which poses a bidirectional contamination risk. This may be repaired if the split is 4.5 cm distal to the hub in the extension pieces (see Video 60.3).

References

1. KDOQI Vascular Access Guidelines. 2006. Retrieved from http://www.kidney.org/professionals/kdoqi/guideline_uphd_pd_va/.
2. Caruana RJ, Raja RM, Zeit RM, Goldstein SJ, Kramer MS. Thrombotic complications of indwelling central catheters used for chronic hemodialysis. Am J Kidney Dis. 1987;9:497–501.
3. Bander SJ, Schwab SJ. Central venous angioaccess for hemodialysis and its complications. Semin Dial. 1992;5:121–8.
4. Depner TA. Catheter performance. Semin Dial. 2001;14(6):425–31.
5. Atherikul K, Schwab SJ, Twardowski ZJ, et al. What is the role of permanent central vein access in hemodialysis patients? Semin Dial. 1996;9:392–403.
6. Fan PY, Schwab SJ. Vascular access: concepts for the 1990s. J Am Soc Nephrol. 1992;3:1–11.
7. Windus DW. Permanent vascular access: a nephrologist's view. Am J Kidney Dis. 1993;21:457–71.
8. Suhocki PV, Conlon Jr PJ, Knelson MH, Harland R, Schwab SJ. Silastic cuffed catheters for hemodialysis vascular access: thrombolytic and mechanical correction of malfunction. Am J Kidney Dis. 1996;28:379–86.
9. Schwab SJ. Assessing the adequacy of vascular access and its relationship to patient outcome. Am J Kidney Dis. 1994;24:316–20.
10. Lok CE, Mokrzycki MH. Prevention and management of catheter-related infection in hemodialysis patients. Kidney Int. 2011;79:587–98.

11. Asif A. Reducing the Morbidity of Tunneled Hemodialysis Catheters—A Symposium. Semin Dial. 2008;21(6):503–90.
12. Schillinger F, Schillinger D, Montagnac R, Milcent T. Post catheterisation vein stenosis in haemodialysis: comparative angiographic study of 50 subclavian and 50 internal jugular accesses. Nephrol Dial Transplant. 1991;6(10):722.
13. Vanholder R, Ringoir S. Vascular access for hemodialysis. Artif Organs. 1994;18:263–5.
14. Merrer J, De Jonghe B, Golliot F, Lefrant JY, Raffy B, Barre E, Rigaud JP, Casciani D, Misset B, Bosquet C, Outin H, Brun-Buisson C, Nitenberg G, French Catheter Study Group in Intensive Care. Complications of femoral and subclavian venous catheterization in critically ill patients: a randomized controlled trial. JAMA. 2001;286(6):700.
15. Maya ID, Allon M. Outcomes of tunneled femoral hemodialysis catheters: comparison with internal jugular vein catheters. Kidney Int. 2005;68(6):2886.
16. Lund GB, Trerotola SO, Scheel Jr PJ. Percutaneous translumbar inferior vena cava cannulation for hemodialysis. Am J Kidney Dis. 1995;25:732–7.
17. Smith TP, Ryan JM, Reddan DN. Transhepatic catheter access for hemodialysis. Radiology. 2004;232(1):246–51. Epub 2004 May 20.
18. Villagrán Medinilla E, Carnero M, Silva JA, Rodríguez JE. Right intra-atrial catheter insertion at the end stage of peripheral vascular access for dialysis. Interact Cardiovasc Thorac Surg. 2011;12(4):648–9. Epub 2011 Jan 10.
19. K/DOQI Clinical Practice Guidelines and Clinical Practice Recommendations 2006 Updates: hemodialysis adequacy, peritoneal dialysis adequacy, vascular access. Am J Kidney Dis. 2006;48(Suppl 1):S1.
20. Kelber J, Delmez JA, Windus DW. Factors affecting delivery of high-efficiency dialysis using temporary vascular access. Am J Kidney Dis. 1993;22:24–9.
21. Agharazii M, Plamondon I, Lebel M, Douville P, Desmeules S. Estimation of heparin leak into the systemic circulation after central venous catheter heparin lock. Nephrol Dial Transplant. 2005;20:1238–40.
22. Vesely TM. Central venous catheter tip position: a continuing controversy. J Vasc Interv Radiol. 2003;14:527–34.
23. Dowling K, Sansivero G, Stainken B, et al. The use of tissue plasminogen activator infusion to re-establish function of tunneled hemodialysis catheters. Nephrol Nurs J. 2004;31:199–200.
24. Savader SJ, Ehrman KO, Porter DJ, Haikal LC, Oteham AC. Treatment of hemodialysis catheter associated fibrin sheaths by rt-PA infusion: critical analysis of 124 procedures. J Vasc Interv Radiol. 2001;12:711–5.
25. Tranter SA, Donoghue J. Brushing has made a sweeping change: Use of the endoluminal FAS brush in haemodialysis central venous catheter management. Aust Crit Care. 2000;13:10–3.
26. Hilleman D, Campbell J. Efficacy, safety, and cost of thrombolytic agents for the management of dysfunctional hemodialysis catheters: a systematic review. Pharmacotherapy. 2011;31(10):1031–40.
27. Raad I, Costerton W, Sabharwal U, Sacilowski M, Anaissie E, Bodey GP. Ultrastructural analysis of indwelling vascular catheters: a quantitative relationship between luminal colonization and duration of placement. J Infect Dis. 1993;168:400–7.
28. Lewis K. Riddle of biofilm resistance. Antimicrob Agents Chemother. 2001;45:999–1007.
29. Forauer AR, Theoharis C. Histologic changes in the human vein wall adjacent to indwelling central venous catheters. J Vasc Interv Radiol. 2003;14(9 Pt 1):1163.
30. Hernández D, Díaz F, Rufino M, Lorenzo V, Pérez T, Rodríguez A, De Bonis E, Losada M, González-Posada JM, Torres A. Subclavian vascular access stenosis in dialysis patients: natural history and risk factors. J Am Soc Nephrol. 1998;9(8):1507.
31. Beathard GA. Central vein stenosis associated with dialysis access. www.UptoDate.com.
32. Wright RS, Quinones-Baldrich WJ, Anders AJ, Danovitch GM. Pleural effusion associated with ipsilateral breast and arm edema as a complication of subclavian vein catheterization and arteriovenous fistula formation for hemodialysis. Chest. 1994;106(3):950.
33. Rose SC, Kinney TB, Bundens WP, Valji K, Roberts AC. Importance of Doppler analysis of transmitted atrial waveforms prior to placement of central venous access catheters. J Vasc Interv Radiol. 1998;9(6):927.
34. Levit RD, Cohen RM, Kwak A, Shlansky-Goldberg RD, Clark TW, Patel AA, Stavropoulos SW, Mondschein JI, Solomon JA, Tuite CM, Trerotola SO. Asymptomatic central venous stenosis in hemodialysis patients. Radiology. 2006;238(3):1051.
35. Surowiec SM, Fegley AJ, Tanski WJ, Sivamurthy N, Illig KA, Lee DE, Waldman DL, Green RM, Davies MG. Endovascular management of central venous stenoses in the hemodialysis patient: results of percutaneous therapy. Vasc Endovascular Surg. 2004;38(4):349.
36. Beathard GA. Percutaneous transvenous angioplasty in the treatment of vascular access stenosis. Kidney Int. 1992;42(6):1390.
37. El-Sabrout RA, Duncan JM. Right atrial bypass grafting for central venous obstruction associated with dialysis access: another treatment option. J Vasc Surg. 1999;29(3):472.
38. Ayarragaray JE. Surgical treatment of hemodialysis-related central venous stenosis or occlusion: another option to maintain vascular access. J Vasc Surg. 2003;37(5):1043.

61 Complications of Maintenance Haemodialysis and How to Avoid Them

Nigel Suren Kanagasundaram

Maintenance haemodialysis (HD) poses some of the greatest technical, logistical and clinical challenges in renal practice. The HD population is highly vulnerable and places a disproportionate strain on hospital resources in comparison to their overall numbers. This chapter will cover some of the most significant complications that can arise in the HD population and how they might be prevented or mitigated. The range of topics covered is by no means comprehensive but have been chosen to reflect those complications that have the greatest impact on the HD population or which require specific considerations to mitigate or manage.

Blood Pressure and Fluid Management

Cardiovascular disease is one of the leading causes of death in HD patients; blood pressure (BP) and fluid management are critical components of this. An added complexity is the cyclical nature of both BP and fluid status over the course of a week; the asymmetric weekly HD schedule not only causes difficulties in interpreting findings but has a real clinical impact with, for instance, highest mortality around the time of the first session of the week, following the longest inter-dialytic gap.

N.S. Kanagasundaram, MBChB, MD, FRCP (Lon)
Renal Services, Newcastle upon Tyne Hospitals
NHS Foundation Trust, Freeman Hospital, High Heaton,
Newcastle upon Tyne, Tyne and Wear NE7 7DN, UK
e-mail: suren.kanagasundaram@nuth.nhs.uk

Aetiology

At least 60 % of HD patients are reported to be hypertensive. As well as pre-existing essential hypertension, salt and water retention, increased activity of the sympathetic and renin-angiotensin-aldosterone systems and arterial stiffness (due to vascular calcification) may play a role. Increased intracellular calcium, due to hyperparathyroidism, and erythropoiesis-stimulating agents may contribute. Of these, salt and water retention is probably the most important.

Evidence in support of this includes the association between high inter-dialytic weight gains and hypertension in some (but not all) studies, a higher prevalence of hypertension at dialysis initiation (volume control presumably improving as therapy progresses) and the finding that drug-free hypertensive control can be achieved by optimising extracellular fluid volumes with long-session HD.

Measurement of BP

Pre- and post-HD BP measurements may not be representative of overall control. The former tend to be higher than mean BP due to increasing salt and water accumulation between sessions, pretreatment patient anxiety and the omission of anti-hypertensive drugs before HD to minimise the risk of intra-dialytic hypotension (IDH). BP tends to fall during HD due to volume removal with post-HD readings, although more representative of inter-dialytic control [1], underestimating mean BP.

Ambulatory BP recording may be the most representative of overall control and may be useful in defining 'systolic load' and in picking up blunted nocturnal dipping [2], but there is still some evidence of intra-individual variability.

Home BP monitoring is a cheap, practical alternative to ambulatory recording and can be useful in qualifying difficult BPs on dialysis days [3].

M. Harber (ed.), *Practical Nephrology*,
DOI 10.1007/978-1-4471-5547-8_61, © Springer-Verlag London 2014

Assessing Volume Status

This is one of the most common clinical challenges in HD and is compounded by different interpretations of what actually defines 'dry weight' – for instance, 'normotension' without symptomatic hypovolaemia, 'normotension' without anti-hypertensive drugs or the absence of clinically detectable oedema. However, there is enough nuance to make a comprehensive definition, problematic. For instance, an oedema-free state does not necessarily mean that dry weight has been reached. Clinically evident peripheral oedema may have other causes – right heart failure, drugs, venous insufficiency, liver failure, etc. – attempts to achieve an oedema-free state may be poorly tolerated. An ultrafiltration (UF) rate that is excessive for an individual patient may cause hypotension even though they remain fluid overloaded. A highly individualised interpretation of dry weight may be needed and will depend on overall BP control, patient tolerability and clinical signs and symptoms.

Bioimpedance plethysmography, inferior vena cava diameter measurement, measurement of atrial and brain natriuretic peptides and blood volume monitoring have all been employed to improve assessment of volume status. Their role in routine clinical practice remains unclear at this stage but is worth considering in problematic patients.

Target BP

Correlation between BP and cardiovascular mortality remains unclear in the HD population although studies of better design and longer duration have tended to show a stronger relationship. For instance, a prospective cohort study of 432 ESRD patients (261 HD) with mean follow-up of 41 months found that each 10 mmHg rise in the averaged mean arterial pressure (MAP) was independently associated with the presence of concentric left ventricular hypertrophy and a deterioration in other echocardiographic indices [4]. An averaged MAP >106 mmHg was also associated with the development of clinical cardiac failure or ischaemic heart disease. In other work, an increased mortality was seen with post-dialysis hypertension (>180 mmHg systolic or >110 mmHg diastolic) [5]. J-shaped mortality curves complicate interpretation of these findings.

In one study, the lowest mortality was found in those with a pre-dialysis systolic BP of 160–189 mmHg [6]. Those with a pre-dialysis systolic BP <110 mmHg and diastolic BP <50 mmHg had the highest risk of death. The relationship seemed strongest in the presence of congestive cardiac failure. A pre-dialysis SBP <120 mmHg for both incident and prevalent patients and achievement of a goal pre-BP <140/90 mmHg [7] were also associated with increased mortality.

Management

It is possible to achieve good BP control solely by correction of extracellular volume overload with long-hours HD. Thrice weekly sessions of 8 h each lower the risk of IDH and allow 90 % of patients to be anti-hypertensive-free [8]. Constrained capacity prevents similar programmes in most units although home, nocturnal or short, frequent HD may circumvent these resource issues. In practice, though, most patients will be receiving 'standard' HD schedules delivered for about 4 h, thrice weekly. Attempts to regain control of the extracellular fluid space can be complex and prolonged.

The first step is to identify patients who might be volume loaded, the only evidence for which might be persisting hypertension. Patients with pre- and post-dialysis BPs consistently >160/90 and/or >140/90, respectively, may benefit from BP control. Others, who may breach these thresholds more intermittently, might benefit from inter-dialytic BP assessment, through primary care, self- or ambulatory BP monitoring. The latter may be beneficial if there is a suspicion of hypotension. If discrete readings are consistently >140/85 or a mean ambulatory reading >130/80 without evidence of hypotension, patients may benefit from augmented BP management.

Salt and Fluid Restriction

The initial steps should be to review the dialysate sodium prescription and dietary salt and fluid intake – see Table 61.1.

A net dialysate sodium gain should be avoided by resetting the dialysate sodium towards the individual's pre-dialysis serum sodium. Sodium profiles should generally be avoided as most result in sodium loading. Where dialysate sodium needs to be reduced, this should be undertaken cautiously to reduce the risks of cramps and hypotension. A unit-wide

Table 61.1 BP and volume control – salt and water management (see text for further details)

Review dialysate sodium prescription	Reduce dialysate sodium towards usual pre-dialysis sodium by 1 mmol/L every 2 weeks Avoid sodium profiling
Review dietary salt intake	Reduce daily sodium intake to 80–100 mmol (a 'no added salt' diet) Beware hidden salt – encourage food label checking Avoid potassium-containing salt substitutes If cardiac failure, aim for tighter restriction
Review fluid restriction	Aim for inter-dialytic weight gain ≤3 % 'active' body weight If nonobese, active and actual body weight are pragmatically equivalent If obese, active body weight = 25 × height^2 (weight in kg, height in metres; 'fat-free' BMI assumed as 25)

reduction in dialysate sodium (from 141 mmol/L to 138) has been associated with improved BP [9] and should be considered where standard prescriptions risk sodium imbalance.

Accounting for urine output, fluid restriction should limit inter-dialytic weight gains to ~3 % of 'active' body weight. This will usually work out at an allowable weight gain of 2.5 kg. Diuretics may help limit the degree of fluid restriction by increasing urine output. Patient education (including dietary sodium restriction of 80–100 mmol/day) (see Table 61.2) is usually delivered by renal dietitians and dialysis nursing staff but should be inculcated into the culture of the unit. The central role of sodium in hypertension, in volume overload and – immediately relevant to the patient – in thirst should be emphasised. It is useful to ask patients to try to differentiate between the sensations of a dry mouth, per se, and thirst as the former may have another cause (see below).

Medical staff play a role in reenforcing the above but also in reviewing drugs that might be contributing to a dry mouth (review anticholinergic agents but check side effect profiles of others, too, in the formulary); consider ACE inhibitors which may ameliorate thirst.

Table 61.2 BP and volume control – salt and water restriction and patient education (see text for further details)

Emphasise key role of sodium in hypertension, volume overload, thirst
Differentiate between sensations of thirst and dry mouth
Review drugs that may be contributing to dry mouth
Patient tips and tricks to manage restrictions
Check sodium content of processed food
Take tablets with food where possible
Use small-volume cups
Sip and savour, don't gulp
Use ice cubes, ice lollies, sweets or gum (n.b. sugar content), mouth washes, artificial saliva
Use pre-filled measuring jug to help guide daily fluid intake

Identification of Goals

Identify a BP/fluid management goal for each stage of management and continue to re-evaluate progress on these goals, ensuring that these are communicated to the patient and amongst all relevant staff. Echocardiography may reveal left ventricular hypertrophy which may require more aggressive BP management using ACE inhibitors or angiotensin-2 receptor blockers.

A number of examples are given in Table 61.3.

The development of hypotensive symptoms, especially during dialysis, should not be assumed to be a result of excessive BP control or overaggressive target weight reduction. Consider the contribution from mistimed or inappropriate anti-hypertensive therapy, excessive ultrafiltration rates and over-rapid reductions in the target weight.

Target Weight Reduction

Cautious reductions in target weight should be the initial step in achieving BP/fluid control (see Table 61.3) unless hypertension or fluid overload are severe. These rates are usually well tolerated but might need to be sustained over a period of weeks to months to take effect. If even these are poorly tolerated, more cautious decrements (e.g. 0.1 kg/week) can be tried. Changes at the end of the weekly dialysis cycle may be better tolerated when patients will have less fluid to lose after the short inter-dialytic gap.

Table 61.3 BP and fluid management – example treatment goals (see text for further details)

Goal	Actions	Trigger for re-evaluation	The next steps
1. Pre- and post-BP consistently <160/90 and <140/90, respectively	Nurse led Reduction of target weight by 0.1 kg/session in 2-week cycles Review of salt and fluid intake – seeking dietetic help if necessary Re-evaluation of control after each 2-week cycle Repeat cycles whilst goals are still not met	Nurse-led feedback if Failure to achieve goals after predefined number of treatment cycles (e.g. 3 or 4) Haemodynamic instability during HD Pre-HD BP <120/50	Medical review of Rate of target weight reduction – consider more cautious/aggressive approach Anti-hypertensive drugs Are timing or dose contributing to haemodynamic instability? Can target weight reduction, alone, achieve goals or is drug treatment necessary? Supplementary measures to reduce haemodynamic instability, e.g. Cooled dialysate Intra-HD blood volume monitoring to guide UF profiling Increased session duration/frequency (if patient willing) Isolated UF with isovolaemic HD Need for inter-dialytic BP measurement to help re-evaluate BP goals

(continued)

Similarly, arthropathy tends to develop after ~10 years and presents with arthralgias and joint stiffness in a symmetrical pattern, starting in the shoulders and spreading to other joints. Symptoms are described as being worse on HD and at night. Effusions can develop, especially of the shoulders and knees, and are usually bilateral. Diagnosis is usually on the basis of the clinical pattern of joint involvement, exclusion of other causes and a typical dialysis vintage. Histological confirmation is often difficult to achieve due to the inaccessibility of deposits, but, where possible, a tissue diagnosis should be considered. There are a number of less common manifestations of dialysis-related amyloidosis. A destructive spondyloarthropathy can develop, usually of the cervical spine, and is often asymptomatic until it causes compressive symptoms such as a radiculopathy. Magnetic resonance imaging can help differentiate this from infectious discitis and will show narrowed disc spaces, erosion of vertebral margins and subchondral sclerosis. A chronic tenosynovitis of the finger flexors can lead to restricted movement, pain and trigger finger. Pathological fractures can occur due to amyloid cyst formation at the ends of long bones. These need to be differentiated from 'brown tumours' (due to severe hyperparathyroidism) and other lesions. A tissue diagnosis may be necessary if there is diagnostic doubt.

Rare extra-articular manifestations include amyloid deposition subcutaneously (near joints) and in the epidural space, gastrointestinal tract and tongue. The presence of cardiac involvement suggests a non-dialysis-related amyloidosis.

Management

Ideally, renal function should be restored with a kidney transplant. The long duration of dialysis associated with the development of dialysis-related amyloidosis usually implies some difficulty with transplantation, though. If it can be performed, however, pain can quickly improve, with a return to mobility following sometime after. There may be some resolution in the size of amyloid deposits, but bone cysts resolve much more slowly.

B2m adsorption columns, used in some units, are not widely available, and their role in routine management remains unclear.

Surgical treatment options include carpal tunnel decompression, synovectomy, curettage or bone grafting of amyloid cysts and joint replacement.

Prevention

High-flux, biocompatible, synthetic dialysis membranes should be used in any likely to be long-term survivors on HD without a realistic prospect of kidney transplantation. Reprocessing of polysulfone membranes may enhance B2M clearance but only when undertaken with bleach and formaldehyde (peracetic acid may reduce adsorption) [17]. Technique changes including longer hours (including nocturnal or daily treatment), haemodiafiltration or haemofiltration should be considered. It should be borne in mind that even with these technique changes, removal will still not completely account for production.

Symptom Control

As well as standard analgesia, intra-articular steroids or oral steroid therapy (e.g. prednisolone 10–20 mg/day) can produce effective symptom control but does risk osteopenia and infection. Dialysis technique and membrane changes should also be undertaken to reduce the risk of further amyloid deposition.

Cardiovascular Disease in the Haemodialysis Patient (See Also Chap. 52)

Cardiovascular disease (CVD) accounts for around 50 % of all deaths on dialysis [18]. Although deaths from myocardial infarction (MI) are more common than in the non-dialysis population, there is a particular preponderance of sudden cardiac arrest and arrhythmia. The incident dialysis population has a higher burden of traditional cardiovascular (CV) risk factors with the individual patient often carrying more than one. Around 40 % of patients enrolled into the HEMO study had a diagnosis of ischaemic heart disease (IHD) [19] with the USRDS reporting a 10 % annual incidence of MI or angina.

Table 61.6 details a number of scenarios where coronary artery disease should be suspected even in the absence of symptoms typical of MI or angina. It should be remembered that the process of HD is a haemodynamic stressor that may

Table 61.6 Possible presentations of coronary artery disease in the HD patient (see text for further details)

Recurrent intra-dialytic hypotension
Persisting inter-dialytic hypotension
Dysrhythmias
Exertional dyspnoea
Persisting symptoms of heart failure despite achievement of assumed target weight
Difficulty achieving dry weight due to hypotension
The incidental finding of ventricular dysfunction (for instance, during renal transplant recipient workup), especially if progressive
The finding of regional wall motion abnormalities on echocardiography

reveal manifestations of coronary artery disease when none may be present between sessions.

In essence, the dialysis team needs to provide a consistent and supportive approach to risk factor modification including smoking. Guidelines for exercise are available from the UK Renal Association, and the culture of the unit should be to encourage regular exercise as the norm (http://www.renal.org/Clinical/GuidelinesSection/CardiovascularDiseaseInCKD.aspx [20]).

Diabetic Management

Attendance for HD thrice weekly detracts from the logistics and (patient) acceptability of non-renal clinic review. This may be especially relevant for routine diabetes management. Close links should be maintained with the patient's local diabetic services, and, where possible, point-of-care assessments should be considered whilst the patient is receiving dialysis. Podiatry interventions (due to intra-dialytic anticoagulation) and retinal screening may not be possible, but the linkage with diabetic services will have been established.

There are two other practical considerations.

Firstly, the insulin prescription should be reviewed in relation to the weekly dialysis cycle as a low dialysate glucose may lower requirements on dialysis days.

Secondly, questions have been raised about the accuracy of the glycosylated haemoglobin (HbA1c) in monitoring diabetics with ESRD. A variety of factors can affect interpretation – interference with assays from carbamylation of haemoglobin in urea-rich environments, reduced red cell life spans, rapid erythropoiesis after augmentation of anaemia management and the effect of blood transfusions. HbA1c levels between 6 and 7 % do, however, appear to reflect the degree of diabetic control although values >7 % may underestimate this:

- However, as yet, it is unclear if good control affects the rate of progression of other microvascular complications of diabetes in HD patients.
- It is also unclear whether this will have any impact on the development of overt cardiovascular disease, particularly given the importance of vascular calcification in aetiology.
- The risk of hypoglycaemia in the more vulnerable patient requires a degree of compromise on overall diabetic control.

Anaemia Management

Recent evidence (discussed elsewhere in this textbook) has removed the impetus for complete correction of anaemia, to within the range of the normal population, but the importance of a robust anaemia management system that avoids see-sawing haemoglobin levels cannot be overemphasised. Sudden anaemia in several patients is suggestive of a systemic problem and may indicate water contamination, e.g. with copper or chloramines.

Sudden Cardiac Death

Sudden cardiac arrest is the most common cause of cardiac death in HD patients. It is more likely to occur around the time of the first HD session of the week [21]. Most episodes are thought to be triggered by myocardial ischaemia in the context of a structurally abnormal heart and produce ventricular dysrhythmias. Risk factors may include coronary artery disease and myocardial structural and functional changes. Features of the dialysis prescription that seem to add to risk include rapid solute shifts and high UF rates. Specifically, a low dialysate potassium (<2 mEq/L [22]), especially when used, inappropriately, when the pre-dialysis serum potassium is well controlled, may be important as may a low calcium dialysate. In addition, a dialysis session duration <3.5 h and ultrafiltration requirements >5.7 % of the post-HD weight were specific associations in DOPPS [23].

For patients with recurrent IDH, there should be a high index of suspicion that episodes might be due to dysrhythmias. Intra-dialytic cardiac monitoring and 24-h ECG recordings should be considered. The finding of a significant dysrhythmia or (survival of) sudden cardiac arrest should prompt a comprehensive evaluation including an assessment for underlying coronary artery disease or cardiac structural abnormality, review of potentially arrhythmogenic drugs, modification of dialysate potassium and calcium settings and alteration of the dialysis prescription to mitigate high UF rates. Appropriate patient education should be undertaken if inter-dialytic fluid gains are excessive and should incorporate review of the dialysate sodium prescription and dietary salt intake. Other measures to ameliorate haemodynamic intolerance of HD are described, above, under 'Intra-dialytic Hypotension', and should include consideration of a transfer to peritoneal dialysis.

Preventative measures should include prescriptions of adequate HD session duration (≥4 h), careful justification of low dialysate potassium and calcium prescriptions (avoiding them where possible by review of drugs, dietary intake, etc.) and attention to inter-dialytic weight gains.

Infection Control

Infection control covers a number of different aspects of HD care and is covered in detail by Collier and Hopkins.

The latter may be a more practical treatment due to its ready availability on most wards. Extravasation is a problem so administration should be via wide-bore vascular access. Some have used hypertonic intravenous saline solutions, but these are of increasingly limited availability due to safety concerns. Recovery should take place between several hours and 24 h after cessation of treatment. If this does not occur, alternative aetiologies should be reconsidered.

Needle Dislodgement

Blood losses may be undetected and potentially fatal. Bleeding from the patient's AV access will occur regardless of whether arterial, venous or both needles are dislodged, and it may be significant if it is not quickly stemmed. Perhaps the biggest danger, though, is of losses through a displaced venous return as venous pressure alarms do not reliably differentiate between atmospheric and downstream venous pressures. With extracorporeal blood flows of 350–400 mL/min, exsanguination may swiftly occur. Arterial needle dislodgement, in isolation, should not lead to significant losses through the extracorporeal circuit; downstream air leak detector alarms should protect the patient from air embolism.

Patients at risk include those who are obtunded or agitated. Others at risk include those with excessive sweating, which may affect the adhesive properties of dressings and tape, and those on long-duration, nocturnal treatment. The needle sites of at-risk patients should be kept under regular surveillance during treatment by dialysis staff. Where dialysis staff are not present (e.g. in the home setting) or where patients are at particular risk, blood leak alarms (similar to nocturnal enuresis pads) may be a valuable adjunct.

All patients should, however, be considered to be at some level of risk, and, where privacy allows, the needled portion of their access should be kept visible (an 'airline seatbelt' policy).

Air Embolism

This rare complication is potentially fatal and requires swift action to save life. On the HD unit, the venous system is the initial route of air entry and is almost universally in the setting of a veno-venous dialysis catheter. Air embolism via AV access is highly unlikely (as vascular >> atmospheric pressures) unless there is an accidental 'push' of air through it. This is likely to be a result of human error rather than a machine problem if air leak detectors in the extracorporeal blood circuit are functioning.

Excluding the risks associated with dialysis catheter insertion or removal, maintenance HD patients are vulnerable to air embolism:

- When sat up (as most are when dialysing) as central venous pressures are lower.
- Through catheter fracture or deliberate/accidental incision.
- Through catheter extrusion – the subcutaneous tunnel may provide a ready portal to the venous system.
- Through loose connections, either of the blood lines at the start of dialysis or of the caps at the end.

A potentially fatal dose has been estimated to be 300–500 mL introduced at >100 mL/s when the filtering capacity of the pulmonary circulation is exceeded and gas enters the arterial circulation. This dose may be much lower if paradoxical embolism, with direct right-to-left communication with the arterial circulation, occurs.

Pathophysiologically, significant venous air embolism that reaches the arterial circulation can cause organ ischaemia including myocardial if the coronary arteries are involved. Further upstream, gas bubbles can cause occlusion of vessels in the pulmonary arterial tree, which will, in turn, increase right heart pressures and ultimately reduce cardiac output due to reduced venous return to the left heart. Smaller gas bubbles in the pulmonary microcirculation can lead to endothelial damage which can, in turn, produce bronchoconstriction, ventilation-perfusion mismatching and noncardiac pulmonary oedema.

The clinical features of air embolism may be:

Organ specific

Depends on the pattern of organ ischaemia when gas enters the arterial tree but can include:

Acute neurology

Livedo reticularis

Coronary insufficiency

Cardiorespiratory

Dyspnoea, wheeze, lung crepitations, tachypnea, tachycardia, central chest pain, hypotension, signs of acute right heart failure.

There may be a 'gasp' reflex, thought to be caused by air entering the pulmonary circulation.

There may be a churning, systolic-diastolic murmur caused by gas trapped within the right ventricle.

The diagnosis of air embolism is largely one of exclusion, but maintaining a high index of suspicion in the correct clinical context is vital as it is a differential diagnosis that is often not considered. As well as the clinical features, described above, aspiration through the most downstream limb of an in situ dialysis catheter (the venous lumen should be closest to the pulmonary circulation) might draw back air if performed swiftly or if the gas bolus is large. A range of investigations (ECG, chest x-ray and urgent echocardiography, if available) should be undertaken to help rule out alternative diagnoses but may also reveal corroborative findings (right heart strain, localised radiographic oligaemia or air in the pulmonary vasculature or ventricle, for instance).

Subsequent investigations, such as CT scanning, may also reveal evidence of vascular gas.

In terms of treatment, the potential source of air entry should be isolated, immediately (e.g. clamp lines or catheter, shut down blood pump, place secure airtight dressing over catheter exit sites). The patient should be placed in the left lateral decubitus head down position to allow gas to accumulate in the right ventricle rather than large pulmonary arteries (in the context of maintenance HD, the initial route into the vasculature will be through the venous system). Aspiration of gas through an in situ dialysis catheter should be attempted immediately after the diagnosis has been entertained and again once the left lateral decubitus head down position has been obtained (using the most downstream lumen). Closed chest massage, in the event of cardiorespiratory arrest, may allow larger gas bubbles to be broken down. Supportive management should be initiated (high-flow oxygen, haemodynamic support, ventilatory support, etc.). Where the diagnosis of air embolism is established and has caused cardiorespiratory or specific organ compromise, particularly neurological, early initiation of hyperbaric oxygen therapy should be considered.

Air embolism can be prevented through secure connection technique of blood lines and caps to dialysis catheter lumens, before and after HD treatment, respectively. Patients with dialysis catheters should be advised on correct care of their access including how to troubleshoot a fractured, open or extruded line – airtight dressings, spare catheter caps and clamps should be readily accessible to the patient when at home or on holiday.

Dialyser Reactions

These may be divided into type A and type B reactions.

Type A reactions usually occur within the first few minutes of dialysis with venous return of blood to the systemic circulation and may be caused by:

- Bacterial fragments, from contaminated water and inadequate sterilisation of reused dialysers
- Chemical products used in dialyser manufacture, sterilisation (e.g. ethylene oxide) or reprocessing (e.g. bleach, hydrogen peroxide, formaldehyde) that have been inadequately rinsed out before use
- Acetate-based dialysate
- The combined use of AN-69 membranes and ACE inhibitors, which enhances bradykinin generation:
  - The use of ACE inhibitors with AN-69 ST membranes, whose electronegative charge is markedly reduced by surface treatment with a biocompatible polymer, carries a significantly lower incidence of anaphylactoid reactions.
  - The combined use of AN-69 membranes and angiotensin-2 receptor blockers (ARBs) has also, rarely, been associated with anaphylactoid reactions, even though these agents do not increase bradykinin levels.

These reactions seem to be more common in those with an allergic tendency.

Symptoms range from the relatively modest (wheeze, urticarial rash, burning at the access needle site, chest or back pains, headaches, gastrointestinal symptoms, flushing, fevers and other allergic manifestations) through to cardiovascular collapse and death.

If a type A reaction is suspected, dialysis must be stopped, and the return of blood prevented by clamping the venous blood line. Blood in the dead space of the dialysis catheter or needles should be aspirated before administering saline flushes or drugs. The reaction should be treated with intravenous hydrocortisone, intravenous antihistamines, nebulised bronchodilators and supportive measures initiated as required (which may include circulatory or ventilatory support).

To investigate possible aetiologies, dialysate should be sent for sensitive culture and endotoxin counts (from the machine's dialysate inlet pipe and from the dialysate outlet of the dialyser). Dialyser rinsing and (if relevant) reprocessing technique should be reviewed. The combined use of ACE inhibitors and AN-69 membrane material should be identified. If no clear cause can be found, at the next session, switch to another membrane material, sterilised using an alternative technique (e.g. gamma irradiation, steam). Ensure the dialyser is well rinsed with at least 2 l of priming fluid before the patient is connected. Keep intravenous steroids and antihistamines to hand. Pretreatment with these agents should be considered if the previous reaction was severe. When starting treatment, keep blood flow low (Qb 50–100 mL/min) until venous return to the systemic circulation has been established for several minutes without incident.

Type B reactions are more common but generally less severe and usually occur later in treatment – between 15 and 30 min after starting. They are thought to be caused by complement activation after exposure of blood to cellulose membrane surfaces with free hydroxyl groups. As these membranes are being superseded by more biocompatible, synthetic materials, it might be anticipated that these reactions will become less and less common. Typical clinical features include chest pain, back pain, nausea and vomiting. Severe, anaphylactoid reactions are rare.

Acute Haemolysis

This should be part of the differential diagnosis of chest pain, back pain or dyspnoea, developing during HD. The potential that acute haemolysis could cause rapid and fatal hyperkalaemia requires a high index of suspicion and swift diagnosis.

Most episodes are due to some aspect of the HD process, itself:

Mechanical trauma from ill-fitting roller pumps, kinked blood lines and narrowed blood line lumens caused by poor manufacture*

Chemical contamination* of dialysate with formaldehyde, bleach, copper (leached from pipework) chloramine and nitrates

Heat mediated due to incorrectly set dialysate temperature

Osmotic injury from hypotonic dialysate caused by incorrect proportioning of concentrates and water

HD may decompensate pre-existing conditions:

For example, cooling of blood in the extracorporeal circuit may exacerbate cold agglutinin disease if temperatures fall low enough.

The diagnosis can be suggested by a port wine appearance of blood in the venous return and can be confirmed, rapidly, by the finding of a pink supernatant in a centrifuged specimen. Point-of-care testing may allow rapid detection of a reduced haematocrit. Corroborative evidence can be found in the FBC and blood film, but these should not be regarded as the initial investigative tools due to the critical delays in obtaining results.

The simultaneous development of symptoms in more than one patient dialysing at the same time should immediately raise the possibility of acute haemolysis of a system-wide aetiology. Examples are asterisked (*), above, but human error or misunderstanding may be propagated across more than one HD machine.

The approach to early discontinuation of HD for the patient developing chest pain or dyspnoea during treatment (see below) should afford some protection whilst assessment is underway. However, if the diagnosis is even suspected, HD must be stopped, immediately, with the venous return clamped to prevent extracorporeal blood from reaching the patient. Treatment should be discontinued, immediately, across the dialysis shift, if a system-wide problem is suspected.

Immediately after clamping, the dead space within dialysis catheter and AV fistula needles should be aspirated then locked. Unless or until alternative vascular access can be established, AV fistula needles should be kept in situ in case of the urgent need to treat hyperkalaemia or transfuse blood. As well as the FBC, biochemistry should also be sent, urgently, along with a group and save sample in case of the need for blood transfusion.

Acute intra-dialytic haemolysis requires the immediate attention of senior medical, nursing and technical staff to investigate aetiology and manage logistics. Contact with other local dialysis units and intensive care units should be made as a contingency in case of a system-wide problem that requires alternative venues for renal replacement therapy.

Differential Diagnosis of Chest Pain Developing *During* Dialysis

Coronary artery disease remains the primary differential due to its prevalence amongst the ESRD population. This may be precipitated by the haemodynamic stress of treatment and may not necessarily be associated with overt intra-dialytic hypotension. Dysrhythmias, to which HD patients are also prone, may manifest as chest pain.

Other alternative diagnoses, with particular relevance to the HD population, include air embolism, pulmonary embolism (for instance, from a clot adherent to a dialysis catheter or from AV access, particularly after an endovascular intervention), acute haemolysis, pneumothorax (after dialysis catheter insertion) and dialyser reactions.

Unless transient and self-limiting, it is probably safer to wash back and discontinue HD whilst the episode is under assessment although this needs to be judged on a case-by-case basis and may depend on the urgency of the need for dialysis (for instance, the dangerously hyperkalaemic patient may need to persist with HD whilst augmenting haemodynamic tolerability by temporarily discontinuing ultrafiltration). If HD is terminated, urgent bloods should be sent to confirm the biochemical safety of early discontinuation of the session.

Differential Diagnosis of Dyspnoea Developing *During* Dialysis

Patients who are fluid overloaded will be dyspnoeic before dialysis is commenced, and this should improve as ultrafiltration progresses. The differential diagnosis of dyspnoea developing or worsening during dialysis includes (a) coronary artery disease, (b) dysrhythmia, (c) air or pulmonary embolism, (d) pneumothorax, (e) dialyser reactions, (f) anaphylaxis due to an administered drug (e.g. intravenous iron), (g) cardiac tamponade, (h) acute haemolysis or (i) bacteraemia.

Systemic HD Care

The chapter, to this point, has focused on some of the most significant complications that can arise in the HD population and specific measures by which they might be prevented or mitigated. This second and final section will examine some of the more important systems that may be put in place that can help augment the quality of HD care as a whole. Rather than addressing individual complications, these measures help ensure a safe environment within which the HD patient can be treated.

Beyond these preventative strategies, all those dealing with HD patients should also be aware of the widespread impact that an isolated breach of process might produce; unusual patterns of clinical presentation or results might just point towards a system-wide problem that requires urgent attention. Although some such problems can be detected and minimised by routine reporting (e.g. staphylococcal bacteraemia rates, water quality feedback), others may require intuition and individual vigilance (e.g. haemolytic complications, iatrogenic hypernatraemia caused by incorrect machine calibration). The importance of a senior, multidisciplinary approach to tackle these problems cannot be overstated.

Convective Therapies

A wide range of toxins may contribute to the uraemic syndrome. The importance of small solute clearance is well established, but middle molecules (500–15,000 Da) might contribute to pathology (the obvious examples being B2M and parathyroid hormone). Larger solutes and protein-bound molecules may, in addition, contribute to the cardiovascular disease that is so prevalent amongst the HD population. The removal of solutes of increasing molecular weight becomes increasingly problematic with conventional diffusion dialysis, with membrane pore size, ultimately, limiting removal. Convective therapies (haemofiltration and haemodiafiltration) are much more effective at removing these larger molecules.

Convection depends on the transmembrane pressure (TMP) and the sieving coefficient (a property of the individual membrane for that solute) = [solute] ultrafiltrate/[solute] plasma. The closer this ratio is to 1, the more complete the removal of that particular solute. Two other factors influence convection. The first of these is protein adsorption to the membrane, which increases resistance to transfer of both water and solutes of all sizes. The second factor is concentration polarisation, caused by the slower movement of larger molecules across the dialysis membrane. This leads to accumulation of these large solutes at the surface of the membrane, impeding the movement of smaller molecules into the dialysate compartment. The large-molecule concentration gradient, developing across the hollow fibre, encourages movement back into the centre of the fibre as well as across the membrane. This phenomenon can be minimised with the use of pre-dilutional fluid replacement, high blood flows and lower UF rates.

Pure convective treatment (i.e. haemofiltration) is less efficient at removing small molecules as it does not have the power of the concentration gradient behind it. This disadvantage is circumvented by the addition of diffusive removal (i.e. with haemodiafiltration). Albumin losses do occur during therapy, but substitution fluid replacement rates of 60–120 mL/min (a maximum of ~25 L/session) should minimise these. Pre- and post-dilutional replacement of substitution fluid have their respective advantages and disadvantages.

The main disadvantage of post-dilutional replacement is haemoconcentration. High transmembrane pressures can also lead to membrane fibre rupture and increased albumin leakage. Transmembrane pressures should, therefore, be kept at less than 400 mmHg. Haemoconcentration should also be limited by keeping the filtration fraction at 50 % or less. The filtration fraction (FF) can be calculated as follows:

FF = ultrafiltration flow rate/plasma flow rate, where plasma flow rate = Qb × (1 – haematocrit) and Qb is the delivered extracorporeal blood flow.

The minimum Qb to keep the FF at 50 % or less can therefore be calculated as:

$$\text{Minimum Qb} = \text{UFR} / 0.5 \times (1 - \text{haematocrit})$$

For example:

(a)

$$\text{Haematocrit} = 0.3, \text{UFR} = 60\,\text{mL}/\text{min}, \text{target FF} = 50\%$$

$$\text{Minimum Qb} = 60 / 0.5 \times 0.7 = 171\,\text{mL}/\text{min}$$

(b)

$$\text{Haematocrit} = 0.4, \text{UFR} = 120\,\text{mL}/\text{min}, \text{target FF} = 50\%$$

$$\text{Minimum Qb} = 400\,\text{mL}/\text{min}$$

The main disadvantage of pre-dilutional replacement is the expense of extra substitution fluid requirements. Mid-dilution HDF is said to minimise the disadvantages and maximise the advantages of the other replacement techniques. Unfortunately, it requires a special filter allowing the infusion of replacement fluid at the midpoint in the dialyser. The substitution fluid required for HDF is now, almost invariably, produced online to ultrapure standards.

In terms of membrane technology, the larger the pore size, the greater the loss of albumin during treatment. However, the use of asymmetric membranes may facilitate the removal of the larger, target molecules (excluding albumin) and also phosphate and beta-2 microglobulin.

There is some evidence, albeit not of RCT standard, that HDF may deliver better small and middle molecule clearances, better phosphate control (although its intracellular compartmentalisation may mean it can take months for any benefit to be realised) and improved haemodynamic stability (perhaps through the sodium loading or cooling effects of fluid replacement). Some evidence points, also, to improved well-being, but there is no clear evidence of benefit in terms of control of BP, anaemia management, regression of cardiac hypertrophy, nutritional status, hospitalisations or survival.

The reduced costs of HDF with the online production of substitution fluid make the technique a much more attractive option despite the current paucity of evidence in favour of its use. Although absolute indications for initiating haemodiafiltration have yet to be defined, the presence or prevention of beta-2 microglobulin amyloidosis, haemodynamic instability or patients with no clear prospect of renal transplantation who are likely to survive 2 years or more would seem like reasonable circumstances to consider the technique.

Water Quality

On a standard treatment schedule, HD patients are exposed to at least 350 L of water per week, separated from their bloodstream only by the semipermeable membrane. For those receiving convective therapies or whose dialysers are reprocessed, water exposure will be direct.

Potential sources of harm include:

- Aluminium intoxication syndrome – aluminium is added to remove colloidal substances from the mains water supply. The syndrome may manifest as encephalopathy, bone disease or erythropoietin resistance but is now much less common since the introduction of reverse osmosis.
- Chloramine-induced haemolysis and methaemoglobinaemia – added to mains water for microbial control. Its removal, and that of chlorine, by HD water treatment processes renders the product water vulnerable to microbial growth.
- Fluoride-induced bone disease – added to mains water; it can be fatal in high concentrations.
- Microbial contamination – can produce pyrogenic reactions when contamination is heavy, but even low levels of bacterial growth may contribute to long-term morbidity. Chronic inflammation (as evidenced by a raised plasma CRP or interleukin-6 level) is common in the chronic HD population and may be associated with an increased risk of long-term morbidity. This may be a consequence of low-level microbial contamination of the dialysate. Bacterial products such as endotoxin fragments, peptidoglycans and bacterial DNA can all induce cytokines and are able to cross even low-flux dialysers.

Quality Assurance

A comprehensive and detailed overview of requirements is given in the joint UK Renal Association – Association of Renal Technologists guideline (www.renal.org/Libraries/Guidelines/RA_and_ART_guideline_final_version_20_01_12_1.sflb.ashx), but a few points need to be drawn out.

Communication

Clear lines of communication should be established with the local water provider to ensure early warning of variations in water content due to both changes in water treatment practice by the supplier and seasonal fluctuations. The biggest threats to the dialysis patient are the deliberate additives to mains water rather than existing contaminants.

Clear lines of communication should also be established with the HD unit institution's own Estates Department to ensure changes in process do not have an impact upon the provision of dialysis water. As an example, *Legionella* preventative practice may involve the use of hydrogen peroxide which can cause both methaemoglobinaemia and haemolysis. Hydrogen peroxide is not well removed by reverse osmosis.

Clear responsibilities should be defined. The monitoring programme should include technical variables (e.g. water plant pressures and conductivity), chemical monitoring and microbiological surveillance. The output from these monitoring programmes should be reported on a regular basis to the clinical lead for HD and 'HD committee'. For all monitored variables, action plans should be available in the event of deviations from expected results. These outputs should, therefore, include documentation of action plans – a good disinfection schedule, for instance, should be reactive to microbial counts with an action level of 50 % of the maximum allowable limit.

Technique

The recommended techniques for monitoring should be used to ensure that they are of sufficient enough sensitivity to detect problems, early. As examples, water culture should use techniques most suited for growing fastidious, water-borne organisms (e.g. membrane filtration) using a low-nutrient medium (e.g. Reasoner's 2A agar) at a lower incubation temperature (e.g. 25 °C) for longer periods (e.g. 7 days). Endotoxin assays should use the limulus amoebocyte lysate assay.

Hardware

The primary water treatment processes are discussed in detail in the joint UK Renal Association – Association of Renal Technologists guideline. A few relevant highlights follow:

- Deionisers provide an excellent environment for microbiological growth so downstream control measures are needed.

- A robust programme of deioniser replacement is required as exhausted resins can release toxic ions (e.g. fluoride) when other ions with higher affinity are present in the supply water.
- Carbon beds (which remove organic compounds, chlorine and chloramines) should be replaced, regularly, to prevent their exhaustion:
  - They should be placed upstream of the reverse osmosis unit as chlorine can cause degradation of the RO membrane.
  - Because of the serious implications of chloramine escape past an exhausted carbon bed, two carbon filtration units are usually placed in series as a safety measure.
- Carbon beds provide a good environment for microbiological growth so downstream control measures will be needed.
- Water softeners are needed in hard water areas to remove both calcium and magnesium – these are best placed upstream of the reverse osmosis unit to prevent degradation of its membrane by these salts.
- An extra filtration step may be needed to help augment microbial control – for instance, point-of-use endotoxin filters at the dialysis machine

Ultrapure Versus Standard Quality Water

The UK guidelines, in keeping with others, suggest the following:

- Standard delivery of water for dialysis:
  - Bacterial colony counts <100 colony-forming units/mL
  - Endotoxin count <0.25 IU/mL
- Ultrapure delivery:
  - Bacterial colony counts <0.1 colony-forming units/mL
  - Endotoxin count <0.03 IU/mL

Some, but by no means all, studies have shown that a switch from standard to ultrapure dialysis may reduce levels of inflammation in chronic HD patients. Its use may improve anaemia management, help prevent dialysis-related amyloidosis and improve nutritional status. There is no clear evidence of benefits in terms of other clinical outcomes, though.

Although ultrapure water is a prerequisite for convective therapies and dialyser reprocessing, it is desirable for all given the relative ease of its provision when water plant hardware and maintenance are already providing good-quality water. There are some practical highlights to consider:

- Maintenance and disinfection programmes should be robust.
- The water pipe connecting the main water delivery circuit to the HD machine is a weak link and vulnerable to contamination – these should be replaced/disinfected on a regular basis.
- Point-of-use, pre-dialyser endotoxin filters should be replaced, regularly, according to manufacturers' instructions but more frequently if downstream water quality deteriorates.
- Care should be taken in the preparation of concentrates, especially bicarbonate concentrates which are especially prone to microbial growth – when using bicarbonate concentrate, as a matter of course, containers should be disposed of at the end of the dialysis unit working day.
- Samples should be tested by the most sensitive, recommended techniques but also when they are likely to yield the worst results (just prior to routine system disinfections and at the far end of the water loop).

It should be remembered, though, that culture and endotoxin assays only detect a proportion of cytokine-inducing substances that many present – yeasts, peptidoglycans and other bacterial fragments will not be picked up.

Care of the Haemodialysis Inpatient

The chronic HD patient suffers more frequent and prolonged hospital admissions than the general hospital population. These inpatient stays place the HD patient at risk for a number of reasons:

- Inappropriate care of vascular access
- Undernutrition
- Inappropriate drug dosing
- The burden of transfer to and from the HD unit for regular sessions, especially if from an outside hospital – opportunities for comprehensive clinical evaluation when an HD inpatient attends, briefly, for their routine session, are limited.

Inpatient care of the HD patient with a non-renal problem should be at least overseen (remotely or in person) by renal services and, where necessary, through joint care. Patients should be advised that if they are admitted, as either an emergency or electively, to another department or hospital, local health-care teams should be making prompt contact with the on-call renal team. They, in turn, should be discussing the need for transfer for renal unit care with the senior nephrologist on duty. It may be better for a patient to transfer their home team (e.g. their general surgical team) than risk the vagaries of remote renal care.

One caveat to transfer of inpatients to the renal unit from outside hospitals is the potential for their arrival with unheralded critical illness. It is our practice for physiological severity scoring of all potential inpatient transfers from other hospitals to allow triage towards either critical care or the renal unit. Even if patients are not diverted for critical care, an understanding of physiological instability can highlight the need for added vigilance and ensure early involvement of critical care outreach teams.

Finally, an under-recognised problem for the inpatient HD patient is the potential for under-prescription and under-delivery of the dose of dialysis. The sicker chronic HD patient may, in urea kinetic terms, be closer to the patient with AKI than their stable, outpatient counterpart. Loss of lean body mass and changes in volume status can affect V (the volume of distribution of urea), and patients can become markedly hypercatabolic. In addition, HD patients admitted with vascular access problems are also, clearly, at risk of inadequate dialysis. For this reason, it is recommended that inpatients on chronic HD, unless entirely clinically stable with documented dialysis adequacy, should have the adequacy of their dialysis prescription and its delivery reviewed at each session.

Organisation of the HD Service

The 'conveyor belt' nature of in-centre HD provision serves the core function of delivering the HD prescription in an efficient and timely fashion. However, care requirements that are divergent from the routine can be vulnerable to these immediate priorities. The challenge for a busy HD service, therefore, is how the complexity of individualised care can be accommodated amongst the logistics of HD delivery and the overarching strategic and organisational goals of the service as a whole. One particular issue is the need to break down those domains of HD care that are traditionally deemed to be exclusively 'nursing' in nature and those deemed to be predominantly 'medical' to ensure that holistic, multidisciplinary care can be delivered.

The HD Clinic

Traditionally viewed as the domain where medical therapy is defined and delivered, this can be vulnerable to a number of factors:

- Inadequate capacity may limit frequent enough follow-up to meet medical care needs. Assuming that most stable HD patients will need review on a 3 monthly basis but that some will need much more frequent follow-up, our own practice is to organise HD clinic capacity to allow an average of five clinic appointments per annum.
- Discordant record keeping – multiple different sources of the clinical record are a risk to patient care. A clear understanding is needed, across the multidisciplinary team as to what are acceptable points of documentation and what are not. Progress towards fully integrated electronic health records will mitigate this problem, but renal-specific functionality is currently delivered by specific software that is not immediately visible within the entirety of the hospital record.
- Non-attendance – coordinating clinic visits with dialysis sessions (before, during or after) can help. Again, enough HD clinic capacity is needed to ensure that there is enough flexibility to allow this degree of coordination – it should be remembered that dialysis shifts rarely coordinate with physicians' routine clinic working patterns.
- Adherence to a strategic 'tick list' – there is much anecdotal and some more robust evidence to suggest that senior allied health-care practitioners are more likely to achieve patient care targets than training grade medical staff. The available resource will clearly dictate how the HD clinic service is staffed (with nurse practitioners, senior medical staff, trainee medical staff under supervision, etc.), but our experience is that a 'tick box' clinic proforma is rarely a satisfactory solution for a deficient strategic drive or inadequate experience. The removal of certain patient care pathways from the domain of the HD clinic (e.g. vascular access surveillance), with the drive provided by health-care professionals dedicated to the task, may be beneficial.
- Communicating the individualised care plan – certain aspects of the care plan will need to be delivered by HD unit nursing staff. Examples include:
  - Once off extra blood tests
  - Regular monitoring with non-standard bloods (e.g. ANCA monitoring in vasculitis patients)
  - Blood pressure and fluid management programmes

  Our own practice uses a dialysis communications section in the HD nursing record that contains all current requirements and can include the need for feedback on the success or failure of a particular course of action. Each HD session requires sign-off that these requirements have been checked. Automated (electronic) alerts would represent a more elegant augmentation to cohesive, multidisciplinary team communications.

The Multidisciplinary Team (MDT) Meeting

The opportunity for MDT discussion of individual patients should be welcomed with some evidence that these produce greater success in achieving treatment goals.

Our practice is for regular meetings of HD medical and nursing staff to discuss individual named patients and with input from other health-care professionals (e.g. renal dietetics, vascular access coordinators). As well as problems, specific to that individual patient, topics covered include BP and fluid management, access to transplantation, urea kinetic modelling (and vascular access) and bloods review. It can also be a useful opportunity to review modality and, for instance, ensure that suitable candidates for HDF, home HD and inpatient, self-care programmes, are identified.

Encouraging participation in in-centre, self-care programmes can yield benefits for both the patient and the service as a whole (for instance, by providing a stepping stone towards home HD).

We also adopt a systemic approach, involving HD medical staff and relevant allied health-care professionals (e.g. anaemia nurses, BP link nurses, renal dietitians) targeted at specific patient care goals including anaemia management, BP control, mineral metabolic control and access to transplantation. Renal IT systems play a critical role in, for instance, identifying outliers who may need more individualised attention.

The 'HD Committee'

As well as individual patient care, provided through the HD clinic and MDT meeting, there is a need to assure safe delivery and development of the service as a whole. The 'HD committee' – whether virtual or real – can be a useful forum for reporting of, for instance, regular infection control audits and water quality results and for discussion of unit developments and new protocols.

Management of Intercurrent Problems

Attendance for thrice weekly session places a heavy burden on patients when transport to and from the dialysis unit and recovery times are factored in. It is therefore unsurprising that main centre HD patients tend to seek the advice of renal unit doctors for unrelated medical problems. It is difficult to offer advice on how this should be managed as this will depend on available staffing resources. However, the use of HD nurses for triaging activities can place them in a difficult position if the wrong call is made. The use of a senior nurse to filter requests for assessment can mitigate the extra burden on a perhaps limited medical resource, but, to some extent, there has to be an acceptance that certain facets of primary care will have to be undertaken on the dialysis unit. Nevertheless, there are key primary care functions (e.g. vaccinations, medication reviews and various screening programmes) that require the relationship between the HD patient and the general practitioner to be maintained. This contact should be strongly encouraged.

References

1. Kooman JP, Gladziwa U, Bocker G, et al. Blood pressure during the interdialytic period in haemodialysis patients: estimation of representative blood pressure values. Nephrol Dial Transplant. 1992;7(9):917–23.
2. Baumgart P, Walger P, Gemen S, et al. Blood pressure elevation during the night in chronic renal failure, hemodialysis and after renal transplantation. Nephron. 1991;57(3):293–8.
3. Agarwal R, Andersen MJ, Bishu K, et al. Home blood pressure monitoring improves the diagnosis of hypertension in hemodialysis patients. Kidney Int. 2006;69(5):900–6.
4. Foley RN, Parfrey PS, Harnett JD, et al. Impact of hypertension on cardiomyopathy, morbidity and mortality in end-stage renal disease. Kidney Int. 1996;49(5):1379–85.
5. Port FK, Hulbert-Shearon TE, Wolfe RA, et al. Predialysis blood pressure and mortality risk in a national sample of maintenance hemodialysis patients. Am J Kidney Dis. 1999;33(3):507–17.
6. Kalantar-Zadeh K, Kilpatrick RD, McAllister CJ, et al. Reverse epidemiology of hypertension and cardiovascular death in the hemodialysis population: the 58th annual fall conference and scientific sessions. Hypertension. 2005;45(4):811–7.
7. Tentori F, Hunt WC, Rohrscheib M, et al. Which targets in clinical practice guidelines are associated with improved survival in a large dialysis organization? J Am Soc Nephrol. 2007;18(8):2377–84.
8. Charra B, Calemard E, Ruffet M, et al. Survival as an index of adequacy of dialysis. Kidney Int. 1992;41(5):1286–91.
9. Thein H, Haloob I, Marshall MR. Associations of a facility level decrease in dialysate sodium concentration with blood pressure and interdialytic weight gain. Nephrol Dial Transplant. 2007;22(9):2630–9.
10. Chen J, Gul A, Sarnak MJ. Management of intradialytic hypertension: the ongoing challenge. Semin Dial. 2006;19(2):141–5.
11. Shoji T, Tsubakihara Y, Fujii M, et al. Hemodialysis-associated hypotension as an independent risk factor for two-year mortality in hemodialysis patients. Kidney Int. 2004;66(3):1212–20.
12. McIntyre CW. Recurrent circulatory stress: the dark side of dialysis. Semin Dial. 2010;23(5):449–51.
13. Poldermans D, Man in 't Veld AJ, Rambaldi R, et al. Cardiac evaluation in hypotension-prone and hypotension-resistant hemodialysis patients. Kidney Int. 1999;56(5):1905–11.
14. Fry AC, Singh DK, Chandna SM, et al. Relative importance of residual renal function and convection in determining beta-2-microglobulin levels in high-flux haemodialysis and on-line haemodiafiltration. Blood Purif. 2007;25(3):295–302.
15. Koch KM. Dialysis-related amyloidosis. Kidney Int. 1992;41(5):1416–29.
16. Jadoul M, Garbar C, Noel H, et al. Histological prevalence of beta 2-microglobulin amyloidosis in hemodialysis: a prospective post-mortem study. Kidney Int. 1997;51(6):1928–32.
17. Diaz RJ, Washburn S, Cauble L, et al. The effect of dialyzer reprocessing on performance and beta 2-microglobulin removal using polysulfone membranes. Am J Kidney Dis. 1993;21(4):405–10.
18. Collins AJ, Foley RN, Herzog C, et al. Excerpts from the US Renal Data System 2009 Annual Data Report. Am J Kidney Dis. 2010;55(1 Suppl 1):S1–420. A426-427.
19. Cheung AK, Sarnak MJ, Yan G, et al. Cardiac diseases in maintenance hemodialysis patients: results of the HEMO study. Kidney Int. 2004;65(6):2380–9.
20. Holt S, Goldsmith D. Renal Association Clinical Practice Guideline on cardiovascular disease in CKD. Nephron Clin Pract. 2011;118 Suppl 1:c125–44.
21. Bleyer AJ, Hartman J, Brannon PC, et al. Characteristics of sudden death in hemodialysis patients. Kidney Int. 2006;69(12):2268–73.
22. Pun PH, Lehrich RW, Honeycutt EF, et al. Modifiable risk factors associated with sudden cardiac arrest within hemodialysis clinics. Kidney Int. 2011;79(2):218–27.
23. Jadoul M, Thumma J, Fuller DS, et al. Modifiable practices associated with sudden death among hemodialysis patients in the Dialysis Outcomes and Practice Patterns Study. Clin J Am Soc Nephrol. 2012;7(5):765–74.
24. Kanagasundaram NS. Hemodialysis adequacy and the hospitalized end-stage renal disease patient–raising awareness. Semin Dial. 2012;25(5):516–9.

Providing a Peritoneal Dialysis Service

62

Stephen G. Holt, Michael X. Cai,
Annabel H. Ryan, and Lawrence P. McMahon

Home-based dialysis better sustains quality of life and allows for flexibility not afforded by centre-based haemodialysis (HD) treatment. Peritoneal dialysis (PD) is an essential part of a thriving home-based dialysis program and, in some places, may be the only practical modality. A key driver for this is that in many parts of the world, PD is considerably cheaper than HD. It is noteworthy that in those places where a 'PD-first' policy has become a government imperative, excellent patient outcomes have followed [1].

One prerequisite for a successful PD program is support from colleagues within the renal department. Perhaps surprisingly, some nephrologists still believe that PD is a second-tier or inadequate treatment option. In such cases, belief in the value of PD may only emerge with evidence of good clinical outcomes and patient satisfaction. Education of all medical and nursing staff that PD is an effective and suitable dialysis choice is critical if the program is to be viable. Equally, however, some patients may be better suited to HD, and it is important to deliver a balanced and objective view of all modalities when advising patients of their options, considering all modalities in the continuum of renal replacement therapy (RRT) experienced by patients over a dialysis career. Nevertheless a 'PD-first' policy is sensible because residual renal function (RRF) is important to the success of PD and loss of native function may render PD more difficult at a later date in the patient's journey through end-stage kidney disease [2]. Some of the barriers preventing consideration of PD, especially for the elderly, can be overcome by using different systems. For example, non-disconnect continuous ambulatory peritoneal dialysis (CAPD) systems, in-centre intermittent automated peritoneal dialysis (IPD) or assisted automated peritoneal dialysis (aAPD) (aka assisted continuous cycling peritoneal dialysis (CCPD)) can be performed, where a peripatetic healthcare professional will assist the patient at home [3].

There are numerous informative and helpful resources and guidelines freely available to help set up a PD service. Some of these are listed in Table 62.1.

Table 62.1 Useful resources with guidelines and training information

Guidelines
http://www.cari.org.au/guidelines.php
http://www.csnscn.ca/site/c.lnKKKOOvHqE/b.8079309/k.799F/Guideline_Document_Library.htm
http://www.european-renal-best-practice.org/content/ebpg-european-best-practice-guidelines-documents
http://www.ispd.org/lang-en/treatmentguidelines/guidelines
http://www.kidney.org/professionals/kdoqi/guidelines_updates/doqi_uptoc.htmL#pd
http://www.renal.org/Clinical/GuidelinesSection/Guidelines.aspx
http://www.kdigo.org/guidelines/topicsummarized/CPG%20Summary%20by%20Topic_Peritoneal%20Dialysis.html
Selected patient and training information
http://kidney.niddk.nih.gov/kudiseases/pubs/peritoneal/
http://www.ispd.org/lang-en/educational-material/materials
http://www.kidneyatlas.org/book5/adk5-04.ccc.QXD.pdf
http://www.renalweb.com
http://www.bjrm.co.uk/patient-information.aspx

S.G. Holt, BSc, MBBS, PhD, FRCP, FRACP (✉) • M.X. Cai, MBBS
Department of Nephrology, Royal Melbourne Hospital,
300 Grattan Street, Parkville, Melbourne, VIC 3050, Australia
e-mail: steve.holt@mh.org.au; mmxcai@gmail.com

A.H. Ryan, RN Div 1
Department of Nephrology, Western Health Sunshine Hospital,
St. Albans, VIC 3021, Australia

L.P. McMahon, MBBS, MD, FRACP
Department of Renal Medicine, Eastern Health and
Eastern Health Clinical School, Monash University,
5 Arnold Street, Box Hill, Melbourne, VIC 3128, Australia
e-mail: lawrence.mcmahon@monash.edu

Electronic supplementary material The online version of this chapter (doi: 10.1007/978-1-4471-5547-8_62) contains supplementary material, which is available to authorized users. Videos can also be accessed at http://www.springerimages.com/videos/978-1-4471-5546-1.

M. Harber (ed.), *Practical Nephrology*,
DOI 10.1007/978-1-4471-5547-8_62, © Springer-Verlag London 2014

Survival on PD vs HD

A number of studies have compared differences in survival between dialysis modalities. Results have been debated at length, but neither modality appears to be able to claim a clear advantage across all age groups. However, there is evidence for an early survival advantage (up to 2–3 years) for some groups of patients who start PD compared to those starting HD, which disappears and may eventually reverse with time. The groups that appear to have the best survival on PD (compared to HD) are young patients (aged below 45 years) and those who subsequently receive a kidney transplant. Elderly diabetics seem to do worst, which may be counterintuitive, as a relatively large proportion of such patients exist within many PD programs [4].

There appears to be a slower decline in RRF for patients starting PD compared to HD [5], and CAPD may be better than APD in this regard [6], although this may relate to membrane transport characteristics and baseline residual renal function [7]. Those patients who are struggling with little or no residual renal function and who face long years on dialysis without transplantation may benefit from extended hours or overnight HD, as the metabolic correction achieved with these techniques is unparalleled, although long-term outcome benefits have yet to be demonstrated [8]. Similarly, any longer-term quality of life or survival benefits of haemodiafiltration (HDF) over PD or standard HD are unclear and might only occur in a subset of patients with high volumes of convective fluid exchange [9]. The simplicity, safety and ease of use of PD therapies are an attraction for many patients. In addition, improvements in quality of life for patients on PD has been repeatedly shown across many age groups [10].

Patient Selection

There are some data suggesting that young, fit patients with meaningful RRF have a survival advantage on PD providing solute clearances are achieved. Most registry studies also agree there are some patients who appear to have worse outlook on PD (e.g. elderly diabetic females). However, the reasons for these differences are not clear, and there are many patients who appear to do very well on PD. Thus, decisions regarding modality should be carefully considered, weighing such aspects as quality of life, daytime activities, technological skills, body habitus, past abdominal surgery and appropriateness of treatment.

Past HD is not a contraindication to PD, but such patients are often anuric and frequently need high-dose APD to obtain sufficient clearance and UF targets above 750 mL [11]. The use of PD as a modality of last resort for patients who have exhausted vascular access options can create additional issues, often compounded by the pressure to succeed. Again, this argues in favour of PD as the initial renal replacement modality so that vascular access options can be preserved until required.

It is important to ascertain whether PD is likely to be successful. There are a few absolute contraindications to peritoneal dialysis, and these are usually related to abdominal suitability (see KDOQI guidelines Table 62.1 for an extensive review of contraindications and relative contraindications). For example, PD is not usually attempted in patients who have a stoma, previous significant abdominal surgery or known intra-abdominal adhesions. Similarly, previous tuberculous or fungal peritonitis and encapsulating peritoneal sclerosis (EPS) are relative contraindications to recommencing PD (although it may be preferable to continue PD whilst the EPS is being treated).

There are currently no diagnostic tools to determine if patients are suitable or trainable for PD, and assessment is largely subjective. However, visual acuity, dexterity, muscle strength (to lift the bags), a clean home environment, family support, a history of poor compliance with treatment, dementia and clinically active psychiatric illness will likely influence the final decision [12]. There are tools currently being evaluated that formalise some of these assessments, but they are time-consuming and neither fully validated nor widely used. The most practical and useful approach often is to obtain the views of experienced PD nursing staff combined with a careful clinical appraisal. The opinion of an experienced physiotherapist or psychologist can also be useful in particular circumstances.

With the right will, many perceived or potential problems can be addressed, including the setting up of assisted PD services or developing overnight in-centre dialysis training facilities.

Obesity

Obesity is sometimes and usually inaccurately cited as a contraindication to PD as many obese patients perform peritoneal dialysis very effectively. Paradoxically we know that obese HD patients have a survival advantage over thinner controls, but not all studies suggest that the same is true for PD [13]. There is no data to indicate that weight loss in obese patients improves outcomes, but it is not clear if this is due to lack of effect or simply lack of evidence. Where studies agree is that being underweight appears to be an adverse prognostic feature on all modalities of renal replacement. Nevertheless, potential problems obese patients face include reduced catheter survival, a more rapid decline in RRF with larger BMI, increased risk of peritonitis and higher intra-abdominal pressures [14].

Weight gain after starting PD is common but appears to be similar in HD patients and perhaps more likely related to loss of uraemia-associated anorexia. PD is often blamed for such weight gain, but the use between 1,000 and 7,000 l of PD fluid per year equates to around

15–150 kg of glucose passing through the abdominal cavity. Importantly, this is not the same as glucose absorption, which depends on dialysate volumes, dialysate concentrations, peritoneal transport characteristics, surface area and dwell time. Nevertheless the average quantity absorbed is an extra ~500 kcal/day (~2 chocolate bars). More frequent use of icodextrin may prevent some of this weight gain [15]. DEXA scanning looking at fat gain in patients starting renal replacement therapy suggested that the gain in HD and PD was equivalent [14], although intra-abdominal fat accumulation is probably higher in PD patients [16]. Interestingly, this may be subject to genetic influences mediated by mitochondrial efficiency [17].

Diabetics

Diabetic status has been linked with higher transport status in some studies, but this has not been substantiated subsequently [18]. Nevertheless the changes in the peritoneum caused by years of exposure to excess glucose in diabetes does change the peritoneum even before PD fluid is used. These changes are similar to those observed by glucose-based PD fluids and generally result in higher transport characteristics, so the reasons that some studies have not reported higher transport characteristics may reflect differences in duration of diabetes and diabetic control. However, there are advantages to using non-glucose solutions (e.g. icodextrin) in diabetic patients with improved fluid status [19], better glucose control [20] and lower incidence of technique failure and all cause mortality [21].

Glucose monitoring on PD is vital, and it is important that diabetic patients receive instruction on how to measure blood sugar and change their diabetic medication at the start of PD. A small amount of icodextrin is absorbed by the peritoneal lymphatic system and metabolised by circulating maltase enzymes, leading to accumulation of maltose in the circulation. This will interfere with blood glucose measurement in monitors using enzymes glucose dehydrogenase-pyrroloquinolinequinone systems, leading to falsely high readings in the face of hypoglycaemia [22]. Such potentially dangerous situations can be avoided by using glucose oxidase-based assay monitors instead.

It should also be noted that icodextrin may lead to low detectable amylase levels, potentially interfering with a possible diagnosis of pancreatitis, and plasma lipase should be used instead [23].

Heart Failure

The community prevalence of congestive cardiac failure (CCF) in western society is increasing due to ageing, associated co-morbidities and improved survival after cardiac events. Many acute hospital admissions involve decompensated heart failure, sometimes resistant to diuretics. This poses a symptom and economic burden on health services which is increasing. Ultrafiltration therapies, in particular PD, appear to have some success in preventing readmission and improving symptomatic classification (e.g. New York Heart Association classification) and quality of life [24]. Icodextrin, possibly an ideal fluid in this situation, has been used successfully to treat resistant CCF [25].

Control of plasma volume related to sodium removal can be difficult in PD. It is often more of an issue in APD compared to CAPD due to the peritoneal transport characteristics associated with each modality. Data on biomarkers of fluid overload (e.g. NT, BNP) in HD compared to PD are conflicting and difficult to interpret with confidence [26].

Cardiac Surgery

Cardiac surgery is common in dialysis patients who have worse outcomes than patients without renal impairment. Many cardiac surgeons suggest that patients will require haemodialysis or haemodiafiltration post-operatively. However, there is no evidence to suggest that continuation of peritoneal dialysis (usually APD) is not equally as successful post-operatively. In fact, there may be advantages to continuing with PD with shorter high-dependency stays [27].

Cirrhotic Patients

Peritoneal dialysis in cirrhotic patients can be successful, although complications do occur. Specific issues include bleeding from abdominal wall collaterals after Tenckhoff catheter insertion, early leakage due to high intra-abdominal pressure and large protein losses. However, if such problems can be managed for the first few weeks, patients often tolerate the process well, and the protein leak, whilst initially high, often reduces with continued treatment [28].

Lung Disease

Conflicting data from small studies suggest either no or small (usually insignificant) changes in lung function testing (FEV_1, FVC, TLC, DLCO) in patients with PD fluid present in the abdomen [29, 30]. Even if changes are identified, it appears lung function can then improve with time [31]. It would seem reasonable to expect patients with mild to moderate airways disease to successfully perform peritoneal dialysis and lung disease per se should not discourage a trial of PD where appropriate and avoiding overfilling the abdomen. Intraperitoneal pressure can be simply measured and keeping maximum filing pressure below 15 mmH_2O may be sensible.

Vascular Access

We advocate a PD-first policy, and there is rarely a need to form a 'backup' arteriovenous fistula (AVF) at the time of PD catheter insertion [32]. However, there is a recent vogue to use PD as a short term 'bridging' therapy, often with assisted or intermittent IPD to allow definitive vascular access with a mature fistula to be established. This is an excellent technique since PD catheters can be used more or less immediately and minimise the very real risk of damage to large veins and bloodstream infection associated with temporary or tunnelled haemodialysis lines [33]. It also means that patients may try peritoneal dialysis, and some may find that they get on well with this technique and have an AVF to fall back on should PD not be successful. There is also increasing interest in combined PD with a weekly HD session to augment clearances and fluid removal [34].

Occasional patients 'run out' of traditional HD access slots and then heroic efforts are made to make grafts and place tunnelled lines via circuitous routes into part of the venous system. These patients sometimes tolerate PD well as access of last resort [35].

Dementia

Patients with dementia can do well on PD providing someone else performs the exchanges. This responsibility usually falls to a spouse, and consideration must be given to respite and support as the demands are on top of what is often a demanding and progressively deteriorating process. Nursing homes sometimes offer a PD service. Alternatively, intermittent thrice-weekly overnight APD may be possible with good residual renal function (5–6 mL/min/1.73 m^2 residual GFR) [36]. Assisted PD programs may also be able to adapt to these circumstances [37].

Diverticular Disease

An incidental finding of diverticular disease (DD) is common, and the incidence increases with age, which can be problematic. In one Swedish study, more than one diverticulum was found in 42 % of patients, and 18 % had more than ten diverticula [38]. The incidence of enteric peritonitis in this study was 26 % at 2 years, and patients who had more than ten diverticulae had the highest risk of peritonitis. In a more recent study in Chinese patients, the finding that diverticular disease was associated with a higher risk of enteric peritonitis was replicated [39]. Both studies showed that the more extensive the diverticular disease, the higher the risk. Patients with diverticulae in the ascending colon appear to be at highest risk, and a history of recurrent problems with diverticulitis should alert the clinician that PD might not be a suitable option. On the other hand, many elderly patients have subclinical diverticular disease, and prospective investigation is likely not to be cost-effective. Our strategy is to disregard a diagnosis of diverticular disease unless a patient has had multiple admissions but to warn the patient of the potential of a problem and to encourage fibre ingestion.

Constipation

This is the most common of all complications experienced in PD patients. It is also the most troublesome in terms of catheter problems (poor drainage, catheter malposition and technique failure). Patients should have one or two soft bowel motions daily, and predisposing factors like hypothyroidism, hypercalcaemia and drugs should be corrected before using laxatives. Opiates, 5HT-3 antagonists, calcium antagonists and iron preparations are common drugs that cause constipation and are to be avoided if possible in PD patients.

The regular use of fibre or bulk-forming laxatives (e.g. methylcellulose, ispaghula) or osmotic laxatives (e.g. macrogols, lactulose or polyethylene glycol) is useful, especially in patients with diverticular disease. Common additions are stool softeners (e.g. docusate) which has a detergent effect, but there is poor evidence for its efficacy. Stimulant laxatives (e.g. senna or bisacodyl) may be used in patients with slowed bowel transit, but this can precipitate peritonitis in some cases due to increasing intraluminal pressure and bacterial translocation. So care is needed. There has been intense debate over whether regular use of senna leads to increased incidence of melanosis coli but this has not been substantiated in humans [40].

Hernias

Hernias are more common in some patients (e.g. age, polycystic kidney disease and raised body mass index), but there is no correlation between dwell volume and hernias. Umbilical hernias are more common than inguinal or incisional and most are present before starting dialysis [41]. Hernias usually worsen with PD fills. It is therefore suggested that, when possible, hernias are repaired extraperitoneally if possible before starting dialysis, and PD is delayed post-operatively for ~4 weeks. Repairing hernias in patients on dialysis can be difficult and sometimes ineffective. Occasionally patients will need transfer to haemodialysis temporarily, but continuing PD with low volumes, long hours on APD is also often possible, but it is wise to discuss this issue with the surgical team prior to planning this [42].

Starting PD

There are no data to support starting any dialysis modality early (according to eGFR) [43, 44]. Rather, the decision to start dialysis should rest on discussions between physician and patient regarding symptoms, volume control and biochemistry. Knowledge of local issues and available catheter insertion techniques will facilitate decision-making. For example, where there is an active catheter insertion service under local anaesthetic, there are often shorter delays in insertion. The Moncrief-Popovich implantation method allows a catheter to be inserted with the distal component buried in a subcutaneous pocket. Prompt externalisation of this portion of the catheter under local anaesthetic is then performed when needed.

Acute PD

A number of studies now indicate that insertion and commencement of PD may be performed rapidly for acute kidney injury (AKI) as well as the initial mode of RRT for patients who are likely to need long-term dialysis (acute start PD, ASPD) [45]. Whilst there can be an increased incidence of mechanical complications with the latter option, no long-term outcome differences have been demonstrated.

For AKI, high-dose dialysis involves APD with fluid volumes up to 44 L over 24 h, with short dwell times (<50 min) and 18–22 exchanges a day. For ASPD, a 7- to 10-day catheter rest is desirable if possible, but, where necessary, low volume APD can be used whilst the patient is supine in bed. An ASPD program includes overnight exchange of ≥12 L of PD fluid for at least 12 h, with fill volumes of 1.2–1.5 L and a high tidal APD (e.g. 50–75 %).

PD Team

The 'PD team' is vital and in many units the PD nurses shoulder the responsibility for day-to-day patient care. Numerous studies validate the advantages of chronic disease management by the nursing team [46]. The late, lamented Dimitrios Oreopoulos suggested that nurses need to have the following qualities, 'compassion, empathy, patience and love', but the benefits of an enthusiastic and experienced nurse who is able to relate to patients and make independent decisions are vital. Peritoneal dialysis is relatively straightforward to teach and to learn, so a lack of previous experience should NOT preclude working on a PD unit. There are published training pathways for PD nurses, teaching the rudiments takes little time and experience is quickly gained [45]. The best PD programs promote a holistic service rather than simply focusing upon dialysis-related problems. An ability to empathise and give advice on other issues (especially diabetes and vascular problems) empowers patients to seek initial advice from the PD team, often about problems that require a multi-professional approach.

Nurses on the ward are frequently required to care for PD patients and to troubleshoot problems out of hours. Thus, adequate training of the ward team is an essential feature of a successful program. It is vital that the ward-based team feels included as part of the home therapies team for patients.

One advantage of PD is that dietary restrictions are often less rigorous. This is particularly with respect to removal of potassium and fluid, although sodium and phosphate removal is often more difficult. However, protein energy malnutrition is widely prevalent in all dialysis patients, regardless of dialysis modality [47]. Thus, dietary advice and direction are important. Since dietetics resources are usually limited, an efficient alternative is for PD nurses and many doctors to provide generic advice (backed up with appropriate written literature), reserving a longer, more focused appointment with the dietician for specific problems. In addition, there are useful roles for the pharmacist, social worker, counsellor and psychologist within the PD team.

Patient Training

The training period will often influence a patient's acceptance of home therapies. A poor experience may well act as a long-term deterrent. Having a well-structured curriculum and consistency of implementation is paramount. The value of retraining or a technique check at intervals, especially after a peritonitis episode, is also helpful. There is a limit to what patients can absorb, and teaching of ~3 key messages a day (certainly <7) can actually facilitate training. The ISPD guidelines set out recommendations for patient [48] and trainee training [49], and there are a variety of Web-based resources available to help (Table 62.2). There is also some evidence that training patients in their own environment is advantageous and that longer training may reduce complications [48].

Whether to start patients on CAPD or APD is largely guided by economics, APD being a more expensive modality. If APD is chosen, confidence can often be enhanced by modest initial aims for clearance and fluid removal.

It is important to recognise that patients (and carers) develop technique fatigue and, if possible, offer some form of respite if this occurs, such as assisting patients (equally their carers) to take a holiday. A CAPD exchange can be performed anywhere that is clean and free from draughts and where there is a place to wash hands. Peritoneal dialysis supplies can easily be transported by car, and heating the PD fluid can be done via a device that plugs into a car 'cigarette lighter' socket if required. CAPD is possible without

Table 62.2 Common key performance indicators

KPI	Common targets
Antibiotic prophylaxis before catheter insertion	100 %
Exit site prophylaxis prescribed (either exit site or nasal prophylaxis)	100 %
Exit site infection	<1 in 40–50 patient months
Peritonitis rate: number of episodes of peritonitis/sum of months on peritoneal dialysis for all patients	<1 in 18–40 patient months
Culture negative peritonitis	<20 %
Primary peritonitis cure rate	>80 %
Adequacy: Kt/V_{urea} >1.7 or total creatinine clearance >50 L/week/1.73 m^2	100 % of those not receiving 'palliative PD'
Haemoglobin: 100–120 g/L (or according to national guidelines)	80 %
Time on therapy: number of months for 50 % of patients to come off PD, excluding transplantation, renal recovery or lost to follow-up	48 months
Peritoneal function (e.g. PET) and adequacy is measured at baseline and then at least yearly or as appropriate.	90–100 %
Technique survival (death and transplant censored)	1 year >80 % (90 %) 3 years >60 % (75 %) 5 years >40 % (65 %)
Patient survival at 1 year (may depend on age and co-morbidity)	>70–90 %

Targets are gleaned from published guidelines or suggested from experience

electricity, even whilst camping. For longer trips, supplies can be ordered in advance and delivered to a holiday address for the cost of delivery.

In a well-adjusted PD patient, dialysis is an accepted part of day-to-day life, and patients can travel, spend nights with their family and friends, work and play sports. Starting, however, is a daunting prospect and many fear their life will change dramatically. Discussing how to fit dialysis around their individual routine helps them understand that PD can be flexible and that they can still enjoy life.

Patients will also be concerned that having a catheter and being on an APD machine will prevent a healthy sex life and an open discussion about sexuality is important. We advise at least a week of abstinence whilst the exit site heals, but thereafter there is no contraindication to having sex either with or without fluid in, on or off an APD machine. It is important to appreciate that sexual dysfunction is common in ~70 % of dialysis patients [50]. Medication can often be the culprit, with beta-blockers commonly implicated. Psychological issues are also important. Thus, referral for psychological, endocrinological, pharmacological or physical treatments is often appropriate [51]. Many female patients on haemodialysis do not menstruate, but it is more frequent with PD. Ovulatory cycles may restart with initiation of dialysis, and this can sometimes be associated with blood in the PD fluid.

Swimming with a catheter is encouraged in well-maintained swimming pools (with precautions) once the exit site has healed. Colostomy bags can be supplied which encase the whole catheter to keep the exit site and catheter dry. After swimming, the patient is advised to ensure the exit site has not been moistened and to perform normal exit site care. Swimming in the sea and fresh water is permitted with the above caveats, but increased gram-negative infection has been reported after this practice, so it is important to be aware of local conditions and obvious pollution risks. Spas or saunas are not recommended.

Patients are encouraged to shower daily, gently washing their exit site and over their PD catheter with soap and water. Drying is performed with a fresh clean cloth every time. Hot baths are discouraged but colostomy bags can be supplied for occasional use.

Other common misperceptions are that alcohol is prohibited, that pets must be given away or destroyed and that young children are not allowed in bed with parents/grandparents who are dialysing. There are some distinctly unhygienic homes where animals are allowed to roam freely and where few surfaces are kept clean. In such environments, any home therapy would be challenging, but only small modifications are usually needed for home therapies to successfully coexist with pets. (To put this in context, zoonotic microorganisms make up only a tiny fraction (<1 %) of all infectious complications [52].) Pets should be kept out of the room when connecting or disconnecting, and the APD machine should always be protected specifically from cats which like lying on the warm fluid and playing with the lines.

Home therapy is eminently suited to patients in regional and rural areas. Whilst the trainer is ideally at the home, a residential training facility can also suffice, where patients can be taught about complications and when and how to seek help. Twenty-four hour assistance and guidance should be available via a home therapy unit, an after-hour backup (e.g. hospital ward or on-call service) or a dialysis company for machine issues. For remote patients, the local or regional medical services can be educated in emergency care of a PD patient with access to a renal centre for after-hour support.

Patients should be supplied with antibiotics, peritonitis policies and contact phone numbers to take to their local medical service. There are a number of new technology-based innovations currently being assessed to improve contact with remote patients, such as internet-based two-way cameras. In the meantime, telephones and e-mail are the usual routes of communication. We have found that e-mail has been a useful aid to communication between patients (especially deaf patients), home therapy nurses and various medical staff. Some patients take an avid interest in their own biochemistry, we encourage this and results can be quickly transmitted via e-mail or Web-based patient view sites.

Catheter Insertion

Techniques

Another essential element to a successful PD program is a catheter insertion service that is readily available and can place a PD catheter when needed. There are a variety of techniques used to insert catheters, none of which have been shown to be superior. These include blind Seldinger techniques and variations (including using radiological guidance), peritoneoscopic or laparoscopic techniques or open surgical techniques such as mini-laparotomy with or without omentectomy.

The physician-inserted local anaesthetic (LAPD) Seldinger insertion [48] is a valuable technique particularly when setting up a PD service. The procedure is relatively simple to learn and quick to perform and improves the capacity of the program to offer home therapies. Rapid decisions on when and how to start patients on PD can replace or at least offer an alternative to the common default option of HD. Additional advantages include the fact that LAPD can generally be done as a day case, which makes it cheaper and generally faster than other techniques. Many of these advantages are shared by similar techniques such as radiologically placed catheters, which have the advantage of real-time imaging.

Peritoneoscopic techniques have become popular in some units and are similar in many ways to the LAPD procedure, except that visual confirmation of positioning is available, although there is a distinctly steep learning curve for those unfamiliar with looking down the scope. Disadvantages are pain from gaseous distension of the abdomen, longer operating times, higher start-up costs (peritoneoscope, light source and other equipment), higher ongoing costs (sterilisation of equipment and more expensive kits) and greater technological demands.

Antisepsis

Prior to insertion, patients should be decolonised by application of nasal mupirocin and an antiseptic wash. The bowel should be emptied by use of a laxative and antibiotics must be given preoperatively [53]. Chlorhexidine in alcohol is extremely irritant to the peritoneum and has been shown to cause chemical peritonitis in animals similar to that seen in encapsulating peritoneal sclerosis, a feared, but rare, complication of PD (see Complications) [54]. However, in a drive towards eradication of hospital-acquired infection, chlorhexidine has achieved widespread use. In PD patients, this antiseptic agent should be used carefully if at all, and no alcoholic chlorhexidine should go near the catheter where it may contaminate the inside of the tube. It is recommended that only aqueous iodine is used on or near the ends of catheters and chlorhexidine is only used for hand hygiene and/or skin preparation but not as a spray around surfaces and equipment.

LAPD (Figs. 62.1, 62.2, 62.3, 62.4 and 62.5 and See Videos 62.1, 62.2, 62.3, 62.4, 62.5 and 62.6)

There are a number of governance and liaison issues before this service can commence.

- Surgical backup is potentially required should unforeseen complications arise. With proper identification of suitable patients, this is not usually a significant problem. However a surgeon should be aware of the procedure and potentially be available to advise if on the rare occasion a bowel perforation occurs.
- Anaesthetic approval for the procedure is important as patients require significant doses of opiates and/or benzodiazepines and are left with an unsupervised airway after the procedure. However, the process involved is very much conscious sedation: patients are rousable, with typical doses of intravenous sedation being 25–50 mg of pethidine and 1–2 mg of midazolam. The procedure can be done without sedation, but both patients and operator are less comfortable in such a situation.
- The infection control unit is keen for the procedure to be done in the sterile environment of an operating theatre. This is not absolutely required, but is welcomed if available. Much more important are adequate anti-infective precautions. Evidence-based recommendations include nasal decolonisation with mupirocin ointment to the nose for some days prior to the procedure, washing with antibacterial soap and bowel cleansing with aperients. Preoperative antibiotics are also important.
- Mark the position of the patient's belt line and the planned exit site with the patient standing. It is important to avoid placing the exit site over the belt line and to ensure it is visible to the patient. The patient is asked to empty their bladder prior to the procedure. An empty bladder should be confirmed by ultrasound. If necessary a urinary catheter (*per urethra*) should be passed.
- The patient does not have to be completely flat (some patients with severe heart failure may be unable to lie completely flat). It is important to be able to feel the midline. If there is a large abdominal apron this can be taped in place centrally to ensure the midline is found.
- Intravenous drugs are then administered, including an antiemetic, antibiotics and sedation, with reversal agents to hand (e.g. flumazenil and naloxone) if needed.
- The abdomen is shaved if necessary and cleaned with chlorhexidine or iodine solution. Locate the insertion site around 2–3 cm below the umbilicus in the midline, and allow this to dry before draping the area. Inject the skin at the insertion site with local anaesthetic and make a 1–2 cm

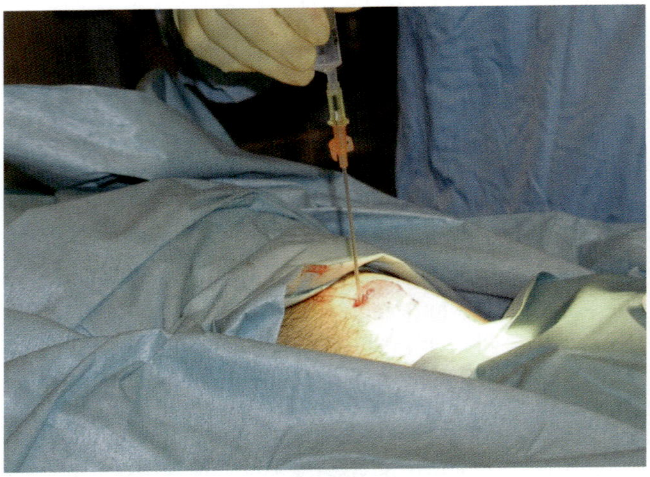

Fig. 62.1 Advancing the blunt sheath, beyond the needle tip and into the peritoneal space

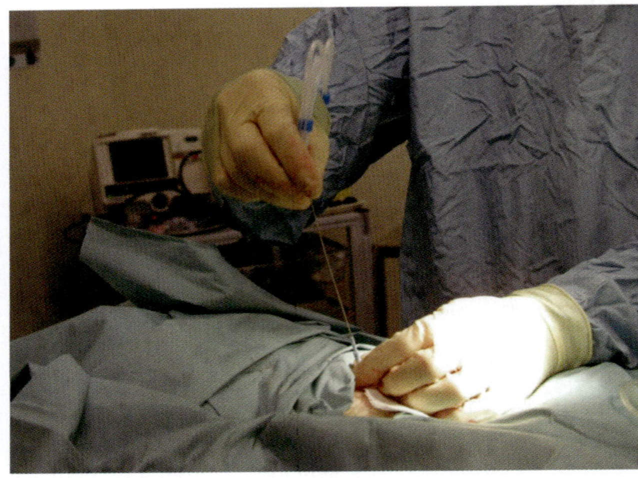

Fig. 62.2 Withdrawing the needle leaving the sheath in situ

horizontal incision in the skin of the abdominal wall. Achieve haemostasis with gauze. Inject local anaesthetic deeper, anaesthetising a tract all the way down to the rectus aponeurosis and, if possible, to the peritoneal surface. Blunt dissect with forceps though the fat layer down to the linea alba to create a tract. Use the same technique to explore the fat space above and lateral to the insertion site where the catheter will turn in the subcutaneous tunnel. Insert the long needle with plastic sheath through the entry wound and down onto the linea alba, which can be appreciated by a smooth, slippery and slightly hard feel at the end of forceps or needle. Using local anaesthetic in this needle, anaesthetise the area around the rectus sheath. Advance the needle gently through the linea alba into the peritoneum. Two distinct 'pops' may be felt as each of these layers is passed. After the second 'pop', *stop*. Do not advance the needle further. Instead, advance the blunt sheath, beyond the needle tip and into the peritoneal space, angling the needle slightly downwards towards the pubic symphysis (Fig. 62.1). Withdraw the needle and leave the sheath in situ. Confirmation that the correct space has been entered can be achieved by flushing fluid under gravity into the abdominal cavity or passing a wire down the needle. It should pass imperceptibly beyond the sheath and deep into the pelvis (Fig. 62.2). If it does not do so, remove and repeat the insertion process or abandon the attempt at this stage.

- Fill the abdomen through the advanced needle with 0.9 % Normal Saline (NS) or PD fluid. (The acidity of NS is said to be potentially harmful to the peritoneal surface, but stickiness of PD fluid may be problematic in itself. It is suggested that a single small volume of NS is unlikely to do damage.) The NS should flow freely into the abdomen under gravity and not need any significant pressure. A further 5–10 mL of lignocaine into this space at this point sometimes assists to ensure that the procedure continues without discomfort. If the patient experiences pain on filling or after <200 mL has been infused, it is likely the pre-peritoneal space has been entered. In that case, stop the infusion, aspirate as much fluid as possible and try to re-enter the peritoneal space by reintroducing the needle slightly caudally or abandoning the procedure in favour of a radiologically assisted or surgical approach. This method is most challenging in very obese subjects or where there is a large abdominal apron that flops to one side. Care should be taken to try to keep the abdominal apron central during insertion. An appreciation that the abdominal fat will move the catheter when the patient stands will enhance catheter placement.
- Once the abdomen is filled with ~700–800 mL of fluid, insert a j-tipped floppy guide wire into the abdominal cavity. Slight discomfort around the rectum or base of the penis sometimes occurs when the wire is in the pouch of Douglas, and some resistance to insertion is often felt here. Overcoming the resistance and inserting more of the wire makes it curve into the pelvis. The tract is then dilated and a peel-away sheath and dilator are advanced along the wire into the peritoneum, angled slightly down into the pelvis. The dilator is removed, leaving the sheath in situ (Fig. 62.3a, b). Before placing the catheter into the abdomen, the cuffs should be soaked in saline (dry cuffs inhibit fibroblast growth, delaying healing). The PD catheter can then be simply fed down the sheath (Fig. 62.4). Push the inner cuff with forceps down to the rectus sheath. The tunnel can then be fashioned by locating the exit site below the incision (so that the exit site is down-facing) and at least 3 cm from the distal cuff. The belt line has been pre-marked and this should be avoided

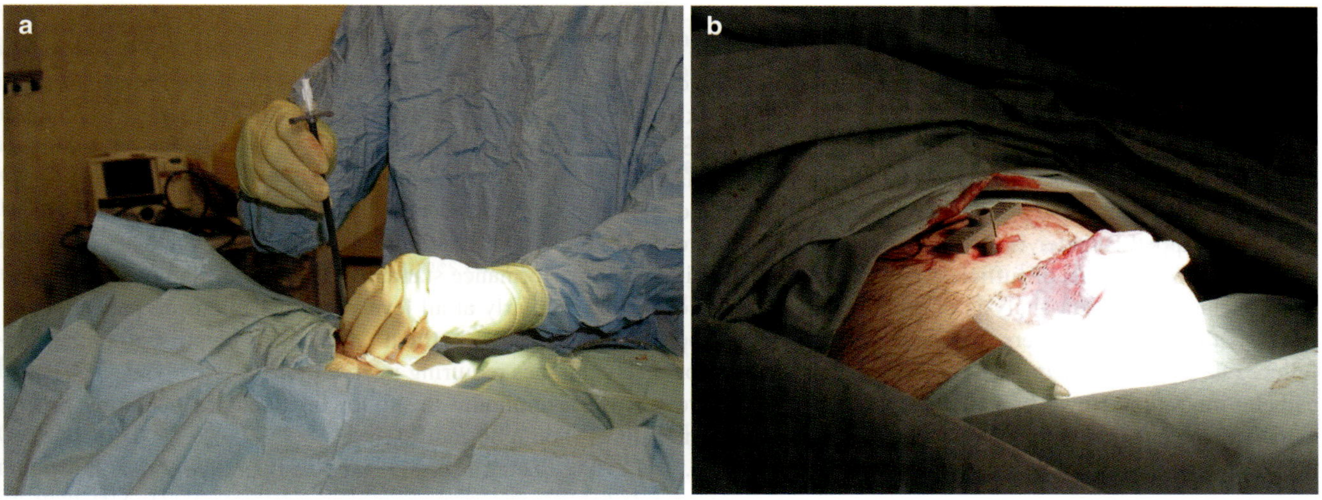

Fig. 62.3 (**a**) The tract is dilated and a peel-away sheath and dilator are advanced along the wire into the peritoneum, angled slightly down into the pelvis. (**b**) The dilator is removed, leaving the sheath in situ

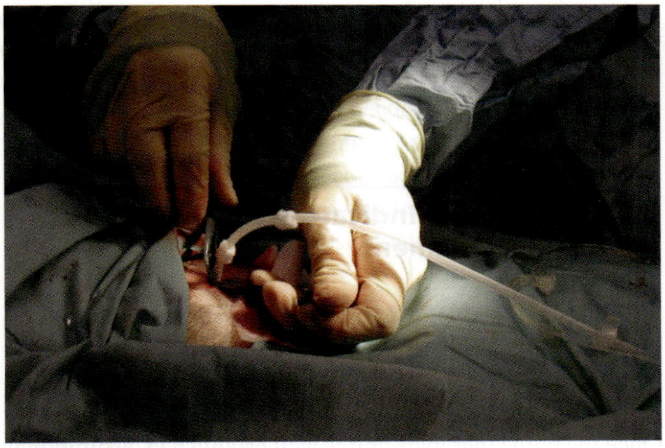

Fig. 62.4 The PD catheter is fed down the sheath

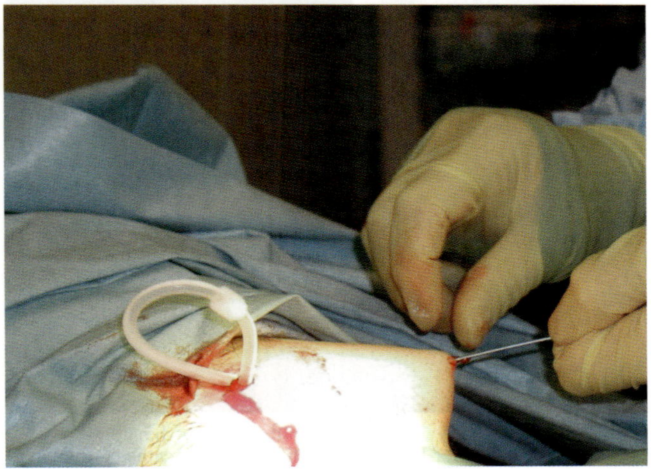

Fig. 62.5 The exit site is made by either a scalpel incision or with a sharp tunnelling tool, and the distal end of the catheter can be pulled through the subcutaneous tunnel and out of the exit site

for the exit site. Once the exit site has been anaesthetised, the subcutaneous tract between the exit site and the incision site can also be infiltrated with lignocaine. The exit site is made either by scalpel incision (Fig. 62.5) or with a sharp tunnelling tool, and the distal end of the catheter can be pulled through the subcutaneous tunnel and out of the exit site. The catheter is then fitted with a plastic or titanium connector for the transfer set, which is then firmly attached. All joints must be carefully tightened, and a cap placed on the transfer set. An absorbent/antibiotic cuff (e.g. Biopatch®) can be placed over the exit site which can usefully absorb any exudate. The catheter should then be immobilised for 2 weeks if possible. Do not put sutures at the exit site if possible, but suture the entry site.

- A Moncrief-Popovich modification for catheter implantation is a useful technique when a patient wishes to do PD, but the time frame for use is unknown, as a catheter can be placed for future use [55]. The process is similar to that described above except that the catheter is brought out through an incision more proximal to the entry site and a pouch is created to keep the (eventually external) portion of the catheter subcutaneous until needed (Fig. 62.6). A further minor procedure is required to externalise the catheter. This involves anaesthetising the skin at the exit site down to the catheter in the subcutaneous layer (avoid puncturing the catheter with the anaesthetic needle). Forceps are used to grab the catheter and pull it out through the anterior abdominal wall. The catheter is immobilised as far as possible to ensure that it moves as little as possible at the exit site, but the catheter may be used immediately.

New Zealand peritoneal dialysis patients. Am J Kidney Dis. 2004;43(3):492–501.
19. Davies SJ, Woodrow G, Donovan K, Plum J, Williams P, Johansson AC, et al. Icodextrin improves the fluid status of peritoneal dialysis patients: results of a double-blind randomized controlled trial. J Am Soc Nephrol. 2003;14(9):2338–44.
20. Paniagua R, Ventura M-J, Avila-Díaz M, Cisneros A, Vicenté-Martínez M, Furlong M-D-C, et al. Icodextrin improves metabolic and fluid management in high and high-average transport diabetic patients. Perit Dial Int. 2009;29(4):422–32.
21. Han SH, Ahn SV, Yun JY, Tranaeus A, Han D-S. Effects of icodextrin on patient survival and technique success in patients undergoing peritoneal dialysis. Nephrol Dial Transplant. 2012;27(5):2044–50.
22. Zhou H, Cui L, Zhu G, Jiang Y, Gao X, Zou Y, et al. Survival advantage of normal weight in peritoneal dialysis patients. Ren Fail. 2011;33(10):964–8.
23. Wang R, Leesch V, Turner P, Moberly JB, Martis L. Kinetic analysis of icodextrin interference with serum amylase assays. Adv Perit Dial. 2002;18:96–9.
24. Floré KMJ, Delanghe JR. Analytical interferences in point-of-care testing glucometers by icodextrin and its metabolites: an overview. Perit Dial Int. 2009;29(4):377–83.
25. Sánchez JE, Ortega T, Rodríguez C, Díaz-Molina B, Martín M, Garcia-Cueto C, et al. Efficacy of peritoneal ultrafiltration in the treatment of refractory congestive heart failure. Nephrol Dial Transplant. 2010;25(2):605–10.
26. Paniagua R, Ventura M-J, Avila-Díaz M, Hinojosa-Heredia H, Méndez-Durán A, Cueto-Manzano A, et al. NT-proBNP, fluid volume overload and dialysis modality are independent predictors of mortality in ESRD patients. Nephrol Dial Transplant. 2010;25(2):551–7.
27. Kumar VA, Ananthakrishnan S, Rasgon SA, Yan E, Burchette R, Dewar K. Comparing cardiac surgery in peritoneal dialysis and hemodialysis patients: perioperative outcomes and two-year survival. Perit Dial Int. 2012;32(2):137–41.
28. Ros Ruiz S, Gutiérrez Vilchez E, García Frías TP, Martín Velázquez TM, Blanca Martos L, Jiménez Salcedo T, et al. The role of peritoneal dialysis in the treatment of ascites. Nefrologia. 2011;31(6):648–55.
29. O'Brien AA, Power J, O'Brien L, Clancy L, Keogh JA. The effect of peritoneal dialysate on pulmonary function and blood gasses in C.A.P.D. patients. Ir J Med Sci. 1990;159(7):215–6.
30. Ulubay G, Sezer S, Ulasli S, Ozdemir N, Eyuboglu OF, Haberal M. Respiratory evaluation of patients on continuous ambulatory peritoneal dialysis prior to renal transplantation. Clin Nephrol. 2006;66(4):269–74.
31. Singh S, Dale A, Morgan B, Sahebjami H. Serial studies of pulmonary function in continuous ambulatory peritoneal dialysis. A prospective study. Chest. 1984;86(6):874–7.
32. K/DOQI. KDOQI clinical practice guidelines and clinical practice recommendations for diabetes and chronic kidney disease. Am J Kidney Dis. 2007;49(2 Suppl 2):S12–154.
33. Fernández-Cean J, Alvarez A, Burguez S, Baldovinos G, Larre-Borges P, Cha M. Infective endocarditis in chronic haemodialysis: two treatment strategies. Nephrol Dial Transplant. 2002;17(12):2226–30.
34. Suzuki H, Hoshi H, Inoue T, Kikuta T, Tsuda M, Takenaka T. Combination therapy with hemodialysis and peritoneal dialysis. Contrib Nephrol. 2012;177:71–83.
35. Solá L, Noboa O, Fleitas G, Laborda R, Quintero V. Transfer to peritoneal dialysis due to vascular access complications. Perit Dial Int. 2007;27(Supplement 3):S18.
36. Guest S, Akonur A, Ghaffari A, Sloand J, Leypoldt JK. Intermittent peritoneal dialysis: urea kinetic modeling and implications of residual kidney function. Perit Dial Int. 2012;32(2):142–8.
37. Dimkovic N, Aggarwal V, Khan S, Chu M, Bargman J, Oreopoulos DG. Assisted peritoneal dialysis: what is it and who does it involve? Adv Perit Dial. 2009;25:165–70.
38. Tranaeus A, Heimbürger O, Granqvist S. Diverticular disease of the colon: a risk factor for peritonitis in continuous peritoneal dialysis. Nephrol Dial Transplant. 1990;5(2):141–7.
39. Yip T, Tse KC, Lam MF, Cheng SW, Lui SL, Tang S, et al. Colonic diverticulosis as a risk factor for peritonitis in Chinese peritoneal dialysis patients. Perit Dial Int. 2010;30(2):187–91.
40. Leung L, Riutta T, Kotecha J, Rosser W. Chronic constipation: an evidence-based review. J Am Board Fam Med. 2011;24(4):436–51.
41. García-Ureña MÁ, Rodríguez CR, Ruiz VV, Hernández FJC, Fernández-Ruiz E, Gallego JMV, et al. Prevalence and management of hernias in peritoneal dialysis patients. Perit Dial Int. 2006;26(2):198–202.
42. Shah H, Chu M, Bargman JM. Perioperative management of peritoneal dialysis patients undergoing hernia surgery without the use of interim hemodialysis. Perit Dial Int. 2006;26(6):684–7.
43. Oh K-H, Hwang Y-H, Cho J-H, Kim M, Ju KD, Joo KW, et al. Outcome of early initiation of peritoneal dialysis in patients with end-stage renal failure. J Korean Med Sci. 2012;27(2):170–6.
44. Cooper BA, Branley P, Bulfone L, Collins JF, Craig JC, Fraenkel MB, et al. A randomized, controlled trial of early versus late initiation of dialysis. N Engl J Med. 2010;363(7):609–19.
45. Gabriel DP, Caramori JT, Martim LC, Barretti P, Balbi AL. High volume peritoneal dialysis vs daily hemodialysis: a randomized, controlled trial in patients with acute kidney injury. Kidney Int. 2008;73:S87–93.
46. Wong FKY, Chow SKY, Chan TMF. Evaluation of a nurse-led disease management programme for chronic kidney disease: a randomized controlled trial. Int J Nurs Stud. 2010;47(3):268–78.
47. Kopple JD. McCollum Award Lecture, 1996: protein-energy malnutrition in maintenance dialysis patients. Am J Clin Nutr. 1997;65(5):1544–57.
48. Bernardini J, Price V, Figueiredo A. Peritoneal dialysis patient training, 2006. Perit Dial Int. 2006;26(6):625–32.
49. Blake PG, Breborowicz A, Han DS, Joffe P, Korbet SM, Warady BA. Recommended peritoneal dialysis curriculum for nephrology trainees. The International Society for Peritoneal Dialysis (ISPD) Standards and Education Subcommittee. Perit Dial Int. 2000;20(5):497–502.
50. Katz A. What have my kidneys got to do with my sex life?: the impact of late-stage chronic kidney disease on sexual function. Am J Nurs. 2006;106(9):81–3.
51. Ayub W, Fletcher S. End-stage renal disease and erectile dysfunction. Is there any hope? Nephrol Dial Transplant. 2000;15(10):1525–8.
52. Broughton A, Verger C, Goffin E. Pets-related peritonitis in peritoneal dialysis: companion animals or trojan horses? Semin Dial. 2010;23(3):306–16.
53. Jose MD, Johnson DW, Mudge DW, Tranaeus A, Voss D, Walker R, et al. Peritoneal dialysis practice in Australia and New Zealand: a call to action. Nephrology (Carlton). 2011;16(1):19–29.
54. Povlsen JV, Ivarsen P. How to start the late referred ESRD patient urgently on chronic APD. Nephrol Dial Transplant. 2006;21 Suppl 2:ii56–9.
55. Brum S, Rodrigues A, Rocha S, Carvalho MJ, Nogueira C, Magalhães C, et al. Moncrief-Popovich technique is an advantageous method of peritoneal dialysis catheter implantation. Nephrol Dial Transplant. 2010;25(9):3070–5.
56. Hoff CM. Experimental animal models of encapsulating peritoneal sclerosis. Perit Dial Int. 2005;25 Suppl 4:S57–66.
57. Xie J, Kiryluk K, Ren H, Zhu P, Huang X, Shen P, et al. Coiled versus straight peritoneal dialysis catheters: a randomized controlled trial and meta-analysis. Am J Kidney Dis. 2011;58(6):946–55.
58. Baboolal K, McEwan P, Sondhi S, Spiewanowski P, Wechowski J, Wilson K. The cost of renal dialysis in a UK setting–a multicentre study. Nephrol Dial Transplant. 2008;23(6):1982–9.
59. Brown EA, Van Biesen W, Finkelstein FO, Hurst H, Johnson DW, Kawanishi H, et al. Length of time on peritoneal dialysis and encapsulating peritoneal sclerosis: position paper for ISPD. Perit Dial Int. 2009;29(6):595–600.

Peritoneal Dialysis Prescription

63

Stanley L. Fan and Nasreen Samad

Peritoneal dialysis (PD) is performed by filling the peritoneal cavity with dialysis fluid, allowing this to dwell before draining the fluid out and repeating the process with fresh dialysate. Solute transfer is by diffusion and convection transport whilst water moves across the osmotic or oncotic gradient.

The rates of solute transport (membrane function) across the peritoneum evolve over time particularly when on peritoneal dialysis. Membrane function is defined by the rate of equilibration of either creatinine or glucose over 4 h (D/Pcr or D_0/D_4glc) and is measured during a Peritoneal Equilibration Test (PET). Osmotic conductance (i.e. the rate of water transfer across an osmotic gradient) can also be defined using modified PETs.

Solute clearance by PD can be optimised by adjusting the dwell size, frequency and duration in accordance to patients' membrane function; the use of automated peritoneal dialysis (APD) is particularly suited for patients who are "high" transporters. However, particularly for incident patients, dialysis prescriptions are usually selected to suit patients' lifestyle and comfort.

This chapter aims to describe the methods of assessing patients and how dialysis prescription can be adjusted during the patients' PD life span to optimise peritoneal solute and fluid clearance.

PD Modalities

Continuous Ambulatory Peritoneal Dialysis (CAPD)

CAPD was introduced in 1976 by Popovich and Moncrief [1]. Patients using this modality usually perform 4 (although this can be 3 or 5) exchanges throughout the day (Fig. 63.1). Each exchange procedure takes approximately 20–40 min depending on how well the PD catheter functions (typically, 20 min drain-out time followed by 10 min drain-in time). The dwell times can be flexible and altered according to patient lifestyle. We usually advise dwell times to be at least 3 h. Day dwells of 6–8 h are acceptable. This permits greater flexibility for patients although as peritoneal membrane transport increases, long day dwells are likely to result in poor ultrafiltration.

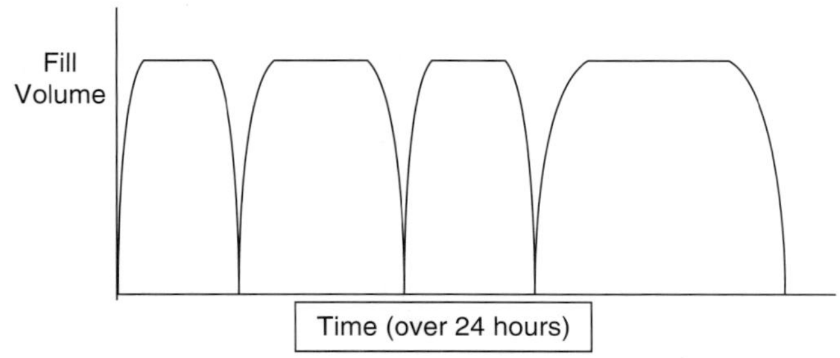

Fig. 63.1 Example of continuous ambulatory peritoneal dialysis (CAPD). Classically, exchanges throughout the day with a longer night dwell. However, great flexibility with timings (daytime dwells can be as short as 3 h)

Types of Automated Peritoneal Dialysis (APD)

Continuous cyclic peritoneal dialysis (CCPD) is the most common form of automated peritoneal dialysis (Fig. 63.2). This modality was introduced in 1981 by Diaz-Buxo [2]. The use of a machine automates the PD exchanges whilst the patient sleeps and leaves a "last fill" at the end of the programme, so patients continue to dialyse during the day. The system gained immediate popularity to treat infants and children. Its use has also grown with adult patients [3] as it allows patients to be free from PD exchanges during the day and larger volumes are also better tolerated in the supine position. CCPD can often achieve greater solute clearance

S.L. Fan, DM and MBBChir (Cantab), FRCP(UK) (✉)
N. Samad, FRCP (UK), MBBS
Renal Unit, Barts Health NHS Trust,
Whitechapel, London E1 1BB, UK
e-mail: s.fan@qmul.ac.uk; nasreen.samad@bartshealth.nhs.uk

M. Harber (ed.), *Practical Nephrology*,
DOI 10.1007/978-1-4471-5547-8_63, © Springer-Verlag London 2014

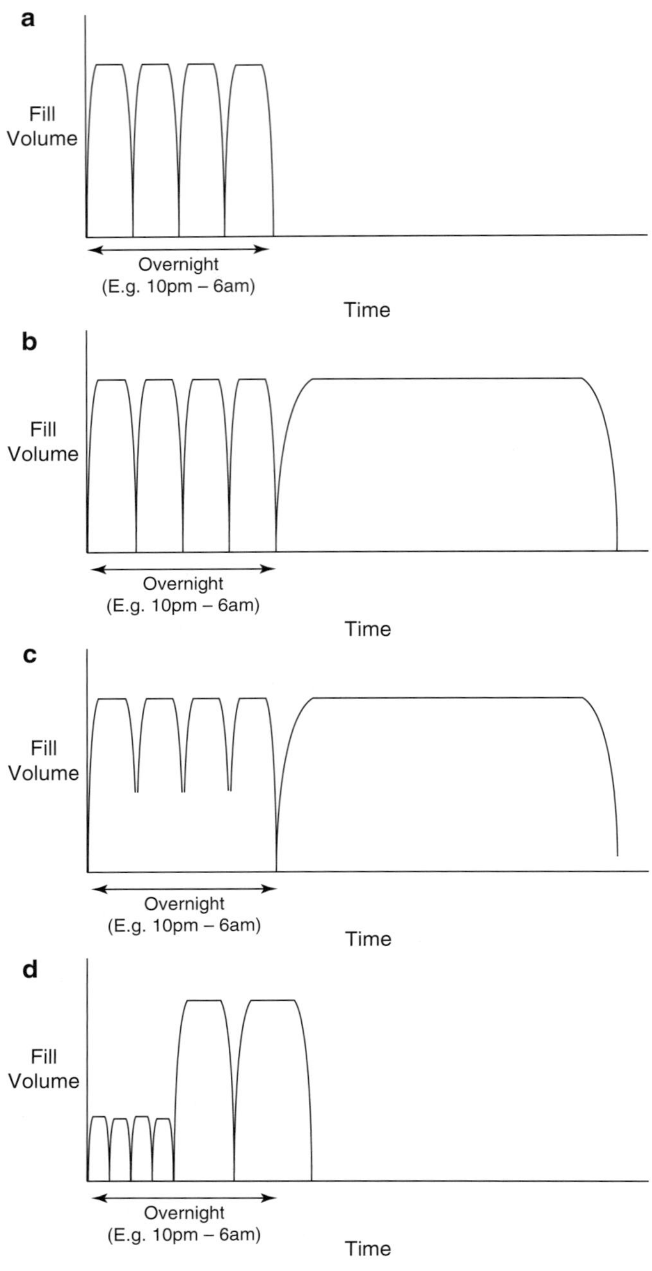

Fig. 63.2 Example of different forms of automated peritoneal dialysis (APD). (**a**) Example of typical night-time intermittent peritoneal dialysis (NIPD). Dialysis occurs only at night (is "dry" during the day). (**b**) Example of typical continuous cyclic peritoneal dialysis (CCPD). Dialysis occurs at night and during day (programmed to have last fill at end on night cycles). (**c**) Example of typical tidal automated peritoneal dialysis. Dialysis occurs at night but machine programmed to cycle without completely emptying peritoneum between cycles. Note initial drain and last fill are not "tidal". (**d**) Example of adaptive automated peritoneal dialysis. Cycles at night are a mixture of short small and large long cycles (Can be with day dwell if required)

than CAPD. To increase dialysis further, day exchanges can be introduced (either manually or by using the APD machine to deliver an exchange in the evening).

Nightly intermittent peritoneal dialysis (NIPD) patients have treatment periods at night but are "dry" during the day. This modality is particularly common for patients that have significant residual renal function. It is therefore popular for incident patients who otherwise feel bloated and nauseous with daytime dwells. Over time, patients tolerate day dwells and "progress" onto CCPD if solute clearances are inadequate.

Tidal peritoneal dialysis consists of exchanges in which the peritoneal cavity always contains some dialysate, a feature that minimises drainage pain or alarms for patients that have PD catheter problems (e.g. malpositioned catheter which results in large residual peritoneal volumes at the end of a drain cycle) [4].

A modified form of APD described as "Adapted APD" has been described recently [5]. During a 9–10-h APD session, the machine is programmed to perform a mixture of short dwells with small fill volumes to promote ultrafiltration and longer dwells and larger fill volume to promote removal of uremic toxins. This has been shown to result in improved dialysis efficiency in terms of UF, KT/V and phosphate and sodium dialytic removal without incurring any extra financial cost.

Assisted Peritoneal Dialysis

This form of PD is suitable for, but not limited to, elderly patients who are unable to perform peritoneal dialysis by themselves [6]. External health-care assistants (HCA) or nurses are employed to connect and disconnect patients to and from a cycler, set up the machine or perform CAPD exchanges. Often, the HCAs also help perform routine monitoring (weight and blood pressure) and inject erythropoiesis stimulating agents (ESAs). Assisted PD can be provided by family members, paid home-care nurses, visiting health-care professionals and staff in rehabilitation centres, retirement homes, nursing homes and chronic-care dialysis units [7].

There remains a debate about the cost-effectiveness of this modality treatment if health-care assistants or nurses are employed to deliver the assistance [8]. A European Survey [9] suggested that the incremental cost associated with providing home-care visits eliminates the savings traditionally associated with PD compared with in-hospital HD, but, of course, the level and cost of providing the assistance can vary widely. Moreover, the cost of transport for elderly dependent patients can be expensive but not always included in the Service Line Reporting Cost for HD [10].

Hybrid (Combination) Peritoneal and Haemodialysis

Combination (hybrid) therapy with peritoneal and haemodialysis has been reported in Japan [11, 12], United States [13] and United Kingdom [14]. From these reports, it is possible to perform simultaneous PD and HD on patients and it has been proposed that this may improve clinical status of patients. Certainly, additional HD sessions (once or twice a week) can be used to increase weekly small solute or water clearance on top of that achieved by PD alone. However, combination treatment has not been widely adopted. Generally, exposing patients to the risks of both HD and PD has deterred adoption of this therapy. However, there are scenarios that are particularly suited for combination treatment. Some patients are unable to perform home HD and refuse to switch to hospital-based HD when they develop insufficient solute clearances or fluid overload. Combination therapy may be an alternative although we would still advise caution; the reason for inadequate solute clearance or ultrafiltration failure may be an early indicator that the peritoneal membrane is damaged and transition to HD is advisable irrespective of whether KDIGO solute clearance targets can be maintained by "top-up" HD.

The reported use of hybrid dialysis is probably the highest in Japan. Interestingly, its use has been promoted as a method to reduce incidence of symptomatic encapsulating peritoneal sclerosis. It is well known that discontinuation of PD can be a trigger that precipitates EPS. Thus, continuing PD even at infrequent exchanges during the transition period may prevent this disease.

Hybrid dialysis can also be considered for patients with primary hyperoxaluria and who are dialysis dependent. Standard thrice weekly HD and PD have been used to treat these patients although oxalate clearances on these modalities are generally lower than oxalate generation [15]. Intensive HD (e.g. daily nocturnal HD) or combination HD and PD can therefore be utilised with some reported success [16].

Choice of PD Modality

Studies suggest no difference in outcomes for death or technique failure resulting from selection of CAPD or APD as initial PD modality. No difference was found from United States Renal Data System on 66,381 incident patients on chronic peritoneal dialysis when adjusted for demographic, clinical, laboratory and dialysis facility characteristics [3]. We have also observed that that whilst there is impairment in quality of life (QoL) both for patients and carers at the start of dialysis therapy, with careful selection of patients, education and support, the Δ of QoL for patients on CAPD vs APD were not different [17]. In fact, it was striking that despite having to help perform PD, there was some improvement in the QoL of caregivers (reflected by an improvement in the social functioning of carers after dialysis was initiated).

Hence, the choice of PD modality depends on several factors which include (Table 63.1):

Table 63.1 Comparison of advantages and disadvantages between CAPD and APD

CAPD	APD
Easy technique	More difficult technique
Daytime exchange can be difficult if working	No or only 1 daytime exchange
Poor UF if patient has high membrane transport characteristic, resulting in fluid overload and inadequate solute clearance. High transport status has been associated with higher technique failure in CAPD	Easier to achieve high UF particularly for patient with high transport status (although the effects of sodium sieving need to be considered). Association between H-transport status and PD technique failure does not appear to exist
Increasing exchange volume increases intraperitoneal pressure when patient ambulant	Intraperitoneal pressure lowers when patient supine, thereby permitting larger dwell volumes
Increased risk of hernia and leaks	If NIPD or small volume dwells used during the day, there is less risk of hernia and leaks
Ease of travel	Can travel with machine but patients often revert to CAPD
6–10 l of fluid used per day	10–15 l of fluid used per day
Less storage space required	More storage space required
Cheaper	More expensive

(a) Social reasons and patient-related factors like employment, need for carer to do PD, housing situation, and the ability to cope with exchanges and cyclers. As APD provides freedom from doing any exchanges during daytime, this tends to be selected by patients with employment and for patients who require assistance with their PD exchanges (e.g. assisted APD). However, some patients may find APD more technically challenging and find their sleep disturbed because of multiple cycler alarms.

(b) Peritoneal membrane characteristics. Patients with high peritoneal membrane transport characteristics particularly benefit from use of APD. There is historical evidence that in an era when APD was not readily available, CAPD patients that are high transporters have higher mortality/technical failure [18]. But this association is no longer true for more recent PD patients where APD utilisation is much higher [19].

(c) Dialysis adequacy including the effect of residual renal function. Residual renal function has an important role in contributing to overall adequacy of dialysis [20]. It may be difficult to provide adequate dialysis to anuric patients on CAPD [21]. But it has been shown that a high proportion of anuric patients can achieve adequate dialysis and ultrafiltration on APD [22].

Empiric Starting PD Prescription

At our institution, dialysis modality is chosen by patients.

For adult patients, empiric prescription for CAPD is generally based on patient size (weight), a typical protocol being:

- If weight >60 kg, start 4 × 2 l exchanges.
- If weight <60 kg, start 4 × 1.5 l exchanges.

For children, fill volume can be chosen by measuring primary pressure [23].

For incident PD patients selecting APD, our PD prescription is determined by patient size (weight) and residual renal function (RRF):

- If weight >60 kg, start with four 2 l fill volume for 8 h.
- If weight <60 kg, start with four 1.5 l fill volume for 8 h.
- If patient is anuric (e.g. patients transferring from haemodialysis), a last fill (1.5–2 l depending on patient size) is included in PD prescription.

It is important to remember that these are set as guidelines, but prescription should be individualised for patients' unique circumstances. The choice of glucose concentration or use of icodextrin is determined by how much ultrafiltration is required to achieve. This is discussed in the following section.

How to Adjust PD Prescription

PD prescription can be adjusted to:

1. Suit changes in patient lifestyle. It is important to remember that switching to CAPD is possible to facilitate patient holidays.
2. Increase solute clearance.
3. Increase ultrafiltration.

Although solute clearance and ultrafiltration are listed separately, they are intricately linked. Increasing ultrafiltration/drain volume will, of course, also increase solute clearance through convection. An important exception is if very short dwells are performed in APD. In this scenario, water clearance via aquaporins can result in water but not solute clearance, and this phenomenon is measured as sodium sieving.

As a rule of thumb, dialysis volume and cycles are adjusted to optimise solute clearance whereas fluid composition (tonicity) is changed to adjust ultrafiltration. The exception is for patients who have a high transport status. These patients lose the osmotic gradient and so dialysis cycles must be adjusted to shorter dwell times like switching the patient from CAPD to APD.

Dialysis Adequacy in Anuric Patients

There continues to be a debate about the effectiveness of PD for anuric patients. CANUSA showed that residual renal function (RRF) is one of the most important determinants of patient survival [20]. However, this does not automatically mean that survival will be prolonged by switching patients to HD (the same relationship between RRF and survival also exists in HD [24]). In the absence of RCT on the subject, we can only interpret the non-randomised observational outcomes. EAPOS showed that >70 % anuric patients can achieve the small clearance target of >60 l/week/1.72 m^2 BSA [25]. In addition, 2-year patient survival was 78 % (although switching to HD according to clinical need was permitted) [22], and this compares favourably with the NECOSAD study of incident PD patients where 2-year survival was 77 % [26].

We conclude that automatic switching of anuric patients to HD is not warranted, but anuria should alert the clinician to carefully consider a transition on an individual basis. Not only will QoL issues be paramount, but particular emphasis should be placed on fluid balance; EAPOS showed a strong association between poor UF (<750 ml/day) and reduced survival. This is also supported by the NECOSAD study where total fluid removal was the only significant predictor of technique survival (RR = 0.79 at 500 ml/day).

Treatment for Hyperkalaemia and Hypercalcaemia

The rate of potassium removal with PD is much slower than with HD and the latter is therefore recommended for patients with severe (life-threatening) hyperkalaemia. Rapid cycles of hypertonic glucose can induce convective loss of potassium and hyperglycaemia that helps drive potassium into cells, thereby lowering serum potassium. Whilst the high ultrafiltration risks cardiovascular instability, this strategy can be useful if there are delays initiating HD.

Commercially available PD solutions contain 1–1.75 mmol/l of calcium. Exchanges with calcium dialysate of 1–1.25 mmol/l will cause net efflux of calcium into dialysis fluid [27]. Successful treatment of acute hypercalcaemia using in-hospital-prepared calcium-free dialysate has also been reported in adult and paediatric populations [28].

Sodium Sieving

Sieving of sodium is defined as the drop in the dialysate-to-plasma ratio of sodium (D/P Na) that occurs during the initial phase of a dialysis exchange with a hyperosmolar dialysis solution.

Water moves across the peritoneal membrane via different "pores". However, sodium cannot follow water through aquaporins, although over a long dwell, sodium concentrations will equilibrate through the other pores. Hence, preponderance of water enters the peritoneal cavity at the beginning of a dwell resulting in a decrease in the dialysate sodium. If dwell times are kept very short, high ultrafiltration is possible but with relative low sodium removal. This may lead to an increased incidence of hypertension [29].

Sodium sieving is measured by the reduction in dialysate Na after 1 h 3.86 % dwell. Reduction in dialysate sodium by >20 mmol or >13 % signifies significant sodium sieving.

Conversely, daytime dwells with icodextrin PD solutions are particularly useful for APD patients [30].

Peritoneal Dialysis Fluid

Glucose

Glucose is the most commonly used osmotic agent and is available in different concentrations. Glucose-based dialysis solutions are at risk of caramelisation (thereby generating glucose degradation products) during heat sterilisation. Sole use of lactate as the buffer in PD solutions also means the infused solutions are acidic. This has led to the development of "biocompatible" solutions. Sodium bicarbonate is kept separated to other constituents of dialysate to avoid precipitation, and the section of the bag containing glucose can now be sterilised at very low pH, minimising the generation of GDPs. Prior to infusing into the patients, the different sections of the bag (containing sodium bicarbonate vs glucose and other constituents) are mixed.

GDPs are potentially toxic to peritoneal membrane and leukocytes in vitro although clinically significant benefits of using "biocompatible solutions" on membrane function and peritonitis rates are not yet conclusively proven [31]. Studies suggest that bicarbonate-/lactate-buffered solutions are safe, well tolerated and physiologically balanced alternatives to conventional lactate-based solutions [32]. They can be particularly useful for patients who develop infusion pain or discomfort when using "standard" glucose bags. The BalANZ study [33] has been recently published. Whilst it did not show a difference in rate of decline of residual renal function between conventional solution and a "biocompatible" solution, there was a significant difference though to the time to anuria and time to first peritonitis episode in favour of the biocompatible solution. Use of biocompatible solutions is likely to depend on assessment of cost-effectiveness.

Glucose Polymer Icodextrin (Extraneal)

Icodextrin has a mean molecular weight of 20,000 and has same osmolality as plasma at 290 mosmol. Icodextrin has high reflection coefficient (σ). Reflection coefficient is described as permeability of solute; where reflection coefficient is greater the permeability of solute is less. This allows the solute to stay longer in the dialysate. Icodextrin has been found to be safe and provides patients with greater fluid removal and small solute clearance [34].

Amino Acids (Nutrineal)

A 1.1 % amino acid mixture is available and has similar osmolality as 1.36 % glucose. Studies indicate that treatment with a daily exchange of this amino acid-based PD solution is safe and may provide nutritional benefit for malnourished PD patients [35]. However, no appreciable improvements were seen in well-nourished patients [36]. Nevertheless, advocates have suggested routine use of this (and icodextrin) permits dialysis regimens that are low in glucose [37] (with potential although not conclusively proven clinical benefits).

PD Clearance Targets

Different organisations have general agreement about PD clearance targets. These are listed in Table 63.2. We direct the reader to the websites that provide justification for these recommendations. However, it is important to understand that peritoneal clearance of solute is not equivalent to residual renal function. Preservation of residual renal function is therefore of utmost importance in the clinical care of patients on peritoneal dialysis.

Equally, achieving the clearance targets is not the sole aim of clinicians looking after PD patients. Increased use

Table 63.2 PD clearance targets set by different Guideline Groups

	CrCl	KT/V	UF	Ref
KDIGO	None	>1.7/week		http://www.kidney.org/professionals/kdoqi/guidelines
EBPG	None except >45 l/week for APD	>1.7/week	1.0 l/24 h in anuric patients	http://www.european-renal-best-practice.org/content/ebpg-european-best-practice-guidelines
UK-RA	>50 l/week	>1.7/week		http://www.renal.org/Clinical/GuidelinesSection/PeritonealDialysis

KDIGO Kidney Disease: Improving Global Outcomes, *EBPG* European Best Practice Guidelines, *UK-RA* UK Renal Association of APD with icodextrin and glucose permits anuric patients to achieve these targets, but if peritoneal membrane is changing, continuing peritoneal dialysis may not be appropriate [38].

Ultrafiltration Targets

The European guidelines setting of ultrafiltration target has been controversial. Perhaps the term "target" is inappropriate, but measuring 24-h UF is extremely important especially if patients are anuric:

1. Overhydrated patients: If UF is <1 l, dialysis prescription is inappropriate. But if UF is >1 l, overhydration may be secondary to noncompliance to salt and fluid restriction.
2. Euvolaemic patient with poor ultrafiltration is at risk of malnutrition resulting from extreme restrictions in diet and fluid intake.

It is important to maintain fluid balance as increased fluid leads to rise in blood pressure, left ventricular hypertrophy and increased mortality [39].

Bioimpedance Assessment of Hydration Status

Bioimpedance analysis (BIA) provides objective information in the assessment of hydration status of the patients. Studies have suggested that bioimpedance analysis is a reliable, consistent, not invasive, simple, portable and relatively inexpensive technique to assess the fluid status of a dialysis patient [40]. A multicentre study of European PD units has shown the majority of prevalent patients were overhydrated when assessed using a multifrequency biompedance machine [41]. Perhaps this emphasises that as clinicians, we need to pay increased focus not only on dialysis prescriptions and ultrafiltration, but on patients' adherence to dietary salt and water restrictions.

Summary

Peritoneal dialysis is an effective method to achieve solute and water clearance. Its utilisation is particularly appropriate for incident dialysis patients with significant residual renal function. Patients can be maintained on PD by adjusting PD modality and prescriptions as described above, thereby permitting many anuric patients to achieve "adequate" ultrafiltration and solute clearances. An elective and planned switch to haemodialysis should be considered for those that appear "underdialysed". However, a holistic approach is important; other aspects of patient well-being, long-term prognosis from other comorbidities and patient perspective should be considered in deciding whether switch from PD to haemodialysis is appropriate.

References

1. Popovich RP, Moncrief JW, Nolph KD, Ghods AJ, Twardowski ZJ, Pyle WK. Continuous ambulatory peritoneal dialysis. Ann Intern Med. 1978;88(4):449–56.
2. Diaz-Buxo JA, Farmer CD, Walker PJ, Chandler JT, Holt KL. Continuous cyclic peritoneal dialysis: a preliminary report. Artif Organs. 1981;5(2):157–61.
3. Mehrotra R, Chiu YW, Kalantar-Zadeh K, Vonesh E. The outcomes of continuous ambulatory and automated peritoneal dialysis are similar. Kidney Int. 2009;76(1):97–107.
4. Juergensen PH, Murphy AL, Pherson KA, Chorney WS, Kliger AS, Finkelstein FO. Tidal peritoneal dialysis to achieve comfort in chronic peritoneal dialysis patients. Adv Perit Dial. 1999;15:125–6.
5. Fischbach M, Issad B, Dubois V, Taamma R. The beneficial influence on the effectiveness of automated peritoneal dialysis of varying the dwell time (short/long) and fill volume (small/large): a randomized controlled trial. Perit Dial Int. 2011;31(4):450–8.
6. Brown EA, Dratwa M, Povlsen JV. Assisted peritoneal dialysis: an evolving dialysis modality. Nephrol Dial Transplant. 2007;22(10):3091–2.
7. Povlsen JV, Ivarsen P. Assisted automated peritoneal dialysis (AAPD) for the functionally dependent and elderly patient. Perit Dial Int. 2005;25 Suppl 3:S60–3.
8. Mendelssohn DC. A skeptical view of assisted home peritoneal dialysis. Kidney Int. 2007;71(7):602–4.
9. Dratwa M. Costs of home assistance for peritoneal dialysis: results of a European survey. Kidney Int Suppl. 2008;108:S72–5.
10. Oliver MJ, Quinn RR, Richardson EP, Kiss AJ, Lamping DL, Manns BJ. Home care assistance and the utilization of peritoneal dialysis. Kidney Int. 2007;71(7):673–8.
11. Fukui H, Hara S, Hashimoto Y, Horiuchi T, Ikezoe M, Itami N, Kawabe M, Kawanishi H, Kimura H, Nakamoto Y, et al. Review of combination of peritoneal dialysis and hemodialysis as a modality of treatment for end-stage renal disease. Ther Apher Dial. 2004;8(1):56–61.
12. Kawanishi H, Moriishi M. Clinical effects of combined therapy with peritoneal dialysis and hemodialysis. Perit Dial Int. 2007;27 Suppl 2:S126–9.
13. Agarwal M, Clinard P, Burkart JM. Combined peritoneal dialysis and hemodialysis: our experience compared to others. Perit Dial Int. 2003;23(2):157–61.
14. McIntyre CW. Bimodal dialysis: an integrated approach to renal replacement therapy. Perit Dial Int. 2004;24(6):547–53.
15. Hoppe B, Graf D, Offner G, Latta K, Byrd DJ, Michalk D, Brodehl J. Oxalate elimination via hemodialysis or peritoneal dialysis in children with chronic renal failure. Pediatr Nephrol. 1996;10(4):488–92.
16. Illies F, Bonzel KE, Wingen AM, Latta K, Hoyer PF. Clearance and removal of oxalate in children on intensified dialysis for primary hyperoxaluria type 1. Kidney Int. 2006;70(9):1642–8.
17. Fan SL, Sathick I, McKitty K, Punzalan S. Quality of life of caregivers and patients on peritoneal dialysis. Nephrol Dial Transplant. 2008;23(5):1713–9.
18. Brimble KS, Walker M, Margetts PJ, Kundhal KK, Rabbat CG. Meta-analysis: peritoneal membrane transport, mortality, and technique failure in peritoneal dialysis. J Am Soc Nephrol. 2006;17(9):2591–8.

19. Johnson DW, Hawley CM, McDonald SP, Brown FG, Rosman JB, Wiggins KJ, Bannister KM, Badve SV. Superior survival of high transporters treated with automated versus continuous ambulatory peritoneal dialysis. Nephrol Dial Transplant. 2010;25(6):1973–9.
20. Bargman JM, Thorpe KE, Churchill DN. Relative contribution of residual renal function and peritoneal clearance to adequacy of dialysis: a reanalysis of the CANUSA study. J Am Soc Nephrol. 2001;12(10):2158–62.
21. Van Biesen W, Vanholder R, Veys N, Lameire N. Peritoneal dialysis in anuric patients: concerns and cautions. Semin Dial. 2002;15(5):305–10.
22. Brown EA, Davies SJ, Rutherford P, Meeus F, Borras M, Riegel W, Divino Filho JC, Vonesh E, van Bree M. Survival of functionally anuric patients on automated peritoneal dialysis: the European APD Outcome Study. J Am Soc Nephrol. 2003;14(11):2948–57.
23. Fischbach M, Terzic J, Laugel V, Escande B, Dangelser C, Helmstetter A. Measurement of hydrostatic intraperitoneal pressure: a useful tool for the improvement of dialysis dose prescription. Pediatr Nephrol. 2003;18(10):976–80.
24. Shafi T, Jaar BG, Plantinga LC, Fink NE, Sadler JH, Parekh RS, Powe NR, Coresh J. Association of residual urine output with mortality, quality of life, and inflammation in incident hemodialysis patients: the Choices for Healthy Outcomes in Caring for End-Stage Renal Disease (CHOICE) Study. Am J Kidney Dis. 2010;56(2):348–58.
25. Brown EA, Davies SJ, Heimburger O, Meeus F, Mellotte G, Rosman J, Rutherford P, Van Bree M. Adequacy targets can be met in anuric patients by automated peritoneal dialysis: baseline data from EAPOS. Perit Dial Int. 2001;21 Suppl 3:S133–7.
26. Jager KJ, Merkus MP, Dekker FW, Boeschoten EW, Tijssen JG, Stevens P, Bos WJ, Krediet RT. Mortality and technique failure in patients starting chronic peritoneal dialysis: results of The Netherlands Cooperative Study on the Adequacy of Dialysis. NECOSAD Study Group. Kidney Int. 1999;55(4):1476–85.
27. Armstrong A, Beer J, Noonan K, Cunningham J. Reduced calcium dialysate in CAPD patients: efficacy and limitations. Nephrol Dial Transplant. 1997;12(6):1223–8.
28. Querfeld U, Salusky IB, Fine RN. Treatment of severe hypercalcemia with peritoneal dialysis in an infant with end-stage renal disease. Pediatr Nephrol. 1988;2(3):323–5.
29. Rodriguez-Carmona A, Fontan MP. Sodium removal in patients undergoing CAPD and automated peritoneal dialysis. Perit Dial Int. 2002;22(6):705–13.
30. Boudville NC, Cordy P, Millman K, Fairbairn L, Sharma A, Lindsay R, Blake PG. Blood pressure, volume, and sodium control in an automated peritoneal dialysis population. Perit Dial Int. 2007;27(5):537–43.
31. Fan SL. Should we use biocompatible PD solutions for all patients? Perit Dial Int. 2009;29(6):630–3.
32. Pecoits-Filho R, Tranaeus A, Lindholm B. Clinical trial experiences with Physioneal. Kidney Int Suppl. 2003;88:S100–4.
33. Johnson DW, Brown FG, Clarke M, Boudville N, Elias TJ, Foo MW, Jones B, Kulkarni H, Langham R, Ranganathan D, et al. Effects of biocompatible versus standard fluid on peritoneal dialysis outcomes. J Am Soc Nephrol. 2012;23(6):1097–107.
34. Wolfson M, Piraino B, Hamburger RJ, Morton AR. A randomized controlled trial to evaluate the efficacy and safety of icodextrin in peritoneal dialysis. Am J Kidney Dis. 2002;40(5):1055–65.
35. Jones M, Hagen T, Boyle CA, Vonesh E, Hamburger R, Charytan C, Sandroni S, Bernard D, Piraino B, Schreiber M, et al. Treatment of malnutrition with 1.1 % amino acid peritoneal dialysis solution: results of a multicenter outpatient study. Am J Kidney Dis. 1998;32(5):761–9.
36. Kopple JD, Bernard D, Messana J, Swartz R, Bergstrom J, Lindholm B, Lim V, Brunori G, Leiserowitz M, Bier DM, et al. Treatment of malnourished CAPD patients with an amino acid based dialysate. Kidney Int. 1995;47(4):1148–57.
37. le Poole CY, van Ittersum FJ, Weijmer MC, Valentijn RM, ter Wee PM. Clinical effects of a peritoneal dialysis regimen low in glucose in new peritoneal dialysis patients: a randomized crossover study. Adv Perit Dial. 2004;20:170–6.
38. Davies SJ, Brown EA, Frandsen NE, Rodrigues AS, Rodriguez-Carmona A, Vychytil A, Macnamara E, Ekstrand A, Tranaeus A, Filho JC. Longitudinal membrane function in functionally anuric patients treated with APD: data from EAPOS on the effects of glucose and icodextrin prescription. Kidney Int. 2005;67(4):1609–15.
39. Ates K, Nergizoglu G, Keven K, Sen A, Kutlay S, Erturk S, Duman N, Karatan O, Ertug AE. Effect of fluid and sodium removal on mortality in peritoneal dialysis patients. Kidney Int. 2001;60(2):767–76.
40. Crepaldi C, Soni S, Chionh CY, Wabel P, Cruz DN, Ronco C. Application of body composition monitoring to peritoneal dialysis patients. Contrib Nephrol. 2009;163:1–6.
41. Van Biesen W, Williams JD, Covic AC, Fan S, Claes K, Lichodziejewska-Niemierko M, Verger C, Steiger J, Schoder V, Wabel P, et al. Fluid status in peritoneal dialysis patients: the European Body Composition Monitoring (EuroBCM) study cohort. PLoS One. 2011;6(2):e17148.

M. Harber (ed.), *Practical Nephrology*,
DOI 10.1007/978-1-4471-5547-8_64, © Springer-Verlag London 2014

of the topic and conclude ...
the best hands probably has the best success rate [10].

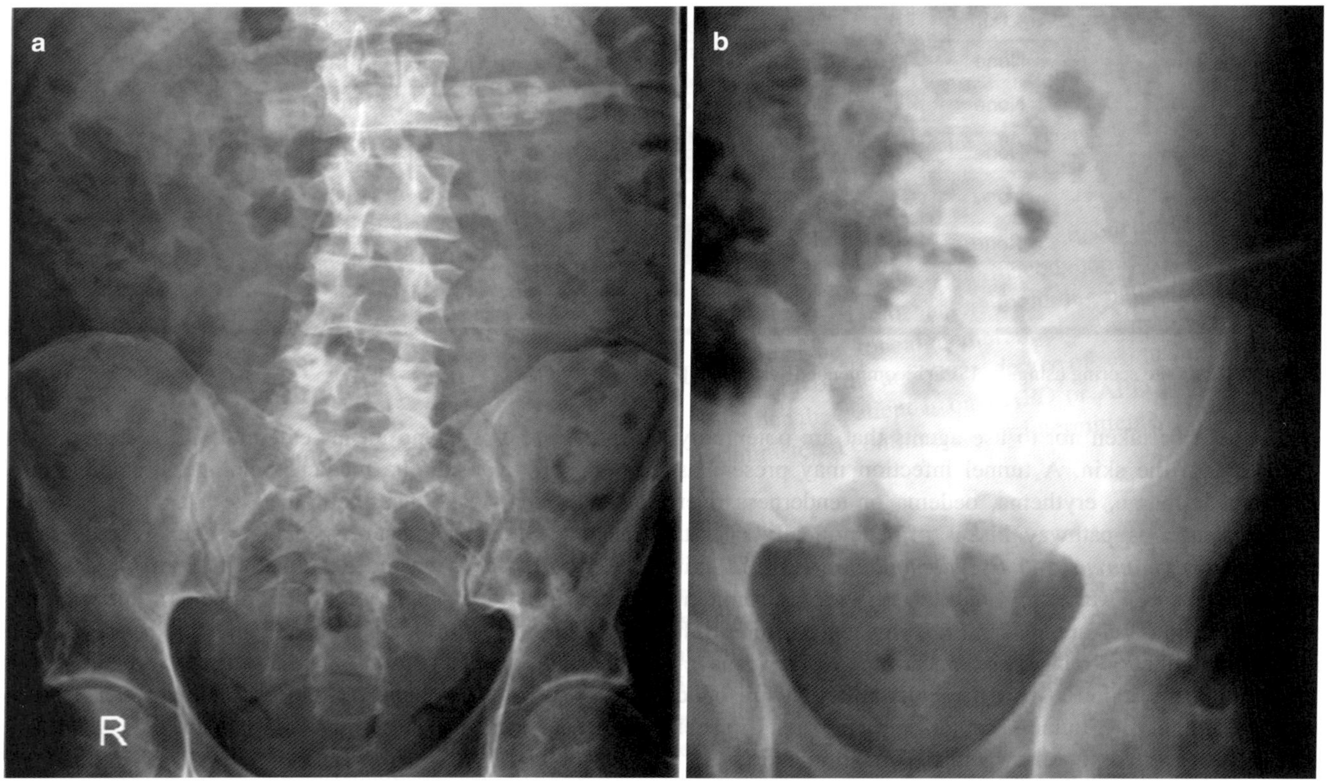

Fig. 64.5 Plain abdominal X-rays demonstrating the PD catheter located in the pelvis (**a**) demonstrating a PD catheter where the tip has migrated out of the pelvis (**b**)

can be diagnosed and treated by laparoscopy. Catheter obstruction may result from fibrin or blood clots which can be resolved by the use of a urokinase lock into the catheter. Of course, catheter dysfunction is not easy to define, being described in practice more by the impact on the patient or nursing staff rather than objective measurements of flow. The most objective measure of the success of catheter placement is whether the patient is using it for their treatment at 1-year post-insertion censored for death, transplantation and other causes of elective transfer from PD.

Patients may complain of pain on inflow or drainage of PD fluid. This may be due to the irritant effect of acidic dialysate, a consequence of negative pressure (suction) particularly in APD or a mechanical consequence of tube position. Techniques available to manage these issues include the use of tidal PD, and it is possible to use the machine software to identify dialysate flow profiles and optimise the tidal prescription. The use of more biocompatible neutral pH dialysates may ameliorate inflow pain possibly due to less chemical irritation of the membrane resulting in reduced stimulation of nociceptors. The position of the tube in the pelvis can lead to mechanical irritation which may be resolved by tube repositioning. If such problems are not resolved promptly, some patients may be discouraged from persisting with PD.

Audit Standards for Catheter Placement

The minimisation of catheter-related complications requires care and attention from the operator in the context of a consistent team-based approach supported by clear guidelines and protocols [7]. These describe the conditions necessary for optimal catheter function with minimisation of complications. The only registry that reports primary catheter function is the French-speaking registry, and this gives really excellent catheter function data [5]. However, in reality, many centres describe results that are considerably lower. The ISPD audit standards for catheter placement include a 1-year catheter survival of at least 80 % and peritonitis within 2 weeks of catheter insertion of less than 5 % [7].

Surgical Complications of PD

The surgical complications related to the insertion of the PD catheter can lead to morbidity, which can seriously compromise outcomes and result in loss of confidence for patients. Early complications include haemorrhage, perforated viscus, wound infection, catheter obstruction and displacement and dialysate leak. Later complications

25. Brown MC, Simpson K, Kerssens JJ, Mactier RA. Encapsulating

include external cuff extrusion, dialysate leaks, hernias, erosion of abdominal organs, haemoperitoneum and chylous effluent. Independent of the insertion technique, the operator must be able to recognise and manage of complications promptly and effectively. Preoperative evaluation and identification of potential risk factors are essential to prevent them [17].

Haemorrhage

Intraperitoneal haemorrhage may arise from trauma to the omental or mesenteric vessels, particularly during closed or blind insertion. This usually presents with blood staining of the effluent, which may be heavy. Slight bleeding may be treated expectantly; however, heavy bleeding, particularly in association with hypotension, will require return to theatre for localisation of the source of the bleeding and haemostasis. Extraperitoneal bleeding may be obvious from the wound edge (main wound or exit site) or an enlarging wound haematoma. Skin edge bleeding can be dealt with using either additional sutures or local injection with a local anaesthetic solution containing adrenaline. Failure to evacuate a haematoma predisposes to delayed wound healing, dehiscence and infection with potential risk of tunnel infection and peritonitis.

Haemoperitoneum

Haemoperitoneum can give a dramatic appearance, but generally settles spontaneously without the patient suffering harm. Many causes exist and have been summarised in an excellent review article [18]. There are rare occasions when it can signify a significant intraperitoneal haemorrhage – for example, following the rupture of a splenic artery aneurysm, although most commonly the cause is a bleed from a peritoneal capillary or due to either ovulation or retroperitoneal menstruation in women. In one series, the incidence of haemoperitoneum was 6 % of all patients on PD. Seventy percent of these did not require any active intervention apart from addition of heparin to the dialysate, with 20 % requiring active intervention for significant haemorrhage and the remaining 10 % having significant intra-abdominal pathology but minor haemoperitoneum [19]. Blood transfusion may be required in severe bleeding due to follicular or ovarian cyst rupture or coagulopathies.

Perforation or Laceration

Perforation of bowel and urinary bladder is a well-recognised complication of closed PD catheter insertion, which rarely occurs with open insertion. Injuries to liver, a polycystic kidney, aorta, mesenteric artery and hernial sac have been reported. Predisposing factors include abdominal adhesions and distensions due to paralytic ileus or bowel obstruction and unconscious, cachectic or heavily sedated patients. The bladder is at risk of injury if it is of high volume, for example, in patients with chronic bladder outflow obstruction, which can be avoided by preoperative voiding or urethral catheterisation if urinary retention is demonstrated on a post-voiding bladder ultrasound scan. Evidence of peritonitis associated with contaminated effluent is an indication for laparotomy and repair of the perforation. Delayed perforation of intestine, bladder and vagina caused by pressure necrosis and erosion from an unused catheter has been described.

Wound Infection

Although rare, this is a serious complication, which may lead to catheter loss. Usual organisms are *Staphylococcus aureus* and *Pseudomonas species*. Contamination of the wound should be prevented by strict adherence to aseptic technique, prophylactic antibiotics and meticulous haemostasis. Treatment of established infection requires antibiotics, surgical drainage and possibly catheter removal for intractable infection involving the catheter. ESI or peritonitis directly as a consequence of catheter placement should be a rare event.

Hernias

It is estimated that between 10 and 20 % of the CAPD population develop hernias due to raised intra-abdominal pressure associated with PD, which can be inguinal, para-umbilical and peri-catheter in location. Part of the preoperative assessment of the prospective PD patient is to assess for the presence of hernias since these can be repaired at the time of catheter placement. However, often these are not present at the time of catheter insertion and develop later, more commonly in patients who use larger intraperitoneal volumes and in patients with adult polycystic kidney disease.

Elective hernia repair should be undertaken if possible and if the peritoneum remains intact and the hernia repair is not extensive, disruption of PD is not required. A small volume and short cycle dwell regimen can be continued post-operatively. However, where the peritoneum is breeched during hernia repair, change to haemodialysis for at least 3 weeks to allow healing of the peritoneum should be considered since leakage of dialysis fluid through the hernia wound encourages infection of mesh used to reinforce the repair. Peri-catheter hernias, which usually occur in the midline, are difficult to manage without removing the catheter. Any

Kidney Int. 1998;54(6):2207–17.

65 Assessment of the Potential Transplant Donor

Gareth Jones

Every good transplant starts with a good operation, and every good transplant operation starts with a good donor. Donor selection is one of the most important factors for long-term graft survival and short-term outcomes in renal transplantation. The offer of a "perfect" donor is rare, and evaluation should be undertaken on the balance of risk and benefit to the recipient. When assessing the donor offer, the clinician should always consider whether the donor is safe to transplant a kidney from and whether the kidney is suitable for the intended recipient. In the case of living donation, the safety and long-term impact of donation on the donor also need to be considered.

The evaluation of donor safety should consider whether transplanting the organ will present a risk to the recipient. The risk appraisal always considers transmissible factors, such as infection and malignancy, but will also consider the organ anatomy and retrieval, where multiple vessels or damage to the organ may confer considerable risk to the recipient. The suitability of the organ for the recipient should take into account both donor and recipient factors. While a young pre-emptive recipient should be matched with a suitably young donor that will provide a high level of graft function for optimal long-term graft survival, an older recipient or patients with high levels of sensitisation or limited dialysis access may consider higher-risk donors where the focus may not necessarily be on optimal long-term graft survival.

When matching the donor to recipient, the potential benefits of transplantation can be overstated, and transplantation at any cost should be avoided. This is particularly relevant in the case of the high-risk recipient where the combination of suboptimal donors with suboptimal recipients often provides a suboptimal result. Contrary to perceived wisdom, the marginal recipient often requires more optimal donor organs to limit the risk of evolving complications, prolonged hospital stay and subsequent poor long-term outcomes.

Selection of the Deceased Donor

The offer of a deceased donor kidney frequently comes at the most inopportune time, and acceptance is usually combined with the pressure of minimising cold ischaemic times. These factors can often lead to the refusal of a donor where careful consideration may uncover a kidney with good long-term outcomes. It is also important to avoid "herd mentality" where the refusal to accept a donor by one unit is followed by refusal in other units on the ground that the previous unit did not want it. Although the reason for refusal may be valid, it is important to take a fresh look at each offer and evaluate the risk of the donor in combination with the circumstances of the recipient. In the case of donors who have been declined by a number of centres and are not suitable for your named recipient, it is always prudent to ask whether the offer would still stand for other recipients within your unit. In this case, the balance of risk may be different for an alternative recipient, and most donor coordination teams would prefer see an organ allocated in a timely fashion rather than discarded.

Achieving a consensus on the suitability of organs for transplantation has always proven difficult. The first attempt at consensus on the contraindications to organ donation in the United Kingdom was by Gore et al. in 1992 [1]. More recent guidance from the United Kingdom on the absolute contraindications to donation is listed below (Table 65.1) [2] and useful tips are on selection of a deceased donor organ are listed in Tables 65.2–65.5.

Donors with Infection

One area where clinical judgement should be exercised is the issue of infection in the donor and, on the whole, undiagnosed or uncontrolled sepsis should be considered as a

G. Jones, MBBS, FRCP, PhD
UCL Centre for Nephrology, Royal Free London NHS Trust, Pond Street, London NW3 2QG, UK
e-mail: gareth.jones14@nhs.net

M. Harber (ed.), *Practical Nephrology*,
DOI 10.1007/978-1-4471-5547-8_65, © Springer-Verlag London 2014

Table 65.1 Contraindications to solid organ donation

General
Age >85 years
Any cancer with evidence of spread outside affected organ (including lymph nodes) within 3 years of donation (however, localised prostate, thyroid, in situ cervical cancer and non-melanotic skin cancer are acceptable)
Melanoma (except completely excised stage 1 cancers)
Choriocarcinoma
Active haematological malignancy (myeloma, lymphoma, leukaemia)
Definite, probable or possible case of human TSE, including CJD and vCJD, individuals whose blood relatives have had familial CJD, other neurodegenerative diseases associated with infectious agents
TB: active and untreated
HIV disease (but not HIV infection)
Renal specific
Chronic kidney disease (CKD stage 3B and below, eGFR < 45)
Long-term dialysis (i.e. not acute relating to acute illness)
Renal malignancy (prior kidney tumours of low grade and previously excised would not exclude donation)
Previous kidney transplant (>6 months previously)

Modified from NHS BT guidance April 2013

Table 65.2 Factors associated with increased risk of graft loss post cadaveric renal transplant, modified from Schold et al. and Panduranga et al

Donor risk score (Schold et al.)	Donor risk index (Panduranga et al.)
Donor-recipient CMV match – positive to negative	Increasing donor age – over 50
African American donor	African American donor
Donor age (below 12 and over 29)	Serum creatinine over 1.5
Cerebrovascular cause of death	Donor hypertension
Increasing HLA mismatches	Donor diabetic
Increasing cold ischaemic time – over 9 h	Cerebrovascular cause of death
History of hypertension	Decreasing donor height below 170 cm
History of diabetes	Decreasing donor weight below 80 kg
	Donation after cardiac death
	Donor HCV positive
	Increasing HLA mismatch
	Cold ischaemic time over 20 h
	Single-kidney transplant
	Non-en bloc transplant

contraindication to donation. Although some centres will consider organs from donors with bacteraemia of known antibiotic sensitivity, it is inadvisable to utilise donors with infection localised to the organ or sepsis from multi-resistant organisms. Fungal sepsis also presents the potential for metastatic infection, and donors with known fungal sepsis, most particularly aspergillus, should not be utilised.

Table 65.3 Suggested minimal investigations for donor assessment

Physical
Office blood pressure measurements × 2
Urinalysis × 2
Full medical history
Physical examination
Haematology
Full blood count
Clotting
Blood group and antibody screen
Biochemistry
Urea, electrolytes, creatinine and eGFR
Calcium and phosphate
Liver function
Fasting glucose and lipids
Urine protein estimation (ACR/PCR or 24-h urine)
Endocrine
Thyroid function
Infection risk – virology
Hepatitis B sAg and cAb
Hepatitis C
HIV
HTLV
CMV
EBV
Infection risk – microbiology
Syphilis
Toxoplasma
Malaria – if from at risk country
Imaging
Chest X-ray
EDTA GFR
CT or MR angiography
(DMSA)
Malignancy risk
PSA – if male
Recent mammography in female over 50
Recent cervical smear
Cardiovascular assessment
ECG
Stress testing in high-risk or elderly donors

Table 65.4 Acceptable GFR by donor age prior to donation

Donor age (years)	Acceptable corrected GFR prior to donation (ml/min/1.73 m^2)
Up to 46	80
50	77
60	68
70	59
80	50

Reproduced from Third edition of UK Guidelines for living donor kidney transplantation [42]

Donors with chronic viral infections or past exposure to viruses may be considered as donors in specific situations. All

Table 65.5 Tips for selecting organs from deceased donors

Most consistent donor indicator of long-term graft outcome	Age
Primary CNS brain tumours	Risk of transmission is low (~1.5 %) with low-grade malignancy and lack of craniotomy/shunting
DCD vs DBD donors	Long-term outcomes are similar in donors aged under 60 years old and cold ischaemic time under 12 h
Creatinine in potential donors	Terminal creatinine is a poor indicator of outcome and admission values may give a better insight eGFR may give a better insight into the function of kidneys in elderly donors
Hepatitis B sAg-positive donors	Can be safely utilised in sAg recipients or patients with prior infection (cAb positive) with sAb levels over 1,000 IU/l
Hepatitis B cAb-positive/sAg-negative donors	Can be safely utilised in sAg-positive recipients or recipients with sAb over 1,000 IU/l through prior exposure or vaccination
Hepatitis C cAb-positive donors	Should only be considered for patients who are hepatitis C PCR positive. In this subgroup, outcome is similar to receipt of hepatitis C-negative kidney
Paediatric donors	Under 2 or less than 10 kg – avoid 2–5 year or 10–15 kg – en bloc transplant 5–10 or 15–35 kg – mainly single transplant Over 10 or over 35 kg – single transplant
Elderly donors	Donors over 60 should be used with caution unless age matched Beware additional comorbidities Consider dual transplant if eGFR < 60 ml/min
Donors not suitable for a named recipient	Ask whether the kidney could be offered to an alternative recipient with your unit

donors in the United Kingdom are currently screened for hepatitis B, hepatitis C, HIV and HTLV. The utilisation of organs from virally infected donors varies according to local policy.

Hepatitis B-Positive Donors

Chronic hepatitis B (hep B sAg positive) has a prevalence of 0.3–1 % in the United Kingdom with significant variation across different communities and higher rates in populations from sub-Saharan Africa and Asia. Although the rate of chronic hepatitis is higher when exposure occurs at a young age, most adults will not develop chronic hepatitis after initial exposure but will have serological evidence of prior exposure (hep B cAb positive, sAg negative). The use of hep B sAg-positive kidneys in naïve recipients leads to universal infection with a high risk of subsequent morbidity and should be avoided. In recipients who are already hep B sAg positive and on antiviral treatment for hepatitis B, the receipt of a sAg-positive kidney can reduce waiting time with a low risk of subsequent complications. The theoretical risk of transmission of resistant hepatitis B strains appears to be low, but recipients should receive antiviral therapy with a lower rate of viral resistance, rather than lamivudine. The utilisation of sAg-positive kidneys donated to patients with a previous exposure to hepatitis (cAb positive) or vaccination is more controversial but appears to have limited complications when combined with a selective programme of repeat vaccination with or without antiviral therapy and hepatitis B immune globulin. A recent review has covered this area in detail [3]. It is important to note that some of the studies did not utilise donors with detectible hepatitis B DNA, although one study used repeated hepatitis B immune globulin in recipients of donors who were found to be DNA positive [4]. This study did not show any transmission of hepatitis B from DNA-positive kidneys, but these recipients had acquired immunity via prior exposure to hepatitis B (i.e. cAb positive prior to transplant). Our local policy is to utilise hepatitis B sAg-positive kidneys for recipients who are sAg positive. If no recipients are found, the kidneys may be offered to patients who have prior exposure to hepatitis B (hep B cAb positive) with adequate levels of sAb (over 500 IU/l). If levels are below 500 IU/l, this can be supplemented with hepatitis B immune globulin. The recipient is also treated with antiviral therapy for 12 months post-transplant. Our policy excludes recipients who have achieved immunity through vaccination, although Jiang et al. [4] did transplant sAg-positive kidneys into cAb-negative/sAb-positive recipients with only a single patient subsequently developing sAg positivity. One note of caution is the rate of false positivity of hepatitis B cAb tests, and a positive result may require confirmation by repeat testing at a local reference laboratory.

Prior infection with hepatitis B (hep B sAg negative, cAb positive) is uncommon in the United Kingdom and only accounts for around 2 % of cadaveric donors, although 11 % of our local end-stage renal failure patients are cAb positive. The rates of cAb seropositivity are much higher in Asia and Africa. The risk of transmission of hepatitis B from a cAb-positive donor is dependent on the organ transplanted, with the risk of transmission highest amongst liver recipients [5] and reducing risk in kidney, heart or lung. The risk of transmission from cAb-positive kidneys has been quoted as 2.4 % based on the experience of Wachs et al. [5]. In this series, 42 patients received kidneys from cAb-positive, sAg-negative

motivation for donation. Although the UK regulatory authorities have removed the mandatory status for psychological evaluation of potential altruistic donors, it is probably best practice for these donors to be evaluated by a person experienced in personal assessment that has sufficient time and skill to explore the motivation for and understanding of altruistic donation. Most donors are motivated to help their fellow human, and some donors may have a previous history of medical altruism, such as blood or bone marrow donation. Caution should be exercised with donors who have recently had major life events, such as significant loss or separation, where donors may be looking for absolution of previous events. In addition, young altruistic donors provide significant vexation for the clinician where a kidney of excellent function is offered but the donor may not be of sufficient emotional maturity or far enough into their "life experience" to fully understand the consequences of donation. It is always important to reaffirm that kidney donation can only be undertaken once and any future partner, child or family member who develops kidney failure would be unable to receive a kidney from this donor if they have already donated to another person.

Assessment of the Potential Live Donor

The assessment of a kidney donor is a complex process that should evaluate the physical health of the donor, their suitability to undergo major abdominal surgery, the suitability of the donor to be left with a single kidney long term, the quality of the donor organ and any risk to the recipient of receiving the organ. It is important to remember that a donor is always giving altruistically and may often be the financial breadwinner of a household. Any workup process should aim to minimise disruption to the work schedules and compact the investigations into as few days as possible. This is particularly relevant when donors have travelled from overseas to donate and may have left families or businesses back in their own country. Overseas donors may be on short visas and any workup should be planned in advance of their arrival.

Current best practice consists of a single day of donor assessment with subsequent medical and surgical review. Donors and recipients should then have time to digest the information before proceeding to independent assessment under the Human Tissue Act. Minimal suggested donor evaluation investigations are listed below in Table 65.3.

Specific Points in the Workup Process

The live donor assessment is rigorous with around 30–40 % of potential donors ruled out during the assessment process. The most common reasons for declining donors after the assessment stage are (1) insufficient renal function, (2) poorly controlled hypertension and (3) anatomic abnormalities with the kidney that are picked up during scanning. The assessment process is multifaceted and each individual donor often presents their own idiosyncratic issues. Most national transplant bodies will provide guidance on the assessment process for living donation and recommendations for acceptability. In the United Kingdom, the British Transplant Society provides guidance for the assessment of donors which are freely available on their website. This guidance is detailed and covers a number of different situations. For the sake of brevity, this chapter will only cover some of the more common problems encountered.

Kidney Function and the Acceptable Level to Donate

The assessment of renal function prior to donation should be undertaken by a referenced measurement of glomerular filtration rate, i.e. Chromium EDTA. Estimated methods such as MDRD or Cockroft and Gault are not sufficiently accurate to predict GFR and should not be relied upon. Although creatinine clearance may give an estimation of renal function and 24-h collections are useful for measuring urinary protein excretion, the variable logistics and room for errors in performing these tests make them unsuitable for the accurate representation of true GFR.

The renal function of a prospective donor must be sufficient for a person to be able to donate a kidney and not be at risk from clinically significant renal failure over their lifetime. The level of GFR at which an individual person can donate their kidney has been achieved by an extrapolation of a number of estimates. In the United Kingdom, the guidance suggests that any person who donates a kidney should be left with sufficient renal function to achieve a GFR of 37.5 ml/min/1.73 m^2 by the age of 80 years. The most recent UK guidance is based on the data from Ibrahim [40] where all donors had to achieve a baseline GFR of at least 80 ml/min/1.73 m^2 and rate of decline post donation was 0.6 ml/min/1.73 m^2 per year. The acceptable rate of decline was then increased to 0.9 ml/min/1.73 m^2 per year to allow for safe variation and further data showing that the rate of decline of renal function in renal donors may be between 0.4 and 0.8 ml/min/1.73 m^2 per year. The last two factors are that renal function is grossly stable until the age of 40 before declining in a predictable fashion, and after donation, there is a compensatory increase in function after donation to achieve a level of 75 % of original function (although this does not necessarily apply to patients over 60). Therefore, until the age of 40, a donor has to achieve a measured GFR of greater than 80 ml/min/1.73 m^2 but after that there is a reduction in this limit by 0.9 ml/min/1.73 m^2 per year (Table 65.4).

Any estimate of a donor's kidney function should also take into account the divided split in function between kidneys. Most centres perform a nuclear medicine scan to assess the divided function of the two kidneys, the presence of scars and the drainage of the kidney (if a dynamic scan is performed). Some units prefer to rely on the length or volume of the kidneys on cross-sectional imaging to guide whether nuclear medicine assessment of divided function is necessary. Either way, the total GFR should be interpreted with the split function to decide the level of function that will be left with the donor and the function to be transplanted to the recipient.

Obesity

Obesity is an increasing problem with donor body mass index slowly increasing with time. Increasing size of the donor is associated with an increase in the rate of surgical complications and the long-term risk post donation from hypertension and proteinuria. In addition, obesity is a significant risk factor for diabetes and its associated long-term complications.

Obese donors should be carefully assessed and counselled about their individual risk with strict weight loss targets given to donors who wish to progress. The risk of regaining weight after donation should also be highlighted, and long-term lifestyle measures should be implemented prior to donation. Some donors have opted for bariatric surgery prior to donation, but the risk of this technique in donors has not been established, and certain procedures may increase long-term renal risk.

Each donor should be assessed individually, with the limits of the body mass index and sex fat distribution (i.e. males tend to have a greater proportion of intra-abdominal fat to females) borne in mind. Although there is no specific cutoff for donation and surgical practice varies between centres, it is wise to counsel and try weight loss techniques in any donor with a BMI over 30 kg/m^2. At a BMI over 35 kg/m^2, most centres would not proceed to donation unless there are extenuating circumstances.

Hypertension

Hypertension is common with around a quarter of the general population lying within the hypertensive range and only one-third of patients adequately treated. Hypertension is a known risk factor for proteinuria and progression of chronic kidney disease. In addition, hypertension can be an indicator of renal disease. The presence of hypertension is a risk for cardiovascular events and patients with hypertension may be at greater risk of cardiovascular events during the perioperative period. Hypertension in the donor may be worsened by a donor nephrectomy and is a recognised risk factor for reduced long-term survival of the transplanted kidney. Donors should be screened for hypertension with office blood pressure readings and treated in accordance with local guidance.

Donors with readings over 140/90 should be assessed with repeated readings and a 24-h ambulatory blood pressure measurement. If found to achieve the diagnostic criteria for hypertension, donors should initiate lifestyle changes and consider pharmacological therapy, if indicated.

Donors with known hypertension should have office and ambulatory blood pressure measurements to assess their level of control. If donors have controlled blood pressure on one or two antihypertensive agents, they may be suitable for donation if they do not have evidence of target end-organ damage but should be counselled for the small risk of worsening hypertension and proteinuria after donation. Lifestyle measures, such as smoking cessation, exercise and weight loss, should be initiated before and after donation to minimise risk. Our local practice is to perform ECG and echo assessments for left ventricular hypertrophy, retinal examination for evidence of hypertensive retinopathy and screen for microalbuminuria. If patients are found to have evidence of target end-organ damage or uncontrolled hypertension, they are advised against donation.

Haematuria

Asymptomatic non-visible haematuria affects 2.5 % of the UK adult male population but the prevalence increases with age and has been estimated to be present in 22 % of males over the age of 60. Although there are national guidelines for the significance and management of haematuria in the general population, the guidance is based on risk assessment and probability of finding significant disease which does not necessarily apply to a potential donor. In living donation, the purpose of the investigation is to rule out any significant transmissible disease while also prognosticating for the future of the donor post-unilateral nephrectomy.

All donors should have at least two urine dipstick analysis performed on two separate occasions. A positive result should be considered at any level of positivity, including trace haematuria. Initial investigations should aim to rule out reversible causes, such as infection, exercise or menstrual contamination. In the event of persistent positive dipstick analysis, donors should undergo further evaluation with urine cytology and renal tract imaging to rule out common urological causes. Cystoscopy should be performed in all patients over 40 with persistent haematuria, especially if they have other risk factors for urothelial malignancy.

All patients with persisting non-visible haematuria will require a renal biopsy to rule out significant glomerular pathology, if they wish to progress as a donor. This investigation is particularly pertinent to donors who are giving to a relative where the underlying cause of kidney failure is undiagnosed or possibly inherited. Given that a native renal biopsy carries a significant risk and non-donor patients in the same situation with normal renal function in the absence of hypertension and proteinuria would not undergo a biopsy, the potential kidney donor is putting themselves at risk purely for the wish to donate. This balance of risk should be explained to the potential donor with full explanation of the potential complications of kidney biopsy, including the small risk of damage to or loss of the kidney. If the donor decides to proceed to a renal biopsy, the kidney that is to be donated should be biopsied in order to reduce any long-term structural risk to the donor in their remaining kidney.

Glomerular pathology has been reported in 8 out of 10 donors who undergo a biopsy for isolated haematuria prior to donation [41] and 46 % of nephrology patients presenting with asymptomatic non-visible haematuria alone. Post-donation, persistent haematuria with dysmorphic red cells on cytology is associated with a higher incidence of proteinuria and declining renal function [43]. Patients who are found to have abnormal renal biopsies, other than thin basement membrane disease, should be ruled out as potential donors due to the risk of progressive renal pathology.

The question of whether patients with thin basement membrane disease should be considered as donors remains a contentious issue. Firstly, the course of thin basement membrane disease may not be entirely benign with 10–20 % of patients developing proteinuria, and 5 % have subsequent renal impairment. Secondly, the diagnosis of thin basement membrane disease can be indistinguishable from early or carrier status of Alport syndrome. In the case of the latter, potential donors with carrier status for X-linked Alport syndrome have a 15 % chance of end-stage renal failure by the age of 60 and should not proceed to donation [44]. For this reason, any mother or sister who intends to donate to a patient with Alport syndrome should be offered genetic counselling, screening for known Alport mutations and a renal biopsy prior to donation. This advice also applies to female extended family members where there is a family history of Alport syndrome. In the case of autosomal recessive Alport syndrome, family members can proceed to donation post biopsy if they have only a single mutation (i.e. heterozygous) of COL4A3 or COL4A4 without proteinuria, hypertension, low GFR or significant chronic damage on their biopsy [44].

Donors who are found to have thin basement membrane disease on biopsy should undergo genetic screening to rule out mutations associated with X-linked Alport syndrome [44]. If the screening is negative, donors may progress to donation in the absence of hypertension, proteinuria, family history of deafness, family history of renal disease and significant scaring on a renal biopsy. A referral to a clinical geneticist should be considered, especially if the underlying cause of renal failure in the recipient is not fully defined or the donor is of Cypriot origin, where higher incidence of renal impairment with thin basement membrane disorder have been reported.

Diabetes

Due to the increased propensity to renal failure, patients with diabetes or those with impaired glucose tolerance have historically been ruled out from donation. A single study from Japan [45] has looked at donors who had impaired glucose tolerance or diabetes when undergoing an oral glucose tolerance test prior to kidney donation. Donors with no evidence of secondary complications, an HbA1c under 6.5 % and no albuminuria were allowed to donate after careful counselling. When compared to donors with normal glucose tolerance, there was no significant difference between the groups in survival to 20 years and renal disease at a median follow-up of 88 months. Although this data is encouraging and may suggest that donation in groups with impaired glucose tolerance or well-controlled diabetes is safe, the follow-up period is relatively short and the cohort of donors with diabetes were newly diagnosed at donation and may not have had sufficient time to develop significant complications. A further study [46] looked at the development of diabetes post donation in donors who had a normal oral glucose tolerance test at the time of donation. After a follow-up of almost 18 years, 5 % of the donors had developed diabetes. The main risk factors were body mass index over 30 kg/m^2 and donating to a relative with type 1 diabetes. At the time of follow-up, there were a greater proportion of donors with hypertension (71 % vs 36 %) and proteinuria (19 % vs 4 %) in the group with diabetes compared to those without diabetes. The rate of decline in renal function post donation was the same in both groups.

Although these studies may suggest that the risk of donation in patients with diabetes is low, it is important to remember that the follow-up time was short and the donors studied were early after the diagnosis of impaired glucose tolerance or diabetes. From epidemiological studies of patients with diabetes, the incidence of end-stage renal disease in type 1 diabetics is between 4 and 17 % at 20 years and 0.8 % at 10 years in the UKPDS type 2 diabetes cohort. In light of the propensity for higher blood pressure and risk of proteinuria post donation, there is likely to be a higher risk of chronic kidney disease or end-stage renal failure in donors with diabetes. Therefore, potential donors with diabetes should generally be ruled out from donation.

The diagnosis of diabetes or impaired glucose tolerance is fairly clear-cut but the issue remains whether the clinician can predict which donors are likely to develop diabetes post donation with a higher long-term risk from chronic kidney failure. The risk of diabetes is increased when a family member has diabetes, which may be pertinent to a donor who is giving a kidney to a family member with end-stage renal failure secondary to diabetic nephropathy. The overall risk of developing diabetes is increased two- to threefold if any first-degree relative has diabetes. If both parents have diabetes, the risk is increased five- to sixfold with some South Asian patients having up to 80 % lifetime risk of developing diabetes in this situation. In addition, certain ethnic groups with higher rates of end-stage renal failure also have higher rates of diabetes, such as South Asian and Caribbean groups. The prospective Nurses' Health study showed that females from an African American, Asian or Hispanic background have a relative risk of 2.2 for developing diabetes when compared to White Americans. Therefore, these at-risk groups should be carefully screened for the presence of diabetes and their lifetime risk considered in conjunction with their lifestyle and anthropometrics.

Women with a history of gestational diabetes are at higher risk of developing type 2 diabetes with the incidence varying between 2.6 and 70 % and the greatest risk occurring within the first 5 years post pregnancy. A further study estimated the risk to be 19 % by 9 years postpartum. Due to this much higher risk of diabetes, donors with gestational diabetes should normally be ruled out from donation. Individual donors with high body mass index or adverse anthropometrics (i.e. waist hip ratios or waist measurements) may also be at greater risk of diabetes.

All donors should be screened for their risk of diabetes with a fasting blood sugar. Donors with normal fasting blood glucose of 5.5 mmol/l or less have a low chance of developing diabetes of around 4 % over 9 years. A fasting glucose of 5.6–6.9 mmol/l indicates impaired glucose tolerance, while a value over 7 mmol/l is indicative of diabetes mellitus. Donors with impaired glucose tolerance and a family history of diabetes have a 30 % 5-year risk of developing diabetes and should probably be ruled out of donation. All patients with fasting values in the impaired glucose tolerance range, a family history of diabetes or obesity should undergo a formal oral glucose tolerance test. Two-hour values over 11.1 mmol/l are indicative of diabetes, and the donor should be ruled out. Two-hour values between 7.8 and 11.0 mmol/l are indicative of impaired glucose tolerance. A meta-analysis of six trials estimated the annual risk of developing diabetes in this group ranges from 3.6 to 8.7 %. Overall, most clinicians would rule out donors with impaired glucose tolerance due to their much greater lifetime risk of developing diabetes, especially if they have other risk factors. If donors still wish to proceed in the face of impaired glucose tolerance, they should be fully cognisant of the risks with full documentation of the discussion.

Although metabolic parameters allow for clear guidance on the risk of donation, young family members of diabetic recipients, such as children, present a greater challenge when considering donation. If a young adult in their twenties presents for donation to a diabetic father, the young donor may well have a normal oral glucose tolerance test and relatively normal anthropometrics. In this situation, the lifetime risk of a diabetes in a donor with a strong family history of diabetes may be up to 80 %. Donation should be cautioned and the long-term risk to the donor made clear with strict adherence to exercise, healthy lifestyle and maintenance of a normal body habitus.

Nephrolithiasis in Potential Donors

The prevalence of symptomatic renal stones in a UK population is around 3–5 % with 5 % of donors found to have asymptomatic renal stones at assessment. The utilisation of cross-sectional imaging techniques for donor evaluation has led to a greater discovery of asymptomatic renal stones.

Any donor with a previous history of renal stones or asymptomatic stones on imaging should undergo full metabolic and urological evaluation to assess the risk of recurrent stone formation. In the event of a significant or uncorrectable abnormality, donation is contraindicated. Donors with bilateral renal stones, a significant stone burden or frequent recurrent stones should also be ruled out from donation. If the chemical composition of the stone is known, donors with struvite, cystine or uric acid stones should be ruled out unless there are obvious reversible causes for the uric acid stones and the urinary urate load is low with a pH over 6.5.

Donors with a previous history of stones or low-volume unilateral stones without an identifiable metabolic cause can be considered as kidney donors. The risk of further stones should be fully discussed with the donor and lifestyle changes or therapy initiated to reduce the risk of future stone formation. The kidney with stones is usually removed for donation, allowing sufficient renal function in the remaining kidney. Our local practice is to remove the stones ex vivo with a small ureteroscope prior to implantation.

Genetic Causes of Kidney Failure

All steps should be undertaken to identify the cause of end-stage renal failure in any potential kidney transplant recipient. In the presence of an inherited cause of renal failure, either monogenic or polygenic, a detailed family history should be elucidated and referral to a clinical geneticist considered. If a genetic abnormality in the recipient has been identified, screening the potential donor for the same defect can be considered to mitigate the risk of donation.

The most common cause of inherited renal failure is adult polycystic kidney disease and any related donors should undergo detailed imaging for cysts in the kidney and other organs. The international diagnostic criteria for polycystic kidney disease should be applied to screen donors whose relatives have adult polycystic kidneys and caution exercised with the offspring and young relatives of polycystic kidney sufferers.

Other inherited conditions where renal failure may occur are:

(Reproduced from the UK Guidelines for living donor kidney transplantation [42])

Autosomal dominant: ADPKD, renal cysts and diabetes, von Hippel-Lindau disease, familial haemolytic uraemic syndrome, familial FSGS, tuberose sclerosis complex, UMOD-associated nephropathy and nail patella syndrome

Autosomal recessive: ARPKD, Alport syndrome and familial nephrotic syndrome

X-linked: Alport syndrome, Fabry disease and Dent's disease

Polygenic: VUR and FSGS

In most cases above, donation should be precluded if a predisposition to the disease is identified. Particular care should be exercised in donors where the recipient has FSGS, HUS or Alport syndrome where the risk of similar disease in the donor is high.

Cardiovascular Suitability for Donation

Live donor nephrectomy is a major intra-abdominal operation which is associated with significant cardiac stress. It is important to preclude any form of cardiac disease that may put the potential donor at significant risk. For this reason, any patient with overt cardiac disease should probably be ruled out from donation to avoid any unnecessary and avoidable cardiac events. All donors should be screened for occult cardiac disease through evaluation of clinical symptoms and scoring of known cardiovascular risk factors. Donors should routinely have an electrocardiogram and cholesterol estimations performed as part of their workup. The donors' exercise tolerance, symptoms of cardiac disease, smoking history and family history of cardiac disease should be recorded to assess risk.

On the whole, most donors who can achieve 4 METS (gentle swimming, gentle cycling or singles tennis) without other risk factors and a normal ECG are usually suitable as donors. The bar for further cardiac evaluation with stress testing should be set low, and our local practice is to perform either exercise testing or stress echocardiography on any potential donor over 50 with other risk factors or an abnormal ECG.

Pregnancy Post Donation

Women of childbearing age are often considered as potential kidney donors. Pregnancy is known to have significant effects on the kidney which may be exacerbated post-unilateral nephrectomy. A number of small series have looked at the effect of donation on pregnancy and have not found any significant effects of kidney donation on pregnancy outcome, hypertension or proteinuria. A further Norwegian registry study found a higher incidence of pre-eclampsia in pregnancies post donation compared to pregnancy prior to donation (5.7 % vs 2.6 %), but no other differences in maternal or foetal outcome were found. Another retrospective postal survey from the United States found a significantly higher rate of foetal loss (19 % vs 11 %), gestational hypertension (5.7 % vs 0.6 %), pre-eclampsia (5.5 % vs 0.8 %) and proteinuria (4.3 % vs 1.1 %) in mothers post donation. Although the data from the last study does suggest an increased risk to the mother and foetus from pregnancy, it should be highlighted that a number of donors did not respond and some who did respond were asked to describe pregnancies that had occurred some decades prior.

When considering all these studies, there is insufficient data to be definitive about the risk of pregnancy post donation, but there does not seem to be a reduction in foetal outcomes. There may be a marginally higher incidence of hypertension, proteinuria and pre-eclampsia, but further detailed studies are required.

Consent and How Much Should the Donor Know?

All donors should be given enough detail to provide full and informed consent to donation. The donor should be aware that they may withdraw their consent and progression to donation at any time, including on the day of transplantation. The provision of information should be in verbal, written and other multimedia formats. This information should focus on the risk of donation and its long-term consequences but should also include detail on the outcomes for the transplanted kidney. This aspect is particularly important when the donor is giving to a recipient with a high risk of recurrent disease, such as HUS, FSGS and dense deposit disease. In addition, donors should be made aware of any issues that might materially affect the lifespan of the transplanted kidney. This situation can lead to significant ethical debate over informed consent and whether the donor should be made aware of significant medical conditions in the recipient, such as HIV and hepatitis C. At present, it is considered best medical practice that the donor is made aware of these issues and the recipient should disclose their status to the donor prior to donation.

Which Kidney to Remove

The choice of kidney to remove should be discussed with the donor and agreed well ahead of the day of surgery. The balance of which kidney is donated is often based on anatomical considerations for donor and recipient, as well as the function of the remaining kidney. The left kidney is most often removed at donor nephrectomy due to the additional length of the vessels, ease of access to the kidney and the overall lower divided function of the left kidney. The presence of renal stones, multiple vessels, multiple ureters and cortical lesions may necessitate the removal of an alternative or functionally larger kidney. In this situation, the function of the remaining kidney should be considered where the single-kidney function is sufficient to maintain long-term kidney function without the risk of significant or symptomatic kidney disease.

Overall, living kidney donation allows the best long-term outcome for patients with end-stage kidney failure. The selection of the donor is crucial to both the long-term outcome of the transplanted kidney and the safety of the procedure. The process of donor evaluation contains a number of clinical and ethical facets, but the final outcome of live donor transplantation is often rewarding for all (Table 65.5).

References

1. Gore SM, et al. Consensus on general medical contraindications to organ donation? BMJ. 1992;305:406.
2. SABTO Guidance on contraindication to donation; 2013.
3. Pilmore H, et al. Hepatitis B positive donors in renal transplantation: increasing the deceased donor pool. Transplantation. 2012;94:2006.
4. Jiang H, et al. Kidney transplantation from Hepatitis B surface antigen positive donors into Hepatitis B surface antibody positive recipients: a prospective nonrandomized controlled study from a single center. Am J Transplant. 2009;9:1853.
5. Wachs ME, et al. The risk of transmission of Hepatitis B from HBsAg(−), HbcAb(+), HBIgM(−) organ donors. Transplantation. 1995;59:230.
6. Satterthwaite R, et al. Risks of transplanting kidneys from Hepatitis B surface antigen-negative, Hepatitis B core antibody-positive donors. Transplantation. 1997;64:432.
7. Madayag RM, et al. Use of renal allografts from donors positive for Hepatitis B core antibody confers minimal risk for subsequent development of clinical Hepatitis B virus disease. Transplantation. 1997;64:1781.
8. Health Protection Agency. Hepatitis C in the UK: 2012 report; 2012.
9. Abbott K, et al. The impact of transplantation with deceased donor Hepatitis C-positive kidneys on survival in wait-listed long-term dialysis patients. Am J Transplant. 2004;4:2032.
10. Morales JM, et al. Long-term experience with kidney transplantation from Hepatitis C-positive donors into Hepatitis C-positive recipients. Am J Transplant. 2010;10:2453.
11. Morales JM, et al. Transplantation of kidneys from donors with Hepatitis C antibody into recipients with pre-transpiantation anti-HCV. Kidney Int. 1995;47:236.
12. Natov SN, et al. Hepatitis C genotype does not affect patient survival among renal transplant candidates. Kidney Int. 1999;56:700.
13. Muller E, et al. Renal transplantation between HIV-positive donors and recipients. N Engl J Med. 2010;362:2336.
14. Desai R, et al. Cancer transmission from organ donors – unavoidable but Low risk. Transplantation. 2012;94:1200.
15. Feng S, et al. Organ donors with positive viral serology or malignancy: risk of disease transmission by transplantation. Transplantation. 2002;74:1657.
16. Kauffman HM, et al. Transplant tumour registry: donor related malignancies. Transplantation. 2002;74:358.
17. Nalesnik MA, et al. Donor-transmitted malignancies in organ transplantation: assessment of clinical risk. Am J Transplant. 2011;11:1140.
18. Brooke NR, et al. Outcomes of transplants from patients with small renal tumours, live unrelated donors and dialysis wait-listed patients. Transplant Int. 2010;23:476.
19. Kauffman HM, et al. Transplant tumor registry: donors with central nervous system tumors. Transplantation. 2002;73:579.
20. Buell JF, et al. Donors with central nervous system malignancies: are they truly safe? Transplantation. 2003;76:340.
21. Watson CJ, et al. How safe is it to transplant organs from deceased donors with primary intracranial malignancy? Am J Transplant. 2010;10:1437.
22. Warrens AN, et al. Advising potential recipients on the use of organs from donors with primary central nervous system tumors. Transplantation. 2012;93:348.
23. Busson M, et al. Analysis of cadaver donor criteria on the kidney transplant survival rate in 5,129 transplantations. J Urol. 1995;154:356.
24. Port FR, et al. Donor characteristics associated with reduced graft survival: an approach to expanding the pool of kidney donors. Transplantation. 2002;74:1281.
25. Schold JD, et al. The broad spectrum of quality in deceased donor kidneys. Am J Transplant. 2005;5:757.
26. Panduranga SR, et al. A comprehensive risk quantification score for deceased donor kidneys: the kidney donor risk index. Transplantation. 2009;88:231.
27. Schmitt R, et al. Recovery of kidney function after acute kidney injury in the elderly: a systematic review and meta-analysis. Am J Kidney Disc. 2008;52:262.
28. Cho YW, et al. Transplantation of kidneys from donors whose hearts have stopped beating. N Engl J Med. 2009;338:221.
29. Nicholson ML, et al. A comparison of the results of renal transplantation from non-heart-beating, conventional cadaveric, and living donors. Kidney Int. 2000;58:2585.
30. Kokkinos C, et al. Outcome of kidney transplantation from non-heart-beating versus heart-beating cadaveric donors. Transplantation. 2007;83:1193.
31. Summers DM, et al. Analysis of factors that affect outcome after transplantation of kidneys donated after cardiac death in the UK: a cohort study. Lancet. 2010;376:1303.

32. Summers DM, et al. Effect of donor age and cold storage time on outcome in recipients of kidneys donated after circulatory death in the UK: a cohort study. Lancet. 2013;381:727.
33. Sharma A, et al. En bloc kidney transplantation from pediatric donors: comparable outcomes with living donor kidney transplantation. Transplantation. 2011;92:564.
34. Kayler LK, et al. Single kidney transplantation from young pediatric donors in the United States. Am J Transplant. 2009;9:2745.
35. Zhang R, et al. Long-term outcome of adults who undergo transplantation with single pediatric kidneys: how young is too young? Clin J Am Soc Nephrol. 2009;4:1500.
36. Bhayana S, et al. Pediatric en bloc kidney transplantation to adult recipients: more than suboptimal? Transplantation. 2010;90:248.
37. Chavalitdhamrong D, et al. Patient and graft outcomes from deceased kidney donors age 70 years and older: an analysis of the Organ Procurement Transplant Network/United Network of Organ Sharing database. Transplantation. 2008;85:1573.
38. Lapointe I, et al. Impact of donor age on long-term outcomes after delayed graft function: 10-year follow-up. Transplant Int. 2013;26:162.
39. Segev D, et al. Perioperative mortality and long-term survival following live kidney donation. JAMA. 2010;303:959.
40. Ibrahim H, et al. Long-term consequences of kidney donation. N Engl J Med. 2009;360:459.
41. Koushik R, et al. Persistent, asymptomatic, microscopic hematuria in prospective kidney donors. Transplantation. 2005;80:1425.
42. United Kingdom guidelines for living donor kidney transplantation, 3rd edn. 2011.
43. Kido R, et al. Persistent glomerular hematuria in living kidney donors confers a risk of progressive kidney disease in donors after heminephrectomy. Am J Transplant. 2010;10:1596.
44. Savige J, et al. Expert guidelines for the management of Alport syndrome and thin basement membrane nephropathy. J Am SocNephrol. 2013;24:364.
45. Okamoto M, et al. The consequences for live kidney donors with preexisting glucose intolerance without diabetic complication: analysis at a single Japanese center. Transplantation. 2010; 89:1391.
46. Ibrahim H, et al. Diabetes after kidney donation. Am J Transplant. 2010;10:331.

66 Assessment of the Potential Transplant Recipient

Albert Power and Peter J. Dupont

Renal transplantation transforms life expectancy in patients with end-stage renal disease (Fig. 66.1). All patients who are considered for renal transplantation require rigorous pre-operative assessment in order to ensure their fitness to undergo surgery under general anaesthesia and to optimise the therapeutic impact of a scarce and precious resource. This chapter will review the practical aspects of delivering such an assessment with reference to available evidence and guidelines [1, 2].

Service Structure

Pre-transplant assessment is best delivered as a streamlined and ideally "one-stop" outpatient service. This will require a multidisciplinary approach with input from a nephrologist, transplant surgeon and clinical nurse specialist. Clinical psychology review can be invaluable for patients with issues with adherence to treatment or adjustment to their diagnosis of end-stage kidney failure.

Patients with complex cardiac histories or positive cardiac screening tests often need input from a cardiologist in determining optimal management. This may be best handled through a regular joint cardiology/nephrology meeting. Medically complex recipients should be reviewed in dedicated multidisciplinary team meetings with input from senior anaesthetic staff and from the patient's primary nephrologist.

For patients with potential live donors, the participation of a specialised live donor coordinator team and an efficient tissue-typing laboratory is vital in reducing the time between patient referral and transplantation.

Once on the transplant list, it is essential that recipient contact details are up-to-date since the transplant offer often occurs outside of normal working hours. In addition there is a need for an awareness of the changing clinical course of each recipient on the transplant waiting list to ensure that those who become medically unfit or who are travelling abroad are suspended from the national deceased donor list in a timely way. A dedicated transplant list coordinator at the transplanting centre ensures that wait-list maintenance is carried out to a high standard and that the local list aligns with that of the national organ allocation service.

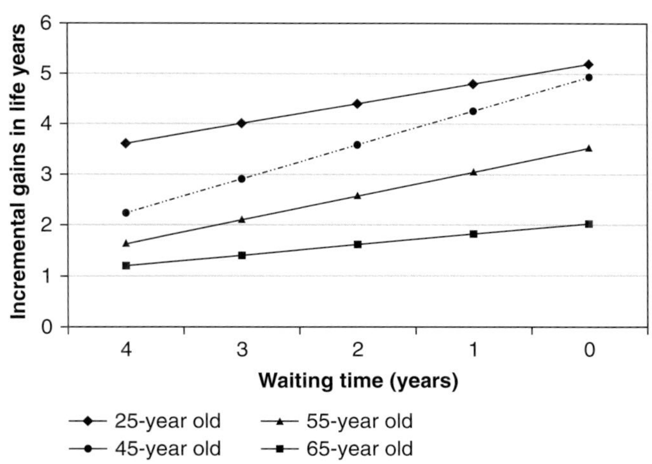

Fig. 66.1 The incremental benefits of transplant wait listing compared to matched non-transplant-listed individuals showing the effects of patient age and waiting time (From Wong et al. [3])

A. Power, MB, BChir, MRCP, MD (✉)
Department of Medicine, Imperial College London, Room 5N8A, Commonwealth Building, Hammersmith Campus, Du Cane Road, London W12 0NN, UK
e-mail: albert.power@nhs.net

P.J. Dupont, PhD, FRCPI
UCL Centre for Nephrology, Royal Free Hospital, Pond Street, London NW3 2QG, UK
e-mail: pdupont@nhs.net

M. Harber (ed.), *Practical Nephrology*,
DOI 10.1007/978-1-4471-5547-8_66, © Springer-Verlag London 2014

When to List?

The European Best Practice Guidelines (2000) recommend transplant wait listing in patients with an eGFR <20 ml/min and predicted to be within 6 months of needing RRT. Judging this latter criterion necessarily involves a degree of subjectivity. Patients with an eGFR <20 ml/min but a slow trajectory may not need to be listed straight away. An exception may be made for those with apparently stable but very poor renal function (e.g. an eGFR <15 ml/min), given that even a small further decline in renal function may precipitate the patient onto dialysis, and such declines often occur in an unpredictable, stepwise fashion.

Cardiovascular Assessment

There are two elements to the assessment of cardiovascular risk for patients undergoing pre-transplant assessment. The first is to ensure that the patient is fit to be subjected to the rigours of general anaesthesia and transplant surgery. The second is to make a judgement as to whether the prospective recipient will survive long enough for post-transplantation to justify allocation of a precious resource. This latter point is relevant because, despite careful preselection, cardiovascular disease remains the most common cause of death with a functioning graft at all times following transplantation (38 % of cases) and particularly within the first 12 months (Fig. 66.2).

There is much controversy surrounding cardiac screening pre-transplantation, and there is scant evidence that screening asymptomatic renal patients for cardiac disease is beneficial in improving outcome. Indeed some would argue that screening tests should serve only to exclude from transplantation those deemed at high risk of peri- and post-operative cardiac events.

In spite of this, most units do screen for cardiac disease although they rarely agree on the best way to do this. Non-invasive tests are often employed including exercise stress testing, echocardiography, dobutamine stress echocardiography (DSE) and nuclear myocardial perfusion scanning (MPS) as well as formal invasive coronary angiography. Non-invasive tests provide important prognostic information but have suboptimal sensitivity and specificity in detecting angiographic coronary artery disease (CAD). Whether the latter point matters is open to debate.

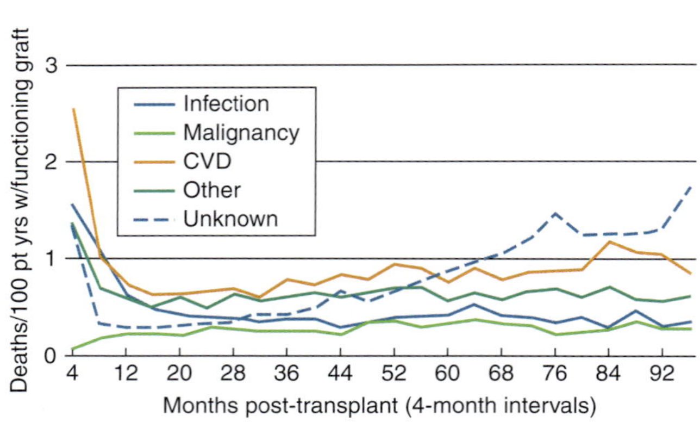

Fig. 66.2 Causes of death following renal transplantation (1997–2006) (From USRDS Annual Data Report 2008)

We provide a suggested algorithm for testing below but there remains no clear consensus regarding the choice and order of tests involved [4].

Non-invasive Cardiac Tests

Conventional transthoracic echocardiography offers an evaluation of cardiac anatomy, assessment of left ventricular function and screens for valvular abnormalities. For younger patients without a cardiac history, a chest X-ray, 12-lead ECG and ± echocardiogram may be quite sufficient.

Older patients and those with a history of cardiac disease, or at high risk for same, should undergo some form of stress testing to screen for inducible myocardial ischaemia. While exercise is a more physiological means of simulating the stress of general anaesthesia and surgery, the high prevalence of poor exercise capacity and motor disability in patients with end-stage renal disease (ESRD) means dobutamine stress echocardiography (DSE) or myocardial perfusion scanning (MPS) may be more appropriate for some. DSE has a pooled sensitivity of 0.8 and specificity of 0.9 in detecting CAD although this performance degrades significantly in patients with diabetes (see below) [4]. Myocardial perfusion scanning similarly has a pooled sensitivity of 0.7 and specificity of 0.8 but was found to perform less well compared to DSE when compared head-to-head [5]. This may relate to the greater degree of subjectivity involved in the interpretation of an MPS as well as the relative reduction in the efficacy of dipyridamole in the uraemic autonomic neuropathy seen in ESRD. Local expertise in these tests should determine the choice of investigation used.

In patients with diabetes and advanced CKD/ESRD, non-invasive testing is less reliable. In a large study of 280 transplant candidates with diabetes, an abnormal MPS was found in 28 % of patients but CAD was diagnosed angiographically in 56 % [6]. Although a positive MPS predicted the presence of CAD (odds ratio 7.2), a negative study was present in half the patients who had overt CAD. In this study CAD diagnosed on angiography was the only independent predictor of major adverse cardiac events. Most centres therefore reserve formal coronary angiography for patients identified at higher risk by non-invasive testing and have lower thresholds in patients with diabetes [7, 8].

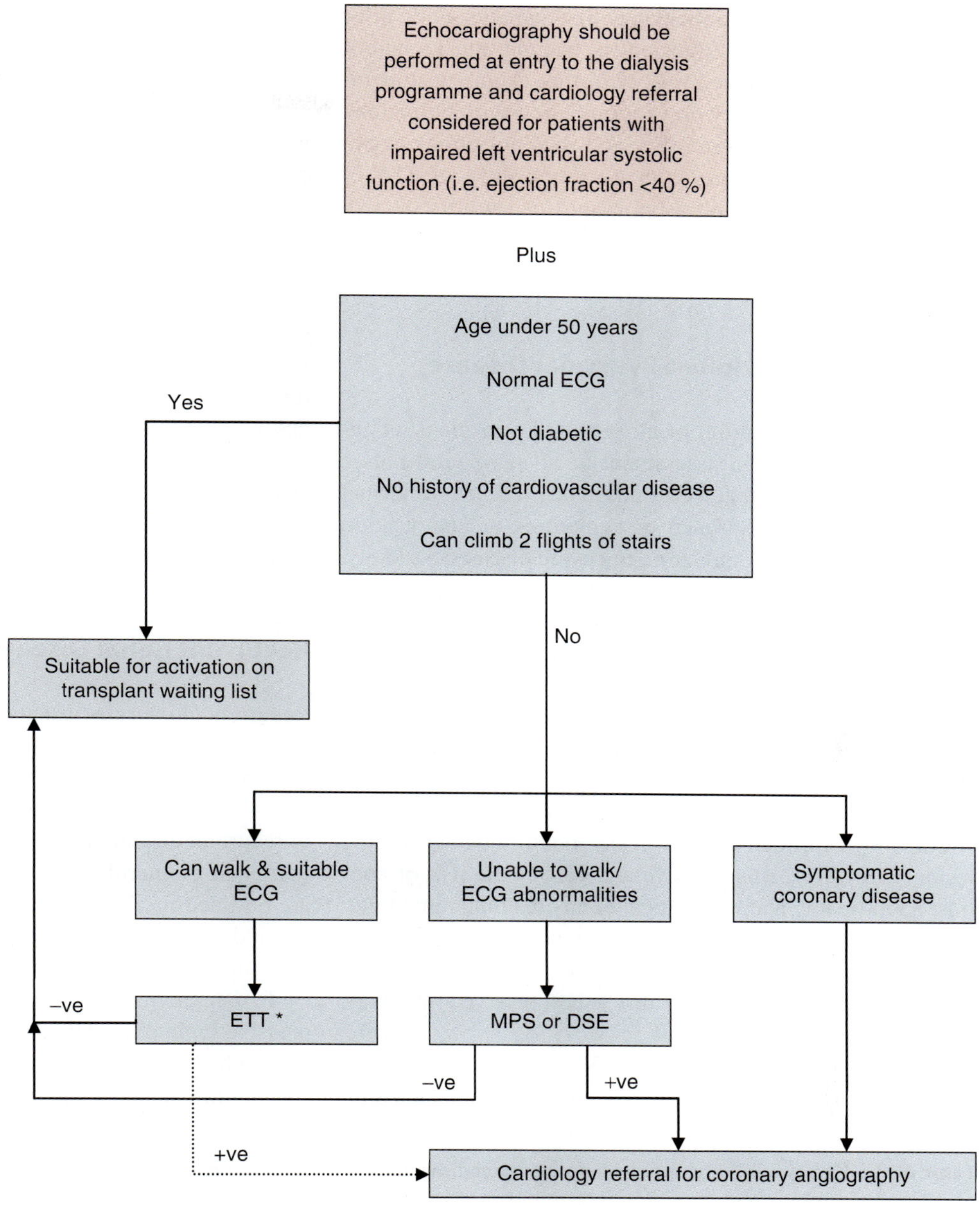

Fig. 66.3 Suggested algorithm for cardiac assessment for transplantation. *Abbreviations*: *ETT* exercise tolerance test, *MPS* myocardial perfusion scan, *DSE* dobutamine stress echocardiogram. *A negative ETT in this context is defined by a truly negative test or completing >6 min or achieving >6 METS

Coronary Angiography

Thresholds for coronary angiography vary widely between units. Advocates of a liberal approach point out that CAD is present in 40–80 % of transplant candidates [9–11], while proponents of a more conservative approach remind us that most patients with ESRD die of sudden cardiac death rather than coronary heart disease. Although angiography remains the gold standard for diagnosing CAD, it can be costly and carries a degree of procedural risk (e.g. vessel trauma, contrast-induced nephropathy). To date randomised trials in the general population have failed to show benefit of revascularisation over modern medical management [12, 13]. There is little robust evidence to support the routine use of this modality in pre-transplant cardiac screening. A suggested algorithm for cardiac assessment is shown in Fig. 66.3 with assessments repeated every 2 years for non-diabetic patients or annually for those with diabetes or known cardiovascular disease.

Assessment for Cerebrovascular Disease

There is little evidence to guide risk assessment for cerebrovascular disease prior to transplantation. It is important to screen patients with polycystic kidney disease and a family history of subarachnoid haemorrhage for cerebral arterial aneurysms. It can be anticipated that patients with prior cerebrovascular events (transient ischaemic attacks and/or strokes) are at heightened risk of further events postoperatively and that secondary prevention (e.g. use of antiplatelet agents, control of hypertension and dyslipidaemia) would be of benefit. In patients with a prior history of TIA or stroke, carotid Doppler ultrasonography can stratify the risk of perioperative stroke but has no role in asymptomatic patients [14].

Assessment of Peripheral Vascular Disease

The physical examination of all potential transplant recipients should include an assessment of all peripheral pulses especially those in the lower limbs. The presence of normal pedal pulses in the absence of symptoms of claudication makes the presence of moderate-to-severe disease less likely. It cannot, however, provide any anatomical information especially as regards haemodynamically significant aorto-iliac lesions. In one study of 152 patients, it was misleading in a third of cases where patients had patent aorto-iliac vessels [15]. As a result, adjunctive vascular imaging is often advocated particularly in higher-risk groups (e.g. older patients, diabetes, smokers, long dialysis duration).

Conventional angiography remains the gold standard test which allows for intervention on any identified flow-limiting lesions. However, it is invasive and carries the risk of contrast nephropathy and impairment of any residual renal function. In addition studies suggest that there is a low incidence of aorto-iliac disease in younger patients (1.9 % in those <40 years old) and that such a modality is best reserved for symptomatic patients [16].

Doppler ultrasonography (USS) is highly operator dependent with variable sensitivity and specificity reaching 91 and 93 %, respectively, in one study [15], while another suggested a positive predictive value of just 60 % [17].

Non-invasive angiography using magnetic resonance angiography (MRA) or CT angiography (CTA) has increased in popularity with the ability to deliver high-quality, three-dimensional imaging of pelvic and lower limb vasculature. CT is the modality of choice to determine the extent of vascular calcification of the pelvic vessels which may inform surgical decisions about allograft placement. Contrast-enhanced angiographic sequences (CTA) can deliver 96 % sensitivity and 97 % specificity but can miss short stenoses. Unlike CT scanning, MRA avoids the use of ionising radiation and has a sensitivity of 97 % and specificity of 99 % but has a higher false-positive rate.

In addition to arterial imaging, an evaluation of venous anatomy with CT or MR venography may be required in patients with a history of difficult vascular access, radiation injury or retroperitoneal fibrosis.

Recurrent Renal Disease

Recurrent glomerular disease remains the third leading cause of long-term allograft failure after chronic allograft nephropathy and rejection with 15 % of all graft failures attributed to recurrent disease in one series [18]. The most common form of recurrent disease is IgA nephropathy although it is not the dominant glomerulopathy responsible for graft loss. These are outlined in Table 66.1 and although they do not always preclude transplantation per se, careful risk determination is very important.

To date there is no evidence that any specific immunosuppressive regime or induction agent affects the risk of recurrent glomerular disease, and therefore, preoperative counselling regarding the risks of graft loss is critical.

Table 66.1 Primary renal diseases associated with significant rates of disease recurrence and which may lead to graft loss

Primary renal disease	Notes
Atypical HUS	Genotypic assessment is essential in stratifying recurrence risk post-transplantation (highest with Factor H and I mutations) [19]. There may be a therapeutic role for plasma exchange or eculizumab post-transplant. Combined liver-kidney transplant may be appropriate for those with factor H deficiency
FSGS	35–55 % recurrence reported in adults although accurate diagnosis is vital especially in distinguishing primary from secondary forms [20, 21]. Predictors include childhood presentation (<15 years old) and aggressive disease (heavy proteinuria, <3 years to reach ESRD). A history of prior recurrence post-transplant conveys an 80 % risk of recurrence in subsequent allografts; early graft loss from recurrent FSGS is considered by some an absolute contraindication to further transplantation. In general, idiopathic forms of FSGS (30 % recurrence risk overall) are much more likely to recur than familial forms. An important exception are those with heterozygous NPHS2 mutations – these are associated with a high risk of recurrence (65 %); homozygous or complex heterozygous have much lesser risk (8 %). It is important to consider the family history when assessing the risks for live-related donors
MPGN	Consider genetic complement disorder, especially with MPGN type 2. Recurrence rates leading to eventual graft failure are quoted as 15 % for type 1, 30 % for type 2 with predictors of recurrence including paediatric presentation and the presence of crescentic GN on original biopsy [22]
Primary hyperoxaluria	Primary hyperoxaluria is an absolute contraindication to renal transplantation unless combined with a liver transplant (100 % recurrence rate leading to graft loss in the absence of a liver transplant). Screening for this disorder should be considered for all young patients with ESRD secondary to stones

Table 66.1 (continued)

Primary renal disease	Notes
Alport's disease	De novo post-transplant anti-GBM disease can occur in up to 5 % patients with underlying Alport's disease. Screening for autoantibody levels postoperatively is advised. Graft loss due to anti-GBM disease in this setting is an absolute contraindication to further transplantation
Systemic sclerosis	Risk of recurrence approximately 3 %. Typically in the 1st year with a prodrome of anaemia and skin disease. ACE inhibitors should be continued perioperatively. CNIs can be used with caution aiming to keep levels as low as possible. High-dose steroids should be avoided due to the risk of provoking a hypertensive crisis (although pulsed methylprednisolone is likely to be needed at induction). 5-year graft survival 57 %. Patient survival 73 % at 5 years
SLE	Although recurrence is uncommon (<5 %) and is an unusual cause of premature graft failure, most clinicians would not list a patient until disease is in clinical remission. Increased risk of thrombotic events in patient with cardiolipin antibodies. Overall burden of immunosuppression needs to be considered when planning post-transplantation regimen
Anti-GBM disease	As a rule does not recur. Allow at least 6-month interval prior to transplantation to allow anti-GBM antibodies to become persistently negative
Vasculitis	Recurrence rate 8–17 %. ANCA positivity at time of transplantation is not predictive. No difference between c- and p-ANCA in terms of recurrence risk. Overall burden of immunosuppression needs to be considered when planning post-transplantation regimen
Membranous GN	Second most common cause of nephrotic-range proteinuria in allograft recipients. High rate of de novo disease (2–9 % at 2 years). Recurrent disease common (3–30 %). Spontaneous remission rare (c.f. native disease). Impact on graft survival unclear
Recurrent UTI/reflux nephropathy	UTIs post-transplantation are common and may contribute to graft injury or loss. Reflux to the native or transplant ureter may be contributory and consideration of native nephroureterectomy may be required. Voiding dysfunction should be ruled out by means of pre- and post-micturition US, flow rate studies, micturating cystourethrography or video-urodynamics as needed. Low-dose nocturnal antibiotic prophylaxis may be needed
Stones	Renal calculi occurring post-transplantation are uncommon (incidence approx 2 %). Composition of stones is similar to the non-transplant population. Predisposing factors include tertiary hyperparathyroidism, foreign body (e.g. ureteric stent), UTI and obstruction
Diabetic nephropathy	Histological changes seen after 2–3 years. Universal recurrence by 5 years. Major contributor to graft failure by 10 years. Arteriolar changes more common than glomerular. SPK protective
IgA nephropathy	Histological recurrence is common (>50 %) but occurs late (>5 years) and rarely causes graft loss (<10 %). Time post-transplantation appears to be the only predictor of risk (rate of recurrence increases with time)
Amyloid	Risk of recurrence of AA amyloidosis is related to the degree activity of the underlying disease. Rates of infection and cardiovascular complications are higher in these patients. AL amyloidosis also recurs and can cause graft failure although a recent series suggests improving outcomes with no graft failures among 22 renal allografts after 48 months follow-up
Multiple myeloma	Previously considered an absolute contraindication to transplantation. Recent advances in therapeutic regimens mean durable remission more likely and transplantation may be appropriate in selected individuals with good prognosis (e.g. good response to chemotherapy with further therapeutic options available or durable complete remission following autologous stem cell transplant). Long-term outcome data are limited
Sickle-cell disease	Limited data on outcomes in the modern era but patient and graft survival likely to be inferior to that in non-sickle-cell recipients. Preoperative transfusion or exchange transfusion to maintain HbS <20 % advised together with 40 % FiO_2 to reduce risk of sickle crisis
Lipoprotein glomerulopathy	Recurrent disease is reported. No proven therapeutic intervention
Collagen III glomerulopathy	Limited data available (single-case report of successful transplantation without recurrence)
Fibrillary glomerulonephritis	Limited data. Recurrence rate around 50 % but relatively benign course

Abbreviations: *HUS* haemolytic uraemic syndrome, *FSGS* focal segmental glomerular sclerosis, *MPGN* membranoproliferative glomerulonephritis, *PH1* primary hyperoxaluria type 1, *GBM* glomerular basement membrane

Malignancy

Dialysis patients have an increased incidence of cancer compared to the general population with particularly high rates of renal cell carcinoma [23]. This phenomenon has been linked to the relative immunoparesis associated with ESRD and its effect on antitumour surveillance. However, at present there is no evidence that transplant wait-listed patients should have increased surveillance compared to their age-matched general population counterparts. The persistent pharmacological immunosuppression required for successful transplantation further disrupts innate antitumour and antiviral surveillance and has been linked to the increase in cancer risk following transplantation. Awareness of the potential for occult malignancy is therefore crucial prior to transplant listing (Table 66.2) and appropriate investigations instituted early.

Table 66.2 Symptoms suggestive of underlying malignancy that warrant directed investigation

Symptoms suggestive of malignancy
Unexplained weight loss (i.e. unrelated to dialysis adequacy, caloric intake)
Erythropoietin resistance
Treatment-resistant iron deficiency
Unexplained fevers (i.e. not related to underlying renal disease, infection, dialyser)
Organ-specific symptoms (e.g. abdominal pain, bleeding per rectum, haemoptysis)

Current UK and European guidelines recommend waiting at least 2 years between successful tumour treatment/remission and transplantation with a 5-year period being recommended for specific malignancies (e.g. colorectal cancer, breast cancer and melanoma). These are based on data showing that 53 % of recurrences occur in transplanted patients within 2 years of their cancer treatment, 34 % within 2–5 years and 13 % if >5 years following treatment [24]. Renal cell carcinomas occur 6 times more frequently in ESRD patients compared to the general population, but appropriately treated, small (<3 cm), non-metastasised lesions do not preclude transplant listing after 2 years of surveillance as the risk of subsequent recurrence is very low.

Previous post-transplant lymphoproliferative disease (PTLD) is not a contraindication to transplant listing, and good outcomes are reported following re-transplantation using conventional immunosuppression [25]. Current UK guidelines advocate a period of at least 1 year from control of PTLD to re-transplantation to minimise recurrence risk and a 10 % recurrence rate is a ballpark figure. It would seem prudent to reimage and check EBV PCR before relisting.

Infection

Infection is the second leading cause of death with a functioning graft. Patients undergoing workup for transplantation should be screened for any occult or latent infection which might be exacerbated by immunosuppression and which may require treatment before transplantation or prophylactic therapy post-transplantation (see Table 66.3 for examples).

Tuberculosis

All transplant candidates should be assessed for a history of prior TB exposure including a full contact (household, institution) and travel history. Heightened awareness is needed for patients deriving from areas of high endemicity (e.g. Africa, South Asia, Eastern Europe). This should be accompanied with an up-to-date chest radiograph to look for any evidence of old, healed TB. Equivocal cases require specialist evaluation with the aid of interferon-based assays (e.g. QuantiFERON-Gold or T-SPOT.TB) and consideration of CT imaging to demonstrate focal disease and/or lymphadenopathy. Conventional tuberculin skin testing performs poorly in patients with ESRD and cannot be relied on to direct diagnosis. UK guidelines recommend a 6-month course of treatment for active TB and consideration for similar treatment in cases of latent TB as directed by specialist review [26]. Following completion of a 6-month course of treatment, surveillance is recommended, but there is no evidence to support further treatment in the absence of disease reactivation [26].

Table 66.3 Principal infections screened for in the pre-transplant assessment

Infection
Tuberculosis (TB) (including past exposure) and *Mycobacterium avium-intracellulare* (MAI)
Hepatitis B
Hepatitis C
Human immunodeficiency virus (HIV)
Herpes simplex virus (HSV)
Human T-cell lymphotropic virus (HTLV)
Cytomegalovirus (CMV)
Epstein-Barr virus (EBV)

Post-transplant chemoprophylaxis (6 months of isoniazid) is advocated for all recipients from areas of high TB endemicity (Table 66.4) but is not needed for patients from low-risk countries or for those who have been previously fully treated for TB.

Atypical Mycobacterial Infection

Mycobacterium avium-intracellulare infection is a rare complication post-transplantation. Treatment is empirical with antituberculous therapy and reduction of immunosuppression. There is no data on the risk of recurrence or reactivation in patients who have suffered MAI previously, e.g. in the context of HIV disease, and who subsequently progress to renal transplantation.

Hepatitis B

All potential transplant recipients should have full hepatitis B virus (HBV) serology performed – hepatitis B surface antigen (HBsAg), hepatitis B core antibody (HBcAb) and hepatitis B surface antibody level (HBsAb). This allows for identification of occult infection as well as stratifying risk of viral reactivation and donor-derived HBV infection.

Patients with evidence of chronic HBV infection require formal hepatological assessment to determine the need for nucleoside/nucleotide analogue treatment prior to transplantation. Monitoring of liver enzymes, HBV DNA and alphafetoprotein levels is recommended every 3–6 months coupled with 6–12 monthly liver USS. Chronic active HBV infection does not preclude transplantation but patients are at risk of

Table 66.4 Countries with a high incidence of TB (>40 cases per 100,000 population)

Africa	Any country	
Asia	Southeast Asia, e.g. Indonesia, Malaysia, Philippines, Thailand, Vietnam, North and South Korea	China
	Mongolia	Afghanistan
	India	Pakistan
	Bangladesh	Sri Lanka
	Saudi Arabia	Iraq
	Countries of the ex-Soviet Union, e.g. Ukraine, Georgia, Lithuania, Latvia	
Europe	Russian Federation	Bosnia and Herzegovina
	Bulgaria	Romania
	Croatia	
Central and South America	Panama	El Salvador
	Brazil	Peru
	Colombia	Venezuela
	Argentina	Honduras

Adapted from the WHO Tuberculosis database. This list is not exhaustive and readers are encouraged to visit the relevant website: http://www.who.int/tb/country/global_tb_database/en/index.html

post-transplant reactivation and require indefinite antiviral therapy [27]. Lamivudine is associated with a high risk of resistance (70 % at 5 years) and the choice of agent (e.g. lamivudine, entecavir, tenofovir) is determined by viral resistance patterns.

By contrast, patients with evidence of past cleared HBV infection (HBsAg –ve, HBV DNA –ve but HBcAb +ve) have a low risk (1–2 %) of reactivation, and post-transplant antiviral prophylaxis and surveillance (e.g. monthly testing for HBsAg for the first 6 months) are both reasonable approaches.

Use of renal allografts from donors who are "core positive" (i.e. HBsAg –ve, HBcAb +ve) is associated with a very low risk of Hep B transmission which is diminished in the face of adequate pre-transplant HBV vaccination. Clinical outcomes in hepatitis B negative recipients of HBcAb+ renal allografts are similar to those of the general transplant population. Antiviral chemoprophylaxis is recommended for all recipients of organs from an HBsAg –ve HBcAb +ve donor for at least 12 months as well as perioperative HBV vaccination and administration of hepatitis B immunoglobulin in HBV nonimmune recipients [28].

Hepatitis C

All potential transplant recipients should be screened for antibody to HCV at time of assessment. Those testing positive should have a HCV RNA and genotypic assay performed. Accelerated HCV-related hepatic fibrosis is seen in immunosuppressed individuals, and overall 10-year survival is approximately 15 % lower in HCV+ renal transplant recipients compared to those who are HCV –ve. However, this is offset by the survival advantage conferred by transplantation compared to remaining on dialysis and HCV per se is not a contraindication to transplantation. Formal hepatological assessment for all HCV+ patients is required and liver biopsy recommended to quantify the degree of fibrosis and guide management. Treatment of HCV using interferon-based regimens post-transplantation is contraindicated due to the significant risk of precipitating acute rejection; therefore, it is very important to try to eradicate hepatitis C where possible prior to transplant listing. The emergence of new interferon-free regimens with agents such as the direct-acting antiviral agents (DAAs) may transform post-transplant management of HCV in the near future [29].

Although use of HCV+ donors for HCV– recipients is not recommended, the use of these kidneys in HCV+ recipients has been performed with equivalent transplant outcomes to HCV– kidneys in HCV+ recipients [30]. However, this carries the risk of infection with a different HCV genotype and disease reactivation, and patients need to be counselled appropriately before proceeding with surgery.

HIV Infection

In the current era of highly active antiretroviral therapy (HAART) and modern transplant immunosuppression protocols, the outcomes of renal transplantation in HIV+ individuals are similar to those in HIV –ve patients [31]. Although HIV infection is not a contraindication to transplantation, disease remission is essential prior to transplant listing (Table 66.5). HIV+ patients have a higher cumulative incidence of acute rejection reaching 31 % in one study [32]. This may relate to the plethora of pharmacokinetic interactions that can occur between HAART and immunosuppressants. The interaction between calcineurin inhibitors (CNIs) and protease inhibitors is extremely potent with significant prolongation of CNI half-life (e.g. some patients only require 0.5 mg tacrolimus weekly). This combination is best avoided where possible and our practice is to move patients to a raltegravir-based regimen when resistance patterns permit, and in the absence of a protease inhibitor, standard doses of CNI can be used. Either way early, close consultation with the treating HIV Medicine team is essential. Some patients may require a dose-finding trial of immunosuppression on some regimens with monitoring of HIV viral load. At present UK guidelines recommend informing live donors of recipient HIV+ status. Some units take the view that it is sufficient to inform the prospective donor that the recipient is at increased risk of complications without disclosing the HIV status.

HTLV Infection

HTLV-1 is endemic in some areas of the world (e.g. Caribbean, Japan). In the general population the

Table 66.5 Criteria for transplant wait listing the HIV+ recipient

Undetectable HIV viral load >6 months
CD4+ T-cell count >200/mm^3 for >6 months
Stable antiretroviral regimen
Availability of further antiretroviral options if resistance develops to the current regimen
Previous progressive multifocal leucencephalopathy usually considered an absolute contraindication

virus is associated with an increased risk of developing spastic paraparesis or T-cell lymphoma (lifetime risk approximately 2 %).

Despite case reports of acute T-cell leukaemia developing within 12 months of transplantation in HTLV+ recipients [33], it remains unclear whether the risk of disease is increased by immunosuppression and increasingly recipient HTLV antibody positivity is felt not to be a contraindication to transplantation. Where available, it is worth considering screening for viral RNA although the impact of transplantation in viraemic patients is not known.

Herpes Simplex (HSV)

Primary HSV infection post-transplantation carries a risk of lethal fulminant hepatitis so it is important to ascertain the immunity of all transplant recipients prior to transplantation. This is particularly important in centres employing a policy of surveillance and pre-emptive treatment rather than prophylaxis for CMV (valganciclovir offers some protection).

Varicella Zoster (VZV)

Around 3 % of patients are not immune and risk a significant mortality if they contract VZV post-transplantation. Patients must be screened pre-transplant and vaccination with two doses of live vaccine seems to offer good protection (Table 66.6). Nonimmune patients receiving a transplant should be given aciclovir prophylaxis.

Epstein-Barr Virus (EBV)

EBV seronegative transplant recipients (10 % of adults, 50 % of children) are at risk of primary EBV infection which conveys a significant risk of subsequent development of PTLD. The role of monitoring of viral load post-transplantation remains unclear (high viral load >10 [5] copies/ml is associated with PTLD but the positive predictive value is poor). Intravenous immunoglobulin and/or antiviral therapy has been suggested as prophylactic strategies but are of unproven value.

Table 66.6 Pre-transplant vaccinations

Vaccine	Comments
Hepatitis B	If nonimmune
Influenza	Annually
Pneumococcus	Every 5 years
Varicella	If nonimmune
Rubella	Women of child-bearing age
Human papilloma virus (HPV)	All sexually active women
Meningococcus	At risk groups (age 16–21 years)
Haemophilus (Hib)	If not previously vaccinated

Strongyloides

Strongyloides stercoralis is an intestinal nematode that can persist in the human host for decades after the initial infection and can progress to fulminant hyperinfection syndrome in immunocompromised hosts. Patients who have resided in endemic regions (South America, Africa, Southeast Asia) should be screened for Strongyloides pre-transplant (serology ± stool) and treated if positive. Ivermectin 200 mcg/kg orally × 2 doses is the current recommended first-line treatment.

Schistosomiasis

Shistosomiasis is a chronic parasitic infection with worms of the trematode family common in Africa, South America and Southeast Asia. Infection can be associated with obstructive uropathy, immune complex GN, amyloidosis and an increased risk of bladder malignancy. Serological screening is indicated for individuals from endemic areas. Treatment is with praziquantel.

Toxoplasma

T. gondii is an intracellular protozoan parasite, with members of the cat family being the definitive hosts. Toxoplasma is rare in the renal transplant population and as a result the diagnosis is often delayed and mortality is concomitantly high. The peak incidence is in the first 3 months post-transplantation with seronegative recipients receiving seropositive kidneys being at greatest risk. The disease can occasionally present many years post-transplantation. Presentation is usually with fever, neurological disturbances and/or pneumonitis. A high index of suspicion is needed. The value of screening recipients for toxoplasma status is controversial but is potentially useful in identifying patients at risk, especially seronegative recipients with seropositive donors, and can help in establishing the diagnosis by showing seroconversion.

Syphilis

Screening for latent syphilis is initially with a rapid plasma reagin (RPR) assay. If the results are positive, the patient should undergo a specific treponemal test (fluorescent treponemal antibody absorption test or microhaemagglutination assay for *Treponema pallidum*) to determine whether the RPR result is biologically false positive. If the RPR result is low-titre and the patient has received appropriate treatment for syphilis in the past, the patient is unlikely to have latent infection. However, any other positive RPR assay result with positive treponemal test results should be considered an indication of active (presumably latent) syphilis and should be treated. Standard treatment is with benzathene penicillin G 2.4 million units IM given weekly for three doses.

Trypanosoma Cruzi (Chaga's Disease)

Trypanosomiasis is endemic in Central and South America. Patients who have resided in endemic areas should be screened (serology) and monitored for reactivation post-transplantation

Coccidioides

Coccidioidomycosis is a fungus endemic in the Southwestern United States. Serological screening and secondary prophylaxis for coccidioidomycosis in transplant recipients are recommended for transplant candidates and recipients as approximately 50 % of coccidioidal infections in transplant recipients are due to reactivation of pre-existing disease.

Histoplasmosis

Histoplasmosis is a fungal infection caused by the dimorphic saprophytic fungus *Histoplasma capsulatum*, which is endemic in the Central United States, South America, the Caribbean, Africa and Asia. In the face of immunosuppression, progressive disseminated disease may develop and is associated with a high mortality rate (20 % or more). Serological screening should be considered to identify patients at risk of reactivation post-transplantation (although the risk is low even in seropositive individuals).

Human Herpesvirus 8

HHV-8 is associated with development of Kaposi's sarcoma. Testing for this virus is not routinely available.

Pre-transplantation Vaccinations

Obesity and Transplant Listing

As well as presenting significant challenges to the surgical team, obesity is associated with a greater risk of delayed graft function, poor wound healing, new-onset diabetes after transplantation (NODAT), premature graft failure and death [34, 35]. Patients with a body mass index (BMI) of >30 kg/m^2 have an increased risk of perioperative complications which rises progressively. Some centres use a BMI cut-off value >35 kg/m^2 as a contraindication to transplantation. In our view, obesity needs to be viewed as another co-morbidity, and in an otherwise fit patient, a rigid BMI cut-off value may not be appropriate. Fat distribution is also relevant and it has been suggested that adoption of waist circumference as a measure of obesity may be a better prognostic marker than BMI. In selected candidates active weight-loss programmes with dietetic input may be required as well as bariatric surgery prior to transplantation although criteria vary across transplant centres. If an obese patient has the potential to have and benefit from a transplant, then the approach to their obesity needs to be decisive; it is common for years to pass while waiting in vain for a dialysis patient to achieve sufficient weight loss.

Other Medical Issues

Patients with poor respiratory function as well as those with multiple co-morbidities represent higher-risk candidates for surgery and formal anaesthetic review may be required.

Drug Pharmacokinetics

Tacrolimus is predominantly absorbed in the first part of the small intestine. Patients with prior small bowel resection will have reduced absorption and so run the risk of subtherapeutic levels in the immediate post-transplant period. A pre-transplant dose-finding trial of immunosuppression is always worth considering as levels may be very low and MPA-based drugs are often poorly tolerated.

Tacrolimus pharmacokinetics are also influenced significantly by CYP3A5 genotype [36]. Specifically, CYP3A5*1 is associated with more rapid tacrolimus metabolism. Such patients require substantially higher tacrolimus doses to achieve therapeutic drug levels. Awareness of the recipient's genetic polymorphism can aid drug dosing in the early peri-transplant period and mitigate CNI toxicity in the long term [37].

16. Brekke IB, Lien B, Sodal G, et al. Aortoiliac reconstruction in preparation for renal transplantation. Transpl Int. 1993;6(3):161–3.
17. AbuRahma AF, Jarrett K, Hayes DJ. Clinical implications of power Doppler three-dimensional ultrasonography. Vascular. 2004;12(5):293–300.
18. El-Zoghby ZM, Stegall MD, Lager DJ, et al. Identifying specific causes of kidney allograft loss. Am J Transplant. 2009;9(3):527–35.
19. Zimmerhackl LB, Besbas N, Jungraithmayr T, et al. Epidemiology, clinical presentation, and pathophysiology of atypical and recurrent hemolytic uremic syndrome. Semin Thromb Hemost. 2006;32(2):113–20.
20. Canaud G, Zuber J, Sberro R, et al. Intensive and prolonged treatment of focal and segmental glomerulosclerosis recurrence in adult kidney transplant recipients: a pilot study. Am J Transplant. 2009;9(5):1081–6.
21. Hickson LJ, Gera M, Amer H, et al. Kidney transplantation for primary focal segmental glomerulosclerosis: outcomes and response to therapy for recurrence. Transplantation. 2009;87(8):1232–9.
22. Little MA, Dupont P, Campbell E, Dorman A, Walshe JJ. Severity of primary MPGN, rather than MPGN type, determines renal survival and post-transplantation recurrence risk. Kidney Int. 2006;69(3):504–11.
23. Shapiro R, Kaplan B. Native renal cysts and dialysis duration are risk factors for renal cell carcinoma in renal transplant recipients. Am J Transplant. 2011;11(1):10.
24. Penn I. The effect of immunosuppression on pre-existing cancers. Transplantation. 1993;55(4):742–7.
25. Johnson SR, Cherikh WS, Kauffman HM, Pavlakis M, Hanto DW. Retransplantation after post-transplant lymphoproliferative disorders: an OPTN/UNOS database analysis. Am J Transplant. 2006;6(11):2743–9.
26. Milburn H, Ashman N, Davies P, et al. Guidelines for the prevention and management of Mycobacterium tuberculosis infection and disease in adult patients with chronic kidney disease. Thorax. 2010;65(6):557–70.
27. Katz LH, Fraser A, Gafter-Gvili A, Leibovici L, Tur-Kaspa R. Lamivudine prevents reactivation of hepatitis B and reduces mortality in immunosuppressed patients: systematic review and meta-analysis. J Viral Hepat. 2008;15(2):89–102.
28. Chung RT, Feng S, Delmonico FL. Approach to the management of allograft recipients following the detection of hepatitis B virus in the prospective organ donor. Am J Transplant. 2001;1(2):185–91.
29. Lee LY, Tong CY, Wong T, Wilkinson M. New therapies for chronic hepatitis C infection: a systematic review of evidence from clinical trials. Int J Clin Pract. 2012;66(4):342–55.
30. Morales JM, Campistol JM, Dominguez-Gil B, et al. Long-term experience with kidney transplantation from hepatitis C-positive donors into hepatitis C-positive recipients. Am J Transplant. 2010;10(11):2453–62.
31. Trullas JC, Cofan F, Tuset M, et al. Renal transplantation in HIV-infected patients: 2010 update. Kidney Int. 2011;79(8):825–42.
32. Stock PG, Barin B, Murphy B, et al. Outcomes of kidney transplantation in HIV-infected recipients. N Engl J Med. 2010;363(21):2004–14.
33. Hoshida Y, Li T, Dong Z, et al. Lymphoproliferative disorders in renal transplant patients in Japan. Int J Cancer. 2001;91(6):869–75.
34. Kovesdy CP, Czira ME, Rudas A, et al. Body mass index, waist circumference and mortality in kidney transplant recipients. Am J Transplant. 2010;10(12):2644–51.
35. Potluri K, Hou S. Obesity in kidney transplant recipients and candidates. Am J Kidney Dis. 2010;56(1):143–56.
36. Renders L, Frisman M, Ufer M, et al. CYP3A5 genotype markedly influences the pharmacokinetics of tacrolimus and sirolimus in kidney transplant recipients. Clin Pharmacol Ther. 2007;81(2):228–34.
37. Gervasini G, Garcia M, Macias RM, Cubero JJ, Caravaca F, Benitez J. Impact of genetic polymorphisms on tacrolimus pharmacokinetics and the clinical outcome of renal transplantation. Transpl Int. 2012;25(4):471–80.
38. Power RE, Hickey DP, Little DM. Urological evaluation prior to renal transplantation. Transplant Proc. 2004;36(10):2962–7.
39. Oliver M, Woywodt A, Ahmed A, Saif I. Organ donation, transplantation and religion. Nephrol Dial Transplant. 2011;26(2):437–44.

67 Tissue Typing, Crossmatch and Antibody Incompatibility in Kidney Transplantation

Henry Stephens, Peter J. Dupont, and Mark Harber

For the majority of suitable patients with end-stage renal disease (ESRD), transplantation offers a significant survival advantage, improved quality of life and a substantial saving in terms of annual medical care. In countries with limited or no chronic dialysis provision, transplantation may offer the only hope of survival for patients with ESRD. However in every country with a transplant programme, the demand for kidney transplants continues to outstrip supply with the consequence that many patients fail to be transplanted in a timely fashion or at all. The two principal immunological barriers to solid organ transplantation (SOT); blood group incompatibility and HLA incompatibility have restricted access to transplantation. In the last two decades, strategies to expand the pool of donors have become increasingly commonplace and include the use of blood group-incompatible (ABOi) transplants, HLA-incompatible transplants (HLAi), acceptable mismatch schemes and paired-exchange programmes.

ABO Compatibility

The ABO blood group locus consists of three alleles A, B and O, of which A and B code for oligosaccharide glycosyltransferase. The O allele does not encode for this glycosyltransferase and thus blood group O patients do not express the antigen. The blood group antigens are expressed almost universally on human tissue, most notably on erythrocytes and endothelial cells. There are a variety of blood group subtypes associated with varying levels of blood group expression, most notably blood group A is divided into A_1 and A_2, the latter having much lower tissue expression and therefore potentially less immunogenicity.

Blood groups might not matter much but for the fact that, from infancy, humans naturally develop anti-blood group (isohaemagglutinins) antibodies (IgG and IgM), probably as a cross-reactivity response to bacteria.

Table 67.1 shows standard blood group compatibilities for renal transplantation.

In the early days of kidney transplantation, some ABOi were done knowingly and there have been unfortunately examples of inadvertent ABOi transplantation since then; in both cases the outcomes were usually disastrous. There are two main consequences of anti-donor blood group antibodies for renal transplantation. The first is that crossing the ABO barrier may result in hyperacute or accelerated rejection and graft loss. In hyperacute rejection anti-blood group antibodies bind to the vascular endothelium, activate complement and platelets resulting in hypoperfusion of the kidney (which may go blue and flaccid on release of clamps). Engorgement of the capillaries occurs (glomerular and peritubular), with aggregation of erythrocytes and thrombosis which then spreads down the vascular tree to include afferent arterioles resulting in interstitial haemorrhage and infarction (Fig. 67.1).

Not all forbidden ABOi transplants meet this fate. A proportion experience initial function but go on to develop accelerated rejection with oliguria within the first few days (rarely beyond 2 weeks post-transplant) as a result of antibody-mediated rejection. Thus for truly ABOi kidney transplantation, the outcome is graft loss or a significant risk of poor function. However, a proportion of apparently ABOi transplants can occur without adverse outcomes if the titre of anti-blood group antibodies either is naturally low or can be rendered low prior to transplant.

H. Stephens, BSc, PhD (✉)
UCL Centre for Nephrology and the Anthony Nolan Trust, Hospital Royal Free London NHS Foundation Trust, Rowland Hill Street, London NW3 2PF, UK
e-mail: h.stephens@ucl.ac.uk

P.J. Dupont, PhD, FRCPI
UCL Centre for Nephrology, Royal Free Hospital, Pond Street, London NW3 2QG, UK
e-mail: pdupont@nhs.net

M. Harber, MBBS, PhD, FRCP
UCL Department of Nephrology, Royal Free London NHS Foundation Trust, Pond Street, Hampstead, London NW3 2QG, UK
e-mail: mark.harber@nhs.net

M. Harber (ed.), *Practical Nephrology*,
DOI 10.1007/978-1-4471-5547-8_67, © Springer-Verlag London 2014

Table 67.1 ABO blood groups and compatibility in renal transplantation

Blood group	Antibody	Compatibility as donor	Compatibility as recipient
A_1	Anti-B	Recipient A	A or O donors
A_2	Anti-B	Recipient A (potentially (O or B))	A or O donors
B	Anti-A	Recipient B	B or O donors (potentially A_2)
AB	Nil	Recipient AB	A, B or O (universal recipient)
O	Anti-A and Anti-B	AB, A, B, O (universal donor)	O (potentially A_2)

There is a window in infancy before anti-AB antibodies are generated and ABOi transplantation have been done in this setting. Although expression of A-Ag is much lower in A_2, their suitability as a donor depends on recipient anti-A titres; high levels still represent a barrier
NB Potentially any blood group combination is compatible for SOT if the recipient anti-blood group Antibody titre is sufficiently low

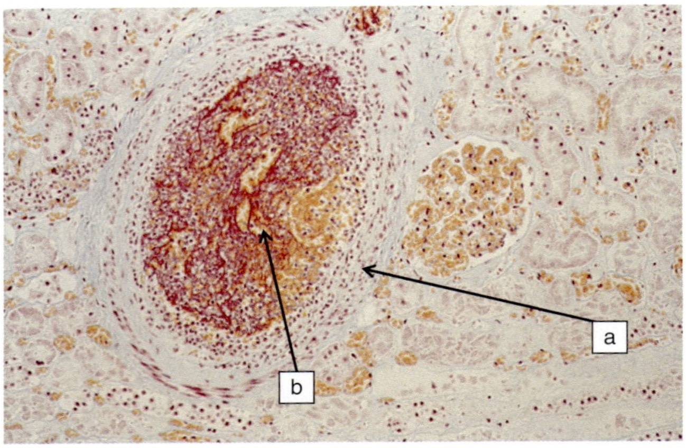

Fig. 67.1 Hyperacute rejection in the setting of ABOi transplantation. Section of an arteriole (*a*) with acute thrombus occluding entire vessel (*b*)

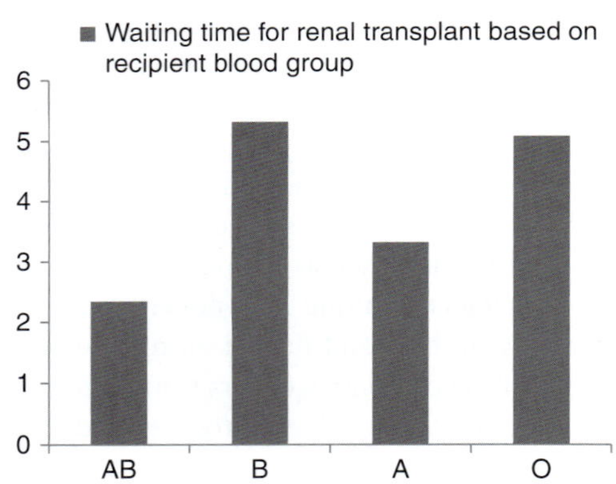

Fig. 67.2 Organ procurement and transplantation network (OPTN) (USA) data showing waiting time in years for different blood groups

The second consequence of the ABO barrier is the impact on waiting times for recipients of different blood groups. The waiting times for patients in the USA are shown in Fig. 67.2 [1] and show a similar pattern to those in Europe, namely, that patients with blood group B and O are likely to wait substantially longer than those with blood group AB or A. Strategies to overcome this disparity and that of having an ABOi live donor are discussed later.

As alluded to above, it has become apparent that ABOi kidney transplants can occur safely if the recipient anti-blood group antibody titres are persistently low (or absent as in infancy). Without preconditioning, anti-A or anti-B titres of 1:4 are deemed by most to be safe.

Human Leukocyte Antigens (HLA) and Tissue Typing

The primary roles of tissue-typing laboratories providing a service to solid organ transplant units are as given below:

1. Facilitate the allocation of transplants by HLA typing and matching recipients and donors.
2. Identify unacceptable donor HLA antigens which could contribute to acute rejection by screening and defining HLA antibodies.
3. Provide a 24 h on-call service.
4. Prevent hyperacute rejection by performing a pre-transplant crossmatch.
5. Post-transplant surveillance of donor-specific HLA antibodies (DSAs).
6. Facilitate live donor transplantation.
7. Provide risk assessments of immunological rejection of renal transplants.

HLA Polymorphism

The genes encoding HLA molecules are the most polymorphic in the human genome, and thousands of molecular variants have now been described (see www.ebi.ac.uk/imgt/hla). There are numerous methods available to define HLA alleles, ranging from serotyping protein phenotypes to genotyping DNA with PCR and sequence-specific primers (SSP) or oligonucleotide probes (SSOPs), as well as direct sequencing of HLA genes [2]. The quickest methods are serotyping and PCR-SSP, which can be performed within 4 h and are suitable for relatively small numbers of test samples and on-call typing of cadaver donors. PCR-SSP typing can also cover all classical class I (HLA-A, HLA-B and HLA-C) and class II (HLA-DR, HLA-DQ and HLA-DP) gene loci. Other techniques using HLA SSOPs ligated to polymer microspheres in solid-phase immunoassays (SPI) or direct sequencing of PCR-amplified HLA genes are more laborious to perform but generate better allele resolution and have the capacity for high-throughput typing.

HLA Nomenclature

The ever-increasing number of molecularly defined HLA alleles has required establishing a rational system of nomenclature. The current international WHO-recognised scheme uses a basic 4-figure system to define alleles that have been typed using DNA-based techniques, with the name of the HLA locus followed by an asterisk and at least 4 digits. The first two digits designate the broad HLA type (e.g. HLA-A*02), roughly equivalent to the serologically defined allotype (HLA-A2); the third, fourth and sometimes fifth digits separated by a colon (e.g. HLA-A*02:01) are used to designate individual amino-acid differences [3]. With some HLA alleles, further digits have been introduced to define non-coding, silent or synonymous nucleotide base changes, as well as intronic, 5′- and 3′-prime polymorphism, if available. Relatively rarely alleles are unexpressed or 'null', while others are low producers or are secreted; these are given the prefixes N (e.g. HLA-A*02:15 N), L or S, respectively [3]. When the molecular HLA typing method does not provide allele-level resolution, a 'string' of HLA alleles are sometimes reported (e.g. HLA-A*02:01/02/03), but these all relate to primary molecular group (HLA-A*02) or allotype (HLA-A2) for the purposes of HLA matching and organ sharing.

HLA Matching

In the UK, the national cadaver donor kidney sharing scheme matches all potential recipients for broad groups of related HLA-A, HLA-B and HLA-DR alleles, largely based on the original serologically defined allotypes which share common structural and genetic features (Table 67.2). Patient selection and organ offers are based on four levels of HLA-A, HLA-B and HLA-DR matching (Table 67.3). These HLA match levels were established from computational modelling of death-censored renal transplant survival data collected in the UK between 1998 and 2004 [4, 5] and are weighted for better matching of HLA-DR and HLA-B (Table 67.3) which have a greater effect on transplant survival [5]. After donor and recipient match levels are established, ranked offers are made on the basis of points allocated for other relevant variables as given in Table 67.3 [5]. Consideration of the HLA-C, HLA-DQ and HLA-DP donor types is also incorporated into the matching algorithm, in order to exclude offers being

Table 67.2 Major HLA-A, HLA-B and HLA-DR antigens or allotypes used for renal transplant matching and their relative frequencies (%) in the UK population

HLA-A		HLA-B		HLA-DR	
Antigen	%	Antigen	%	Antigen	%
A1	34	**B5** (B51, B52)	19	**DR1**	19
A2	50	**B7**	27	**DR2** (DR15, DR16)	29
A3	26	**B8**	25	**DR3**	27
A9 (A23, A24)	17	**B12** (B44, B45)	33	**DR4**	35
A10 (A25, A26, A34, A66)	9	**B13**	4	**DR5** (DR11, DR12)	16
A11	12	**B14** (B64, B65)	7	**DR6** (DR13, DR14	23
A19 (A30, A31, A32, A33, A74)	19	**B15** (B62, B63, B75, B76, B77)	12	**DR7**	26
A29	8	**B16** (B38, B39)	5	**DR8**	4
A28 (A68, A69)	7	**B17** (B57, B58)	9	**DR9**	2
		B18	8	**DR10**	1
		B21 (B49, B50)	4	**DR51**	29
		B22 (B54, B55, B56)	4	**DR52**	58
		B27	9	**DR53**	57
		B35	13		
		B37	3		
		B40 (B60, B61)	13		
		B41	1		
		B47	1		
		B53	1		
		B70 (B71, B72)	1		
		Bw4	62		
		Bw6	86		

HLA allotypes used in matching renal transplants are given in bold with relevant related subtypes in parentheses. HLA allotype frequencies are derived from 10,000 UK deceased solid organ donors collected between 1994 and 2009 (see www.organdonation.nhs.uk/statistics). Other HLA-A and HLA-B allotypes that are included in the UK matching algorithms but occur at <1 % frequency are A36, A43, A80, B42, B46, B48, B59, B67, B73, B78, B81, B82 and B83

Table 67.3 HLA-A, HLA-B and HLA-DR matching for cadaver renal transplants used in the UK organ sharing scheme since 2006

HLA match level	HLA-A, HLA-B, HLA-DR mismatch (mm)	Possible HLA-A, HLA-B, HLA-DR (mm) combinations
1	000	000
2	0DR + 0/1B	100, 010, 110, 200, 210
3	0DR + 2B or 1DR + 0/1B	020, 120, 220, 001, 101, 201, 011, 111, 211
4	1DR + 2B or 2 DR	021, 121, 221, 002, 102, 202, 012, 112, 212, 022, 122, 222

The UK matching algorithm is also weighted to allocate points for recipient age, waiting time, balance of exchange between transplant units, age difference, level of HLA matchability for rare HLA antigens, level of HLA sensitisation as well as organ donor vs recipient location [5]

made to recipients with preformed antibodies to any potential mismatched antigens encoded by these class I and II loci.

There is considerable variation in HLA allele frequencies between different ethnic groups. The UK organ donor pool is highly representative of northern European populations, while the transplant waiting lists of patients in end-stage renal failure can have a mixed ethnic composition of Caucasoids, Africans and Asians, particularly in large contemporary urban centres such as London. To compensate for any lack of accessibility of well-matched organs, the UK sharing scheme has introduced a rational HLA matching default system, whereby alleles common in Africans such as HLA-B53 are considered a match for B51 because of structural similarities or DR9 which is common in Oriental populations is now considered a match for DR4 which is similar and much more common in Caucasoids [5].

HLA Antibody Screening

Antibodies directed against mismatched donor HLA can induce transplant rejection and until relatively recently have been difficult to characterise, let alone quantify [6]. Antibody screening and crossmatching with complement-dependent lymphocytotoxicity (CDC) and the more sensitive flow cytometry use cellular targets. However, commercially available SPI utilising HLA molecules bound to polystyrene microspheres or bead arrays are now being universally used to characterise HLA antibodies with small footprint fluoroanalysers or Luminex. Thus, both HLA typing of test DNA and semi-quantitative antibody binding to HLA proteins can be performed on the same Luminex platform, with binding of HLA probes or antibody expressed as a mean fluorescence intensity (MFI) of a reporter signal. Single-antigen Luminex bead panels covering all major classical class I (HLA-A, HLA-B and HLA-C) and class II (HLA-DR, HLA-DQ and HLA-DP) antigens are particularly useful in determining the full range of HLA antibody profiles in renal patients being considered for renal transplants [6]. However, the final MFI levels detected on beads represent the amount of antibody bound relative to the total HLA antigen present on a given bead, which varies between beads and should not be necessarily considered a measure of antibody titre. Nevertheless, the ability of Luminex single-antigen beads to identify epitope-specific antibodies that react with groups of HLA antigens or cross-reactive groups (CREG), as well as antibodies to HLA-C, HLA-DQ and HLA-DP which are known to contribute to transplantation rejection [6], has helped in evaluating risk of rejection of renal transplants allocated on the basis of HLA-A, HLA-B and HLA-DR matching.

The rapid uptake of SPI by tissue-typing laboratories has greatly enhanced their capacity to identify HLA antibodies. However, these technologies are highly sensitive and it is still difficult for transplant physicians to fully comprehend the clinical relevance of these antibodies. Various correlations between MFI, antibody level, crossmatch results and clinical outcomes have been described [6]. However, standardised cut-off MFI values for HLA antibodies and antigens to be reported as unacceptable have yet to be established. In response to this dilemma, consensus guidelines have recently been developed by an international group of experts in the field [6], as summarised below:

1. SPI must be used for detecting pre-transplantation HLA antibodies, in particular the use of single-antigen bead assays to detect antibodies to HLA-A, HLA-B, HLA-C, HLA-DRB1, HLA-DRB3, HLA-DRB4, HLA-DQA1, HLA-DQB1, HLA-DPA1 and HLA-DPB1 gene products.
2. The use of SPI should be supplemented with cell-based CDC and flow cytometry to examine correlations between all three methods, and the likelihood of a positive crossmatch and risk categories should be established.
3. Donor-specific HLA antibodies (DSAs) detected by CDC and a positive flow crossmatch should be avoided due to their strong correlation with antibody-mediated rejection and graft loss.
4. A renal transplant can be performed in the absence of a prospective crossmatch if single-antigen bead screening for antibodies to all class I and II HLA loci is negative (virtual crossmatch see below), if agreed with clinical users and regulatory bodies.
5. High-risk transplant recipients (with preformed DSA and positive crossmatch before desensitisation) should be monitored post-transplant with SPI and protocol biopsies performed in the first 3 months post-transplantation.
6. Intermediate risk transplant recipients (with historic DSA but currently negative) should be monitored with SPI in the first month post-transplant, and if DSAs emerge, a biopsy should be performed.
7. Low-risk patients (unsensitised, first transplant) should be screened for DSA with SPI at least 3–12 months after transplant, and if DSAs emerge, a biopsy should be performed.
8. Auditing crossmatch results conducted in the presence of Luminex-defined donor-specific HLA antibodies can assist in determining which MFI levels are likely to correlate with positive crossmatches, with most laboratories reporting HLA antibodies >2,000 MFI as being unacceptable, although this is case variable and dependent on the overall antibody profiles and CREGS detected.

Crossmatching

This is the definitive pre-transplantation cell-based test which together with information derived from HLA antibody

Table 67.4 Interpretation of allogeneic and autologous crossmatch (CDC or flow cytometry)

Allogeneic T Recipient sera + Donor T cells	Allogeneic B Recipient sera + Donor B cells	Autologous T Recipient sera + Recipient T cells	Autologous B Recipient sera + Recipient B cells	Crossmatch interpretation
–	–	–	–	–ve
–	–	+	+	–ve
–	–	+	–	–ve
–	–	–	+	–ve
+	+	+	+	–ve or +ve[a]
–	+	–	+	–ve or +ve[a]
+	+	–	–	+ve
–	+	–	–	+ve
+	–	–	–	–ve or +ve[b]

[a]Recipient sera reactive with autologous cells may mask genuine alloreactive HLA DSAs; immediate review of historic HLA antibody screening and recent sensitisation events are advised before overall interpretation of crossmatch is given

[b]Recipient sera reactivity with donor T cells alone indicates non-HLA antibodies which may be irrelevant, but a review of historic HLA antibody screening and any recent sensitisation events is essential

screening provides a comprehensive assessment of the immunological risk of graft rejection. The target cells in a crossmatch are donor lymphocytes derived from peripheral blood, spleen or lymph node. T cells are used for the detection of donor HLA class I-specific antibodies and B cells for both class I and II antibodies. The CDC crossmatching detects both HLA-specific and non-HLA-specific complement-fixing antibodies of IgG and IgM classes. By contrast, crossmatching with flow cytometry is more sensitive and specific and is generally used to identify both complement-fixing and non-complement-fixing IgG. Both tests can be performed concurrently with fresh and selected recipient sera to provide a more comprehensive risk assessment of rejection. Autoreactive antibodies bind to both autologous and allogeneic lymphocytes but are largely irrelevant to transplant outcome and can be identified and excluded by performing an autologous crossmatch of recipient cells with relevant historic recipient sera, in addition to the allogeneic crossmatch of recipient sera with donor cells (Table 67.4). The interpretation of crossmatch is complex and relies on careful selection and inclusion of positive and negative control sera, comparing test results with pre-established cut-offs of serum reactivity, consideration of sensitising events (previous transplants, recent blood transfusions and infections) and the selected recipients known HLA antibody profiles as determined with SPI, together with the HLA class I and II mm between potential donor and recipient [7].

Virtual Crossmatch

A standard pre-transplant crossmatch takes 4–6 h and this tends to contribute to prolonging cold-ischaemia time (CIT). This is particularly important in kidneys that are not local and are already at risk of long CIT and those from donors that have died a cardiac death (DCD). If the crossmatch turns out to be positive, the process has to start again for the next recipient who, through no fault of their own, will receive a kidney with an even longer CIT and statistically less good outcome. There are several ways to improve the system and reduce CIT including declaration of unacceptable antigens (so avoiding inappropriate allocation) and in unsensitised patients omitting the crossmatch. This is known as performing a 'virtual crossmatch' where the recipient antibody profile has been comprehensively documented and potential sensitisation events excluded. It is more difficult to predict the crossmatch result in highly sensitised patients and these (and moderately sensitised patients) are excluded. The usual inclusion criteria for virtual crossmatch are shown in Table 67.5.

Table 67.5 Suggested criteria for virtual crossmatch

(a) Well-documented anti-HLA antibody profile including historical sensitisation
(b) No recent sensitising events (e.g. transplantation or withdrawal of IS in a failed transplant, pregnancy, transfusion or recent infection)
(c) Up-to-date antibody screening with samples twice monthly (for at least the last 6 months)
(d) If anti-HLA antibodies are present, then stable and declining levels with the exclusion of current MFI >1,500 (conservative) or >2,000 (less so)
(e) Close liaison between tissue typing and clinicians

Some schemes exclude women of child-bearing age but it is only those who are at risk of becoming pregnant, i.e. sexually active and not using reliable contraception, that are at risk of sensitisation, so a fairer approach uses an individualised assessment

Taylor and colleagues reported on more than 10 years' experience of virtual crossmatch. In over 600 deceased donor transplants, 247 (42 %) proceeded without waiting for the

Table 67.6 Non-HLA antigens associated with rejection in renal transplant

Anti-angiotensin 1 receptor antibodies	Activating IgG engage AT1 receptor and cause both accelerated hypertension and vascular rejection [13]
Anti-endothelial cell antibodies (AECA)	Associated with higher rejection and poorer outcome if de novo
MICA antibodies (MICA)	Associated with acute rejection and worse outcome in some studies
Anti-prelecan (anti-LG3) antibodies	Associated with vascular rejection
Anti-vimentin antibodies	*Predominantly associated with heart transplant but documented in renal transplants*

Table 67.7 Risk factors for sensitisation following transplantation

1. Blood transfusion	This is probably still significant despite the protective effect of IS
2. Young recipient	Vigorous immune system
3. Multiple mismatches	Consistent finding
4. Sensitised patient	High CRF (PRA) to non-donor HLA prior to transplant
5. Deceased donor transplant	Possible also delayed graft function
6. HLA class II mismatch	DQ mismatch may be a particular risk
7. Acute rejection episodes	Significant risk factor
8. Withdrawal of immunosuppression	Following failure of transplant or in context of infection/malignancy
9. Non-compliance	A perennial problem causing AR and chronic low level sensitization

crossmatch (which was subsequently negative in all of these patients). The CIT was roughly 2.5 h less in the virtual crossmatch group and delayed graft function was reduced [8]. Large-scale retrospective studies have shown that negative virtual crossmatches have an excellent predictive value of negative crossmatch, whereas positive virtual crossmatches are associated with substantial risk of graft loss [9].

Other Non-HLA Antibodies

A variety of non-HLA antibodies have been identified in the setting of rejection (see Table 67.6). The role and frequency of non-HLA antibodies in renal transplantation are not clear, but there are occasionally patients who get what appears to be AMR in the absence of anti-HLA antibodies. Furthermore outcome of HLA-identical transplants is worse if the recipient is highly sensitised implying a role for non-HLA antibodies [10].

In one study the presence of donor-reactive AECA was associated with a rejection rate of 46 % vs 12 % for those without [11, 12]. Stimulatory anti-angiotensin receptor antibodies were beautifully described by Dragun and colleagues, as causing both severe vascular rejection and malignant hypertension [13]. Pre-transplant major histocompatibility complex class I-related chain A (MICA) antibodies (present in around 10–15 %) have been associated with worse graft outcome. Zou et al. reported an 88 % 1-year graft survival in patients with MICA antibodies vs 93 % in those without [14] although a study of a large European cohort found no adverse effect of MICA antibodies. There are commercially available kits for some of these non-HLA antibodies, but the place of screening is yet to be established. The one group worth considering for screening are those patients with early or aggressive antibody-mediated rejection (AMR) despite adequate immunosuppressive levels and with no identifiable donor-specific anti-HLA antibodies (DSA). These patients are relatively rare but potentially at risk with a second transplant if the cause is not identified.

Sensitisation

Individuals become sensitised to foreign donor HLA primarily by transplantation, pregnancy and transfusion. Less frequently sensitisation may occur following exposure to microorganisms and allergens, presumably due to cross-reactivity. These antibodies are more commonly IgM.

Transplantation is a very important contributor; DSAs appear in 11 % of previously unsensitised patients in the first year and 20 % by 5 years (with 25 % of these grafts failing within 3 years) [15]. In the UK, 52 % of re-transplants are sensitised compared with 15 % on the waiting list who have never received a transplant. Risk factors for sensitisation following transplantation are shown in Table 67.7.

Loss of a graft is an even more significant risk factor. In a review of nearly 16,000 patients from the Scientific Renal Transplant Database comparing panel-reactive antibody (PRA) prior to the first transplant with PRA on relisting for the second transplant, it was noted that 50 % of patients had become sensitised (PRA > 30 %) and 34 % highly sensitised. Risk factors include younger age of recipient, episodes of acute rejection, number of HLA mismatches and weaning of immunosuppression on return to dialysis. Those matched for HLA-A and HLA-B were at relatively low risk (10 %) [16]. Several studies have reported a significant increase in donor-specific antibodies following transplant nephrectomy. This may be because the transplanted kidney operates as a sink for donor-specific antibodies or because nephrectomy is often performed due to a late flare of rejection following immunosuppression withdrawal [17]. This late effect was highlighted in another study showing a 70 % sensitisation rate following graft loss, but for 80 % of these patients, sensitisation was not apparent until sometime later [18].

Blood, platelet or buffy coat transfusions have long been known to be an important risk factor for allosensitisation. In one study where anti-HLA antibodies were recorded pre- and post-3-unit whole blood transfusion, 30 % of the patients became sensitised [19]. The introduction and erythropoietin

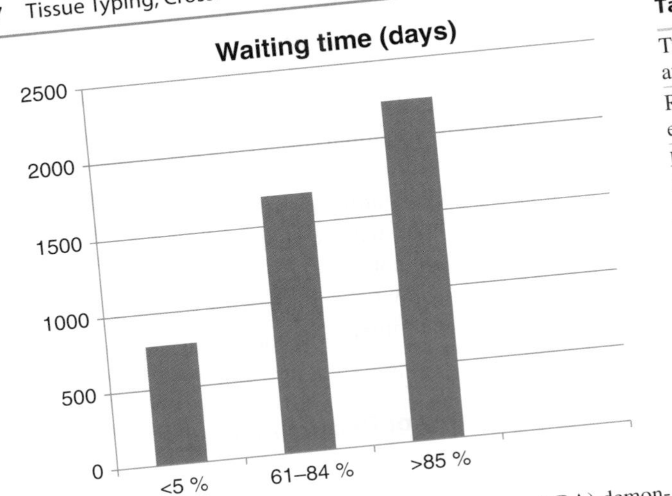

Fig. 67.3 Waiting time in days based on sensitisation (PRA) demonstrating a tripling of waiting time in the highly sensitised population (From Fuggle [22])

and subsequent reduction in transfusions roughly halved the rate of sensitisation secondary to transfusion. Further, universal leukodepletion has been implemented in many countries in part to reduce the risk of infections such as CMV, prion transmission and transfusion reaction. A spin-off is reduced rates of allosensitisation in potential transplant recipients. However, sensitisation does still occur, and in the UK one retrospective analysis demonstrated 17 % sensitisation of male patients receiving at least one unit of leukodepleted blood [20]. Other studies also suggest a relative risk of roughly 1 in 5 following transfusion. Although it does not prove causality, a review of over 2,000 transplants in Ireland demonstrated a significantly worse 1-year graft survival (83 % vs 94 %) in those who received a blood transfusion at the time of transplant compared with those who did not [21].

Pregnancy is also an important risk factor for sensitisation. On the UK waiting list, the male to female sensitisation rates are 17 and 33 %, respectively. It is often difficult to define these events as subclinical pregnancies/early miscarriages can result in sensitisation but are often not acknowledged or recorded. This is a clinically relevant issue for units adopting a virtual crossmatch policy as significant AMR has occurred in this setting.

The penalties of sensitisation are very significant in terms of waiting time, graft survival and, as a consequence, patient survival. In the UK, approximately a quarter of the patients on the waiting list are sensitised. In terms of waiting time, a UK-based study demonstrated a trebling of waiting time for transplantation for highly sensitised patients (see Fig. 67.3).

There is a strong association between PRA and acute rejection rate (as well as graft survival). In one study, 50 % of those with a PRA >50 % had acute rejection. In another study of over 5,300 patients, 2-year graft survival was significantly lower at 76.5 % in those with anti-HLA Ab to class I and II pre-transplant (but negative CDC crossmatch) compared to 87.5 % in those with no antibodies [23]. Thus sensitised patients not only face longer waits but also suffer worse outcomes. De novo donor-specific antibodies also augur poor outcomes with a six- to ninefold greater risk of graft loss. A quarter of such grafts are lost within 3 years of the appearance of DSAb, with Chronic rejection the mechanism in 76 % [15].

A graft lost early for avoidable or unavoidable reasons with subsequent sensitisation to common antigens may very substantially impact on a patient's survival and quality of life. For this reason prevention of sensitisation is paramount, and policies to reduce sensitisation need to be embedded in unit policy and culture.

Table 67.8 Strategies for avoiding allosensitisation

Transfusion policy avoiding transfusion	Compelling evidence that overall transfusions can be reduced
Recipient-specific elective transfusion	Transfusions matched for HLA class I (A and B)
Post-transfusion immunosuppression	2 weeks of immunosuppression with CNI where appropriate
Autologous blood transfusion	Intraoperative blood harvesting, pre-emptive autologous storage
Avoidance of pregnancy in patients with significant risk of ESRD	Where possible and appropriate, the importance of contraception should be emphasised in all women of child-bearing age likely to receive a transplant
Avoidance of rejection	An important cause of sensitisation and a risk of protocols focusing on minimal immunosuppression as well as patients at risk of poor compliance
Continued immunosuppression in failed grafts	Weaning IS has a significant risk of sensitisation, maintenance seems to be preventative therefore worth considering in a patient likely to be re-transplanted soon
Graft nephrectomy	To be considered if risk to benefit ratio in favour of IS wean and further transplant considered

Prevention of Sensitisation

The management of the sensitised patient is discussed later, but it is utterly irrefutable that in this setting prevention is better than cure and that a patient's prospects are likely to be enhanced in a unit with a thoughtful approach to avoiding sensitisation. Strategies that should be considered for prevention are shown in Table 67.8.

Transfusion Avoidance

As discussed above, even with universal leukodepletion, transfusion risks sensitisation. In many circumstances, this is unavoidable but systematic and careful ESA use and iron management have been demonstrated repeatedly transfusion

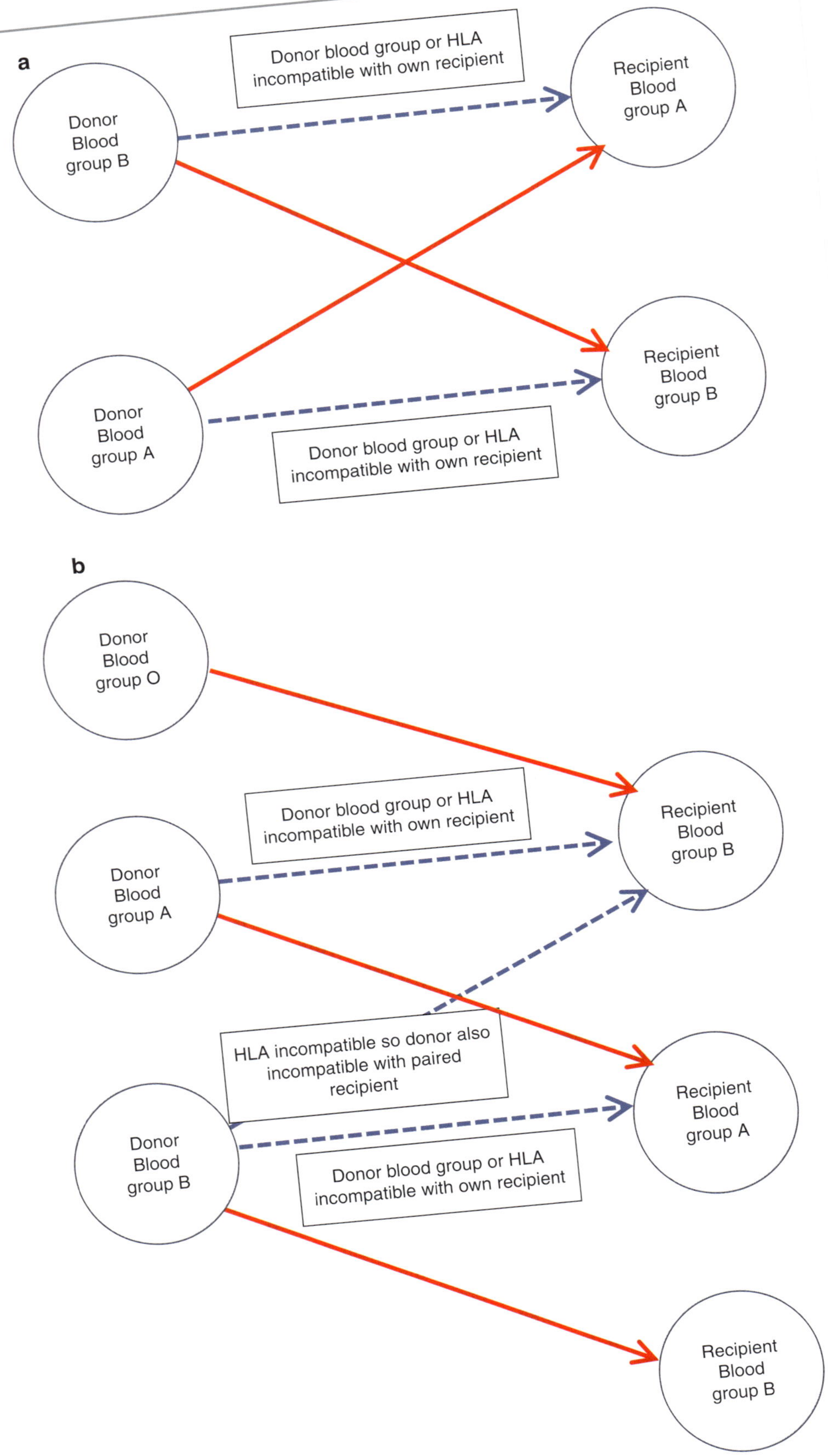

Fig. 67.4 (**a**) Example of standard two-way paired exchange between two recipients with incompatible donors. (**b**) Example of domino paired exchange with a single altruistic donor permitting three live donor transplants

Table 67.10 Common protocols for ABOi

Splenectomy/PE/ augmented IS	Splenectomy now superseded by less invasive medical treatments
Rituximab*/PE/ augmented IS	Rituximab usually given a month before transplant (14 days before antibody removal), *final crossmatch needs to be done *before* rituximab
Rituximab*/ immunoabsorption	Immunoabsorption more expensive than plasma exchange but avoids perturbing coagulation
Standard treatment plus PE	ABOi transplants are being done for medium to low titres with only PE as additional treatment or with IVIg plus plasma exchange but without rituximab

Protocols using plasma exchange (PE) must monitor clotting and fibrinogen, correcting with fresh frozen plasma before surgery or invasive procedures

Most protocols aim to keep anti-blood group titres down to acceptable levels for the first two weeks using post-transplant antibody removal if necessary. Beyond this, 'accommodation' seems to occur whereby ABOi antibodies appear not to cause graft damage possibly through isotype switching

Table 67.11 Options for the sensitised patient

Institutional strategies	
Paired donation	Combined with ABOi transplant programmes
Acceptable mismatch programs	For example, Eurotransplant programme defining non-sensitised antigens
Desensitisation	
Increased immunosuppression	Potent induction agents (e.g. ATG) with higher maintenance IS
Reduction in B cells	Rituximab (role unclear) (crossmatch needs to be done *before* rituximab)
IV immunoglobulin	Low-dose IVIg 100 mg/kg, high-dose 2 g/kg plus or minus plasma exchange
Antibody removal	Plasma exchange, protein A or Ig-Therasorb®
Proteosome inhibition	Bortezomib
Complement inhibition	Eculizumab
Combined liver-kidney transplant	
Combined stem cell transplant	Mixed chimerism to prevent rejection of live donor kidney in highly sensitised

and techniques. The commonest technique (of several) is erythrocyte isohaemagglutination using donor serum in serial dilutions but even this has considerable inter-observer variation. More recently some labs are using flow cytometry of formalin fixed A or B erythrocytes, incubated with recipient serum and then with anti-human IgM or IgG FITC-conjugated antibodies.

As high-titre ABOi have such an adverse outcome, it is critical to have a close relationship with the lab providing ABO Ab titres. Stringent governance processes must be established for audit and delivery of reliable titres. In addition, an ABOi programme requires access to same-day anti-A/B titres to plan further Ab removal peritransplant or postpone the transplant if titre has not reached minimum pre-agreed threshold. In practical terms regimens using antibody removal usually, but not always, employ augmented immunosuppression commencing before, or at the time of, initial plasma exchange (see Table 67.10). It is helpful to monitor anti-blood group titres pre- and post-removal session of each antibody to predict achievement of target titre and quantify rebound in antibody levels. The decision to proceed with transplant is usually made on the antibody titre post-removal either the day before transplant or on the morning of the transplant if the assay turnaround time is swift.

Strategies for the Management of the HLA and Non-HLA Sensitized Patient

There are several approaches to facilitate transplanting of highly sensitised patients which broadly fall into two groups (Table 67.11). The first are organisational approaches usually through national allocation bodies to find a donor without forbidden antigens. The second approach is to desensitise the patient by a combination of antibody removal and reduction in production. For either approach it is critical to have an accurate picture of the patient's sensitisation including database of historical peak antibody levels, sensitising events and a robust system for DSAb screening (minimum monthly) and post sensitising event (usually at 14 days). It is worth bearing in mind that historically positive T or B cell CDC crossmatches associated with anti-HLA, even if negative at the time of transplant, are associated with a very poor outcome [27].

Institutional Strategies for Transplanting Sensitised Patients

For sensitised patients, there are several organisational strategies that advantage the patient and avoid the need and risk of augmented immunosuppression. Paired-exchange programmes offer highly sensitised patients with a live donor the potential for a low-immunological-risk transplant. As stated above, highly sensitised patients are less like to achieve an offer in the pairing runs, but particularly for those with blood group O donors, this is a highly desirable option that also benefits other patients. For those on the deceased donor list, allocation is often skewed in favour of highly sensitised patients via a point scheme, but such patients still face a very considerable wait. A more proactive adopted by Eurotransplant characterises HLA antigens to which a highly sensitised patient is not sensitised and records these as acceptable mismatches. This successful programme resulted in 60 % of recruited patients being transplanted within 2 years and is a cheaper solution with better outcome than desensitisation programmes [28].

Desensitisation Strategies

A variety of desensitisation studies have been published over the last 15 years. Almost all suffer from being single centre, numerically small, non-randomised, retrospective and with only short-term follow-up. Twenty-one studies published between 2000 and 2010 are nicely reviewed by Marfo et al. [29] and illustrate that positive crossmatches can often be overcome with reasonable short-term outcomes but at the expense of acute rejection (AR) rates of 36 % and acute AMR rates of 25 %. In another review of a desensitisation programme, 119 crossmatch-positive transplants with baseline DSAb had AMR rejection rates of 25 % with MFI below 10,000 and 50 % in those with pretreatment levels of >10,000 (with a HR of graft loss at 7.7). Furthermore transplant glomerulopathy (TG) rates of 40 % were recorded in patients with DSAb [30].

Given the increasing association between acute AMR, subsequent chronic AMR, TG and overall poor outcome, such strategies need to be approached with caution.

Increased Immunosuppression

One approach for crossmatch-negative but B-cell flow-positive transplants is to merely augment immunosuppression, usually by increasing induction. This is most commonly through the use of anti-thymocyte globulin (ATG) particularly in patients with current allo-flow-positive crossmatch or historical B-cell-positive crossmatch or in those with current or historical donor-specific antibodies in the face of negative crossmatch. These patients are undoubtedly at increased risk of antibody-mediated rejection and early graft loss, but the data guiding how much immunosuppression to give to whom is very weak, and a significant increase in IS is not without its risks. In short if the transplant is felt to be a good kidney and an acceptable immunological risk, then increased immunosuppression is probably essential but needs to be accompanied by appropriate long-term prophylaxis and a discussion of the risks and benefits with the patient.

Reduction in Anti-HLA Antibody Production

Depleting antibodies such as ATG and Campath-H1 (alemtuzumab) will markedly reduce the number of helper T cells and B cells and hopefully DSAb as a consequence. In addition, rituximab, a humanised anti-CD20 mAb, is highly effective at depleting B cells and is often used as preconditioning in live donor ABOi and HLAi transplants. Used as an alternative to splenectomy, ABOi outcomes with rituximab seem to be just as good while being less invasive. Efficacy of depletion can be easily monitored by staining for co-expressed CD19. However, mature plasma cells (the source of DSAb) do not express CD20, so the precise role of rituximab (apart from removing potentially allogeneic naïve B cells) remains unclear, and the efficacy of rituximab in ABOi and HLAi has never been tested in formal randomised controlled trials (RCTs).

An alternative approach has been to use the proteasome inhibitor bortezomib which induces apoptosis of active plasma cells and is licensed for the treatment of multiple myeloma. This approach has been used to treat AMR and lower anti-HLA Abs. However as the plasma cells need to be active for bortezomib to work, it is probably not effective at reducing anti-HLAb in those awaiting a transplant. Bortezomib is also expensive and has significant side effects including neuropathy, and there are not as yet any RCTs to support its use in desensitisation protocols.

Intravenous Immunoglobulin (IVIg)

IVIg has a variety of immunomodulatory effects including induction of apoptosis in B cells, inhibition of complement activation (C3b and C4b) and neutralisation (C3a and C5a), up-regulation of FcϒIIB inhibitory receptors on B cells, neutralisation of anti-HLA Ab via anti-idiotype effect and binding of Fc® receptors on other immune cells. The fact that IVIg is not grossly immunosuppressive and contains protective antibodies against common microbes is obviously appealing. IVIg has been used in two ways – high dose or repeated low doses. The high-dose approach uses 2 g/kg of IVIg combined with plasma exchange (PE) with transplant proceeding under a variety of other induction agents if the crossmatch becomes negative. This approach has also permitted relative desensitisation of sensitised patients on the deceased donor list. In a rare RCT, monthly IVIg × 4 doses resulted in a doubling of the transplant rate for such patients (from 17 to 39 %) [31]. Various groups have adopted this approach with some success but typically encountered very high acute rejection rates with AMR in excess of 20 %. Short-term outcomes look promising but long-term data is lacking. Furthermore another group recently reported no improvement in PRA following high-dose IVIg [32].

The low-dose approach involves giving lower doses of IVIg (100 mg/kg) repeatedly after PE as part of pre-transplant desensitisation protocol. While it seems counter-intuitive to give IVIg and then PE this expensive agent out again, there is evidence that IVIg alone is much less effective. Similarly antibody removal with PE alone tends to up-regulate antibody production, whereas IVIg administration has a suppressive

Table 67.12 Comparison of plasma exchange (PE) and immunoabsorption (IA) techniques

Plasma exchange	
Advantages	Cheap, readily available and local know-how
Disadvantages	Removal of clotting and complement factors, thrombocytopenia, anaemia, monitoring of clotting and fibrinogen with need to reverse anticoagulation prior to surgery, reactions to fresh frozen plasma if required (especially if IgA deficient), moderate efficacy
Immunoabsorption	
Advantages	Highly efficient, no interference with clotting, complement, platelets or erythrocytes
Disadvantages	Expensive, specialised columns and expertise, limited availability

feedback effect on antibody production. This approach is usually combined with augmented IS, particularly depleting antibodies for induction. Short-term graft survival rates are acceptable, but AR and AMR rates remain very high, and there is concern about long-term outcomes.

Although IVIg is not significantly immunosuppressive, it is not completely without risk. In particular, high-dose IVIg can cause AKI and arterial and venous thrombosis. Allergic reactions are also fairly frequent and can be severe if the patient is IgA deficient.

Removal of Anti-HLA Antibodies

The half-life of antibodies is approximately a month, thus any desensitisation strategies that merely target production risk early AMR from pre-existing antibodies. Therefore antibody removal is now almost universally part of any desensitisation and ABOi programmes where the peak titre is above threshold and is probably essential in this setting. The majority of programmes use PE as it is readily available and cheap. Immunoabsorption (IA) used to a degree in Japan and Europe is much more expensive but cleaner and more efficient. A comparison between the techniques is shown in Table 67.12.

Both techniques have been used acutely in highly sensitised patients offered deceased donor kidneys to render the crossmatch negative (usually followed by ATG induction and further antibody removal post-transplant). In one study using IA, 5-year graft survival and death-censored graft survival were 63 and 76 %, respectively; however, 25 % of patients still incurred AMR.

Complement Inhibition

An alternative approach to antibody removal is to disrupt the terminal cascade of complement and thus hope to prevent the pathological effect of DSAb. Eculizumab, an anti-C5a monoclonal antibody licensed for the treatment of paroxysmal nocturnal haemoglobinuria, has been shown in one non-randomised retrospective study to dramatically reduce the rate of AMR and TG in live donor crossmatch-positive transplants from 41 and 36 % to 8 and 7 % at 1 year in historical vs eculizumab treated, respectively [33]. However despite this remarkable effect, the same group has subsequently reported high rates of chronic AMR despite C5a-inhibition. The inhibition of complement approach remains appealing, but currently eculizumab is obscenely expensive, the duration of treatment unknown, it impairs immunity to encapsulated bacteria and there are no RCTs to recommend its use.

Combined Liver-Kidney Transplant (CLK)

This strategy has been employed with some success in very limited numbers [34] following the observation that anti-HLA antibodies reduce following a liver transplant possibly because the liver acts as a 'sink'. However a review of nearly 2,500 CLK transplants done for other reasons demonstrated significantly reduced patient and graft survival for sensitised patients [35]. Furthermore there are significant risks associated with CLK and ethical issues related to using liver transplants for this purpose, limiting this approach to sensitised patients who require a liver transplant for other reasons.

Stem Cell Transplant

Chimerism has been documented to occur post-transplant and to correlate with significantly reduced rejection. Haemopoietic stem cell transplantation (HSCT) has recently been combined with HLAi kidney transplantation [36]. Sensitised patients with HLAi-incompatible donors were given non-myeloablative treatment, including total body irradiation, then donor stem cell transplant contemporaneous with live donor kidney transplant. The outcome was apparently durable chimerism, minimal AMR in the face of minimal maintenance immunosuppression. Although tolerance in this setting is a highly desirable outcome, the long-term outcomes remain unknown and the place of combined HSCT and kidney transplant is yet to be determined. Nevertheless this approach is worth considering in patients with a suitable donor and another indication for HSCT such as myeloma or sickle cell disease.

Summary

One argument for desensitisation is the better survival with a transplant than on haemodialysis, and this may be true depending on the degree of immunological risk; however returning to dialysis following a failed transplant results in a significant survival disadvantage compared with wait-listed patients [37]; in addition, treatment of antibody-mediated rejection is difficult, hazardous and sorely lacking in an evidence base.

The immunological rules of engagement in SOT have been learned by trial and quite a lot of error; breaching these rules enters 'tiger territory' and should not be done lightly or without due governance.

Tips and Tricks

Prevention of sensitisation is extremely important therefore identify and flag any patient (particularly young) likely suitable for a transplant and ensure measures are put in place to avoid sensitisation.

Establish a thoughtful transfusion policy including responsive ESA and iron dosing and transfusion avoidance, and consider HLA-compatible elective transfusion, autologous transfusion and intraoperative erythrocyte salvage.

Consider transplant nephrectomy under IS in recipients with failed transplants who are suitable for further transplantation and a policy of encouraging contraception in women of child-bearing age with CKD.

Paired-exchange and acceptable mismatch programmes are much cheaper and likely to have better patient and graft survival than desensitisation programmes. Therefore patients with incompatible live donors should be encouraged to enter paired-exchange programmes for blood group- and HLA-incompatible donors, especially where the recipient is young. Some donors feel uncomfortable with the paired-exchange concept, and it is often helpful to have donors who have had good experience with paired-exchange talking at patient education sessions.

Close ties with the tissue-typing department are essential for virtual crossmatch programmes as well discussing safety and interpretation of crossmatch.

For any ABOi or desensitisation programme, it is essential to have a good service-level agreement for screening and rapid turnaround times.

References

1. Kidney. SRTR & OPTN annual report, 2011. http://srtr.transplant.hrsa.gov/annual_reports/2011/flash/01_kidney/index.html
2. Bunce M, Young NT, Welsh KI. Molecular HLA typing—the brave new world. Transplantation. 1997;64:1505–13.
3. Marsh SGE, Albert ED, Bodmer WF, Bontrop RE, Dupont B, Erlich HA, Fernández-Viña M, Geraghty DE, Holdsworth R, Hurley CK, Lau M, Lee KW, Mach B, Maiers M, Mayr WR, Müller CR, Parham P, Petersdorf EW, Sasazuki T, Strominger JL, Svejgaard A, Terasaki PI, Tiercy JM, Trowsdale J. Nomenclature for factors of the HLA system. Tissue Antigens. 2010;75:291–455.
4. Fuggle SV, Johnson RJ, Bradley JA, Rudge CJ, Kidney Advisory Group of NHS Blood and Transplant. Impact of the UK 1998 National Allocation Scheme for deceased heartbeating donor kidneys. Transplantation. 2010;89:372–8.
5. Johnson R, Kidney Advisory Group of NHS Blood and Transplant. New UK 2006 National Kidney Allocation Scheme for deceased heart-beating donor kidneys. Transplantation. 2010;89:387–94.
6. Tait BD, Süsal C, Gebel HM, Nickerson PW, Zachary AA, Claas FH, Reed EF, Bray RA, Campbell P, Chapman JR, Coates PT, Colvin RB, Cozzi E, Doxiadis II, Fuggle SV, Gill J, Glotz D, Lachmann N, Mohanakumar T, Suciu-Foca N, Sumitran-Holgersson S, Tanabe K, Taylor CJ, Tyan DB, Webster A, Zeevi A, Opelz G. Consensus guidelines on the testing and clinical management issues associated with HLA and non-HLA antibodies in transplantation. Transplantation. 2013;95:19–47.
7. Howell WM, Harmer A, Briggs D, Dyer P, Fuggle SV, Martin S, Sinnott P, Smith J, Taylor CJ, Vaughan R, British Society for Histocompatibility & Immunogenetics; British Transplantation Society. British Society for Histocompatibility & Immunogenetics and British Transplantation Society guidelines for the detection and characterisation of clinically relevant antibodies in allotransplantation. Int J Immunogenet. 2010;37:435–7.
8. Taylor CJ, Kosmoliaptsis V, Sharples LD, Prezzi D, Morgan CH, Key T, Chaudhry AN, Amin I, Clatworthy MR, Butler AJ, Watson CJ, Bradley JA. Ten-year experience of selective omission of the pretransplant crossmatch test in deceased donor kidney transplantation. Transplantation. 2010;89(2):185–93.
9. Caro-Oleas JL, Gonzalez-Escribano MF, Gentil-Govantes MA, Acevedo MJ, Gonzalez-Roncero FM, Bernal-Blanco G, Nunez-Roldan A. Influence of donor specific HLA antibodies detected by Luminex in kidney graft survival: a multivariate analysis. Hum Immunol. 2013;74(5):545–9.
10. Opelz G, Collaborative Transplant Study, 9470. Non-HLA transplantation immunity revealed by lymphocytotoxic antibodies. Lancet. 2005;365:1570–6.
11. Breimer ME, Rydberg L, Jackson AM, Lucas DP, Zachary AA, Melancon JK, Von Visger J, Pelletier R, Saidman SL, Williams Jr WW, Holgersson J, Tyden G, Klintmalm GK, Coultrup S, Sumitran-Holgersson S, Grufman P. Multicenter evaluation of a novel endothelial cell crossmatch test in kidney transplantation. Transplantation. 2009;87(4):549–56.
12. Sun Q, Cheng Z, Cheng D, Chen J, Ji S, Wen J, Zheng C, Liu Z. De novo development of circulating anti-endothelial cell antibodies rather than pre-existing antibodies is associated with post-transplant allograft rejection. Kidney Int. 2011;79(6):655–62.
13. Dragun D, Muller DN, Brasen JH, Fritsche L, Nieminen-Kelha M, Dechend R, Kintscher U, Rudolph B, Hoebeke J, Eckert D, Mazak I, Plehm R, Schonemann C, Unger T, Budde K, Neumayer HH, Luft FC, Wallukat G. Angiotensin II, type 1-receptor activating antibodies in renal-allograft rejection. N Engl J Med. 2005; 352(6):558–69.
14. Zou Y, Stastny P, Susal C, Dohler B, Opelz G. Antibodies against MICA antigens and kidney-transplant rejection. N Engl J Med. 2007;357(13):1293–300.
15. Everly MJ, Rebellato LM, Haisch CE, Ozawa M, Parker K, Briley KP, Catrou PG, Bolin P, Kendrick WT, Kendrick SA, Harland RC, Terasaki PI. Incidence and impact of de novo donor-specific alloantibody in primary renal allografts. Transplantation. 2013;95(3):410–7.
16. Meier-Kriesche HU, Scornik JC, Susskind B, Rehman S, Schold JD. A lifetime versus a graft life approach redefines the importance of HLA matching in kidney transplant patients. Transplantation. 2009;88(1):23–9.
17. Augustine JJ, Woodside KJ, Padiyar A, Sanchez EQ, Hricik DE, Schulak JA. Independent of nephrectomy, weaning immunosuppression leads to late sensitization after kidney transplant failure. Transplantation. 2012;94(7):738–43.

18. Scornik JC, Kriesche HU. Human leukocyte antigen sensitization after transplant loss: timing of antibody detection and implications for prevention. Hum Immunol. 2011;72(5):398–401.
19. Raftery MJ, Lang CJ, O'Shea JM, Varghese Z, Sweny P, Fernando ON, Moorhead JF. Controlled trial of azathioprine and cyclosporin to prevent anti-LHA antibodies due to third-party transfusion. Nephrol Dial Transplant. 1988;3:671–5.
20. Balasubramaniam GS, Morris M, Gupta A, et al. Allosensitization rate of male patients awaiting first kidney grafts after leuko-depleted blood transfusion. Transplantation. 2012;93:418–22.
21. O'Brien FJ, Lineen J, Kennedy CM, Phelan PJ, Kelly PO, Denton MD, Magee C, Conlon PJ. Effect of perioperative blood transfusions on long term graft outcomes in renal transplant patients. Clin Nephrol. 2012.;77(6):432–7.
22. Fuggle SV, Martin S. Tools for human leukocyte antigen antibody detection and their application to transplanting sensitized patients. [Review]. Transplantation. 2008;86(3):384–90.
23. Susal C, Dohler B, Opelz G. Presensitized kidney graft recipients with HLA class I and II antibodies are at increased risk for graft failure: a Collaborative Transplant Study report. Hum Immunol. 2009;70(8):569–73.
24. Magee BA, Martin J, Cole MP, Morris KG, Courtney AE. Effects of HLA-matched blood transfusion for patients awaiting renal transplantation. Transplantation. 2012;94(11):1111–6.
25. Knight MG, Tiong HY, Li J, Pidwell D, Goldfarb D. Transplant nephrectomy after allograft failure is associated with allosensitization. Urology. 2011;78(2):314–8.
26. Shimmura H, Tanabe K, Ishikawa N, Tokumoto T, Takahashi K, Toma H. Role of anti-A/B antibody titers in results of ABO-incompatible kidney transplantation. Transplantation. 2000;70(9):1331–5.
27. Ten Hoor GM, Coopmans M, Allebes WA. Specificity and Ig class of preformed alloantibodies causing a positive crossmatch in renal transplantation. The implications for graft survival. Transplantation. 1993;56(2):298–304.
28. Claas FH, Rahmel A, Doxiadis II. Enhanced kidney allocation to highly sensitized patients by the acceptable mismatch program. [Review]. Transplantation. 2009;88(4):447–52.
29. Marfo K, Lu A, Ling M, Akalin E. Desensitization protocols and their outcome. [Review]. Clin J Am Soc Nephrol. 2011;6(4):922–36.
30. Gloor JM, Winters JL, Cornell LD, Fix LA, DeGoey SR, Knauer RM, Cosio FG, Gandhi MJ, Kremers W, Stegall MD. Baseline donor-specific antibody levels and outcomes in positive crossmatch kidney transplantation. Am J Transplant. 2010;10(3):582–9.
31. Jordan SC, Tyan D, Stablein D, McIntosh M, Rose S, Vo A, Toyoda M, Davis C, Shapiro R, Adey D, Milliner D, Graff R, Steiner R, Ciancio G, Sahney S, Light J. Evaluation of intravenous immunoglobulin as an agent to lower allosensitization and improve transplantation in highly sensitized adult patients with end-stage renal disease: report of the NIH IG02 trial. J Am Soc Nephrol. 2004;15(12):3256–62.
32. Alachkar N, Lonze BE, Zachary AA, Holechek MJ, Schillinger K, Cameron AM, Desai NM, Dagher NN, Segev DL, Montgomery RA, Singer AL. Infusion of high-dose intravenous immunoglobulin fails to lower the strength of human leukocyte antigen antibodies in highly sensitized patients. Transplantation. 2012;94(2):165–71.
33. Stegall MD, Diwan T, Raghavaiah S, Cornell LD, Burns J, Dean PG, Cosio FG, Gandhi MJ, Kremers W, Gloor JM. Terminal complement inhibition decreases antibody-mediated rejection in sensitized renal transplant recipients. Am J Transplant. 2011;11(11):2405–13.
34. Gutierrez A, Crespo M, Mila J, Torregrosa JV, Martorell J, Oppenheimer F. Outcome of simultaneous liver-kidney transplantation in highly sensitized, crossmatch-positive patients. Transplant Proc. 2003;35(5):1861–2.
35. Askar M, Schold JD, Eghtesad B, Flechner SM, Kaplan B, Klingman L, Zein NN, Fung J, Srinivas TR. Combined liver-kidney transplants: allosensitization and recipient outcomes. Transplantation. 2011;91(11):1286–92.
36. Leventhal J, Abecassis M, Miller J, Gallon L, Tollerud D, Elliott MJ, Bozulic LD, Houston C, Sustento-Reodica N, Ildstad ST. Tolerance induction in HLA disparate living donor kidney transplantation by donor stem cell infusion: durable chimerism predicts outcome. Transplantation. 2013;95(1):169–76.
37. Kaplan B, Meier-Kriesche HU. Death after graft loss: an important late study endpoint in kidney transplantation. Am J Transplant. 2002;2(10):970–4.

68 Surgical Aspects of Kidney and Pancreas Transplantation

Chris J. Callaghan and Christopher J.E. Watson

Kidney transplantation is the preferred treatment of end-stage renal failure for the majority of patients suffering from this disease, with prolonged life expectancy and improved quality of life when compared to other forms of renal replacement therapy [1, 2]. Selected patients with renal failure due to diabetes also benefit from combined pancreas and kidney transplantation, while a subgroup of patients with diabetes without concomitant renal failure can undergo pancreas transplantation alone. However, transplantation of these organs has a higher incidence of death and morbidity in the short term, and it is therefore crucial that potential recipients are adequately assessed preoperatively in order to minimise risks and determine those likely to benefit from transplantation. As part of this process, careful assessment of surgical considerations is essential.

Organ transplantation is a complex process, and good recipient outcomes are reliant on a carefully orchestrated and interrelated chain of events. This begins with assessment of a potential donor and continues on with meticulous donor surgery, appropriate organ preservation and storage, and timely organ implantation. From a surgical perspective, this process continues with recipient post-operative care and the detection of surgical complications, the majority of which present within 3 months of transplantation.

C.J. Callaghan, PhD, FRCS (✉)
Renal and Transplant Surgery, Guy's Hospital, Great Maze Pond, London SE1 9RT, UK
e-mail: christopher.callaghan@gstt.nhs.uk

C.J.E. Watson, MA, MD, BChir, FRCS
University Department of Surgery, Addenbrooke's Hospital, Hills Road, Cambridge CB2 0QQ, UK
e-mail: cjew2@cam.ac.uk

Deceased Donor Kidney and Pancreas Procurement

In most Western countries, deceased donors provide the majority of transplanted kidneys. Even with increasing live donation rates, deceased donors will remain an essential source of organs due to the ability to transplant two kidneys from one donor. Importantly, the technical difficulties and morbidity associated with live donor pancreas procurement make deceased donors the most appropriate source of pancreata for transplantation.

Procurement Techniques

The evidence base for procurement techniques is lacking, and therefore there is significant variability between surgeons. The description given below is of a technique favoured by the authors, though many other acceptable approaches have been described. Iatrogenic damage to kidneys occurs in approximately 7 % of organs recovered and is less likely to take place when the donor is young, slim, and female and when procurement is performed by experienced multi-organ retrieval teams [3]. Kidney damage is more common during procurement from donation after circulatory death (DCD) donors [3].

Procuring kidneys from donation after brain death (DBD) donors is performed via a midline laparotomy and median sternotomy. Methodical inspection of the abdominal and thoracic viscera is necessary to identify any donor pathology. The right and left colon and duodenum are mobilised medially. An arterial cannulation site is dissected out (e.g. the right common iliac artery or distal abdominal aorta), taking care to identify and preserve any right-sided lower polar renal arteries. Further dissection of the liver hilum or peri-pancreatic tissues is then performed, as necessary (see below).

M. Harber (ed.), *Practical Nephrology*,
DOI 10.1007/978-1-4471-5547-8_68,

Once these preparations have been completed, systemic heparinisation of the donor is achieved with a bolus of 300 IU/kg of heparin intravenously. When the heparin has circulated adequately, a large cannula (e.g. 20 Fr diameter) is introduced into the arterial cannulation site, and secured. The donor's descending thoracic aorta is cross-clamped, preservation fluid is started via the arterial cannula, and blood and preservation fluid exits the circulation via a venting site, either an incision in the right atrium of the heart or a separate cannula in the inferior vena cava. The abdomen and peri-renal areas are packed with saline ice slush to ensure rapid cooling of the kidneys, pancreas, and liver.

After 3–4 L of preservation fluid have run through, the kidneys can be explanted. The left renal vein is divided at its confluence with the inferior vena cava (IVC) and reflected laterally. The abdominal aorta is then split in the midline from the bifurcation to just above the origin of the superior mesenteric artery. Both ureters are identified at the pelvic brim and divided. On the left, the entire lateral patch of abdominal aorta is dissected posteriorly and laterally, leaving the patch intact to preserve any unrecognised polar arteries. A plane is then developed posterior and lateral to the kidney, and a 2–3 cm cuff of peri-ureteric tissue is included with the ureter to prevent damage to the ureteric blood supply. On the right, the IVC is divided inferiorly at the level of the confluence of the common iliac veins and superiorly between the infra-hepatic IVC and the confluence of the left renal vein. The right abdominal aortic patch and entire IVC are then removed with the right kidney, as above. Once removed, kidneys are placed in bowls of saline ice slush to prevent rewarming and enable back-table inspection.

Safe procurement of the pancreas is a more challenging procedure due to the fragile nature of the organ, its complex vascular anatomy, and its proximity to the liver and major vascular and gastrointestinal anatomical structures. Prior to heparinisation, and in addition to the above dissection, the DBD pancreas donor requires dissection of the hepatic hilum to identify the gastroduodenal and splenic arteries, as well as the portal vein. The common bile duct should be ligated and divided in this phase of the procedure. Aortic cannulation, heparinisation, cross-clamping, perfusion, and venous venting should proceed as above, and the lesser sac and peri-pancreatic tissues should be packed with iced saline.

The pancreas should be explanted before the kidneys. The gastroduodenal artery should be ligated after the pancreas is perfused, and the splenic artery transected near its origin. The portal vein is divided at the level of the gastroduodenal artery, leaving a 1 cm length with the pancreas. The duodenum should be stapled just distal to the pylorus. Using the spleen as a handle, the pancreas is mobilised medially. The proximal jejunum is stapled, the origin of the transverse mesocolon divided, and the root of the mesentery stapled and divided. Finally, the superior mesenteric artery is transected at its origin on the aorta and the pancreas removed. The right common, external, and internal iliac arteries and veins should be removed to enable vascular reconstruction of the pancreas.

Table 68.1 Maastricht categories of DCD donors

Category	Description
I	Dead on arrival in the emergency department
II	Unsuccessful resuscitation
III	Cardiac arrest after planned withdrawal of treatment
IV	Cardiac arrest of a brain-dead patient
V[a]	Unexpected cardiac arrest in hospital

Adapted from Kootstra et al. [4]
Categories I, II, and V are termed uncontrolled DCD donors, while categories III and IV are known as controlled donors
[a]New addition proposed by Sanchez-Fructuoso [34]

Procurement of pancreases or kidneys from controlled (Maastricht category III or IV [4]) (Table 68.1) DCD donors uses a 'super-rapid' retrieval technique to minimise warm ischaemic damage. The abdomen is entered rapidly, and cannulation of the right common iliac artery is performed before median sternotomy, cross-clamping of the descending thoracic aorta, venous venting, and packing the abdomen with ice. Although some centres insert a double-balloon triple-lumen catheter via the femoral artery to perfuse the kidneys in a kidney-only DCD donor, results appear to be inferior to the open cannulation technique [5]. Explanting the organs should begin immediately after the preservation fluid has run through. Although the basic principles of retrieval of organs from DCD and DBD donors are similar, the lack of arterial pulsation in the DCD donor makes identification of vascular structures difficult, and surgical injuries are more likely to occur [3].

Organs from DCD donors inevitably undergo a period of warm ischaemia, and prolonged warm ischaemia is expected to lead to poor subsequent graft outcomes. Warm ischaemic limits vary between organs and are likely to vary between donors. Although guidelines for acceptable warm ischaemic thresholds exist [6], the evidence base supporting these is very limited. The authors' opinions on these issues are detailed below.

Organ Assessment

Once explanted, the organs should be placed in a bowl of ice saline slush to facilitate further cooling and inspection. The kidneys and pancreas are assessed for quality of perfusion, anatomy, the presence of damage, and pathology (e.g. renal tumours). Kidneys from DCD donors are often patchily perfused and require additional perfusion on the back-table. The pancreas should be inspected to determine the degree of fat infiltration, and the jejunum should be opened to enable flushing with preservation fluid and then re-stapled shut. Organs should then be packed in bags containing preservation fluid and stored in ice boxes. The role of machine perfusion techniques is expanding and is discussed below.

Any damage, perfusion defects, anatomical abnormalities, or pathology must be clearly documented and communicated to the implanting team. Decisions regarding usability or the need for complex reconstruction are best made by an experienced implanting surgeon.

Organ Preservation and Storage

Scientific Basis of Organ Preservation Techniques

Organ preservation techniques are used to maintain organ function before transplantation and thus enable organ transport, cross-matching, and recipient preoperative preparations. In the absence of warm oxygenated blood, cells convert to anaerobic metabolism, leading to progressive cellular damage through loss of cellular energy substrates, failure to maintain cell wall integrity via the Na^+/K^+-ATPase, accumulation of free radicals, progressive cellular acidosis, and activation of cellular autolysis.

Organ preservation aims to inhibit this process and can be broadly categorised into either cold storage or machine perfusion techniques. Cold storage is currently the predominant technique due to its simplicity, efficacy, and relatively low cost. Machine perfusion is an artificial means by which to maintain perfusion of an organ and involves attaching the organ to a perfusion machine through which preservation fluid or blood is cycled.

Preservation fluids used for cold storage are perfused at 4 °C as soon as possible after cessation of circulation. There are numerous types of preservation fluids, but in the UK the most commonly used are University of Wisconsin (UW) solution (ViaSpan, SPS-1, Belzer-UW), Marshall's hypertonic citrate solution (Soltran), histidine-tryptophan-ketoglutarate solution (Custodiol-HTK), and Celsior solution. Their principles of action are similar, namely, (1) cooling, to reduce cellular metabolism (10 % of normal at 4 °C); (2) use of an osmotic agent (e.g. lactobionate, mannitol) to reduce cellular oedema; (3) presence of a buffer to reduce intracellular acidosis (e.g. phosphate, bicarbonate); and (4) use of electrolytes to maintain the intracellular ionic composition (Table 68.2).

Use of Preservation Fluids for Cold Storage

The choice of preservation fluid is dictated by many factors including efficacy, the organs procured, expected cold ischaemic time, type of donor, cost, availability, and ease of use. All fluids are perfused via intravascular cannulae at 4 °C as soon as possible after loss of organ circulation in the donor.

Surprisingly, given the importance of organ preservation fluids to the field of transplantation, the evidence base for their use is relatively sparse. A recent meta-analysis has demonstrated that for cold storage of deceased donor kidneys the rates of delayed graft function post-transplantation are similar with UW, HTK, and Celsior [7]. Insufficient data were available to comment on other outcome measures such as primary non-function, acute rejection, and graft survival. There were no randomised controlled trials that compared Soltran with alternative fluids. When cold ischaemic times exceed 20 h, renal graft survival decreases, with a 4 % increase in the risk of graft failure at 1 year post-transplant with every additional hour of cold storage [8]. Some studies have suggested that perfusion with UW may be advantageous if cold ischaemic time is expected to exceed 24 h [9].

The evidence for pancreas preservation fluids is even more limited. UW is currently the most common preservation fluid in both the USA and the UK, but HTK is becoming increasingly popular. Only one randomised trial has been conducted comparing HTK and UW preservation of pancreases, and although this showed equivalent graft outcomes, the study was underpowered [10]. However, a recent large risk-adjusted US registry analysis showed that use of HTK as

Table 68.2 Common preservation fluids and their composition

Preservation fluid	Ionic composition	Buffer	Osmotic agents	Additional constituents
UW (ViaSpan; SPS-1; Belzer-UW)	Low Na^+, high K^+	Phosphate	Hydroxyethyl starch, lactobionate, raffinose	Glutathione[a], allopurinol[a], adenosine[b], insulin, dexamethasone
Marshall's hyper-osmolar citrate (Soltran)	Medium Na^+ and K^+	Sulphate, citrate	Mannitol	
Bretschneider's HTK (Custodiol-HTK)	Low Na^+ and K^+	Histidine	Mannitol	Tryptophan[c], ketoglutarate[b]
Celsior	High Na^+, low K^+	Histidine	Lactobionate, mannitol	Glutathione[a], glutamate[c]

Adapted from Saeb-Parsy et al. [8]
[a]Antioxidant
[b]Metabolic substrate
[c]Amino acid

a preservation fluid instead of UW was associated with poorer pancreas graft survival [11]. Small randomised trials have demonstrated that pancreas graft outcomes after perfusion with Celsior are equivalent to those with UW, especially when cold ischaemic times are short.

Machine Perfusion Techniques

The ability to perfuse organs via a machine prior to transplantation has been present for many decades, but interest in these techniques has undergone a resurgence due to the increasingly poor quality of organs from deceased donors and higher rates of delayed graft function due to rising DCD donor numbers. Anticipated physiological advantages of machine perfusion include thorough blood washout, removal of metabolic waste, provision of nutrients, vascular access for the administration of immunomodulatory or cytoprotective drugs, and assessment of organ viability.

Machine perfusion can be divided into hypothermic and normothermic techniques. Oxygen can be delivered to the organ via either hypothermic or normothermic machine perfusion, but in the clinical setting has only been used with the normothermic approach. Normothermic perfusion has theoretical advantages over hypothermic machine perfusion (HMP), due to the expected restoration of aerobic metabolism and cellular energy stores. It is more complex and costly due to the need for a warming circuit and oxygenator. With both techniques, the main expected benefit would be reduced delayed graft function rates. The latest generation of hypothermic perfusion machines are portable, relatively simple to use, and require minimal maintenance. They remain costly and complex when compared to cold storage.

Two large trials have recently compared HMP to cold storage in deceased donor kidney transplantation [12, 13]. Moers et al. conducted a randomised controlled trial in continental Europe, including kidneys from both DBD and DCD donors. Overall, delayed graft function was significantly reduced in machine-perfused kidneys, with similarly beneficial effects in kidneys from both types of deceased donors. Follow-up has shown superior 3-year graft survival in machine-perfused kidneys from DBD donors, but not those from DCD donors [14]. HMP had an especially beneficial effect on 3-year graft survival in kidneys from extended criteria donors (donor age >60 years or age 50–60 years with at least two of the following characteristics: history of hypertension, death due to cerebrovascular cause, terminal serum creatinine >132 μmol/L).

In contrast, a randomised controlled trial from the UK of HMP in kidneys from controlled (Maastricht category III) DCD donors only, showed no improvement in delayed graft function rates when compared to cold storage [13]. The discrepant results between the two trials may be explained by the following: (1) the European study did not have a standardised protocol for either the cold storage preservation solution or recipient immunosuppression; (2) the rate of delayed graft function was surprisingly high in the European DCD cold storage group (70 %); (3) in the UK trial the kidneys were placed on machine perfusion after arriving at the implanting centre, while in the European trial they were placed on the machine at the retrieving centre.

Normothermic perfusion of organs can be performed in vivo (in DCD donors) or ex vivo. The in vivo technique involves rapid placement of large cannulae in a major artery and vein of a DCD donor and perfusing the donor's abdominal organs via a cardiopulmonary bypass circuit. Restoration of warmed, oxygenated blood flow to abdominal organs is expected to allow the return of depleted intracellular energy stores and reversal of intracellular acidosis. Although technically challenging and costly, this technique is increasingly used in Spain and France and is currently undergoing clinical evaluation in the UK.

In contrast to the in vivo technique, ex vivo normothermic machine perfusion involves placing arterial and venous cannulae into an isolated organ and attaching it to a cardiopulmonary bypass machine. This is far less technically daunting than the in vivo approach and has the advantage of enabling the organ to be transported while warm, oxygenated blood continues to circulate [15].

In contrast to renal transplantation, ex vivo pancreatic machine perfusion (both hypothermic and normothermic) remains experimental. The pancreas is not readily amenable to back-table perfusion due to the complexity and delicacy of its arterial supply. However, transplantation of pancreases from DCD donors treated with in vivo normothermic perfusion has been performed, though numbers are small.

Deceased Donor Kidney Transplantation

Donor Selection

The assessment of potential deceased donors is often challenging due to time constraints, lack of access to preoperative imaging, difficulties obtaining medical records out of hours, alterations in donor physiology due to brain death or post-resuscitation, and co-morbidities associated with an ageing deceased donor population. Deceased donor selection criteria are dependent on the local waiting list lengths, perception of risk by the assessing clinicians, recipient characteristics, and unit experience. Donor selection issues are complex, with a spectrum of risks that are difficult to accurately assess. The authors' views are presented, but it remains the responsibility of the implanting team (and the informed recipient) to decide whether the risks associated with organ donation outweigh the benefits of using that organ. General

Table 68.3 Contraindications to organ donation

Contraindications to organ donation
Age >85 years
HIV disease (not well-controlled HIV infection, as these donors may be suitable for HIV + recipients)
Cancer within the last 3 years (excluding non-melanoma skin cancers, localised prostate or thyroid cancer, and in situ cervical cancer)
Definite, probable, or possible transmissible spongiform encephalopathy, including CJD and vCJD, family history of familial CJD, and other neurodegenerative diseases associated with infectious agents
Malignant melanoma (other than local and completely excised cancers)
Choriocarcinoma
Active haematological malignancy (myeloma, lymphoma, leukaemia)
Active and untreated TB
Contraindications to kidney donation
The need for long-term dialysis (not acute renal failure requiring dialysis/filtration)
Chronic renal impairment (eGFR <45 mL/min/1.73 m^2)
Renal malignancy (excluding history of low-grade and completely excised tumours)
Previous kidney transplant >6 months previously
Contraindications to pancreas donation
Insulin-dependent diabetes (excluding ICU-associated insulin requirements)
History of pancreatic malignancy
Acute or chronic pancreatitis
Significant pancreatic trauma

Adapted from the NHSBT ODT Directorate document 'Contraindications to Organ Donation' 2012

and kidney-specific contraindications to donation are listed in Table 68.3. There is controversy regarding the use of donors with high-grade primary intracranial malignancies (e.g. glioblastoma multiforme), though a recent review has recommended cautious use of these donors after careful recipient assessment and counselling [16].

Donor history, examination findings, and relevant investigations are collected by the donor co-ordinator or specialist nurse in organ donation (SN-OD). Factors particularly relevant to kidney transplantation include donor age, cause of death, baseline and pre-retrieval renal function, virology, and donor past medical history (e.g. hypertension, diabetes, malignancy, significant systemic disease). A recent review of UK kidney transplant outcome data showed that (a) donor age, (b) history of hypertension, (c) increased body weight, (d) longer hospital stay before death, and (e) use of adrenaline are associated with reduced graft function post-transplant [17]. Surprisingly, donor terminal creatinine (taken immediately pre-retrieval) was *not* associated with poor graft function.

The authors have the same selection criteria for DBD and controlled (Maastricht III & IV [4]) DCD kidney donors. Recent UK data demonstrates that adults receiving a first kidney transplant from DCD donors have equivalent graft survival to those receiving a kidney from a DBD donor [18]. Many units will decline potential controlled DCD kidney donors that do not progress to cardiac arrest within 1 or 2 h of treatment withdrawal. The authors believe that it is reasonable to wait for up to 4 h; in addition, post-withdrawal donor cardiorespiratory parameters appear not to have a significant deleterious impact on subsequent renal graft survival [19].

Some units advocate routine histological assessment of kidneys from older deceased donors (e.g. those over 65 years old) with the aim of identifying kidneys with underlying age-related impairment prior to transplantation. Kidneys with moderate age-related disease may be suitable for implantation into one recipient, i.e. double kidney transplantation. As the age of deceased donors increases, this has the advantage of potentially increasing the donor pool, though prospective randomised data supporting double kidney transplantation is currently lacking. This approach relies on access to histopathology expertise out of hours and is not available in most transplant units.

Surgical Aspects of Recipient Selection

The main issues to consider when determining if a potential recipient is surgically suitable for kidney transplantation are the presence of iliac vessel vasculopathy, sufficient space in an iliac fossa for a graft, coagulopathy, peritoneal diseases, and the state of the bladder.

Unexpected inability to implant a kidney is a deeply upsetting event for both the potential recipient and the surgeon and usually occurs because of unrecognised severe iliac arterial disease. It is therefore essential that risk factors for arterial disease are identified and that patients with possible arterial disease are thoroughly evaluated to prevent inappropriate listing. These risk factors include age, smoking, diabetes, renal failure due to renovascular disease or hypertension, known peripheral vascular disease (intermittent claudication), long duration of haemodialysis, and poor calcium and phosphate control. All patients should have careful clinical assessment of their groin pulses, and those with risk factors or abnormal examination findings should undergo duplex scanning of the iliac arteries and/or a non-contrast CT scan, depending on the index of suspicion. If a sufficient segment of disease-free common or external iliac artery cannot be identified, transplantation is usually precluded, though innovative techniques to solve this problem have been described [20]. Intraperitoneal placement on to the abdominal aorta and IVC may be another option in those with severe iliac arterial disease.

A history of previous DVT or PE or a previous long-term femoral dialysis catheter requires an iliac vein duplex to ensure that the veins are patent. The presence of thrombus in the common or external iliac veins is a contraindication to placement of a kidney on that side, and a previous femoral vein thrombosis a relative contraindication to ipsilateral transplantation.

Patients with polycystic kidney disease should be assessed carefully to make sure that there is sufficient space in at least one iliac fossa for a proposed kidney transplant. The presence of a palpable kidney well below the level of the anterior superior iliac spine (ASIS) on both sides suggests that pre-listing native nephrectomy is required. Patients with kidneys just below the ASIS may be managed by puncturing the lower pole cysts at the time of transplant, though in general this should be avoided due to the small risk of introducing infected cyst fluid into the transplant operative field. CT scanning of the abdomen and pelvis can be used to assess native kidney size in patients with polycystic kidney disease where the examination findings are unclear. Other indications for native nephrectomy prior to listing for kidney transplantation include recurrent haematuria or pyelonephritis and severe uncontrollable proteinuria or hypertension.

Those with a previous kidney transplant in situ can have a subsequent graft placed in the opposite side, assuming that there are no other surgical contraindications. Patients with grafts in both sides require transplant nephrectomy in one iliac fossa before listing; occasionally, there may be sufficient space below a proximally placed shrunken graft to enable transplantation without nephrectomy, but radiological confirmation with a CT scan is required first.

Long-term anticoagulation requires reversal at the time of transplant, and a protocol for managing this should be in place at listing. Patients who have lost a graft due to venous or arterial thrombosis should be investigated for the presence of procoagulant states before relisting and also need careful consideration of the need for post-operative anticoagulation. Advice from haematology colleagues is essential. In general, a previous thrombosis without a clear cause identifies the recipient at high risk for future thrombotic events, and management should be adjusted accordingly. On admission for transplantation, reversal of warfarin can be achieved with small doses of vitamin K, fresh frozen plasma, or clotting factor concentrates (e.g. Octaplex, Beriplex). The INR should be below 1.6 before starting surgery, and further clotting factors and additional units of cross-matched blood should be available intraoperatively. Anticoagulation with an intravenous heparin infusion can be started during surgery, but it is usually best to defer this for a couple of hours after completion of surgery, though this depends on the underlying indication for anticoagulation and the degree of bleeding encountered during surgery. Patients receiving heparin infusions are at high risk of post-operative bleeding and often require a return to theatre in the early post-operative period; close monitoring on the ward or high dependency unit is essential.

Patients with severe peritoneal diseases such as encapsulating peritoneal sclerosis (EPS) require careful assessment pre-listing. Extraperitoneal placement of kidney grafts is essential due to the difficulties in entering the intraperitoneal space, but separating the thickened, diseased peritoneum from the extraperitoneal tissues can be challenging. The extra time required to achieve this should be factored into the expected cold ischaemic time of the graft, and kidneys with prolonged ischaemic times prior to implantation (>24 h) should be avoided in this patient group. The presence of non-absorbable mesh in the abdominal wall can make extraperitoneal graft placement difficult, and patients with a previous mesh inguinal hernia repair should have the kidney placed on the opposite side. Beware of the patient who has had a laparoscopic inguinal hernia repair; meshes placed via this approach are often large, may cover both inguinal regions, and the scar gives no indication of the side of the operation. The original operation note must be reviewed.

Most transplant units do not require formal assessment of bladder capacity and urodynamics prior to listing for kidney transplantation, as this is difficult in patients with oligo-anuria and bladder adaptation usually occurs post-transplant. In patients with urological abnormalities contributing to their renal failure, close liaison with urological colleagues may be necessary to plan the best method of achieving urinary outflow from a proposed graft. There is usually a relatively straightforward technique to achieve this, e.g. anastomosis of the transplant ureter to an ileal conduit, intra-operative placement of a suprapubic catheter in those with known bladder outflow obstruction, or cutaneous ureterostomy in patients with previous cystectomy without reconstruction.

Implantation Techniques

Kidneys retrieved from deceased donors often require extensive surgical preparation (benchwork) before they are suitable for implantation. Fat is removed from the surface of the kidney to check the adequacy of parenchymal perfusion and identify any possible tumours. The arterial patch should be inspected for vascular disease and the presence of accessory renal arteries. Dissection of the renal vein and artery is then performed to identify aberrant vascular anatomy and repair any damage that might have occurred during retrieval. A cuff of tissue should be left around the ureter to prevent damage to the ureteric blood supply. After benchwork, the kidney is returned to cold storage or machine perfusion, awaiting the recipient.

The recipient is placed supine on the operating table, and a urethral catheter is inserted into the bladder. Prophylactic

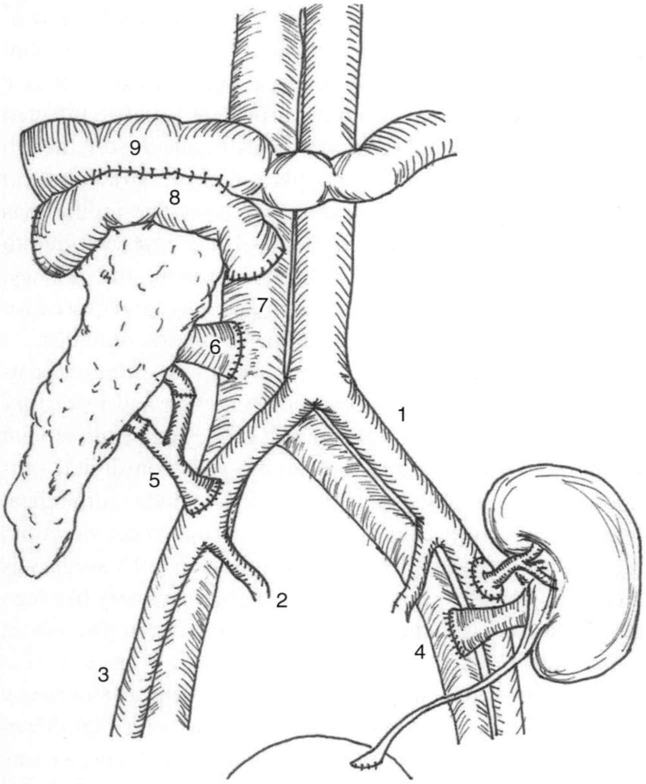

Fig. 68.1 Surgical anatomy of pancreas and kidney transplantation. Diagram of the authors' preferred technique for deceased donor pancreas and kidney transplantation. *1* common iliac artery, *2* internal iliac artery, *3* external iliac artery, *4* external iliac vein, *5* donor iliac 'Y'-graft anastomosed to the superior mesenteric artery and splenic artery, *6* portal vein, *7* inferior vena cava, *8* donor duodenum, and *9* recipient small bowel (Image courtesy of Mr Simon Harper, Cambridge Transplant Unit, with permission)

antibiotics should be given prior to knife-to-skin. In adult recipients, the standard implantation technique is an extraperitoneal approach via a groin incision. Not only is this the simplest approach to the iliac vessels and bladder, but it also facilitates post-operative percutaneous biopsy as intraperitoneal structures such as the bowel are pushed medially. After the extraperitoneal plane is developed, the external iliac artery and vein are dissected free, with ligation of neighbouring lymphatic vessels. After the vein is clamped, and the kidney is wrapped in a cold swab in the correct orientation (ureter caudally), an end-to-side anastomosis between the renal vein and the external iliac vein is performed with a continuous non-absorbable monofilament suture. The external iliac artery is clamped, and the aortic patch containing the renal artery (or arteries) is anastomosed end-to-side, again with a continuous non-absorbable monofilament suture. Alternative arterial inflow sites include the common iliac artery (end-to-side) or the internal iliac artery (end-to-end) (Fig. 68.1). The venous and arterial anastomoses take approximately 30–40 min; once completed the vascular clamps can be released, and the kidney is perfused with recipient blood. The sight of copious volumes of urine emanating from the transplant ureter is especially gratifying, but unfortunately is uncommon in deceased donor kidney transplantation. As long as renal perfusion is good, with excellent blood flow palpable in the renal artery, the presence or absence of urine at this stage is immaterial.

Once haemostasis has been achieved, the ureteric anastomosis to the bladder can be performed. Identification of the bladder can be facilitated by inflating the bladder with coloured saline, e.g. methylene blue. There are many different ureteric anastomotic techniques, but most transplant surgeons favour an extravesical anastomosis, e.g. the Lich-Gregoir technique. This involves dissecting through the muscular layer of the bladder, making a small (7–10 mm diameter) hole in the mucosa, and performing an anastomosis between the spatulated ureter and the bladder mucosa. Routine placement of a ureteric stent reduces the rate of urine leaks and ureteric stenosis by approximately 75 %, but the optimal duration of catheter and stent placement is unknown. Once the ureteric anastomosis is complete, perfusion and haemostasis of the kidney should be reassessed. If both are satisfactory, optional further steps include biopsy of the kidney and placement of a drain.

When both kidneys are available from a deceased donor, and the expected function of a single kidney transplant is unacceptably low, double kidney transplantation can be performed. The technique favoured by the authors is described. Both kidneys can be implanted into one iliac fossa in order to reduce operative (and cold ischaemic) time and to preserve the contralateral iliac fossa for any future transplant. The right iliac fossa is favoured due to the ease of access to the inferior vena cava and common iliac vein, if required.

The incision is slightly larger for double kidney transplantation, but otherwise the initial dissection is identical to single kidney transplantation. Both kidneys can usually be implanted on to the external iliac artery and vein, but in small recipients, or when both kidneys are large, dissection and control of the common iliac artery and vein (and occasionally the inferior vena cava) are required. The first kidney to be implanted should be placed as cranially (proximally) as possible. The choice of which kidney to implant first is dictated predominantly by the length of the available ureter (the kidney with the longest ureter should be implanted first), though when both kidneys have long ureters then vascular anatomy should be considered. The venous and arterial anastomoses are performed in the usual manner, and the kidney re-perfused. The distal vein and artery can then be clamped and the second kidney implanted while the proximal kidney remains perfused. The authors favour two separate vesicoureteric anastomoses.

Post-operative Surgical Complications

Complications that require surgical interventions after kidney transplantation include bleeding (5–10 %), renal artery/vein thrombosis (2–3 %), infected deep and superficial wound collections (5–10 %), lymphocele (5–10 %), renal artery stenosis (1–2 %), and major urinary complications (leak/stenosis) (2–3 %). Their frequency is highly variable and is dependent upon many factors such as the quality of the donor organs, presence of recipient co-morbidities, surgical technique, and the intensity of perioperative immunosuppression.

Blood loss during kidney transplantation is inevitable, with an average haemoglobin drop of about 2 g/dL (in part due to volume expansion and haemodilution). Ongoing significant post-operative bleeding presents as a spectrum of disorders ranging from a gentle drifting down of haemoglobin concentrations in the days after the operation, to progressive haemodynamic instability, to catastrophic exsanguination leading to cardiac arrest. Any suspicion of bleeding mandates prompt resuscitation and surgical review. Bleeding is a clinical diagnosis, and suspicion should lead to a return to theatre. CT scanning to detect perinephric haematomas may be of use in patients with subtle haemoglobin drops, but ultrasonography is generally misleading for the investigation of bleeding. Drains can become blocked with clot, and the lack of a bloody drain output does not exclude bleeding.

Renal artery/vein thromboses usually present with 5–10 days of the operation with a sudden drop in urine output. Venous thromboses also lead to graft tenderness and haematuria. Ultrasound or contrast-enhanced CT scanning may detect the thrombus, and emergency return to theatre is warranted, though the condition is almost always irreversible and graft nephrectomy is the most likely outcome. Technical failings are thought to be the underlying cause, though hypercoagulable states should be considered.

Infected superficial wound infections (outside the muscle layer) can present with wound cellulitis, discharge, and occasionally graft dysfunction. Diagnosis is clinical, though a contrast-enhanced CT scan is useful to exclude a deep component. Treatment requires laying open of the wound (either on the ward or in theatre), evacuation of the abscess cavity, and appropriate intravenous antibiotics. When a deep (perinephric) collection is present, graft dysfunction and malaise are more common, though immunosuppressed patients can have often surprisingly large collections with minimal symptoms or signs. The authors generally favour operative washout of deep collections rather than radiologically guided drains, as open surgery enables thorough lavage, closure of fascial defects, and open graft biopsy if needed. Intravenous antibiotics are also needed.

Collections of lymphatic fluid around the kidney (lymphoceles) are common post-transplant and may come from disrupted donor or recipient lymphatics. These are often detected on post-operative ultrasound scans and do not require treatment unless they are associated with graft dysfunction or significant compression of vital structures (e.g. iliac or renal veins). Radiologically guided aspiration and fluid biochemistry and culture are essential to differentiate between a lymphocele, urinoma (urine leak), and an infected deep collection. Simple aspiration may be successful, though recurrent lymphoceles require placement of a radiological drain. Instillation of sclerosants (e.g. povidone-iodine) has been described, but the authors avoid this approach due to the risk of introducing infection around the kidney. Laparoscopic or open surgical drainage may be required for lymphoceles failing to respond to percutaneous drainage.

Renal artery stenosis presents weeks to months post-operatively with deteriorating renal function and refractory hypertension. The diagnosis may be suggested by ultrasound scanning, but the definitive diagnosis relies on digital subtraction angiography. Treatment options include radiological angioplasty or stenting, or surgical vascular reconstruction. Angioplasty has a high risk of recurrence, whilst surgery is technically challenging. Treatment preferences vary between surgeons and cases should be discussed between disciplines before intervention.

Major ureteric complications (ureteric stenoses or urinary leaks) are rare post-operatively, but can be a significant source of morbidity and even graft loss. Contributing factors include poor surgical technique, damage to lower polar renal arteries (which supply the transplant ureter), BK virus infection, and failure to use a ureteric stent. Urine leaks commonly manifest within days of transplantation with leakage of straw-coloured fluid through the wound with high creatinine content on biochemical analysis. Occasionally, fluid aspirated from deep collections turns out to be urine on analysis. The patient should have a urethral catheter inserted to decompress the bladder, and imaging should be performed to identify the site of the leak (e.g. cystogram or nephrostogram). Leaks from the ureteric anastomosis are best treated with a return to theatre and ureteric reimplantation. Ureteric stenoses present with graft dysfunction with a dilated pelvicalyceal system on ultrasonography. A nephrostomy should be inserted and a nephrostogram performed to locate the stenotic area (usually at the site of the ureteric anastomosis). Blood and urine should be sent for BK viral loads and decoy cells, respectively. Distal ureteric stenoses can be treated with a variety of techniques including ureteric reimplantation, Boari flap, bladder mobilisation and bladder hitch, and anastomosis of the native ureter to the transplant renal pelvis.

Pancreas Transplantation

Donor Selection

Selection criteria for pancreas donors are more restrictive than kidney donors, with an upper age limit of approximately 60 years of age. General and specific contraindications to pancreas donation are listed in Table 68.3. High body mass index (BMI) is strongly associated with reduced pancreas graft survival, and the majority of pancreas donors have a BMI less than 30.

A large US registry analysis identified the following donor risk factors for 1-year pancreas graft loss: (a) increasing age, (b) male sex, (c) non-white race, (d) high BMI, (e) low height, (f) cerebrovascular accident as cause of death, (g) prolonged cold ischaemic time, (h) DCD donor, and (i) elevated serum creatinine [21]; in the UK, only increasing age and cold ischaemic time have been shown to be adverse factors. Surprisingly, donor serum amylase/lipase, smoking or alcohol history, and cocaine use were not associated with poorer pancreas graft outcomes, though this may be because current clinical practice restricts the use of grafts from donors with some of these characteristics.

Most transplant surgeons avoid using pancreases from donors with a heavy alcohol history, though accurate estimation of alcohol intake in deceased donors is difficult. In young donors with a history of heavy alcohol use with otherwise favourable characteristics, the authors recommend that the gland be recovered and then inspected by an experienced implanting surgeon to determine usability.

Simultaneous pancreas and kidney transplants from DCD donors have similar graft survivals to those from DBD donors, with equivalent donor selection criteria [22]. Acceptable warm ischaemic limits for controlled DCD donors have not yet been fully defined, but most centres would decline pancreases after more than 30 min of severe hypotension or hypoxia after withdrawal of life-supporting treatment.

Perhaps the most important factor in donor pancreas selection, and also the most difficult to quantify at present, is the appearance and 'feel' of the gland. Pancreases with significant intrapancreatic fat infiltration or fibrosis are believed to have poor outcomes if transplanted, though objective evidence quantifying this risk is lacking. Assessment by an experienced surgeon is a key component in successful pancreas transplantation.

Surgical Aspects of Recipient Assessment

The assessment of potential candidates for pancreas transplantation is highly complex. Major issues in assessment include determining the patient's cardiorespiratory fitness and selecting the appropriate type of transplant from the myriad of options available. The surgical aspects of recipient assessment prior to pancreas transplantation include assessment of vasculopathy, investigating procoagulable states, and consideration of the ability to close the abdomen post-transplant (i.e. BMI and abdominal girth). Broad acceptance criteria for candidates for simultaneous pancreas-kidney (SPK) transplantation, pancreas-after-kidney (PAK) transplantation, and pancreas transplantation alone (PTA) are outlined in Table 68.4.

Table 68.4 Recipient selection for pancreas transplantation

Patients are considered for pancreas transplantation on the following basis:
PTA: patients with life-threatening hypoglycaemia (requiring third-party assistance) but normal or near-normal renal function
SPK transplant: patients with renal failure (GFR < 20 mL/min/1.73 m^2 or on dialysis) and insulin-dependent diabetes
PAK transplant: patients with stable, functioning kidney transplants and insulin-dependent diabetes
The majority of patients have type I diabetes, but some insulin-dependent type II diabetes patients of low BMI (<30 kg/m^2) may also be suitable
Relative contraindications to pancreas transplantation
BMI > 30 kg/m^2
Insulin requirements >1.5 units/kg/day
Extensive aorto-iliac disease

Pancreas transplantation is a major undertaking, with operations lasting from 4 to 12 h and blood losses of 1–2 L or more. Adequate cardiorespiratory reserve is therefore necessary to cope with these intraoperative demands, and the physiological stresses that post-operative complications may place on the recipient. Thorough cardiac assessment is especially important given the high rate of asymptomatic coronary artery disease in the diabetic population; investigations should therefore include an echocardiogram and cardiac stress test (e.g. myocardial perfusion scan or dobutamine stress echo), with lung function tests in those with respiratory symptoms. Cardiology advice is often necessary and coronary angiography is frequently required pre-listing.

Patients with insulin-dependent diabetes and renal failure have a variety of choices and careful assessment and counselling are required. These choices include SPK transplantation, kidney transplantation alone (deceased or live donor, if available), and PAK transplantation. In this patient group, long-term survival after SPK or live donor kidney transplantation is superior to that following deceased donor kidney transplantation [23]. Patient survival after SPK transplantation compared to that of pancreas after live donor kidney (PALK) transplantation is reasonably similar, with superior pancreas graft survival in the SPK group [24, 25]. The availability of a suitable live donor, the requirement for glycaemic control, local waiting times for pancreas transplantation, difficulties with vascular access, and the characteristics of the potential live donor are factors to be considered when deciding between these options.

Other issues must also be considered before listing a potential recipient for pancreas transplantation. Meticulous examination of the lower limbs is necessary to detect peripheral vascular disease and foot ulcers. The presence of peripheral vascular disease should prompt radiological investigation of the aorto-iliac system to exclude significant disease that might prevent organ implantation. Foot ulcers must be healed before listing to prevent sepsis post-transplantation. Implantation of a pancreas and a kidney into recipients with a BMI more than 30 kg/m^2 may make abdominal closure difficult and is associated with an increased incidence of abdominal sepsis. Potential recipients with BMI >30 kg/m^2 and significant central obesity should not be listed until they lose weight.

Pancreas allograft thrombosis occurs in 5–10 % of patients post-transplant and is the most common cause of early graft loss. Careful evaluation of the potential recipient is necessary to detect procoagulant states. Detection of clotting abnormalities, or a history of thromboembolic disease, may not preclude listing for transplantation, but should prompt the use of a more aggressive anticoagulation regimen post-transplant.

Implantation Techniques

It is essential that the pancreas is assessed by the implanting surgeon as soon as it arrives at the implanting centre; cold ischaemic time has a strong influence on graft survival, and preparation of the pancreas for implantation often takes more than an hour. The pancreas is a delicate organ with a complex blood supply, and damage during procurement is common; repair is often needed. Implantation requires vascular reconstruction with donor vessels (usually the bifurcation of the common iliac artery), and these are commonly diseased or may also be damaged during procurement. Assessment of the degree of fatty infiltration of the pancreatic parenchyma is important, as fatty pancreases have a high rate of reperfusion pancreatitis and poor graft survival. These complexities at least partly explain the high rate of discard of procured pancreases (up to 50 %).

Preparation of the pancreas prior to implantation begins with removal of the spleen and ligation of the splenic hilar vessels, removal of extrapancreatic fat, and shortening of the attached duodenum/jejunum. The portal vein must be dissected free of tissue, and an extension graft of donor iliac vein may be needed if it is too short, though many surgeons prefer to avoid these due to concerns about thromboses at the suture line. The standard arterial reconstruction technique is to anastomose the donor external iliac artery to the pancreatic superior mesenteric artery stump, and the donor internal iliac artery to the splenic artery. This 'Y-graft' reconstruction enables a single, larger arterial anastomosis between the donor common iliac artery and the recipient vessel on implantation.

Pancreatic implantation techniques are highly variable and depend primarily on the means by which the pancreatic venous and exocrine secretions are drained. The pancreatic venous outflow can go directly into the systemic circulation (e.g. via a pancreatic portal vein anastomosis with the IVC, right common or external iliac vein), or via the portal circulation by anastomosis of the pancreatic portal vein with the recipient's superior mesenteric vein. Portal drainage is technically challenging, though it has the advantage of enabling physiological first-pass metabolism of insulin in the liver. This was thought to improve post-transplant lipid profiles and graft survival, though this has not been borne out in practice. The overwhelming majority of UK surgeons therefore prefer systemic venous drainage (Fig. 68.1).

The exocrine secretions of the pancreas can be drained into either the gut or the bladder; both are technically straightforward. Bladder drainage enables the monitoring of graft function by measuring urinary amylase (early rejection leads to a drop in urinary amylase by more than 25 % from baseline), but secretion of bicarbonate-rich fluid and activated enzymes into the bladder can lead to acidosis, dysuria, and reflux pancreatitis. Disabling symptoms lead to a significant proportion of patients with bladder-drained pancreatic grafts requiring conversion to enteric drainage. The disadvantages of enteric drainage include inability to monitor exocrine function and leakage of small bowel contents if the anastomosis between the donor duodenum and the small bowel breaks down. There appears to be no difference between the two techniques in terms of graft or patient survival, and therefore the preferred approach varies between surgeons and centres. Most UK surgeons currently prefer enteric drainage for SPK transplants as early pancreatic rejection is usually associated with renal allograft dysfunction and is marked by rising serum lipase and amylase levels. Bladder drainage of PAK and PTA transplants is attractive due to the difficulties detecting early rejection in enteric-drained grafts. Bladder-drained pancreases are placed 'head down' as opposed to the 'head up' position as seen in Fig. 68.1.

A common approach for implantation of a systemic-enterically drained pancreas as part of a SPK is as follows. A long midline laparotomy is performed, and the right colon mobilised medially. The IVC and right common iliac artery are dissected free. An end-to-side anastomosis between the pancreatic portal vein and lower IVC is performed. The arterial Y-graft is then anastomosed end-to-side with the right common iliac artery. Reperfusion characteristically results in significant graft bleeding, and the surgeon, anaesthetist, and theatre team must be appropriately prepared. The recipient's insulin infusion should be stopped at reperfusion as graft insulin is produced almost immediately. Once haemostasis is achieved, the recipient's small bowel can be anastomosed side to side with donor duodenum, either directly or as a Roux-en-Y loop. After further haemostasis, the kidney can be implanted; this can be placed intraperitoneally or extraperitoneally in the left iliac fossa.

Post-operative Surgical Complications

Early complications (within 1 month) after pancreas transplantation are common, with up to one-third of recipients requiring a return to theatre during their index admission. The common causes of re-laparotomy include bleeding, pancreatic leaks, peri-pancreatic collections, and leakages of gastrointestinal contents. Late complications that require surgery include those associated with bladder drainage. Graft thrombosis is common after pancreas transplantation (5–10 %) and can present at any point after implantation, although it most frequently occurs within the first month.

Intra-abdominal bleeding is common due to the friable nature of the pancreas, the multiple anastomoses required for perfusion, and the need for anticoagulation to prevent graft thrombosis. As with kidney transplantation, bleeding can present with a gradual, progressive drop in haemoglobin concentration over a number of days, sudden catastrophic hypovolaemic shock, or variations between the two. Again, bleeding is a clinical diagnosis, but CT scanning may be useful in subtle cases. Resuscitation and return to theatre for re-laparotomy, washout, and haemostasis are essential. Do not rely on drain output; drains can block. Enteric-drained pancreases can present with GI bleeding; these most commonly come from the anastomosis to the donor duodenum or the entero-enterostomy of a Roux-en-Y loop and require the anastomosis to be taken down and the bleeding controlled.

A number of complications after pancreas transplantation present in similar ways, with abdominal pain over the graft, fever, vomiting, and raised serum amylase/lipase and inflammatory markers. Differential diagnoses include graft pancreatitis, leakage of enzyme-rich pancreatic fluid, and the presence of an infected peri-pancreatic collection. Raised blood glucose is uncommon with these disorders. A contrast-enhanced CT scan may identify an infected collection amenable to radiological drainage, but often the radiological findings are indistinct. Severe abdominal pain that does not settle rapidly with non-operative management (i.e. gut rest, intravenous fluids, analgesia, and antibiotics), is an indication for re-laparotomy, washout, sampling of intra-abdominal fluid, and placement of drains. If the pancreas has been drained via the enteric route, all GI anastomoses must be checked carefully for the presence of an enteric leak. A significant enteric leak in a septic patient may also be an indication for graft pancreatectomy, especially if the leak is not amenable to repair.

Graft thrombosis (either venous or arterial) presents with abdominal pain, raised blood glucose, and characteristically normal serum amylase. Other causes for a raised blood glucose such as steroids, total parenteral nutrition, and elevated tacrolimus levels should be considered, but with a low threshold for urgent contrast-enhanced CT scanning to check the perfusion of the graft. In a patient with significant abdominal pain, any perfusion defects on CT should prompt a return to theatre to inspect the graft. The presence of significant graft ischaemia requires graft pancreatectomy. Patients with small perfusion defects and minimal pain can be fully anticoagulated, and occasionally graft function settles.

As discussed in the above section, bladder drainage of pancreatic exocrine secretions leads to the loss of enzyme- and bicarbonate-rich fluid in the urine, leading to significant dysuria and acidosis in 20–30 % of patients. Also, urinary tract infections can lead to severe reflux pancreatitis. Inability to control these symptoms with simple measures such as antibiotics, oral bicarbonate, or urinary catheterisation is an indication for re-laparotomy to convert to enteric drainage.

Live Donor Kidney Transplantation

Donor Selection

Deceased donor and living donor assessments are very different. As there is no physical benefit to the live donor in donating an organ, the priority with live donor assessment is to minimise donor risk. This includes the short-term risks associated with major surgery (with estimated mortality of 1 in 3,000 [26]) and the long-term implications of living with one functioning kidney [27]. Also, the additional time and resources available make investigation and quantification of expected live donor graft function more complete. From a potential recipient's perspective, the advantages of transplantation with a live donor kidney include superior graft survival, the opportunity for pre-emptive transplantation, antibody-incompatible or paired-exchange techniques, and planned preoperative optimisation. Selected specific surgical issues of live donor assessment are discussed below; comprehensive guidelines for live donor assessment are available elsewhere (www.bts.org.uk).

Deciding which kidney to remove can be challenging, but the basic principle of minimising harm to the donor (rather than maximising graft outcome in the recipient) should be adhered to. Investigation of anatomy requires cross-sectional imaging with either CT or MRI. Multiple renal arteries and veins are common. Singles vessels are preferable, but not essential. When single vessels are present, the left kidney is preferred due to its longer vein and increased ease of implantation in the recipient. Kidneys with two or three renal arteries can be used with good outcomes, though specialised arterial reconstruction techniques may be necessary (see below). Small lower polar arteries that are unlikely to be able to be reconstructed are a relative contraindication to donation, as lower polar vessels supply the ureter and an increased rate of ureteric complications in the recipient is expected. The presence of a large lumbar vein or retroaortic vein is not a contraindication to donation. Quantifying split function is not necessary in all cases, but DMSA scanning should be requested if there is a significant size differential, stones are present, or if anatomical parenchymal abnormalities are noted. The kidney with superior function should remain with the donor.

The presence of renal calculi is not a contraindication to donation, though careful assessment and review by a urologist is essential. As mentioned, DMSA scanning is recommended to detect renal scarring and to quantify split function, and a metabolic screen should be performed to identify underlying metabolic abnormalities. Kidneys with small stones (less than 1 cm diameter) in donors with no metabolic abnormalities can be donated. The stone can usually be removed using endoscopic techniques after donation and should be sent for analysis. If the stone is unable to be removed, then careful follow-up of the recipient is required. Metabolic abnormalities of the donor require a specialist opinion; donation is not necessarily precluded.

Renal cysts are common, with 10 % of those over 50 years of age having one or more simple cysts. Potential donors with a family history of polycystic kidney diseases require careful consideration, and potential donors under 40 years old with one or more cysts should undergo genetic testing. Polycystic disease is unlikely in those aged 40–59 years if they have less than two cysts in each kidney. Over 59 years, up to four cysts in each kidney are acceptable [28].

Surgical Aspects of Recipient Assessment

The principles of assessing potential recipients of live donor kidneys are the same as those for deceased donor kidneys. Recipients with significant surgical risks or major cardiorespiratory morbidities are better candidates for implantation with live donor kidneys rather than deceased donor kidneys, as transplantation can be performed on an elective basis. This enables preoperative medical and anaesthetic optimisation and risk reduction.

Live Donor Nephrectomy Techniques

Until the late 1990s, live donor nephrectomy was an open procedure, most commonly performed via a flank incision through the retroperitoneum. Since then, the introduction of laparoscopic technology has seen a marked expansion in the number of available donor nephrectomy techniques. Laparoscopic options now include totally laparoscopic, hand-assisted transperitoneal (when one of the operator's hands is present throughout the procedure), and hand-assisted nephrectomy via a retroperitoneal approach. Right nephrectomy, donor obesity, and kidneys with multiple vessels are no longer a contraindication to laparoscopic surgery.

Meta-analyses of studies comparing open and laparoscopic techniques have shown that operative and warm ischaemic times are lower with open nephrectomy, but that blood loss is less with the laparoscopic approach [29, 30]. There were early concerns that the raised intra-abdominal pressure necessary for laparoscopic surgery would result in poorer graft outcomes due to reduced renal blood flow, but these have proven to be unfounded. The most significant advantages of laparoscopic nephrectomy are a shorter hospital stay, a faster return to work (by 2.5 weeks), and less pain post-operatively (including chronic wound pain). Conversion to open surgery is needed in approximately 1 % of laparoscopic procedures. Mini-incision open nephrectomy does not appear to be superior to laparoscopic surgery.

New techniques continue to be developed. Abdominal scarring can be minimised by utilisation of a totally laparoscopic approach with extraction of the kidney via the vagina or by using a single port in the umbilicus through which the laparoscope and working instruments are placed. Robot-assisted laparoscopy has also been described, though lengths of stay were similar to a traditional laparoscopic method [31]. Given that the only robot currently on the market costs approximately £1 million, it seems unlikely that this approach will become widespread.

Ultimately, the central tenet of live donor surgery is to protect the safety of the donor. Reassuringly, laparoscopic nephrectomy is not associated with an increased rate of post-operative complications [29, 30]. Because patient mortality after live donor nephrectomy is extremely rare lack of statistical power has meant that mortality differences have not been able to be detected between the two techniques. The decision on which donor nephrectomy technique is used should therefore be determined by the experience and preference of the surgeon.

Implantation Techniques

The technique of live donor kidney implantation is very similar to that of deceased donor kidney transplantation, with a few notable exceptions; the renal vein is shorter, and the renal artery has no aortic patch (and hence is also shorter). As a result, vascular anastomoses are more technically challenging.

To overcome these obstacles, many surgeons favour mobilising the common and external iliac arteries and veins. This requires dissection, ligation, and division of the internal iliac vein, enabling the common and external iliac veins to be elevated considerably. When one large renal artery is present, either an end-to-side anastomosis with the external iliac artery or an end-to-end anastomosis with the divided end of the internal iliac artery can be performed. When multiple renal arteries are present, the authors favour using the excised distal internal iliac artery and its major branches as a graft for back-table reconstruction, with subsequent implantation on to the remaining proximal end of the internal iliac artery [32].

Post-operative surgical complications are very similar to those of deceased donor kidney transplantation, except in limited regards. Rates of bleeding are higher in live donor kidney recipients undergoing antibody-removal protocols for ABO- or HLA-incompatible grafts, and lymphocele rates may also be higher.

Patient Safety Systems in Organ Transplantation

Systems to improve patient safety in organ transplantation can be categorised into organisational, data monitoring, and perioperative systems.

Organisational systems include the reconfiguration of local organ retrieval teams into consultant-led National Organ Retrieval Service teams in April 2010. This occurred in response to the publication of the Organ Donation Taskforce Report in 2008. As part of this process, data on injuries to organs at procurement are collected at a national level, and teams involved in organ procurement are contracted to the Service on the basis of maintaining low rates of damage. It is still too early to determine if this reconfiguration has resulted in lower rates of damage.

Data monitoring on graft and patient survival is carried out by NHSBT for every UK transplant unit. Those units with high rates of graft or patient loss are required to explain the clinical reason behind such results, and consistently poor results may lead to an inspection. Unit closure may be recommended if remedial measures are not undertaken. Outcome monitoring is undertaken by the Scientific Registry of Transplant Recipients in the USA (www.srtr.org).

Perioperative systems designed to improve patient safety include the use of the World Health Organisation (WHO) checklist [33]. Checklists vary between NHS Trusts, but all have three basic components. The first occurs prior to anaesthesia and aims to determine if the correct patient is present, and that they have been consented and marked appropriately for the correct operation. After anaesthesia but before surgery starts, the surgical and anaesthetic teams again check that the correct patient is present and that the necessary instruments and other equipment are in place. Plans for antibiotic and venous thromboembolic prophylaxis are also checked. Before the patient leaves theatre, the team should check that swab and instrument counts are correct and that any special instructions for staff in anaesthetic recovery areas have been clearly documented. For organ transplantation, the operating surgeon should also ensure that the correct organ is in theatre and that virology, ABO-compatibility, and tissue-typing cross-match results are appropriate.

Despite having these systems in place, errors can occur. This is of particular concern in transplantation, where patient safety errors can have life-threatening consequences for multiple patients. It is expected that systems to reduce the likelihood of these mistakes occurring will continue to evolve.

References

1. Wolfe RA, Ashby VB, Milford EL, Ojo AO, Ettenger RE, Agodoa LY, et al. Comparison of mortality in all patients on dialysis, patients on dialysis awaiting transplantation, and recipients of a first cadaveric transplant. N Engl J Med. 1999;341(23):1725–30.
2. Valderrabano F, Jofre R, Lopez-Gomez JM. Quality of life in end-stage renal disease patients. Am J Kidney Dis. 2001;38(3):443–64.
3. Ausania F, White SA, Pocock P, Manas DM. Kidney damage during organ recovery in donation after circulatory death donors: data from UK National Transplant Database. Am J Transplant. 2012;12(4):932–6.
4. Kootstra G, Daemen JH, Oomen AP. Categories of non-heart-beating donors. Transplant Proc. 1995;27(5):2893–4.
5. Wind J, Snoeijs MG, van der Vliet JA, Winkens B, Christiaans MH, Hoitsma AJ, et al. Preservation of kidneys from controlled donors after cardiac death. Br J Surg. 2011;98(9):1260–6.
6. Reich DJ, Mulligan DC, Abt PL, Pruett TL, Abecassis MM, D'Alessandro A, et al. ASTS recommended practice guidelines for controlled donation after cardiac death organ procurement and transplantation. Am J Transplant. 2009;9(9):2004–11.
7. O'Callaghan JM, Knight SR, Morgan RD, Morris PJ. Preservation solutions for static cold storage of kidney allografts: a systematic review and meta-analysis. Am J Transplant. 2012;12(4):896–906.
8. Saeb-Parsy K, Watson C, Bradley JA. Organ preservation in renal transplantation. Br J Renal Med. 2007;12(4):1–6.
9. Opelz G, Dohler B. Multicenter analysis of kidney preservation. Transplantation. 2007;83(3):247–53.
10. Schneeberger S, Biebl M, Steurer W, Hesse UJ, Troisi R, Langrehr JM, et al. A prospective randomized multicenter trial comparing histidine-tryptophan-ketoglutarate versus University of Wisconsin perfusion solution in clinical pancreas transplantation. Transpl Int. 2009;22(2):217–24.
11. Stewart ZA, Cameron AM, Singer AL, Dagher NN, Montgomery RA, Segev DL. Histidine-tryptophan-ketoglutarate (HTK) is associated with reduced graft survival in pancreas transplantation. Am J Transplant. 2009;9(1):217–21.
12. Moers C, Smits JM, Maathuis MH, Treckmann J, van Gelder F, Napieralski BP, et al. Machine perfusion or cold storage in deceased-donor kidney transplantation. N Engl J Med. 2009;360(1):7–19.
13. Watson CJ, Wells AC, Roberts RJ, Akoh JA, Friend PJ, Akyol M, et al. Cold machine perfusion versus static cold storage of kidneys donated after cardiac death: a UK multicenter randomized controlled trial. Am J Transplant. 2010;10(9):1991–9.
14. Moers C, Pirenne J, Paul A, Ploeg RJ. Machine perfusion or cold storage in deceased-donor kidney transplantation. N Engl J Med. 2012;366(8):770–1.
15. Hosgood SA, Nicholson ML. First in man renal transplantation after ex vivo normothermic perfusion. Transplantation. 2011;92(7):735–8.
16. Warrens AN, Birch R, Collett D, Daraktchiev M, Dark JH, Galea G, et al. Advising potential recipients on the use of organs from donors with primary central nervous system tumors. Transplantation. 2012;93(4):348–53.
17. Watson CJ, Johnson RJ, Birch R, Collett D, Bradley JA. A simplified donor risk index for predicting outcome after deceased donor kidney transplantation. Transplantation. 2012;93(3):314–8.
18. Summers DM, Johnson RJ, Allen J, Fuggle SV, Collett D, Watson CJ, et al. Analysis of factors that affect outcome after transplantation of kidneys donated after cardiac death in the UK: a cohort study. Lancet. 2010;376(9749):1303–11.

19. Reid AW, Harper S, Jackson CH, Wells AC, Summers DM, Gjorgjimajkoska O, et al. Expansion of the kidney donor pool by using cardiac death donors with prolonged time to cardiorespiratory arrest. Am J Transplant. 2011;11(5):995–1005.
20. Frost J, Thiyagarajan UM, Bagul A, Nicholson ML. Renal transplantation with arterial inflow from an axillofemoral graft. Transplantation. 2011;92(4):e20–2.
21. Axelrod DA, Sung RS, Meyer KH, Wolfe RA, Kaufman DB. Systematic evaluation of pancreas allograft quality, outcomes and geographic variation in utilization. Am J Transplant. 2010;10(4):837–45.
22. Qureshi MS, Callaghan CJ, Bradley JA, Watson CJ, Pettigrew GJ. Outcomes of simultaneous pancreas-kidney transplantation from brain-dead and controlled circulatory death donors. Br J Surg. 2012;99(6):831–8.
23. Salvalaggio PR, Dzebisashvili N, Pinsky B, Schnitzler MA, Burroughs TE, Graff R, et al. Incremental value of the pancreas allograft to the survival of simultaneous pancreas-kidney transplant recipients. Diabetes Care. 2009;32(4):600–2.
24. Poommipanit N, Sampaio MS, Cho Y, Young B, Shah T, Pham PT, et al. Pancreas after living donor kidney versus simultaneous pancreas-kidney transplant: an analysis of the OPTN/UNOS database. Transplantation. 2010;89(12):1496–503.
25. Wiseman AC. Pancreas transplant options for patients with type 1 diabetes mellitus and chronic kidney disease: simultaneous pancreas kidney or pancreas after kidney? Curr Opin Organ Transplant. 2012;17(1):80–6.
26. Segev DL, Muzaale AD, Caffo BS, Mehta SH, Singer AL, Taranto SE, et al. Perioperative mortality and long-term survival following live kidney donation. JAMA. 2010;303(10):959–66.
27. Ibrahim HN, Foley R, Tan L, Rogers T, Bailey RF, Guo H, et al. Long-term consequences of kidney donation. N Engl J Med. 2009;360(5):459–69.
28. Pei Y, Obaji J, Dupuis A, Paterson AD, Magistroni R, Dicks E, et al. Unified criteria for ultrasonographic diagnosis of ADPKD. J Am Soc Nephrol. 2009;20(1):205–12.
29. Nanidis TG, Antcliffe D, Kokkinos C, Borysiewicz CA, Darzi AW, Tekkis PP, et al. Laparoscopic versus open live donor nephrectomy in renal transplantation: a meta-analysis. Ann Surg. 2008;247(1):58–70.
30. Wilson CH, Sanni A, Rix DA, Soomro NA. Laparoscopic versus open nephrectomy for live kidney donors. Cochrane Database Syst Rev. 2011;(11):CD006124.
31. Gorodner V, Horgan S, Galvani C, Manzelli A, Oberholzer J, Sankary H, et al. Routine left robotic-assisted laparoscopic donor nephrectomy is safe and effective regardless of the presence of vascular anomalies. Transpl Int. 2006;19(8):636–40.
32. Firmin LC, Nicholson ML. The use of explanted internal iliac artery grafts in renal transplants with multiple arteries. Transplantation. 2010;89(6):766–7.
33. Haynes AB, Weiser TG, Berry WR, Lipsitz SR, Breizat AH, Dellinger EP, et al. A surgical safety checklist to reduce morbidity and mortality in a global population. N Engl J Med. 2009;360(5):491–9.
34. Sánchez-Fructuoso A, Prats D, Torrente J, Pérez-Contín MJ, Fernández C, Alvarez J, et al. Renal transplantation from non-heart beating donors: a promising alternative to enlarge the donor pool. J Am Soc Nephrol. 2000;11(2):350–8.

Management of the Acute Transplant

69

Rawya Charif, Jack Galliford, David Game, and Adam McLean

In only a little over a single working lifetime from the late 1950s, kidney transplantation has moved from a startlingly novel, exciting, and dangerous new therapy for the then-terminal diagnosis of end-stage renal failure to become a routine and common operation throughout the developed world and in many developing countries. The charismatic surgical pioneers of the early decades have given way, as the health and economic benefits of successful transplantation have become apparent, to a dense superstratum of protocols, guidelines, and legal requirements constraining activity within the highly ethically complex landscape of deceased donor organ retrieval and allocation and live donor directed (and undirected altruistic) kidney donation.

Outside a few marginal geographical sites, where the wild old ways of unregulated activity persist, all kidney transplants will therefore take place within the fairly tight constraints of national or regional legislation below which sit the local institutional protocols within which units strive to drive up the now startlingly high success rates of this procedure.

No text can conform to all the different protocols in current use in the UK, let alone further abroad, so this chapter is focussed on identifying the underlying principle involved along with universal practical considerations so that practitioners can understand and implement the local regimen of the institution where they find themselves looking after the recent recipients of kidney transplants in an effective manner.

Because surgical and medical practice in renal transplantation are now highly developed and successful, the overwhelming majority of renal allografts proceed without complications with 1-year survival with functioning grafts >90 % in UK deceased donor programmes and >95 % for live donor transplants [1]. There remain a small number of rare but important adverse events however (principally haemorrhage or vascular thrombosis related to the transplant vessels and aggressive early antibody-mediated rejection) which can threaten the survival of the graft or patient so that even in apparently straightforward and uncomplicated cases, a high degree of vigilance is required to anticipate, prevent, identify, and reverse severe complications.

Preoperative Management

Calling in Potential Recipients

Issues around when and who to call in to hospital as the potential recipient of a deceased donor kidney transplant revolve around the desirability of minimising cold ischaemic time (CIT – when the organ has been retrieved, flushed with cold perfusion fluid, and stored, usually on ice, for transport to the implanting centre). Prolonged CIT is associated with increased ischaemia-reperfusion injury to the graft, and increased risk of delayed graft function, and (especially in extended criteria donors) with poor long-term outcomes in terms of graft survival [2]. CIT will be significantly increased if a recipient is unexpectedly found to have a positive cross-match against a particular kidney and (the relevant organ allocation scheme allowing) an alternative recipient has to be called up and undergo pre-transplant checks and an appropriate period of preanaesthetic starvation. Because of this, it has

R. Charif, MRCP, MD (Res)
Imperial College Kidney and Transplant Centre, Imperial College Healthcare NHS Trust, Hammersmith Hospital, Du Cane Road, London W14 9A, UK
e-mail: rawya.charif@imperial.nhs.uk

J. Galliford, MBBS, FRCP
Imperial College Kidney and Transplant Centre, Hammersmith Hospital, Du Cane Road, London W12 0HS, UK
e-mail: jack.galliford@imperial.nhs.uk

D. Game, MA, PhD, FRCP
Department of Nephrology and Transplantation, Guy's Hospital, Great Maze Pond, London SE1 9RT, UK
e-mail: david.game@gstt.nhs.uk

A. McLean, MA, MBBS, FRCP, DPhil (✉)
Imperial College Kidney and Transplant Centre, Hammersmith Hospital, Imperial College Healthcare NHS Trust, 4th Floor Ham House, Du Cane Road, London W12 0HS, UK
e-mail: adam.mclean@imperial.nhs.uk

M. Harber (ed.), *Practical Nephrology*,
DOI 10.1007/978-1-4471-5547-8_69,

is increasing, as is interest in the detection of non-HLA antibodies, although none of the potentially useful systems has yet made its way into standard practice.

Virtual Cross-Matching (See Chapter 67)

The high sensitivity of solid-phase/recombinant target platforms has allowed the confident recognition of the complete absence of HLA-specific antibodies in unsensitised individuals, allowing the transplant procedure to go ahead without a formal cross-match (so-called virtual cross-matching), potentially reducing cold ischaemic time for deceased donor transplant recipients [8].

Immunosuppression (See Chapter 70)

The choice of immunosuppressive drugs used for the initial post-transplant period will be determined by local protocols, often with different regimens aiming to address different levels of immunological risk. Improvements in immunosuppressive strategies and the associated reduction in allograft rejection and minimisation of side effects have been central to the improved survival seen in renal transplantation. Because of the range of drugs available and possibly the different stakeholders in each transplant unit, there is considerable variation of immunosuppression protocols between units, despite the UK National Institute for Health and Clinical Excellence (NICE) guidelines [9]. The commonly used drugs are described here briefly.

Calcineurin Inhibitors (CNIs)

Within the modern era of renal transplantation, CNIs have become the mainstay of immunosuppression, and their use can be credited with decreased rates of rejection and better short- and long-term survival in the last decade. The pharmacokinetics of CNIs can be monitored with 12 h trough values. Elevation or depression of immunosuppressive drug concentrations can be toxic and predispose to graft dysfunction, infection, and neurotoxicity; subtherapeutic values can predispose to rejection. Therefore it is important to remember that a number of other drugs can interfere with the (cytochrome P450) metabolism of CNIs.

The last 20 years of clinical research in transplant immunosuppression have been dominated by a still-unresolved debate about the extent to which the undoubted short-term benefits of CNI use (in terms of acute rejection and graft survival) are undermined by the long-term consequences of chronic CNI toxicity. High-dose cyclosporin-based regimens are undoubtedly associated with essentially universal medium- and long-term graft dysfunction associated with histological changes attributable to CNI toxicity [10], but it is not clear whether the moderately more effective and less nephrotoxic agent tacrolimus suffers from the same long-term disadvantages, and attempts to develop CNI-free regimens (at least those based on sirolimus plus MMF) have been broadly unsuccessful in terms of high rejection rates and poor graft survival [11].

Ciclosporin or Cyclosporin (CsA or CyA)

Ciclosporin binds to cyclophilin and this complex inhibits calcineurin phosphatase and T cell activation. The modern formulation Neoral is a microemulsion and provides more reliable absorption from the gastrointestinal tract. Long-term side effects specific to ciclosporin are hirsutism, hypertension, dyslipidaemia, and gum hypertrophy (especially in conjunction with calcium antagonists).

Tacrolimus (FK506)

The mechanism of tacrolimus action is similar to that of CyA. It is more effective in preventing acute rejection than CyA [12, 13], and the improved graft survival associated with the low-dose tacrolimus regimen in the highly influential SYMPHONY study [14] has led to its adoption as the de facto CNI agent of choice.

Tacrolimus binds to FK-binding proteins creating a complex that inhibits interleukin 2 (IL-2) transcription and T cell activation. Although tacrolimus is widely accepted as having a preferable cardiovascular profile to CyA in terms of blood pressure and lipids, it is associated with new onset diabetes after transplantation (NODAT) due to peripheral insulin resistance. This problem can be diminished by the avoidance of long-term steroid exposure; 12 h trough values are more predictable which may be why the potential for long-term toxicity is lessened. A non-generic, modified release version of tacrolimus (Advagraf) and an expanding range of generic slow-release versions offer once-daily dosing regimens.

Antiproliferative Agents

Azathioprine

Azathioprine is derived from 6-mercaptopurine which interferes with DNA synthesis. Together with corticosteroids, it provided the mainstay immunosuppressive agent until the introduction of CyA in the 1980s and subsequently became part of standard triple therapy immunosuppression with both steroids and CyA thereafter. Despite NICE recommendations for azathioprine use in low-risk transplantation (NICE 2004), it has been abandoned by many units in favour of mycophenolate mofetil.

Mycophenolic Acid (MPA/MMF/Myfortic)

Mycophenolic acid (MPA) is a non-competitive and selective antagonist to inosine monophosphate dehydrogenase, which is an enzyme important in the de novo synthesis of purines. The concentrations of MPA, although not commonly measured, can be monitored with 12 h tough levels (easy) or with longer area under the curve sampling and calculation to avoid side effects (leucopenia, infection, and gastrointestinal) while maintaining effective immunosuppression. The routine use of MPA is not recommended by NICE in the absence of a perceived immunological risk (NICE 2004). Despite this, and the absence of formal demonstration of benefit over azathioprine in terms of graft survival, most units seem persuaded that the fact that MMF is associated with reduced acute rejection [15, 16] justifies its use. The inclusion of MMF in the optimum arm of the SYMPHONY study [14] has cemented its widespread in regimens including an antiproliferative agent.

mTOR inhibitors (Rapamycin: Sirolimus and Everolimus)

Rapamycin also binds to FK-binding protein and inhibits cytokine-induced signal transduction pathways by impairment of progression through the G1 phase of the cell cycle. Consequently it inhibits the proliferation of T cells. Because it does not produce the long-term nephrotoxicity associated with CNIs, rapamycin has been used as a replacement for CNIs in both the acute and chronic settings. It has also been used in association with CNIs in place of antiproliferative drugs. Although the predominant benefit is the reduction of calcineurin toxicity, it has been shown to be superior to CyA and steroids (both with and without azathioprine) in the prevention of acute rejection [17, 18], but this may be associated with an increased risk of infection (especially infections associated with delayed wound healing) [19].

Blocking mTOR has been shown to reduce tumorigenesis in vitro, and anecdotal reports do exist in vivo such as in Kaposi's sarcoma. Side effects include hyperlipidaemia; proteinuria with associated focal glomerular sclerosis; marrow suppression (mostly erythropoietin-requiring anaemia), especially when used in combination with MPA; lymphocoele formation; poor wound healing; testicular atrophy in men; and cystic ovaries. In some patients with a low glomerular filtration rate (GFR), rapamycin has been associated with proteinaceous bronchiolitis. In addition, poor wound healing has made this drug difficult to use in the immediate postoperative period.

Corticosteroids (Prednisolone, Methylprednisolone)

Corticosteroids act as agonists of glucocorticoid receptors at low doses, but at higher doses their effects become non-specific and receptor independent. It is a great pity that corticosteroids, which have been the mainstay of immunosuppression throughout the evolution of transplantation, are associated with deleterious side effects such as susceptibility to infection, weight gain, NODAT, hypertension, hyperlipidaemia, and osteopenia. The increased cardiovascular risk and death associated with steroid side effects have led many transplant centres to reduce or avoid steroid exposure in the immediate postoperative period or alternatively to withdraw steroids at a later date after successful transplantation.

Attempts to run long-term steroid-free maintenance regimens from CyA-based immunosuppressive platforms were associated with inferior graft survival [20], but the availability of tacrolimus and MMF has allowed the development of steroid-free long-term regimens with excellent outcomes [21] despite the slightly increased rejection risk associated with early steroid withdrawal, even under 'modern' immunosuppression [22].

Induction Agents: Monoclonal and Polyclonal Antibodies

Antibody therapy is becoming increasingly popular in transplantation for both the induction phase and treatment of rejection and can be categorised as depleting or nondepleting. These are covered in the Chap. 70 on transplant immunosuppression, but depleting antibodies are not risk-free, and while units will have well-developed protocols, it is important to consider the pros and cons of these agents for the individual due to be transplanted (ideally as part of transplant workup).

Data Collection

Once the renal transplant recipient is discharged to outpatient follow-up in the transplant clinic, it is important that baseline information is easily available. If not already recorded in the local renal data system, a clear record needs to be available of the donor details (age, cause of death, comorbidity, hypertension, diabetes, vascular disease), baseline and pre-mortem renal function, and donation details (DCD vs DBD). The recipient's primary renal diagnosis; renal replacement therapy history; CMV, EBV, and VZV serological status; and state of sensitisation to HLA antigens should also be reviewed and recorded. The available data should be reviewed preoperatively and any samples required for missing information sent. Postoperatively, a clear record of the cold and warm ischaemic time and the vascular and urological anatomy of the transplant should be clearly and accessibly recorded; see Table 69.1.

In Recovery

In the immediate postoperative period, the recipient should undergo a careful volume status assessment including a chest X-ray and review of anaesthetic charts for fluids in and out during surgery.

Table 69.1 Data collection

Recipient details
Primary renal diagnosis
Renal replacement therapy timeline (include positive confirmation if pre-emptive transplant)
CMV, EBV, HIV, VZV status
Hypertension history (including drugs)
Vascular history (coronary/cerebral, peripheral)
Dry weight pre-transplant
Donor details
Live vs deceased donor
Donor age
Donor comorbidity (hypertension, diabetes, renal impairment)
Deceased after cardiac death (DCD) vs deceased after brain death (DBD)
Cold ischaemic time
Surgical warm ischaemic time (and pre-agonal WIT for deceased donors with prior out-of-hospital arrest)
Agonal WIT for DCDs
Number of arteries and veins
Surgical comment on on-table perfusion
Surgical comment on any vessels sacrificed
Surgical comment on bladder
Presence of (and plan for) ureteric stent
Infections bacterial or viral
Transplant details
HLA matching (A:B:DR)
Presence of any repeat mismatches
Any known antibody incompatibility (ABO, HLA) and what/ whether desensitisation undertaken
Induction immunosuppressive therapy (if used)
Maintenance immunosuppression used (and planned)
Prompt vs delayed graft function
Problems or issues with wound
Rejection episodes
Discharge details
Creatinine at discharge
Weight at discharge
Drug levels (including trend) at discharge
Prophylaxis for opportunistic infection given
Dialysis access (venous lines/PD catheter) action and plan

Distal perfusion of the leg on the side of the transplant should be checked and the presence or absence of foot pulses recorded.

If consistent with local institutional practice, an ultrasound of the graft in recovery is extremely useful as establishing a baseline and allowing prompt return to theatres for reexploration in the (extremely rare) event of impaired perfusion following wound closure, caused by direct compression of the graft or vessels in recipients who have had a large kidney implanted into a narrow pelvis or where torsion of the vessels has occurred. This may be particularly helpful if the recipient has a native urine output as augmentation of this with osmotic diuretic, loop diuretics, or dopamine intra-operatively, as has commonly been a dogma from the dawn of surgical approaches to transplantation, may cloud assumed allograft output and thereby the implication of adequate perfusion.

An urgent potassium is essential to determine dialysis requirement, especially if no urine is forthcoming.

When there is primary graft function, initial urine output is often high (it is not uncommon for loop diuretics and or mannitol to be administered in theatre despite the complete lack of evidence suggesting any benefit) after the release of vascular clamps. Attention should be paid to blood loss from surgical drains, and the patient should be haemodynamically stable prior to return to the transplant ward.

The First 24 h

Recipients with primary graft function are usually straightforward to manage during the initial post-transplant period with the focus being on maintaining satisfactory fluid balance, administration of immunosuppression, and vigilance for early surgical complications. Common practice is to provide intravenous fluid (usually crystalloid) to match the urine output, but care must be taken to factor in the volume of other fluids being administered intravenously (blood, other colloids, and intravenous drugs) or by mouth, since overenthusiastic fluid administration leading to overload is a common problem. As soon as the patient is able to mobilise, daily weights are a helpful check on the tendency to overfill the recently transplanted (and can be compared to the pre-transplant weight or dialysis target dry weight).

Autoregulation of renal blood flow is impaired after even short periods of cold ischaemia, so the graft needs to be protected from hypoperfusion by ensuring an adequate blood pressure (aiming for mean arterial pressure of at least 65 mmHg). If this cannot be achieved with the establishment of adequate intravascular fluid volume, then pressor agents may be used; some units still use dopamine (at or slightly above the traditional 'renal' dose of 2–5 μg/kg/h), although the formal evidence that this agent has any renal protective effect other than the promotion of diuresis in this context is limited [23, 24].

Recipients who remain oliguric post-transplant or whose urine output declines steadily after an initial period (typically of 2–6 h) of reasonable urine output require careful management. An ultrasound of the graft and chest X-ray should be arranged, and after a careful clinical assessment of fluid balance and assessment for evidence of bleeding, a fluid challenge (usually 250–500 ml colloid) should be given. *If* the recipient is adequately filled and not bleeding, a furosemide infusion may help manage hyperkalaemia and avoid acute dialysis but does not shorten the AKI, and it is important to ensure intravascular volume is adequately maintained.

The First Week

Obsessive attention should be paid to urine output, haemoglobin, serum creatinine, and clinical examination directed towards the wound and fluid balance in the first week after transplantation, with monitoring of all of these likely to occur several times a day and night. Ideally the creatinine should fall by 50 % on a daily basis and failing that fall by >10 % which may be considered therefore to be more than the variability of the laboratory analyser. Should creatinine not fall, or worse rise, then addressing the volume status is paramount. It is an unfortunate paradox that CNIs have a narrow therapeutic window and are nephrotoxic at high doses so drug levels should be performed daily (12 h trough). A transplant USS will ensure that perfusion is adequate and exclude obstruction. If all of these are addressed systematically and the creatinine remains suboptimal, then renal allograft biopsy remains the gold standard for diagnosis and is performed as either an open or percutaneous procedure according to time from transplantation and local protocols. A post-perfusion biopsy in theatre is often very helpful in determining the severity of AKI and degree of chronic damage.

Baseline samples should be taken during the early post-transplant for analysis of proteinuria and the presence of anti-HLA antibodies, as these may be invaluable in establishing a time frame if subsequent problems with recurrent proteinuric disease or antibody-mediated rejection occur.

In the case of delayed graft function (DGF), it can be several weeks before independent kidney function is achieved, and regular dialysis may be required during this period. This can be a frustrating time for patients and physician alike, but be cautious in assuming that the pathology will not change as rejection can superimpose meaning that regular allograft biopsies (approximately weekly) should be performed to guide therapy. Meanwhile vigilance must be maintained with regard to urine output, fluid balance/weight, ensuring allograft perfusion with regular imaging, and drug therapeutic monitoring.

Early Graft Dysfunction

Early complications are predominantly based around poor or reducing urine volumes (Table 69.2), the failure of the creatinine to fall at a desirable rate, wound infections, catheter problems, and fluid balance difficulties. The catheter is usually removed in the first few days after transplantation, although this is often prolonged if intra-operatively there are surgical concerns about the bladder anastomosis and/or bladder wall thickness.

Local infection control protocols need to be carefully thought out and diligently implemented with the use of prophylactic antibiotics and guidance on first line treatments in the face of urinary tract or wound infections.

Table 69.2 Early oliguria post-renal transplant

Clinical symptoms suggestive of bleeding or graft thrombosis such as pain over graft/abdomen	
Risk factors – difficult anastomosis, multiple vessels, procoagulant state, patient with small pelvis	
Clinical signs suggestive of hypovolaemia, bleeding, or graft thrombosis such as hypotension, tachycardia, graft tenderness, and frank haematuria	
Exclude blocked catheter and clot retention	
Urgent ECG, CXR, bloods	
Cross-match 4 units	
Venous gas K and Hb	
With hypotension Resuscitate IV colloids If evidence of bleeding with falling Hb, transfuse If deranged clotting or thrombocytopenia, consider FFP and platelets	*Without hypotension* Fluid challenge if clinical evidence of hypovolaemia Treat hyperkalaemia if present Bladder washout +/– change of catheter if in clot retention by surgical team
Urgent USS/CT for perfusion and evidence of haematoma and exclude obstruction (e.g. compression from haematoma)	Urgent USS for graft perfusion and patency of vessels and exclude obstruction
Evidence of bleeding Contact surgical team Prepare for theatre if necessary to control haemorrhage and evacuate haematoma	Evidence of graft thrombosis Contact surgical team Prepare for theatre immediately If graft thrombosis with reverse flow in diastole is seen on USS
If hypovolaemia and bleeding excluded, consider other causes for hypotension such as cardiac causes	If reduced cortical perfusion/no flow in diastole with patent large vessels, consider intraparenchymal pathology such as AMR Check for DSA and pro-thrombotic screen

Chest expansion is rarely complete intra-operatively so deep breathing and, if possible, chest physiotherapy will assist with the avoidance of atelectasis and pneumonias postoperatively. Opiates may promote a postoperative ileus (remember the operation is conventionally extra-peritoneal, so there is no surgical bowel manipulation) that can be uncomfortable for the patient and interfere with the metabolism of some medications. The recipient should be sat out as soon as sensible and mobility encouraged; this will improve chest expansion and promote a return to normal gut motility.

Delayed Graft Function

Failure of the transplanted kidney to function promptly as a consequence of ATN/acute tubular injury is common, occurring (albeit only occasionally) in live donor kidneys with minimal cold ischaemia and more frequently than not in grafts exposed to extended, combined, warm, and cold ischaemia in the more extreme types of donation after circulatory death. The graft will be perfused (but with the completely non-specific finding of a raised resistive index) on ultrasound scan. It is not uncommon for oliguria to develop progressively after a few hours of urine production postoperatively (presumably as a result of the onset of the reperfusion phase of ischaemia-reperfusion injury).

Care must be taken to avoid overfilling the oliguric recipient, instituting dialysis in a timely fashion if required and careful, repeated assessment of the graft to give an indication of other causes of graft dysfunction which may supervene before the onset of function. This will usually entail daily ultrasound scans and regular biopsies (standard practice being to undertake a biopsy on postoperative day 7 and then at weekly intervals until function is established).

A common reaction to DGF is to delay or reduce the exposure to CNIs, although evidence that this is effective is marginal [25, 26].

Thrombosis and Anticoagulation

Transplant arterial or venous thrombosis remains a rare but difficult to manage complication. Patients at risk include those with a known pro-thrombotic tendency (although the predictive value of standard tests for thrombophilia is low [27], the anatomical situation of a kidney compressed by being transplanted into a narrow pelvis or by surrounding haemorrhage, and prolonged cold ischaemic time. Prophylaxis with low-dose aspirin is known to be effective [28], although this carries an increased risk of bleeding should early biopsy be required, so heparin (usually subcutaneously as unfractionated or LMW) is more frequently used with due appreciation needing to be given to the effects of low-GFR on the clearance of LMW heparins. The initiation of anticoagulation is a matter for careful discussion with the surgeons involved in the procedure (who will definitely have an opinion) and should be based on the amount of intra-operative or postoperative haemorrhage and an assessment of the patient's risk of thrombosis based on their past history of haemorrhage or thrombosis, the anatomy of the graft, and the early postoperative platelet count.

Main or intra-graft arterial thrombosis may be accompanied by platelet consumption with peripheral thrombocytopenia and can be identified by absence of parenchymal perfusion on ultrasound scan.

Renal transplant vein thrombosis may be accompanied by macroscopic haematuria and sudden onset of a painful and swollen graft. The ultrasound will show reversal of flow in diastole. In both situations, the availability of a prior baseline ultrasound is extremely helpful to allow assessment of the extent to which factors such as body habitus, juxtaposition of vessels, and existing variation in regional perfusion and pulse pressure may influence the reliability of ultrasound-derived information. The assessment of graft perfusion by CT scan with contrast provides more objective information that can be derived from ultrasound, but risks precipitating or prolonging AKI. More importantly it may delay the crucial intervention of surgical exploration of the graft with critical ischaemia. Contrast enhanced ultrasound may offer a rapid, bedside test with greater sensitivity than doppler ultrasound.

Acute Cellular Rejection

The increasing use of biological induction therapy (with mono- or polyclonal agents) combined with the use of high-efficacy agents such as tacrolimus and mycophenolate has been associated with a sharp reduction in the incidence of early acute cellular rejection (Fig. 69.1) [14]. This does however still occur, even in recipients not obviously at high risk as a result of prior sensitisation, history of previous immunological graft loss, low CNI levels, or young recipient age. In grafts with immediate function, the onset of graft dysfunction due to cellular rejection can vary from the indolent (over several days) to the very rapid, with rising creatinine and falling urine volume. Despite several decades of endeavour, no non-invasive test has proved to have sufficient predictive value to replace the creatinine as screening modality, and transplant biopsy as the definitive investigation, for cellular rejection [29].

The timing of transplant biopsy in the early postoperative period is largely determined by the desirability of maintaining anticoagulation in the initial post-transplant period and the potential difficulty of managing post-biopsy haemorrhage in a potentially unstable early postoperative window. Seven days post-transplant is generally considered a safe time-point for percutaneous biopsy. Prior to this, and especially in the first 3–4 days, consideration should be given to open biopsy as the safest method of obtaining a definitive tissue diagnosis for graft dysfunction, with the added benefit of allowing direct examination of the graft and vessels which will encompass important parts of the differential diagnosis of early graft dysfunction (Table 69.3 and Figs. 69.1 and 69.2).

Table 69.3 Differential diagnosis of cellular infiltrates in transplant biopsies, see [30, 31]

T cell rejection (ACR)	Tubulitis (Fig. 69.1) with or without vascular (Fig. 69.2) and glomerular involvement. Typically interstitial infiltrate is lymphocytic but may also contain eosinophils, neutrophils, and macrophages. More likely in under patients who are immunosuppressed, commonest cause of interstitial infiltrate
Polyoma virus nephropathy	BKV (95 %) or JC (≤5 %), interstitial infiltrate typically rich in plasma cells, enlarged atypical tubular nuclei but may be indistinguishable from ACR thus *SV40 large T antigen stain critical in all presumed ACR.* BKV is more likely in over immunosuppressed
Post-transplant lymphoproliferative disorder	More common in the graft early on EBV D+/R-, monotonous diffuse infiltrate suggestive, immunohistochemistry (EBNA) staining critical
Cytomegalovirus nephropathy	A rare cause of interstitial nephritis, other end-organ damage usually apparent before renal involvement. Viral inclusion bodies may be seen in glomerular and tubular cells with enlarged 'owl's eye' effect. Extensive infiltrate uncommon
Bacterial Pyelonephritis	Neutrophil casts in tubules highly suggestive but may coexist with ACR. Positive urine culture helpful but can frequently occur in the absence of positive MSU, especially after short course of antibiotics. Cellular infiltrate pleomorphic including neutrophils and the second commonest cause and more likely in those with recent UTIs especially if recurrent, diabetes, abnormal bladder, and stent in situ
Mycobacterial infection	Ethnicity and country of origin may indicate high risk, often associated with granulomas (acid-fast bacilli rarely seen)
Recurrent disease	Important to consider in patients with an original disease associated with acute interstitial nephritis such as sarcoid, vasculitis, SLE but all unusual in the early stages of a transplant due to augmented immunosuppression
Allergic interstitial nephritis	Common transplant drugs such as septrin, proton pump inhibitors, azathioprine, and penicillins may all cause an interstitial nephritis confused with ACR

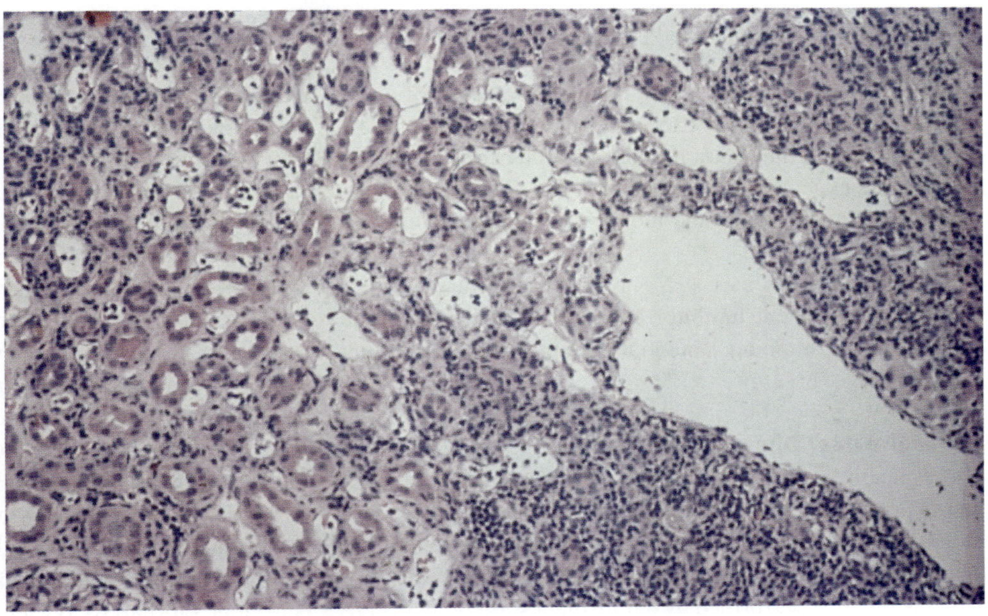

Fig. 69.1 Low-powered view of acute cellular rejection showing cellular infiltrate with lymphocytes invading tubules (tubulitis). Differential diagnosis is shown in Table 69.3

Acute Antibody-Mediated Rejection

Acute antibody-mediated rejection remains a rare complication except in the context of planned (or unwitting) transplantation against a pre-existing donor-specific antibody barrier, whether to HLA and non-HLA protein or ABO-blood group antigens, but the reducing incidence of cellular rejection makes this a proportionately increasingly important cause of early graft dysfunction [32]. The presentation may often be dramatic, with sudden onset anuria, often presaged by macroscopic haematuria. Classically, graft dysfunction will be preceded by the development of rapidly rising levels (as assessed by fluorescence intensity on solid-phase bead-based Luminex assay) of donor-specific antibodies.

With improvements in tissue typing, much of which has occurred alongside the development of solid-phase antibody assays, there has been improved detection of both preformed and de novo anti-HLA antibody which is associated with AMR. Controversy remains regarding the practical importance of these tests in the absence of a positive flow or cytotoxic cross-match, but undoubtedly their presence should raise suspicion of AMR. A renal allograft biopsy remains the gold standard for diagnosis (Fig. 69.2), either open (surgeon performed intra-operatively) or percutaneous

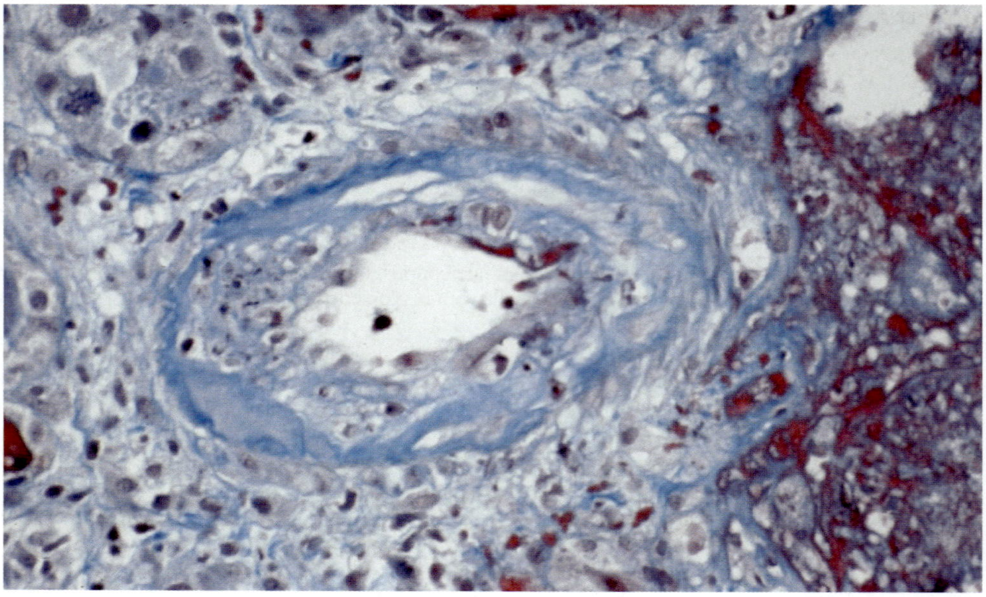

Fig. 69.2 Vascular rejection: arteriole showing lymphocytic infiltrate under the endothelium of the vessel

according to time from transplantation and local protocols, but if this is unsafe (proximity in time to surgery, overlying bowel, patient fitness, anticoagulation, risk of graft rupture), then presumptive therapy may be advised. Most protocols use a combination of intravenous corticosteroids and plasma exchange with or without the addition of intravenous immunoglobulin and mono- or polyclonal antibody therapy.

In the presence of early AMR refractory to standard therapy, the complement inhibitor eculizumab and proteasome inhibitor bortezomib are potential therapies still undergoing evaluation.

Urine Outflow Obstruction

If the patient is catheterised, then always ensure the catheter is not blocked, by external pressure (lying on catheter or clamped accidentally) prior to consideration of clot retention. The latter will require either a catheter change or flushing which should be performed by a transplant surgeon with care not to impact on the vesicoureteric anastomosis. Irrigation of the bladder can not only jeopardise the bladder anastomosis but make fluid balance incredibly difficult to record and can be complicated by hyponatraemia. Instrumentation of a renal patient's urethra, which often has not had urine passage, is not straightforward and can lead to false passages which should also be considered in terms of catheter placement. In elderly anuric men on dialysis, prostatic obstruction may only declare itself after renal transplantation and should be anticipated.

Hypotension

The crucial differential diagnosis for the hypotensive patient in the early post-transplant period lies between haemorrhage and sepsis. In the former case, the patient will usually be peripherally shutdown and cold, while in the latter they will be vasodilated and hot. Beyond basic clinical examination, including close attention to the contents of surgical drains, an ultrasound will demonstrate peri-transplant haematoma, but cannot easily detect retroperitoneal haemorrhage. CT scan will demonstrate this clearly (with the disadvantage of exposing the recently transplanted kidney to a contrast load) but should be undertaken if the recipient is clearly bleeding and does not stabilise promptly with administration of appropriate blood products (the alternative intervention being urgent surgical reexploration, which may be mandated by the clinical urgency of the apparent haemorrhage). When a CVP line is present, the response of the central venous pressure to fluid bolus administration can be used to gauge adequacy of filling, although the common complications in dialysis patients of thoracic vein stenosis or thrombosis and cardiac ventricular dysfunction/poor ventricular compliance may need to be borne in mind. It is often helpful to discuss the patient's prior behaviour on dialysis (in terms of the BP response to fluid loading) with the physician who looked after them on dialysis.

Patients with diabetes (or other primary renal diseases associated with autonomic dysfunction) will often have marked postural falls in BP in the early transplant period, and care must be taken on their initial postoperative mobilisation to avoid significant hypotensive episodes which may be sufficient to cause falls or compromise graft perfusion.

Cyto-depleting induction therapies, whether monoclonal (alemtuzumab, OKT3) or polyclonal (anti-thymocyte globulins), may be associated with a cytokine release syndrome presenting with hypotension, rigours, thrombocytopenia, and occasionally a brisk spike in temperature. If not already given as part of the induction regimen, IV steroids (100 mg hydrocortisone) and IV antihistamines will usually control the reaction which is relatively short lived (1–3 h).

Hypertension

The almost universal tendency to want to maintain a high urine output during the initial post-transplant period makes fluid overload with associated hypertension an extremely common phenomenon in the first few days post-transplant. Beyond attempting to avoid the all-too-common scenario of a patient with high blood pressure after intravenous administration of 10 L of excess fluid, patients will often require staged reintroduction (or commencement) of antihypertensive medication. ACE inhibitors and angiotensin receptor blockers are often viewed with anxiety in the early postoperative period because of the theoretical risk of interfering with intrinsic homeostatic responses to volume stress in a kidney in the process of recovering from ischaemia-reperfusion injury, but the definite long-term benefits of agents which interrupt the renin/angiotensin system in renal transplant recipients [33] do make them attractive agents even in the early postoperative period. The suggestion (popular in the late 1980s) that non-dihydropyridine calcium channel antagonists such as verapamil and diltiazem had a protective effect against CNI toxicity and has made these popular agents for use in early post-transplant hypertension. In any event, agents which are very long acting and renally excreted (such as atenolol) or liable to produce sharp drops in BP on first administration (such as standard-release nifedipine) should be avoided.

A proportion of recipients (especially the young and often in patients of Afro-Caribbean ethnic origin) will respond to volume depletion with a marked vasoconstrictor response accompanied by significant arterial hypertension. In this context, carefully controlled vasodilatation (with low-dose nitrates or other vasodilators) accompanied by cautious fluid replacement ('dilate-and-fill') will result in resolution of the hypertension, the vasoconstriction, and (hopefully) the associated hypoperfusion of the graft.

Careful attention to fluid balance with gradual reversion to a euvolaemic state (which may require careful use of loop diuretics) after any overenthusiastic initial fluid loading will usually bring the blood pressure under control, although the vasoconstrictor effects of calcineurin inhibitors mean that most transplant recipients require long-term antihypertensive medication.

Accelerated-Phase Hypertension/Thrombotic Microangiopathy (TMA)

Hypertension associated with failure of microvascular endothelial homeostatic protection mechanisms is a rare but always challenging and complex event early post-transplantation. The differential diagnosis includes the extreme manifestation of CNI toxicity (which is often invoked but rarely encountered), recurrence of underlying atypical HUS/complement regulatory disease, and antibody-mediated rejection. Although moderate degrees of thrombocytopenia are common after cyto-depleting induction therapies, any fall in platelet count should trigger a request for examination of a peripheral blood film, LDH, and whatever serves as the local haemolysis screen, since the presence of RBC fragments or evidence of haemolysis give early warning of microangiopathy. Consideration should also be given to the primary renal diagnosis since atypical HUS is difficult to diagnose and will frequently be labelled as 'hypertensive nephropathy'. Onset at a young age and a positive family history are important clues.

In the presence of established thrombotic microangiopathy, careful attention to CNI levels, an urgent search for donor-specific and anti-phospholipid antibodies, evidence of lupus or lupus-associated autoimmune disease, and the consideration of the possibility of recurrent atypical HUS or active hepatitis C should all be undertaken. If correction of fluid overload and control of hypertension using renin/angiotensin blockade do not result in resolution of the TMA, then plasma exchange with FFP infusion should be considered. The recently licensed (for paroxysmal nocturnal haemoglobinuria) and very expensive, terminal component complement inhibitor eculizumab has been reported to be highly effective in a range of acute post-transplant microangiopathies.

Heparin-induced thrombocytopenia (HIT) may mimic the clinical presentation of post-transplant TMA but is an even rarer entity. Most of transplant recipients (with the exception of those pre-emptively transplanted) will have had ample heparin exposure prior to transplantation, and the absence of catastrophic reaction to heparin when stable on dialysis means that the many alternative causes of thrombocytopenia in the early post-transplant period are overwhelmingly more likely than HIT to be the explanation of a low platelet count in this situation.

Sepsis

Significant CMV disease prior to 3 months post-transplant remains rare and is easily diagnosed and treated using modern PCR-based diagnostics and the highly orally active agent valgancyclovir. Local protocols may involve the administration of prophylactic antiviral therapy after determination of risk by donor and recipient CMV status or may avoid prophylaxis in favour or serial monitoring of post-transplant recipient CMV PCR levels. It is usual for prophylaxis to *Pneumocystis jirovecii* (previously known as *Pneumocystis carinii* or PCP) to be used universally with septrin or inhaled pentamide. TB prophylaxis should be considered and usually instituted in patients with previous history of TB and in patients deemed at high risk of developing TB post-transplant such as those of Indoasian ethnic origin. Together with these approaches, the progressive reduction in the amount of corticosteroid administered during the early post-transplant period over the last 3 decades (even in those regimens not focussed on steroid avoidance) has altered the landscape of early post-transplant sepsis, with herpes virus reactivation and fungal sepsis becoming much less common (and resulted in the abandonment of the previously standard practice of requiring total dental clearance or prophylactic cholecystectomy prior to transplantation). Current immunosuppressive regimens are highly potent and effective, but leave patients a relatively low risk of significant early sepsis, except in the context of recipients at risk of chronic or recurrent urosepsis (such as those with polycystic kidney disease or abnormal lower urinary tract anatomy), respiratory tract sepsis (bronchiectasis, pulmonary scarring secondary to pulmonary-renal inflammatory disease, or, most dangerously, lung transplant recipients with their risk of fungal or multi-resistant bacterial colonisation) or those exposed to de novo infection from contaminated organs. Positive perfusion fluid culture results should be treated with great seriousness, as representing a very high-risk situation.

Common sources of sepsis during the primary admission will usually respond to broad-spectrum antibiotics.

Proteinuria

Moderate (presumably predominantly tubular) proteinuria is very common in the immediate post-transplant period as a consequence of the tubular injury during the cold ischaemic phase, but persistent, significant early proteinuria (protein/creatinine ratio >100 mg/mmol) indicates major glomerular pathology, with recurrent focal and segmental glomerulosclerosis (FSGS) the most important underlying cause. Membranous nephropathy and complement-abnormality-associated MPGN can recur post-transplant, but usually with a timescale presenting beyond the initial transplant admission. When associated with delayed graft function, this can be a difficult diagnosis to establish. Early biopsy may not detect focal glomerular scarring at an early stage, and electron microscopy may be required to identify the associated podocytopathy.

In the presence of established, or probable, recurrent FSGS, the main current therapeutic option is aggressive plasma exchange, with recent case reports suggesting that anti-CD 20 monoclonal antibody (rituximab) may have a therapeutic or even prophylactic role [34].

Discharge Planning

Patients facing discharge after successful kidney transplantation have to cope with a range of important challenges and tasks.

The first of these will be a new and often complex drug regimen which will often include agents with a narrow therapeutic index and important toxicities. The discharge drug combination must be reviewed carefully with the patient to ensure they understand what the different drugs are for and how they should be taken. Particular attention should be paid to immunosuppressive agents with regard to the importance of taking these in a regular manner, not missing doses, and when to delay morning doses of twice-daily drugs to allow measurement of trough drug levels. Patients need to know not to take additional drugs without prior discussion with the transplant unit because of the risk of drug interactions.

The recently transplanted kidney often takes several weeks to acquire the ability to regulate urine concentration adequately, and patients will often be discharged during a polyuric phase with high volume, low concentration urine. They need to understand the importance of identifying and reacting to developing fluid depletion (or overload) which can be most accurately anticipated after discharge by asking patients to check a daily weight and adjust their salt and water intake accordingly. Recipients who were oliguric or anuric prior to transplantation (especially if they have been on dialysis for many years) will often find it difficult to cope with the sudden switch from fluid restriction to having to drink several litres daily, often with associated reduced appetite and urinary frequency, and need to be warned about this.

Patients transplanted pre-emptively need to understand that the early post-discharge period will involve much more frequent hospital attendance with disruption to their day-to-day activities than they were experiencing in the pre-transplant period (those who were on dialysis when transplanted will be able to set this intensity of supervision off against the time they gain from being dialysis independent), but need to understand that early surveillance in the transplant clinic may be much less predictable and regular than dialysis treatments.

A clear and brief summary of the postoperative course, including whether graft function was immediate or delayed; details of any surgical complications, rejection episodes, or infections; and the patient's weight, graft function, and CNI trough levels at discharge, is necessary to ensure effective transfer of care to the transplant clinic.

Tips and Tricks: Five Common Mistakes and How to Avoid Them

1. Missing retroperitoneal haemorrhage

   Ultrasound is the main traditional form of imaging for the recent renal transplant, providing confirmation of graft perfusion, early (if non-specific) warning of problems from changes in resistive index, and identification of lymphocoeles and other surgically related fluid collections. It is not however a sensitive modality for the identification of retroperitoneal haemorrhage which, if progressive, can lead to pressure on the renal vessels (with associated risk of venous thrombosis or in extreme cases avulsion of the vascular anastomoses) or circumferential pressure on the graft itself with associated reduced function.

   In cases where the patient's Hb is dropping without an obvious reason, a CT scan with contrast is required to exclude significant haemorrhage around or behind the graft. This is not an easy request to submit because (especially in the context of delayed or suboptimal graft function) of the risk of nephrotoxicity from X-ray contrast.

Remember, contrast nephrotoxicity is a transient phenomenon; kidney transplant vein thrombosis is usually forever.

2. Failing to anticipate changes in Tacrolimus absorption

   Tacrolimus is absorbed throughout the GI tract (even from the oral mucosa, although this is not a reliable route). As well as first-pass metabolism in the liver, there is significant degradation of tacrolimus within small bowel mucosa, so that intercurrent events which prevent the drug from reaching the small intestine, or reduce the time it spends there, will lead to increased tacrolimus levels. Two common scenarios are:

   (i) A postoperative ileus following transplantation is associated with high tacrolimus levels due to reduced transit of the drug through to its sites of metabolism in the small bowel combined with efficient absorption from the gastric mucosa. This leads to reduction in the dose around postoperative day 4–5, just as the ileus is resolving. The patient then goes home about day 7 with tacrolimus levels which are falling sharply and is underdosed during the second post-transplant week, a period of high risk of acute cellular rejection in grafts undertaken without the cover of induction therapy.

   (ii) Diarrhoeal episodes are frequently associated with decreased tacrolimus breakdown (due to reduced exposure to the small intestinal mucosa combined with efficient absorption within the large intestine). When combined with the metabolic consequences of intravascular volume depletion, this may commonly present with significant hyperkalaemia (overriding the effects of gastrointestinal K^+ loss) and significant graft dysfunction.

   Cyclosporin is predominantly absorbed from the small intestine and is less prone to these effects than tacrolimus.

3. Not knowing important interactions with Calcineurin inhibitors

   Calcineurin inhibitors (cyclosporin and tacrolimus) have a narrow therapeutic index and are principally metabolised by the cytochrome P450 3A4 enzymes, and drugs which affect this system can significantly alter blood levels.

   The commonest interactions leading to high levels and toxicity are from CYP 3A inhibition by macrolide antibiotics (especially erythromycin, with clarithromycin exerting a smaller but still significant effect), azole antifungal agents (most commonly fluconazole), and the now rarely prescribed Cimetidine. There is a clinically significant effect of co-administration of CNI's with grapefruit juice (presumably via inhibition of enteric CYP3A4).

   Less commonly, reduction in CNI levels can follow induction of cytochrome P450 by phenytoin, carbamazepine, or rifampicin.

4. Overfilling the recipient with delayed graft function

   Delayed graft function is not a life-threatening complication of transplantation. Fluid overload in a renal patient, who may well have impaired cardiac performance commonly due to coronary vascular disease or chronic uraemic myocardial dysfunction (often diastolic ventricular relaxation impairment), rapidly results in pulmonary oedema which is life-threatening and in this context will require dialysis/ultrafiltration as an emergency which is always best avoided postoperatively. Less medically concerning, although uncomfortable for the recipient, is severe peripheral tissue salt and water accumulation as a result of overenthusiastic fluid administration in pursuit of a reassuringly high initial urine volume.

5. Failure to react fast enough to sudden oligoanuria

   The first rule of thumb is always get a US as it rarely proves unhelpful and often is reassuring if not diagnostic.

   (i) Obstruction.

   (ii) Antibody-mediated rejection. Can be detected clinically with pain over the allograft and/or macroscopic haematuria. More prevalent in sensitised recipients (commonest causes of sensitisation being pregnancy and previous transplantation, particularly when retransplantation occurs across a repeat mismatch) and associated with graft loss as well as suboptimal outcomes both acute and chronically.

   (iii) Renal artery or vein thrombosis. A relatively rare but highly important cause of allograft loss and more commonly seen in those with a prothrombotic tendency (be wary if arteriovenous access for dialysis has proved difficult to maintain or previous other thrombotic events occurred). Early anticoagulation is likely to be protective but this needs careful consideration and negotiation with the surgical team postoperatively. Often its presentation is dramatic with sudden anuria and only suspicion (with or without the assistance of a Doppler USS revealing reversed flow in diastole) may result in the correct management which is immediate surgical exploration and examination of the venous anastomosis.

References

1. NHS Blood and Transplant. Organ donation and transplantation. Activity report 2011/12. http://www.organdonation.nhs.uk/statistics/transplant_activity_report/current_activity_reports/ukt/activity_report_2011_12.pdf.
2. Siedlecki A, Irish W, Brennan DC. Delayed graft function in the kidney transplant. Am J Transplant. 2011;11(11):2279–96. PMID: 21929642.
3. Cravedi P, Kopp JB, Remuzzi G. Recent progress in the pathophysiology and treatment of FSGS recurrence. Am J Transplant. 2013;13(2):266–74. doi:10.1111/ajt.12045. PMID: 23312002.

4. Patel R, Terasaki PI. Significance of the positive crossmatch test in kidney transplantation. N Engl J Med. 1969;280(14):735–9. PMID: 4886455.
5. Gebel HM, Bray RA, Nickerson P. Pre-transplant assessment of donor-reactive. HLA-specific antibodies in renal transplantation: contraindication vs. risk. Am J Transplant. 2003;3(12):1488–500. PMID: 14629279.
6. Tait BD, Süsal C, Gebel HM, Nickerson PW, Zachary AA, Claas FH, Reed EF, Bray RA, Campbell P, Chapman JR, Coates PT, Colvin RB, Cozzi E, Doxiadis II, Fuggle SV, Gill J, Glotz D, Lachmann N, Mohanakumar T, Suciu-Foca N, Sumitran-Holgersson S, Tanabe K, Taylor CJ, Tyan DB, Webster A, Zeevi A, Opelz G. Consensus guidelines on the testing and clinical management issues associated with HLA and non-HLA antibodies in transplantation. Transplantation. 2013;95(1):19–47. PMID: 23238534.
7. Amico P, Hönger G, Bielmann D, Lutz D, Garzoni D, Steiger J, Mihatsch MJ, Dragun D, Schaub S. Incidence and prediction of early antibody-mediated rejection due to non-human leukocyte antigen-antibodies. Transplantation. 2008;85(11):1557–63. PMID: 18551059.
8. Taylor CJ, Kosmoliaptsis V, Summers DM, Bradley JA. Back to the future: application of contemporary technology to long-standing questions about the clinical relevance of human leukocyte antigen-specific alloantibodies in renal transplantation. Hum Immunol. 2009;70(8):563–8. PMID: 19445992.
9. TA85 immunosuppressive therapy for renal transplantation in adults. National Institute for Health and Clinical Excellence (NICE) 2004. http://guidance.nice.org.uk/TA85/Guidance/pdf/English.
10. Nankivell BJ, Borrows RJ, Fung CL, O'Connell PJ, Allen RD, Chapman JR. The natural history of chronic allograft nephropathy. N Engl J Med. 2003;349(24):2326–33. PMID: 14668458.
11. Srinivas TR, Schold JD, Guerra G, Eagan A, Bucci CM, Meier-Kriesche HU. Mycophenolate mofetil/sirolimus compared to other common immunosuppressive regimens in kidney transplantation. Am J Transplant. 2007;7(3):586–94. PMID: 17229066.
12. Pirsch JD, Miller J, Deierhoi MH, Vincenti F, Filo RS. A comparison of tacrolimus (FK506) and cyclosporine for immunosuppression after cadaveric renal transplantation. FK506 Kidney Transplant Study Group. Transplantation. 1997;63(7):977–83.
13. Vincenti F, Jensik SC, Filo RS, Miller J, Pirsch J. A long-term comparison of tacrolimus (FK506) and cyclosporine in kidney transplantation: evidence for improved allograft survival at five years. Transplantation. 2002;73(5):775–82. PMID: 11907427.
14. Ekberg H, Tedesco-Silva H, Demirbas A, Vítko S, Nashan B, Gürkan A, Margreiter R, Hugo C, Grinyó JM, Frei U, Vanrenterghem Y, Daloze P, HalloranDaloze PF, ELITE-Symphony Study. Reduced exposure to calcineurin inhibitors in renal transplantation. N Engl J Med. 2007;357(25):2562–75. PMID: 18094377.
15. Halloran P, Mathew T, Tomlanovich S, Groth C, Hooftman L, Barker C. Mycophenolate mofetil in renal allograft recipients: a pooled efficacy analysis of three randomized, double-blind, clinical studies in prevention of rejection. The International Mycophenolate Mofetil Renal Transplant Study Groups. Transplantation. 1997;63(1):39–47. PMID: 9000658.
16. Mathew TH. A blinded, long-term, randomized multicenter study of mycophenolate mofetil in cadaveric renal transplantation: results at three years. Tricontinental Mycophenolate Mofetil Renal Transplantation Study Group. Transplantation. 1998;65(11): 1450–4. PMID: 9645801.
17. Kahan BD. Efficacy of sirolimus compared with azathioprine for reduction of acute renal allograft rejection: a randomised multicentre study. The Rapamune US Study Group. Lancet. 2000;356(9225):194–202. PMID: 10963197.
18. MacDonald AS, RAPAMUNE Global Study Group. A worldwide, phase III, randomized, controlled, safety and efficacy study of a sirolimus/cyclosporine regimen for prevention of acute rejection in recipients of primary mismatched renal allografts. Transplantation. 2001;71(2):271–80.
19. Alangaden GJ, Thyagarajan R, Gruber SA, Morawski K, Garnick J, El-Amm JM, West MS, Sillix DH, Chandrasekar PH, Haririan A. Infectious complications after kidney transplantation: current epidemiology and associated risk factors. Clin Transplant. 2006;20(4):401–9. PMID: 16842513.
20. Kasiske BL, Chakkera HA, Louis TA, Ma JZ. A meta-analysis of immunosuppression withdrawal trials in renal transplantation. J Am Soc Nephrol. 2000;11(10):1910–7. PMID: 11004223.
21. Borrows R, Chan K, Loucaidou M, Lawrence C, Van Tromp J, Cairns T, Griffith M, Hakim N, McLean A, Palmer A, Papalois V, Taube D. Five years of steroid sparing in renal transplantation with tacrolimus and mycophenolate mofetil. Transplantation. 2006;81(1):125–8. PMID: 16421488.
22. Woodle ES, Peddi VR, Tomlanovich S, Mulgaonkar S, Kuo PC, TRIMS Study Investigators. A prospective, randomized, multicenter study evaluating early corticosteroid withdrawal with Thymoglobulin in living-donor kidney transplantation. Clin Transplant. 2010;24(1):73–83.
23. Dalton RS, Webber JN, Cameron C, Kessaris N, Gibbs PG, Tan LC, Walters MA, Sadek SA, Datta AK. Physiologic impact of low-dose dopamine on renal function in the early post renal transplant period. Transplantation. 2005;79(11):1561–7. PMID: 15940046.
24. Grundmann R, Kindler J, Meider G, Stöwe H, Sieberth HG, Pichlmaier H. Dopamine treatment of human cadaver kidney graft recipients: a prospectively randomized trial. Klin Wochenschr. 1982;60(4):193–7. PMID: 7040782.
25. Andrés A, Budde K, Clavien PA, Becker T, Kessler M, Pisarski P, Fornara P, Burmeister D, Hené RJ, Cassuto-Viguier E, SENIOR Study Team. A randomized trial comparing renal function in older kidney transplant patients following delayed versus immediate tacrolimus administration. Transplantation. 2009;88(9):1101–8. PMID: 19898206.
26. Wilson CH, Brook NR, Gok MA, Asher JF, Nicholson ML, Talbot D. Randomized clinical trial of daclizumab induction and delayed introduction of tacrolimus for recipients of non-heart-beating kidney transplants. Br J Surg. 2005;92(6):681–7. PMID: 15856479.
27. Ghisdal L, Broeders N, Wissing KM, Saidi A, Bensalem T, Mbaba Mena J, Lemy A, Wijns W, Pradier O, Hoang AD, Mikhalski D, Donckier V, Cochaux P, El Housni H, Abramowicz M, Vereerstraeten P, Abramowicz D. American Journal of Transplantation. 2010;10(1):99–105.
28. Robertson AJ, Nargund V, Gray DW, Morris PJ. Low dose aspirin as prophylaxis against renal-vein thrombosis in renal-transplant recipients. Nephrol Dial Transplant. 2000;15(11):1865–8. PMID: 11071979.
29. Williams WW, Taheri D, Tolkoff-Rubin N, Colvin RB. Clinical role of the renal transplant biopsy. Nat Rev Nephrol. 2012;8(2):110–21. PMID: 22231130.
30. Mengel M, Sis B, Haas M, Colvin RB, Halloran PF, Racusen LC, Solez K, Cendales L, Demetris AJ, Drachenberg CB, Farver CF, Rodriguez ER, Wallace WD, Glotz D, Banff meeting report writing committee. Banff 2011 Meeting report: new concepts in antibody-mediated rejection. Am J Transplant. 2012;12(3):563–70.
31. Solez K, Colvin RB, Racusen LC, Haas M, Sis B, Mengel M, Halloran PF, Baldwin W, Banfi G, Collins AB, Cosio F, David DS, Drachenberg C, Einecke G, Fogo AB, Gibson IW, Glotz D, Iskandar SS, Kraus E, Lerut E, Mannon RB, Mihatsch M, Nankivell BJ, Nickeleit V, Papadimitriou JC, Randhawa P, Regele H, Renaudin K, Roberts I, Seron D, Smith RN, Valente M. Banff 07 classification of renal allograft pathology: updates and future directions. Am J Transplant. 2008;8(4):753–60. PMID: 17352710.
32. Willicombe M, Roufosse C, Brookes P, Galliford JW, McLean AG, Dorling A, Warrens AN, Cook TH, Cairns TD, Taube D. Antibody-

mediated rejection after alemtuzumab induction: incidence, risk factors, and predictors of poor outcome. Transplantation. 2011;92(2):176–82. PMID: 21637139.

33. Paoletti E, Bellino D, Marsano L, Cassottana P, Rolla D, Ratto E. Effects of ACE inhibitors on long-term outcome of renal transplant recipients: a randomized controlled trial. Transplantation. 2013;95(6):889–95. PMID:23380881.

34. Ponticelli C, Glassock RJ. Posttransplant recurrence of primary glomerulonephritis. Clin J Am Soc Nephrol. 2010;5(12):2363–72. PMID: 21030574.

Immunosuppression for Kidney Transplantation

70

Iain A.M. MacPhee

General Principles

Acute rejection tends to occur during the first 3 months after transplantation and is uncommon later than this, unless compliance is poor or immunosuppressive therapy is reduced excessively. This drives the general principle of more intensive immunosuppression during the early period after transplantation with minimisation in the longer term to reduce toxicity but aiming to effectively suppress chronic rejection. The allograft response is mediated by immune mechanisms designed to clear intracellular pathogens. Inhibition of this response was never going to come at no expense. The main complications of the immunosuppressed state are caused by direct infection with intracellular pathogens, most commonly viruses, and virally induced malignancy.

Therapeutic Drug Monitoring (TDM)

The immunosuppressive drugs all have a narrow therapeutic index with wide variation between individuals in the blood concentration achieved by a given dose. This has led to routine use of TDM for the calcineurin inhibitors and mTOR inhibitors while use for mycophenolate is controversial. Area under the concentration-time curve (AUC) predicts efficacy. The correct term for quantity of drugs in blood is 'concentration' rather than 'level' (see Aronson, *BMJ* for an erudite explanation of this issue) [1]. The usual sample required is EDTA-anticoagulated blood to allow assay in whole blood or plasma. Clinicians should know which assay their laboratory uses to measure drug concentrations and understand the performance characteristics. Assays based on high-performance liquid chromatography (HPLC) tend to give less variable results than immunoassays and only measure the parent drug, while some immunoassays also measure cross-reacting metabolites. In general, it is easier to set up a system for same-day reporting of results using an immunoassay where samples are processed in parallel rather than in sequence. Initial setup costs are higher for HPLC and running costs are higher for immunoassay.

I.A.M. MacPhee, DPhil, FRCP
Division of Clinical Sciences: Renal Medicine,
St. George's, University of London, Cranmer Terrace,
London SW17 0RE, UK
e-mail: imacphee@sgul.ac.uk

Generic Immunosuppression

Recently, the patents for a number of the widely used immunosuppressive drugs have expired leading to the availability of less costly generic preparations. Regulatory approval for generic drugs requires single dose bioequivalence studies in normal human volunteers with no requirement for testing in renal transplant recipients. The generic preparations are not tested for bioequivalence to each other, and patients should not be sequentially changed from one preparation to another as this may lead to fluctuations in drug exposure. The calcineurin inhibitors should be prescribed by brand. This is less of an issue for the other generic drugs with the exception of ensuring that mycophenolate mofetil and enteric-coated mycophenolate sodium are not interchanged.

Specific Drugs

An excellent review on the immunosuppressive drugs is provided in Ref. [2].

Induction Agents

The term induction agent is used for therapeutic antibodies given to most patients around the time of the transplant when the risk of rejection is greatest. These agents either block cell receptors (non-lytic induction) or deplete cells (lytic induction).

M. Harber (ed.), *Practical Nephrology*,
DOI 10.1007/978-1-4471-5547-8_70, © Springer-Verlag London 2014

Anti-CD25 Antibody

The reduction in incidence of acute rejection without an increase in the infectious complication rate when the CD25 antibodies were introduced is almost unique in the development of immunosuppression, although it is less clear whether this translates into improved long-term outcome [3]. Basiliximab, the only currently available drug in this class, is a chimeric antibody that binds to the alpha chain of the interleukin-2 (IL-2) receptor which is only expressed on activated T-lymphocytes. Two doses of 20 mg are given intravenously, prior to revascularisation of the transplant and then 4 days later. There is concern that generation of human anti-chimeric antibody (HACA) precludes the reuse of basiliximab in subsequent transplants, but there are no strong supporting data for this view. Basiliximab is not an effective treatment for acute rejection.

Lytic Induction

Polyclonal Anti-T-Lymphocyte Antibodies

Antithymocyte globulin (ATG) is produced by immunisation of rabbits with human thymocytes and anti-lymphocyte globulin (ALG) in horses immunised with human lymphocytes. The resulting immunoglobulin preparations have a broad range of specificities and deplete most haematopoietic cells. They also contain antibody to intercellular adhesion molecules that may explain the observed inhibition of ischaemia-reperfusion injury, although this has not been shown to translate into improved transplant outcome. ATG and ALG are effective agents for both induction and the treatment of severe or steroid-resistant acute rejection. They are potently immunosuppressive with increased incidence of infectious and malignant complications. Exposure to these foreign proteins can generate anaphylactic reactions and neutralising antibodies that preclude redosing with the same agent, as well as serum sickness 1–2 weeks following reexposure. Cross-linking of cellular receptors after the first dose can activate cells prior to lysis causing cytokine release syndrome which can be minimised by giving intravenous steroid and antihistamine prior to the first dose and infusing the ATG slowly over at least 6 h.

For induction therapy with ATG, 1–1.5 mg/kg/day is infused intravenously for 3–9 days after transplantation and 1.5 mg/kg/day for 7–14 days to treat acute rejection, based on ideal rather than actual weight. Infusion through a central venous cannula is recommended, but a large peripheral vein is an acceptable alternative. A 0.22 μm in-line filter should be used to remove particulate material. Therapy is best monitored by the extent of depletion of CD3-positive peripheral blood lymphocytes (T lymphocytes). The normal range is 1–30 cells/μL with a suggested algorithm for pre-dose count: <10 cells/μL, omit dose; 10–20 cells/μL, 50 % usual dose; and >20 cells/μL, full dose. In the event of severe haematological toxicity: platelet count $<50\times10^9$/L or white blood cell count $<2\times10^9$/L omit dose and platelet count $50–75\times10^9$/L or white blood cell count $2–3\times10^9$/L give 50 % usual dose [4]. Mycophenolate or azathioprine may need to be discontinued during ATG treatment to avoid severe haematological toxicity.

Alemtuzumab

Alemtuzumab (previously known as Campath-1H) is a humanised monoclonal antibody specific for CD52 that causes sustained depletion of a broad spectrum of peripheral blood mononuclear cells including T and B lymphocytes and natural killer (NK) cells. Low rates of acute rejection and low financial cost have driven widespread use. Peripheral blood lymphocyte counts take between 3 months and 1 year to return to normal. A single intravenous dose of 30 mg delivered lower rates of acute rejection than basiliximab in low immunological risk patients treated with tacrolimus and mycophenolate and early steroid withdrawal (5 % vs 17 % $p<0.001$ at 1 year) balanced by increased incidence of infection. Efficacy and safety in high-risk patients were equivalent to ATG [5]. Subcutaneous administration reduces the risk of cytokine release syndrome. Late episodes of acute rejection beyond the initial 3-month period are more frequent in alemtuzumab-based regimens than with other induction agents. Planned follow-up schedules need to take account of this to avoid late diagnosis of episodes of acute rejection. Antibody-mediated autoimmunity, including haemolytic anaemia, thrombocytopaenia and hyperthyroidism, is a rare complication of alemtuzumab therapy. There are some data to suggest an increased propensity to antibody-mediated rejection in alemtuzumab-treated patients, perhaps suggesting loss of regulation of B lymphocytes.

Rituximab

Rituximab, a chimeric monoclonal antibody specific for CD20 that depletes B lymphocytes but not plasma cells, has been used primarily as an induction agent in antibody-incompatible transplantation. Typically, a single dose of 375 mg/m^2 given 2–4 weeks before transplantation results in depletion of circulating B lymphocytes for 6–9 months without significant hypogammaglobulinaemia [6]. Rituximab given at the time of transplantation has no impact on acute rejection. Use in heavily immunosuppressed patients leads to increased incidence of infectious complications including the rare but serious progressive multifocal leucoencephalopathy [7]. Binding of rituximab to B lymphocytes can cause a false-positive B-cell lymphocytotoxic or flow cytometry crossmatch which can be overcome by removing the CD20 antibody with pronase.

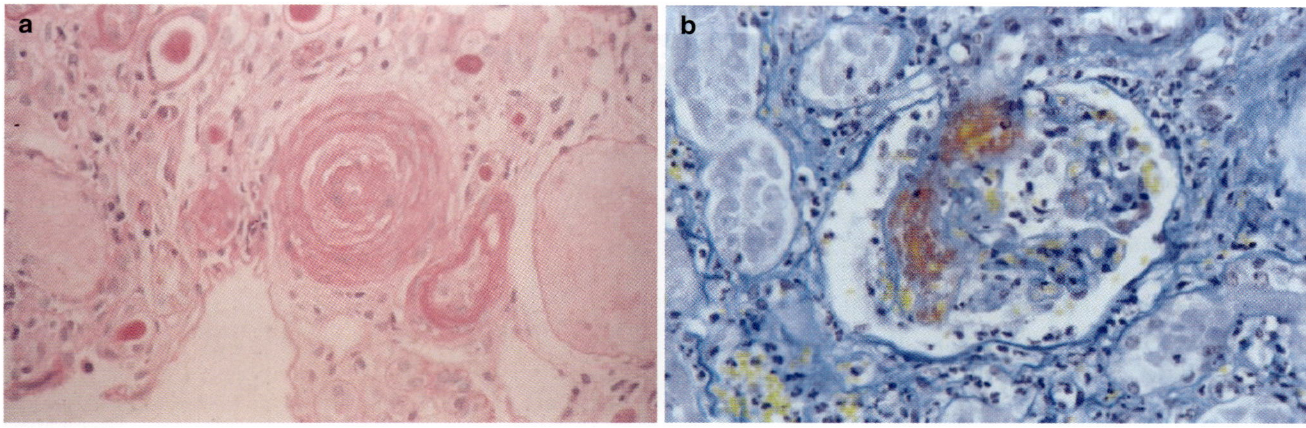

Fig. 70.1 (**a**) Severe arteriopathy in a patient with sustained high blood concentrations of ciclosporin. (**b**) Showing a glomerulus with thrombosis in the capillary loops

MuromonabCD3 (OKT-3)

This murine monoclonal antibody to the CD3 component of the T-lymphocyte receptor complex activates and then depletes T lymphocytes often causing severe cytokine release syndrome with pulmonary oedema. It is an extremely effective immunosuppressant with a consequent high incidence of infectious and malignant complications that has led to a decline in use. A typical regimen would be 5 mg daily given intravenously for 7–14 days, monitored as described above for ATG [8].

Small Molecule Drugs (Maintenance Immunosuppression)

Calcineurin Inhibitors

The calcineurin inhibitors (CNI), ciclosporin and tacrolimus, are the mainstay of most current immunosuppressive regimens. Toxicity, in particular nephrotoxicity, has led to a widespread aspiration to avoid CNIs, but their effective control of early acute rejection has maintained their place in the absence of equally effective alternatives. They bind to intracellular proteins, cyclophilin for ciclosporin and FK-binding protein 12 for tacrolimus, and the resultant complex inhibits the phosphatase calcineurin that is required to activate the transcription factor nuclear factor of activated T lymphocytes (NF-AT). Inhibition of NF-AT blocks the production of IL-2. Tacrolimus has generally been found to be more effective than ciclosporin in preventing rejection, but there are published studies showing equal efficacy to microemulsion ciclosporin. Nephrotoxicity is manifest both as a reversible renal vasospastic response without histological change that may be ameliorated by the co-prescription of calcium channel blockers and a more chronic arteriopathy (Fig. 70.1a) with renal fibrosis. Acute tubular toxicity may be manifest as tubular vacuolation, and haemolytic uraemic syndrome can develop secondary to CNIs (and mTOR inhibitors) (Fig. 70.1b). The CNIs are probably equally nephrotoxic. While it might be considered logical, delayed introduction of CNI in patients with delayed graft function does not improve outcomes [9]. The CNIs are diabetogenic, tacrolimus more so than ciclosporin with approximately twofold higher incidence of new-onset diabetes after transplantation (NODAT) [10].

The CNIs are metabolised in the enterocyte and liver by the oxidative enzymes cytochrome P450 (CYP) 3A4 and 3A5 with metabolites excreted in bile and are transported by P-glycoprotein (P-gp) encoded by the *ABCB1* gene (previously known as *MDR1*). Oral bioavailability is only 25–30 %, in part due to the active barrier to drug absorption formed by drug metabolism and transport out of the enterocyte [11]. As a consequence, equivalent exposure when given intravenously requires 30 % of the oral dose for ciclosporin and 20 % for tacrolimus. Inhibitors of these proteins, e.g. macrolide antibiotics (erythromycin, clarithromycin) and imidazole antifungals (fluconazole, ketoconazole), increase the oral bioavailability by approximately twofold. Inducers of CYP and P-gp, e.g. rifampicin, carbamazepine and phenytoin, reduce CNI exposure. If possible, interacting drugs should be avoided. If their use is essential, a 50 % change in CNI dose with careful monitoring and return to the original dose on stopping therapy usually maintains blood concentrations in the therapeutic range. Patients taking CNIs should avoid grapefruit which significantly inhibits CYP3A leading to increased CNI exposure. This advice on interacting agents also applies to the mTOR inhibitors (see below).

Ciclosporin

Ciclosporin was initially formulated in corn oil as Sandimmun™ with subsequent development of microemulsion preparations such as Neoral™ (confusingly branded as Sandimmun Neoral™ in some countries) to reduce variability

Table 70.1 Algorithms for calculating AUC for MPA from blood samples collected at 0, 0.5 and 2 h after drug administration

1. For fasted adults on MMF + tacrolimus:	
$AUC = 7.75 + 6.49 \times C0 + 0.76 \times C0.5 + 2.43 \times C2$	$r^2 = 0.862$
2. For fasted adults on MMF + CsA:	
$AUC = 11.34 + 3.1 \times C0 + 1.102 \times C0.5 + 1.909 \times C2$	$r^2 = 0.752$
3. For not fasted paediatric patients on MMF and tacrolimus:	
$AUC = 10.01391 + 3.94791 \times C0 + 3.24253 \times C0.5 + 1.0108 \times C2$	$r^2 = 0.800$
4. For fasted paediatric patients on MMF and CsA:	
$AUC = 18.609 + 4.309 \times C0 + 0.536 \times C0.5 + 2.148 \times C2$	$r^2 = 0.72$

Algorithms used in the FDCC study [26]

weekly during the first month of treatment, twice monthly during the second and third months and then monthly throughout the first year. Dose reduction should be considered when the white blood cell count falls below 4×10^9/L or platelets below 100×10^9/L.

Azathioprine

While azathioprine has been largely superseded by mycophenolate for de novo transplants, it remains a well-tested and useful agent. Azathioprine is a prodrug that is metabolised to the purine analogue 6-mercaptopurine that inhibits DNA synthesis inhibiting the proliferation of rapidly dividing cells. There is also inhibition of intracellular signalling via the CD28 co-stimulatory pathway [27]. In the early post-transplant period, mycophenolate is more effective than azathioprine in preventing acute rejection, but longer-term benefit is less clear. Azathioprine offers a well-tolerated, once daily treatment option after the immediate post-transplant period. The primary toxicities are dose-dependent myelosuppression and idiosyncratic hepatotoxicity. Full blood count and liver blood tests should be monitored weekly for at least the first 4 weeks after initiation followed by a reduced frequency but not less than every 3 months. Dose reduction should be considered with white blood cell counts below 4×10^9/L or platelets below 100×10^9/L or evidence of hepatic injury.

Azathioprine is well absorbed orally with no need to adjust the dose for intravenous administration. Azathioprine is metabolised by 6-thiopurine-S-methyltransferase (TPMT). 6-Mercaptopurine has a short half-life of 38–114 min, but the 6-thioguanine nucleotides persist in the tissues allowing once daily dosing. A typical initial daily dose is 1–3 mg/kg body weight with dose adjusted according to toxicity. One in 300 individuals carry homozygous mutant alleles for the TPMT gene resulting in loss of enzyme activity and accumulation of azathioprine leading to toxicity [28]. In some specialties, testing for erythrocyte TPMT content (avoiding assay within 30–60 days of blood transfusion) or genotyping for mutant alleles has become standard practice prior to initiating azathioprine treatment. This practice has not been adopted widely for transplantation, possibly due to very close monitoring around the time of starting treatment that allows timely dose reductions in response to haematological toxicity. Measurement of azathioprine in blood is not useful, but measurement of 6-thioguanine nucleotides has been used for TDM.

One of the most important drug interactions in immunosuppressed patients is the inhibition of metabolism of azathioprine by allopurinol used to treat gout, a common complication in renal transplant recipients. While some would advocate the use of low-dose azathioprine in this situation, avoidance of the combination is the safest option with use of mycophenolate in patients with gout.

Leflunomide

Leflunomide is an orally active pyrimidine synthesis inhibitor with a long elimination half-life that is licensed for treatment of rheumatoid arthritis. A derivative FK-778 was tested in renal transplant recipients and found to have equivalent efficacy to mycophenolate but development was discontinued. Leflunomide has activity against BK polyomavirus, offering an option in refractory cases [29].

Mammalian Target of Rapamycin (mTOR) Inhibitors

The mTOR inhibitors (sirolimus and everolimus) inhibit a transcription factor that is at a pivotal point in a number of intracellular signalling pathways including the response of T-lymphocytes to cytokines and pro-fibrotic processes such as wound healing. They come with the advantages of not being nephrotoxic or causing hypertension but do seem to be as diabetogenic as tacrolimus. Medium-term (3–5 years) graft function and histological changes on protocol biopsy were better in sirolimus- than in ciclosporin-treated patients [30]. They are less potent than CNIs in de novo patients. They bind to the same immunophilin, FKBP-12, as tacrolimus but do not compete functionally with tacrolimus, as was initially feared would be the case. This is a difficult class of agent to use due to tolerability with 30 % of patients in most trials of sirolimus discontinuing the drug due to toxicity. They are metabolised by CYP3A4 and CYP3A5, so the advice on interacting drugs provided for the CNIs also applies to the mTOR inhibitors.

Sirolimus

Sirolimus, previously known as rapamycin, has a long elimination half-life of around 60 h that may be perceived as a benefit in allowing once daily dosing with simplicity potentially improving compliance. A counter argument is that achieving steady state after a dose change takes several days and leads to slow response to TDM. The half-life in children is much shorter (closer to 10 h), and twice daily dosing may be appropriate. While sirolimus is not nephrotoxic itself, inhibition of P-gp enhances entry of the CNIs to renal tubular epithelial cells, potentiating CNI nephrotoxicity [31]. Although not directly nephrotoxic, the antiproliferative activity of the mTOR inhibitors delays recovery from acute tubular necrosis, so they are not an ideal agent in patients with delayed graft function.

Most patients become hyperlipidaemic due to changes in lipid distribution. While it is uncertain whether this confers increased atherosclerotic risk, it is likely to trigger prescription of lipid-lowering treatment. Haematological toxicity including thrombocytopaenia and anaemia is common, particularly in patients taking another antiproliferative agent. Proteinuria is often exacerbated, probably through inhibition of vascular endothelial growth factor (VEGF), and mTOR inhibitors should be avoided when 24-h urinary protein exceeds 800 g [32]. Mouth ulcers, rashes and ankle oedema are common. Mouth ulcers probably occur more frequently in patients not on steroid treatment. Dose reduction and topical dental steroid paste can help with healing. Severely disabling lymphoedema is a rare complication that does not always resolve on drug discontinuation. Pneumonitis is a rare but serious complication presenting with dyspnoea, dry cough, fever or generalised fatigue that can mimic a number of other opportunistic infections or malignancy leading to delayed diagnosis. mTOR inhibitors should be avoided in individuals with pre-existing lung disease where the incidence is increased. Late switch and significantly impaired renal function have also been identified as risk factors for pneumonitis. Typical investigation findings are bronchiolitis obliterans, organising pneumonia and lymphocytic alveolitis. Diagnosis is based on a high index of suspicion with thoracic CT scanning and possibly bronchoscopy to confirm the diagnosis. Pneumonitis usually resolves on drug discontinuation, and it is best to discontinue mTOR inhibitors in patients with respiratory pathology of uncertain aetiology [33]. Reduced fertility in both sexes has been reported.

The therapeutic range for sirolimus, 24 h post-dose (trough), measured in whole blood is probably 10–15 ng/mL during the first 3 months after transplantation and then 5–10 ng/mL [34]. The high rate of acute rejection for sirolimus-treated patients in the Symphony study suggests that a target of 4–8 ng/mL is insufficient for de novo patients [13]. *CYP3A5* expressers have reduced exposure to sirolimus but not everolimus [35] which may explain the higher sirolimus dose requirement in Black patients.

Everolimus

Everolimus was derived from sirolimus by conjugation of a 2-hydroxyethyl group resulting in a molecule with a shorter elimination half-life of 18–35 h requiring twice daily dosing. While there are suggestions from clinical trials that tolerability may be better than for sirolimus, this may just reflect lower target drug exposure (whole blood 12 h after dosing trough concentration 3–8 ng/mL), and it would be anticipated that it will share the benefits and problems of sirolimus. While the European license for sirolimus indicates use instead of a CNI, clinical trials with everolimus aim to use it with low-dose CNI.

The Place of mTOR Inhibitors in the Immunosuppressive Regimen

Use in de novo renal transplant recipients without a CNI has fallen from favour due to increased rate of acute rejection when compared to CNI-based regimens and impaired wound healing, particularly in obese patients, and increased incidence of lymphoceles [34].

Alternative strategies involve de novo use of low-dose mTOR inhibitor along with a CNI or initial use of a CNI with later switch to an mTOR inhibitor. The optimal time to switch from CNI to mTOR inhibitor is probably between 6 weeks and 6 months after transplantation as late conversion, beyond 1 year after transplantation, does not result in improved renal function [36]. An abrupt switch from CNI to mTOR inhibitor reduces the risk of infection due to overimmunosuppression noted in early studies where the therapies were overlapped. Consideration should be given to discontinuing mTOR inhibitors prior to elective surgery and substituting a CNI, followed by reinstatement after 6 weeks to allow wound healing.

Incidence of malignancy is reduced by treatment with sirolimus. Treatment with sirolimus often causes regression of Kaposi's sarcoma [37] and reduces the rate of recurrence of non-melanoma skin cancer [38]. This is probably the immunosuppressive class of choice in patients with previous malignancy. The mTOR inhibitors inhibit

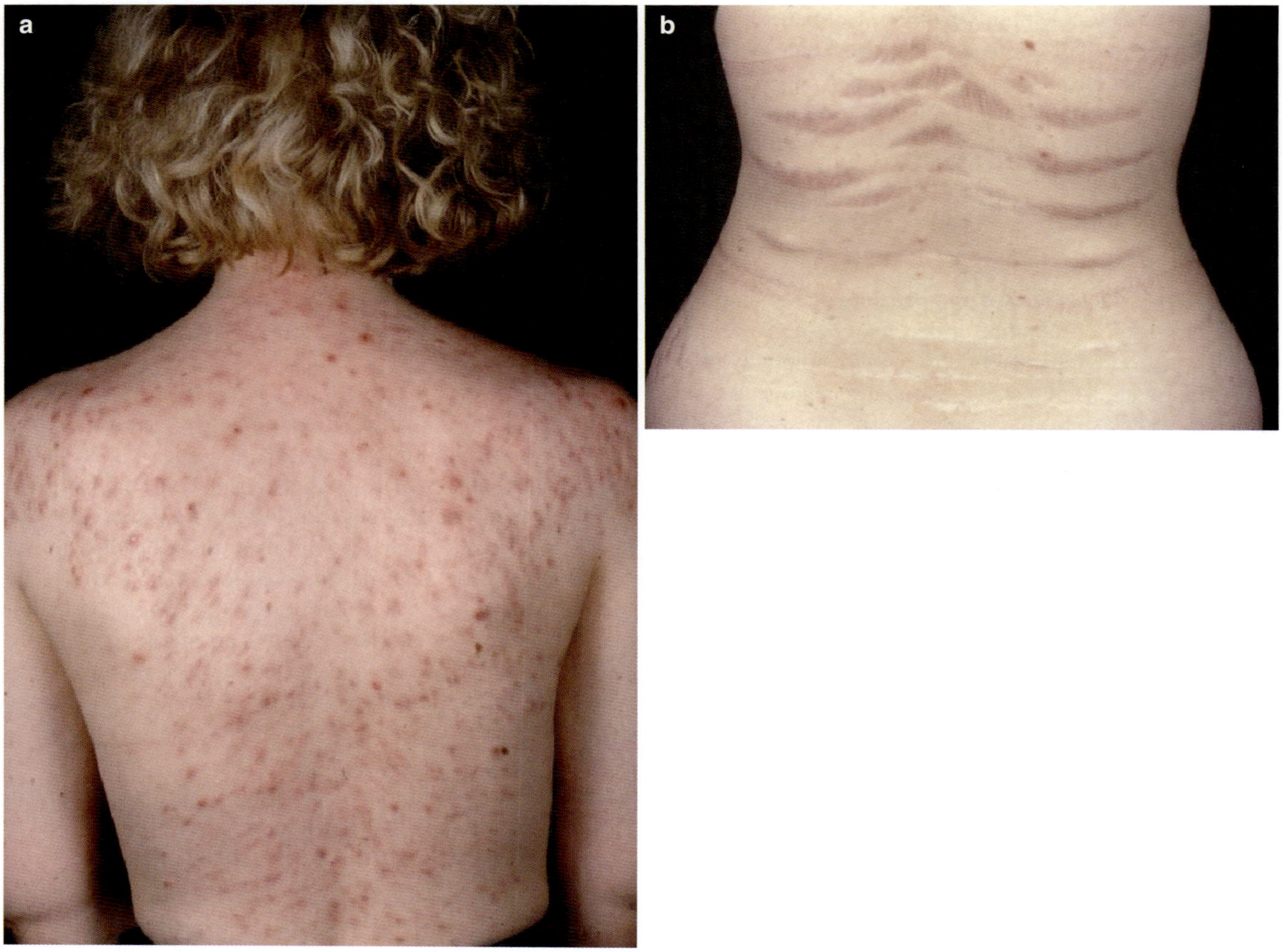

Fig. 70.6 (**a**) Extensive acne eruption in a patient on steroids. (**b**) Striae following high-dose oral steroids

cyst growth in patients with autosomal dominant polycystic kidney disease, in particular the growth of hepatic cysts which may be helpful in patients suffering significant symptoms due to mass effect [39].

Corticosteroids

Corticosteroids are part of the physiological mechanism to control inflammation and reduce the risk of autoimmunity in times of stress or trauma. As such, corticosteroids have a broad spectrum of anti-inflammatory and immunosuppressive activity that inhibits the innate immune response to ischaemia-reperfusion injury in the peri-transplant period. Data from steroid withdrawal studies suggest that steroids may help to control chronic rejection, perhaps by regulating the response to episodic inflammatory stimuli such as infection. The wide-ranging toxicity of steroids has led to progressive reduction in their use over time. They have an adverse influence on cardiovascular risk factors, including glucose intolerance, hypertension, an adverse impact on lipid profile and increased appetite predisposing to obesity. Osteoporosis, cosmetic effects due to redistribution of body fat and acne are feared by patients, and striae commonly cause long-term cosmetic distress (Fig. 70.6).

Administration of steroid in the morning rather than in the evening can reduce the tendency to sleep disturbance when high doses are given. Most immunosuppressive regimens include a bolus of high-dose intravenous steroid at the time of transplantation followed by oral prednisolone. In a study of steroid minimisation with the aim of reducing the risk of NODAT, there was only a statistically significant reduction in the group given no steroid, including omission of the intravenous bolus at the time of surgery and not in the group where steroid was discontinued after day 7, and this came at the expense of an increased rate of acute rejection [40]. When steroids were withdrawn after 7 days in tacrolimus-treated patients, fewer patients required insulin therapy, but there was no difference in the overall incidence of NODAT and there was more acute rejection [41].

Prednisolone is well absorbed with maximum blood concentration at 1–2 h after dosing and an elimination half-life of 2.5–4.5 h. The current standard maintenance dose of prednisolone is 5 mg once daily, which is only marginally higher than what would be considered replacement for physiological glucocorticoid requirement. This does raise the question as to whether a meaningful therapeutic effect is being delivered. However, prednisolone exposure in renal transplant recipients is up to 50 % greater for a given dose than in normal control subjects which may explain the apparent therapeutic effect of a 5 mg dose [42]. Enteric-coated prednisolone should be avoided as it has little impact on the risk of peptic ulceration and leads to reduced and unpredictable drug absorption. The following doses of other steroids have equivalent glucocorticoid effect to 5 mg prednisolone: hydrocortisone 20 mg, methylprednisolone 4 mg or dexamethasone 0.75 mg. A key point to remember in managing patients on long-term steroid therapy is the suppression of the hypothalamic-pituitary-adrenal axis. The steroid dose must be increased at times of physiological stress, including surgery.

Belatacept

Belatacept, a fusion protein between a modified CTLA4/CD152 molecule and a human immunoglobulin domain, blocks the co-stimulatory signal delivered to T-lymphocytes via CD28. Clinical trials testing it as an alternative agent to CNI in de novo renal transplant recipients found better renal function and less interstitial fibrosis with tubular atrophy in protocol biopsies than in ciclosporin-treated patients but at the expense of more acute rejection and post-transplant lymphoproliferative disorder (PTLD). Most of the patients with PTLD were Epstein-Barr virus naive leading to the recommendation to avoid belatacept in this patient group [43]. Provision of facilities for monthly intravenous infusions is an important consideration.

Choosing the Optimal Drug Combination

With the array of immunosuppressive drugs available, there will never be a clinical trial comparing all possible permutations, and a number of different approaches that may be equally effective are employed by different transplant centres. The most influential recent trial is the Symphony study which concluded that a regimen based on CD25 antibody induction, low-dose tacrolimus, mycophenolate and steroid was the most effective regimen on the basis of a low rate of acute rejection and the best preserved renal function when compared to similar regimens based on ciclosporin or sirolimus rather than tacrolimus. An important caveat that tends to be 'glossed over' in discussions of the study is that the low-dose tacrolimus group had significantly more NODAT than the other groups [13].

There are several important drug interactions between the immunosuppressive drugs. High-dose steroid therapy reduces the oral bioavailability of tacrolimus (and possibly ciclosporin but not sirolimus), most likely through induction of CYP3A. Tacrolimus dose may need to be increased during treatment for rejection to maintain therapeutic blood concentrations. It is sometimes necessary to reduce tacrolimus dose following steroid withdrawal. Ciclosporin but not tacrolimus increases sirolimus exposure. Sirolimus reduces tacrolimus exposure.

Treatment of Rejection

Acute T-Lymphocyte-Mediated Rejection

Most cases of T-lymphocyte-mediated acute cellular rejection (Banff grade I) respond to high-dose steroid. The route of administration does not impact on efficacy, but dyspeptic problems with oral regimens based on starting doses of 200 mg prednisolone daily have led to limited current use. The conventional dose of intravenous methylprednisolone is 500–1,000 mg daily for 3 days. There is no evidence that daily doses greater than 500 mg add any benefit but do carry the theoretical risk of increased toxicity. More severe rejection with vascular involvement (Banff grade II or III) is often treated with a more potent agent such as ATG. However, the evidence for this approach is lacking, and severe rejection is often steroid responsive. An alternative approach is to treat with steroid and reserve the more potent agent for biopsy-confirmed ongoing rejection after 5 days.

Acute Antibody-Mediated Rejection (AMR)

AMR is more challenging to treat than T-lymphocyte-mediated rejection. Treatment is aimed at removal of circulating donor-specific antibody and prevention of resynthesis. Most antibody removal regimens comprise plasma exchange and intravenous immunoglobulin (IVIG) [44]. Rituximab and ATG are used to deplete B lymphocytes aiming to prevent ongoing antibody secretion. Agents that specifically target antibody-secreting plasma cells have been a deficiency in the immunosuppressive armamentarium that has recently been addressed by the introduction of bortezomib with promising preliminary data on treatment of AMR. Eculizumab, an antibody to the C5 component of complement, inhibits formation of the membrane attack complex and has been effective in reversal of AMR but is extremely financially expensive.

Chronic Antibody-Mediated Rejection (CAMR)

There is no well-established treatment for CAMR. Deterioration in renal function may be slowed or prevented by optimising immunosuppression with tacrolimus,

1

18

19.

20.
1
3

71 Infectious Complications of Transplantation

Rhys Evans, Sanjay Bhagani, Tanzina Haque, and Mark Harber

Post-transplant infection is a common cause of graft deterioration, morbidity and mortality. It is also responsible for delayed discharge, multiple, often prolonged admissions and thus a significant clinical challenge. Infections can be donor derived, pre-existing in the recipient, nosocomial and opportunistic. For each of these categories, it is often possible to significantly reduce the hazard and thus the adverse consequences by first identifying patients at high risk. As always, clinical vigilance is vital, but equally important is the establishment of robust clinical systems for prevention, screening and rapid treatment.

Donor Infections

A variety of infections can be transmitted from the donor to the recipient of a kidney transplant with outcomes that range from mildly troublesome to fatal. To avoid this unpleasantness, transplant programmes institute a variety of screening procedures (see Table 71.1), but this screening is not watertight. Therefore, careful clinical assessment is critical and interpretation of risk is key; recipient serology is also crucial in assessing risk. Serum accompanies the donor organ and thus can be tested by the receiving unit for any serology felt to be relevant.

R. Evans, MBBS, MRCP (✉)
UCL Centre for Nephrology, Royal Free Hospital, Pond Street, London NW3 2QG, UK
e-mail: rhys.evans3@nhs.net

S. Bhagani, BSc (Hons), MBChB, FRCP (UK)
Department of Infectious Diseases/HIV Medicine, Royal Free Hospital, Pond Street, London NW3 2QG, UK
e-mail: s.bhagani@nhs.net

T. Haque, MBBS, PhD, FRCPath
Department of Virology, Royal Free Hospital, Pond Street, London NW3 2QG, UK
e-mail: thaque@nhs.net

M. Harber, MBBS, PhD, FRCP
UCL Department of Nephrology, Royal Free London NHS Foundation Trust, Pond Street, Hampstead, London NW3 2QG, UK
e-mail: mark.harber@nhs.net

M. Harber (ed.), *Practical Nephrology*,
DOI 10.1007/978-1-4471-5547-8_71, © Springer-Verlag London 2014

Recipient Infections Pre-transplant: Treatment, Vaccination and Prophylaxis

For the same infectious agent, there tends to be a hierarchy of virulence post-transplant with primary infections being worse than reinfections, which are more virulent than reactivations. Risk stratification is therefore highly important; identification and eradication or control of infection as well as vaccination pre-listing and appropriate prophylaxis post-transplant is not always done as well as it might be.

Table 71.2 shows infections that should be treated or controlled pre-transplant and vaccinations either recommended or to be considered on the grounds of common sense. In addition, non-specific clinical features such as unexplained splenomegaly, lymphadenopathy, persistently raised CRP, eosinophilia, polyclonal gammopathy (in the absence of autoimmunity) all need explaining before listing. In patients who have previously received high doses of immunosuppression or chemotherapy or in those with recurrent viral (e.g. herpes) or bacterial infections, it is important to check immunoglobulin levels and lymphocyte subsets. It is worth noting that immunosuppression post-transplant reduces seroconversion rates to around 50 % of that achieved by control patients, and the evidence suggests that a second dose of vaccine such as H1N1 offers no benefit [1]. Nonetheless, it is clear that vaccination has benefit, saves lives and should be built into any transplant programme [2]. Whenever possible vaccinations should be undertaken predialysis; in particular live or attenuated vaccines must be given before immunosuppression as cannot be given post-transplant.

There are several sets of guidelines recommending post-transplant prophylaxis, and Table 71.3 illustrates the main recommendations. As with pre-transplant vaccinations, units are frequently inconsistent about some areas of post-transplant prophylaxis such as TB prevention, culture of

Table 71.1 Donor screening

History of donor	At risk behaviour, country of origin and travel
History from donor hospital	Presenting illness (NB: beware undiagnosed meningoencephalitis or flaccid paralysis[a]), evidence of undiagnosed nosocomial infection (CRP, WBC), treated nosocomial infection (UTI, pneumonia, bacteraemia – virulent vs. non-virulent, antibiotic history and duration – discuss with microbiology in donor hospital if not clear). Blood cultures, MSU/CSU, respiratory viral PCR screen, line and wound swabs, post-mortem findings
CXR	Active consolidation (or previous TB). Review other imaging
Minilaparotomy	Mostly to exclude malignancy but also gross infection/lymph nodes
Perfusion fluid	Cheap and important test especially if virulent organism (e.g. candida or Staphylococcus aureus is cultured – may lead to mycotic aneurysm)
Viruses:	
1. HIV 1 and 2 Ab	Seroconversion window – HIV RNA not routinely available. Some HIV donors may be suitable for HIV recipients if infection is controlled and resistance history readily available
2. Hepatitis B surface and core Ab	Seroconversion window – hepatitis B DNA not routinely available
3. Hepatitis C Ab	Seroconversion window – hepatitis C RNA not routinely available potential donors for Hepatitis C recipients
4. HTLV 1 and 2 Ab	Proviral DNA or RNA not routinely available. NB: caution if Ab positive and signs of disease
5. CMV Ab	Routinely checked on all donors
6. EBV Ab	Not routinely done, assume >95 % adult donors positive (can be done at recipient centre)
7. HSV Ab	Not routinely done but essential if encephalitis (check for HSV DNA in CSF)
8. VZV Ab	Assume >95 % adult donors positive
9. HHV-8 Ab	Not routinely done, possible merit in donors from endemic regions (e.g. North African countries)
10. HHV-6 Ab	Not routinely done
11. BKV serology	Not routinely done, assume 70 % seropositive
12. West Nile virus (WNV)	Consider screening (nucleic acid testing) in endemic areas, especially if undiagnosed encephalitis
Bacteria:	
1. Syphilis serology	Old vs. current infection vs. yaws, if in doubt treat
2. Tuberculosis	Inferferon-gamma release assays rarely done on donors but worth considering in live donors if from endemic regions
Fungi:	
1. Histoplasmosis cruzi Ab	Consider in donors from endemic regions: Africa, Australia, Eastern Europe, North America
2. Coccidioides Ab	Consider in donors from endemic regions: Central, South America, Southern USA
Parasitic:	
1. Toxoplasma Ab	Routine screening
2. Strongyloides Ab	Consider in endemic regions: sub-Saharan Africa, Southeast Asia, Central and S. America, Eastern Europe
3. Trypanosoma cruzi Ab	Consider in donors from endemic regions: Central and South America
4. Leishmania	Consider screening donors from endemic regions
5. Malaria	Consider screening donors in or recently from endemic regions

Communication between recipient hospitals: a unit identifying an infection acquired from a donor has a duty to relay this rapidly to other recipient units
Ab antibody
[a]Donor transmission of rabies, WNV, and LCMV has an extremely poor outcome

perfusate and hepatitis B follow-up. A robust system to ensure that patients are appropriately considered for post-transplant prophylaxis in line with local policy is critical to ensure patient safety.

Timeline for Post-transplant Infections

Although not absolute there is a clinically helpful timeline for infections post-transplant expounded by Rubin [3].

0–2 weeks: infections are mostly a direct result of surgery, i.e. chest and wound infection, line-associated sepsis and occasionally bacterial infection derived from the donor (positive perfusate culture, donor UTI, donor bacteraemia or unexplained meningoencephalitic illness).

1–4 weeks: predominantly nosocomial infections related to stay and hospitalisation, i.e. UTI, line- and PD catheter-associated infection, and *Clostridium difficile*. Oral and oesophageal candidiasis is also common at this stage especially in patients on steroids. Of the herpes viruses, primary HSV is unusual in presenting at this early stage. Other viruses such as transmitted WNV can also present at this time.

4–26 weeks: this is the period dominated by opportunistic infections related to the heaviest period of

Table 71.2 Pre-treatment and vaccination

Hepatitis C RNA positive	Erstwhile attempt to eradicate infection with pegalated interferon and ribavirin before listing. Consider newer direct-acting antivirals pre-transplant
Hepatitis B	Universal vaccination of nonimmune CKD patients (and ESRD), pre-listing assessment and stable virological control of hepatitis B with antivirals
HIV Ab positive	Undetectable viral load and CD4+ >200 for 6 months prior to listing
VZV Ab negative	Vaccination (live vaccine) of the 3 % of ESRF population negative for VZV with live vaccine. Prophylaxis with acyclovir if transplanted within 2 weeks of vaccination
Influenza and H1N1	Annual vaccination
MMR (live vaccine)	If not previously vaccinated, vaccinate 1 month pre-transplant. Testing and vaccination of all women of child-bearing age pre-listing if rubella IgG negative
Diptheria, tetanus and pertussis	If not previously vaccinated vaccinate pre-transplant and routine boosters 5–10 yearly
Polio (inactivated)	Routine vaccination if not given, can be given post-transplant but *not live vaccine*
Human papillomavirus	Girls eligible for local vaccination programme should be strongly encouraged. No evidence yet for a benefit in older females to prevent CIN or prevent anogenital warts in women or men, but worth considering especially in those likely to receive high levels of immunosuppression
CMV	Early vaccine studies looking encouraging, large-scale studies pending
Pneumococcal	Vaccination according to national guidelines ideally pre-transplant
Haemophilus influenzae B	Consider pre-transplant in those with pulmonary pathology (can also be given post-transplant)
Meningococcal meningitis B&C	Vaccination according to national guidelines
Recurrent UTI	Patients with recurrent UTI before transplantation are highly likely to have significant urosepsis after transplantation; where possible the cause should be identified and treated pre-listing. NB: persistent pyuria also needs explaining even if not associated with overt sepsis
Tuberculosis	Screening in patients with ESRF by Mantoux or interferon-ϒ assays often negative due to diminished T-cell response
Strongyloides Ab positive	If treatment history not clear, especially if eosinophilia, treat with two doses of ivermectin 200 mch/kg/day for 2 days
Schistosomiasis Ab positive	Treat with two doses of praziquantel

immunosuppression. Most herpes viruses (reactivation and primary infection), e.g. CMV (in the absence of prophylaxis typically at 40 days), EBV, HSV, VZV (shingles) and HHV-8/7/6. Respiratory viruses may present with chest involvement. Invasive fungal infections such as candida or aspergillus tend to present in this period as may mycobacterium TB. Parasitic infections such as reactivation of strongyloides or toxoplasmosis tend to occur early. UTIs remain very common and, in the absence of prophylaxis, PCP presents in this period.

>26 weeks: periodic viral reactivation of HSV or VZV (shingles) can occur at any stage, and a small proportion of patients develop very high levels of EBV viraemia often many years post-transplant. Viral warts are also common in the first year. Late-onset CMV presents usually within the 8 weeks following cessation of prophylaxis (orogenital HSV may also recur). Incidental infections such as listeria, legionella and respiratory viral infection can occur at any time. CMV-, EBV-, VZV- and HSV-negative patients can acquire primary infection many years post-transplant particularly if they have a young family or become exposed to young children. MTB tends to present relatively early in the course of a transplant, while Non-tuberculous mycobacteria (NTM) tends to present later. Cryptococcus tends to present late and PCP can occur at any stage, although risk diminishes with time. NB: hepatitis B and C reactivation can occur at any time especially after cessation of prophylaxis in hepatitis B and can be promoted by the use of steroids.

Urinary Tract Infection

UTI post-transplant is very common and associated with a significant morbidity, hospitalisation and graft loss and by definition constitutes 'complicated UTI'. UTI post-transplant is covered in more detail in Chap. 34, but it is worth emphasising that (a) patients with abnormal anatomy and recurrent UTI pre-transplant are likely to have significant problems with urosepsis post-transplant unless the underlying cause is resolved; (b) as transplant UTIs are by definition 'complicated', short courses of antibiotics may result in partially treated and recurrent infections (with high risk of generating multiple admissions and highly resistant organisms); and (c) patients with recurrent or severe urosepsis need prompt assessment in a urolo-radio nephrology MDT.

Table 71.3 Infection prophylaxis post-renal transplantation

CMV	Pre-emptive monitoring or prophylaxis (see text). Valgancyclovir 900 mg daily if normal renal function (450 mg possibly as effective and less side effects), dose adjusted if GFR <60
HSV Ab negative	*Essential* if not receiving valgancyclovir prophylaxis for CMV. Valacyclovir 500 mg twice a day or acyclovir 200 mg three times a day for 1 month regardless of donor HSV status
HSV Ab positive	If history of recurrent cold sores pre-transplant, likely to be worse post-transplant. Acyclovir 200 mg o.d. prophylaxis
VZV Ab negative	Administer varicella zoster immunoglobulin if significant exposure to chicken pox or shingles (within 7 days of exposure)
Hepatitis B core Ab positive donor	HBV immunoglobulin (HBIG) at transplant (HBIG 4,000 IU IV stat and measure HBs Ab levels at day 7 and repeat dose if levels are <500 IU/L); start lamivudine 2–3 days before or at least on the day of transplant; monitor HBsAg regularly
Hepatitis B core Ab positive recipient	Lamivudine prophylaxis 2–3 days before or immediately after transplantation. Monitor HBsAg regularly
Hepatitis B surface Ag positive donor	HBV vaccination for recipients pre-transplant. HBIG (HBIG 4,000 IU IV stat) at transplant, measure HBsAb levels at day 5 and repeat dose if levels are <500 IU/L. Monitor HBsAb levels weekly and repeat HBIG to maintain levels >500 IU/L during the first month post-RT. Start antiviral prophylaxis 2–3 days before or immediately after transplantation. Preferred drug is entecavir. Obtain donor HBV treatment status if available and modify antiviral prophylaxis accordingly if there is a risk of drug resistance. Monitor HBsAg regularly
Hepatitis B surface Ag positive recipient	Start antiviral therapy preferably 2–3 weeks prior to or at least immediately after transplantation. Entecavir is the preferred option if no concerns about resistance
Wound prophylaxis	Local policy
UTI prophylaxis	Septrin (as part of universal *Pneumocystis jirovecii* prophylaxis), some units give additional UTI prophylaxis (see Chap. 35)
Bacterial growth in perfusate	Treatment on the basis of culture, but consider long course if virulent organism, e.g. *Staphylococcus aureus*, *Pseudomonas*
Mycobacterium	6 months of isoniazid 300 mg o.d. and pyridoxine 10–25 mg o.d. in high risk, no need to treat those who have fully completed treatment course. Prophylaxis against NTM not currently recommended
Pneumocystis jirovecii	First choice: trimethoprim-sulphonamide 480 mg o.d. or 960 mg 3× per week for 3–6 months or until CD4$^+$ count >200 if depleting antibodies or late immunosuppression (*also gives co-prophylaxis against toxoplasmosis, nocardia, listeria and UTI*). Allergy to TMP-SM/s second line (no norcardia/UTI prophylaxis afforded by these agents): monthly nebulised pentamidine 300 mg, dapsone 50–100 mg daily (if not G6PD deficient) (addition of pyrimethamine 50–75mg/week to dapsone provides toxoplasm prophylaxis), atovaquone 1,500 mg daily (also has anti-toxoplasma activity). Prophylaxis is recommended for recipients exposed to cases of PCP
Candida sp.	Fluconazole 200–400 mg daily, itraconazole 200 mg twice a day, voriconazole 200 mg twice a day
Coccidioides immitis	Fluconazole 200–400 mg if past history or positive serology

NB: perfect aseptic technique for line/catheter insertion, prompt line drain and catheter removal, chest physiotherapy and early mobilisation, as well as appropriate isolation and infection control measures for inpatients

A robust system is needed for identifying patients with communicable infections such as shingles and viral respiratory tract infections and for seeing them in isolation in outpatients

Specific Infectious Agents: Guidelines [4]

HHV-5 Cytomegalovirus (CMV)

CMV is a beta herpes virus and the most common opportunistic infection post-transplant: about 40–50 % of renal transplants develop viraemia, and it represents a significant challenge in some organ transplant recipients.

CMV has a seroprevalence of 45–100 % with higher rates in Africa, lower rates in Northern Europe and USA, and increasing prevalence with age. Transmission can be via saliva, urine, sexual contact, breast-feeding, placental transmission, blood transfusion or transplantation. In the immunocompetent host primary infection is usually asymptomatic, although it can present as a mononucleosis-like illness, following which the virus undergoes a prolonged period of latency but can become reactivated by a variety of mechanisms including 'stress', sepsis and immunosuppression. For example, TNF-alpha released by rejection or infection can activate the major immediate early promoter (MieP) of CMV and induce intracellular replication. Transplant recipients (and occasionally, it is worth remembering, patients immunosuppressed for autoimmune conditions) can have a primary infection (D+/R−), reinfection (with a different strain) (D+/R+) or reactivation (D−/R+).

The risk of viraemia is very strongly associated with D+/R− status, but in addition the use of depleting antibody induction, acute rejection, poor graft function and older donor age are known risk factors. In renal transplants predominantly induced with anti-IL2-R mAb and no prophylaxis,

Table 71.4 Clinical characteristics of CMV infection post-transplant

CMV viraemia	Often asymptomatic. Commonly associated with leucopenia or myelosuppression before developing CMV syndrome
CMV syndrome	Temperature >38 °C for at least 2 days in the absence of another cause, plus CMV DNA viraemia and either neutropenia, thrombocytopenia, lymphocytosis, myalgia, headache or arthralgia
Pneumonitis	Interstitial pneumonitis with early desaturation. Can be rapidly progressive and may have co-infections such as PCP
Upper GI	Gastritis/duodenitis common symptoms in early primary infection, mouth ulcers and oesphagitis
Lower GI	Colitis – often bloody and may be fulminant
Hepatitis	Raised transaminases and flu-like illness
Pancreatitis	Asymptomatic with raised amylase to fulminant pancreatitis
Encephalitis/meningitis	Usually late feature
Retinitis	Usually a late manifestation in profoundly immunocompromised patients
Myocarditis	Usually late
Nephritis	Relatively rare but can result in graft failure or native kidney loss. May have characteristic 'owl's eye' appearance in biopsy
Cystitis	Relatively rare following SOT but can occur post-BMT

NB: peripheral blood is usually, but not always, positive for CMV DNA in the presence of end-organ disease

viraemia occurred in 70 % of D+/R−, 53 % D+/R+, 44 % of D−/R+and none of the D−/R−. The peak viral load is also significantly higher in the D+R− patients [5].

Clinical characteristics: many patients who have viraemia are asymptomatic, but there is a strong correlation between viral load and symptoms. The clinical characteristics of CMV infection in the immunocompromised are shown in Table 71.4. Viraemia and clinical features usually occur between 4 and 12 weeks (typically 6) post-transplant, but it is easy to be caught out by disease occurring outside this period (a) following treatment of late rejection, (b) cessation of prophylaxis (c) and in D−/R− transplants following primary exposure sometimes years later.

The kinetics of viral replication has clinical relevance; primary infection is associated with a doubling time of 1.5 days vs. 2.7 days for reactivation. This means that a CMV naïve patient can go from asymptomatic with a low detectable viral load to significant end-organ disease within a week. A patient with primary infection often presents with the so-called CMV syndrome (high fever without localising physical signs) that can progress rapidly to gastritis, colitis (often bloody), pneumonitis and other end-organ involvement. This is usually associated with very high viral loads. Patients with reactivation or reinfection *may* have a less fulminant course with isolated colitis or pneumonitis without an obvious full-blown viral syndrome. Either way, end-organ damage can progress rapidly and can occur with only low-level viraemia or very rarely in the absence of viraemia; therefore, a high index of suspicion is required. CMV is immunosuppressive in its own right and often 'opens the door' to other opportunistic infections such as HHV-6 and HHV-4 (EBV) and PCP.

The clinical characteristics of CMV infection Table 71.4.

The diagnosis of CMV infection is based on the detection of virus either by antigenaemia or detection and quantification of CMV nucleic acid testing by real-time quantitative PCR. In practice most laboratories now use real-time PCR and should adhere to universal diagnostic standards. This technique is highly reproducible, and concerns that PCR would result in false positives have not been our experience.

Although viraemia is common, with modern management clinical disease affects only about 8 % of renal transplant recipients, and the vast majority of this is CMV syndrome; however, when end-organ disease occurs, it can be devastating and rapidly progressive. Pneumonitis may present with shortness of breath and oxygen desaturation post-exercise and may progress swiftly from mild dyspnoea to marked desaturation particularly after mild exertion. Chest X-ray (see Fig. 71.1) or CT scan may show signs of an interstitial lung disease, but there is a wide differential so it is essential to get samples, rapidly, (ideally a bronchoalveolar lavage) where possible or treat blindly (covering CMV) or both. It is important to note that CMV infection predisposes to other infections, and viral pneumonitis can coexist with *Pneumocystis* pneumonitis. Meningitis and encephalitis may present with classic symptoms and signs, or epilepsy and impaired cognition. It can be diagnosed from PCR on CSF, so ensuring the appropriate sample is taken at the time of lumbar puncture is important. Where possible, with tissue-invasive disease such as gastritis, colitis (Fig. 71.2) and nephritis (Fig. 71.3), biopsy, culture and PCR are critical. However, the pancreas and retina are less-appealing biopsy targets: ophthalmologists can normally make a firm clinical diagnosis, and CMV pancreatitis is usually, therefore, a presumptive diagnosis based on viraemia and clinical findings.

In short, it is important to have a high index of suspicion in any transplant with end-organ disease, with rapid requesting and processing of blood or any other tissue for CMV PCR, and if possible/appropriate, ensure that a biopsy is sent to virology as well as histopathology departments.

Beyond the direct effects of the virus, CMV infection has been implicated in several indirect consequences including

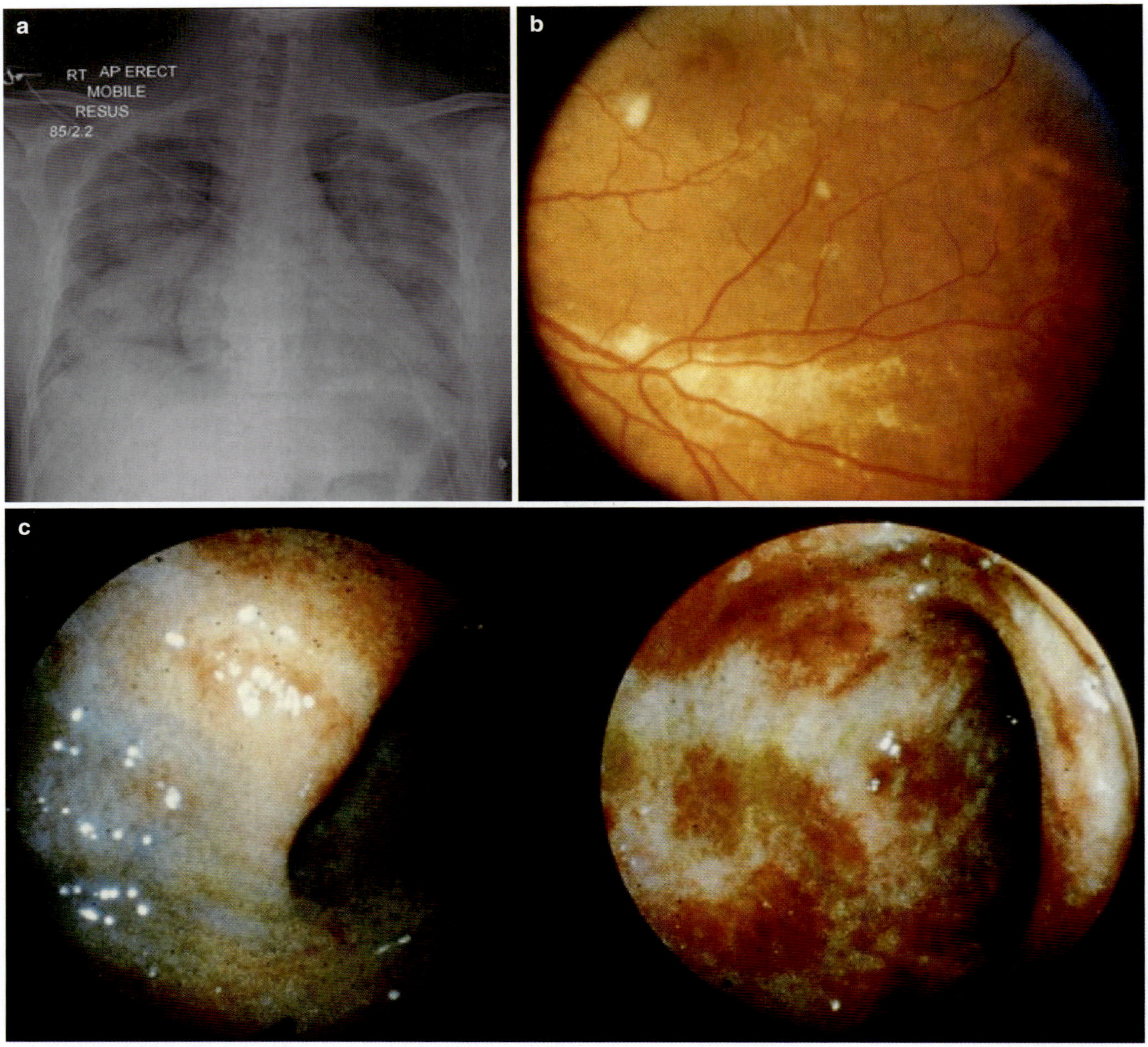

Fig. 71.1 (**a**) CMV pneumonitis in a renal transplant recipient. The patient had minimal constitutional illness, a dry cough and presented severely hypoxic. The differential is large including pulmonary oedema, but the peripheral sparing goes against this despite the cardiomegaly. There were very low levels of CMV viraemia, but BAL was positive and there was a very rapid improvement in clinical condition with IV gancyclovir. (**b**) Early CMV retinitis. (**c**) CMV colitis in a renal transplant recipient presenting with abdominal pain and bloody diarrhoea. This patient also had only low levels of viraemia and the diagnosis was made on biopsy

(a) increased cellular rejection, (b) increased infection by other microbes, (c) increased mortality and (d) worse graft survival [6, 7]. This is not without controversy. For instance, studies showing an association with acute cellular rejection have not always differentiated cause of effect, and a significant proportion (80 % in our experience) of acute rejection precedes CMV viraemia, so much of this association may simply be a response to increased immunosuppression. CMV viraemia is immunomodulatory and predisposes to EBV and HHV-6 viraemia, as well as an increase in fungal infections, although again CMV viraemia may also be a biomarker of over immunosuppression. Some studies have shown increased mortality, and worse 4-year graft survival has also been shown [8]; however, a UK study based on serology in 10,000 transplants showed no effect on patient or allograft survival [9]. A detailed analysis is beyond the scope of this chapter, but what is clear is that overt CMV disease is nasty and best avoided.

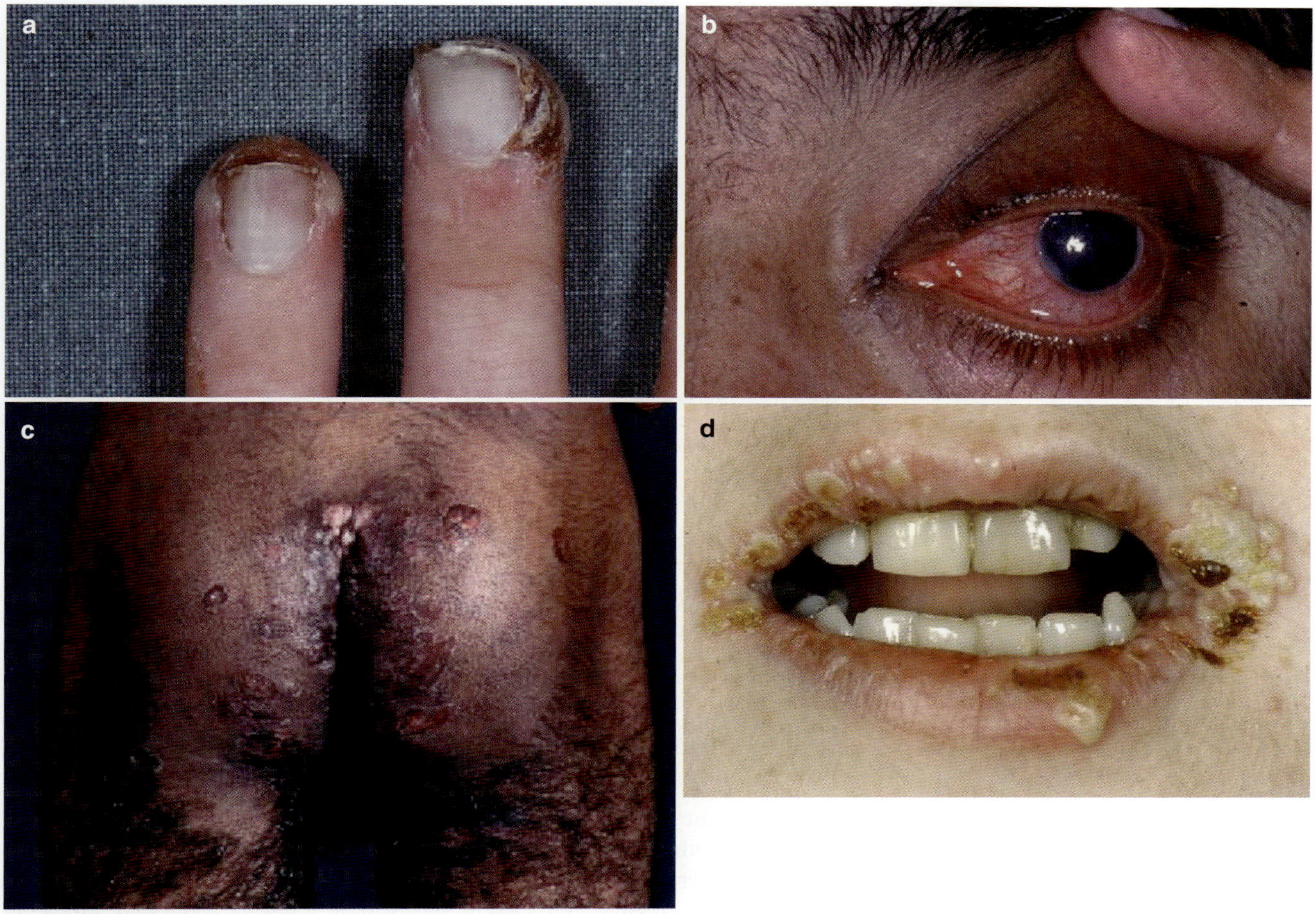

Fig. 71.2 Herpes simplex virus (**a**) herpetic whitlow, (**b**) herpes ophthalmitis, (**c**) perineal HSV and (**d**) extensive labial HSV

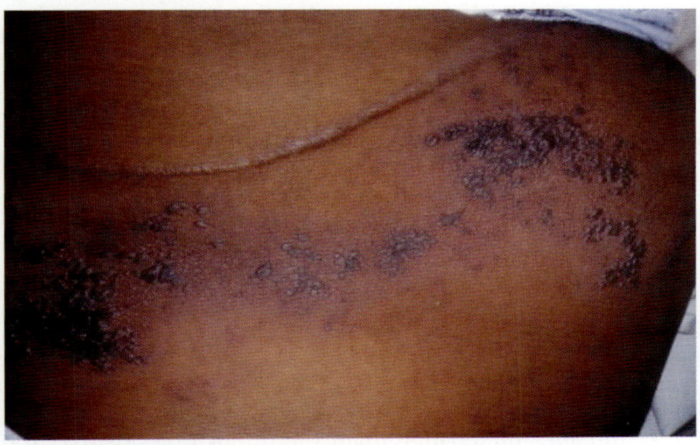

Fig. 71.3 Herpes zoster reactivation (shingles)

There are a variety of recommendations on the prevention and treatment of CMV post-transplant [4, 10, 11], and the 2011 BTS guidelines nicely summarise the current evidence [12]. For kidney transplantation most guidelines favour universal prophylaxis (for D+/R− or any positive recipients), especially following depleting antibodies. This is, in part based on meta-analyses of prophylaxis studies demonstrating a benefit in all cause mortality with prophylaxis [13]. Most of the studies in the meta-analyses have short follow-up and very few patients in the pre-emptive arm. Guidelines mostly acknowledge that pre-emptive therapy is probably equally appropriate if the logistics can be robustly managed (the case for pre-emptive over prophylaxis is eloquently argued by Thomas Reischig [14]) and there is some suggestion that the prevailing opinion is moving towards equal recommendation for pre-emptive and prophylaxis.

The main advantages of universal prophylaxis include ease of administration and co-prophylaxis against viruses (such as primary HSV), with disadvantages including drug side effects (especially leucopenia) and the concern of late-onset disease. The advantages of pre-emptive approach include limiting drug exposure to those that need it, encouraging immunity, and the near complete absence of late disease. The disadvantages of pre-emptive therapy include the extra vigilance required and the lack of co-prophylaxis.

Table 71.5a Universal prophylaxis (especially if received depleting antibodies). Valgancyclovir 900/450 mg daily (dose adjusted for GFR)

D+/R−, D+/R+ and D−/R+: 200 days for D+/R−, 100 days for R+	Late-onset disease biggest hazard. Ensure robust monitoring on cessation of prophylaxis. Resistant CMV and non-compliance may rarely result in disease in prophylactic period if no routine monitoring. Leucopenia common side effect
Partial prophylaxis (if not received depleting antibodies)	
D+/R− 200 days, no prophylaxis for R+	Numerically, D+/R + and D−/R + account for more viraemia than D+/R- so requires good monitoring of CMV PCR for R + group and the ability to safely run two different approaches
D−/R−	No prophylaxis for CMV, but HSV-negative recipients must have at least 1 month of anti-HSV prophylaxis and irradiated blood products

Table 71.5b Pre-emptive therapy

D+/R−, D+/R+ and D−/R+: no prophylaxis	1. HSV prophylaxis in HSV-negative recipients for at least 1 month (e.g. valacyclovir) 2. Robust monitoring (guidelines at least weekly) ideally twice weekly especially in D+/R− and those receiving depleting antibodies for the first 3 months from transplant or treated rejection episode. Rapid turnaround time and reporting (e.g. e-mail alerts to transplant pool) 3. Twice weekly monitoring for those with viraemia and in those successfully treated 4. System to ensure patients admitted to other hospitals or units are identified and monitored appropriately 5. Issue patients with 3-day starter pack of valgancyclovir to take if develops viraemia 6. Start treatment at any positive for D+/R− and at local threshold for R+ (e.g. 3,000 copies per ml)
Hybrid (if received depleting antibodies or high immunological risk)	
D+/R−: no prophylaxis initially, prophylaxis following treatment of viraemia	D+/R− patients with primary infection following depleting antibody are highly likely to relapse following treatment as are those who have had rejection and cannot safely tolerate ISR. For these patients it may be worth considering prophylaxis after successful treatment

To summarise the current guidelines [4, 10–12] on prevention, most recommend prophylaxis with valgancyclovir (superior to acyclovir, valacyclovir or oral gancyclovir) starting within 10 days of transplant for D+/R− and R+ patients. Based on the findings of the IMPACT study [15] which showed a reduced rate of late-onset CMV disease with 200 compared to 100 days treatment (16 % vs. 37 %), the guidelines tend to favour treatment for 200 days in D+/R− and in those who have received depleting antibodies such as ATG. The dose recommended for those with normal renal function is 900 mg per day, but 450 mg appears to be as effective, causes much less leucopenia but potentially increases the risk of resistance [16]. Further dose reduction for renal impairment is required. The risk of CMV disease in D−/R− is so low as to not require CMV prophylaxis but does therefore mandate anti-HSV prophylaxis. Clinicians need to be vigilant to CMV post-prophylaxis and have a system of monitoring patients at this time as well as being alert to the possibility of viral resistance or non-compliance during prophylaxis.

Our experience of the pre-emptive approach has been very positive with CMV syndrome developing in only 4.9 %, end-organ disease in approximately 1 % and only 2.3 % of late-onset viraemia (first episode after 90 days) [5]. There are some important cautions included in Table 71.5a and 71.5b. Pre-emptive therapy relies on robust monitoring and reporting as well as a good relationship with your virology department. Because of the rapid doubling time of primary infection, we ensure twice weekly CMV monitoring for the first 8 weeks (longer if there has been an episode of viraemia) and weekly for a further 4 weeks. An e-mail reporting service to the transplant team, with clear lines of responsibility, works well and we give D+/R− patients 3 days of valgancyclovir on discharge to start if viraemia is detected as an outpatient. Patients admitted to other hospitals or under other teams may be at risk as monitoring and reporting can breakdown, and it is important to have a strategy for these patients.

Finally, it is clear that some patients such as those D+/R− who have viraemia after depleting antibodies or who are high immunological risk (i.e. have had early rejection) and therefore cannot risk immunosuppression reduction (ISR) are highly likely to have recurrent viraemia after completion of treatment, and it may be worth considering converting to prophylaxis after treatment with the advantage that the recipient will have developed some immunity with the first viraemia.

Treatment. In asymptomatic serologically positive R+ patients with viral counts below 3,000 genomes/ml, our practice is to reduce the overall burden of immunosuppression (CNI if level high, anti-proliferative if not). We treat reactivation if viraemia is >3,000 genomes/ml or if there is evidence of end-organ disease. As a unit that practises pre-emptive therapy, CMV naïve patients with a positive donor are discharged with 3 days of valgancyclovir (starter pack)

Table 71.6 Risk factors for the development of Kaposi's sarcoma post-transplant

Serostatus of donor/recipient	Data suggesting that both reactivation and primary infection at transplant are significant risk factors
Geographical location	Mediterranean, Middle East, Eastern Europe and sub-Saharan Africa
Burden of immunosuppression	Overall burden of immunosuppression is important especially depleting mAb
Age of recipient	>50 years
Homosexual males	Multiple partners
Transfusion	In high-prevalence areas

to take if there is a single positive PCR of any level to avoid delay in treatment (also worth considering post-prophylaxis).

First-line treatment of significant viraemia or CMV disease should be with valgancyclovir or IV gancyclovir (especially the latter if any doubt about absorption) dose adjusted for eGFR (see Table 71.6). In patients who have not recently undergone rejection, it is advisable to reduce any anti-proliferative agent or consider stopping altogether if serious disease. Treatment of CMV disease should be continued for at least 2 weeks even if early elimination of viraemia and our practice is to continue treatment until two negative PCRs in everyone. Relapse is common, especially in the D+/R− and in those who have received depleting antibodies. There is insufficient evidence to support the use of IVIg (CMV Ab enriched or otherwise), which is expensive and a scarce resource, but it is likely to be relatively harmless and might be worth considering in a tight corner if the patient is not responding to antivirals. It is important to ensure PCP prophylaxis continues, and GCSF can be helpful in the face of neutropenia.

Viral resistance is much more common in the D+/R− subgroup (up to 10 %) with prolonged treatment and the use of depleting antibodies. Apart from this high-risk group, a strong indication of resistance is failure to clear the virus by 3 weeks, and mutation analysis should be requested in this setting. Mutations of UL97 kinase and UL54 DNA polymerase are the currently recognised markers of resistance, and it is important to note that as gancyclovir, cidofovir and foscarnet all target UL54 DNA polymerase, resistance to gancyclovir can lead to cross resistance to cidofovir and foscarnet. The latter two drugs are reserved as second-line drugs and generally reviled by nephrologists because of their high rate of nephrotoxicity. Nonetheless they can be life-saving in extreme disease (doses for both need to be carefully adjusted for GFR and pre-hydration essential).

Leflunomide and mTOR inhibitors theoretically both have anti-CMV properties, and there are case reports of some success using leflunomide to treat resistant CMV in SOT. However, there is likely to be reporting bias, and as yet no RCTs to support the use of leflunomide as treatment.

The circumstantial evidence in favour of a clinically relevant anti-CMV effect of mTOR inhibitors is more convincing, and there are many studies that show significantly reduced rates of CMV infection in de novo kidney transplants receiving mTOR inhibitors [17]. The evidence that mTOR inhibitors are helpful in treatment of CMV infection again degenerates to anecdote with small cases series. Our experience, and a niche that may prove important, is in those patients with persistent or resistant CMV who cannot tolerate further reduction in immunosuppression. Swapping tacrolimus for sirolimus or adding sirolimus to tacrolimus in high immunological risk patients with dose reduction of the CNI can be effective as clearing CMV and simultaneously avoiding rejection.

With modern management, CMV disease (the majority being CMV syndrome) affects only about 8 % of renal transplants. In our experience of a pre-emptive approach, treatment was required in 63 % of D+/R−, 22 % of D+/R+ and 18 % of D−/R + for viraemia, and end-organ disease occurred in only 1 %.

Herpes Simplex Virus: HSV 1 and 2

Reactivation of HSV in the form of nasolabial cold sores or genital ulcers is relatively common but can be very aggressive in the significantly immunocompromised (see Fig. 71.2). Patients may give a history of previous cold sores and, if frequent pre-transplant, are highly likely to recur post-transplant. This can be prevented with ready access to topical acyclovir or low-dose oral acyclovir prophylaxis (e.g. 200 mg daily). Treatment with oral acyclovir, valacyclovir or famcyclovir is highly effective but should start early, and dose adjustment for GFR is important. HSV can also affect the cornea and conjunctiva presenting as a red eye/keratitis and progressing to a dendritic ulcer with potential sight loss (Fig. 71.2), and any painful red eye should have viral swabs and rapid ophthalmology review.

Very rarely, seronegative patients can develop a fulminant primary HSV infection. This has been reported with both HSV1 and HSV2 and has a very high mortality. A high fever is universal, but skin lesions are present in only half the patients, which may explain delay in diagnosis. The patient may seem better than their fever would imply initially, but without treatment pancytopenia, gastric ulceration and acute hepatitis (CT imaging may appear as abscesses) rapidly progress to encephalopathy, coagulopathy and death. The diagnosis can be made by detecting HSV DNA in blood, CSF, swabs and biopsies. However, onset to death is short, so a high index of suspicion is important and early empirical treatment critical. CMV prophylaxis with valgancyclovir is essentially protective against primary HSV, but in those HSV-negative patients not having CMV, prophylaxis should be given either as acyclovir or valacyclovir (regardless of donor status). There is no consensus on duration of prophylaxis, but our practice is to give valacyclovir 500 mg b.i.d for the first month of transplant. HSV is very sensitive to acyclovir and, as mentioned above, any suspicion of fulminant HSV should prompt rapid IV treatment (10–12.5 mg/kg t.i.d.), reduction in anti-proliferatives and placement on a high dependency unit.

HHV-3 (Varicella zoster virus (VZV))

Reactivation with herpes zoster (shingles) is markedly more common in transplant recipients (10×) than the general population, occurring in roughly 10 % of patients in the first 5 years (Fig. 71.3) [18] but more commonly still in those receiving lymphocyte-depleting antibodies. As neuralgia precedes the rash, the diagnosis can be initially missed and should be considered in anyone with new onset severe, otherwise unexplained pain. Treatment is with acyclovir or valacyclovir for 7 days, analgesia, surveillance for secondary infection and usually reduction in anti-proliferatives.

Primary infection is potentially life-threatening in solid-organ transplant recipients, and about 3 % of the adult population are VZV naïve; others bear a similar risk if hypogammoglobulinaemic. Identification of naïve patients on the waiting list is mandatory, and vaccination should be robustly embedded in any pre-transplant programme, although the evidence is that as a community we are very poor at doing this. The vaccine is usually given as two doses, 4–8 weeks apart, and as it is a live vaccine, we offer acyclovir to any patient receiving a transplant within 2 weeks of the vaccination. Patients unlucky enough to get primary varicella infection while under the influence of significant immunosuppression can present with pneumonitis, hepatitis, ulcerative gastritis and colitis. Pancreatitis, encephalitis, meningitis and DIC can follow swiftly and have a mortality of 30 %. Treatment of primary chickenpox should be with rapid initiation of IV acyclovir (10–12.5 mg/kg t.i.d. adjusted for GFR) for 7–10 days, usually until all the lesions have crusted over. Treatment may need to be continued longer (2–3 weeks) for CNS involvement or disseminated infection. Of course, it is more desirable to avoid the risk of a primary infection so that seronegative patients should be identified pre-transplant, advised to avoid exposure and given clear (written) advice on what to do if exposed either to chickenpox or shingles (often unwittingly in the transplant clinic waiting room). If pre-transplant serostatus is not known, an urgent VZV IgG test is required to establish VZV immune status.

1. Attend hospital within 24 h (up to 7 days of exposure) for varicella zoster immune globulin (VZIG; 1,000 mg IM adult dose). If a second exposure occurs after 3 weeks, a further dose may be required.
2. If VZIG is unavailable or the exposed patient cannot be given an IM injection (contraindicated in bleeding disorders), IVIg can be used (0.2 g per kg body weight).
3. Consider acyclovir/valacyclovir or famcyclovir prophylaxis in household contacts.

HHV-4 Epstein-Barr Virus (EBV)

EBV is gamma-herpes virus with 95 % world seroprevalence, mostly acquired asymptomatically in childhood or as infectious mononucleosis (IM) in 25 % during puberty. It immortalises B-cell lines and remains mostly latent with occasional lytic cycles and shedding mostly in saliva in healthy individuals. Given the prevalence of EBV infection, primary infection following transplantation is common in a seronegative recipient. Viraemia is common post-transplant occurring in roughly 50 % of all patients, but this is usually asymptomatic. Occasionally patients may present with IM or non-specific viral illness, but the greatest concern is the propensity for EBV to induce post-transplant lymphoproliferative disorder (PTLD). Ninety percent of early PTLDs are EBV positive, and a primary infection post-transplant confers a 10–75-fold risk of PTLD (greater still if concomitant CMV infection and/or the use of depleting antibodies). There is also data to support EBV viraemia preceding development of PTLD; however, recent guidelines make the reasonable point that there is no evidence to support the routine monitoring of EBV levels post-renal transplant [19].

The Renal Association Guidelines [20], however, do recommend EBV PCR monitoring in D+/R- patients for the first year and following treatment for rejection. Despite the lack of evidence, risk stratification is key and it is worth considering monitoring: (1) D+/R− patients (especially if they received depleting antibodies), (2) patients who are viraemic pre-transplant (usually previous transplants), (3) those with previous EBV +ve lymphoma, (4) following treatment of rejection and (5) possibly at annual review as a surrogate marker of over immunosuppression – a small percentage of patients develop very high levels asymptomatically with increasing time post-transplant. In the absence of convincing evidence, it is our practice to monitor the above groups. Stable patients with viraemia are monitored as follows:

Levels of <10,000 monitor 3 monthly
Levels of 10,000–50,000 monitor 6–8 weekly and consider immunosuppression reduction
Levels of >50,000 gentle ISR monitor 4 weekly

While it is common sense, and our practice, to reduce immunosuppression in the presence of persistent high-level EBV viraemia, there is negligible evidence to support ISR in the absence of lymphoma and there is a risk of late rejection so it should be undertaken cautiously. There is no convincing evidence in favour of antiviral prophylaxis.

The management of post-transplant lymphoproliferative disorder requires a specialist multidisciplinary approach and is discussed in chapter 70.

HHV-6

The prevalence of HHV-6 infection is very high with >90 % of the population infected in early childhood. Reactivation of HHV-6 is very common in the early post-transplant period often as a co-infection with CMV and HHV-7 [21] with clinical manifestations from asymptomatic viraemia, self-limiting viral illness, to a more disseminated disease with pneumonitis, encephalitis lymphadenopathy and bone marrow suppression. As most units do not screen for HHV-6 and the vast majority of patients are either asymptomatic or settle spontaneously, treatment is not usually required, but there are case reports of death secondary to HHV-6, and it is worth considering as a diagnosis in a patient with unexplained viral illness. Treatments if required are gancyclovir or valgancyclovir, exclusion of co-existent CMV and reduction in ISR.

HHV-7

Reactivation of childhood-acquired virus may occur early post-transplant either asymptomatically or with a non-specific viral illness, but severe disease is extremely rare. Management involves exclusion of more likely infections, then immunosuppression reduction and, if necessary, treatment with foscarnet or cidofovir.

HHV-8

The main clinical manifestation of HHV-8 primary infection, reactivation or reinfection in solid-organ transplants is the development of Kaposi's sarcoma. Although HHV-8 infection does occur sporadically, there is a significant geographical bias in the seroprevalence of HHV-8 with the Mediterranean, Eastern Europe, the Middle East and sub-Saharan Africa having high rates. The role of immunosuppression is profound in that the prevalence of KS in SOT is 500 times that of the general population, occurring in 0.5 % of transplant recipients from North-West Europe and up to 5 % of transplant recipients in Saudi Arabia. Known risk factors for post-transplant KS are shown in Table 71.6 [22].

Clinical presentation is predominantly cutaneous involvement with red/purple/black nodules (see Fig. 71.4) typically on the lower body, initially often associated with lower limb oedema which may precede the development of skin lesions. Visceral involvement may also occur including lymphadenopathy, pulmonary nodules, chylous pleural effusions and gastrointestinal involvement. Clinical presentation is usually within the first year, but it is not unusual for the diagnosis of visceral KS to be delayed particularly in the setting of GI involvement. The mortality associated with KS particularly with visceral involvement is around 10 %, and graft loss is common as a consequence of ISR.

Serology is rarely helpful in the diagnosis and donors are not currently screened; however, it might be worth considering donor and recipient screening in high-prevalence areas to identify risk. Histology is the gold standard for diagnosis; any suspicious lesion should be biopsied, and a high index of suspicion is important particularly for gastrointestinal involvement. PCR for HHV-8 may be considered as a tool to monitor response to treatment for visceral KS, although it will not be helpful in the absence of viraemia.

Treatment is with reduction in immunosuppression or complete cessation if life-threatening visceral involvement or progressive disease. The reduction of immunosuppression required to induce remission often results in graft loss, and conversion from CNI to mTOR inhibitor (which possesses anti-VEGF activity) has had some significant success [23], although this is not universal. With aggressive, unresponsive disease, antivirals (foscarnet, cidofovir) and chemotherapy such as bleomycin, adriamycin and taxols have been tried with variable success.

Our practice is to stop the anti-proliferative agents initially and if no response within 2–4 weeks or significant visceral involvement convert non-proteinuric patients from their CNI to an mTOR inhibitor. If intolerant of mTOR inhibitor, then proceed with a stepwise reduction in CNI, ideally with slow small cuts rather than large cuts, if the disease permits [24].

KS has a high risk of recurrence in a second transplant; we aim to avoid heavy induction and plan for an early switch to an mTOR inhibitor if possible.

Polyoma Viruses: Polyomavirus hominis 1 (BK) and 2 (JC)

BK and JC are usually picked up in childhood remaining latent in the presence of a normal immune system but can cause significant nephropathy (polyoma virus-associated nephropathy, PVAN) in renal transplant (although very rarely in other transplants), and JC virus is the causative agent in multifocal leucoencephalopathy.

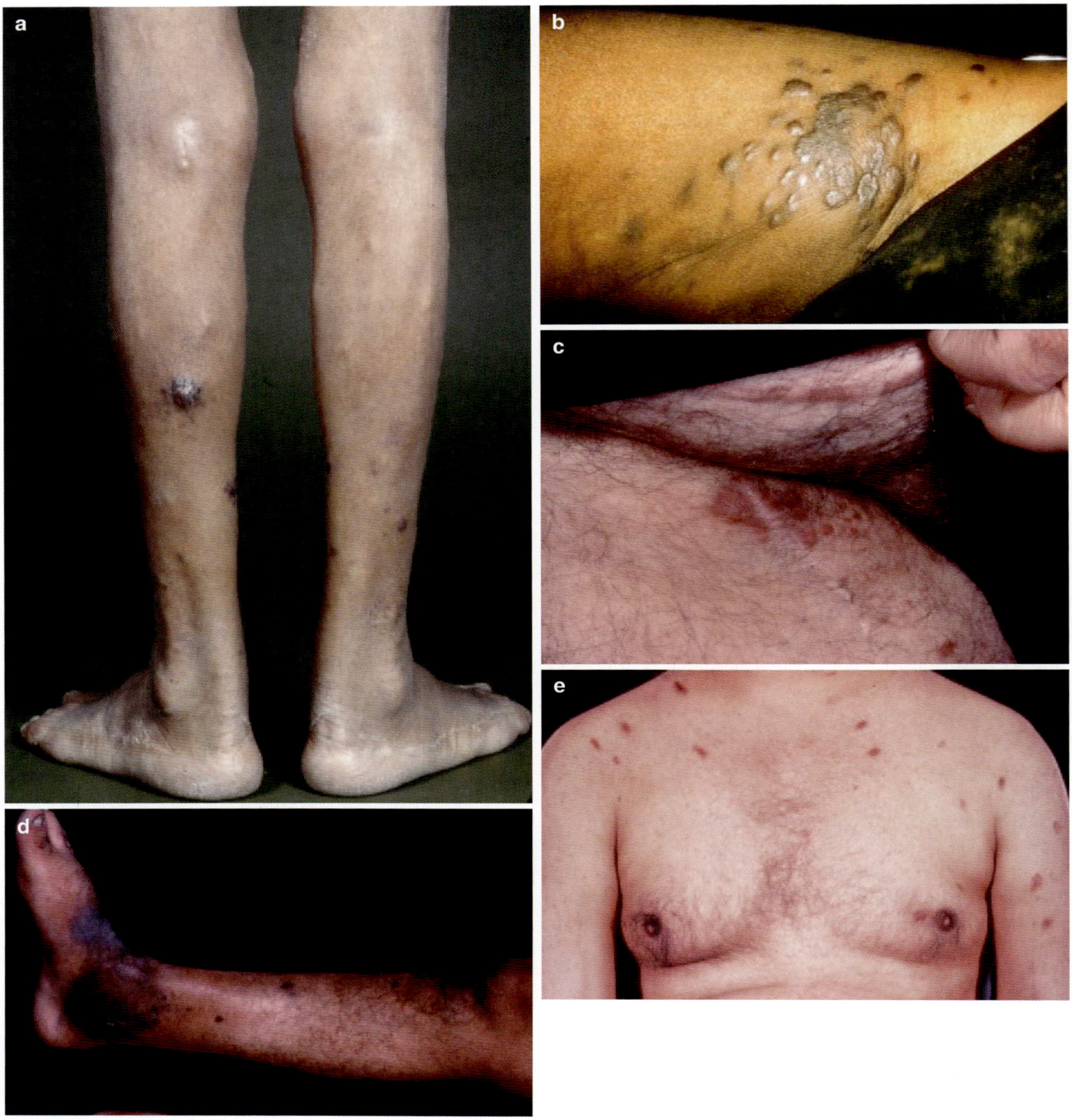

Fig. 71.4 (**a**–**e**) Multiple cutaneous manifestations of Kaposi's sarcoma

BKV

It is a double-stranded DNA virus, acquired mostly in childhood with seroprevalence in excess of 85 %. It remains latent in the renal tract, and 5–10 % of immunocompetent individuals intermittently shed virus, but there is no evidence of pathological consequences of BK infection in the general population. In RTR, infection results in nephropathy in 1–10 % of recipients with high risk of graft loss, as well as causing ureteric strictures and haemorrhagic cystitis (usually in BMT).

The incidence of PVAN seems to have genuinely increased in the last 30 years, and registry data from the US organ procurement and transplant network suggests current rates of 6 % PVAN by 5 years (the vast majority occurring in the first

2 years) [25]. The main risk factor appears to relate to the total burden of immunosuppression (use of depleting antibodies, treatment of acute rejection and combination of tacrolimus and mycophenolic acid). However, it is extremely rare to get PVAN in other SOT with much higher levels of IS in part because the renal tract is the site of latency for BKV. In addition, other known risk factors such as D+R−, episodes of acute rejections, deceased donor, ureteric stent and viral co-infection may all contribute to infection and tubular cell injury/division necessary for BKV growth. It is also possible that some serotypes are more virulent and may cause a reinfection. There is a clinically important natural history to PVAN; 20–40 % of RTRs have viruria which precede the 5–15 % of those that get viraemia by 4–6 weeks and diagnosis of PVAN by 12 weeks [26], thus offering a window for detection and prevention.

There are usually no clinical features associated with BKV infection in RTR except a deterioration in renal function or ureteric obstruction, so screening and biopsy are critical.

Urine PCR for BKV DNA has a sensitivity of about 50 % but given the high rates of viruria lack specificity for PVAN. In plasma $>10^4$copies/ml of BKV DNA is a sensitive and specific marker of PVAN with a high negative predictive value. Consequently the KDIGO guidelines recommend screening plasma for BKV DNA, monthly for 3 months, followed by 3 monthly for 12–24 months [4]. An alternative to plasma DNA is to use urine cytology (Papanicolaou stain) to identify the viral cytopathic effect in 'decoy cells' (detached tubular epithelial cells with viral nuclear inclusions). This has a lower positive predictive value than viraemia (similar to DNA screening of urine) but is cheaper than nucleic acid testing [27]. Urine positive for viral cytopathic effect should prompt plasma BKV DNA screening. Plasma BKV DNA screening should also be done in the context of an unexplained rise in creatinine or ureteric obstruction. Not everyone with viraemia develops PVAN so the gold standard for diagnosis is histological evidence of polyoma virus with viral cytopathic changes, nuclear inclusion, interstitial infiltrate and tubulitis. Granulomas may also be present (Fig. 71.5). It is confirmed by positive simian virus large T-antigen staining (SV40). However, the infection is patchy and the disease may be missed early on especially if the biopsy is small or superficial. In addition, initial views of the biopsy may appear identical to the tubulitis of acute cellular rejection so all biopsies with a cellular infiltrate should be stained for SV40 with urgency to avoid increasing IS when reduction is necessary.

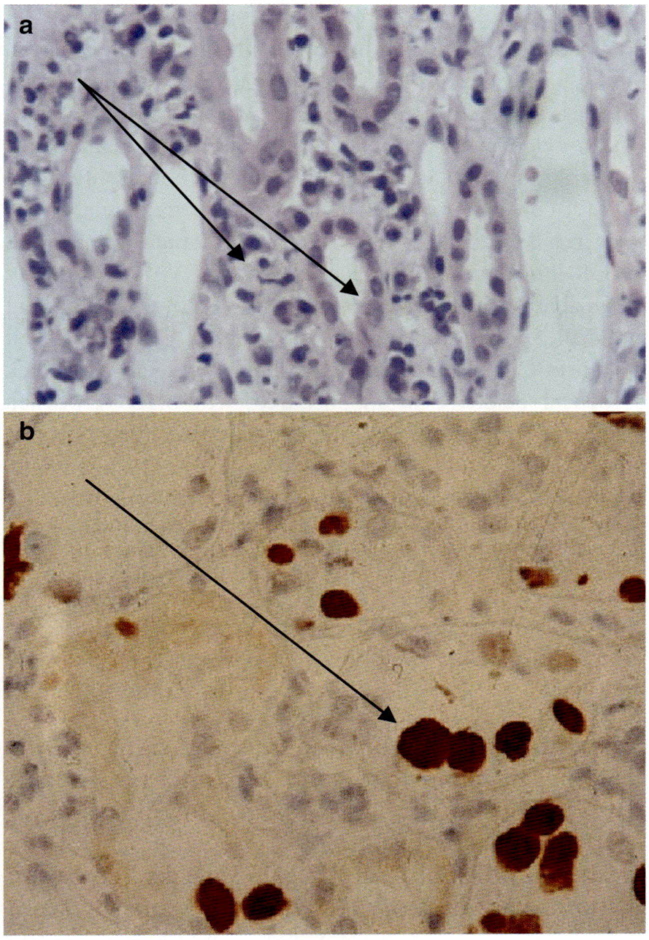

Fig. 71.5 BKV. Nephropathy showing cellular infiltrate and nuclear inclusions (**a**). Diagnosis of BKV confirmed by positive SV40 staining (**b**)

Treatment

It is important to note that there is no substantial data in support of any treatment of PVAN apart from ISR. Although not the subject of a RCT, pre-emptive ISR has been associated with viral clearance in 80–95 % and a reduction in death-censored graft survival. A variety of protocols have been suggested for ISR in the face of viraemia [26, 28], but essentially start with halving either mycophenolic acid or azathioprine, and if no reduction in viraemia, then either reduction in CNI or stopping the anti-proliferative altogether. Rapid and abrupt cuts in IS are more likely to be associated with rejection, and differentiating the main pathological process even with SV40 staining can be very difficult.

A variety of drugs have been tried on the basis of theoretical or in vitro anti-polyoma activity and reported mostly as small case series and nonrandomised trials [26, 29]. These include leflunomide (usually at a dose of 20–60 mg/day), cidofovir (0.25 mg/kg with probenecid every 2 weeks), fluoroquinolones, IVIg and mTOR inhibitors. The use of leflunomide is out of the comfort zone for most nephrologists; drug monitoring is not available to most units and judging the appropriate dose is therefore tricky. Cidofovir has very considerable nephrotoxicity, pre-hydration with IV fluids is necessary, and the subsequent deterioration in renal function causes further diagnostic difficulty. There is a little evidence that fluoroquinolones reduce viraemia, but no evidence currently of improved clinical outcomes. Given the high prevalence of BKV infection, IVIg would seem a harmless therapeutic option, but it is a scarce resource without an evidence base, and it is not clear what significance humoral immunity has in clearing an intracellular virus. The data for conversion to mTOR inhibitors as treatment is also poor, but there is quite a lot of circumstantial evidence that mTOR inhibition may reduce the risk of PVAN by roughly a half that of other IS regimens [25] possibly by inhibiting cell cycle progression and not disabling BKV-specific T-cell responses to the same degree. In short there is a severe lack of decent evidence to support treatment of PVAN when appropriate ISR has failed. Our practice and that of some others [28] if PVAN persists following ISR or there has been a rejection episode is to introduce an mTORi (if proteinuria <0.5 g/l), ultimately aiming for mTORi monotherapy.

Original reports recounted grim outcomes in terms of graft survival, and roughly 50 % of grafts with PVAN were lost; however, greater awareness and better screening seem to be improving the outcome. A histological grading system (A–C) for PVAN has been devised based on the amount of cellular involvement and the extent of interstitial fibrosis and atrophy (reviewed in 28). The take-home message is that grade A is associated with 13 % graft loss, but grade C 100 % graft loss, i.e. early detection and ISR are likely to be dramatically more helpful than applying toxic medication for advanced disease. Limited data suggests a recurrence rate of about 20 %, but loss of second graft seems rare. There seems no evidence to remove the failed graft, but persistent viraemia is a likely risk factor, and removal of IS until an immune response suppresses viraemia would seem very prudent.

JC viral infection is commonly acquired asymptomatically early in life reaching 50 % seroprevalence by middle age, viruria can be detected in normal individuals, and viraemia has been detected in 5 % of transplant patients. Despite this, clinically apparent reactivation in the form of progressive multifocal leucoencephalopathy (PML) is very rare in transplantation. A caveat here is that the risk of PML is clearly related to the burden of immunosuppression; cases have been reported in patients with SLE following rituximab and in transplants following belatacept as well as less-specific depleting antibodies. PML has a wide differential and may be confused with CNI toxicity. The treatment is with staged immunosuppression reduction mindful of immune reconstitution syndrome (IRIS) with rapid withdrawal resulting in a vigorous immune response and worsening of clinical features as a consequence. Cidofovir has been used with limited success. The issue of re-transplantation is a moot point, often PML from whatever cause is an absolute contraindication, but it might be considered once there is good evidence of immune recovery in the absence of further depleting antibodies and following counselling.

Respiratory Viruses

A number of respiratory viruses infecting RTR (see Table 71.7) can cause asymptomatic or minor infection sometimes with prolonged shedding, but can also result in devastating respiratory illness and death. For most of these viruses, there is either no effective antiviral, or antivirals that have only modest efficacy. Management therefore relies on good housekeeping in terms of annual influenza vaccination (measles vaccination if not previously done), ensuring staff and patient hand hygiene is taught (and practised) and the ability to isolate potentially infectious patients. Rapid nucleic testing of nasopharyngeal swabs or aspirates is important to avoid inappropriate antibiotics and admitting an infectious patient into an open transplant ward.

Table 71.7 Respiratory viruses in renal transplant recipients

Respiratory syncytial virus (paramyxovirus)	Common respiratory infection post-SOT can progress to pneumonitis/bronchiolitis. Ribavirin (IV or inhaled) can be used (no RCTs) alone or with IVIg and reduction in immunosuppression. Consider palivizumab
Coronavirus (SARS coronavirus)	Coronavirus can cause URTi and LRTi, relevant in heavily immunosuppressed patients. SARS coronovirus carries a significant risk of ARDS and mortality. Currently no treatment for coronaviridae infections so emphasis on avoidance, ISR and supportive care
Adenovirus	May be shed for long periods from upper airway. Serotypes 1 and 2 associated with pneumonia. Supportive and reduction in IS (cidofovir can be used for disseminated infection)
Rhinovirus	Predominantly URTi but can cause LRTi, currently no effective treatment
Parainfluenzae virus	URT and LRT infection as well as asymptomatic shedding, no effective treatment
Influenza A and B (orthomyxovirus)	Influenza A H1N1 2009 pandemic responsible for considerable morbidity among SOT. Vaccination effective in SOT (less so in first 6 months post-transplant) and should be offered annually. Widespread resistance to M2 inhibitors (amantadine and rimantadine), some resistance to neuraminidase inhibitors (oseltamivir and zanamivir), but primary treatment oseltamivir 75 mg b.i.d. for 5 days. Prophylaxis should be considered for significant RTR contacts (oseltamivir 75 mg o.d. for 10 days)
Metapneumovirus	URTi and LRTi currently no effective treatment
Bocovirus	URTi, clinical relevance unclear
Enteroviruses	URTi and LRTi as well as meningitis and encephalitis

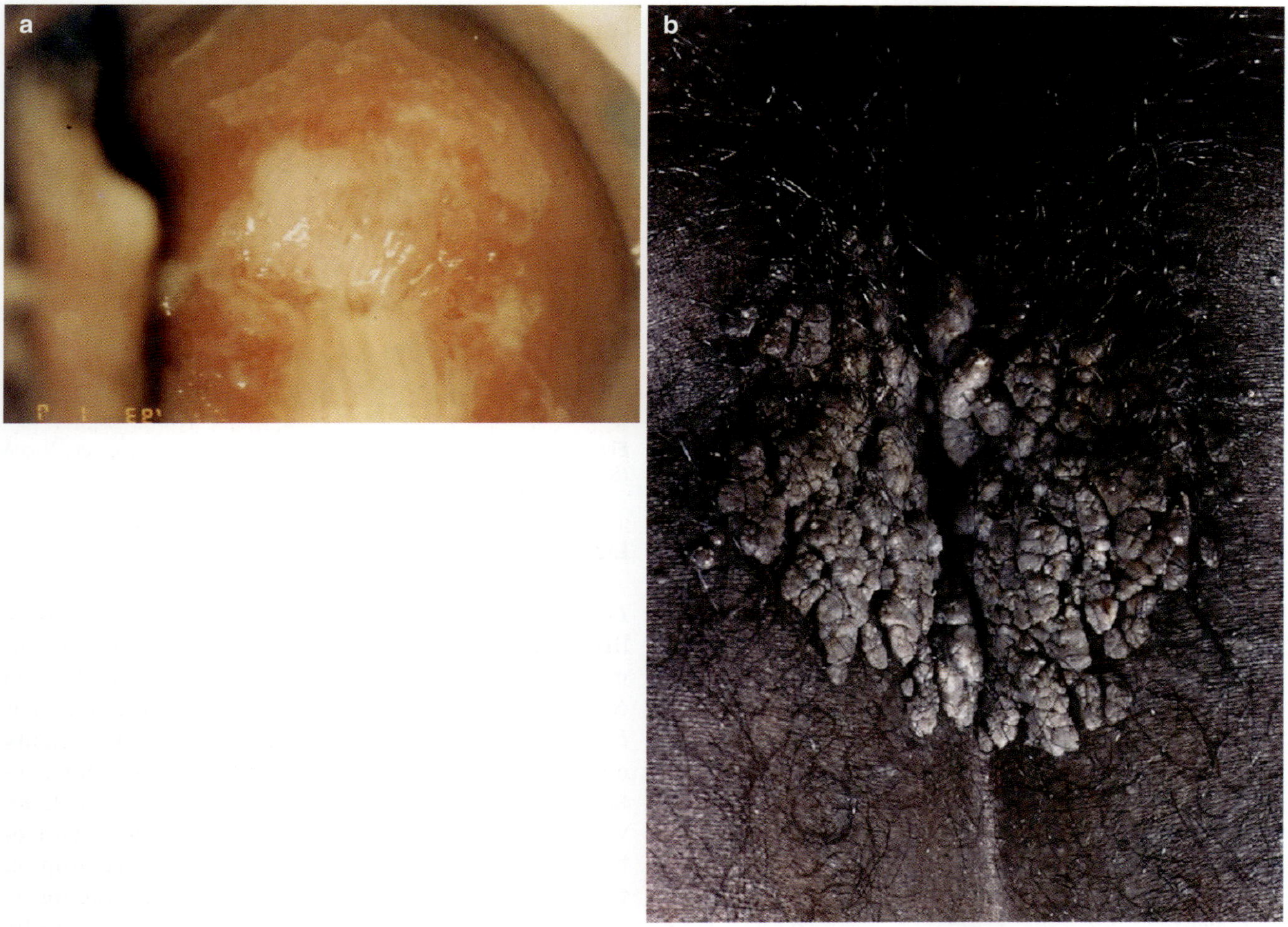

Fig. 71.6 (**a**) Colposcopy showing CIN3 in a 30-year-old renal transplant patient with human papillomavirus infection. (**b**) Perianal warts secondary to human papillomavirus infection in a renal transplant recipient

Beyond specific antivirals therapy is supportive care, treating secondary bacterial infections and immunosuppression reduction. IVIg has been used in patients with severe infections and worth considering in patients with severe infections and worth considering in life-threatening disease.

Parvovirus B-19

Parvovirus B-19 is a single-stranded DNA virus acquired by respiratory transmission, although it can be transmitted via transfusion or with the donor organ. Acute infection is with fever, arthritis and rash and sometimes with an acute aplastic crisis with marked anaemia (thrombocytopenia and leucopenia also common). Nephrotic syndrome secondary to a collapsing focal segmental glomerulopathy is also reported. Diagnosis can be made serologically with IgM, but PCR for viral DNA is more sensitive and permits monitoring of response. Viraemia can persist and treatment of aplastic anaemia or glomerulonephritis is with IVIg 0.4 g/Kg over 5 days.

Human Papillomavirus HPV

It is an important cause of morbidity post-transplant both in terms of viral cutaneous and anogenital warts as well as skin, vulval and perianal malignancy (Fig. 71.6). The skin manifestations and management of viral warts are discussed in chapter on renal skin disease, and it is worth remembering that HPV has been detected in the majority of post-transplant squamous cell and basal cell carcinomas [30]. Post-transplant patients have much higher incidence of HPV infection with pro-oncogenic serotypes 16 and 18. Registry data shows a substantial excess of cervical and anal precancer (approximately ×10) and a 50–100-fold increase in vulval premalignancies; most alarmingly the average age of vulval premalignancy in this group is 37, almost 25 years earlier than the general population. HPV vaccination of school girls may help reduce the incidence in women, but as yet there is no data to support the routine vaccination of patients on the waiting list. Many countries have guidelines recommending annual cervical screening post-transplant, but in the UK the evidence is that the uptake is extremely poor at around 10 % and is something we could improve [31].

Hepatitis E

Hepatitis E is an RNA virus transmitted by the faecal oral route, particularly from undercooked meat (predominantly genotype 3 in Western countries) and associated with high mortality with acute hepatic failure in patients with preexisting chronic liver disease or pregnancy. Recent data suggests, however, that it may be associated with chronic subclinical hepatitis in solid-organ transplants. In France the seroprevalence pre-transplant is 14 %, but reactivation has not been demonstrated. >50 % of de novo cases post-transplant are asymptomatic with the rest having hepatitis. Approximately 40 % of these patients clear the virus spontaneously, but 60 % do not and go on to have chronic infection with abnormal LFTs but occasionally rapid progression to cirrhosis. However, the overall prevalence of chronic infection is not known, and making the diagnosis is important as clearance of the virus may prevent cirrhosis and, if suspected, the diagnosis can be made on RNA from blood or stool. Treatment is with ISR or, failing that, success has been reported with pegalated interferon or ribavirin [32].

Bacteria

Legionella

Cell-mediated immunity appears particularly important in the defence against *Legionella pneumophila*, and consequently SOT recipients are at substantial risk if exposed (usually from contaminated air-conditioning systems or water tanks and in outbreaks). High fever and cough with flu-like symptoms are the norm. The CXR may show focal, nodular, lobar or diffuse consolidation sometimes with cavitation. Urine legionella antigen testing is quick (but does not detect the 10–30 % of serogroups that are not pneumophila such as micdadei) unlike paired legionella serology which is rarely helpful in real time. As with mycoplasma and chlamydia, PCR for legionella can be done on BAL samples.

Treatment is with macrolides (ideally azithromycin as it causes less inhibition of cytochrome p450), fluroquinolones, rifampicin (marked inducer of cytochrome p450) or dual therapy in sick patients.

Since tests may not be diagnostic, 'atypical' pathogen cover should be considered (ideally with a macrolide) for SOT recipients with a lower respiratory tract infection.

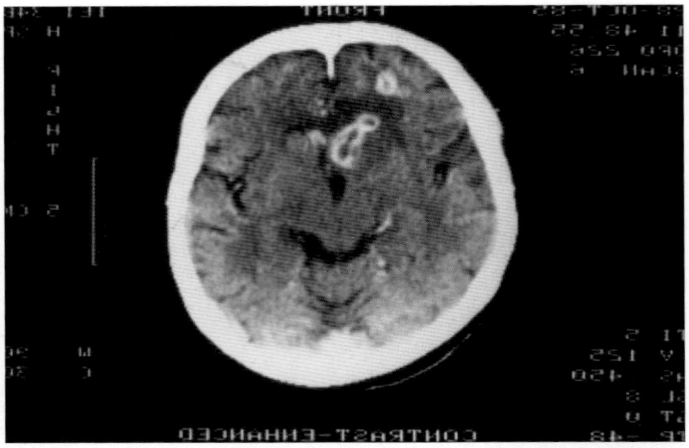

Fig. 71.7 Listeria causing a ring-enhancing space occupying lesion (SOL) in a recipient 6 years post-transplant

Listeriosis

Listeria monocytogenes is an environmental gram-positive bacillus, contracted orally from pets, domestic animals or unpasteurised or poorly kept foods and consequently can occur in outbreaks as well as sporadically. Listeria infection is associated with a high mortality especially in the immunocompromised as it is intracellular and normally eradicated by cell-mediated immunity which is disabled in SOT. It is the most common cause of bacterial meningitis in SOT and in addition has tropism for brain parenchyma. Incubation is within 24 h of ingestion, and symptoms develop within a week. Clinically presentation is non-specific: fever possibly following a diarrhoeal illness, malaise, meningitis (50 %) or encephalitis with abscess (10 %) (Fig. 71.7) [33]. Diagnosis is typically made on blood culture or examination of CSF.

Treatment is with intravenous ampicillin (2 g every 4 h). Gentamycin (3 mg/kg in three divided doses) is usually added in for immunocompromised patients. Trimethoprim-sulphamethoxazole (septrin) is an alternative for penicillin-allergic patients.

Nocardia

Nocardia is a rare but serious opportunistic infection post-transplant caused by actinomycetes nocardia species, mostly acquired by inhalation, occasionally via skin inoculation. The incidence in the reported literature is around 1 %, but this probably represents reporting bias, and the evidence is that it is less common in part because of universal prophylaxis with septrin. A review of the English literature case reports following renal transplantation shows a huge variation in onset from 4 weeks to 22 years [34].

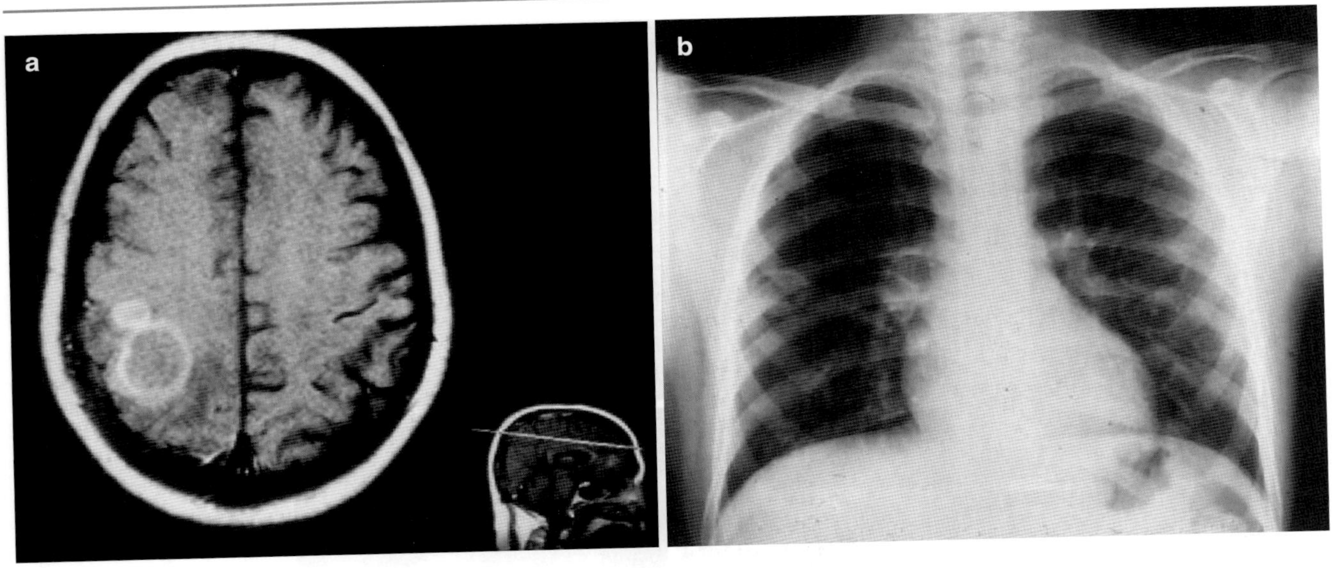

Fig. 71.8 Nocardia causing a ring-enhancing SOL on CT (**a**) and multiple cavities on CXR (**b**)

The vast majority of cases present with or have primary pulmonary involvement, and a significant proportion of these go on to have disseminated disease with a predilection for brain and cutaneous involvement (Fig. 71.8). Pulmonary involvement does not typically present as classical pneumonia, but fever, lung nodules and cavities are common. Cerebral involvement may be insidious and non-specific with headaches, confusion, focal neurological signs and is also associated with a fever [34].

Norcardia, especially disseminated disease, is associated with a significant mortality (17 %), and early diagnosis with biopsy of unexplained skin nodules or other accessible lesions is essential. Treatment for early pulmonary disease is with sulphonamides usually trimethoprim-sulphamethoxazole 15 mg/kg/day. For severe pulmonary or any cerebral involvement, imipenem and amikacin are added in, with the caveat that some nocardia species have resistance, and biopsy with culture and sensitivities is very important. Treatment must be prolonged to 6–12 months for pulmonary and 9–12 for cerebral involvement [35].

Mycobacteria: TM and Non-tuberculous Mycobacterium (NTM)

The incidence of active TB in renal transplants in Western countries is between 0.3 and 1 % which is 20–70× higher than the general population, and in Asia rates of 5–15 % have been reported. Apart from country of origin, diabetes, chronic liver disease and the burden of immunosuppression (e.g. the use of depleting antibodies) are significant risk factors [36, 37]. Screening pre-transplant is difficult as tuberculin skin tests, e.g. Mantoux test, while helpful if positive, often result in false negatives in patients with ESRD, and patients with previous BCG may have false positives. CXR with signs of previous TB are clearly helpful, and interferon gamma release assays may be helpful but do not distinguish between previous exposure and active disease, but again can be negative in patients with ESRD or post-transplant [38].

Clinical presentation occurs at an average of about 10–12 months post-transplant with the majority of infections thought to be reactivation with roughly 10 % due to primary infection (a very small percentage of which are donor derived). Fever appears to be a prominent feature occurring in 70 % with weight loss and asthenia. Strikingly, two-thirds of patients present with extra-pulmonary disease (compared to 15 % in the general population) (Fig. 71.9) [39], and consequently tissue biopsy and ensuring procedurists send a sample for culture are important in making the diagnosis. In immunocompromised patients, mycobacterial burden is often high and mycobacterial blood cultures may be helpful, especially in the setting of disseminated atypical mycobacterial infections (e.g. *Mycobacterium avium-intracellulare* complex infections – see below).

Management for MTB in SOT is the standard anti-TB treatment but presents issues in terms of drug interactions, the main one being the induction of cytochrome p450 by rifampicin resulting in marked reduction in CNI levels. It is usual to have to triple the dose of CNI within the first 2 weeks of rifampicin-based therapy. Importantly, the converse is true when rifampicin is stopped with the need for significant dose reduction. It is critical therefore to have close liaison between the infectious disease team and the nephrologist. Treatment is often accompanied by ISR, but this needs to be done with

suspicion is required: at lumber puncture, high opening pres-

least 12 months (or lifelong if peripheral blood CD4 cells remain <200).

First-line treatment for PCP is septrin at 120 mg/kg/day in divided doses [44]; this requires a large volume of IV

5 mg) as is clotrimazole or oral fluconazole 50 mg o.d.

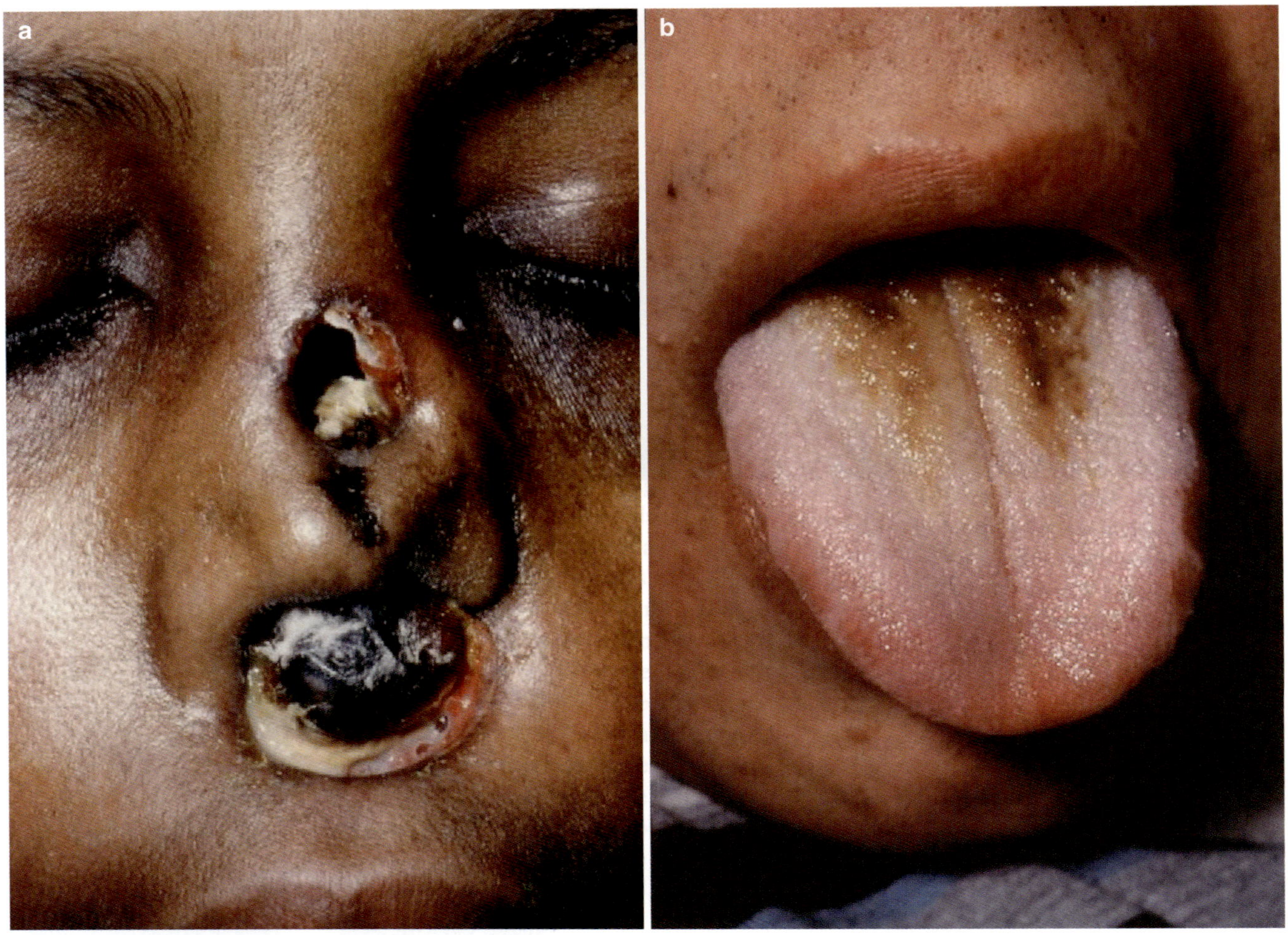

Fig. 71.12 Aspergillus infection. (**a**) Invasive nasopalatal aspergillus infection. (**b**) *Aspergillus niger* infection of the tongue

Morbidity and mortality in cryptococcal meningitis is mainly associated with raised intracranial pressure (as a result of CSF absorption blockade), and repeated lumber punctures to remove CSF are required in the first 2 weeks of therapy.

Mucormycosis

Mucormycosis is a rare opportunistic fungal infection most commonly documented in debilitated and poorly controlled diabetics but also documented in renal transplants (1 % of invasive fungal infections). Risk factors include prolonged neutropenia, diabetes and iron-chelation therapy as well as immunosuppression. Mucocutaneous, particularly orofacial, rhinocerebral and pulmonary involvement are the most common, and because of the propensity to invade vessel, a fatal outcome from pulmonary haemorrhage and dissemination is common (Fig. 71.13). Treatment is with IV liposomal amphotericin (with posaconazole as an alternative or dual therapy), and surgical resection of pulmonary and extra-pulmonary tissue is important. The mortality from mucormycosis in RTR remains the highest of any fungal infection at over 50 %.

Histoplasmosis capsulatum and *Coccidioidomycosis immitis*

These are endemic fungi that are responsive for <4 % of invasive fungal infections in SOT but with a very high mortality. Both fungi occur in SW USA, Central and South America, but histoplasma is also reported in Europe, Asia and Africa. Outbreaks of both conditions have been described in RTRs, and rare cases of donor-derived infection have also been reported; however, the majority of infections appear to be reactivation (occurring within 6 months) or primary infections (occurring at any stage).

The main exposure risk for histoplasma is bird or bat guano. Histoplasmosis in RTR may present with fever, cellulitis, mouth ulcers and oronasopharynx, pulmonary or meningeal involvement [48]. Fungal cultures may take weeks, and as with other fungal infections biopsies can be

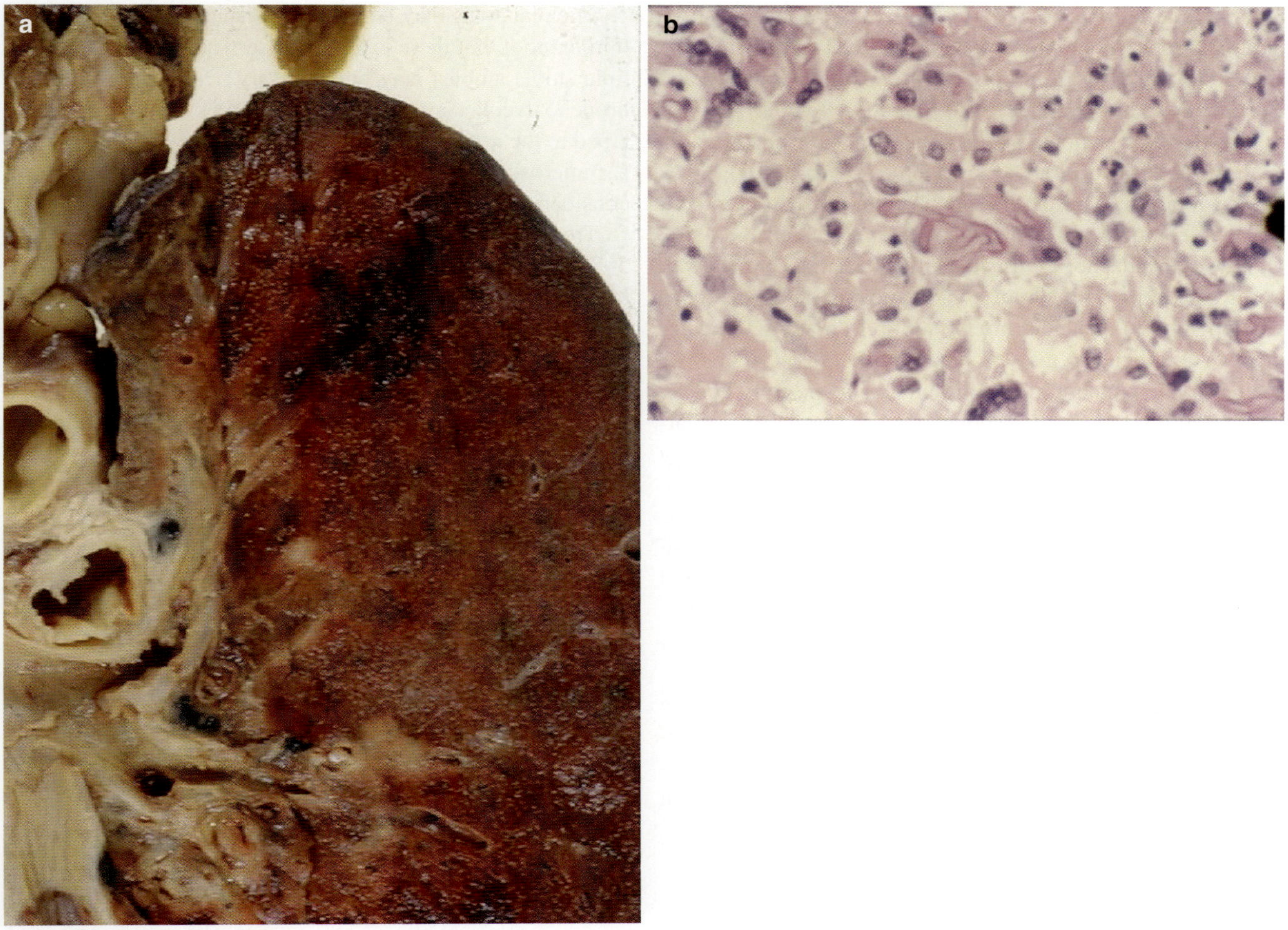

Fig. 71.13 (**a**) Post-mortem specimen showing the lung with haemorrhage secondary to vessel involvement of a transplant patient with mucormycosis. (**b**) Biopsy showing invasive mycelium

very helpful. Urine antigen screening has a high (>90 %) sensitivity but is not widely available. Histopathological examination may show characteristic intracellular organisms.

In immunocompetent individuals coccidioidomycosis almost exclusively causes pulmonary involvement, but in SOT 75 % is extra-pulmonary, commonly involving liver, bone marrow and meninges [49]. Guidelines do not recommend serological screening, but some authors advocate this for donor and recipient in endemic regions.

First-line treatment for both fungi is with liposomal amphotericin, with itraconazole as second line for histoplasmosis, fluconazole or caspofungin for coccidioidomycosis and accompanied by ISR. As fatal relapses can occur, it is usual to treat with an azole for at least a year, and after meningeal involvement, usually for life.

Cryptosporidiosis

Cryptosporidium parvum (associated with drinking water, swimming pools and livestock) can cause a chronic disabling diarrhoea in RTR which is watery/mucoid and associated with abdominal pain. In most individuals it is a self-limiting illness patients are not normally screened but in one study of SOTs with diarrhoea 20 % of cases were attributed to cryptosporidium, so it is probably underdiagnosed in most practice [50]. Cryptosporidium Ag testing by ELISA is highly sensitive with a good specificity and worth considering in any RTR with culture-negative diarrhoea not responsive to replacement of the usual suspect medications. There is no specific treatment, spiramycin, nitazoxanide and paromomycin have been tried with some success but relapses can occur.

Parasites

Toxoplasmosis

Toxoplasma gondii is an opportunistic parasite which can cause disease in RTR through reactivation, primary infection and occasionally through donor transmission. Risk factors include seronegative status of recipient, seropositive donor, burden of immunosuppression (CD4 counts below 200), lack of septrin prophylaxis and exposure to cats. Reactivation and donor-derived infection tend to present within the first 3 months of a transplant with pneumonitis (two-thirds) or neurological involvement (two-thirds) (90 % at post-mortem), and cardiac involvement is also common. Fever is common but neurological symptoms are non-specific with headache, confusion and ultimately coma [51]. Serology is only really helpful in diagnosing risk as seroconversion is often slow and rarely helpful in making the diagnosis. The diagnosis may be made by contrast CT or MRI scanning showing multiple ring-enhancing lesions and an appropriate radiological response after 2–3 weeks of treatment. CNS ring-enhancing lesions in SOT recipients may be due to a number of causes, and if an appropriate response to treatment is not seen, a stereotactic brain biopsy may be required. When safe to do so, a CSF examination with CSF Toxoplasma DNA detection by PCR is highly sensitive and specific for CNS toxoplasmosis.

Septrin prophylaxis for PCP is very effective at preventing toxoplasmosis, but reactivation can occur on stopping. Treatment is with pyrimethamine 200 mg loading dose followed by 50–75 mg daily and folinic acid plus sulphadiazine 4–6 weeks or septrin 5 mg/kg for 30 days. The mortality remains high at 50–65 %, those with primary infection being particularly at risk [52].

Strongyloides stercoralis

Strongyloidiasis in the setting of SOT is a very rare but serious condition with mortality of around 50 %. Strongyloides is endemic in large areas of the tropics and subtropics. Initial infection is via larval penetration of the skin and is usually asymptomatic. Larvae migrate to the pulmonary vessels and then via swallowed sputum to the duodenum and jejunum where mature female larvae shed eggs. Importantly infection can remain quiescent for over 30 years so a history of living in an endemic area is as important as being transplanted in an endemic area.

Reactivation and hyper-infestation can occur in those with previous exposure once significantly immunocompromised, usually within 6 months, sometimes within the first month, but occasionally years after a transplant. Presentation tends to be predominantly respiratory and gastrointestinal with abdominal pain, diarrhoea, nausea, vomiting and abdominal distension and may lead to ileus. Respiratory involvement is with tachypnoea, dyspnoea, fever and cough and ARDS occurs in about two-thirds of cases. The CXR is usually abnormal with diffuse or patchy infiltrates. Eosinophilia, although a very helpful clue, is often not present [53] although may well have been present but missed on pre-transplant bloods.

The diagnosis may be made by visualising larvae in sputum or stool, but there is a high false-negative rate and multiple stool samples may be necessary. Duodenal aspiration, bronchoalveolar lavage and the Enterotest (a piece of string taped to the nose passing into the duodenum then withdrawn for microscopy) all have their supporters and are all worth considering if there is clinical suspicion.

Treatment is with ivermectin (200 mcg/kg often for 5–7 days in hyper-infestation or 2 days in others) along with broad-spectrum antibiotics and repeat treatment if there is evidence of gut translocation. Patients can deteriorate very rapidly with hyper-infestation either via ARDS or recurrent gram-negative septicaemia as the larvae burrow into the gut. Early identification is therefore critical, and a sensible approach is to check strongyloides serology of all patients from endemic areas pre-listing. If positive, or with unexplained eosinophilia, stool should be screened for ova cysts and parasites and an ID opinion should be sought with regard to blind eradication.

Trypanosomiasis

Chagas disease (*Trypanosoma cruzi*) endemic in Central and South America can cause disease in RTR by reactivation (20 % of seropositive patients) or donor-derived infection (20 % of seropositive donors) [54]. Infection results in fever, myocarditis, meningoencephalitis or cutaneous involvement such as panniculitis typically within a year of transplant [55]. Pre-transplant serology or treatment is not currently recommended in part because of the toxicity of treatment but close surveillance post-transplant for D+ or R+. The diagnosis, management and treatment of trypanosomiasis should be undertaken with the infectious diseases team. Benzinidazole is the treatment of choice (with nifurtimox as an alternative) for 8 weeks in the context of parasitaemia.

Scabies

This can result in hyper-infestation and severe secondary bacterial infection (Fig. 71.14), but the pruritis may be subdued and source of the cellulitis not immediately apparent.

Syndromes

There are a variety of clinical scenarios in the immunocompromised with a wide differential diagnosis. Tables 71.8, 71.9, 71.10, 71.11 and 71.12 show the differential diagnosis for diarrhoea, chest infiltration, nodules, CNS space occupying lesions and meningoencephalitis.

28. Suwelack B, et al. The influence of immunosuppressive agents on

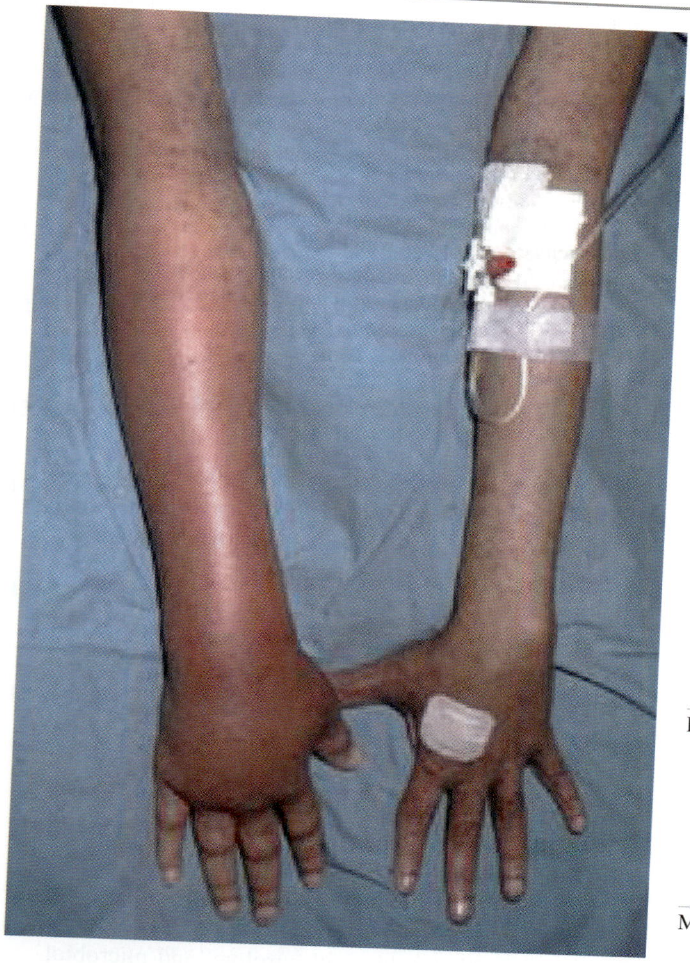

Fig. 71.14 Hyper-infestation with Norwegian scabies

Table 71.8 Differential diagnosis of diarrhoea in SOT recipients

Medication:	
Immunosuppression	Mycophenolic acid (may develop overtime), tacrolimus (NB: diarrhoea increases tacrolimus levels), mTORi
Antibiotics	
Miscellaneous	Laxatives, colchicine, metformin
Infectious opportunistic:	
Viral:	
CMV[a]	Usually but not always, associated with CMV viraemia, diarrhoea often bloody
Norovirus	Seasonal, nausea and vomiting prominent
Rotavirus	
Coxsackie[a]	
HSV[a]	
Adenovirus[a]	
Bacterial:	
Clostridium difficile	
Listeria[a]	
MAI[a]	
Salmonella[a]	
Yersinia[a]	
E. coli[a]	
Campylobacter	
Parasitic:	
Cryptosporidium	
Microsporidium[a]	
Isospora belli	
Giardia lamblia	
Strongyloides[a]	
Entamoeba histolytica[a]	

[a]Can result in disseminated disease

Table 71.9 Differential diagnosis of pulmonary infiltrates in SOT recipient

Infection:	
Bacteria	Conventional bacteria, mycobacteria, nocardia
Viruses	CMV, community respiratory viruses (influenza, parainfluenza, RSV)
Fungi	Aspergillus, pneumocystis, cryptococcus
Fluid:	
ARDS	Sepsis, allergic reaction to anti-CD25mAb, ATG, OKT-3, Campath-H1
Fluid retention/ cardiac failure	Left ventricular failure, diastolic dysfunction, transplant renal artery stenosis (flash pulmonary oedema)
Pulmonary haemorrhage	
Medication:	
mTOR inhibitor	mTORi-induced pneumonitis; opportunistic infection less likely if CD4+ count >200 (if in doubt stop mTOR and treat with steroids)
Others	Azathioprine, cyclophosphamide, nitrofurantoin

Table 71.10 Differential diagnosis of pulmonary nodule in SOT recipient

Infective:	
Bacterial abscess	Nocardia, legionella, gram positive (*Staph. aureus*, *Rhodococcus equi*), gram negative (Enterobacteriaceae, *Pseudomonas aeruginosa*, *Klebsiella pneumoniae*), anaerobes and septic emboli
Mycobacteria	Mycobacterium tuberculosis and non-TB mycobacteria
Fungal	Aspergillus, cryptococcus, histoplasmosis, coccidioidomycosis and paracoccidioidomycosis, PCP
Malignancy:	
PTLD	May or may not be associated with EBV viraemia
KS	Usually multiple, may be associated with chylous effusion HHV-8 PCR positive
Donor-derived malignancy	

52. Martina MN, et al. Toxoplasma gondii primary infection in renal transplant recipients. Two case reports and literature review. Transpl Int. 2011;24(1):e6–12.
53. DeVault Jr GA, et al. Opportunistic infections with Strongyloides stercoralis in renal transplantation. Rev Infect Dis. 1990;12(4):653–71.
54. Riarte A, et al. Chagas' disease in patients with kidney transplants: 7 years of experience 1989–1996. Clin Infect Dis. 1999;29(3):561–7.
55. Kocher C, et al. Skin lesions, malaise, and heart failure in a renal transplant recipient. Transpl Infect Dis. 2012;14(4):391–7.

Coccidioides

72 Long-Term Management of Kidney Transplant Recipients (KTRs)

Richard J. Baker

The first successful renal transplant was carried out between identical twins in Boston, USA, in 1954. Despite this early success, until the mid-1980s, approximately half of all renal transplants were lost within the first year, primarily due to refractory acute rejection. The advent of ciclosporin markedly improved outcomes, and by 1990 the 1-year graft survival rate approached 90 %.

Anecdotal evidence suggested that a renal transplant usually provided a better outcome for a given patient, and this was confirmed in longitudinal studies looking at the functional performance and quality of life in KTRs. More recently robust evidence has emerged that patients who undergo renal transplantation not only enjoy a better quality of life, which is dialysis-free, but also live longer as shown in Fig. 72.1 for patients in the USA (although the outlook for dialysis patients in Europe may be better due the comparatively high mortality rates in the USA) [1]. One of the principal benefits of successful renal transplantation seems to be a reduction in the rate of cardiac events when compared to the wait-listed population [2].

Although the transplant will fail in about 50 % of all KTRs, the other half will die with a functioning transplant (Fig. 72.2). The principal causes of death are vascular disease, neoplasia and infection. For this reason it is essential to provide lifelong follow-up in clinics which specialise in both preventing and treating these diseases. There are detailed guidelines available from KDIGO and the Renal Association [3, 4].

The marked improvement in short-term graft survival has in turn generated a welcome new challenge – the problem of maximising long-term transplant outcomes. This involves three principal concerns in addition to standard general medical care:

- Optimising the survival of the graft by preventing and treating the pathological processes that cause graft damage
- Preventing premature patient morbidity and mortality due to cardiovascular disease, neoplasia and infection, all which are exacerbated by immunosuppressive drugs
- Managing the failing transplant with appropriate introduction of medications and timely discussion of options for renal replacement therapy including re-transplantation if applicable

Optimising Graft Function

Optimising the survival of the graft starts prior to transplantation and forms one of the cornerstones of low clearance care. In particular early discussion of potential living donors is required. Patients will generally obtain better outcomes in the following circumstances:

1. Living donor kidneys – Potential related and unrelated living donors should be actively sought prior to transplantation. This may involve use of the living donor paired exchange pool
2. Pre-emptive transplantation
3. Accurate and frequent determination of sensitisation status

Monitoring Graft Function

Meticulous monitoring of graft function is an essential component of transplant care particularly in the first few months after the operation. Despite extensive efforts to develop other techniques (see Table 72.1), serum creatinine remains the gold standard for measuring transplant function. Many clinics use one of the MDRD equations to estimate glomerular filtration rate (eGFR) for their transplant patients which helps to communicate function to KTRs, but these equations have not been fully validated in the transplant population.

R.J. Baker, MBBChir, MA, FRCP, PhD
Renal Medicine, St James's University Hospital, Lincoln Wing, Beckett Street, Leeds LS9 7TF, UK
e-mail: richard.baker@leedsth.nhs.uk

M. Harber (ed.), *Practical Nephrology*,
DOI 10.1007/978-1-4471-5547-8_72,

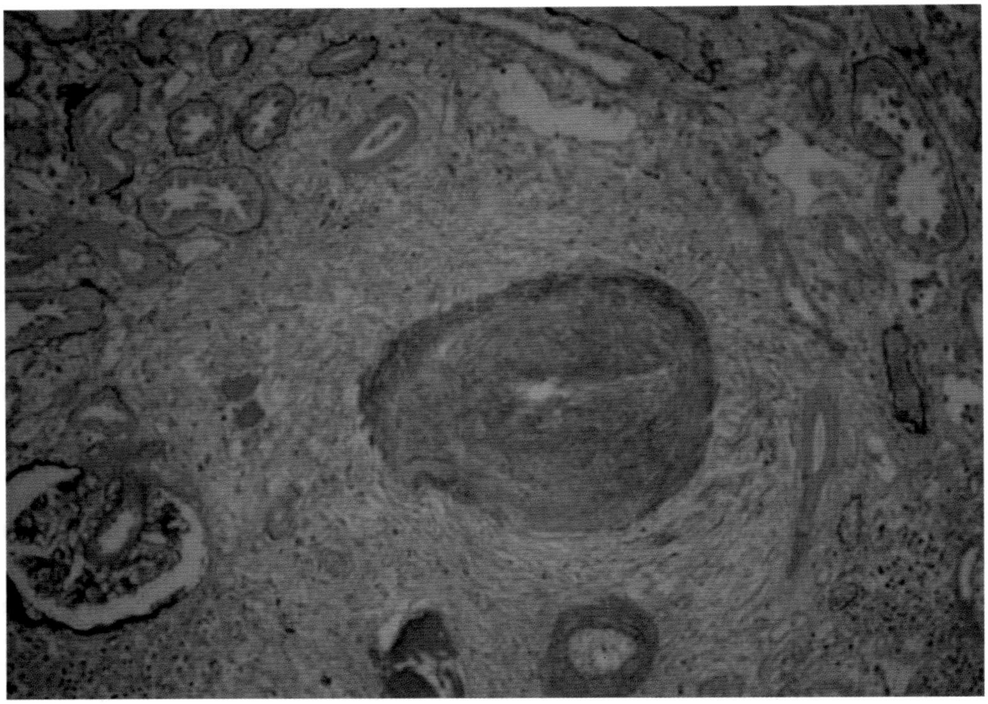

Fig. 72.5 Vascular fibrointimal hyperplasia

Evidence suggests that chronic antibody mediated rejection causes damage in the microcirculation which is manifested in the biopsy by peritubular capillaritis ("ptc" lesions) and glomerulitis ("g" lesions). The changes in the peritubular capillaries are demonstrated clearly on electron microscopy as multilayering of the tubular basement membrane. Over a prolonged period this damage causes thickening of the glomerular basement membrane without immune complex deposition ("cg" lesions) and mesangial matrix expansion ("mm" lesions). This morphological picture on the biopsy is usually associated with the development of anti-HLA antibodies in the circulation, which can be detected with increased sensitivity by solid-phase assays. The original descriptions of CAMR detailed the covalent deposition of complement products at the site of antibody action illustrated by C4d staining in glomerular and, in particular, peritubular capillaries. However more recent evidence suggests that C4d-negative CAMR is common and accounts for at least half of all CAMR. It has been proposed that CAMR is the major cause of chronic graft loss and that the principal cause of this process is poor adherence to IS medication, an assertion that requires further study.

The recognition of CAMR is generally based on the following criteria:

- Evidence of chronic graft damage – morphological features (2 out of 4)
  - IFTA
  - Vascular fibrointimal hyperplasia ("cv" lesions)
  - Transplant glomerulopathy ("cg" lesions)
  - Peritubular capillary multilayering on electron microscopy
- C4d staining
- Donor-specific antibodies (DSAs)

This pattern of graft damage is being increasingly recognised in biopsies of KTRs with deteriorating graft function and is usually associated with significant proteinuria (PCR > 50). Most clinicians will increase the IS in this setting. This involves continuing CNI medications (tacrolimus level 5–10 ng/ml, ciclosporin 100–150 ng/ml), maximising the dose of antiproliferative agent and adding maintenance steroids (0.1 mg/kg/day) (see Table 72.6). In practice this approach is successful in some KTRs although the immunosuppressant change usually coincides with multiple other interventions (e.g. attention to blood pressure and lipids). Other IS approaches have been attempted in small uncontrolled studies such as bortezomib, rituximab, intravenous immunoglobulins, high-dose intravenous steroids and plasma exchange. So far none of these expensive and labour-intensive approaches have been found to be beneficial.

Cardiovascular Risk

Half of all KTRs will die with a functioning transplant, and approximately half of these deaths (i.e. 25 % overall) will be due to vascular disease. It is important that the renal transplant clinic actively promotes good vascular health. Healthy living should be encouraged with exercise, weight loss, smoking cessation and patient-specific dietary advice. There are comprehensive guidelines available for this purpose [3, 4].

Epidemiological studies in KTRs suggest that risk factors for vascular disease are similar to the general population including diabetes, cigarette smoking and hyperlipidaemia. Recent evidence suggests that renal function may be the strongest determinant of cardiovascular risk [29]. In this study once the eGFR dropped below 45 ml/min/1.73 m^2, there was a 15 % increase in both the death rate and the incidence of cardiovascular disease with each 5 ml/min drop in eGFR. Intriguingly this suggests that absolute transplant function may be more important than pre-existing comorbidities.

Hypertension

Hypertension occurs in approximately 70 % of KTRs due to a number of reasons:

- Suboptimal graft function
- The presence of native kidneys with activation of the RAS and overactive sympathetic activity
- IS medications, especially CNIs and steroids
- High BMI
- Transplant renal arterial disease
- Allografts from hypertensive donors

Higher blood pressures are not only linked to graft loss but also vascular events. Furthermore, registry data suggests that when blood pressure control improves, then this will result in decreased rates of vascular events as well as improved long-term graft outcome [9]. Clinic readings are often high, and it is essential to develop methods for regular and accurate BP measurement. For this purpose home blood pressure monitoring and 24-h continuous ambulatory monitoring may be useful, especially in cases of white coat hypertension.

Treatment consists of lifestyle modification and drug treatment. Unfortunately there is a dearth of high-quality trial data in this area. A meta-analysis of the existing trial evidence suggested that there was little to choose between agents with perhaps a slight advantage to calcium channel blockade. It should be noted that trials have not been carried out in specific subgroups such as diabetics or KTRs with proteinuria. The clinical priority should be achieving the target by whatever means is best tolerated (Clinic blood pressure <130/80 mmHg or 125/75 if proteinuric [PCR>50]). UK Renal Registry data suggests that compliance with this standard in the UK is currently poor.

Immunosuppressive drugs such as corticosteroids, ciclosporin and tacrolimus contribute to hypertension, and modification of IS may benefit blood pressure control. However such considerations will usually be secondary, and the effective use of antihypertensive agents remains the cornerstone of treatment.

Transplant renal artery stenosis is an important cause of hypertension in KTRs and usually occurs between 3 months and 2 years after transplantation. It should be suspected in patients with refractory hypertension, and there may be clinical evidence of salt and water retention. Ultrasound Doppler studies are more useful than in native kidneys and may show the typical "parvus tardus" waveform. MRA scans are also useful, and although they tend to be too sensitive, they do have a high negative predictive value. Definitive treatment requires angiography with angioplasty +/– stenting.

New-Onset Diabetes After Transplantation (NODAT)

The development of new-onset diabetes after transplantation (NODAT) is an increasing problem and is associated with significantly increased morbidity and mortality [30, 31]. In the USA up to 40 % of adult KTRs develop NODAT within 3 years of transplantation. Risk factors for NODAT include:

1. Increasing donor age – older donors increase risk
2. Obesity – higher BMIs increase risk possibly related to increased secretion of adiponectin
3. Previous gestational diabetes
4. Ethnicity – more common in Asian and black recipients
5. Certain HLA types (HLA-B13, B15, B27 and B42) and other genetic polymorphisms
6. Family history of diabetes
7. HLA matching and donor characteristics
8. Viral infection – up to four times more common in HCV +ve KTRs, probably since HCV decreases hepatic insulin sensitivity
9. Type of underlying native renal disease – commoner in ADPKD
10. Medications – associated with steroid usage, sirolimus and CNIs especially tacrolimus

Five-year patient survival drops from 93 to 87 % for those KTRs who develop NODAT, and median graft survival also falls from 11 to 8 years.

Prevention involves identifying susceptible individuals using the risk factors above and counselling regarding lifestyle modification. Predictive risk scores have been proposed based on preoperative characteristics but they lack precision. Random glucose measurements should be checked before listing for transplantation, and if necessary fasting readings or a glucose tolerance test should be performed. Both high glucose levels prior to transplantation and high levels during the first seven postoperative days are associated with the subsequent development of NODAT after transplantation. Whether screening waiting list patients with a glucose tolerance test is cost effective remains to be evaluated. In certain cases it may be justified to modify the IS regime to minimise the future risk of NODAT, e.g. steroid avoidance or switching the CNI from tacrolimus to ciclosporin. An interesting strategy under investigation is the early introduction of hypoglycaemic agents such as vildagliptin and pioglitazone in KTRs with early hyperglycaemia. Recent trial evidence has

References

1. Wolfe RA, Ashby VB, Milford EL, Ojo AO, Ettenger RE, Agodoa LY, et al. Comparison of mortality in all patients on dialysis, patients on dialysis awaiting transplantation, and recipients of a first cadaveric transplant. N Engl J Med. 1999;341(23):1725–30.
2. Meier-Kriesche HU, Schold JD, Srinivas TR, Reed A, Kaplan B. Kidney transplantation halts cardiovascular disease progression in patients with end-stage renal disease. Am J Transplant. 2004;4(10):1662–8.
3. KDIGO clinical practice guideline for the care of kidney transplant recipients. Am J Transplant. 2009;9 Suppl 3(3):S1–155.
4. Baker R, Jardine A, Andrews P. Renal Association Clinical Practice Guideline on post-operative care of the kidney transplant recipient. Nephron Clin Pract. 2011;118 Suppl 1(1):c311–47.
5. Tullius SG, Tran H, Guleria I, Malek SK, Tilney NL, Milford E. The combination of donor and recipient age is critical in determining host immunoresponsiveness and renal transplant outcome. Ann Surg. 2010;252(4):662–74.
6. Giral M, Foucher Y, Karam G, Labrune Y, Kessler M, de Ligny BH, et al. Kidney and recipient weight incompatibility reduces long-term graft survival. J Am Soc Nephrol. 2010;21(6):1022–9.
7. Hariharan S, McBride MA, Cherikh WS, Tolleris CB, Bresnahan BA, Johnson CP. Post-transplant renal function in the first year predicts long-term kidney transplant survival. Kidney Int. 2002;62(1):311–8.
8. Mange KC, Cizman B, Joffe M, Feldman HI. Arterial hypertension and renal allograft survival. JAMA. 2000;283(5):633–8.
9. Opelz G, Dohler B. Improved long-term outcomes after renal transplantation associated with blood pressure control. Am J Transplant. 2005;5(11):2725–31.
10. Shah T, Kasravi A, Huang E, Hayashi R, Young B, Cho YW, et al. Risk factors for development of new-onset diabetes mellitus after kidney transplantation. Transplantation. 2006;82(12):1673–6.
11. Hricik DE. Metabolic syndrome in kidney transplantation: management of risk factors. Clin J Am Soc Nephrol. 2011;6(7):1781–5.
12. Cherukuri A, Welberry-Smith MP, Tattersall JE, Ahmad N, Newstead CG, Lewington AJ, et al. The clinical significance of early proteinuria after renal transplantation. Transplantation. 2010;89(2):200–7.
13. Halimi JM, Laouad I, Buchler M, Al-Najjar A, Chatelet V, Houssaini TS, et al. Early low-grade proteinuria: causes, short-term evolution and long-term consequences in renal transplantation. Am J Transplant. 2005;5(9):2281–8.
14. Ojo AO, Held PJ, Port FK, Wolfe RA, Leichtman AB, Young EW, et al. Chronic renal failure after transplantation of a nonrenal organ. N Engl J Med. 2003;349(10):931–40.
15. Nankivell BJ, Borrows RJ, Fung CL, O'Connell PJ, Allen RD, Chapman JR. The natural history of chronic allograft nephropathy. N Engl J Med. 2003;349(24):2326–33.
16. El-Zoghby ZM, Stegall MD, Lager DJ, Kremers WK, Amer H, Gloor JM, et al. Identifying specific causes of kidney allograft loss. Am J Transplant. 2009;9(3):527–35. doi:10.1111/j.1600-6143.2008.02519.x.
17. Holdaas H, Fellstrom B, Jardine AG, Holme I, Nyberg G, Fauchald P, et al. Effect of fluvastatin on cardiac outcomes in renal transplant recipients: a multicentre, randomised, placebo-controlled trial. Lancet. 2003;361(9374):2024–31.
18. Briganti EM, Russ GR, McNeil JJ, Atkins RC, Chadban SJ. Risk of renal allograft loss from recurrent glomerulonephritis. N Engl J Med. 2002;347(2):103–9.
19. Hariharan S, Johnson CP, Bresnahan BA, Taranto SE, McIntosh MJ, Stablein D. Improved graft survival after renal transplantation in the United States, 1988 to 1996. N Engl J Med. 2000;342(9):605–12.
20. Cole EH, Johnston O, Rose CL, Gill JS. Impact of acute rejection and new-onset diabetes on long-term transplant graft and patient survival. Clin J Am Soc Nephrol. 2008;3(3):814–21.
21. Famulski KS, Einecke G, Sis B, Mengel M, Hidalgo LG, Kaplan B, et al. Defining the canonical form of T-cell-mediated rejection in human kidney transplants. Am J Transplant. 2010;10(4):810–20.
22. Wiebe C, Gibson IW, Blydt-Hansen TD, Karpinski M, Ho J, Storsley LJ, et al. Evolution and clinical pathologic correlations of de novo donor-specific HLA antibody post kidney transplant. Am J Transplant. 2012;12(5):1157–67.
23. Sellarés J, de Freitas DG, Mengel M, Reeve J, Einecke G, Sis B, et al. Understanding the causes of kidney transplant failure: the dominant role of antibody-mediated rejection and nonadherence. Am J Transplant. 2012;12(2):388–99.
24. Loupy A, Hill GS, Jordan SC. The impact of donor-specific anti-HLA antibodies on late kidney allograft failure. Nat Rev Nephrol. 2012;8(6):348–57.
25. Mengel M, Sis B, Haas M, Colvin RB, Halloran PF, Racusen LC, et al. Banff 2011 Meeting report: new concepts in antibody-mediated rejection. Am J Transplant. 2012;12(3):563–70.
26. Farris AB, Colvin RB. Renal interstitial fibrosis: mechanisms and evaluation. Curr Opin Nephrol Hypertens. 2012;21(3):289–300.
27. Ekberg H, Tedesco-Silva H, Demirbas A, Vitko S, Nashan B, Gurkan A, et al. Reduced exposure to calcineurin inhibitors in renal transplantation. N Engl J Med. 2007;357(25):2562–75.
28. Sharif A, Shabir S, Chand S, Cockwell P, Ball S, Borrows R. Meta-analysis of calcineurin-inhibitor-sparing regimens in kidney transplantation. J Am Soc Nephrol. 2011;22(11):2107–18.
29. Weiner DE, Carpenter MA, Levey AS, Ivanova A, Cole EH, Hunsicker L, et al. Kidney function and risk of cardiovascular disease and mortality in kidney transplant recipients: the FAVORIT trial. Am J Transplant. 2012;17(10):1600–6143.
30. Sarno G, Muscogiuri G, De Rosa P. New-onset diabetes after kidney transplantation: prevalence, risk factors, and management. Transplantation. 2012;3:3.
31. Yates CJ, Fourlanos S, Hjelmesaeth J, Colman PG, Cohney SJ. New-onset diabetes after kidney transplantation-changes and challenges. Am J Transplant. 2012;12(4):820–8.
32. Hecking M, Haidinger M, Doller D, Werzowa J, Tura A, Zhang J, et al. Early basal insulin therapy decreases new-onset diabetes after renal transplantation. J Am Soc Nephrol. 2012;23(4):739–49.
33. Engels EA, Pfeiffer RM, Fraumeni Jr JF, Kasiske BL, Israni AK, Snyder JJ, et al. Spectrum of cancer risk among US solid organ transplant recipients. JAMA. 2011;306(17):1891–901.
34. Euvrard S, Morelon E, Rostaing L, Goffin E, Brocard A, Tromme I, et al. Sirolimus and secondary skin-cancer prevention in kidney transplantation. N Engl J Med. 2012;367(4):329–39.
35. Parker A, Bowles K, Bradley JA, Emery V, Featherstone C, Gupte G, et al. Management of post-transplant lymphoproliferative disorder in adult solid organ transplant recipients – BCSH and BTS Guidelines. Br J Haematol. 2010;149(5):693–705.
36. Dantal J, Hourmant M, Cantarovich D, Giral M, Blancho G, Dreno B, et al. Effect of long-term immunosuppression in kidney-graft recipients on cancer incidence: randomised comparison of two cyclosporin regimens. Lancet. 1998;351(9103):623–8.
37. Stavroulopoulos A, Cassidy MJ, Porter CJ, Hosking DJ, Roe SD. Vitamin D status in renal transplant recipients. Am J Transplant. 2007;7(11):2546–52.
38. Gwinner W, Suppa S, Mengel M, Hoy L, Kreipe HH, Haller H, et al. Early calcification of renal allografts detected by protocol biopsies: causes and clinical implications. Am J Transplant. 2005;5(8):1934–41.
39. Yabu JM, Winkelmayer WC. Posttransplantation anemia: mechanisms and management. Clin J Am Soc Nephrol. 2011;6(7):1794–801.
40. Vlahakos DV, Marathias KP, Agroyannis B, Madias NE. Posttransplant erythrocytosis. Kidney Int. 2003;63(4):1187–94.
41. Deshpande NA, James NT, Kucirka LM, Boyarsky BJ, Garonzik-Wang JM, Montgomery RA, et al. Pregnancy outcomes in kidney transplant recipients: a systematic review and meta-analysis. Am J Transplant. 2011;11(11):2388–404.
42. Sibanda N, Briggs JD, Davison JM, Johnson RJ, Rudge CJ. Pregnancy after organ transplantation: a report from the UK Transplant pregnancy registry. Transplantation. 2007;83(10):1301–7.
43. Kendrick EA, Davis CL. Managing the failing allograft. Semin Dial. 2005;18(6):529–39.

International Health Partnerships

73

Stacey Mearns

There are gross inequalities and inequities in health and healthcare around the world. A male born in Malawi can expect to live until the average age of 44 compared to 80 if born in Japan [1]. Child mortality in the World Health Organisation (WHO) Africa region is estimated at 119 per 1,000 live births, compared to 14 per 1,000 live births in the WHO European region [1]. Ninety-nine percent of all maternal deaths occur in developing countries [2]. It is estimated that Africa has 2.3 health workers per 1,000 population, compared with the Americas, where there are 24.8 healthcare workers per 1,000 population [3]. Closing the gap on such inequalities requires access to essential health services, which in itself requires stronger health systems with appropriate infrastructure, medicines and equipment, as well as trained health workers.

What Are Health Partnerships?

Health partnerships, also known as health links, are long-term reciprocal partnerships between health institutions in developed countries and their counterparts in developing countries. Partners can vary from hospitals, training institutions, health authorities and professional networks. Health linking is becoming an important feature of the development landscape and provides an opportunity to strengthen health systems in some of the world's poorest countries, helping to close the inequality gap. An example of health partnership is the Sister Renal Center Program supported by the International Society of Nephrology [4]. This programme links emerging renal units in developing countries to centres of excellence in developed countries, with the aim of promoting long-term partnership enabling the advancement of the practice of nephrology in developing countries through the sharing of education, training and disease prevention strategies.

Health links are designed to build capacity through a wide range of activities. The majority of health partnership activities focus on training and education in order to increase numbers of skilled health workers. However, there are a variety of activities that a health partnership may engage with (see Table 73.1), such activities will be dependent on the expertise and resources available within the partnership. Health links can offer an opportunity for a wide range of staff to be involved from academics and clinical staff to managers, support staff and students.

Health link projects can play an important role in strengthening health systems, leading to significant improvements and impact. A health link between Kambia District Health Management Team (Sierra Leone) and Gloucestershire Hospital NHS Foundation Trust (UK) provides a clear example of the power of health links to lead to substantial change. As part of an International Health Links Funding Scheme (IHLFS) project, multiple training courses on managing obstetric emergencies were given to 90 health workers within the district over 3 years. The project resulted in improved skills, confidence and motivation of staff within Kambia, as well as a reduction in the maternal mortality rate by a third between the beginning and end of the project [5]. As a result of the ISN Sister Renal Center Program, the Ilorin teaching

Table 73.1 Activities of health links

Activities
Training
Capacity building
Curriculum development
Facilitating research
Mentoring
Provision of equipment
Visitor exchanges
Service development

S. Mearns, BSc, MBChB, DTMH, MRCP
General Medicine, Royal Free Hospital,
Hampstead, London NW3 2QG, UK
e-mail: staceymearns@gmail.com

M. Harber (ed.), *Practical Nephrology*,
DOI 10.1007/978-1-4471-5547-8_73, © Springer-Verlag London 2014

Table 73.2 Benefits of health links

Benefits for developing country partner
Clinical education and training
Build institutional capacity
Staff development
Clinical service development and improvement
Introduction of research activities
Benefits for developed country partner
Personal and professional development of staff, building skills that are directly transferable in the home health institution
Enable understanding of healthcare from a different perspective
Improved motivation
Improved cultural experience and global health knowledge
Introduction of research activities

hospital in Nigeria through collaboration with multiple centres in Europe has shown growth in facilities, training activities and research and has introduced the provision of hemodialysis. The hospital has also gone on to establish a renal research group, rolled out a chronic kidney disease prevention programme and received accreditation for subspecialty training in nephrology [6].

Health links are intended to be mutually beneficial and allow for the reciprocal exchange of knowledge and skills leading to health system strengthening for both parties involved. There are many benefits to health partnerships (see Table 73.2), but at best they can:

- Inspire a desire for positive change both globally and locally
- Cultivate an openness to new ideas and thinking
- Generate enthusiasm and motivation
- Lay strong foundations for global citizenship

The above benefits are not a guarantee, and it is not enough to assume that if a health link exists, then it is a good thing. For health links to have real value, they must be carefully planned and considered. There needs to be equality within the partnership, ensuring both parties participate in vision setting and decision making and that activities are jointly managed. Further elements of successful partnerships include effective communication and information sharing, as well as openness to learning and development from both ends. In addition health links are more likely to be successful when they build upon and utilise existing structures and strengths, rather than create parallel services, and where possible align their activities with local and national health plans.

The Tropical Health and Education Trust (THET) is a UK-based organisation that supports the establishment and development of international health partnerships. A huge range of support is available from THET including guides of best practice, case studies of partnerships and training through their conferences. For anyone interested in starting a health partnership, THET is an excellent place to start (see support to health links).

How to Set Up a Health Partnership

The following steps are suggested as a guide to developing new health partnerships. The Tropical Health and Education Trust has produced a health links manual, which is an excellent and detailed resource for initiating a link (see useful resources).

Preparing for Partnership

When preparing for partnership you should firstly create a group of interested individuals within your organisation, who are committed and motivated to making the link work, and establish a health link committee. Whilst links often start between individuals, it is important to move to involve your wider organisation, as this will improve the sustainability of the partnership. As a group it is helpful to explore the potential value for a long-term partnership for your institution, explore and clarify your motives for partnership, and most importantly review what is already happening and what you can learn from others. The Tropical Health and Education Trust (THET) supports the development and work of health links; they are a very useful resource of information and can provide contacts for existing health links.

Choosing a Partner

Many health links often start through personal contacts. Ask around within your organisation, as there are likely to be many people who have worked overseas and whom have contacts. THEt also has an e-health bay, which contains a database of contacts in developing countries looking to start a partnership.

When selecting a partner it is important to ensure that there is clear need, as well as organisational support from both ends. Health links often work best when they are locally driven (bottom-up); in other words, there is a clear need and want from the developing country end to link; this will ensure much better co-operation and co-ordination of activities. Before choosing a partner it is critical to visit the institution and perform a feasibility visit.

Feasibility Visit

A feasibility visit involves visiting potential partner institutions in order to jointly identify rationale for partnership and scope of activities. Establishing projects and priorities within the health partnership should be done through a consultative process involving a needs assessment. Through this process, partnership activities can be planned with clear parameters and objectives. When conducting a needs assessment, the following should be considered:

- Be clear about what your organisation can offer.
- Start with the simple question of how can we help.
- Jointly agree priorities and partnership activities.

It is important to note that needs assessment should be an ongoing process throughout the partnership period rather than a one off activity. This will help to ensure that your health partnership remains dynamic, growing and adapting activities as both institutions develop and contexts change. It is helpful to develop a partnership agreement (memorandum of understanding), which lays out what the responsibilities and expectations of both parties, as well as the intended partnership activities.

Designing a Health Link Project

After completing a feasibility visit and needs assessment, you should have enough information to begin to design projects within your partnership. The initial design phase of any project should begin with determining the goals and objectives of the project, utilising SMART principles (specific, measurable, attainable, relevant and time-bound), going on to then outline the main activities of the project. Accompanying this it is important to have an implementation plan, outlining key time frames and responsibilities for both partners.

It is also useful to from the outset to define a monitoring and evaluation plan for your project. Monitoring and evaluation helps to track project progress and measure subsequent impact, as well as facilitate learning amongst other key stakeholders. In addition monitoring and evaluation information can be used to inform future decisions regarding your projects and partnership and provide key information for attracting funding and publicising your work.

Project monitoring and evaluation planning can be done using a variety of different tools (see useful resources); in its simplest form start with two key questions:

- What would success look like if your project were successful?
- What are the methods through which this success can be measured?

Working through this process will enable greater understanding of your project and partnership from the start.

Funding a Health Link

In order to acquire funds for health partnerships and subsequent projects, it is important to develop a detailed budget and proposal, which will be easier to do after working through the above steps in designing a health link project.

There are several sources of potential funding available for health partnerships including grants from THET's Health Partnership Scheme [7] and the International Society of Nephrology [4], to donations and sponsorships from individuals and within your trust. There is ever growing interest locally, nationally and internationally in health partnerships, which will result in more potential sources of funding becoming available. Effective fundraising requires time and effort, thus it is useful to have a dedicated fundraising strategy and team within your partnership.

Summary

Health partnerships have the capacity to make significant contributions to health systems in developing countries. Establishing a successful, long-lasting partnership takes time, and it is of critical importance to be flexible and realistic from the outset. Above all health partnerships should be based on genuine need and build on local strengths.

Huge advances and innovations have occurred across the field of medicine in the last century, revolutionising health and healthcare as we now know it. However, growing global inequalities have resulted in the benefit of such advances not reaching the poorest in the world, who arguably need them the most. As clinicians we can all have a role to play in changing the current status quo, and through health partnerships, we can begin to turn the tide on such inequities.

Useful Resources

Health Links

- Gedde M. The International Health Links Manual: a guide to starting up and maintaining long-term international health partnerships. THET. 2009.
- Crisp L. Global Health Partnerships: the UK contribution to health in developing countries. London: Central Office of Information; 2007. Available at: http://www.dh.gov.uk/prodconsumdh/groups/dhdigitalassets/@dh/@en/documents/digitalasset/dh065359.pdf.
- UK Department of Health. Global Health Partnerships: the UK contribution to health in developing countries. The Government response. London: Central Office of Information; 2008. Available at: http://www.dh.gov.uk/prodconsumdh/groups/dhdigitalassets/@dh/@en/documents/digitalasset/dh083510.pdf.

Monitoring and Evaluation

- Gordon M, Potts C. What difference are we making: a monitoring and evaluation toolkit for Health Links. London: THET; 2008.
- A guide for project M&E. Managing for impact in rural development by the International Fund for Agricultural Development. Available at: http://www.ifad.org/evaluation/guide/.
- Evaluation of links between North and South Healthcare Organisations. Available at: http://www.build-online.org.uk/.

Support to Health Links

- THET: www.thet.org.
- BUILD (Building Understanding through International Links for Development): www.build-online.org.uk.
- Partnerships in Health Information (Phi): http://www.partnershipsinhealthinformation.org.uk.
- Country level initiatives
  - Scotland-Malawi partnership: http://www.scotland-malawipartnership.org.
  - The Wales for Africa Health Links Group: http://www.wales.nhs.uk/sites3/home.cfm?orgid=834.
- Specialty initiatives
  - Vision 2020 Links Programme: www.iceh.org.uk.
  - International Society of Nephrology (ISN): www.theisn.org.

References

1. WHO. World Health Statistics 2012. WHO report. 2012. Available at: http://www.who.int/gho/publications/world_health_statistics/en/index.html.
2. WHO. Maternal mortality. Fact sheet No. 348. Geneva: World Health Organisation; 2012. Available at: http://www.who.int/mediacentre/factsheets/fs348/en/index.html.
3. Working Together for Health. WHO report. 2006. Available at: http://www.who.int/whr/2006/en/index.html.
4. The International Society of Nephrology. Global Outreach Sister Renal Center Program. Available at: http://www.theisn.org/src.
5. Dowling J, Holmes D, Kallon H, Sesay T. IHLFS Large grant completion report. The Kambia Appeal. 2013.
6. The International Society of Nephrology Sister Renal Center Program Success Stories. Available at: http://www.theisn.org/isn-information/news-success-stories/itemid-504.
7. Health Partnership Scheme. Tropical Health and Education Trust. Available at: http://www.thet.org/hps/.

Appendix: Resources for Patients and Carers and Physicians

Patient and Carer Resources

Kidney disease is complex, and there are many aspects to diagnosis and management that are not a part of general knowledge. In part because it is impossible to have printed information leaflets on every disease in every clinical environment, the provision of user-friendly patient information beyond the consultation is often variable and an overlooked area of patient care. Increasingly patients will turn to the Internet for information but may be confronted with erroneous and unhelpful results.

The table below contains useful websites that can be recommended as useful starting points. The table is designed to be downloaded, added to and modified for local needs and languages. If this or similar patient information is available on all unit computers, then it greatly facilitates patient and doctor access and helps ensure web addresses can be added to patient letters.

General	**Chronic kidney disease, its complications and treatment**
How your kidney works www.howstuffworks.com/search.php?terms=kidney	Patient.co.uk http://www.patient.co.uk/health/Chronic-Kidney-Disease
National Kidney Disease Education Programme www.nkdep.nih.gov/index.shtml	Renal Association http://www.renal.org/whatwedo/InformationResources/CKDeGUIDE.aspx
The Kidney Patient Guide www.kidneypatientguide.org.uk/contents.php	National Kidney Federation http://www.kidney.org.uk/help/medical-information-from-the-nkf-/medical-info-ckd-info-index/
Baxter Renal Info www.renalinfo.com/us/	NHS Choices http://www.nhs.uk/Conditions/Kidney-disease-chronic/Pages/Introduction.aspx
National Kidney Federation www.kidney.org.uk	A Guide for Primary Care www.ckdonline.org
Royal Infirmary of Edinburgh Renal Unit www.edren.org	**Procedures**
The British Kidney Patient Association www.britishkidney-pa.co.uk/patient-info	Kidney Biopsy http://kidney.niddk.nih.gov/kudiseases/pubs/biopsy/
Kidney Research www.kidneyresearchuk.org	**Vascular access**
British Renal Society www.britishrenal.org	Edinburgh Royal Infirmary Renal Information http://www.edren.org/pages/handbooks/unit-handbook/vascular-access.php
Renal Association www.renal.org	Arteriovenous FISTULAFIRST http://www.fistulafirst.org/Patients/PatientEducationalMaterials.aspx
Choosing dialysis	Peritoneal Dialysis Access http://www.renalinfo.com/us/treatment/end_stage_kidney_failure/peritoneal_dialysis/peritoneal_dialysis_access.html
Kidney Options http://kidneyoptions.com/therapyoptions.html	**Transplantation**
ERA-EDTA www.era-edta.org/images/8_ERBPinformation_for_patients_What_sort_of_dialysis_should_I_choose.pdf	British Transplantation Society www.bts.org.uk

(continued)

This document can be downloaded from Extra Materials http://extras.springer.com/

M. Harber (ed.), *Practical Nephrology*,
DOI 10.1007/978-1-4471-5547-8, © Springer-Verlag London 2014

Dialysis: Types of	NHS Blood and Transplant www.organdonation.nhs.uk
Kidney Dialysis Information Centre http://www.kidneydialysis.org.uk/	Transplant Support Network www.transplantsupportnetwork.org.uk
Choosing not to have dialysis: conservative care	Talking about Transplanting www.talktransplant.com
Ending Dialysis http://www.renalresource.com/booklets/wfdt.php#ending	Transplant Trust www.thetransplanttrust.org.uk
NHS Kidney Care http://www.kidneycare.nhs.uk/our_work_programmes/improving_choice_for_kidney_patients/end_of_life_care_for_akd/	The Transplantation Society http://www.tts.org/
Haemodialysis	European Society for Transplantation www.esot.org
Home haemodialysis www.kidney.niddk.nih.gov/kudiseases/pubs/pdf/*homehemodialysis.pdf*	Kidney Patient Guide: Kidney Transplant Animation http://www.kidneypatientguide.org.uk/TRAanim.php
Peritoneal dialysis	**Organ donation**
International Society for Peritoneal Dialysis www.ispd.org	British Organ Donor Society http://body.orpheusweb.co.uk/index.html
Travelling on dialysis	**Living kidney donation**
NKF UK Holiday Pages www.kidney.org.uk Dialysis at Sea www.dialysisatsea.com Fresenius Holiday Dialysis www.hditravel.com Global Holiday Dialysis Facilities www.globaldialysis.com	Organ Donation http://www.organdonation.nhs.uk/how_to_become_a_donor/living_donation/
Keeping active	**Renal dietetics**
Transplant Sport www.transplantsport.org.uk	Leicester Nutrition and Dietetic Service www.lnds.nhs.uk
European Transplant and Dialysis Sport Federation www.etdsf.org	Culinary Kidney Cooks www.culinarykidneycooks.com
World Transplant Games Federation www.wtgf.org	Davita (US) www.davita.com/recipes Recipes for Diabetics www.diabetic-recipes.com www.diabetesdaily.com
Condition specific information	**Condition specific information**
Alport's disease www.alportsyndrome.org	**Minimal change** http://www.edren.org/pages/edreninfo/minimal-change-disease.php
Amyloidosis Foundation http://www.amyloidosis.org/index.html	**Membranous** http://www.edren.org/pages/edreninfo/membranous-nephropathy.php
ANCA Associated Vasculitis Foundation http://cureanca.com/	**Membranoproliferative GN**
Bartter's syndrome www.barttersite.org/bartters-syndrome	MPGN www.mpgn.org.uk
Cystinosis	**Myeloma**
Cystinosis Foundation www.cystinosis.org.uk	Myeloma Bone Cancer www.myeloma.org.uk
Diabetic nephropathy	EuLite Renal Myeloma Study www.myeloma.org.uk/patient-information/clinical-trials/hcp-trial-tracker/eulite-study/
Diabetes UK http://www.diabetes.org.uk/Guide-to-diabetes/Complications/Kidneys_Nephropathy/	**Nephrotic Syndrome Support** www.nephroticsyndromesupport.org
Diabetes.co.uk www.diabetes.co.uk/diabetes-complications/kidney-disease.html	**Pregnancy and kidney disease** http://www.emrn.org.uk/documents/Kidney%20Disease%20&%20Pregnancy.pdf
Fabry's disease www.fabry.org/FSIG.nsf/Pages/Fabry	http://www.kidney.org/atoz/content/pregnancy.cfm

Fanconi's disease

Fanconic Anemia Research Fund
www.fanconi.org

Fanconi Anaemia Family Support
www.fanconisupport.info

Fanconi Hope
www.fanconi.org.uk

FSGS

Edinburgh Royal Infirmary
www.edren.org/pages/edreninfo/fsgs.php

Nephcure
www.nephcure.org/fsgs-facts

Goodpasture's disease

National Kidney and Urologic Diseases Information Clearinghouse (NKUDIC)
http://kidney.niddk.nih.gov/kudiseases/pubs/goodpasture/

GPA/Wegner's granulomatosis

Wegener's Granulomatosis Support Group
http://www.wegeners.org.nz/

Vasculitis-Patient.com
http://wegenersgranulomatosis.net/15_about_wegeners.php

Haemolytic uraemic syndrome

Atypical HUS

UK aHUS Patient/Family *Support Group*
www.ahus.org.uk

HUS

Patient.co.uk Website
www.patient.co.uk/doctor/Haemolytic-Uraemic-Syndrome.htm

Henoch Schonlein Purpura Support Group
www.hspsupport.co.uk

IgA nephropathy

National Kidney federation (NKF)
http://www.kidney.org.uk/help/medical-information-from-the-nkf-/kidney-diseases-index/medical-info-kidney-disease-iga/

Interstitial nephritis

Patient.co.uk Website
*www.*__patient__*.co.uk/doctor/*__Interstitial__*-Nephritides-and-Nephrotoxins.htm*

Kidney stones

The British Association of Urological Surgeons
http://www.baus.org.uk/patients/urology-is/stones

Kidney Stoners
http://www.kidneystoners.org/

Liddle's syndrome
www.syndrome.org/liddles-syndrome

Loin pain haematuria syndrome

Patient.co.uk Website
www.patient.co.uk/leaflets/loin_pain_and_hematuria_syndrome.htm

Polyarteritis nodosa

Vasculitis Foundation
www.vasculitisfoundation.org/education/forms/polyarteritis-nodosa

Polycystic kidney

Polycystic Kidney Disease
www.pkdcharity.co.uk

Pyelonephritis

Patient.co.uk Website
www.patient.co.uk/doctor/pyelonephritis

Reflux nephropathy

National Kidney Foundation
http://www.kidney.org.uk/help/medical-information-from-the-nkf-/kidney-diseases-index/medical-info-kidney-disease-reflux-index/medical-info-reflux-cause/

Renal artery stenosis

National Kidney and Urologic Diseases Information Clearinghouse (NKUDIC)
http://kidney.niddk.nih.gov/kudiseases/pubs/RenalArteryStenosis/

Renal cancer

Kidney Cancer Care
www.kcuk.org

Prostate Cancer Charity
www.prostate-cancer.org.uk

National Charity for prostate Cancer
www.prostateuk.org

Prostate Cancer Support
www.prostatecancersupportin.co.uk

Renal tubular acidosis

National Kidney and Urologic Diseases Information Clearinghouse (NKUDIC)
http://kidney.niddk.nih.gov/kudiseases/pubs/tubularacidosis/

Scleroderma

Raynaud's and Scleroderma Association
http://scleroderma.org.uk/

Scleroderma Foundation
http://www.scleroderma.org/site/PageServer#.Uf6lMhFwbIU

Scleroderma Society
http://www.sclerodermasociety.co.uk/AboutUs2.php

Scleroderma crisis

Scleroderma Society
http://www.sclerodermasociety.co.uk/Theheartandscleroderma1.php

Urinary tract infections

NHS Choice
http://www.nhs.uk/conditions/Urinary-tract-infection-adults/Pages/Introduction.aspx

National Kidney and Urologic Diseases Information Clearinghouse (NKUDIC)
http://kidney.niddk.nih.gov/kudiseases/pubs/utiadult/

Vasculitis

(continued)

Lupus/SLE	Vasculitis UK www.vasculitis.org.uk/about/support-us
Lupus www.lupus.org.uk/ www.lupus.org.uk/ *Lupus Patients Understanding & Support (LUPUS)* www.lupus-support.org.uk **Lupus nephritis** National Kidney and Urologic Diseases Information Clearinghouse (NKUDIC) http://kidney.niddk.nih.gov/kudiseases/pubs/lupusnephritis/	Vasculitis Foundation www.vasculitisfoundation.org/support

Physician Resources

A huge number of helpful guidelines, standards and resources have been generated in recent years. The table below covers a few of the English language websites that cover a large body of kidney disease and its management. As with the patient and carer resources table, it is designed to be downloaded to unit computers, edited and modified as required.

Associations

American Society of Nephrology www.asn-online.org	International Society for Peritoneal Dialysis www.ispd.org
American Society of Transplantation www.myast.org	International Society for Renal Nutrition and Metabolism www.renalnutrition.com
Australian and New Zealand Society of Nephrology http://www.nephrology.edu.au/renalresources/index.asp	Kidney Health Australia http://www.kidney.org.au/KidneyDisease/KidneyHealthPrograms/tabid/617/Default.aspx
British Renal Society www.bristishrenal.org	National Kidney Foundation(US) www.kidney.org
British Transplantation Society www.bts.org.uk	NHS Blood and Transplant www.organdonation.nhs.uk
European Renal Association-European Dialysis and Transplant Association www.era-edta.org	Renal Association www.renal.org
European Society for Organ Transplantation www.esot.org	The Transplantation Society www.tts.org
International Society for Hemodialysis www.ishd.net	Renal Society of Australasia http://www.renalsociety.org/
International Society for Nephrology www.nature.com/isn/index.html	Vascular Access Society http://vascularaccesssociety.com/

Guidelines

Australia and New Zealand Dialysis and Transplant Registry http://www.anzdata.org.au/	Guidelines for the European Best Practice Groups of ERA-EDTA www.ndt-educational.org
Australia and New Zealand Organ Donation Registry http://www.anzdata.org.au/anzod/v1/indexanzod.html	K/DOQI Guidelines (USA) Kidney Disease Outcomes Quality Initiative www.kidney.org/professionals/kdoqi/index.cfm
British Transplantation Society Guidelines www.bts.org.uk/standards.htm	Kidney Disease: Improving Global Outcomes (KDIGO) www.kdigo.org
Collaborative Transplant Study www.ctstransplant.org	Renal Association (UK) Clinical Practice Guidelines www.renal.org/Clinical/GuidelinesSection/Guidelines.aspx
Dialysis Outcomes and Practice Patterns Study DOPPS Study www.dopps.org	UK Renal Registry www.renalreg.com
European Renal Registry www.era-edta-reg.org/index.jsp	United States Renal Data System www.usrds.org
Eurotransplant www.transplant.org	United States Transplant Registry www.srtr.org

Further Information Resources

Cochrane Renal Group www.cochrane-renal.org	National Institute for Health and Care Excellence www.nice.org.uk
Resource Centre http://www.renalresource.com/	Advanced Renal Education Programme http://www.advancedrenaleducation.com/Home/tabid/36/Default.aspx

Index

A

AA Amyloidosis, 10, 300, 312–315, 317–320, 759
Abdominal compartment syndrome, 51, 52
Ablative therapies, 458, 459, 463
ABO blood group compatibility, 768
ABO incompatible transplant, 775
Absorption, 13, 32, 103, 112, 116–120, 127, 141, 177, 251, 416, 419, 422, 521, 556, 571, 572, 581, 584, 617, 622, 629, 631, 707, 733, 763, 800, 809, 815, 816, 818, 819, 823, 825, 837, 850
Acanthocytes, 22
Accelerated-phase hypertension, 807–808
Acceptable mismatch, 767, 777, 780
A-class drugs, 147, 149–151
Acne, 240, 531, 822
Acquired obstruction, 441
Acquired perforating dermatosis, 14, 257, 526
ACTN4, 172
Actue ventricular failure, 152
Acute kidney injury (AKI),
Acute leukaemias, 59, 342
Acute peritoneal dialysis, 79, 114
Acute tubular injury, 3, 21, 22, 39, 51, 55–57, 94, 95, 162, 176, 258, 260, 261, 266, 267, 269, 270, 273, 283, 286, 298, 325, 444, 446, 634, 804
Addison's disease, 6, 9, 112, 113, 115, 121
Adenine phosphoribosyl-transferase deficiency, 26, 415
ADH. *See* Antidiuretic hormone (ADH)
ADPKD. *See* Autosomal dominant polycystic kidney disease (ADPKD)
Adynamic bone disease, 115, 583, 585, 872
Aetiology, 6, 13, 40, 94, 97, 115, 171–172, 183, 189, 190, 197, 203, 210, 220, 235, 270, 281, 283, 285, 286, 288, 292–294, 299, 311, 323, 324, 327, 332, 346, 382–384, 392, 470–471, 475, 477, 478, 481, 498, 534, 592–593, 595, 596, 606, 685, 693, 698, 733, 821, 861
Agenesis, 430, 431, 433
Air embolism, 690, 696–698
AL amyloidosis, 54, 303, 305, 307, 313–315, 320, 759
Alcohol, 13, 67, 76, 89, 95, 120, 124, 125, 130, 131, 147, 155, 261, 264, 419, 432, 527, 570, 618, 637–639, 710, 711, 791
Alcoholic ketoacidosis, 123, 130
Alemtuzumab, 373, 778, 806, 814, 870
Alkaline diuresis, 67, 69
Allergic interstitial nephritis, 805
Allopurinol, 59, 65, 67, 239, 240, 252, 284, 339, 415, 425, 426, 634, 785, 816, 820, 825, 873
Allosensitisation, 772–774, 860, 862–863
Alopecia, 7, 14, 55, 178, 236, 241, 526, 530
α-Actinin-4, 172
α-1 antitrypsin deficiency, 184, 192, 382
α-blockers, 142, 445, 446, 689
Alpha-3 chain, 230
Alpha-galactosidase A, 509, 511
α-Microglobulin, 26
5-α Reductase inhibitors, 446
Alport's disease, 209, 232, 759
Alport syndrome, 40, 205, 497–504, 506, 750, 751
Alternative pathway, 189, 191–193, 196–202, 264, 326, 327
Altruistic donor, 746, 747, 775, 776
Aluminium-based binders, 585
Amanita phalloides, 52
Ambulatory blood pressure measurement, 138–139, 749
Aminoaciduria, 26, 27, 110, 111, 129, 274
Aminoglycoside nephrotoxicity, 67
Ammonium urate stones, 426, 427
Amyloid, 5, 10, 13, 14, 40, 52, 56, 87, 111, 161, 257, 262, 263, 266, 269, 275, 300, 311–321, 340, 341, 544, 551, 632, 692, 759, 798
Amyloid arthropathy, 316
Amyloidosis, 10, 11, 41, 54, 107, 165, 175, 298, 300, 301, 303–305, 307, 311–321, 526, 529, 530, 552, 690, 692, 700, 701, 733, 759, 762
Anaemia, 2, 5, 15, 16, 68, 154, 163, 172, 227, 229, 236, 245, 264, 266, 270, 276, 287, 293, 297, 305, 309, 323, 324, 331, 332, 334–338, 360, 365, 366, 371, 398, 406, 453, 466, 486, 494, 512, 518, 543, 549, 550, 557–559, 569–578, 605, 607, 616, 617, 627, 691, 693, 699, 701, 703, 759, 779, 801, 814, 821, 843, 873, 875
Analgesic nephropathy, 9, 287, 398, 418, 431, 441, 466, 543
Anaphylatoxins, 81, 86, 201, 202
Anatomy, 15, 32, 35, 42–43, 365, 398, 402, 403, 409, 410, 421, 422, 431, 442, 476, 486, 658–660, 680, 739, 756, 758, 784, 788, 789, 793, 799, 801, 804, 808, 831
ANCA associated systemic vasculitis, 215, 216, 239
Anderson-Fabry's, 10, 11, 14, 25, 509–513, 526, 530, 543, 798
Angiofibromas, 14, 475, 526
Angiokeratoma, 14, 510, 526, 530, 543
Angiokeratomata, 510
Angiomyolipomas, 456, 457, 466, 475–477, 485
Anion gap, 125–126, 129–132, 415, 422
Ankylosing spondylitis, 14, 184, 300–301, 314
Annual review clinics, 869, 875
Anterior lenticonus, 500
Anti-β2-glycoprotein-1, 244
Antibiotic prophylaxis, 37, 38, 95, 96, 186, 250, 309, 397, 402, 407, 433, 638, 677, 710, 726, 759
Antibody-associated proliferative glomerulonephritis, 192, 195
Antibody mediated rejection, 324, 767, 770, 772, 774, 780, 797, 799, 803, 805–807, 809, 814, 823–824, 859, 862, 865–866
Anti-cardiolipin antibodies, 191, 245, 369, 378
Anti-CD25 antibody, 814
Anticholinergics, 7, 9, 51, 435, 441, 444, 551, 687
Anticoagulation, 55, 81, 83–86, 88, 186, 245, 288, 371, 372, 391–393, 596, 600, 606, 608, 611, 652, 653, 678, 679, 693, 695, 779, 788, 792, 793, 804, 806, 809

M. Harber (ed.), *Practical Nephrology*,
DOI 10.1007/978-1-4471-5547-8, © Springer-Verlag London 2014

Antidiuretic hormone (ADH), 27, 92, 93, 103–107, 482, 483, 485, 607
Anti-glomerular basement membrane antibody, 503
Antiglomerular basement membrane disease, 51, 55, 227–232, 525
Anti-lymphocyte globulin, 814
Antineutrophil cytoplasmic antibody, 367
Antineutrophil cytoplasmic antibody glomerulonephritis, 51
Antiphospholipid antibodies, 236, 244, 245, 369, 370
Antiphospholipid syndrome, 191, 235–245, 369, 378
Anti-PLA2R1, 185
Antiproliferative agents, 800, 801, 819–821, 866, 869–871, 873, 875
Anti-retrovirals, 25, 269–271, 273, 274, 423, 600, 761, 762, 824
Anti-retroviral therapy, 25, 269–271, 274, 761
Anti RNA Polymerase III Antibody, 294
Anti-Ro/SSA antibodies, 369
Anti-thrombin III, 162
Antithymocyte globulin (ATG), 777–779, 806, 814, 815, 823, 825, 836, 853
Anti-VEGF antibody, 461
Anus, 868
Aorta, 49, 52, 141, 143, 152, 381, 384, 393, 544, 680, 731, 783, 784, 787
Aortic dissection, 9, 152, 154
Aortitis, 52, 284, 447–450, 543
Apolipoprotein A-1 Amyloidosis (AApoAI), 316, 320
Apolipoprotein A2 Amyloidosis (AApoA2), 316
Argatroban, 84, 85, 611
Aristolic acid, 21
Arteriopathy, 815
Arteriovenous fistulae, 42, 608, 610
Arteriovenous malformation, 8, 41, 456, 466
ARVD. *See* Atheromatous renovascular disease (ARVD)
Ash-leaf spots, 475
Aspirin overdose, 131
Assisted peritoneal dialysis, 675, 718
Asymptomatic bacteruria, 365
Atazanavir, 270, 274
ATG. *See* Antithymocyte globulin (ATG)
Atheromatous renovascular disease (ARVD), 383–386, 388–390
Atherosclerotic renal artery stenosis, 37, 52, 388, 551
Atopy, 33, 172
Atrial natriuretic peptide, 165, 168, 361
Atypical haemolytic uraemic syndrome, 198–200, 326–328, 798
Audit, 43, 45, 47, 63, 64, 67, 72, 155, 226, 638, 641, 654, 655, 694, 703, 714, 725, 726, 729, 730, 770, 774, 777
Autoimmune, 7, 53–55, 107, 116, 128, 183–185, 190, 192, 194–195, 200, 215, 217, 218, 220, 227, 229, 235, 261, 264, 283, 284, 288, 291, 294, 324, 329, 330, 336, 396, 420, 503, 542, 543, 643, 644, 807, 832, 871
Automated eGFR reporting, 548–549
Automated peritoneal dialysis, 705, 717–718, 734
Autonomic bladder, 51, 52, 397, 404
Autonomic neuropathy, 315, 316, 441, 689, 691, 756
Autosomal dominant hypocalcaemia, 415
Autosomal dominant hypophosphataemic rickets, 117, 118
Autosomal dominant polycystic kidney disease (ADPKD), 107, 365, 398, 404, 474, 481–488, 491, 493, 498, 751, 822, 867
Autosomal recessive hypophosphataemic rickets, 117
Autosomal recessive polycystic kidney disease, 11, 485, 492–493
Avascular necrosis, 237, 587, 872
Azathioprine, 52, 67, 178, 208, 212, 223–225, 237–239, 244, 251–254, 284, 298, 300, 369, 373, 375, 376, 449, 570, 634, 800, 801, 805, 814, 816, 819, 820, 824, 825, 841, 853, 864, 865, 869, 871, 873

B

Bacterial cystitis, 396–397
Bacterial endocarditis, 215, 314, 392
Bacterial pyelonephritis, 257, 805
Bacteria virulence, 398
Balanitis, 395–396
BANFF classification, 44, 862, 863, 865
Bardet-Biedl Syndrome, 11, 14, 494
Bartter syndrome, 9, 107, 109, 120, 127, 132, 415
Basal cell carcinoma, 14, 314, 531–533, 843
Base excess, 126, 127
Basiliximab, 814
Beer potomania, 102
Behcet's disease, 215, 314
Belatacept, 373, 774, 823, 842, 870
Bence jones proteinuria, 22, 55, 115, 305, 544
Benign prostatic hyperplasia (BPH), 399, 439, 444, 446
Beta-2 microglobulin, 26, 27, 79, 111, 282, 311, 313–315, 319, 332, 632, 690, 699, 700
Bicarbonate losses, 125
Bilateral agenesis, 430
Bioimpedance plethysmography, 686
Biopsy, 6, 39, 52, 66, 94, 158, 161, 173, 183, 189, 203, 218, 228, 237, 252, 260, 270, 281, 293, 308, 316, 325, 333, 347, 366, 391, 408, 415, 440, 458, 476, 495, 501, 509, 520, 526, 542, 552, 569, 583, 605, 734, 749, 758, 770, 789, 803, 820, 833, 859
Birt hogg dube syndrome, 472, 477
Black water fever, 338
Bladder contractility, 434, 435
Bladder exstrophy, 433–435
Bladder outflow obstruction, 54, 432, 434, 439, 441, 442, 552, 731, 788
Bladder tumour, 35, 51
Blood borne viruses, 10, 13, 53, 269–279, 635, 641–643, 693
Blood clot, 8, 51, 441, 448, 730
Blood pressure, 3, 40, 55, 64, 86, 93, 109, 135, 147, 161, 175, 186, 193, 209, 244, 260, 271, 293, 315, 345, 359, 381, 419, 433, 447, 473, 484, 504, 542, 548, 573, 590, 605, 625, 668, 685, 718, 747, 800, 860
Blood transfusion, 36, 85, 128, 332, 333, 335, 336, 356, 486, 557, 569, 570, 574–577, 605, 693, 698, 731, 771–773, 820, 832, 862
Body potassium, 108, 109, 112–114, 361
Bone, 15, 33, 54, 66, 114, 127, 163, 179, 192, 222, 231, 239, 250, 261, 274, 285, 304, 313, 329, 339, 365, 413, 436, 457, 475, 485, 493, 518, 544, 549, 570, 581, 591, 616, 625, 642, 653, 690, 747, 839, 859
Bone marrow transplantation, 54, 329, 518
Bone mineral density and prophylaxis, 250, 586, 587, 871
Bortezomib, 307, 309, 777, 778, 806, 823, 866
BPH. *See* Benign prostatic hyperplasia (BPH)
BP-lowering drugs, 147–151
Brain injury, 85–86, 596
Brain natriuretic peptides, 103, 313, 388, 594, 686
Breast feeding, 244, 824, 832, 874
Bronchiolitis, 801, 821, 842

C

Ca channel, 172, 297
Cadmium, 111, 129, 287, 454, 650
Calcidiol, 581
Calcimimetic, 115, 585, 587
Calcineurin inhibitor induced bone pain, 873
Calcineurin inhibitors, 10, 14, 67, 97, 98, 113, 120, 152, 161, 163, 179, 187, 250, 324, 373, 534, 587, 600, 761, 800, 807, 809, 813, 815, 818, 825, 861, 873
Calciphylaxis, 14, 119, 526, 527, 583, 584, 586, 587

Calcitriol, 117, 299, 581, 582, 585, 586
Calcium-based binders, 585
Calcium disorders, 113–114
Calcium oxalate, 24, 25, 131, 299, 414–422, 425, 493, 519–521
Calcium stone, 27, 416, 418–420, 425, 493
Campath-1H, 814
CAMR. *See* Chronic antibody mediated rejection (CAMR)
c-ANCA, 55, 218, 219
Cancer, 29, 53, 64, 109, 186, 194, 235, 286, 303, 329, 333, 350, 406, 423, 441, 453, 469, 483, 492, 525, 544, 574, 740, 759, 787, 797, 821, 843, 868
Cancer screening, 286, 287, 869, 871, 875
Candida, 163, 263, 266, 273, 396, 406, 409, 410, 637, 680, 830–832, 848, 854
CAPD. *See* Continuous ambulatory peritoneal dialysis (CAPD)
Carbonic anhydrase 2 mutations, 129
Cardiac failure, 3, 27, 31, 50, 66, 86, 96, 103, 112, 125, 264, 296, 320, 350, 353, 551, 589, 658, 686, 707, 733, 853
Cardiac tamponade, 690, 698
Cardiorenal syndrome, 86–88, 544
Cardiovascular, 3, 41, 50, 66, 78, 96, 116, 135, 147, 161, 186, 205, 244, 270, 346, 359, 384, 413, 459, 485, 509, 518, 538, 548, 565, 569, 584, 589–600, 608, 616, 621, 658, 685, 686, 720, 733, 747, 756–758, 800, 822, 857
Cardiovascular risk, 15, 16, 136–138, 140, 143, 144, 155, 161, 186, 205, 207, 211, 244, 354, 355, 413, 511, 542, 545, 548, 550, 556, 589, 600, 752, 756, 801, 822, 866–867, 875
Carnitine deficiency, 57, 575
Carnitine palmitoyltransferase deficiency, 57
Carpal tunnel syndrome, 315–317, 690
Castleman's disease, 314, 339, 340
Cast nephropathy, 54, 59, 66, 303–308, 340
Catastrophic APLS, 245
Catecholamine associated crisis, 152
Catheter associated UTI, 407
CD46 mutations, 327, 328
C4d staining, 862, 864, 866
Cellular rejection, 804–805, 809, 823, 834, 841, 859, 862, 863
Cellular variant, 177
Central nervous system (CNS), 104, 124, 245, 285, 314, 324, 434, 471, 473, 474, 485, 585, 618, 630, 680, 742, 753, 838, 848, 852, 854, 869, 870
Central pontine myelinolysis (CPM), 104
Central venous dialysis, 675
Cerebral salt-wasting, 103
CFHR5 nephropathy, 11, 196, 199–200, 543, 544
C3 glomerulonephritis, 196, 198–200
C3 glomerulopathies, 189, 190, 196, 199, 200, 544
C3 glomerulopathy, 189–202
Charcoal haemoperfusion, 67
Chemotherapy, 26, 59, 64, 285, 303, 307–309, 313, 318–320, 324, 333, 339, 450, 460, 544, 547, 551, 759, 829, 839, 871
Chest pain, 5, 143, 152, 484, 696–698, 732, 849
Childhood minimal change disease, 177
Chlamydia, 27, 259, 266, 284, 396, 407, 441, 844
Chloride transporter, 167
CHOIR study, 574
Cholesterol emboli, 7, 14, 51, 52, 55, 390–392, 526, 544, 551
Chronic antibody mediated rejection (CAMR), 823–824, 859, 863–866
Chronic graft failure, 858–859
Chronic kidney disease (CKD), 5, 25, 31, 48, 63, 79, 91, 131, 135, 165, 186, 244, 270, 281, 314, 328, 331, 345, 359, 391, 415, 429, 475, 481, 491, 509, 525, 537, 547, 563, 569, 581, 589, 606, 622, 630, 647, 658, 740, 861, 878
  staging, 538
Chronic kidney disease mineral and bone disorder, 581–587
Churg-strauss, 53, 215
Churg-strauss syndrome, 53
Chvostek's sign, 116
Chylous effusion, 853
Ciclosporin, 178–181, 600, 634, 800, 815–820, 823–825, 857, 861, 862, 865–867, 869–871
Citrate, 27, 83–86, 88, 89, 112, 113, 120, 128, 129, 415, 417, 420, 422, 425, 476, 493, 516, 520, 611, 617, 639, 678, 785
Classical pathway, 195, 197, 200, 201, 236
Clinical features, 33, 41, 59, 92–94, 101–102, 105, 110, 111, 114, 116, 118–121, 128, 171, 174, 185–186, 193, 199, 204–205, 210–211, 216, 218, 224, 227, 245, 259, 264–265, 281, 292, 304, 314–315, 324, 327–329, 332, 348, 398–401, 408, 421, 440–441, 471, 475, 477, 478, 483–484, 494, 499, 500, 503–504, 506, 509–510, 544, 551, 696, 697, 735, 736, 829, 833, 841, 842
Clinical manifestations, 9, 110, 165, 193, 216, 220, 245, 275, 277–278, 282, 283, 291, 293, 304, 315, 316, 323, 337, 433, 471, 472, 506, 510, 522, 581, 604, 690–692, 839
Clinical markers, 59, 339, 340, 609
Clinicopathologic, 177, 189, 270–271, 863
CLL leukaemia, 342
C3 nephritic factor, 197, 199, 200, 798
CNI toxicity, 763, 800, 807, 842, 854, 859–861, 863, 865
CNS. *See* Central nervous system (CNS)
Coarctation, 14, 109, 141, 143
Cocaine, 10, 13, 14, 66, 128, 141, 152, 218, 219, 293, 791
Cogan syndrome, 494
Cold ischaemic time, 739, 743–745, 753, 785, 786, 788, 789, 791, 792, 797, 800, 802, 804, 875
Collagenofibrotic glomerulopathy, 341
Collapsing variant, 176, 265, 332
Compensation, 123–124, 131
Complications, 1, 36, 39, 41, 48, 68, 75, 91, 107, 152, 161, 173, 211, 222, 230, 236, 250, 262, 270, 282, 291, 313, 332, 345, 359, 385, 404, 420, 430, 444, 458, 471, 481, 492, 503, 517, 525, 538, 547, 569, 586, 589, 603, 625, 637, 662, 675, 685, 707, 725, 739, 759, 783, 790, 797, 813, 829, 872
Concordance, 8, 389, 564, 566, 764
Congenital adrenal hyperplasia, 109, 113, 142
Congenital anomalies of the kidney and urinary tract, 429–437
Congenital magnesium wasting, 120
Congenital nephrotic syndrome, 158, 172, 263, 506
Congo red staining, 317, 340
Consent, 10, 36–38, 42–44, 249, 596, 664, 667, 746, 752, 764, 765, 795
Continuous ambulatory peritoneal dialysis (CAPD), 486, 632, 640, 705–707, 709, 714, 715, 717–720, 728, 729, 731, 734
Continuous quality improvement, 652, 656, 714–715, 726
Continuous renal replacement therapy, 70, 76, 117, 119
Continuous veno-venous haemofiltration, 77
Contraception, 255, 368, 371, 373, 376–378, 557, 771, 773, 780, 874
Contra-indications, 41, 67
Contrast-induced AKI, 57, 65, 66
Contrast-induced nephropathy, 65, 385, 757
Contrast nephropathy, 27, 52, 57, 386, 758
Copper, 20, 129, 377, 378, 675, 676, 693, 698
Cornea verticillata, 510
Coronary artery disease, 384, 388, 389, 510, 692, 693, 698, 756, 791, 799
Corticosteroids, 59, 172, 174, 175, 178, 181, 195, 196, 208, 209, 212, 222, 230, 237–242, 244, 252–254, 270, 271, 273, 274, 285, 286, 299, 300, 381, 392, 476, 526, 555, 600, 643, 800, 801, 806, 807, 822–824, 867, 871
C1q nephropathy, 177

Cranial diabetes insipidus, 9, 107, 108
CREATE study, 574
Crescentic glomerulonephritis, 204, 209, 211, 216, 227–229, 232, 252, 300, 503, 862
Crescentic IgA, 53, 252
Criteria, 43, 48, 71–72, 76, 91, 149, 174, 215, 216, 245, 298, 304–305, 307, 308, 313, 323, 327, 354, 389, 407, 419, 420, 450, 462, 463, 467, 470, 471, 474–478, 487, 492, 501, 526, 528, 609, 610, 618, 623, 678, 735, 742–745, 749, 751, 762, 763, 771, 786, 787, 790, 791, 797, 860, 863, 866
Cross-match(ing), 15, 767–780, 785, 788, 795, 797–800, 803, 805, 814
Cryoglobulinaemia, 39, 51, 53, 55, 190, 192–194, 211, 257, 262, 263, 265–267, 275–277, 298–300, 340, 342, 544
Cryoglobulinaemic vasculitis, 215, 237, 266, 276
Crystal nephropathy, 24, 25, 27, 53, 56, 64, 69, 440
CT urogram, 422–424, 442, 443
Cuff extrusion, 731–733
Cushing's syndrome, 105, 108, 109, 139, 142, 143
CYCAZAREM trial, 224, 254
CYCLOPS vasculitis regimen, 249
Cyclosporine, 14, 186, 187, 230, 239, 296, 329, 369, 373, 375, 376, 570, 774
CYP3A5, 763, 818, 821
Cysteine, 21, 24, 26
Cystinosis, 14, 26, 111, 117, 126, 515–519, 543, 563
Cystinuria, 26, 414, 415, 420, 421, 425
Cystitis, 10, 13, 27, 178, 239, 249, 255, 261–263, 285, 342, 395, 396, 398–405, 407–410, 423, 441, 833, 840
Cytochrome P450, 13, 800, 809, 815, 824, 825, 844, 845, 848
Cytokine release syndrome, 806, 814, 815
Cytomegalovirus nephropathy, 805
Cytotoxic Cell-Dependant-Cytotoxicity, 799

D

Danaparoid, 84, 611
Darbepoetin alfa, 574, 575
Day case, 39, 43, 249, 427, 679, 711
Deceased after brain death, 802
Deceased after cardiac death, 802
Defective cobalamin metabolism, 324, 329
Delayed graft function, 15, 404, 521, 743–745, 763, 772, 785, 786, 797, 799, 802–804, 808, 809, 815, 821
Dense deposit disease, 14, 191, 196–200, 544, 752
Dent's disease, 25, 111, 117, 414, 415, 420, 427, 543, 548, 751
Dermatitis herpetiformis, 184
Dermatomyositis, 184, 295, 298
Dermatoses in transplantation, 531
Desmopressin, 41, 106, 108, 605–607
Diabetics
- insipidus, 6, 9, 21, 50, 105–108, 282, 286, 299, 433, 501, 543
- ketoacidosis, 20, 21, 117, 118, 120, 124, 125, 129, 130

Diabetogenic, 815, 818, 820
Diagnosis, 1, 20, 29, 39, 47, 64, 91, 101, 127, 135, 150, 161, 171, 183, 189, 203, 215, 227, 235, 252, 258, 269, 281, 293, 303, 313, 323, 337, 346, 364, 381, 395, 415, 431, 439, 454, 469, 483, 492, 497, 509, 515, 526, 542, 547, 566, 571, 586, 610, 618, 623, 637, 671, 680, 690, 707, 727, 749, 755, 790, 797, 814, 833, 864, 881
Dialyser membrane reaction, 690
Dialysis, 1, 29, 33, 41, 47, 65, 75, 97, 114, 131, 155, 209, 223, 228, 250, 265, 278, 282, 291, 303, 313, 334, 345, 367, 387, 408, 420, 446, 454, 484, 491, 498, 511, 521, 525, 537, 549, 564, 569, 582, 592, 605, 613, 621, 632, 635, 647, 658, 675, 685, 705, 717, 725, 739, 756, 767, 787, 798, 817, 829, 857, 878, 881
Dialysis related amyloidosis, 314–316, 690, 692, 701
Didanosine, 125, 270, 274
Dietary assessment, 419
Dietary salt intake, 166, 554, 686, 693
Diethylene glycol, 125
Differential diagnosis, 25, 26, 55, 94, 95, 102, 129, 175, 183, 189–191, 205, 211, 219, 227, 261, 266, 268, 273, 283, 341, 383, 392, 400, 414, 431, 433, 484–485, 500, 504, 506, 509, 543, 586, 690, 694–698, 727, 793, 804–807, 852–854
Diffuse Infiltrative Lymphocytosis Syndrome (DILS), 273
Dilated, 7, 35, 41, 177, 271, 361, 423, 424, 427, 431, 432, 435, 440, 442–444, 446, 492, 493, 512, 529, 682, 712, 713, 790
DILS. *See* Diffuse Infiltrative Lymphocytosis Syndrome (DILS)
Direct radiation nephritis, 338
Direct thrombin inhibitors, 84, 245, 611
Disconnect system, 726
Dissecting aortic aneurysm, 152
Disseminated intravascular coagulopathy, 51, 259
Distal renal tubular acidosis, 109, 125, 128, 352, 414–416, 493, 501
Distal tubular disorders, 141–142
Diuretic renography, 443
Donation, 32, 40, 371, 376, 382, 427, 465, 493, 502, 503, 521, 547, 739–740, 742–753, 775, 777, 783, 786, 787, 791, 793–795, 797, 801, 804, 875, 879
Donation after brain death, 743, 744, 753, 783, 784, 786, 787, 791, 801, 802, 860, 875
Donation after circulatory death, 783, 795, 804
Donor derived damage, 859–860
Donors after cardiac death, 743
Donor selection, 739, 786, 790–791, 793–794
Donor specific antibodies, 15, 184, 187, 191, 192, 772, 773, 778, 798, 799, 805, 866
Duplex ureter, 431, 432
Dysfunction, 1, 28, 34, 40, 47, 86, 91, 107, 141, 152, 157, 168, 199, 224, 257, 260, 270, 286, 294, 311, 323, 332, 364, 384, 404, 429, 434, 442, 459, 492, 503, 510, 518, 544, 548, 571, 582, 594, 604, 621, 662, 676, 689, 710, 729, 743, 759, 790, 798, 817, 853, 858
Dyslipidaemia, 15, 556, 598, 599, 622, 734, 758, 800
Dysmorphic red blood cells, 22
Dysplasia, 5, 10, 14, 37, 107, 116, 141, 172, 384, 430–433, 436, 494, 544
Dyspnoea, 3, 5, 8, 87, 616, 617, 690, 692, 696–698, 732, 821, 833, 847–849, 852

E

Early graft dysfunction, 803–805
ECD. *See* Extended criteria donors (ECD)
Eclampsia, 53, 151, 152, 154, 191, 245, 363, 367
Ecstasy, 13, 102–104
Ectopic kidney, 35, 430
Eculizumab, 200, 325, 328, 330, 338, 758, 777, 779, 806, 807, 823
Electron microscopy, 25, 40, 45, 175, 176, 183, 185, 189, 191, 193, 206, 209, 219, 220, 237, 265, 267, 271, 272, 274, 275, 312, 317, 340, 341, 497, 501, 504, 511, 808, 859, 864, 866
Embolisation, 38, 43, 44, 50, 55, 388, 390–392, 458, 466, 476, 848
Emphysematous pyelonephritis, 20, 397, 400, 401, 403
Encapsulating peritoneal sclerosis, 706, 711, 719, 725, 735–736, 788
End stage liver disease, 96, 275
Endurance sports, 12, 103, 104

Enteric-coated mycophenolate sodium, 813, 819
Enteric hyperoxalosis, 7, 67
Enteric hyperoxaluria, 416, 422, 551
Enzyme replacement therapy, 511–512
Eosinophiluria, 24, 282
Epidemiology, 47–61, 101, 102, 183, 190, 203, 210, 217–218, 227–229, 235, 244, 264, 267, 269, 281, 291, 313, 331, 336, 345, 396, 408, 409, 413, 439, 454, 463, 470, 474, 481, 498, 503, 509, 537–545, 589, 614, 736, 858–859
Epithelial sodium channel, 110, 142, 165–167
Epoetins, 569, 573–575
Erythrocyte TPMT content, 820
Erythropoiesis stimulating agent, 334, 569, 573, 575, 576, 685, 689, 718
Escherichia coli, 56, 259, 324, 397, 728
Essential thrombocythaemia, 342
Ethylene glycol, 25, 67, 70, 89, 125, 126, 130, 131, 416, 634
Eurolupus regimen, 249
Everolimus, 373, 461–463, 488, 801, 820, 821, 871
Exit site Infection, 636, 637, 639, 640, 644, 679, 680, 682, 710, 726–729, 733
Exogenous mineralocorticoid excess, 142
Extended criteria donors, 742–745, 786, 797, 860
Extended criteria donors (ECD), 742–744, 786, 797, 860
Extended duration dialysis, 76
Extracorporeal shock wave lithotripsy, 426, 427, 476, 521
Extra-renal loses, 103, 108, 121

F

Factor H, 191, 192, 197–199, 201, 202, 326–328, 330, 758
Factor I, 199, 202, 326–328, 330
Failing allograft, 874–875
Failure, 3, 21, 31, 40, 47, 66, 75, 91, 101, 124, 135, 151, 161, 165, 171, 199, 206, 216, 227, 236, 251, 259, 270, 281, 291, 303, 311, 323, 332, 345, 362, 381, 399, 418, 429, 440, 454, 470, 485, 494, 497, 515, 525, 537, 547, 563, 570, 581, 589, 604, 618, 628, 629, 636, 647, 657, 675, 686, 707, 719, 727, 740, 755, 770, 783, 797, 824, 833, 858
False positive, 6, 7, 20, 21, 218, 219, 236, 266, 399, 423, 439, 758, 763, 814, 833, 845
Familial distal renal tubular acidosis, 414, 415
Familial hypomagnesaemia, 120, 415
Fanconi syndrome, 25–27, 40, 109–112, 117, 118, 129, 274, 278, 285, 287, 336, 420, 509, 515, 517, 518, 543
Fasting, 21, 124, 125, 130, 150, 733, 747, 750, 751, 816, 867, 868, 875
Fatty liver, 53, 56
Femoral, 37, 92, 316, 587, 590, 638–640, 659, 661, 676, 677, 681, 682, 784, 787, 788, 799, 872
F-Flurodeoxyglucose PET, 447
FGF-23, 117, 118, 581–583
Fibrillary, 192, 257, 263, 266, 271, 275, 303, 307, 340–342, 498, 759
Fibrillary GN, 263, 266, 271, 275, 303, 307, 340, 341
Fibrinogen A Alpha Chain Amyloid, 316
Fibrinoid necrosis, 152, 191, 220, 221, 294, 339
Fibroblast Growth Factors, 117, 600
Fibromuscular disease, 381–383, 391
Fibronectin glomerulopathy, 341
Finnish type, 158
Flexible ureterorenoscopy, 426, 427, 521
Flow cross-match, 798
Focal segmental glomerulosclerosis, 11, 157, 171–181, 298, 300, 332, 340, 501, 627, 798, 808, 862
Fondaparinux, 84, 611
Fungal peritonitis, 640, 706
Fungal urinary tract infections, 409

G

Galactosaemia, 111, 129
Gas transfer coefficient, 229
Gastrointestinal content leakages, 793
GBM. *See* Glomerular basement membrane (GBM)
Gelsolin amyloidosis, 316
Genetic, 30, 111, 118, 120, 127, 128, 157, 158, 171–173, 185, 198–200, 228, 235, 270, 278, 294, 312, 317, 324, 326, 327, 338, 346, 382, 414, 415, 418–420, 427, 434, 436, 453, 461, 467, 469–471, 473–478, 481, 485, 487, 488, 492, 494, 495, 497–506, 510, 511, 515, 519–522, 540, 543, 544, 655, 707, 746, 750, 751, 758, 763, 769, 794, 798, 817, 867
Genitourinary TB, 408
GFR. *See* Glomerular filtration rate (GFR)
GI acid loss, 127
Gingival hyperplasia, 816
Gitelman syndrome, 109, 110, 113, 120, 127, 132
Glomerular basement membrane (GBM), 9, 10, 22, 33, 39, 40, 51, 55, 69, 157, 171–173, 175, 189–191, 193, 196–199, 206, 220, 223, 224, 227–232, 236, 242, 249–252, 254, 264, 338, 497–506, 544, 558, 759, 863, 866
Glomerular filtration rate (GFR), 47, 75, 94, 137, 140, 166, 236, 293, 317, 325, 331, 332, 349, 360, 388, 391, 405, 410, 429, 430, 522, 538, 541, 542, 547, 582, 590, 708, 748, 801, 836, 838, 857
Glomerular lesion, 13, 22, 25, 53, 161, 220, 228, 262, 263, 265, 266, 273, 275, 278, 282, 298, 431, 555
Glomerulonephritis, 1, 22, 40, 51, 69, 95, 152, 157, 163, 177, 183, 189, 203, 215, 227, 235, 249, 257, 270, 281, 296, 304, 333, 354, 369, 418, 448, 486, 503, 542, 551, 606, 634, 759, 798, 843, 859
Glomerulus, 21, 44, 176, 183, 184, 189, 191, 192, 194–197, 199, 207, 215, 220, 221, 237, 240–242, 252, 265, 274, 299, 300, 324, 325, 346, 440, 475, 509, 630, 631, 690, 815, 863
Glucocorticoid-remediable aldosteronism, 142
Glucocorticoid remedial hyperaldosteronism, 111
Glucocorticoids, 105, 108, 109, 111, 112, 141–143, 163, 216, 220, 249, 250, 369, 587, 801, 823
Glucose-6-phosphate dehydrogenase deficiency, 336, 338
Glutathione synthetase deficiency, 125
Glycogen storage diseases, 111
Glycogen storage type 1, 129
Glycolate, 126, 131, 415, 520
Glycosuria, 20, 21, 26, 27, 110, 111, 129, 274, 351, 399
Gold, 10, 34, 113, 141, 171, 184, 254, 300, 382, 391, 392, 420, 422, 423, 471, 493, 539, 634, 657, 757, 758, 760, 803, 805, 839, 841, 857, 859, 863
GOMMID, 304
Gonorrhoea, 21, 27, 263, 396, 407
Goodpasture's disease, 55, 227–229, 503
Goodpasture's syndrome, 40, 53, 54, 69, 71, 227, 544
Gordon's syndrome, 8, 113, 142
Gout, 10, 11, 419, 484, 485, 494, 543, 816, 820, 873
Governance, 38, 225, 647, 654, 656, 711, 714–715, 777, 780
Graft failure, 209, 758, 759, 763, 785, 799, 833, 858–860, 862, 875
Graft function, 15, 336, 404, 521, 628, 739, 743–745, 763, 772, 785–787, 792, 793, 797–799, 802–804, 808, 809, 815, 820, 821, 832, 857, 858, 860, 861, 863, 866, 867, 872, 874
Graft thrombosis, 606, 744, 793, 803
Granulomatosis, 10, 14, 55, 215, 223, 284, 396, 526, 528
Granulomatosis with polyangiitis, 10, 14, 215, 223, 284
Granulomatous interstitial nephritis, 269, 283, 285, 299

H

Haemangioblastomas, 471–474
Haematological, 54, 112, 114, 194, 236, 249, 309, 319, 323, 328, 331–342, 518, 570, 575, 655, 740, 787, 814, 820, 821, 868, 873–874
Haematological toxicity, 814, 820, 821
Haematuria, 7, 21, 35, 39, 40, 54, 69, 91, 162, 174, 185, 193, 204, 216, 227, 235, 258, 272, 282, 298, 304, 315, 333, 348, 365, 392, 399, 413, 447, 466, 483, 491, 497, 538, 548, 604, 749, 774, 788, 803, 883
Haemglobinuria, 23
Haemodiafiltration, 77–79, 81–83, 86–89, 319, 575, 622, 632, 651, 692, 695, 699, 700, 706, 707
Haemodialysis, 2, 31, 67, 76, 97, 114, 131, 265, 308, 334, 345, 370, 404, 454, 486, 491, 511, 521, 525, 549, 569, 585, 591, 605, 622, 630, 638, 647, 657, 685, 705, 707, 718, 725, 779, 787, 798, 882
Haemodialysis in-patient, 82, 266, 371, 372, 492, 525, 569, 572, 573, 575, 596, 598, 605, 610, 622, 638, 639, 647, 652, 657–672, 692
Haemofiltration, 3, 76, 77, 79, 80, 82, 86, 114, 119, 521, 632, 692, 695, 699
Haemoglobin, 6, 24, 36, 41, 49, 51, 126, 184, 231, 305, 323, 331, 332, 334–337, 368, 372, 456, 553, 560, 569, 570, 572, 574–577, 605, 693, 710, 790, 793, 803, 861
Haemoglobinopathies, 331–333, 336, 338, 570, 575
Haemolytic anaemia, 245, 264, 270, 293, 297, 323, 324, 336–338, 365, 814
Haemolytic uraemic syndrome, 51, 54, 56, 191, 198–200, 324, 326, 331, 544, 570, 571, 759, 798, 815, 862
Haemolytic uraemic syndrome (HUS), 7, 40, 51–54, 56, 71, 191, 198–200, 251, 257, 263, 323–331, 544, 570, 751, 752, 758, 759, 798, 807, 815, 862
Haemoperfusion, 67, 89
Haemoperitoneum, 727, 731
Haemosiderin, 22, 333, 336, 337
Haemosiderosis, 337
Hairy cell leukaemia, 314, 342
Hand hygiene, 635–636, 638, 641, 644, 711, 842
Hantavirus, 12, 52, 53, 258–260, 285
Haptoglobin, 293, 337, 571
Health links, 877–879
Health partnerships, 877–879
Heat stroke, 54, 57
Heavy chain deposition disease, 340, 341
Heavy metals, 11–14, 25, 40, 51, 111, 129, 286–287, 543
Heme oxygenase-1, 332
Henderson-hasselbalch equation, 123
Henoch-schönlein purpura, 14, 51, 53, 203–212, 215, 526, 528, 529
Heparany sulphate proteoglycan, 497, 498
Heparin-induced thrombocytopenia, 84, 609, 610, 807
Heparinoids, 84, 611
Hepatitis, 10, 36, 52, 91, 183, 192, 205, 215, 240, 252, 257, 269, 284, 341, 526, 543, 636, 649, 693, 740, 760, 807, 813, 830
Hepatitis B, 10, 11, 52, 53, 55, 95, 183, 184, 192, 205, 215, 257, 259, 263, 265, 266, 269, 271, 272, 274, 276–278, 284, 527, 543, 544, 636, 641, 649, 693, 740, 741, 747, 753, 760–762, 830–832
Hepatitis C, 11, 36, 53, 184, 192–194, 242, 259, 263, 266, 271, 274–277, 284, 341, 526, 636, 641, 740, 741, 747, 752, 753, 760, 807, 830, 831
Hepatorenal baroreflex, 92
Hepatorenal syndrome (HRS)
  type 1, 91–93, 96, 97
  type 2, 91, 92, 96, 97
Hereditary angiopathy aneurysms and cramps, 11, 506
Hereditary fructose intolerance, 111, 129
Hereditary hypophosphataemic rickets, 117, 415
Hereditary leiomyomatosis, 470, 478
Hereditary systemic amyloidosis, 314
Hernia, 719, 731, 732, 788
Herpes simplex, 259, 284, 396, 760, 762, 835, 837–838
Hibernating parenchyma, 389
High anion gap acidosis, 125, 126
High transporter, 717, 719
High-turnover bone disease, 872
Hirudin, 84, 85, 89, 611
Histological classification, 235
Histopathology, 55, 94, 171, 175–176, 235–236, 295, 511, 566, 787, 833
HIV-associated nephropathy, 11, 172, 270–273
HIV-associated thrombotic microangiopathy, 270
HIV immune complex kidney disease (HIVICK), 269, 271, 272
Hodgkin lymphomas, 59
Hodgkin's disease, 171, 172, 314
Horseshoe kidney, 14, 41, 419, 430, 493
House dust, 171
HTLV. *See* Human T cell lymphotrophic virus (HTLV)
Human immunodeficiency virus (HIV), 5, 10, 11, 36, 40, 53, 55, 102, 152, 172, 176, 184, 192, 194, 207, 219, 229, 257, 259, 263, 265, 266, 269–274, 276, 278, 284, 285, 324, 329, 341, 378, 454, 526, 527, 530, 538, 543, 544, 600, 636, 641, 643, 693, 740, 741, 747, 752, 760–762, 765, 787, 802, 825, 830, 831, 848
Human leukocyte antigen (HLA), 228, 768
  antibody screening, 765, 770–771, 859, 875
  incompatible transplant, 767
  matching, 769–770, 802, 860, 862, 867
  nomenclature, 769
  polymorphism, 768–769
Human T cell lymphotrophic virus (HTLV), 278, 643, 740, 741, 747, 760–762, 765, 830
Hungry bone syndrome, 116, 120, 586
HUS. *See* Haemolytic uraemic syndrome (HUS)
Hyaline casts, 25, 176
Hydronephrosis, 35, 361, 365–366, 374, 408, 409, 421, 432, 435, 439, 466, 552
Hydrotetracarbon, 52
Hydroxycarbamide, 333
Hydroxychloroquine, 238, 241, 242, 245, 251, 369, 528
Hyeruricaemia, 53
Hyper-acute antibody-mediated rejection, 79
Hypercalcaemia, 7, 9, 10, 51, 53, 54, 57, 59, 67, 69, 70, 76, 88, 107, 108, 114–116, 121, 283, 286, 299, 305, 308–309, 339, 414, 418, 419, 544, 551, 581, 584, 585, 708, 720, 872
Hypercalciuria, 27, 111, 117, 120, 128, 299, 414–416, 418–420, 422, 493, 520
Hyperchloraemic acidosis, 83, 109, 126, 286
Hyperemesis gravidarum, 53, 56
Hyperfibrinogenaemia, 162
Hyperfiltration, 172, 173, 332–334, 347, 360, 431, 436, 440, 554, 627, 859–860, 874
Hyperkalaemia, 1, 9, 36, 55, 67, 68, 70, 71, 75, 76, 95, 97, 108, 112–114, 121, 142, 270, 339, 352, 353, 446, 447, 555–557, 594–598, 625, 630, 633, 667, 689, 697, 698, 720, 802, 803, 809, 817
Hyperlipidaemia, 102, 103, 163, 174, 175, 177, 181, 425, 463, 483, 801, 821, 860–862, 867, 868
Hypernatraemia, 76, 88, 105–107, 694, 695, 699
Hyper-osmolar states, 102, 103
Hyperoxalosis, 7, 25, 40, 67, 70, 543
Hyperoxaluria, 27, 69, 414–416, 418–420, 422, 425, 427, 519–522, 551, 719, 758, 759, 798
Hyperparathyroid bone disease, 583

Hyperparathyroidism, 114–118, 121, 142, 274, 286, 415, 418, 526, 549, 550, 575, 581–583, 585, 587, 589, 592, 618, 685, 692, 759, 872
Hyperphosphataemia, 55, 59, 70, 76, 116, 117, 119, 332, 340, 581, 584, 589, 600, 618
Hyperphosphaturia, 418
Hypertension, 2, 37, 40, 52, 70, 81, 91, 105, 127, 135, 147, 161, 175, 185, 191, 205, 236, 260, 269, 282, 291, 304, 316, 324, 332, 346, 360, 381, 419, 429, 454, 474, 481, 492, 504, 511, 518, 540, 549, 581, 589, 605, 627, 667, 679, 685, 721, 733, 743, 758, 772, 786, 798, 816, 859
Hypertensive crises, 151, 152, 154, 264
Hypertensive encephalopathy, 152, 154, 291, 292, 296, 695
Hypertrichosis, 14, 179, 527, 531, 816
Hyperuricaemia, 14, 59, 69, 70, 76, 340, 414, 417, 425, 485, 494, 553, 816, 860, 873
Hyperuricosuria, 27, 414, 420, 520
Hypoadrenalism, 103, 104, 315, 824
Hypoalbuminaemia, 8, 52, 71, 125, 162, 165, 172, 175, 186, 606, 629, 727, 870
Hypocalcaemia, 9, 55, 59, 66, 70, 116, 117, 119–122, 131, 231, 340, 415, 515, 585, 586, 695
Hypochloraemic alkalosis, 83
Hypocitraturia, 27, 414, 416, 418, 420
Hypokalaemia, 9, 66, 105, 107–112, 120, 121, 128–130, 132, 142, 168, 231, 261, 287, 425, 515, 516, 625, 627
Hypomagnesaemia, 108, 110, 112, 116, 119, 120, 122, 415, 495
Hypomagnesuria, 414
Hyponatraemia, 11, 13, 76, 88, 94, 97, 101–107, 175, 515, 694, 806
Hypoperfusion, 6, 22, 50–52, 70, 94, 95, 124, 125, 153, 154, 162, 408, 589, 767, 802, 807
Hypophosphataemic nephrolithiasis, 415
Hypophosphataemic osteoporosis, 415
Hypoplasia, 430, 492, 494, 500, 501
Hypotension, 2, 3, 6, 8, 15, 39, 50, 56, 59, 64, 65, 67, 68, 70, 75, 78–83, 85–89, 92, 93, 97, 121, 122, 138–141, 143, 154, 155, 162, 258, 261, 315, 317, 320, 340, 353, 360, 372, 425, 445, 446, 484, 551, 555, 592, 595, 596, 662, 685–687, 689–696, 698, 731, 791, 803, 806, 824
Hypothermic machine perfusion, 786
Hypothyroidism, 103, 104, 121, 142, 163, 462, 466, 518, 570, 708
Hypovolaemia, 3, 6, 31, 49, 50, 52–54, 56, 64, 87, 102, 103, 105, 107, 109, 125, 128, 152, 165, 174, 175, 177, 261, 269, 270, 287, 557, 685, 803

I

Ideal body weight, 623, 631
Idiopathic, 57, 107, 116, 183, 184, 192, 196, 219, 236, 239, 241, 243, 287–288, 414, 415, 422, 447–449, 518, 552, 618, 758
Idiopathic rhabdomyolysis syndrome, 57
IgA, 7, 11, 13, 26, 40, 53, 94, 95, 157, 162, 176, 177, 186, 190, 191, 194–196, 203–212, 229, 230, 236, 245, 252, 253, 262–264, 266, 267, 271, 272, 278, 300, 301, 342, 500, 504, 544, 551, 758, 759, 779, 798, 862
IgA nephropathy, 7, 11, 13, 94, 157, 177, 186, 195, 203–212, 236, 252, 264, 267, 271, 301, 500, 504, 551, 758, 759, 798, 862
IgG-4, 14, 447, 448, 543
IgM nephropathy, 177, 195
IHD. *See* Intermittent haemodialysis (IHD)
Ileal conduit, 19, 27, 397, 435, 436, 788, 798
Immune complex, 53, 190, 192, 193, 195, 203, 205–207, 212, 215, 235, 236, 250–252, 257, 263, 264, 266, 267, 269–272, 275, 276, 284, 298, 300, 762, 866
Immune complex kidney disease, 269, 271–272
Immune reconstitution inflammatory syndrome (IRIS), 269, 273–274, 842, 846, 849
Immunizations, 171
Immunoglobulin A nephropathy, 203, 300
Immunological graft loss, 804, 862
Immunosuppression, 14, 162, 179, 186, 200, 209, 219, 229, 240, 249, 276, 285, 319, 329, 342, 373, 404, 448, 473, 530, 550, 600, 641, 733, 759, 772, 786, 800, 813, 829, 859
Immunosuppressive drug, 16, 172, 800, 813, 819, 823, 824, 857, 861, 867–869, 874, 875
Immunotactoid, 192, 257, 271, 275, 304, 307, 340, 341
Immunotherapy, 162, 226, 312, 321, 460, 462
Impaired kidney function, 5, 589, 592, 594–596, 599, 630–632
Implantation techniques, 788–789, 792, 794
IMPROVE trial, 224
Inappropriate ADH, 103, 104
Indications, 1, 3, 22, 27, 34, 36, 37, 39–41, 44, 45, 67, 70, 75, 76, 97, 135, 139, 190, 209, 270, 278, 288, 320, 348, 353, 362, 388, 389, 407, 413, 426, 427, 442, 475, 483, 484, 486, 493, 520, 532, 538, 547, 577, 585, 594–596, 608, 621, 633, 700, 728, 731, 733, 763, 779, 788, 793, 804, 837
Indinavir, 53, 64, 269, 270, 273, 274, 417
Induction agents, 254, 758, 777, 778, 801, 813, 814, 870
Infection,
Infection stones, 426
Infectious diseases, 187, 193, 194, 253, 257–268, 281, 285, 401, 597, 765, 845, 847, 852, 854
Infective endocarditis, 13, 14, 39, 52, 53, 219, 253, 258, 266, 642
Informed consent, 664, 667, 746, 752
Ingested acid, 125
Inherited phosphate wasting disorders, 117
Injury, 2, 21, 31, 39, 47, 63, 75, 91, 102, 131, 152, 157, 162, 173, 184, 193, 203, 215, 227, 235, 252, 257, 269, 281, 291, 303, 323, 331, 347, 364, 385, 419, 432, 444, 475, 481, 550, 576, 587, 592, 603, 625, 633, 648, 670, 677, 698, 709, 731, 743, 758, 797, 814, 841, 860
Inpatient procedure, 43
Insect bites, 8, 336
Insect stings, 171
Insertion, 15, 37, 38, 80, 92, 106, 267, 366, 407, 638–641, 659, 660, 662, 666, 675–679, 681, 690, 696, 698, 707–712, 714, 726, 727, 729–732, 832
Interferon-α, 171, 271, 276, 460, 463
Intermittent haemodialysis, 70, 76–79, 81, 83, 86, 88, 97, 632, 798
Intermittent haemodialysis (IHD), 70, 76–79, 81–84, 86, 88, 97, 594, 607, 632, 692, 695, 798
Interstitial
  cystitis, 262, 263, 396, 410, 441
  fibrosis, 10, 176, 195, 196, 206, 207, 271, 284, 286, 287, 440, 522, 823, 842, 861, 863–865
  nephritis, 11, 24, 27, 39, 44, 52–55, 67, 69, 95, 111, 162, 171, 257–259, 261–263, 266, 269, 275, 281–286, 298, 299, 392, 448, 466, 551, 552, 557, 634, 805, 864
Intra-atrial, 677
Intracranial aneurysm, 484
Intra-dialytic hypertension, 82, 689
Intra-dialytic hypotension, 2, 15, 78–80, 82, 83, 85, 87, 372, 662, 685, 687, 689–695, 698
Intrarenal abscess, 398
Intravascular haemolysis, 7, 23, 49, 54, 56, 67, 113, 118, 119, 258, 293, 331, 336, 337, 551
Intravenous immunoglobulin, 225, 309, 762, 778, 806, 823, 866
Intrinsic acute kidney injury, 50, 51

Investigations, 4, 20, 34, 40, 47, 69, 94, 102, 135, 152, 175, 184, 191, 205, 218, 240, 253, 259, 281, 307, 316, 323, 333, 348, 367, 382, 400, 418, 429, 459, 471, 483, 491, 501, 510, 519, 539, 550, 566, 570, 586, 592, 603, 623, 636, 680, 696, 708, 745, 756, 774, 787, 798, 821, 858
Iron chelation, 336, 850
Iron deficiency absolute, 571
Iron deficiency functional, 571
Iron supplementation, 569, 572–573, 577
Isolated dominant hypomagnesaemia, 120
Iso-osmolar state, 103
IVC thrombosis, 52, 161

J
Joubert's syndrome, 494

K
Kaposi's sarcoma, 14, 526, 530, 534, 763, 801, 821, 837, 839, 840, 868, 871
Kappa, 191, 303
KDIGO classification, 47, 48
Ketamine, 13, 396, 407
Ketoacidosis, 20, 21, 109, 117, 118, 120, 124, 125, 127, 129–130, 356
Key performance indicators, 710, 714–715
Kidney
  disease,
  failure, 61, 87, 199, 303, 631, 745, 747, 749–752, 755
  function, 5, 6, 16, 47, 51, 54, 70, 158, 303, 305–309, 328, 334, 338, 345, 360, 361, 367, 373, 374, 432, 483, 539, 542, 547, 549, 550, 552, 554–557, 559, 560, 572, 589, 592–600, 621, 625, 627, 630–632, 743–745, 748, 752, 803
  injury, 2, 22, 31, 39, 47, 63, 75, 91, 119, 131, 152, 193, 204, 215, 227, 257, 269, 281, 291, 303, 323, 336, 350, 385, 475, 481, 550, 593, 605, 625, 633, 677, 685, 709, 743

L
Lactate dehydrogenase deficiency, 57
Lactic acidosis, 31, 76, 83, 124, 125, 127, 130, 270, 350
Laminin, 313, 497, 498, 506
Lanthanum carbonate, 584
Laparoscopic renal biopsy (LRB), 44
Lead, 6, 20, 37, 48, 80, 92, 106, 127, 138, 147, 157, 165, 173, 189, 207, 216, 227, 235, 259, 283, 292, 312, 326, 336, 350, 359, 382, 414, 432, 454, 470, 482, 502, 515, 526, 542, 548, 566, 583, 592, 603, 630, 637, 650, 663, 685, 707, 721, 727, 739, 756, 784, 798, 813, 830, 859, 877
Lecithin-cholesterol acyltransferase deficiency, 512
Leflunomide, 820, 837, 841
Left internal jugular, 676, 677, 680
Left renal vein entrapment syndrome, 393
Legionnaire's disease, 52, 53
Leptospirosis, 12, 48, 52, 54, 95, 259–261, 285
Leucocyte Alpha-GAL-A Activity, 510
Leukocytes chemotactic factor 2 Amyloidosis (ALECT2), 311, 314, 316
Liddle's syndrome, 42, 141, 883
Light chain
  cast nephropathy, 340
  nephropathy, 53, 66, 67
Light chain deposition disease (LCDD), 111, 303, 340
Lipids, 354, 531, 603, 733, 747, 800, 863, 866, 868, 869
Lipoprotein glomerulopathy, 512, 759
Lithium, 6, 9, 67, 70, 76, 80, 89, 107, 108, 115, 121, 171, 172, 184, 286, 543, 544, 549, 618, 634
Live donor
  kidney transplantation, 745, 779, 791, 793
  nephrectomy techniques, 794
Livedo reticularis, 14, 55, 245, 391, 526, 696
Liver transplantation, 76, 91, 96, 97, 328, 415, 521, 523
Lobar nephronia, 398
Locks, 639, 655, 676, 678, 679, 694, 730
Loop Diuretics, 67, 105, 110, 114–116, 121, 128, 141, 162, 166–168, 284, 308, 320, 390, 443, 595, 598, 802, 807
Loss, 3, 37, 41, 47, 66, 68, 79, 93, 102, 124, 141, 158, 162, 166, 172, 197, 209, 216, 227, 244, 250, 258, 271, 285, 314, 326, 336, 347, 361, 383, 398, 414, 440, 461, 469, 482, 492, 499, 515, 529, 539, 548, 564, 569, 584, 599, 613, 621, 640, 661, 679, 696, 705, 720, 725, 743, 758, 767, 785, 802, 814, 831, 858
Lower urinary tract abnormalities, 798
Lowe syndrome, 111, 129
Low molecular weight heparins, 41, 84, 556, 594, 633
Low solute intake, 103, 104
Low Transporter,
Lupus glomerulonephritis, 235–237, 239
Lupus-like nephritis, 271–273
Lupus nephritis, 10, 185, 191, 195, 196, 205, 235–244, 251–253, 272, 368–370, 377, 378, 552, 884
Lupus vasculopathy, 236
Lymphangioleiomyomatosis, 475
Lymphocele, 790, 795, 821
Lymphocytic leukemia, 53, 171, 339, 340, 342, 805, 806, 821
Lymphoedema, 530, 821
Lymphoma, 7, 10, 14, 51, 53, 59, 107, 115, 172, 184, 219, 251, 269, 273, 275, 317, 331, 339, 340, 342, 432, 441, 448, 449, 466, 552, 727, 733, 740, 742, 762, 787, 838, 839, 868–870
Lytic induction, 813, 814

M
Maastricht category, 743, 784, 786
Machine perfusion, 785, 786, 788
Macroglobulinaemia-monoclonal Igm, 340
Macroglossia, 14, 315–317, 544
Magnesium, 108–110, 115–121, 125, 166, 261, 364, 415–417, 420, 422, 425–427, 436, 447, 495, 515, 516, 617, 649, 701
Magnesium disorders, 119–120
Maintenance therapy, 154, 223–225, 237–239, 241, 244, 251, 253, 254
Malakoplakia, 399, 406, 441, 456
Malaria, 12, 48, 54, 56, 184, 192, 257, 258, 263, 265, 331, 336, 338, 747, 830, 874
Malignancy, 7, 10, 11, 15, 16, 21, 40, 51, 53, 54, 59, 104, 114–116, 124, 125, 161, 171, 178, 183, 184, 186, 187, 205, 215, 217, 249, 309, 324, 329, 338, 339, 342, 392, 396, 406, 439–442, 446, 448, 450, 453, 456, 464–466, 469, 483, 485, 486, 491, 527, 530–532, 538, 544, 551, 569, 575, 623, 727, 733, 739, 741–742, 747, 749, 753, 756, 759–760, 762, 765, 772, 774, 787, 813, 816, 821, 830, 843, 853, 854, 868, 869, 871
Malignant hyperthermia, 57
Malignant skin conditions, 532–533
Maltese Cross, 24, 25, 510, 543
Mammalian target of rapamycin inhibitors (mTORIs), 462–463, 875
Management, 1, 19, 29, 39, 47, 63–72, 75, 94, 102, 123, 140, 147–155, 158, 161–163, 165–168, 177, 183, 205, 215, 230, 239, 250, 258, 270, 288, 292, 303, 311, 333, 345, 359, 383, 395, 416, 429, 439, 463, 473, 481, 493, 511, 526, 538, 547–561, 569–578, 584, 589, 603, 613, 622, 633, 638, 653, 657, 679, 685, 709, 725, 749, 755, 773, 788, 797, 816, 833, 857–875, 877

Mannose binding lectin pathway, 201
Masked hypertension, 139, 140
Mastocytosis, 184
Maternal outcomes, 367, 371, 373–374
Mcardle's, 57
Meckel-gruber syndrome, 14, 494
Medial fibroplasia, 382
Medial hyperplasia, 382
Medical therapy, 3, 37, 70, 76, 383, 384, 386, 388–390, 393, 442, 512, 585, 594, 702, 765
Medication, 7, 37, 39, 51, 64, 103, 139, 148, 168, 183, 184, 224, 238, 250, 258, 270, 282, 296, 308, 320, 334, 346, 368, 383, 407, 418, 435, 441, 476, 515, 527, 542, 550, 564, 595, 614, 625, 633, 636, 668, 707, 764, 804, 824, 842, 857
Medullary cystic disease, 25, 107
Medullary sponge kidney, 36, 414, 416, 419, 421, 422, 493
Megacalyx, 431
Megaureter, 262, 431–433
Melanoma, 184, 466, 531, 532, 534, 740, 742, 760, 787, 821, 868, 869
Membranoproliferative glomerulonephritis, 95, 177, 189–202, 298, 333, 340, 759, 798
Membranoproliferative glomerulonephritis (MPGN), 14, 162, 171, 189–202, 261–263, 265–267, 275–278, 299, 333, 340, 342, 544, 758, 759, 798, 808
Membranous GN, 53, 162, 261, 263, 266, 271, 275, 277, 278, 296, 298–300, 342, 759
Membranous nephropathy, 808, 862
MEPEX trial, 223
6-Mercaptopurine, 375, 800, 820
Mercury, 20, 111, 129, 184, 287
Merkel cell carcinoma, 531, 534
Mesangial hypercellularity, 176, 177, 189, 191, 206, 207, 235, 236, 267
Mesangial hypercellular variant, 177
Mesangial IgM, 176
Mesangiocapillary glomerulonephritis, 40, 189, 862
Metabolic
  acidosis, 55, 70, 76, 83, 85, 86, 97, 109, 111, 113, 123–132, 415, 420, 426, 435, 436, 515, 556, 586, 623, 695
  alkalosis, 85, 109–111, 123, 126–128, 130, 132
  screening, 418, 419, 426, 794
  syndrome, 413, 417, 420–422, 425, 733, 860
Metabolism, 21, 83, 89, 117, 130, 131, 299, 324, 329, 373, 378, 416, 423, 436, 485, 512, 519, 522, 523, 539, 581, 582, 600, 614, 616, 622, 623, 629–631, 633, 653, 654, 695, 733, 745, 763, 785, 786, 792, 798, 800, 804, 809, 815, 819, 820, 825, 874
Metformin, 31, 76, 89, 124, 125, 349–350, 355, 633, 853, 860
Methanol, 80, 89, 125, 126, 130–131
Methoxypolyethylene glycol epoetin beta, 574, 575
Methylmalonic acidaemias, 522–523
Microangiopathy, 10, 51, 53, 55, 155, 190, 191, 198, 236, 245, 260, 263, 265, 266, 269, 270, 275, 276, 287, 323, 324, 333, 339, 364, 807, 859, 863
Microscopic haematuria, 11, 26, 40, 94, 174, 175, 185, 193, 194, 197, 199, 216, 220, 236, 239, 260, 264, 266, 267, 272, 273, 275, 277, 298, 304, 348, 493, 497, 503, 544
Microscopic polyangiitis (MPA), 53, 55, 215–220, 222, 251, 266, 267, 373, 763, 800, 801, 819, 820, 825
Micturating cystourethrogram, 759
Middle aorta syndrome, 52
Midogen, 482
Migration, 331, 458, 475, 486, 665, 676, 677, 679, 714, 727, 729, 733, 764
Mineral, 113, 128, 141, 250, 365, 413, 417, 436, 485, 499, 518, 560, 581–587, 592, 600, 627, 653, 654, 691, 703, 871
Mineralocorticoid deficiency, 112, 113
Mineralocorticoid excess, 108, 109, 111, 112, 127, 142
Minimal change disease, 165, 168, 171–181, 209, 237, 275, 298, 300, 555
Minimal change nephropathy (MCN), 157–159, 171, 180, 340, 342
Mitochondrial disorders, 11, 111
Mixed connective tissue disease, 298
Molecular adsorbent recirculating system, 97
Moncrief-Popovitch implantation method, 709
Monoclonal deposits, 304
Monoclonal gammopathies, 313
Monoclonal gammopathy, 197, 198, 304, 313, 340, 351
Monoclonal immunoglobulin deposition diseases, 340
Monoclonal Light Chain, 303, 318
Mouth Ulcers, 14, 55, 236, 241, 258, 821, 833, 850
MR urography, 369, 424, 443
mTOR inhibitors, 461, 466, 476, 477, 488, 801, 813, 815, 819–822, 824, 827, 839, 841, 842, 853
Muehrcke's bands, 14, 174
Multicystic dysplasia, 430
Multidisciplinary education programme, 557
Multidrug resistant organisms, 635–638, 642
Multiple myeloma, 7, 49, 59, 64–67, 111, 115, 193, 194, 303–309, 319, 331, 339, 340, 759, 778
Muromonabcd3, 815
Mushroom poisoning, 52, 54, 67
Mycobacterial infection, 273, 274, 760, 805, 845
Mycophenolate, 16, 179, 181, 186, 200, 208, 223, 224, 230, 237, 240, 253, 254, 369, 373, 376, 449, 529, 570, 800, 804, 813, 814, 816, 819, 820, 823–825
Mycophenolate mofetil, 186, 196, 200, 208, 223, 224, 230, 237, 240, 251, 253, 254, 369, 373, 376, 449, 529, 800, 813, 819
Mycophenolic acid, 373, 376, 449, 800–801, 819, 841, 853, 871
Mycoplasma, 27, 192, 259, 263, 264, 284, 396, 407, 642, 844
Mycosis fungoides, 171, 342
Myelodysplasia, 184, 340
Myelofibrosis, 342
Myeloma, 7, 40, 49, 53–55, 59, 64–67, 95, 102, 111, 125, 129, 193, 194, 229, 303–311, 313, 319, 331, 339, 340, 547, 551, 571, 740, 759, 778, 779, 787
Myelomonocytic leukaemia, 342
Myeloperoxidase, 218, 296
Myelosuppression, 373, 819, 820, 833
Myoadenylate deaminase deficiency, 57
Myocardial infarction, 52, 86–88, 135, 149, 152, 388, 413, 589, 592, 594, 600, 609, 690, 692, 799
Myocardial ischaemia, 87, 152, 154, 292, 294, 592, 689, 693, 756
Myoglobin, 20, 23, 24, 49, 51, 57, 69, 257
Myoglobinuria, 7, 23, 55, 57
Myophosphorylase deficiency, 57

N

Nafamostat, 84, 85
Nail patella syndrome, 498, 504–506, 543, 751
National confidential enquiry into patient outcome and death (NCEPOD), 63, 64, 89
Natriuresis, 93, 94, 105, 115, 154, 167, 168, 332, 594, 595
Needle dislodgement, 690, 696
Nephrectomy, 43, 161, 172, 181, 393, 401, 403–406, 408, 427, 456, 458–459, 463–467, 472, 473, 486, 518, 544, 605, 689, 749, 751, 752, 765, 772–774, 780, 788, 790, 794, 875
Nephrin, 158, 172
Nephrocalcinosis, 27, 111, 114, 120, 128, 129, 299, 415, 417–418, 493, 519–521, 543
Nephrogenic diabetes insipidus, 9, 105–107, 282, 286, 299, 443, 543
Nephrogenic systemic fibrosis, 33, 385, 386, 526–527

Nephrolithiasis, 7, 10, 11, 111, 270, 274, 299, 397, 406, 409, 415, 441, 476, 485, 551, 751
Nephronophthisis, 9, 14, 286, 485, 494, 543
Nephron-sparing, 457–459, 465, 473, 476, 477
Nephrostogram, 446, 790, 859
Nephrostomy, 37, 366, 401, 426, 427, 444, 446–450, 466, 552, 790, 859, 864
Nephrotic syndrome, 2, 40, 49, 103, 158, 161–163, 165, 171, 183, 190, 204, 239, 263, 272, 282, 299, 304, 315, 332, 366, 425, 506, 511, 548, 599, 606, 622, 629, 751, 843
Nephrotoxicity, 58, 59, 65–67, 179, 319, 521, 550, 557, 801, 808, 809, 815, 819, 837, 841, 861
Nephrotoxins, 65–67, 95, 266
Neurogenic pulmonary oedema, 104
Neuroleptic malignant syndrome, 57
Neuropathic bladder, 7, 432–434
Neuropathic pain, 510, 616
Neurotoxicity, 118, 121, 800, 816–818, 854
New onset diabetes after transplantation (NODAT), 763, 800, 815–818, 822, 823, 860, 867–868
Nightly intermittent peritoneal dialysis (NIPD), 718, 719
Nodular prurigo, 525
Non-calcium renal stone disease, 414, 415
Non-dilated kidney, 440
Non-HLA antibodies, 771, 772, 799–800
Non-Hodgkin lymphoma, 59, 342, 868, 869
Non-immunological causes, 859–862
Non inflammatory necrotising vasculopathy, 236
Non-obstructed kidneys, 440
Non-peptide vasopressin receptor antagonists, 104
Non pharmacological management, 147, 614
Non-steroidal anti-inflammatory drugs, 108, 110, 113, 141, 282
Normothermic perfusion, 786
Nuclear medicine renography, 443
Nucleoside reverse transcriptase inhibitors, 125
Nutrition, 70, 76, 94, 163, 297, 520, 569, 621–628, 653, 654, 734, 793

O

Obesity, 14, 41, 43, 44, 66, 124, 140, 144, 172, 345, 347, 386, 413, 416, 417, 419, 421, 427, 454, 494, 526, 542, 544, 548, 552, 553, 575, 587, 621, 627, 628, 631, 706–707, 746, 748–749, 751, 763, 792, 794, 822, 860, 867
Obliterans, 821
Obstetric AKI, 54
Obstructed, 37, 41, 50, 69, 262, 263, 401, 403, 432, 433, 440, 441, 443, 444, 446–448, 483, 543, 729, 868
Obstructive sleep apnoea, 8, 143
Occlusion, 3, 4, 6, 8, 9, 37, 50, 295, 323, 324, 377, 382, 383, 385, 389, 391, 392, 551, 590, 592, 594, 658, 676, 678, 679, 681, 682, 696
Oedema, 2–4, 6–8, 38, 53, 55, 56, 67, 70, 76, 85, 86, 92, 93, 101, 104, 107, 131, 141, 152, 161, 165, 167, 168, 174, 175, 177, 179, 186, 211, 227, 260, 261, 264, 270, 277, 281, 292, 293, 297, 360, 362, 363, 388, 391, 446, 447, 530, 534, 590, 594–598, 616, 629, 661, 680, 682, 686, 695, 696, 729, 732, 785, 809, 815, 821, 834, 839, 853, 873
Older donors, 744–745, 832, 867
Oliguria, 5, 9, 39, 43, 75, 76, 86, 92, 152, 193, 261, 293, 409, 767, 803, 804
Open renal biopsy (ORB), 43–44
Organic anion transporter, 166, 167
Organic osmolytes, 104
Organ preservation, 783, 785–786
Organ storage, 783, 785
Osteomalacia, 110, 116–119, 128, 274, 436, 872
Osteoporosis, 15, 16, 102, 237, 350, 377, 378, 414, 415, 420, 822, 872
Overactive bladder complex, 396
Oxalate
  comprising, 126
  nephropathy, 10, 52
Oxalosis, 25, 415, 418, 522, 862
Oxford classification, 207

P

Paediatric donors, 744, 753
Page kidney, 6, 9, 42, 43, 109, 141
Paired exchange, 767, 775–777, 780, 793, 857
p-ANCA, 55, 218, 219, 759
Pancreas, 42, 127, 356, 375, 448, 471, 472, 474, 484, 783–795, 833, 848, 861, 868
Pancreas transplantation, 356, 783–795
Pancreatic leaks, 793
Papillary necrosis, 7, 27, 36, 51, 52, 107, 287, 333, 398, 406, 408, 413, 418, 431, 441, 544
Paracentesis, 52, 93, 95, 96
Parathyroidectomy, 115, 116, 120, 526, 585–587, 872
Parathyroid hormone, 6, 116, 420, 576, 618, 699
Paroxysmal cold haemoglobinuria, 336
Paroxysmal nocturnal haemoglobinuria, 54, 129, 200, 336–337, 779, 807
Partial lipodystrophy, 198, 199, 544
Partial nephrectomy, 427, 458–459, 463, 464, 473
Parvovirus B19, 265, 332
Pathogenesis, 65, 92, 171–173, 183–185, 203–204, 207, 210, 215, 221, 222, 225, 250, 264, 270, 281, 292–294, 305–306, 311–312, 331–332, 336–338, 346, 406, 408, 433, 463, 470–471, 475, 491, 493, 498–500, 523, 589, 690, 869
Pathophysiology, 50, 91–93, 130, 151–152, 165, 189–191, 193, 197–198, 235, 409, 414–416, 422, 429–430, 440, 482–483, 509, 512, 525, 581, 585, 589, 604, 605, 608, 609, 621, 622, 863, 864
Patient selection, 32, 320, 460, 706, 729, 769
Patient training, 709–710, 726
Pauci immune vasculitis, 264
PD Peritonitis, 726–728
Peginesatide, 570, 574
Pelvic kidney, 430
Pelvic malignancy, 7, 51, 441, 450
Pelviureteric junction obstruction, 431, 432, 435
Percutaneous nephrolithotomy, 426, 427, 476, 521
Periaortitis, 447–450
Perimedial fibroplasia, 382
Perinephric abscess, 41, 398, 400, 406
Periodic Fevers, 314, 317
Peri-pancreatic collections, 793
Peripheral vascular disease, 3, 52, 549, 596, 657, 758, 787, 791, 799
Perirenal haematoma, 43
Peritoneal dialysis
  catheters, 486, 675, 729
  clearance target, 721–722
  prescription, 717–722
  service, 705–715
  team, 709
  ultrafiltration target, 722
Peritoneal equilibration test, 717, 734
Peritoneal leak, 80, 732
Peritoneal membrane characteristics, 719, 728
Peritonitis, 49, 52, 80, 81, 92–96, 162, 174, 371, 373, 486, 624, 632, 636, 640, 644, 706, 708–711, 714, 721, 725–731, 733, 735
Peritubular capillary multilayering, 866
Periungual fibromas, 14, 475, 526

Persistent hyperparathyroidism, 872
Personal protective equipment, 635, 636
Phaeochromocytoma, 8, 11, 139, 142, 143, 471, 473, 474, 479
Pharmacodynamics, 165–168, 629, 630, 728
Pharmacology, 135, 147, 629–634, 819
Pharmacotherapy, 389, 424, 425
Phosphate
  binders, 117, 119, 526, 557, 558, 570, 572, 584, 585, 617, 618, 629
  disorders, 117
Phosphatonins, 117
Phosphaturia, 20, 26, 27, 110, 129, 274, 418, 582
Phospholipase A2 receptor, 184
Phospholipase Ce1, 172
Phosphorylase kinase deficiency, 57
Phosphorylase mutase deficiency, 57
Physician-inserted local anaesthetic, 711
Pierson syndrome, 498, 506
Pigment nephropathy, 21, 23, 27, 56, 67
PKD1, 475, 481–485, 487
PKD2, 481–484, 487
Plasma catecholamines, 143
Plasma cell leukaemia, 304
Plasma exchange, 173, 181, 200, 209, 211, 222, 223, 231, 232, 251, 252, 254, 266, 270, 276, 307, 308, 325, 327–330, 758, 775, 777–779, 798, 806–808, 823, 824, 859, 866
Plasma free metanephrines, 139, 143
Plasmapheresis, 128, 212, 229, 230, 250–252, 308
Pneumococcal pneumonia, 53
Pneumonitis, 273, 463, 761, 821, 825, 833, 834, 838, 839, 842, 848, 852, 853
Podocin, 158, 172
Podocyte
  foot process effacement, 158, 175
  foot process fusion, 172, 175
POEMS, 340
Poisoning, 7, 11, 14, 20, 25, 40, 52, 54, 67, 69, 76, 80, 81, 88–, 89, 106, 111, 117, 125, 130, 131, 287, 630
Pollens, 171
Polyangiitis, 10, 14, 53, 55, 215, 223, 284, 300
Polyarteritis nodosa, 8, 14, 51, 53, 216, 263, 266, 278, 314, 526, 528
Polyclonal anti-T-lymphocyte antibodies, 814
Polycythaemia rubra vera, 342
Polymyositis, 295, 298
Polyoma virus nephropathy, 805
Ponticelli regimen, 186
Poor adherence, 139, 140, 860, 862, 866
Poor graft function, 787, 832, 860, 861
Porphyria cutanea tarda, 14, 526–528
Post-biopsy monitoring, 43
Posterior reversible encephalopathy syndrome, 152
Postinfectious glomerulonephritis, 10, 51, 55, 191, 193, 237, 253, 264
Postinfective, 51
Post-micturition residual, 441, 450, 451
Post-obstructive diuresis, 3, 120, 447
Post-obstructive haemorrhage, 447
Post-operative hyponatraemia, 103
Post-operative surgical complications, 790, 792–793, 795
Post-perfusion biopsy, 803
Postrenal acute kidney injury, 50, 51
Post-transplant lymphoproliferative disease, 760, 869–871
Post-transplant lymphoproliferative disorder (PTLD), 53, 341, 760, 762, 774, 805, 823, 838, 839, 853, 854, 859, 864, 868
Potassium disorders, 108
Potter's syndrome, 430
Preconception counselling, 209, 359, 361, 366, 371, 372, 376, 874
Pre-eclampsia, 12, 56, 121, 191, 330, 359, 362–365, 367–374, 376, 484, 752
Pregnancy, 7, 21, 30, 41, 53, 55, 103, 209, 230, 239, 251, 324, 353, 359–378, 393, 395, 422, 434, 440, 476, 535, 542, 750, 771, 809, 824, 844, 862
Pregnancy outcomes, 359, 361, 362, 365, 367–374, 376, 518, 752
Pre-malignant skin conditions, 532–535
Pre-renal acute kidney injury, 2
Presentation, 1, 26, 33, 40, 51, 53, 63, 101, 110, 129, 158, 162, 171, 173, 183, 193, 210, 215, 228, 235, 259, 270, 282, 291, 303, 312, 323, 362, 381, 404, 413, 431, 440, 458, 477, 483, 493, 509, 515, 526, 538, 558, 586, 592, 604, 637, 654, 690, 725, 748, 758, 798, 825, 839
Prevalence, 5, 59, 110, 139, 183, 235, 258, 269, 288, 291, 314, 331, 345, 362, 383, 404, 413, 470, 493, 498, 509, 525, 537, 550, 590, 605, 614, 627, 630, 636, 649, 658, 675, 690, 707, 735, 740, 756, 832, 861
Primary central nervous system tumours, 742
Primary focal segmental glomerulosclerosis, 172–174
Primary FSGS, 171, 174, 176–177
Primary hyperoxaluria, 414–416, 420, 422, 425, 427, 519, 522, 719, 758, 759, 798
Prognosis, 39, 40, 47, 59, 91, 94, 97, 98, 138, 158, 161, 174, 176, 177, 180, 183, 186, 187, 189, 195, 199, 205, 206, 208, 209, 236, 237, 244, 257, 258, 260, 265, 266, 271, 277, 285, 294, 296, 305, 307, 324, 325, 328, 332, 334, 339, 384, 392, 393, 450, 454–456, 462, 463, 465, 467, 474, 478, 484, 499, 500, 503, 504, 509, 520, 521, 526, 529, 534, 540, 541, 548, 551, 561, 613, 617, 621, 722, 736, 759, 863, 864, 869
Proliferative GN, 189–196, 199, 263, 266, 301, 304
Prolonged intermittent renal replacement therapy, 76, 77, 81
Prophylaxis, 12, 37, 39, 51, 64, 103, 139, 148, 168, 183, 184, 224, 238, 250, 258, 270, 282, 296, 308, 320, 334, 346, 368, 383, 407, 418, 435, 441, 476, 515, 527, 542, 550, 564, 595, 614, 625, 633, 636, 668, 707, 764, 804, 824, 842, 857
Propylene glycol, 125
Prostacyclin, 84, 85, 89, 154, 605
Prostatic hypertrophy, 51, 440, 441, 551
Prostatitis, 27, 395, 396, 409
Protamine, 84
Proteinase 3, 218
Proteinuria, 1, 26, 33, 40, 51, 53, 63, 101, 110, 129, 158, 162, 171, 173, 183, 193, 210, 215, 228, 235, 259, 270, 282, 291, 303, 312, 323, 362, 381, 404, 413, 431, 440, 458, 477, 483, 493, 509, 515, 526, 538, 558, 586, 592, 604, 637, 654, 690, 725, 748, 758, 798, 825, 839
Proximal renal tubular acidosis, 125, 129
Prune belly syndrome, 14, 56, 433, 435
Pseudohyperkalaemia, 112, 113
Pseudohypoaldosteronism, 112, 113, 142
Pseudohypoaldosteronism Type II, 113, 142
Pseudohypokalaemia, 109
Pseudohyponatraemia, 102, 103
Psychogenic polydipsia, 9, 102, 103, 106
Pulmonary oedema, 2, 4, 6, 8, 38, 53, 55, 70, 76, 93, 104, 131, 141, 152, 165, 174, 292, 293, 297, 364, 388, 391, 446, 594–596, 616, 687, 696, 809, 815, 834, 853
Pulmonary renal syndrome, 10, 53, 216, 227
Purpura, 14, 51, 53, 56, 191, 194, 203–212, 215, 216, 241, 267, 275, 316, 323, 328, 340, 391, 526, 528–530
Pyelonephritis, 5, 8, 9, 12, 20, 26, 35, 36, 40, 41, 51–53, 56, 107, 257, 258, 262, 281, 285, 314, 361, 365, 392, 395–407, 414, 430–432, 441, 456, 457, 466, 493, 543, 551, 788, 805, 863
Pyonephrosis, 69, 400, 401, 403, 406, 414, 442, 446
Pyuria, 10, 24–27, 39, 40, 69, 273, 274, 282, 298, 395, 396, 402, 406–409, 543, 544, 551, 831

Q

Quinine, 258, 284, 324, 329, 338, 694

R

Radiation, 7, 27, 29–35, 38, 51, 53, 59, 191, 287, 338, 339, 365, 386, 396, 400, 421, 423, 441–443, 448, 454, 456, 532, 544, 758
Radiation cystitis, 396
Radiation fibrosis, 51, 441
Radiation nephritis, 287, 338, 339, 544
Radical nephrectomy, 458, 463–465
Radio contrast, 29, 51
Rapamycin inhibitors, 462–463
Rapidly progressive glomerulonephritis, 24, 25, 69, 215, 218, 223, 227, 229, 251, 252, 264, 360
R:A Ratio, 142
Rasburicase, 59, 65, 67, 338, 340
Raynaud's phenomenon, 236, 526, 529, 530
Recipient selection, 745, 787, 791
Recombinant urate oxidase, 65, 340
Recurrent(ce)
  disease, 34, 40, 173, 181, 187, 209, 210, 459, 486, 543, 746, 752, 758, 759, 798, 805, 858–860, 862, 864
  IDH, 690, 693
  posttransplantation, 196
Recurrent UTI, 21, 365, 369, 396, 400, 402, 405–407, 410, 414, 450, 543, 551, 759, 831
Red blood cell cast, 22
Redistributive hypokalaemia, 109
Rejection, 8, 66, 80, 95, 116, 128, 200, 222, 230, 250, 267, 288, 307, 319, 371, 403, 427, 440, 455, 474, 486, 521, 533, 585, 592, 607, 614, 623, 631, 636, 651, 661, 677, 685, 707, 718, 728, 752, 774, 786, 797, 823, 832
Relapse, 2, 16, 96, 162, 163, 172–174, 177–181, 187, 221, 222, 224, 225, 227, 229, 230, 237–240, 242, 243, 249, 252, 254, 276, 285, 313, 325, 328, 329, 396, 400, 402, 405, 410, 534, 836, 837, 851
Relapsers, 178–180
Removal, 8, 66, 80, 95, 116, 128, 200, 222, 230, 250, 267, 288, 307, 319, 371, 403, 427, 440, 455, 474, 486, 521, 533, 585, 592, 607, 614, 623, 631, 636, 651, 661, 677, 685, 707, 718, 728, 752, 774, 786, 797, 823, 832
Renal abscesses, 261, 266, 406, 409
Renal acid loss, 127
Renal allograft biopsy, 803, 805
Renal artery imaging, 385
Renal artery stenosis, 6, 8, 36–38, 50, 52, 108, 109, 139, 141, 300, 339, 346, 381–391, 393, 551, 552, 555, 790, 853, 859, 867
Renal artery thromboembolism, 392
Renal artery thrombosis, 227, 245
Renal biopsy, 39, 55, 66, 94, 158, 175, 183, 190, 203, 218, 228, 237, 252, 260, 271, 281, 293, 318, 325, 337, 347, 366, 440, 501, 511, 520, 552, 569, 606, 749, 859
Renal bone disease, 583, 871
Renal causes, 7, 12, 70, 91, 108, 118, 120, 140–141, 154
Renal cell carcinoma, 314, 392, 453, 455–456, 464, 465, 470, 473, 476, 478, 485, 486, 491, 492, 759, 760, 871
Renal colic, 274, 365, 369, 413, 418, 421, 423, 440
Renal coloboma syndrome, 14, 494–495
Renal complications, 274, 333, 354, 384
Renal cysts, 14, 405, 431, 454, 456, 464, 470, 472, 473, 475, 476, 481, 483, 485, 487, 491, 494, 496, 506, 552, 751, 794
Renal disease, 12, 19, 37, 48, 80, 92, 106, 127, 138, 147, 157, 165, 173, 189, 207, 216, 227, 235, 259, 283, 292, 312, 326, 336, 350, 359, 382, 414, 432, 454, 470, 482, 502, 515, 526, 542, 548, 566, 583, 592, 603, 630, 637, 650, 663, 685, 707, 721, 727, 739, 756, 784, 798, 813, 830, 859, 877
Renal failure, 1, 19, 29, 39, 47, 63–72, 75, 94, 102, 123, 140, 147–155, 158, 161–163, 165–168, 177, 183, 205, 215, 230, 239, 250, 258, 270, 288, 292, 303, 311, 333, 345, 359, 383, 395, 416, 429, 439, 463, 473, 481, 493, 511, 526, 538, 547–561, 569–578, 584, 589, 603, 613, 622, 633, 638, 653, 657, 679, 685, 709, 725, 749, 755, 773, 788, 797, 816, 833, 857–875, 877
Renal insults, 39, 63, 64, 186, 266, 554
Renal losses, 49, 52, 103, 108, 109, 113–115, 118, 120, 125
Renal lymphangiomatosis, 393
Renal medullary carcinoma, 333, 453
Renal papillary necrosis, 333
Renal paraenchymal disease, 139–141
Renal replacement modality, 77, 81, 632
Renal replacement therapy, 1, 3, 14, 48, 59, 68–71, 75–89, 96, 97, 111, 113–115, 117, 119, 171, 193, 195, 197, 218, 260, 270, 316, 319, 325, 334, 339, 354–356, 378, 386, 434, 473, 475, 481, 484–486, 491, 504, 511, 522, 526, 537–538, 542, 555, 557, 558, 599, 613, 614, 621, 632, 633, 635, 643, 658, 695, 698, 705, 707, 783, 801, 802, 857, 864
Renal scarring, 12, 34, 35, 195, 294, 400, 405, 430, 431, 433, 794
Renal sinus cysts, 510, 511
Renal tuberculosis, 408, 418
Renal tubular acidosis, 21, 26, 109, 113, 125, 128, 129, 132, 270, 274, 282, 284, 286, 287, 298, 299, 304, 333, 352, 414–417, 421, 493, 501, 522, 556
Renal vasculature, 32, 258, 286, 324
Renal vasculitis, 22, 37, 205, 217, 224, 236, 263
Renal vein stenosis, 393
Renal vein thrombosis, 6, 51, 52, 162, 186, 236, 242, 392, 551, 606
Renin:aldosterone ratio, 142
Repair, 30, 158, 159, 185, 397, 440, 653, 664, 670, 682, 708, 731, 732, 788, 792, 793, 868
Reproductive function, 874
Residual renal function, 78, 87, 616, 664, 689, 690, 705, 706, 708, 718, 719, 721, 722, 725, 728, 734–736, 758, 824
Resistant hypertension, 139, 140, 142, 143, 390, 746
Respiratory
  acidosis, 123, 124, 126, 131
  alkalosis, 117, 118, 123, 124, 131, 361
Reticulocyte count, 323, 570, 571, 574–576
Retinal angiomas, 474
Retinol binding protein, 25, 26, 111, 274, 420, 548
Retrieval technique, 784
Retroperitoneal fibrosis, 51, 284, 432, 440–442, 447–450, 543, 758
Retroperitoneal haemorrhage, 476, 806, 808
Rhabdomyolysis, 7, 12, 13, 23, 49, 54–58, 67, 113, 115–119, 121, 261, 263, 298, 466, 475, 551
Rheumatoid arthritis, 10, 14, 137, 184, 186, 192, 215, 236, 243, 295, 300, 314, 317, 549, 820
Rheumatological, 184, 291–301, 544, 644
RIFLE criteria, 48, 76
Right internal jugular, 676, 677, 680, 681
Rigid ureteroscopy, 427
Risk factor, 5, 21, 30, 49, 63, 97, 101, 135, 147, 162, 183, 228, 244, 258, 270, 291, 334, 345, 367, 384, 396, 414, 447, 456, 475, 483, 491, 526, 537, 548, 587, 588, 605, 627, 638, 649, 669, 692, 716, 725, 742, 772, 787, 803, 821, 832, 858
Rituximab, 159, 178, 179, 181, 187, 200, 222–225, 230, 238, 239, 242–245, 251–254, 276, 329, 369, 777, 778, 808, 814, 823, 824, 842, 866, 870, 871
Ross fused ectopia, 430

S

Salicylate, 64, 67, 69, 70, 89, 117, 125, 131, 284, 630
Salt-losing nephropathies, 6, 103, 105

SAP scintigraphy, 317
Sarcoid, 7, 14, 39, 40, 283, 299, 300, 544, 551, 805
Sarcoidosis, 10, 51, 53, 115, 184, 283, 299, 300, 418, 419, 798
SCC. *See* Squamous cell carcinoma (SCC)
SCD. *See* Sickle cell disease (SCD)
Schistosoma haematobium, 11, 24, 26
Schistosomiasis, 7, 10, 184, 192, 257, 258, 262–263, 439, 441, 543, 544, 762, 765, 831
Scleroderma, 10, 14, 154, 184, 192, 236, 291–295, 297, 298, 526, 529, 530
Scleroderma renal crisis (SRC), 10, 154, 291–298
SCN. *See* Sickle cell nephropathy (SCN)
Secondary FSGS, 172, 174, 181, 440
Secondary hyperaldosteronism, 109
Secondary hypertension, 8, 111, 135, 139–143
Secondary I_gAN, 205, 207
Secondary vasculitis, 215
Selection, 32, 78, 101, 136, 139, 270, 320, 372, 388, 460, 657, 676, 706, 719, 729, 739, 741, 745–747, 752, 769, 771, 786–788, 790–791, 793–794
Selectivity Index, 175
Seniour-Loken syndrome, 14, 494
Sensitization, 772, 875
Sensory Neuropathy, 315
Sepsis, 3, 4, 7, 12, 31, 39, 48–50, 52, 54, 55, 59, 64–68, 70–72, 79–81, 93–96, 116, 118, 125, 225, 243, 257–260, 266, 269, 270, 320, 335, 336, 338, 339, 342, 399, 400, 402–404, 409, 410, 427, 432, 445, 450, 466, 491, 493, 541, 544, 551, 555, 557, 569, 586, 633, 635, 639, 642, 661, 667, 668, 677, 682, 690, 695, 727, 739, 740, 774, 791, 792, 806–808, 830–832, 853
Septic abortion, 53, 56
Septic shock, 53, 56, 57, 68, 95
Serotonin, 605, 610, 618
Serotype O157, 324
Serum Amyloid P Protein, 311, 317
Serum FLC immunoassays, 305
Serum Sickness, 215, 264, 277, 278, 814
Sevelamer, 584
Severe post-partum haemorrhage, 56
Sezary syndrome, 342
Shared decision making, 557–558
Sharps disposal, 635, 636, 641
Shiga toxin, 324, 325
Shiga Toxin-Associated HUS, 324
Shigella dysenteriae, 324
Sickle cell disease (SCD), 54, 107, 184, 331–335, 392, 398, 441, 544, 759, 779
Sickle cell nephropathy (SCN), 11, 287, 331–335, 544
Simultaneous pancreas kidney (SPK), 375, 759, 791, 792
Sirolimus, 330, 373, 388, 461–463, 476, 482, 488, 531, 534, 570, 600, 800, 801, 816, 818–821, 823–825, 837, 861, 867, 869, 871, 873, 874
Sjogren's Syndrome, 14, 107, 111, 184, 194, 236, 275, 283, 284, 298–299, 544
Sjögren Syndrome, 128, 192
Skin, 4, 30, 49, 83, 106, 174, 203, 215, 236, 258, 282, 291, 315, 340, 391, 408, 448, 462, 469, 485, 502, 521, 525, 586, 605, 618, 635, 658, 680, 711, 729, 740, 759, 787, 821, 868
Skin cancer, 465, 525, 532–535, 740, 742, 787, 821, 869, 871
SLE. *See* Systemic lupus erythematosus (SLE)
SLED. *See* Sustained low-efficiency dialysis (SLED)
Snake bite, 7, 48, 51, 54, 67, 336
Sodium-potassium-2, 166, 167
Solute transfer, 717, 734
Spina bifida, 14, 434, 435, 441
SPK. *See* Simultaneous pancreas kidney (SPK)
Squamous cell carcinoma (SCC), 14, 114, 115, 297, 531–534, 869
SRC. *See* Scleroderma renal crisis (SRC)
Staging of renal cell carcinoma, 455
Starvation ketoacidosis, 125
Stavudine, 125
Steroid-resistant nephrotic syndrome, 40, 158, 171
Stewart hypothesis, 126–127
Striae, 14, 174, 531, 822
Stroke, 8, 54, 70, 85, 124, 135, 138–140, 147–150, 152, 216, 245, 292, 296, 297, 332–334, 349, 353, 359, 388, 474, 510, 574, 578, 589, 596, 598, 600, 608, 679, 758
Stroke prevention, 149–150, 333
Subclavian, 4, 382, 638, 677, 680
Sub-Periosteal Erosions, 583
Surgical warm ischaemic time, 802
Surreptitious vomiting, 132
Surveillance, 7, 108, 259, 263, 270, 286, 366, 373, 374, 459–460, 463–465, 467, 471, 474, 477, 479, 492, 535, 623, 635–637, 643, 653, 657, 662–667, 671, 672, 694–696, 700, 702, 741, 759–762, 768, 775, 808, 838, 852
Sustained low-efficiency dialysis (SLED), 76, 82
SV40 *large-*T *antigen stain*, 805
Sympathetic crisis, 152
Systemic Lupus Erythematosis, 314
Systemic lupus erythematosus (SLE), 11, 14, 16, 40, 55, 128, 186, 192, 215, 235–238, 241–245, 249, 251–254, 267, 271, 272, 283, 284, 298, 330, 341, 378, 526, 528, 542, 544, 759, 805, 842

T

Tacrolimus, 14, 178, 179, 181, 187, 191, 251, 329, 369, 373, 375, 376, 529, 600, 634, 761, 763, 793, 800, 801, 804, 809, 814–820, 822–825, 837, 841, 853, 861, 865–867, 870
Takayasu's Aortitis, 52, 141, 449
Takayasu's Arteritis, 10, 11, 14, 314, 381, 382
Tamm-Horsfall protein, 399, 494
TBI. *See* Total body irradiation (TBI)
T cell lymphoma, 342, 762
T cell rejection, 805
TDM. *See* Therapeutic drug monitoring (TDM)
Tenofovir, 25, 53, 111, 117, 118, 129, 269, 270, 273, 274, 278, 761
Tension pneumothorax, 124, 690
Terlipressin, 87, 96
Terminal pathway, 201–202
Thalassaemia, 336, 570
Therapeutic drug monitoring (TDM), 251, 813, 816, 819–821, 825
Thiamine deficiency, 163
Thiazide diuretics, 103, 104, 108, 110, 113, 117, 120, 128, 132, 149, 151, 166, 167, 353, 390, 416, 425, 426, 493, 556, 598, 634
Thiazides, 67, 102–105, 108–110, 113–115, 117, 120, 128, 132, 141, 142, 149, 151, 162, 166–168, 284, 320, 353, 390, 416, 420, 425, 426, 493, 556, 595, 598, 634
Thin basement membrane disease, 40, 205, 749, 750
Thin basement membrane nephropathy (TMN), 11, 498, 500–506
Thomsen-Friedenreich antigen, 326
Thrombectomy, 392, 393, 659, 667–668, 678, 679
Thromboembolism, 161, 162, 175, 186, 245, 392, 574, 600, 603, 606, 608, 610, 667
Thrombosis, 6, 9, 15, 51–53, 84, 152, 161, 162, 174, 177, 186, 227, 236, 242–245, 325, 337, 339, 341, 342, 378, 392–393, 448, 551, 606–611, 659, 661–664, 667, 668, 672, 675–680, 689, 744, 767, 779, 788, 790, 792, 793, 797, 803, 804, 806, 808, 809, 815
Thrombotic microangiopathic anaemia, 154
Thrombotic microangiopathies, 56, 152, 189, 323–330
Thrombotic microangiopathy (TMA), 7, 10, 51, 53, 55, 56, 155, 189–191, 198, 236, 245, 260, 263, 265, 266, 269, 270, 275, 276, 287, 323–330, 333, 338, 339, 341, 544, 807, 859, 863

Thrombotic thrombocytopenia purpura (TTP), 323, 324, 328–330, 340
TIN. *See* Tubulointerstitial nephritis (TIN)
TIO. *See* Tumor-induced osteomalacia (TIO)
TIPS. *See* Transjugular intrahepatic portosystemic shunt (TIPS)
TLS. *See* Tumour lysis syndrome (TLS)
T-lymphocyte mediated rejection, 823
TMA. *See* Thrombotic microangiopathy (TMA)
TMN. *See* Thin basement membrane nephropathy (TMN)
Toluene, 13, 117, 125
Total body irradiation (TBI), 339, 779
Toxin, 56, 67, 69, 82, 184, 324–325, 371
Transition, 304, 313, 355, 365, 429, 563–566, 581, 613, 652, 715, 719, 720, 862
Transition clinics, 564–566, 862
Transjugular, 41, 43, 44, 92, 93, 96–98
Transjugular intrahepatic portosystemic shunt (TIPS), 92, 93, 96–97
Transluminal angioplasty, 383
Transplant, 9, 29, 39, 94, 157, 172, 184, 209, 215, 259, 275, 281, 297, 307, 319, 328, 334, 371, 396, 419, 440, 486, 493, 503, 511, 518, 525, 537, 554, 564, 587, 599, 613, 624, 631, 635, 655, 692, 706, 729, 739, 755, 767, 783, 797, 813, 829, 857
Transplant arterial, 804
Transplantation, 10, 34, 40, 54, 76, 91, 111, 161, 172, 187, 196, 209, 231, 263, 269, 296, 307, 319, 324, 334, 345, 371, 393, 395, 415, 441, 456, 473, 485, 491, 499, 511, 517, 525, 551, 576, 583, 589, 621, 643, 692, 706, 730, 739, 753, 755, 767, 797, 813, 829, 857
Transplant glomerulopathy, 157, 184, 778, 859, 861–863, 866
Transplant recurrence, 173, 181, 199
Transthyretin Met 30 Amyloidosis, 313
Transtubular potassium gradient (TTKG), 108, 109, 113
Transvenous renal biopsy (TVRB), 44
Treatment thresholds, 135–138
TREAT study, 574, 575, 577
Trousseau's sign, 116, 120
TSC. *See* Tuberous sclerosis complex (TSC)
TTKG. *See* Transtubular potassium gradient (TTKG)
TTP. *See* Thrombotic thrombocytopenia purpura (TTP)
Tuberculosis (TB), 7, 10, 11, 14, 27, 39, 40, 51, 53, 115, 219, 224, 257–259, 262, 263, 283–285, 314, 406, 408, 418, 431, 439–441, 448, 543, 570, 575, 636, 642, 644, 727, 740, 760, 761, 787, 807, 825, 829–831, 845, 846, 853, 854
Tuberous sclerosis complex (TSC), 11, 14, 470, 474–477, 485, 487
Tubular abnormalities, 8, 40, 273, 299, 332–333, 336
Tubular atrophy, 176, 206, 207, 223, 287, 298, 347, 494, 522, 823, 863–865
Tubular injury, 3, 15, 21, 22, 25, 39, 50, 51, 55–57, 94, 95, 109, 120, 131, 162, 176, 258, 260, 261, 266, 267, 269, 270, 273, 283, 286, 287, 298, 325, 436, 444, 446, 483, 634, 804, 808
Tubular proteinuria, 25, 26, 111, 129, 274, 287, 420, 543, 808
Tubuloglomerular feedback, 50, 361, 554
Tubulointerstitial disease, 7, 11, 235, 236, 271, 273, 299
Tubulointerstitial nephritis (TIN), 10, 11, 13, 14, 25, 26, 40, 94, 236, 258, 261–263, 266, 267, 269, 270, 273–276, 281–288, 298, 300, 408, 494, 522, 543, 548, 552, 554
TubuloInterstitial Pathology, 273
Tumor-induced osteomalacia (TIO), 117–119
Tumour lysis syndrome (TLS), 7, 10, 25, 49, 53, 54, 59, 65, 67, 70, 76, 113, 116, 117, 119, 339, 340, 418, 551
Type 2 diabetes, 149, 150, 345–354, 484, 543, 550, 552, 555, 750
Type IV collagen, 230, 232, 497, 498, 500, 502, 504, 506
Type IV renal tubular acidosis, 113, 333
Typhoid, 54, 874
Tyrosinaemia, 111, 129
Tyrosine kinase inhibitors (TKIs), 462, 466

U

Ultrapure, 77, 79, 649, 699, 701
Unacceptable donor antigens (UDAs), 798
Uncomplicated, 59, 362, 397, 400, 407, 484, 521, 680, 797
Uncomplicated UTI, 395, 396, 401–404, 410
Uraemic pruritis, 525, 526
Urate, 4, 10, 49, 51, 55, 65–67, 76, 103, 104, 119, 126, 339, 340, 360, 361, 364, 414, 417, 418, 420, 422, 426, 427, 494, 543, 751, 873
Ureteric stenosis, 408, 789, 859
Ureterosigmoidostomy, 435, 436
Urethral stricture, 7, 51, 56, 397, 441, 446
Urethral syndrome, 396
Urethritis, 395, 396, 402, 407, 441
Uric acid, 21, 24, 27, 59, 69, 274, 333, 339, 340, 415, 417, 419–422, 425, 426, 522, 600, 751, 873
Uric acid stone, 415, 417, 420, 421, 425, 426, 751
Uricosuria, 26, 27, 110, 129
Urinary catecholamines, 143
Urinary complications, 790
Urinary fractionated metanephrines, 143
Urinary leaks, 9, 41, 43, 54, 450, 790
Urinary PH, 69, 109, 274, 417, 420–422, 426, 493
Urinary total metanephrines, 143
Urinary Tract Infection, 21, 25–27, 204, 262, 273, 365, 395–410, 413, 420, 429, 433, 491, 493, 554, 637, 764, 793, 831–832
Urinary tract obstruction, 7, 54, 55, 257, 365, 409, 413, 418, 421, 439–450
Urine albumin
  creatinine ratio, 22
Urine protein
  creatinine ratio, 22
Urodynamics, 407, 433–435, 442, 450, 544, 759, 788
Uromodulin, 10, 11, 305, 399, 416, 494
Uromodulin gene (UMOD), 494, 751
Urosepsis, 42, 52, 56, 129, 395, 403–405, 410, 439–441, 551, 764, 808, 831
Urticarial vasculitis, 184

V

Vaccine preventable disease, 635, 643–644
Vaginitis, 395, 396, 402, 407
Vanillylmandelic acid (VMA), 143
Vascular calcification (VC), 119, 421, 582–584, 586, 606, 685, 693, 758
Vascular fibrointimal hyperplasia, 866
Vascular thrombosis, 245, 339, 378, 497
Vasculitides, 10, 211, 215, 314, 528, 586
Vasculitis, 10, 22, 37, 39, 40, 51, 95, 141, 184, 194, 203, 215, 227, 236, 249, 257, 275, 283, 299, 339, 381, 441, 526, 544, 550, 702, 759, 805
Vasculopathy, 191, 235, 236, 292, 295, 734, 787, 791
VC. *See* Vascular calcification (VC)
VDR. *See* Vitamin D receptor (VDR)
Venous anatomy, 15, 659, 758, 799
Venous thrombosis, 9, 162, 244, 245, 337, 341, 606, 779, 804, 808
Virtual cross-matching, 800
Visceral glomerular epithelial cells, 157
Vitamin B6 deficiency, 163
Vitamin D, 111, 114–119, 224, 274, 283, 299, 414–416, 418–420, 518, 521, 526, 544, 581–587, 622, 630, 872
  deficiency, 116–119, 274, 872
Vitamin D receptor (VDR), 582, 585, 586
  agonists, 585

Von Gierke disease, 129
Von Hippel-Lindau disease, 453, 454, 470, 471, 485, 751, 871
Von Willebrand factor (vWF), 41, 162, 328, 603–605, 607, 608
Vulva, 868

W
Waldenstroms, 339, 340
Waldenstrom's macroglobulinaemia, 192–194, 304, 339, 340, 342
Warm ischaemia, 784
Water deficit, 107
Water deprivation, 106, 332
Water intoxication, 103
Water quality, 699–701, 703
WCH. *See* White coat hypertension (WCH)
Wegener's granulomatosis, 215, 284, 528
Weight gain, 15, 87, 163, 179, 350, 425, 587, 600, 627, 685–687, 689, 693, 706, 707, 801, 860, 863
Whitaker test, 444
White coat hypertension (WCH), 139–140, 867
Wilm's tumour, 184, 493
Wilson's disease, 111
Wound collections, 790
Wound healing, 467, 731, 763, 801, 820, 821

X
Xanthine oxidase inhibitor, 65, 339, 425
Xanthine stones, 425, 426
Xanthinuria, 415, 425
Xanthogranulomatous pyelonephritis (XPN), 8, 397, 406, 410, 414, 456, 466
Xerosis, 14, 525, 526
X-linked hypophosphataemic rickets, 117

Z
Zebra bodies, 511